Clinical Otology

4th Edition

Myles L. Pensak, MD, FACS, CEO
Senior Associate Dean for Clinical Affairs
Senior Vice President, UC Health
H.B. Broidy Professor and Chairman
Department of Otolaryngology–Head and Neck Surgery
University of Cincinnati Academic Health Center
Cincinnati, Ohio

Daniel I. Choo, MD, FACS
Professor and Director
Division of Pediatric Otolaryngology
University of Cincinnati College of Medicine
Department of Otolaryngology–Head and Neck Surgery
Cincinnati Children's Hospital Medical Center
Cincinnati, Ohio

Thieme
New York • Stuttgart • Delhi • Rio de Janeiro

Thieme Medical Publishers, Inc.
333 Seventh Ave.
New York, NY 10001

Executive Editor: Timothy Y. Hiscock
Managing Editor: J. Owen Zurhellen, IV
Editorial Assistant: Mohammad Ibrar
Senior Vice President, Editorial and Electronic Product
   Development: Cornelia Schulze
Production Editor: Sean Woznicki
International Production Director: Andreas Schabert
International Marketing Director: Fiona Henderson
Director of Sales, North America: Mike Roseman
International Sales Director: Louisa Turrell
Vice President, Finance and Accounts: Sarah Vanderbilt
President: Brian D. Scanlan
Printer: Asia Pacific Offset

Library of Congress Cataloging-in-Publication Data

Clinical otology (Hughes)
Clinical otology / [edited by] Myles L. Pensak, Daniel I. Choo. – Fourth
edition.
     p. ; cm.
Preceded by: Clinical otology / [edited by] Gordon B. Hughes, Myles L.
Pensak. 3rd ed. 2007.
Includes bibliographical references and index.
ISBN 978-1-60406-753-8 (hardcover) – ISBN 978-1-60406-913-6
(e-book)
I. Pensak, Myles L., editor. II. Choo, Daniel I., editor. III. Title.
[DNLM: 1. Ear Diseases. 2. Ear–physiology. 3. Hearing Disorders.
WV 200]
  RF120
  617.8–dc23
                 2014016258

Copyright © 2015 by Thieme Medical Publishers, Inc.
Thieme Publishers New York
333 Seventh Avenue, New York, NY 10001 USA
+1 800 782 3488, customerservice@thieme.com

Thieme Publishers Stuttgart
Rüdigerstrasse 14, 70469 Stuttgart, Germany
+49 [0]711 8931 421, customerservice@thieme.de

Thieme Publishers Delhi
A-12, Second Floor, Sector-2, Noida-201301
Uttar Pradesh, India
+91 120 45 566 00, customerservice@thieme.in

Thieme Publishers Rio, Thieme Publicações Ltda.
Argentina Building 16th floor, Ala A, 228 Praia do Botafogo
Rio de Janeiro 22250-040 Brazil
+55 21 3736-3631

Printed in China   5 4 3 2 1

ISBN 978-1-60406-753-8

Also available as an e-book:
eISBN 978-1-60406-913-6

Important note: Medicine is an ever-changing science undergoing continual development. Research and clinical experience are continually expanding our knowledge, in particular our knowledge of proper treatment and drug therapy. Insofar as this book mentions any dosage or application, readers may rest assured that the authors, editors, and publishers have made every effort to ensure that such references are in accordance with **the state of knowledge at the time of production of the book.**

Nevertheless, this does not involve, imply, or express any guarantee or responsibility on the part of the publishers in respect to any dosage instructions and forms of applications stated in the book. **Every user is requested to examine carefully** the manufacturers' leaflets accompanying each drug and to check, if necessary in consultation with a physician or specialist, whether the dosage schedules mentioned therein or the contraindications stated by the manufacturers differ from the statements made in the present book. Such examination is particularly important with drugs that are either rarely used or have been newly released on the market. Every dosage schedule or every form of application used is entirely at the user's own risk and responsibility. The authors and publishers request every user to report to the publishers any discrepancies or inaccuracies noticed. If errors in this work are found after publication, errata will be posted at www.thieme.com on the product description page.

Some of the product names, patents, and registered designs referred to in this book are in fact registered trademarks or proprietary names even though specific reference to this fact is not always made in the text. Therefore, the appearance of a name without designation as proprietary is not to be construed as a representation by the publisher that it is in the public domain.

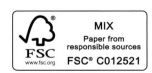

To Penny and our growing family; and to William Fussinger who has advised and supported staff, residents, and faculty of the Department of Otolaryngology–Head and Neck Surgery at UC for forty years.

—*MLP*

For Kim, Alayna, and Natalie, who make all things worthwhile.

—*DC*

Contents

Management

Foreword

When a person is asked to offer introductory remarks in a book, comments about the authors usually concern the later phases of their careers. However, my role in the lives of the two editors of this fourth edition of *Clinical Otology* occurred even before they embarked on training in otolaryngology–head and neck surgery.

I first met Myles Pensak while he was a general surgery resident in Syracuse spending his rotation in otolaryngology. As he became aware of the full range of disorders affecting the head and neck, in particular the special senses, he quickly recognized that this was the surgical specialty for him. The time period was prior to the matching system in ORL, so it was too late to formally apply to a residency program. As fate would have it, a vacancy was available in the program at Yale with Clarence Sasaki. The rest is history, as the ORL world knows well.

Daniel Choo was a student at the medical school in Syracuse and we were fortunate to have him match to our program in ORL. His medical school record was outstanding, including a basic science research project that earned first place recognition by the Academy of ORL. His commitment to academic otolaryngology was carefully planned with a clin-ical fellowship in Sarasota, FL followed by several years at the National Institutes of Health where he became trained in molecular medicine. Of course his scientific contributions have been widely recognized in pediatric otology where he is making a solid presence nationally and internationally.

Why have these two leaders in our specialty succeeded so exceptionally when their primary exposure in otolaryngology was identical to others who practice good otology but are not known for any particular contribution to our body of knowledge? I believe that the reason is genetic and that it is manifest in those who demonstrate curiosity of the mind and the desire to push the frontiers of our body of knowledge. Leo Rosten said "Happiness comes only when we push our brains and hearts to the farthest reaches of which we are capable."

This fourth edition of *Clinical Otology* represents the editors' skill and understanding of all aspects of otologic practice that are essential for the trainee as well as practicing surgeons. The chapters are inclusive, clearly presented, and exhaustively referenced.

Richard R. Gacek, MD

Preface

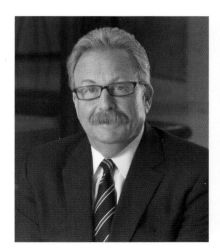
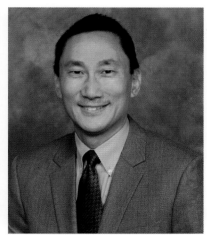

Myles L. Pensak   *Daniel I. Choo*

Since the publication in 2007 of the third edition of *Clinical Otology*, the political and economic landscape wherein clinical medicine is practiced underwent significant change, and continues to do so. These transformational environmental actions compel us to continually enhance our clinical knowledge base in order to improve the effectiveness and efficiency of our healthcare delivery while remaining unflinchingly focused on providing compassionate and patient-focused care. This updated fourth edition of *Clinical Otology* embraces newly discovered molecular and electrophysiologic understandings of otologic pathology. Moreover, chapters addressing assessment and management incorporate many of these new findings in establishing a contemporary algorithm for the practitioner to incorporate into a clinical paradigm.

The book is again divided into four major sections to include basic science, diagnostics, management, and rehabilitation. The editors appreciate the continued contributions by seasoned authors; and acknowledge the contributions from a number of new contributors. As with prior editions, all chapters are accompanied by a detailed contemporary bibliography for further self-study. In addition, while not actively participating in the production of this fourth edition, we acknowledge the fundamental work done by Gordon B. Hughes, MD, without whom this book would not have come to fruition.

The editors take special pride in acknowledging the continued contributions of Eiji Yanagisawa, who is joined by his son Ken in providing outstanding photographic illustrations for the book. The editors further appreciate the close collaboration of our publisher, Thieme, in particular J. Owen Zurhellen, Timothy Hiscock, and Kristi Goldade.

It is our sincerest hope that students and colleagues will find this text to be a foundational component in their otologic learning and that the information, principles and management concepts introduced in the text will spur not only an appreciation of the elegant intricacies of otologic medicine, but also a curiosity to ask, "How can we understand this better? How can we do this better?" Questions such as these will serve as the basis for the future of otology and of *Clinical Otology*.

Contributors

Zubair M. Ahmed, PhD
Dept. of Otorhinolaryngology–Head and Neck Surgery
University of Maryland School of Medicine
Baltimore, Maryland

Kelly S. Beaudoin, MSPT
Balance Solutions Physical Therapy Inc.
University Heights, Ohio

Dennis I. Bojrab, MD
CEO and Director of Research,
Michigan Ear Institute
Professor of Otolaryngology,
Oakland University William Beaumont School of Medicine
Clinical Professor of Otolaryngology and Neurosurgery,
Wayne State University
Royal Oak, Michigan

Laura Brainard, MD
Ear Associates
Albuquerque, New Mexico

Jason A. Brant, MD
Resident Physician
Department of Otorhinolaryngology–Head and Neck Surgery
Hospitals of the University of Pennsylvania
Philadelphia, Pennsylvania

David K. Brown, PhD, FAAA
Associate Professor and Director, AuD SIMLab
School of Audiology
Pacific University
Hillsboro, Oregon

Kevin D. Brown, MD, PhD
Assistant Professor
Department of Otolaryngology–Head and Neck Surgery
Weill Cornell Medical College
New York, New York

Douglas A. Chen, MD, FACS
Pittsburgh Ear Associates and
Director, Division of Neurotology-Department of
  Neurosurgery
Allegheny General Hospital
Pittsburgh, Pennsylvania

Daniel I. Choo, MD, FACS
Professor and Director, Division of Pediatric Otolaryngology
University of Cincinnati College of Medicine
Department of Otolaryngology–Head and Neck Surgery
Cincinnati Children's Hospital Medical Center
Cincinnati, Ohio

John Greer Clark, PhD
Associate Professor and Audiology Clinic Director
Department of Communication Sciences and Disorders
University of Cincinnati
Cincinnati, Ohio
President, Clark Audiology, LLC
Middletown and Hamilton, Ohio

Kathleen D. Coale, PT
Addison Gilbert Hospital
Beverly, Massachusetts

Rebecca S. Cornelius, MD, FACR
Professor of Radiology & Otolaryngology
Department of Radiology, Neuroradiology Division
University of Cincinnati Medical Center
Cincinnati, Ohio

Marcia Dewey, AuD, CCC/A
Audiology Coordinator, Tinnitus Team Leader
Department of Otolaryngology and Communication Sciences
Froedtert & The Medical College of Wisconsin
Milwaukee, Wisconsin

David R. Friedland, MD, PhD
Professor and Vice Chairman
Chief, Division of Otology and Neuro-otologic Skull Base
  Surgery
Chief, Division of Research
Department of Otolaryngology and Communication Sciences
Medical College of Wisconsin
Milwaukee, Wisconsin

Bruce J. Gantz, MD, FACS
Professor and Head
Department of Otolaryngology—Head and Neck Surgery
University of Iowa Hospitals and Clinics
Iowa City, Iowa

Joel A. Goebel, MD, FACS, FRCS
Professor and Vice Chairman
Director Dizziness and Balance Center
Department of Otolaryngology–Head and Neck Surgery
Washington University School of Medicine
Saint Louis, Missouri

John H. Greinwald Jr., MD, FAAP
Professor of Otolaryngology and Pediatrics
Ear and Hearing Center
Cincinnati Children's Hospital
Cincinnati, Ohio

Christine H. Heubi, MD
Department of Otolaryngology–Head and Neck Surgery
University of Cincinnati Academic Health Center
Cincinnati, Ohio

Lisa W. Hilbert, AuD, CCC-A, FAAA
Clinical Program Manager
Division of Audiology
Cincinnati Children's Hospital Medical Center
Cincinnati, Ohio

Todd A. Hillman, MD
Pittsburgh Ear Associates
Pittsburgh, Pennsylvania

Keiko Hirose, MD
Associate Professor
Washington University School of Medicine
Otolaryngologist-in-Chief
St. Louis Children's Hospital
St. Louis, Missouri

David B. Hom, MD, FACS
Professor and Director
Division of Facial Plastic and Reconstructive Surgery
Dept. of Otolaryngology–Head and Neck Surgery and
  Dermatology
University of Cincinnati College of Medicine
Cincinnati Children's Hospital Medical Center
Cincinnati, Ohio

May Y. Huang, MD, FACS
Neurotology and Otology
Northwest Ear Inc.
Seattle, Washington

Lisa L. Hunter, PhD, F-AAA
Scientific Director, Audiology
Communication Sciences Research Center
Associate Professor, Otolaryngology and Communication
  Sciences and Disorders
University of Cincinnati
Cincinnati, Ohio

Robert K. Jackler, MD
Professor of Otolaryngology-Head and Neck Surgery and
  Neurosurgery
Stanford University
Stanford, California

Daniel R. Jensen, MD
Pediatric Otolaryngologist, Children's Mercy Hospital
Assistant Professor, Department of Pediatric Surgery
University of Missouri–Kansas City School of Medicine
Kansas City, Missouri

Robert W. Keith, PhD
Professor Emeritus of Otolaryngology
University of Cincinnati College of Medicine
Cincinnati, Ohio

Bradley W. Kesser, MD
Associate Professor and Director, Division of Otology/
  Neurotology
Dept. of Otolaryngology–Head and Neck Surgery
University of Virginia School of Medicine
Charlottesville, Virginia

Matthew L. Kircher, MD
Dept. of Otolaryngology–Head and Neck Surgery
Loyola University Health System
Maywood, Illinois

Ilkka Kivekäs, MD, PhD
Research Fellow in Otolaryngology
Boston Children's Hospital and Harvard Medical School
Boston, Massachusetts
Assistant Professor in Otorhinolaryngology
Tampere University Hospital and the University of Tampere
Tampere, Finland

Jeffery J. Kuhn, MD, FACS
Associate Professor and Director
Division of Otology/Neurotology and Skull Base Surgery
Dept. of Otolaryngology–Head and Neck Surgery
University of Cincinnati College of Medicine
Cincinnati, Ohio

Arvind Kumar, MD
Professor Emeritus of Otolaryngology
University of Illinois
Chicago, Illinois

John F. Kveton, MD, FACS
Clinical Professor of Surgery/Otolaryngology and
  Neurosurgery
Section of Otolaryngology
Yale University School of Medicine
New Haven, Connecticut

Paul R. Lambert, MD
Professor and Chair
Dept. of Otolaryngology–Head & Neck Surgery
Medical University of South Carolina
Charleston, South Carolina

John P. Leonetti, MD
Professor
Dept. of Otolaryngology–Head and Neck Surgery
Loyola University Health System
Maywood, Illinois

Stephanie R. Lockhart, MA, CCC-A, F-AAA
Audiology Director
UC Health Otolaryngology-Head and Neck Surgery
Cincinnati, Ohio

Lawrence R. Lustig, MD
Howard W. Smith Professor and Chair,
Dept. of Otolaryngology–Head and Neck Surgery
Columbia University Medical Center
New York, New York

Sam J. Marzo, MD
Professor and Residency Program Director
Dept. of Otolaryngology–Head and Neck Surgery
Loyola University Health System
Maywood, Illinois

John S. McDonald, DDS, MS, FACD
Volunteer Professor,
Departments of Anesthesia and Pediatrics
University of Cincinnati College of Medicine
Cincinnati, Ohio

Michael J. McKenna, MD
Massachusetts Eye and Ear Infirmary
Boston, Massachusetts

Cliff A. Megerian, MD, FACS
The Julius McCall Professor and Chairman
Dept. of Otolaryngology–Head and Neck Surgery
Case Western Reserve University
Richard and Patricia Pogue Endowed Chair
Director Ear, Nose and Throat Institute
University Hospitals Case Medical Center
Cleveland, Ohio

Aaron C. Moberly, MD
Assistant Professor of Otolaryngology-Head and Neck
  Surgery
Division of Otology, Neurotology, and Cranial Base Surgery
The Ohio State University Wexner Medical Center
Columbus, Ohio

Edwin M. Monsell, MD, PhD
Professor
Dept. of Otolaryngology–Head and Neck Surgery
Wayne State University School of Medicine
Detroit, Michigan

Humberto Morales, MD
Assistant Professor of Radiology
Department of Radiology, Neuroradiology Division
University of Cincinnati Medical Center
Cincinnati, Ohio

Brendan O'Connell, MD
Dept. of Otolaryngology–Head and Neck Surgery
Medical University of South Carolina
Charleston, South Carolina

Benjamin H. Pensak, JD
Partner, Morgan Lewis & Bockius LLP
San Francisco, California

Myles L. Pensak, MD, FACS, CEO
Senior Associate Dean for Clinical Affairs, Senior Vice Pres-
  ident, UC Health, and H.B. Broidy Professor and Chairman,
Dept. of Otolaryngology–Head and Neck Surgery
University of Cincinnati Academic Health Center
Cincinnati, Ohio

Angel J. Perez, MD
Medical Corps, United States Navy
Resident Physician
Dept. of Otolaryngology–Head and Neck Surgery
Naval Medical Center
Portsmouth, Virginia

Dennis S. Poe, MD, PhD
Associate Professor, Dept. of Otology & Laryngology
Harvard Medical School
Dept. of Otolaryngology and Communications Enhancement
Boston Children's Hospital
Boston, Massachusetts

Matthew J. Provenzano, MD
Dept. of Otolaryngology–Head and Neck Surgery
Cincinnati Children's Hospital Medical Center
Cincinnati, Ohio

Lesley A. Rabach, MD
Yale University School of Medicine
Department of Surgery, Section of Otolaryngology–Head and
  Neck Surgery
Yale New Haven Hospital
New Haven, Connecticut

Jennifer A. Ratigan, AuD, CCC-A
Legacy Research and Technology Center
Portland, Oregon

Saima Riazuddin, PhD, MPH, MBA
Dept. of Otorhinolaryngology–Head and Neck Surgery
University of Maryland School of Medicine
Baltimore, Maryland

Elodie M. Richard, PhD
Dept. of Otorhinolaryngology–Head and Neck Surgery
University of Maryland School of Medicine
Baltimore, Maryland

Pamela C. Roehm, MD, PhD
Dept. of Otolaryngology–Head and Neck Surgery
Temple University School of Medicine
Philadelphia, Pennsylvania

Michael J. Ruckenstein, MD, MSc, FACS, FRCS
Professor, Vice Chairman, Residency Program Director
Dept. of Otorhinolaryngology–Head and Neck Surgery
Director, Implantable Hearing Device Center
Medical Director, Balance Center
University of Pennsylvania
Philadelphia, Pennsylvania

Leonard P. Rybak, MD, PhD, FACS
Professor of Surgery
Division of Otolaryngology
Southern Illinois University School of Medicine
Springfield, Illinois

John M. Ryzenman, MD
Director, The Ohio Ear Institute
Columbus, Ohio

Ravi N. Samy, MD, FACS
Associate Professor
Department of Otolaryngology
Program Director, Neurotology Fellowship
University of Cincinnati
Cincinnati Children's Hospital Medical Center
Cincinnati, Ohio

Peter L. Santa Maria, MD
Dept. of Otolaryngology–Head and Neck Surgery
Stanford University
Stanford, California

Mitchell K. Schwaber, MD
Nashville Ear Nose & Throat Clinic
Nashville, Tennessee

Samuel H. Selesnick, MD, FACS
Professor and Vice Chairman
Dept. of Otolaryngology–Head & Neck Surgery
Weill Cornell Medical College
New York, New York

Maroun Semaan, MD
Associate Director, Otology Neurotology and Balance
  Disorders
University Hospitals Case Medical Center
Cleveland, Ohio

Nael M. Shoman, MD, FRCSC
Clinical Assistant Professor
Division of Otolaryngology–Head and Neck Surgery
Royal University Hospital
Saskatoon, Saskatchewan, Canada

Aristides Sismanis, MD, FACS
Professor of Otorhinolaryngology
University of Athens
Director of the A′ ORL Clinic
Hippokration Hospital
Athens, Greece

Eric L. Slattery, MD
Neurotology and Skull Base Surgery Fellow
Michigan Ear Institute
Farmington Hills, Michigan

Shan Tang, MD
Dept. of Otolaryngology–Head and Neck Surgery
Weill Cornell Medical College
New York, New York

Peter C. Weber, MD, MBA
Dept. of Otolaryngology–Head and Neck Surgery
Medical University of South Carolina
Charleston, South Carolina

D. Bradley Welling, MD, PhD, FACS
Walter Augustus LeCompte Chair,
Dept. of Otology and Laryngology
Harvard Medical School
Chief of Otolaryngology,
Massachusetts Eye and Ear Infirmary
Chief of Otolaryngology,
Massachusetts General Hospital
Boston, Massachusetts

Judith White, MD, PhD
Associate Professor of Surgery, Lerner College of Medicine
Departments of Otolaryngology- Head and Neck Surgery and
  Neurology
Head, Vestibular Section, Head and Neck Institute
Medical Director, Dizziness Balance and Fall Prevention
  Center
Cleveland Clinic
Beachwood, Ohio

Cameron C. Wick, MD
Resident
Ear, Nose, and Throat Institute
University Hospitals Case Medical Center
Case Western Reserve University
Cleveland, Ohio

Eiji Yanagisawa, MD, FACS
Clinical Professor
Section of Otolaryngology
Department of Surgery
Yale University School of Medicine
New Haven, Connecticut

Ken Yanagisawa, MD, FACS
Southern New England Ear Nose Throat & Facial Plastic
   Surgery Group, LLP
Assistant Clinical Professor of Surgery, Yale University School
   of Medicine
Section Chief of Otolaryngology, Saint Raphael Campus, Yale
   New Haven Hospital
New Haven, Connecticut

Rizwan Yousaf, PhD
Dept. of Otorhinolaryngology–Head and Neck Surgery
University of Maryland School of Medicine
Baltimore, Maryland

Part 1

Basic Science

1 Anatomy and Embryology of the Ear

John M. Ryzenman and Arvind Kumar

1.1 Introduction

The complexity of the anatomy of the ear and temporal bone is well recognized. Consequently, surgery of this area is challenging. It is therefore incumbent upon the otologic/neurotologic surgeon to possess a three-dimensional familiarity with the structure of the temporal bone and the relationship of the individual components within it and its intracranial environs. Because diagnosis of temporal bone disorders and surgery can be complicated by aberrant development, an understanding of normal embryogenesis and familiarity with common developmental disorders is critical.

This chapter presents the anatomy of the temporal bone in a traditional descriptive form punctuated with clinically and surgically relevant pearls, and then as sequential cross sections of anatomic dissections with their corresponding high-resolution computed tomography (CT) images. Such a review, when combined with cadaver dissection of fresh temporal bones, will prepare the otologic surgeon for live surgery.

1.2 Anatomy of the Ear

The temporal bone is composed of the tympanic, squamous, mastoid, and petrous bones, as well as the styloid process. The temporal bone anatomic structures are commonly divided into the external, middle, and inner ear.

The external ear consists of the pinnae, the external auditory canal, and the tympanic membrane. The middle ear is defined as the air-containing space between the medial surface of the tympanic membrane and the promontory (floor of the middle ear), which is traversed by the ossicular chain. The inner ear is dense bone encasing the membranous labyrinth structures of the cochlea, vestibule, utricle, saccule, and three semicircular canals.

1.2.1 External Ear Anatomy

Pinna

The pinna is a cartilaginous framework covered in squamous keratinizing epithelium that functions primarily to collect, amplify, and funnel sound, directing it to the auditory canal. This structure is covered in greater detail in Section 1.3.1, below.

External Auditory Canal

The lateral third of the external auditory canal (EAC) is cartilaginous in nature whereas the medial two thirds are osseous. The lateral cartilaginous part is C-shaped and lined with stratified squamous keratinizing epithelium, ceruminous glands, and normal adnexa that are also found elsewhere in the body. The osseous canal is composed of the tympanic bone anteriorly, inferiorly, and posteriorly, and the squamous bone superiorly. The skin of this portion is thin and has no adnexa.

The length of the EAC is 25 to 31 mm; its width is 6 to 9 mm, and it is typically ovoid in cross section. The curvature of the canal is such that the most anterior region of the tympanic

membrane may not be visible endaurally, due to the prominence of the anterior canal wall (or posterior wall of the glenoid fossa). The sensory innervation of the ear is derived from cervical nerves 2 and 3 and cranial nerves V and X.

Tympanic Membrane

The tympanic membrane (TM) forms the medial "wall" of the EAC, and is approximately 0.1 mm thick, with a total vibrating surface area of 55 square millimeters. The trilaminar membrane is formed by an outer squamous keratinizing epidermis, a middle fibrous lamina propria, and an inner mucosal layer. Two important landmarks are the lateral process and the manubrium (handle) of the malleus (▶ Fig. 1.1).

The manubrium is enveloped in periosteum and terminates at the umbo. From the lateral process, the anterior and posterior malleolar folds stretch to the respective extremities of the tympanic sulcus of the temporal bone. These folds separate the small triangular pars flaccida from the larger pars tensa. The pars flaccida (also known as the Shrapnell membrane) is also trilaminar, but has a lamina propria composed of elastic collagen fibers as opposed to the regularly arranged collagen fibers pars tensa. This membrane attaches directly to the tympanic notch of the superior wall of the EAC.

The fibrous annulus is the thickened periphery of the tympanic membrane, and it is lodged in the tympanic sulcus, both of which are deficient superiorly at the notch of Rivinus (tympanic incisure).

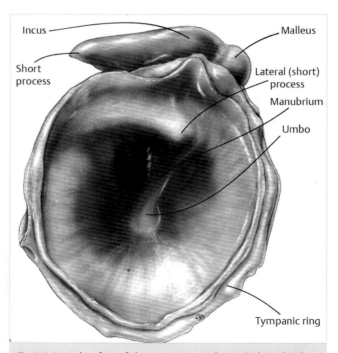

Fig. 1.1 Lateral surface of the tympanic membrane. (Adapted with permission from Anson BJ, Donaldson JA. Surgical Anatomy of the Temporal Bone. New York: Raven Press, 1992.)

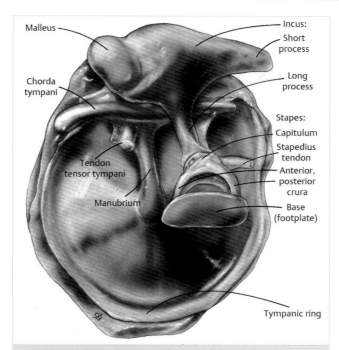

Fig. 1.2 Medial surface of the tympanic membrane and ossicular chain. (Adapted with permission from Anson BJ, Donaldson JA. Surgical Anatomy of the Temporal Bone. New York: Raven Press, 1992.)

1.2.2 Middle Ear Anatomy

The middle ear is a sagittally oriented cleft that is pneumatized by the eustachian tube, traversed by the ossicular chain (described in detail below), and lined by cuboidal epithelial mucosa and goblet cells. The middle ear space is also traditionally further partitioned.

Mesotympanum

The mesotympanum represents the bulk of the middle ear space and is bounded by an imaginary line circumferentially from the tympanic sulcus (or most medial edge of the auditory canal) to the floor of the middle ear. Superiorly the compartment is limited by a horizontal plane drawn from the scutum to the tympanic segment of the facial nerve (fallopian) canal. This space has lateral, medial, and posterior "walls," and is bordered by three spaces: the protympanum (anteriorly), the epitympanum (superiorly), and the hypotympanum (inferiorly). Within the mesotympanum are found the manubrium, the long process of the incus, the stapes, and the chorda tympani nerve (▶ Fig. 1.2).

- The lateral wall is formed by the tympanic membrane.
- The medial wall is formed largely by the promontory. There are two openings into the inner ear on this surface: the oval window and the round window niche.
- Posteriorly, the most prominent feature of the mesotympanum is the pyramidal eminence (from which emerges the stapes tendon). Lateral and medial to this eminence are two recesses: the facial recess (suprapyramidal) and the sinus tympani (infrapyramidal), respectively (▶ Fig. 1.3).

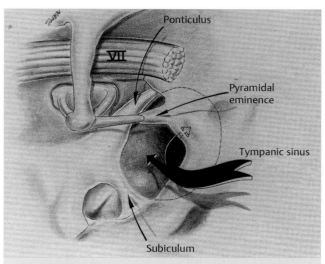

Fig. 1.3 Infrapyramidal recess (sinus tympani). Note that the facial recess (not depicted here) is lateral to the facial nerve (which has been cut away). VII, cranial nerve VII. (Adapted with permission from Gulya AJ, Schuknecht HF. Anatomy of the Temporal Bone with Surgical Implications. New York: Parthenon Publishing, 1995:88.)

- The boundaries of the facial recess are as follows: medially, the pyramidal eminence and the vertical facial nerve canal; laterally, the chorda tympani nerve in its canal; and superiorly, the fossa incudis. This recess may communicate with the mastoid space via its air cells, or be filled with solid bone.
- The boundaries of the sinus tympani are as follows: superiorly, the ponticulus, running between the pyramidal eminence and the promontory; inferiorly, the subiculum, which extends from the styloid eminence to the round window niche; laterally, the vertical facial nerve canal; and medially, the posterior semicircular canal. The extent of this recess is variable but it does not routinely communicate with the mastoid air cells. It may harbor pathology such as cholesteatoma, and is not readily visible through the canal. It can be visualized with angled endoscopes, or from the mastoid space via a "fallopian bridge" dissection (drilling the bone between the facial nerve and the posterior semicircular canal).

Epitympanum

The epitympanum is bordered superiorly by the bone of the tegmen tympani and contains the aditus ad antrum (which communicates posteriorly with the mastoid antrum). The inferior limit of the epitympanum is the horizontal facial nerve canal. The lateral wall of the epitympanum is the superior canal wall/scutum and pars flaccida. A vertical crest of bone on the medial wall extending from the tegmen to the cochleariform process is frequently referred to as the "cog." It partitions the epitympanum posteriorly and anteriorly. As described by Sheehy,[1] the cog serves as a marker for identifying the facial nerve during surgery. The other markers are the semicanal for the tensor tympani, the cochleariform process, and the groove on the promontory for the Jacobson nerve. The posterior partition contains the head of the malleus and the body of the incus. On the medial wall of the posterior epitympanum, it is possible to visualize the horizontal semicircular canal and the horizontal

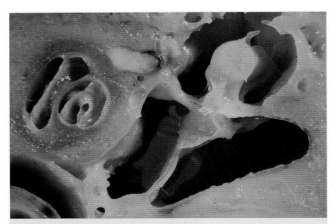

Fig. 1.4 Coronal fresh section of the temporal bone at the cochleariform process, superior to which is the posterior epitympanic space (that contains the head of malleus).

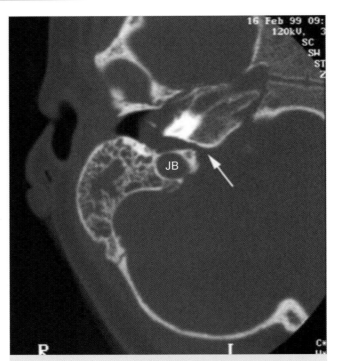

Fig. 1.5 Example of high jugular bulb (JB), seen in same axial plane as the cochlea. Also note the bulging eardrum due to a cerebrospinal fluid leak attributed to a persistent Hyrtl's fissure (*arrow*). (Used with permission from Jégoux F, Malard O, Gayet-Delacroix M, et al. Hyrtl's fissure: a case of spontaneous cerebrospinal fluid otorrhea. AJNR Am J Neuroradiol 2005;26:963–966.)

facial nerve canal, extending from the cochleariformis process to the second genu (▶ Fig. 1.4). On the floor of the anterior epitympanum (or supratubal recess) are found the geniculate ganglion and the semicanal of the tensor tympani muscle. This space opens anteriorly into the protympanum.

Hypotympanum

The hypotympanum is the space below the plane of the inferior wall of the EAC. Its pneumatization can vary from a shallow sulcus to extensive air cell tracks. Rarely, this space may contain a dehiscent, high-riding jugular bulb or an aberrant carotid artery. Laceration of an exposed jugular bulb can occur with ventilating tube placement or during elevation of the eardrum. Typically, a plate of bone is seen overlying and protecting the jugular bulb. A persistent tympanomeningeal fissure (Hyrtl's fissure) can be a pathway between the middle ear and the subarachnoid space of the posterior cranial fossa (▶ Fig. 1.5).

Anteriorly the hypotympanum contains the vertical segment of the petrous carotid canal, which extends superiorly through the protympanum to the osseous eustachian tube orifice. If the hypotympanic pneumatization is adequate, access to the petrous apex via the infracochlear route is facilitated by drilling between the carotid canal, the jugular bulb, and the basal turn of the cochlea (▶ Fig. 1.6).

Protympanum

The protympanum, located anterosuperiorly in the middle ear cleft, communicates with the eustachian tube. Its anterior-medial wall, under the anterior tympanic sulcus, contains the aforementioned vertical petrous carotid canal, typically encased in bone as it turns into a horizontal plane forming the medial wall of the osseous eustachian tube.

The Ossicular Chain

Sound pressure is conveyed via the ossicular chain as a mechanical displacement from the tympanic membrane to the cochlea, and consists of the malleus, incus, and stapes. The malleus is the lateralmost ossicle composed of a head and manubrium

(handle), which are connected by a "neck," as well as the lateral and anterior processes. The lateral process has a cartilaginous tip that imperceptibly blends with, and thus is densely adherent to, the pars propria of the tympanic membrane. At the umbo, dense adherence is afforded by the splitting of the pars propria periosteum to encircle the tip of the manubrium. The anterior process is attached to the anterior tympanic spine by the anterior mallear ligament. Ossification of this ligament (more commonly than other supportive ligaments) can cause a conductive hearing loss that mimics otosclerosis.[2] This attachment, together with the posterior incudal ligament, establishes the ossicular axis of rotation. The tendon of the tensor tympani muscle sweeps through the cochleariformis process and attaches to the medial aspect of the neck and manubrium. Ordinarily, the medial pull of the tensor tympani muscle is opposed by the tympanic membrane. In cases of long-standing perforation, however, the tensor tympani acts unopposed, and can medially displace the manubrium, rendering myringoplasty and ossiculoplasty more difficult by contracting the middle ear space. Forcible lateralization of the malleus, or sectioning of the tendon, may be required to perform these procedures.

The incus is the largest of the ossicles, composed of a body and three processes: short, long, and lenticular. The body rests in the epitympanum articulating with the head of the malleus via the incudomallear joint. The short process of the incus occupies the incudal fossa, anchored by the posterior incudal ligament. The long process stretches inferiorly, paralleling posterior to the manubrium, terminating in the medially oriented lenticular process, which articulates with the head of the stapes. The

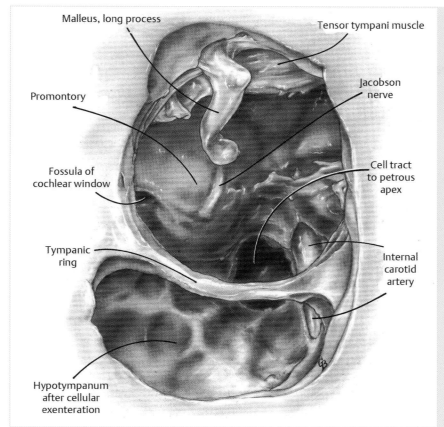

Malleus, long process

Tensor tympani muscle

Jacobson nerve

Promontory

Fossula of cochlear window

Cell tract to petrous apex

Tympanic ring

Internal carotid artery

Hypotympanum after cellular exenteration

Fig. 1.6 The tympanic membrane has been excised, with the tympanic ring left intact. Bone has been removed inferior to the tympanic ring, demonstrating the extent of the hypotympanic pneumatization and the proximity of the vertical petrous carotid artery. (Adapted with permission from Anson BJ, Donaldson JA. Surgical Anatomy of the Temporal Bone. New York: Raven Press, 1992.)

lenticular process is particularly susceptible to osteitic resorption associated with medially retracted tympanic membranes.

The stapes is the most medial and smallest of the ossicles, composed of a head (capitulum), anterior and posterior crura, and the footplate. The footplate is encircled by the annular ligament, which serves as a "joint," sealing the footplate (like an O-ring around a piston) in the oval window. Ossification of this ligament occurs in otosclerosis. The stapedius tendon stretches anteriorly from the pyramidal eminence to attach to the superior aspect of the posterior crus, just inferior to the capitulum.

1.2.3 Eustachian Tube and Temporal Bone Pneumatization

The degree of pneumatization of the temporal bone is variable and may serve as a predictor of eustachian tube function. Five main tracts of pneumatization are recognized: the posterosuperior cell tract (running at the juncture of the posterior and middle fossa plates of the temporal bone), the posteromedial cell tract (paralleling and running inferior to the posterosuperior tract), the subarcuate tract (running through the arch of the superior semicircular canal), the perilabyrinthine tracts (running superior and inferior to the bony labyrinth), and the peritubal tract (surrounding the eustachian tube).

The eustachian tube itself is singularly significant in the maintenance of normal middle ear function and hearing. It consists of a fibrocartilaginous segment located anteromedially and an osseous segment located posterolaterally (▶ Fig. 1.7). The junction of these segments, the isthmus, is the narrowest

portion of the eustachian tube. The total length of this tube averages 35 mm.

The fibrocartilaginous eustachian tube (▶ Fig. 1.8) has a shepherd's crook cross section, with a larger medial and a smaller lateral lamella. The inferior margin of the medial lamella has a groove for the levator palatini muscle, whereas the tensor veli palatini muscle attaches to the tip of the lateral lamella. Active opening of the upper half of the type, which ventilates the tympanic cavity, is accomplished by contraction of the tensor veli palatini muscle.[3] The mucociliary clearance function is located in the lower half of the type, which has an abundance of mucociliary cells. The lateral fat pad (of Ostmann) contributes to the resting closure of the tube and helps protect the tympanic cavity.[3] Loss of this fat pad is thought to be related to patulous eustachian tube syndrome.

1.2.4 Inner Ear Anatomy

Bony Labyrinth

The bony labyrinth serves as a protective covering for the membranous structures of the inner ear, and comprises the vestibule, the semicircular canals, and the cochlea. The bone is trilaminar, with an inner (endosteal) layer, an outer (periosteal) layer, and a middle mixed layer of intrachondrial and endochondral bone, characterized by globuli interossei or islands of cartilage. Both the middle and endosteal layers demonstrate poor reparative capacities, and thus fractures of the labyrinth tend to heal only by the formation of fibrous tissue, with some bony repair by the periosteal layer.

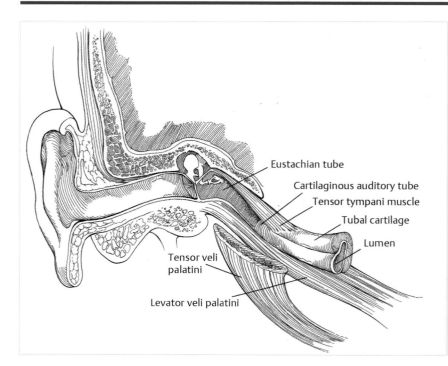

Fig. 1.7 The eustachian tube and its associated muscles. (Adapted with permission from Bluestone CD, Stool CE, eds. Pediatric Otolaryngology. Philadelphia: WB Saunders, 1990:320.)

Eustachian tube

Cartilaginous auditory tube

Tensor tympani muscle

Tubal cartilage

Lumen

Tensor veli palatini

Levator veli palatini

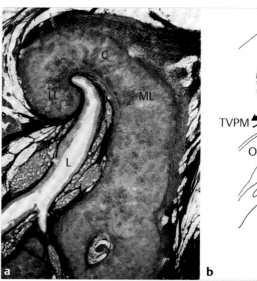
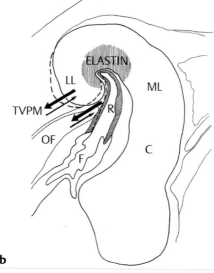

Fig. 1.8 (a) Vertical section through the fibrocartilaginous (C) eustachian tube of an adult, illustrating the medial lamella (ML), the lateral lamella (LL), and their relation to the lumen (L). (b) Line drawing of a fibrocartilaginous (C) eustachian tube, illustrating the hypothesized functional areas. Tensor veli palatini muscle (TVPM) contraction causes lateral movement (*thick arrows*) of the lateral lamella (LL) with respect to the medial lamella (ML) from its resting position (*solid outline*) to its new position (*dashed line*). The elastin in the hinge portion mediates a return to resting position (*thin arrows*). R, roof; F, floor; OF, lateral fat pad of Ostmann.

Vestibule

The vestibule is an approximately 4-mm central chamber of the bony labyrinth, and it is dominated by depressions housing the utricle (the elliptical recess), the saccule (the spherical recess), and the basal end of the cochlear duct (the cochlear recess). The cribrose areas are perforations through which the nerve bundles gain access to the inner ear. The endolymphatic duct, housed within the bony vestibular aqueduct, originates at the posteroinferior aspect of the vestibule.

Cochlea

The cochlea is a 32-mm bony spiral that spirals 2½ turns about its central axis, the modiolus, to a total height of 5 mm. The base of the cochlea abuts the fundus of the internal auditory canal

(IAC), and is perforated (the cribrose area) by its cochlear nerve fibers. The osseous spiral lamina also winds about the modiolus, partially subdividing the cochlear canal into the scala tympani and the scala vestibuli. The interscalar septum separates the cochlear turns (▶ Fig. 1.9).

Semicircular Canals

There are three semicircular canals: lateral (horizontal), posterior (posterior vertical), and superior (anterior vertical). These canals are orthogonally oriented to one another, measure 1 mm in diameter (expanding to 2 mm at the ampullae), and describe a 240-degree arc. Each of the three ampullae opens into the vestibule, as does the nonampullated end of the lateral canal. The nonampullated ends of the posterior and superior canals

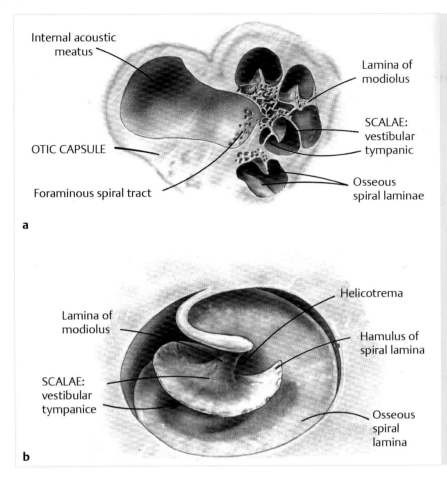

Fig. 1.9 Osseous structure of the cochlea. (a) Relationship with internal auditory canal. (b) Communication of the vestibular and tympani scalae at the helicotrema. (Adapted with permission from Anson BJ, Donaldson JA. Surgical Anatomy of the Temporal Bone. New York: Raven Press, 1992.)

fuse to form the crus commune, and thus complete their communication with the vestibule.

Internal Auditory Canal

The IAC is an osseous channel that is traversed by the superior vestibular, inferior vestibular, cochlear, facial nerves, the nervus intermedius, and the labyrinthine artery and vein. The dimensions of the canal display substantial variability with the diameter averaging 3.7 mm and the length averaging 8 mm.[4]

The porus acusticus is the medial terminus of the bony canal, whereas the lateral end is referred to as the fundus. At the fundus of the canal, the vestibular, facial, and cochlear nerves are consistently identified in their typical anatomic locations as determined by the falciform (horizontal) crest and the vertical crest (Bill's bar). Progressing medially in the canal toward the brainstem, the cochlear and vestibular nerve branches undergo fusion into the eighth cranial nerve,[5] and rotate about the facial nerve, such that the facial nerve assumes a position anterior to the eighth nerve bundle, and the vestibular nerve assumes a position superior to the cochlear nerve (▶ Fig. 1.10).

Knowledge of the medial anatomic relations at the nerve root entry to the brainstem are critical in vestibular nerve sectioning, but are less reliable in tumor extirpation of the cerebellopontine angle, where considerable displacement by a tumor can distort the expected anatomy.

The *perilymphatic labyrinth* is composed of perilymph spaces located between the bony labyrinth and the delicate membranous labyrinth. It includes the vestibule, the scalae tympani and vestibuli, the perilymphatic spaces of the semicircular canals, and the periotic duct.

Membranous Labyrinth

The membranous labyrinth (▶ Fig. 1.11), consisting of the cochlear duct, the otolithic organs (the utricle and the saccule), the three semicircular ducts and their ampullae, and the endolymphatic duct and sac, is housed within the bony labyrinth, with the connective tissue, blood vessels, and fluid of the perilymphatic space interposed. The membranous labyrinth is filled with endolymph, with the vestibular and cochlear portions of the inner ear being connected by the utricular and saccular ducts, and the ductus reuniens.

Cochlear Duct

The cochlear duct or scala media (▶ Fig. 1.12) is an epithelial duct that spirals from the vestibular cecum in the vestibule to the cupular cecum at the apex of the bony cochlea. The epithelium of the cochlear duct is dominated by the organ of Corti, which rests on the basilar membrane. The inner and outer hair cells are the primary auditory receptors. In the human, there is

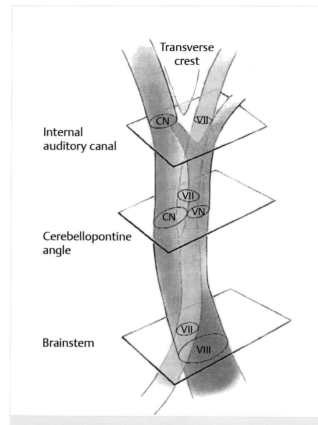

Fig. 1.10 Illustration of the rotation of the nerves in the internal auditory canal. CN, VII, cranial nerve; IVN, inferior vestibular nerve; SVN, superior vestibular nerve; VIII, vestibular nerve. (Used with permission from Nadol JB Jr, Schuknecht HF, eds. Surgery of the Ear and Temporal Bone. New York: Raven Press, 1993.)

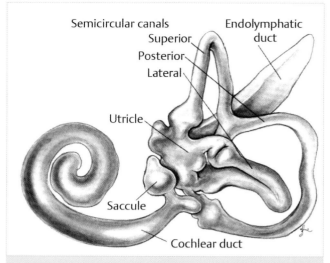

Fig. 1.11 The adult membranous labyrinth as viewed from medially. (Adapted with permission from Anson BJ, Donaldson JA. Surgical Anatomy of the Temporal bone and Ear. Philadelphia: WB Saunders, 1973.)

a single row of inner hair cells and three rows of outer hair cells that form a precisely ordered cellular mosaic. The hair cells are partially enveloped by the synaptic terminations of cochlear nerve fibers and are associated with several types of supporting cells. The spiral ligament is a specialized layer of periosteum in the outer wall of the bony cochlea, upon which rests the stria vascularis, a band of specialized tissue that is composed of three layers of cells with a rich capillary and secretory network. The Reissner membrane forms the anterior wall, or roof, of the cochlear duct, and extends from the spiral limbus to the spiral ligament at the vestibular crest. The tectorial membrane is a gelatinous leaf that extends from the vestibular lip of the limbus to end in the border net, blanketing the organ of Corti.

Utricle

The utricle is an elliptical tube that sweeps inferiorly from the elliptical recess. Its macula, oriented in the horizontal plane, is the sensory organ of the utricle, containing its hair cells, and is divided into two regions by the striola. The otolithic membrane is the otoconia-studded gelatinous blanket into which the cilia of the macular hair cells project.

Saccule

The saccule is a flattened sac, and its macula lies in the spherical recess inferior to the utricle, predominantly in the vertical plane. The saccule is characterized by a reinforced area, and its endolymphatic space communicates with that of the cochlea by means of the ductus reuniens.

Semicircular Ducts

The semicircular ducts run in the periphery of their bony canals; at the ampullae are the cristae ampullares, mounds of sensory neuroepithelium, connective tissue, and blood vessels surmounted by a gelatinous dome, the cupula.

Endolymphatic Duct and Sac

The endolymphatic duct runs in a bony channel, the vestibular aqueduct, from its sinus, located in the posterolateral wall of the vestibule, to the endolymphatic sac, which lies on the posterior surface of the petrous pyramid. The course of the aqueduct initially parallels the crus commune, but then makes a turn to parallel the posterior semicircular canal for the remainder of its course. The total length of the vestibular aqueduct is determined by peri- and infralabyrinthine pneumatization.[6]

The endolymphatic sac (ES) lies about 10 mm posterolateral to the porus of the IAC in a slight depression called the endolymphatic fossette, which is covered by the operculum. The ES is believed to have both resorptive and immunologic functions.[7,8] A surgical landmark for the sac is the Donaldson line, derived by extending the plane of the lateral semicircular canal perpendicular to and bisecting the posterior semicircular canal through to the posterior fossa dura; the sac lies inferior to this line, but in some ears with Ménière disease it may be located more inferiorly and medial to the facial nerve.[6]

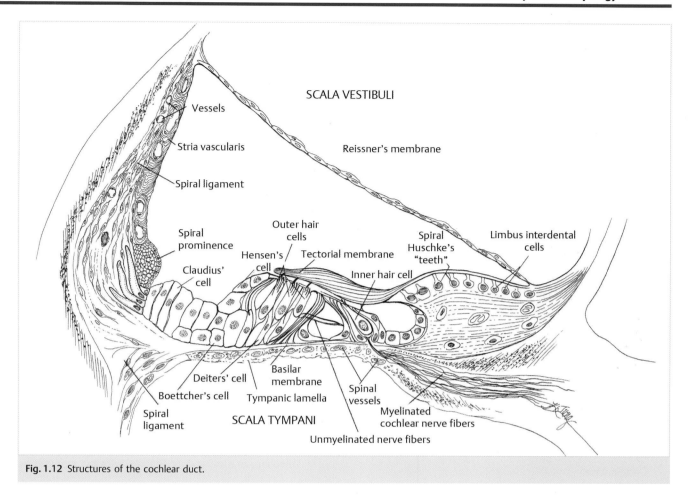

Fig. 1.12 Structures of the cochlear duct.

Utriculoendolymphatic Valve

The utriculoendolymphatic valve (of Bast) is located in the anteroinferior wall of the utricle at the orifice of the utricular duct, and is believed to act in a passive manner to release excess endolymphatic pressure.[9] The cochlear aqueduct carries the periotic duct from its origin at the basal turn of the scala tympani to the medial surface of the jugular fossa. As such it can transmit solutes and pressure from the subarachnoid space to the cochlea. The duct itself is filled with loose connective tissue or obliterated with bone, but if patent, can allow for the transmission of fluid, particles, and thus intracranial pressure between the subarachnoid space and the scala tympani (▶ Fig. 1.13).

The cochlear duct is a useful surgical landmark in translabyrinthine dissection of the IAC, serving both as early release of cerebrospinal fluid and an indicator of the proximity of lower cranial nerves. In some patients a patent cochlear aqueduct or dehiscence of the cochlear modiolus could result in a "perilymphatic gusher" during stapes surgery or transmit intracranial pressure mimicking Ménière disease.

1.2.5 The Facial Nerve

Although the facial nerve is neither an auditory nor a vestibular apparatus, its normal anatomic course through the ear makes it exquisitely relevant to ear disease and ear surgical management. As the nerve of the second branchial arch, the facial nerve innervates the structures derived from Reichert cartilage. Its trunk is made up of five types of fibers: (1) branchial efferent fibers supplying the muscles of facial expression—the stapedius, stylohyoid, and digastric muscles; (2) special visceral efferent fibers to the lacrimal gland, and the seromucinous glands of the nasal cavity and submaxillary and sublingual glands; (3) special sensory (taste) fibers from the anterior two thirds of the tongue, tonsillar fossae, and the posterior palate; (4) somatic sensory fibers from the external auditory canal and the conchal region; and (5) visceral afferent fibers from the mucosa of the nose, pharynx, and palate.

There are three nuclei related to the facial nerve. The motor nucleus of the facial nerve is in the caudal pons. The superior salivatory nucleus, located dorsal to the motor nucleus, conveys parasympathetic secretory stimuli to the submaxillary, sublingual, lacrimal, nasal, and palatine glands. The nucleus of the solitary tract is in the medulla oblongata and receives the taste, proprioceptive, and cutaneous sensory fibers of the facial nerve.

The course of the facial nerve is divided into five segments (▶ Fig. 1.14). The intracranial segment extends some 24 mm from the pons to the porus of the IAC. The intracanalicular segment runs in the IAC for 8 mm, joined at the fundus by the nervus intermedius, where the facial nerve occupies the anterosuperior quadrant. The nerve enters the fallopian canal at the meatal foramen that represents the narrowest part of the whole canal. The labyrinthine segment is the shortest and narrowest,

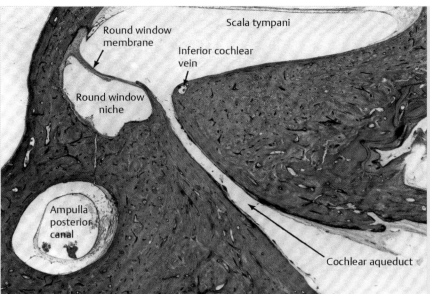

Fig. 1.13 Illustration of both the widely patent cochlear aqueduct and the microfissure between the posterior semicircular canal and the round window niche in a 67-year-old man. (Used with permission from Schunknecht HF, Seifi AE. Experimental observations on the fluid physiology of the inner ear. Ann Otol Rhinol Laryngol 1963;72:687.)

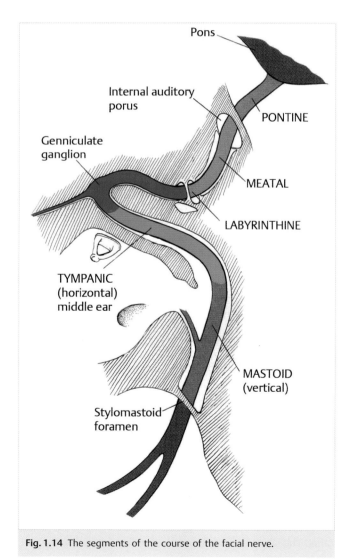

Fig. 1.14 The segments of the course of the facial nerve.

4 mm in length from the entrance to the fallopian canal to the geniculate ganglion, and approximately 0.8 mm in diameter. The fourth, or tympanic, segment covers approximately 13 mm in the medial wall of the tympanic cavity, superior to the cochleariform process and the oval window. At the sinus tympani, the facial nerve turns inferiorly, marking the beginning of the mastoid segment, which extends some 20 mm to the stylomastoid foramen.

The fallopian canal commonly demonstrates numerous gaps, or dehiscences, that expose the facial nerve to potential insult. Baxter[10] found dehiscences of ≥ 4 mm in over half the specimens studies; the most common site, comprising 66% of all dehiscences, was the tympanic segment near the oval window. Dehiscences can also occur in the medial wall of the epitympanum, superior to the geniculate ganglion, in the facial recess, and adjacent to the tensor tympani tendon. On occasion, the facial nerve can herniate through the dehiscence mimicking a middle ear mass (▶ Fig. 1.15).[11]

There are three branches of the facial nerve that arise in the temporal bone. The greater superficial petrosal nerve, carrying preganglionic parasympathetic and sensory fibers, originates from the anterior aspect of the geniculate ganglion and emerges onto the floor of the middle cranial fossa via the facial hiatus. The nerve to the stapedius muscle arises from the mastoid segment of the facial nerve near the pyramidal eminence.

The chorda tympani nerve composes the sensory bundle of the facial nerve, constituting some 10% of its cross-sectional area. The chorda separates from the main trunk a few millimeters superior to the stylomastoid foramen, although it may occasionally arise distal to the foramen, or as high as at the level of the lateral semicircular canal. The chorda takes a vertical course through the temporal bone, anterior and lateral to the mastoid segment of the facial nerve, and enters the tympanic cavity at the iter chordae posterius. The chorda passes lateral to the long process of the incus and medial to the malleus typically passing above the tensor tympani tendon before exiting the tympanic cavity through the iter chordae anterius (canal of Huguier) to enter the petrotympanic (glaserian)

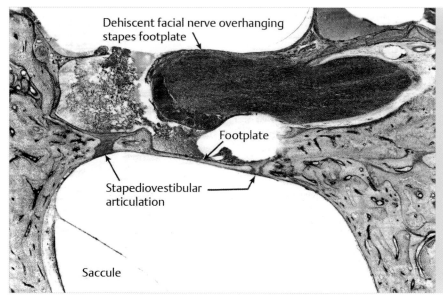

Dehiscent facial nerve overhanging
stapes footplate

Footplate

Stapediovestibular
articulation

Saccule

Fig. 1.15 In this 51-year-old man, the facial nerve not only is dehiscent in the area of the oval window but also herniates over the footplate. (Used with permission from Gulya AJ, Schuknecht HF. Anatomy of the Temporal Bone with Surgical Implications, 2nd ed. Pearl River, NY: Pantheon Press, 1995.)

fissure. Variations in the location of the chorda tympani nerve can occur and are of surgical significance. In addition to the aforementioned variations in its vertical segment, the chorda may pass lateral, rather than medial, to the tympanic membrane, and may pass lateral, rather than medial, to the malleus, or inferior to the tensor tympani.

The nervus intermedius (nerve of Wrisberg) is the sensory component of the facial nerve, and it carries taste, secretory, and sensory fibers. In the IAC, the nervus intermedius runs between the superior vestibular and facial nerves, whereas in the tympanic segment it rests dorsally in the facial nerve. In the mastoid segment, the sensory bundle is found in the lateroposterior portion of the facial nerve, and it finally exits anteriorly as the chorda tympani nerve.

1.2.6 Sensory Innervation of the Middle Ear

The middle ear mucosa, including the medial surface of the tympanic membrane, are innervated by the tympanic branch of the glossopharyngeal (Jacobson nerve). The Jacobsen nerve originates from the inferior ganglion of cranial nerve IX in the petrosal fossula at the jugulocarotid crest, and enters the tympanic cavity by the inferior tympanic canaliculus, accompanied by the inferior tympanic artery; it mediates referred otalgia from pharyngeal disorders. It traverses the promontory joined at the tympanic plexus by caroticotympanic nerves (sympathetic fibers from the pericarotid plexus), coalescing in a groove that terminates at the cochleariform process, where it enters the semicanal of the tensor tympani. From this canal it emerges onto the middle fossa surface of the petrous temporal bone as the lesser superficial petrosal nerve (▶ Fig. 1.16).

The auricular branch of the vagus nerve (the Arnold nerve) consists of seventh, ninth, and tenth cranial nerve fibers. It originates in the jugular foramen and enters the lateral wall of the jugular fossa via the mastoid canaliculus. The auricular branch of cranial nerve X supplies sensation to the skin of the posterior pinna and external auditory canal and portions of the outer layer of the tympanic membrane. Arnold's nerve mediates herpetic involvement of the external auditory canal in herpes zoster oticus, as well as the coughing reflex elicited by touching the skin of the external auditory canal.

The auriculotemporal branch arises from the mandibular branch of the fifth cranial nerve, and supplies sensation to the temporal mandibular joint, tragus, anterior external auditory canal wall, and tympanic membrane. Referred pain from the jaw joint can thus at times be indistinguishable from auricular pain.

1.2.7 Vestibular Nerves

The superior and inferior vestibular nerves occupy the posterior half of the IAC. The superior vestibular nerve innervates the superior and lateral semicircular canal cristae, the macula of the utricle, and the superior portion of the saccular macula. The inferior vestibular nerve innervates the inferior portion of the saccular macula and the posterior semicircular canal. The nerve to the posterior ampulla (the singular or posterior ampullary nerve) separates from the inferior vestibular nerve trunk a few millimeters lateral to the porus acusticus and passes to the posterior canal ampulla via the singular canal.

1.2.8 Cochlear Nerve

The cochlear nerve originates from spiral ganglion neurons. At the fundus of the IAC, the cochlear nerve rests in the anteroinferior quadrant. It enters the brain a few millimeters caudal to the root entry zone of the fifth cranial nerve.

1.2.9 Sections of the Temporal Bone

Horizontal Cross Sections of the Right Temporal Bone

▶ Fig. 1.17 demonstrates a superior view of the right temporal bone. In situ, the base of this bone is slotted between the great-

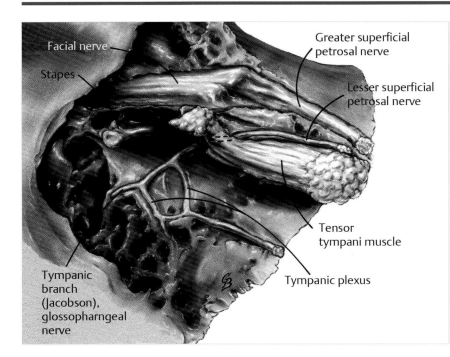

Fig. 1.16 The course of the Jacobson nerve in the middle ear. (Adapted with permission from Anson BJ, Donaldson JA. Surgical Anatomy of the Temporal Bone. New York: Raven Press, 1992.)

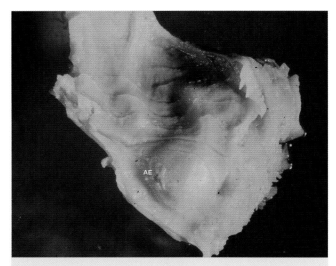

Fig. 1.17 Superior view of the right temporal bone. AE, anterior epitympanic recess.

er wing of the sphenoid anteriorly and the occipital bone posteriorly. The bone has three surfaces: superior, posterior, and inferior. In ▶ Fig. 1.17 we see the superior surface that constitutes the floor of the middle cranial fossa. In this specimen, the dura is attached, and it is important to know that the outer layer of the dura is the firmly attached periosteum of the base of the skull. It is this thick fibrous inner layer of dura that is seen here.

Important surface landmarks on this superior surface are the arcuate eminence and facial hiatus. Underneath the arcuate eminence is the superior semicircular canal, and the semicircular canal lies at right angles to the long axis of the petrous temporal bone. In the middle fossa approach to the internal auditory meatus, this canal is identified as one reference landmark for the IAC.

The facial hiatus, located anterior to the arcuate eminence, marks the exit of the greater superficial nerve from the geniculate ganglion. Another way of locating the roof of the IAC is by tracing the greater superficial petrosal nerve back to the geniculate ganglion and then following the labyrinthine portion of the facial nerve back to the fundus of the IAC.

▶ Fig. 1.18 shows a section made just below the superior arch of the superior semicircular canal (SSC). An axial CT image showing the corresponding structures is included.

The salient features of this cross section are as follows:

- The plane of the SSC is at right angles to the plane of the posterior surface of the petrous pyramid.
- The tentorium cerebelli is attached to the edge of bone, delineating the middle fossa surface from the posterior fossa surface.
- The superior petrosal sinus runs along this edge of bone and lies in the tissue plane between the outer and inner layers of dura. This venous channel connects the cavernous sinus with the transverse/sigmoid sinus.
- The petrous apex lies anteromedially.
- Air cells extend laterally from the superior semicircular canal.
- If the superior canal is found to be unroofed in vivo (▶ Fig. 1.19) the symptoms of SSC syndrome can result (vertigo, hearing loss, pulsatile tinnitus, autophony).

▶ Fig. 1.20 shows a section taken 2 mm inferior to the previous section. An axial CT image shows the corresponding structures.

The epitympanum and the antrum are unroofed and the important structures are labeled.

- The fossa incudis marks the level of the aditus ad antrum.
- The subarcuate artery (or its remnant) passes between the limbs of the superior canal, via the subarcuate air cell tract.
- The two limbs of the superior semicircular canal are open.
- The horizontal canal, covered by bone, forms the medial wall of the aditus.

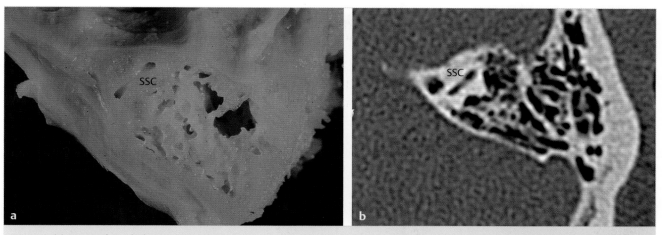

Fig. 1.18 (a) Section through the superior arch of the superior semicircular canal (SSC). (b) Axial CT depicting the SSC. Note the plane of the SSC is perpendicular to the posterior surface of the petrous pyramid.

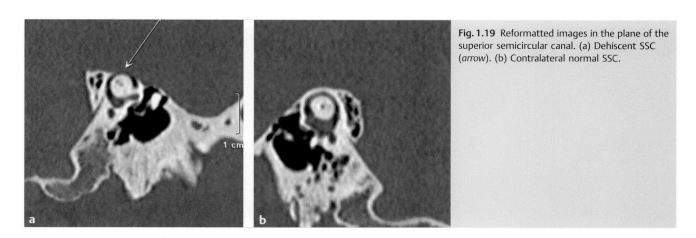

Fig. 1.19 Reformatted images in the plane of the superior semicircular canal. (a) Dehiscent SSC (*arrow*). (b) Contralateral normal SSC.

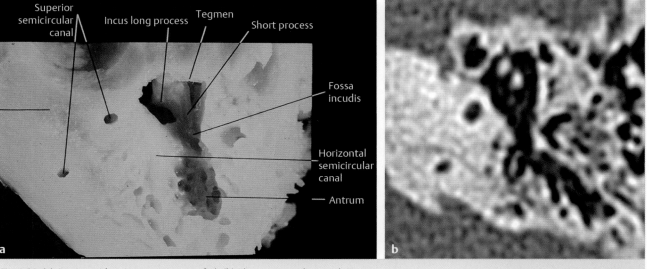

Fig. 1.20 (a) Section with epitympanum unroofed. (b) The corresponding axial CT.

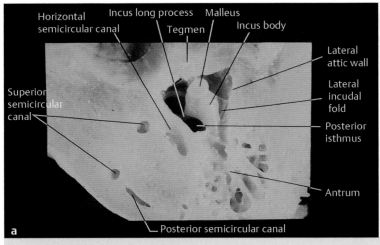
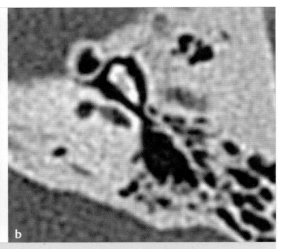

Fig. 1.21 (a) Axial section through fossa incudis and horizontal semicircular canal. (b) Corresponding axial CT.

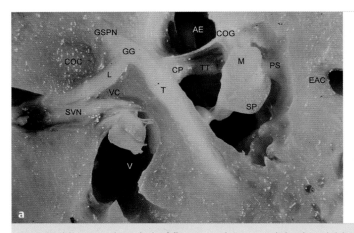
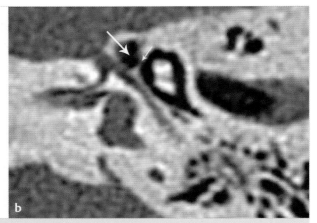

Fig. 1.22 (a) Section through the fallopian canal. From medial to lateral: labyrinthine (L) segment of the facial nerve; geniculate ganglion (GG); the greater superficial petrosal nerve (GSPN) exiting from it; and tympanic (T) segment of the facial nerve. (b) Axial CT scan of the right temporal bone shows a single-celled anterior epitympanic recess (*long arrow*). The anterior attic bony plate, or cog (*short arrow*), separates the anterior epitympanum from the posterior epitympanum.

▶ Fig. 1.21 shows a section 2 mm inferior to the previous section and exposes the roughly triangular shape of the epitympanum in the horizontal plane. The apex of the triangle lies at the fossa incudis.

- The lateral attic wall forms the lateral arm of this triangle.
- The medial wall (depicted as the horizontal facial nerve) forms the other limb of this triangle.
- The horizontal semicircular canal is open, and the ampullated end of the superior canal lies anteriorly.
- The posterior branch of the superior canal joins the crus commune within this 2 mm section.
- The posterior semicircular canal extends posterolaterally from the crus commune.

▶ Fig. 1.22 shows a section cut 2 mm inferior to the previous one, with its corresponding axial CT scan, which demonstrate the following from lateral to medial:

- The roof of the external auditory canal (EAC)

- Prussak's space (PS), located lateral to the neck of the malleus and the body of the incus. Its lateral wall is formed by the outer attic wall.
- The head of the malleus (M) and the short process (SP) of the incus.
- The cochleariform process (CP) is clearly seen in relation to the tympanic segment of the facial nerve. Laterally the tendon of the tensor tympani (TT) muscle emerges from the lumen of the cochleariform process and is attached laterally to the neck of the malleus.
- The spaces adjacent to the medial wall of the middle ear from anterior to posterior are (1) the anterior epitympanic recess (AE), anterior to the cochleariform process (CP); (2) the isthmus anticus anterior to the long process of the incus; and (3) the isthmus posticus.
- The fallopian canal from the meatal foramen medially (proximally) to the second genu laterally (distally). Thus, we can clearly see, from medial to lateral, the labyrinthine segment

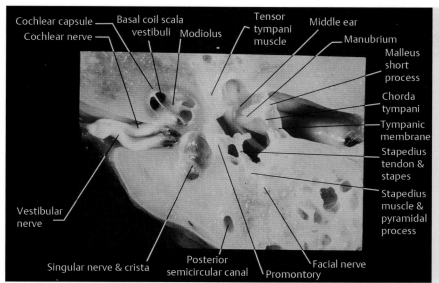

Cochlear capsule — Basal coil scala vestibuli — Modiolus — Tensor tympani muscle — Middle ear — Manubrium — Cochlear nerve — Malleus short process — Chorda tympani — Tympanic membrane — Stapedius tendon & stapes — Stapedius muscle & pyramidal process — Vestibular nerve — Singular nerve & crista — Posterior semicircular canal — Promontory — Facial nerve

Fig. 1.23 Section at the level of the external and internal auditory canals, which are roughly parallel to each other.

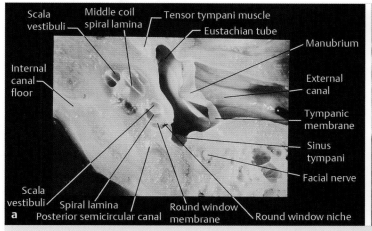

Scala vestibuli — Middle coil spiral lamina — Tensor tympani muscle — Eustachian tube — Manubrium — Internal canal floor — External canal — Tympanic membrane — Sinus tympani — Facial nerve — Scala vestibuli — Spiral lamina — Posterior semicircular canal — Round window membrane — Round window niche

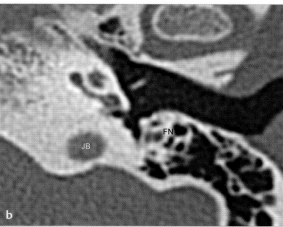

JB · FN · b

Fig. 1.24 (a) Fresh section in axial plane showing all sectioned turns of the cochlea. (b) Axial CT showing a high jugular bulb (JB) medial to the vertical facial nerve (FN).

of the facial nerve, the geniculate ganglion, the greater superficial petrosal nerve exiting from it, and the tympanic segment of the facial nerve.

- Anterior to the labyrinthine segment of the facial nerve is the basal turn of the cochlea (COC).
- Posterior to the labyrinthine segment is the superior vestibular nerve (SVN).
- The triangular bone between the facial and superior vestibular nerves is the vertical crest (VC), also commonly referred to as "Bill's bar." This bony separator can be clearly seen when the fundus of the IAC is viewed through the canal under magnification.
- The vestibule (V) is seen in this section medial to the tympanic segment of the facial nerve and, within it, the macula of the utricle.
- Medially, the whole length of the IAC has been unroofed at this level, exposing the facial and superior vestibular nerves. The medial opening into the IAC is called the porus acusticus.

▶ Fig. 1.23 shows a section at the level of the external and IACs. The structures seen from lateral to medial are as follows:
- The floor of the bony EAC
- The tympanic membrane forms the lateral wall of the middle ear. The handle of the malleus is embedded in it.
- The tensor tympani muscle lies anteriorly, forming the upper part of the medial wall of the middle ear.
- More posteriorly, the promontory forms the medial wall of the middle ear.
- A portion of the anterior crus of the stapes and stapes head are attached to the stapedius tendon, which passes through the pyramidal process to the stapedius muscle. This muscle lies anterior to the vertical descending portion of the facial nerve.
- The space between the pyramidal process and the tympanic annulus anterolaterally is a recess of variable depth, depending on the pneumatization. This recess is called the facial recess or the suprapyramidal recess.

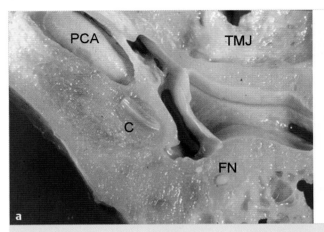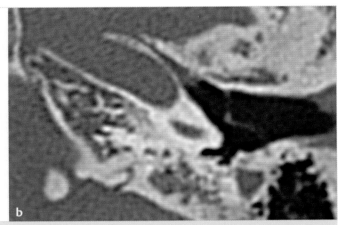

Fig. 1.25 (a) Section at the level of the horizontal petrous carotid artery. (b) Corresponding axial CT.

- This section of the IAC contains the cochlear nerve anteriorly and the inferior vestibular nerve posteriorly. The cochlear nerve enters the base of the modiolus.
- The basal and middle cochlear turns are opened.
- The macula of the saccule lies on the anteromedial wall of the vestibule.

▶ Fig. 1.24 shows a section 2 mm below the previous section, and its corresponding axial CT.

The structures seen from lateral to medial are as follows:
- EAC
- TM with the manubrium embedded in it
- The middle ear extends from the shallow sinus tympani posteriorly, to the eustachian tube anteriorly.
- The important features of the medial wall of the middle ear are the tensor tympani muscle anteriorly and the promontory posteriorly. The basal turn of the cochlea lies deep to the promontory. The round window niche is seen in this section.
- The vertical portion of the facial nerve is seen posterolateral to the sinus tympani. The stapedius muscle is medial to the facial nerve.
- The round window membrane and the cochlea, which is sectioned through all three turns. The spiral lamina separates the scala tympani from the scala vestibuli.
- The ampulla of the posterior semicircular canal is marked. The vertical facial nerve at this level is 2 mm lateral to the ampulla of the posterior semicircular canal, which is important to remember while drilling medial to the facial nerve.

▶ Fig. 1.25 shows a section 2 mm below the previous section and its corresponding axial CT.

The structures seen from lateral to medial are as follows:
- EAC
- Tympanic membrane
- Posteriorly is the vertical portion of the facial nerve (FN) as it exits toward the stylomastoid foramen.
- Anteriorly is the temporomandibular joint (TMJ).
- The horizontal petrous carotid artery (PCA) has been unroofed. Note its position medial and parallel to the bony eustachian tube.
- The inferior portion of the basal turn of the cochlea (C) is seen just posterior to the petrous carotid artery.

Coronal Sections of the Left Temporal Bone from Anterior to Posterior

▶ Fig. 1.26 shows the left temporal bone sectioned through the horizontal petrous carotid, with its corresponding coronal CT scan taken at this level. The salient features of this cross section from lateral (right) to medial (left) are as follows:
- Capitulum of the mandible and the temporomandibular joint (TMJ)
- Bony portion of the eustachian tube (ET)
- The tensor tympani (TT) muscle lies in the medial wall of the eustachian tube.
- The bony lateral wall of the carotid canal forms the medial wall of the eustachian tube.
- The atherosclerotic petrous carotid artery (PC) lies within the carotid canal.

▶ Fig. 1.27 shows a section 4 mm posterior to the previous section, with its corresponding coronal CT image. The structures seen here are as follows:
- The EAC, which is the lateral-most structure
- The lateral attic wall and pars flaccida are labeled.
- The malleus head lies in the epitympanum.
- Posteriorly the body of the incus can be seen.
- The space between the outer attic wall and the head of the malleus and the body of the incus is referred to as the Prussak space.
- In this specimen there is adequate space between the tegmen and the top of the ossicular chain.
- Medial to the cochleariformis process we see the geniculate ganglion.
- Laterally, the tendon of the tensor tympani emerges from the cochleariformis process to attach to the neck of the malleus.
- The three turns of the coils of the cochlea are open and we see the helicotrema in the apical coil.

▶ Fig. 1.28 shows a section posterior to the previous section, with its corresponding coronal CT scan. The structures seen from lateral to medial are as follows:
- EAC

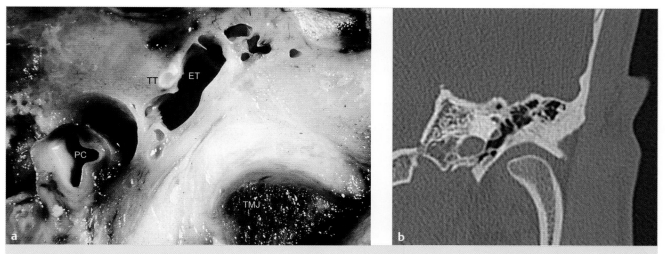

Fig. 1.26 (a) Left temporal bone sectioned through horizontal petrous carotid. (b) Corresponing coronal CT of the temporal bone.

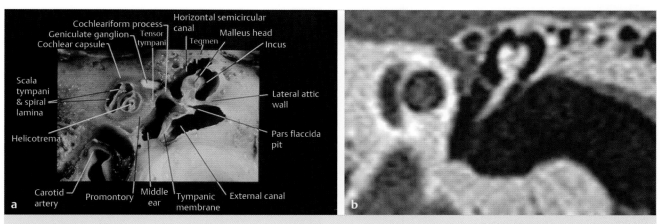

Fig. 1.27 (a) Coronal fresh section through the malleus and cochleariform process. (b) Corresponding coronal CT of the temporal bone.

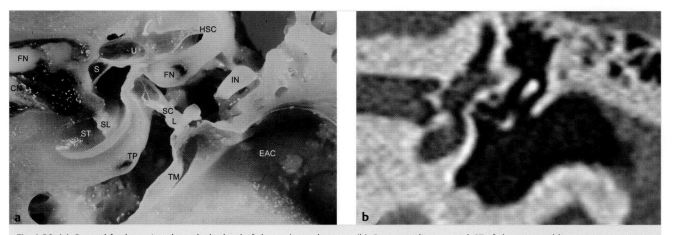

Fig. 1.28 (a) Coronal fresh section through the level of the umbo and stapes. (b) Corresponding coronal CT of the temporal bone.

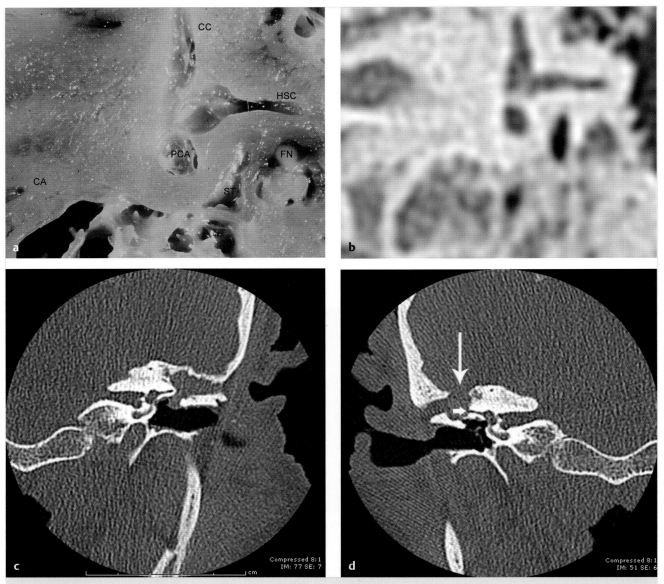

Fig. 1.29 (a) Section taken through the crus commune, the horizontal semicircular canal, and the distal most part of the tympanic facial nerve. (b) Corresponding coronal CT of the temporal bone. (c,d) Coronal CT depicting cholesteatoma with intact horizontal canal (c), fistulized HSC (d, *small arrow*), and eroded tegmen mastoideum with dehiscence of middle fossa floor (d, *large arrow*).

- The tympanic membrane (TM) is transected at the level of the umbo.
- The body of the incus (IN) is seen in the epitympanum.
- The bony horizontal semicircular canal (HSC) projects into the posterior epitympanum and aditus.
- The ampullated end of the superior canal is situated in close proximity to the ampullated end of the horizontal canal.
- The incus lenticular (L) process (shown sectioned from body of incus) articulates with the stapes capitulum (SC).
- The basal turn of the cochlea with the scala tympani (ST) exposed and spiral lamina (SL)
- This section is sectioned through the IAC such that the contents of the anterior compartment are readily seen. Directly

below the horizontal semicircular canal is the tympanic segment of the facial nerve.
- Below this segment of the facial nerve is the oval window with the superstructure of the stapes (ST) and the footplate in place.
- Note the thickness of promontory bone overlying the scala tympani with the grove for the tympanic plexus (TP).

▶ Fig. 1.29a shows the posteriormost cross section taken through the crus commune (CC), the horizontal semicircular canal (HSC), posterior canal ampulla (PCA), sinus tympani (ST), cochlear aqueduct (CA), and the distalmost part of the tympanic facial nerve (FN). The coronal CT image (▶ Fig. 1.29b) demonstrates the corresponding structures radiographically.

1.3 Embryology of the Ear

The embryology of the ear and temporal bone is regarded by most students as complicated and difficult to understand. The subject is considerably simplified if the development of individual parts of the ear and temporal bone are studied separately. The figures illustrate the basic concepts. Before we consider the steps of embryogenesis, it is worthwhile to define the terminology of development. Jackler et al[12] suggested that the understanding of developmental anomalies is best clarified by defining these three terms:

1. Aplasia: complete lack of development.
2. Hypoplasia: incomplete development. Thus, a congenitally narrowed EAC should not be labeled as "stenotic" but rather "hypoplastic." Stenosis is an acquired narrowing of a lumen by inflammation, trauma, or neoplasm.
3. Dysplasia: aberration in development.

1.3.1 Pinna

The pinna develops from the mesoderm of the first and second branchial arches at 4 weeks of gestation. Within 2 weeks the six hillocks of His appear on the mandibular and hyoid arches. These numbered hillocks progressively fuse to form the pinna (▶ Fig. 1.30). The adult configuration is achieved by the fifth month, independent of developmental processes in the middle and inner ears.

1.3.2 External Auditory Canal

In the adult the EAC is made up of a lateral fibrocartilaginous segment and the medial osseous segment. The fibrocartilaginous segment develops from the dorsal part of the first branchial groove. In the course of development, this groove progressively deepens so that its ectoderm transiently abuts the endoderm of the first pharyngeal pouch. In the sixth week, a mesodermal ingrowth breaks this contact and it subsequently forms the lamina propria (meatal plate) of the tympanic membrane. After 9 weeks, a cord of epithelial cells grows medially, terminating at the meatal plate. This epithelial cord begins to recanalize from medial to lateral. The skin lining the recanalized EAC forms the external layer of the TM and the lining of the EAC (▶ Fig. 1.31).

The bony segment of the EAC (the tympanic ring) develops from four ossification centers surrounding the lamina propria or the meatal plate. These ossification centers fuse by 10 weeks, forming a C-shaped ring that opens superiorly (notch of Rivinus). Incomplete fusion inferiorly and its persistence in adulthood creates a patent foramen of Huschke. Lateral growth of the tympanic ring with the otic capsule begins after the eighth month of gestation, a process not completed until after birth. The squamous temporal bone forms the roof of the bony EAC (▶ Fig. 1.32).

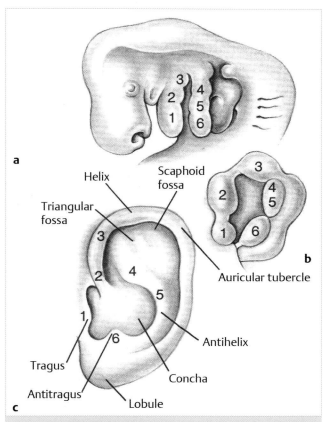

Fig. 1.30 Drawings of the human ear origin from the first and second branchial arches, illustrating the development of the six hillocks, and their contribution to the final adult structure. (a) Approximately 6 weeks. (b) Approximately 7 weeks. (c) Adult. (Adapted with permission from Anson BJ, Donaldson JA. Surgical Anatomy of the Temporal Bone and Ear. Philadelphia: WB Saunders, 1973.)

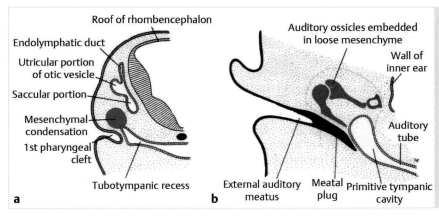

Fig. 1.31 (a) Transverse section of a 7-week embryo in the region of the rhombencephalon, showing the tubotympanic recess, the first pharyngeal cleft, and mesenchymal condensation, foreshadowing development of the ossicles. (b) Middle ear showing the cartilaginous precursors of the auditory ossicles. Thin yellow line in the mesenchyme indicates future expansion of the primitive tympanic cavity. Note the meatal plug extending from the primitive auditory meatus to the tympanic cavity. (Adapted with permission from Sadler TW. Langman's Medical Embryology. Philadelphia: Lippincott Williams and Wilkins, 2004.)

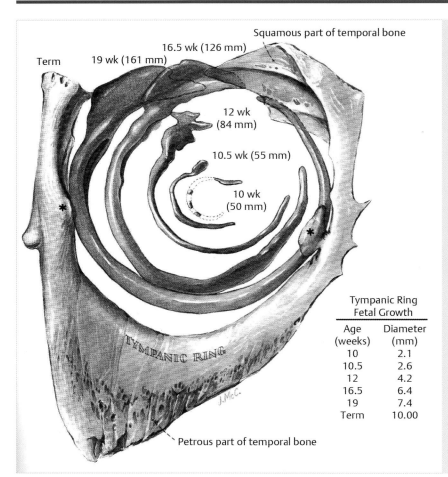

Fig. 1.32 Tympanic ring: developmental anatomy shown by reconstructions and a specimen. (Adapted with permission from Anson BJ, Donaldson JA. Surgical Anatomy of the Temporal Bone. New York: Raven Press 1992.)

Tympanic Ring Fetal Growth	
Age (weeks)	Diameter (mm)
10	2.1
10.5	2.6
12	4.2
16.5	6.4
19	7.4
Term	10.00

1.3.3 The Middle Ear and Mastoid Compartment

The tympanomastoid compartment develops as an outpouching of the first pharyngeal pouch (the tubotympanic recess). The endodermal tissue of the dorsal end of this pouch gives rise to the eustachian tube and tympanic cavity. The terminal end of the pouch buds into four sacci that progressively pneumatize the tympanomastoid compartment. By 30 weeks, the development of the tympanic cavity is essentially complete.

1.3.4 Ossicular Chain

At 4 weeks the upper ends of the first and second branchial arches are connected by a bridge of mesenchyme that eventually gives rise to the malleus and incus (▶ Fig. 1.33). The stapes develops from the second branchial arch except for the footplate and annular ligament, both of which are of otic capsule origin. By 15 weeks, the ossicles have attained adult size and ossification begins, first in the incus and last in the stapes.

1.3.5 Membranous Labyrinth

The first indication of the developing ear is a thickening of the surface ectoderm on each side of the rhombencephalon (▶ Fig. 1.34). These thickenings, the otic placodes, rapidly

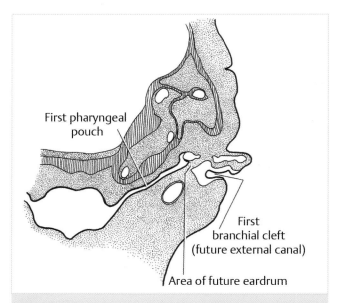

Fig. 1.33 Drawing depicting the development of the human external auditory canal.

invaginate to form the otic vesicles (▶ Fig. 1.35). With further development, each vesicle divides into a ventral compartment that gives rise to the saccule and a dorsal compartment that forms the utricle.

The endolymphatic appendage is the first to appear from both these sacs. The lateral (horizontal) duct, the superior semicircular duct, and the utricular macula are phylogenetically the oldest parts of the inner ear and develop from the utricular sac. The posterior semicircular duct, the macula of the saccule, and the cochlear duct develop from the ventral sac (▶ Fig. 1.36). During the sixth week of organogenesis, the semicircular ducts appear as outpocketings or canal plates expanding from the dorsal otic vesicle. The central regions of these canal plates appose each other with the contacting epithelium undergoing apoptosis. The loss of this central region of the canal plates leaves behind the loop-like structure of the three semicircular ducts (▶ Fig. 1.37). One end of each duct dilates to form the ampulated end of each duct.

Differentiation of the cristae ampularis and maculae of the utricle and saccule: Cells of each ampulla differentiate into a specialized structure—the crista ampullaris. Similar sensory areas, the maculae acusticae, develop into specialized sensory cells in the walls of the utricular and saccular sacs.

Development of organ of Corti: In the sixth week of development, the inferior portion of the otic vesicle evaginates and extends ventrally, giving rise to the cochlear duct that penetrates the surrounding mesenchyme in a spiral fashion. By the eighth week it completes 2.5 turns. Initially the epithelial cells of the cochlear duct are alike. With further development, they form two ridges—an inner ridge and an outer ridge (▶ Fig. 1.38).

The outer ridge forms one row of inner and three rows of outer hair cells. The inner ridge gives rise to the spiral limbus (▶ Fig. 1.39).

1.3.6 Perilymphatic Labyrinth

At 8 weeks, the mesenchyme surrounding the cochlear duct differentiates into cartilage. In the tenth week this cartilaginous shell undergoes vacuolization and two perilymphatic spaces, the scala vestibule and the scala tympani, are formed (▶ Fig. 1.38c).

1.3.7 Otic Capsule

The initial step in the development of the otic capsule occurs at the end of the fourth week, as the cell density of the mesenchyme enveloping the membranous labyrinth increases, this mesenchyme differentiates into cartilage. According to Bast and Anson,[13] the first ossification center appears in the region of the cochlea. The following five features in the development of the otic capsule are unique:
- Origin from 14 ossification centers, appearing within a period of 6 weeks, beginning with the 15th week
- Fusion of the centers peripherally without intermediate zones of epiphyseal growth or suture lines (21 weeks)
- Trilamilar structure of each center and consequently of the entire capsule
- Independent timetable of growth for each layer of every center and individual pattern of histogenesis
- Lifelong retention of fetal architecture in the total absence of those processes that elsewhere convert fetal into haversian bone

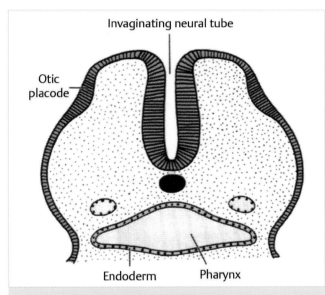

Fig. 1.34 Region of the rhombencephalon showing the otic placodes in a 22-day embryo. (Adapted with permission from Sadler TW. Langman's Medical Embryology. Philadelphia: Lippincott Williams and Wilkins, 2004.)

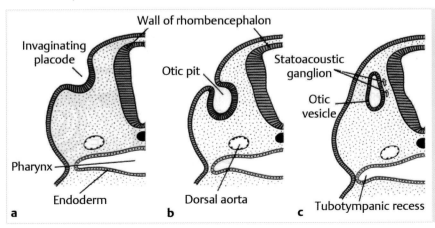

Fig. 1.35 Transverse sections through the region of the rhombencephalon showing formation of the otic vesicles: (a) 24 days; (b) 27 days; (c) 4.5 weeks. Note the statoacoustic ganglia. (Adapted with permission from Sadler, TW. Langman's Medical Embryology. Philadelphia, PA: Lippincott Williams and Wilkins, 2004.)

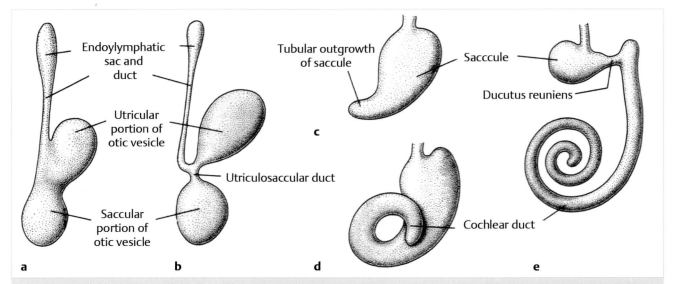

Fig. 1.36 (a,b) Development of the otocyst showing a dorsal utricular portion with the endolymphatic duct and a ventral saccular portion. (c,d,e) Cochlear duct at 6, 7, 8 weeks, respectively. Note formation of the ductus reunions and the utriculosaccular duct. (Adapted with permission from Sadler TW. Langman's Medical Embryology. Philadelphia: Lippincott Williams and Wilkins, 2004.)

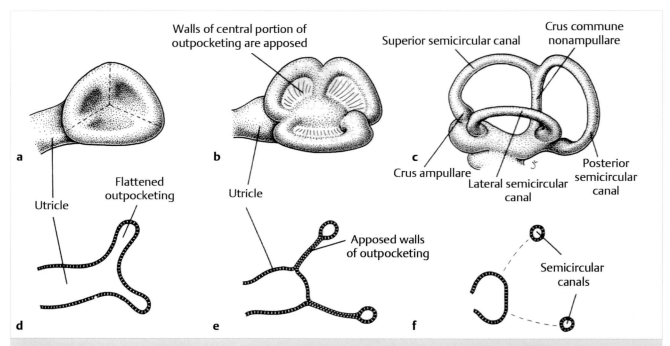

Fig. 1.37 Development of the semicircular canals. (a) 5 weeks. (c) 6 weeks. (e) 8 weeks. (b,d,f) Apposition, fusion, and disappearance, respectively, of the central portions of the walls of the semicircular outpocketings. Note the ampullae in the semicircular canals. (Adapted with permission from Sadler TW. Langman's Medical Embryology. Philadelphia: Lippincott Williams and Wilkins, 2004.)

Three layers of bone emerge from ossification of the cartilaginous otic capsule (▶ Fig. 1.40):

- The endosteal layer does not significantly change throughout adult life, except that it may proliferate in response to infection (labyrinthitis ossificans).
- The periosteal layer in contrast does change by lamellar addition of bone and by pneumatization until early adult life.
- Enchondral bone is sandwiched between the endosteal and periosteal layers. It is made up of intrachondral and endo-

chondral bone. The endochondral layer undergoes little change throughout life and has minimal reparative capabilities, healing by fibrous union at best.

1.3.8 Cochlear Modiolus

The modiolus arises independently from membrane bone beginning at 20 weeks, and ossification is complete by 25 weeks.

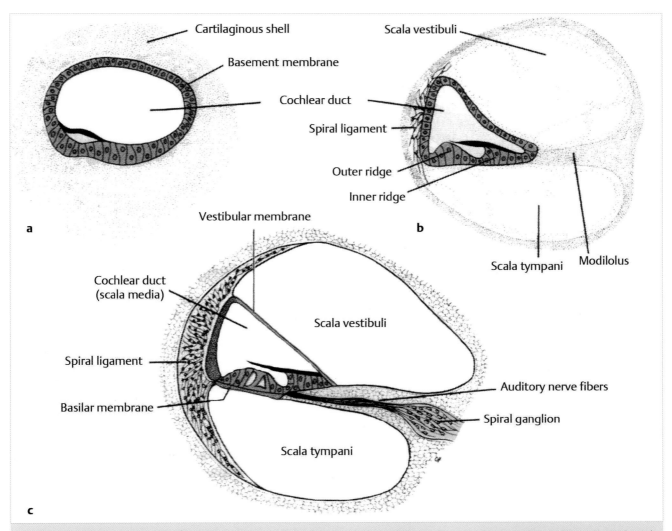

Fig. 1.38 Development of the scala tympani and scala vestibuli. (a) The cochlear duct is surrounded by a cartilaginous shell. (b) During the 10th week large vacuoles appear in the cartilaginous shell. (c) The cochlear duct (scala media) is separated from the scala tympani and the scala vestibule by the basilar and vestibular membranes, respectively. Note the auditory nerve fibers and the spiral (cochlear) ganglion. (Adapted with permission from Sadler TW. Langman's Medical Embryology. Philadelphia: Lippincott Williams and Wilkins, 2004.)

1.3.9 Neural Differentiation

Scarpa Ganglion and Spiral Ganglion

During formation of the otic vesicle, a small group of cells delaminate from the dorsomedial wall and form the statoacoustic ganglion. The ganglion subsequently splits into cochlear and vestibular portions.

Facial Nerve

According to Gasser et al,[14] at about 4 weeks "the facial nerve primordium arises from the rhombencephalon" as a column of neutral crest cells and "extends ventrally to contact the epibranchial placode of the second arch," a thickened area of ectoderm just caudal to the dorsal aspect of the first groove. The geniculate ganglion forms at the area of contact.

By approximately 6 weeks, there is a distinguishable geniculate ganglion, and the facial crest has evenly divided into caudal and rostral segments; the caudal segment becomes the main trunk of the facial nerve, and the rostral segment becomes the chorda tympani nerve, the first branch of the facial nerve to form.

The greater superficial petrosal nerve, the second branch of the facial nerve to form, appears at the seventh week of gestation from the ventral aspect of the geniculate ganglion, and the main trunk of the facial nerve established its intratemporal anatomic relationship in the cartilaginous otic capsule.

The fallopian canal begins formation at the end of 20 weeks' gestation as the apical cochlear ossification center gives rise to two projections of bone that eventually are to encircle the anterior tympanic segment of the facial nerve.

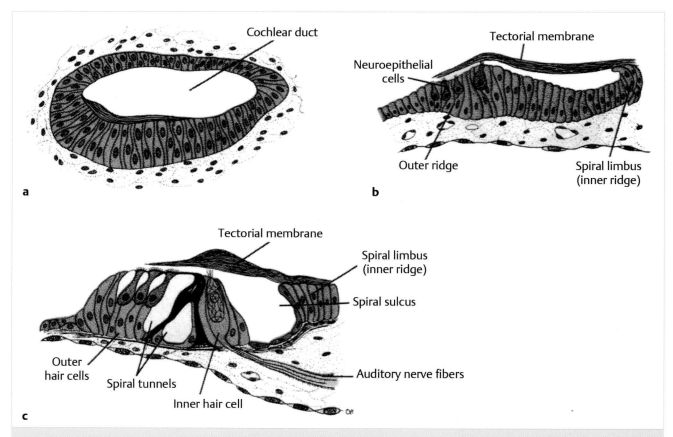

Fig. 1.39 Development of the organ of Corti. (a) 10 weeks. (b) Approximately 5 months. (c) Full-term infant. Note the appearance of the spiral tunnels in the organ of Corti. (Adapted with permission from Sadler TW. Langman's Medical Embryology. Philadelphia: Lippincott Williams and Wilkins, 2004.)

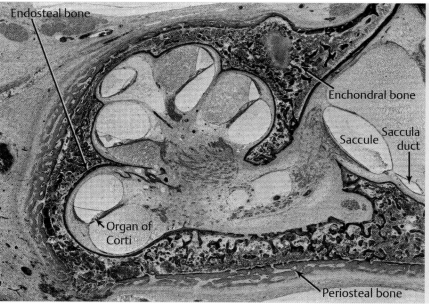

Fig. 1.40 In the fetus of 16 weeks, the three layers of otic capsule bone are clearly demarcated. (Used with permission from Gulya AJ, Schuknecht HF. Anatomy of the Temporal Bone with Surgical Implications, 2nd ed. Pearl River, NY: Pantheon Press, 1995.)

References

[1] Sheehy JL. The facial nerve in surgery of chronic otitis media. Otolaryngol Clin North Am 1974; 7: 493–503

[2] Fisch U. Malleus fixation. In: Tympanoplasty, Mastoidectomy, and Stapes Surgery. New York: Thieme, 2008:238–239

[3] Sando I, Takahashi H, Matsune S, Aoki H. Localization of function in the eustachian tube: a hypothesis. Ann Otol Rhinol Laryngol 1994; 103: 311–314

[4] Olivares FP, Schuknecht HF. Width of the internal auditory canal. A histological study. Ann Otol Rhinol Laryngol 1979; 88: 316–323

[5] Silverstein H. Cochlear and vestibular gross and histologic anatomy (as seen from postauricular approach). Otolaryngol Head Neck Surg 1984; 92: 207–211

[6] Arenberg IK, Rask-Andersen H, Wilbrand H, Stahle J. The surgical anatomy of the endolymphatic sac. Arch Otolaryngol 1977; 103: 1–11

[7] Parker DA, Schindler RA, Amoils CP, Lustig LR, Hradek GT. Hyaluronan synthesis in the adult guinea pig endolymphatic sac. Laryngoscope 1992; 102: 152–156

[8] Wackym PA. Histopathologic findings in Menière's disease. Otolaryngol Head Neck Surg 1995; 112: 90–100

[9] Schuknecht HF, Belal AA. The utriculo-endolymphatic valve: its functional significance. J Laryngol Otol 1975; 89: 985–996

[10] Baxter A. Dehiscence of the fallopian canal. An anatomical study. J Laryngol Otol 1971; 85: 587–594

[11] Johnsson L-G, Kingsley TC. Herniation of the facial nerve in the middle ear. Arch Otolaryngol 1970; 91: 598–602

[12] Jackler RK, Luxford WM, House WF. Congenital malformations of the inner ear: a classification based on embryogenesis. Laryngoscope 1987; 97 Suppl 40: 2–14

[13] Bast TH, Anson BJ. The Temporal Bone and the Ear. Springfield, IL: Charles C. Thomas, 1949

[14] Gasser RF, Shigihara S, Shimada K. Three-dimensional development of the facial nerve path through the ear region in human embryos. Ann Otol Rhinol Laryngol 1994; 103: 395–403

2 Principles of Clinical Audiology and Assessment of Auditory Physiology

Robert W. Keith, Jennifer A. Ratigan, and Daniel I. Choo

2.1 Introduction

The physiology of the auditory system is complex, and our understanding of how the system functions is not yet complete. Chapter 1 discussed the anatomy of the auditory system, but a complete understanding of the auditory system also requires knowledge of the nature of sound and the function of the structures. Only with this comprehensive understanding can we have the greatest impact on patients with hearing loss.

This chapter addresses the breadth of the basic principles of auditory physiology, with an emphasis on the scientific concepts that form the underlying mechanisms by which we clinically evaluate and manage ear and hearing disorders. Developing a deeper fund of knowledge regarding the physiological basis for audition is particularly important today when considering the ever-growing and diversifying battery of evaluation tools available to the clinician. Irrespective of the novel technologies and instruments that emerge, the fundamental physiological principles of the auditory system are likely to remain relevant.

2.2 Acoustics

Acoustics is the science that is concerned with the production, control, transmission, reception, and effects of sound. Sound is energy: mechanical radiant energy that is transmitted through pressure waves in a material medium (e.g., air, water, metal). In the case of hearing, sound is the sensation perceived by the ear. This sound energy is captured by the outer ear, transformed by the middle ear, and transduced by the inner ear. Sound is described in terms of its basic physical attributes: frequency, intensity, and time/phase of the vibration.[1] These physical attributes also have psychological correlates, which are pitch, loudness, and quality, respectively. These terms are often used interchangeably, thus leading to misunderstanding and misuse, which is especially true for frequency and intensity.

People often mistakenly refer to the pitch of a tone when they really mean its frequency and to the loudness of a tone when they mean its intensity. The pitch of a tone is perceived by the listener, whereas one can quantifiably measure the frequency of the same tone with an oscilloscope. A tone with a frequency of 1,000 Hz may fluctuate in frequency by a few hertz (cycles per second) either up or down over a period of time, which can be measured by the oscilloscope. However, the normal-hearing listener is not able to perceive such small changes in pitch. Changes in pitch are what we detect when the frequency of a tone changes and are measured in a unit called the mel. There is little correlation between the two except that mels increase and decrease with frequency. For example, when we play the scale on the piano from middle C (256 Hz) to the C above middle C (512 Hz), we are moving up an octave; every time we move up an octave, the frequency doubles. As we move from one C to the next C, however, the units on the mel scale do not double[2] because pitch, although highly correlated with frequency, is subjective and influenced by both the frequency and the intensity of the sound.

Loudness is the psychological correlate of intensity. Changes in the intensity of a sound may or may not result in a perceived change in loudness. Loudness is a subjective analysis of the sound by the listener. It is affected by the duration and frequency of the sounds that are present, and a unit of loudness level is the phon. The smallest change in a physical parameter of sound (such as frequency or intensity) that results in a perceived change (of pitch or loudness) is called a just noticeable difference (JND).

2.2.1 Frequency

A single-frequency sound, or pure tone, is the standard used in the assessment of auditory sensitivity (threshold). Frequency is a physical attribute of a sound and is defined as the number of cycles per unit of time. For example, if a metronome were to move back and forth 1,000 times in 1 second, it would have 1,000 cycles per second. One cycle, therefore, is defined as one complete event and has occurred when a particle has completed all its variations, returned to its original point of rest, and is about to begin the same variations again. Although measured in cycles per second, frequency is reported in hertz (Hz). As in the above example, the result would be a 1,000-Hz tone because it completed 1,000 cycles per second. A sound can be visualized in the time domain, as shown in ▶ Fig. 2.1, which describes tones of different frequencies.

Period refers to the amount of time it takes for one cycle to occur; therefore, period is the reciprocal of frequency (period = 1/frequency). This 1,000-Hz tone would have a period of 1/1,000 seconds. Wavelength (λ) is the distance sound travels in one period and is reported in centimeters, feet, or miles, depending on how the velocity is recorded. Velocity is the speed in which the sound travels from the source to a distant point and is determined by the density of the medium. Because sound is transmitted mainly through the air, the velocity would be 344 m (or 1,130 feet) per second. Therefore, wavelength is the speed at which the sound travels divided by the frequency of the sound (λ = velocity/frequency). Given a 1,000-Hz tone, the period and the wavelength can be computed, as shown in ▶ Table 2.1.

A single-frequency sound is a simple sound or pure tone. However, sounds in the real world are seldom simple and are made of more than one frequency; these are called complex sounds. If the variations of a sound are repetitive over time, the sound is periodic. Both simple (pure tones) and complex (voice) sounds may be periodic. Sounds that are not repetitive over time are aperiodic (e.g., noise).

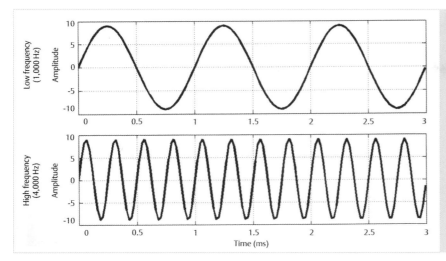

Fig. 2.1 Graphs of two sine waves of different frequencies plotted over time. The top graph is a low frequency (1,000 Hz) and the bottom is a higher frequency (4,000 Hz) as denoted by the number of cycles in the same time window.

Table 2.1 Frequency, Period, and Wavelength of a 1,000-Hz Tone

Frequency	Period	Wavelength (λ)
$\text{Frequency} = \dfrac{\text{Velocity}}{\text{Wavelength}}$	$\text{Period} = \dfrac{1}{\text{Frequency}}$	$\lambda = \dfrac{\text{Velocity}}{\text{Frequency}}$
$\text{Frequency} = \dfrac{344\,\text{m/s}}{0.344\,\text{m}} = 1,000\,\text{Hz}$	$\text{Period} = \dfrac{1}{1,000\,\text{Hz}}$ $= 0.001\,\text{second}\,(1\,\text{millisecond})$	$\lambda = \dfrac{344\,\text{m/s}}{1,000\,\text{cycles/s(Hz)}} = \lambda = 0.344\,\text{m}$

Noise is defined as an aperiodic, complex sound. There are several types of noise, such as white noise, speech, and narrow-band noise. White noise is a broadband noise that is complex and aperiodic. Its name is derived from the fact that it contains all the frequencies in the audible spectrum, randomly distributed, just as white light contains all the colors of the visual spectrum. White noise is not often used in audiometry as it is too broad in its spectrum. However, the other noises, speech and narrow-band noise, are derived from this white noise with a narrower band or frequency response than white noise.

Speech noise refers to a band of noise that has had the frequencies below and above the speech frequencies (3 to 300 kHz) filtered out. Speech noise is most often used for masking during speech audiometry. Narrow-band noise (NBN) is actually white noise with certain frequencies (above and below a given center frequency) filtered out. The result of the filtering is a frequency range of noise smaller than broadband white noise but broad enough to effectively mask the tested frequency. Narrow-band noise is most often used for masking in pure-tone testing.

2.2.2 Intensity

The number of times an object vibrates determines its frequency, but how far the object moves determines its intensity. Intensity or amplitude then becomes another physical attribute of sound. Intensity relates to the strength of a sound as shown in ► Fig. 2.2; the distance a mass moves from the point of rest is the amplitude of the sound. Intensity is usually measured in decibels (dB), after the renowned Alexander Graham Bell. There

are five descriptors of the decibel: it is (1) a relative unit of measure; (2) a ratio; (3) logarithmic; (4) nonlinear; and (5) expressed in terms of various reference levels.[2] An often-overlooked aspect of the decibel is that it is a relative unit of measure that needs to be described with a reference or it loses its meaning. For example, dB SPL is related to sound pressure level, dB HL is related to hearing level, and dB SL is related to the sensation level, where the tone is presented at above that amount above the threshold. The use of the term *dB* without a referent is meaningless and should be avoided.

In the simplest terms, the decibel represents a difference between two sounds: a referent and the sound being described. The formula for dB (pressure) is dB = 20 log R, where R is the ratio between the referent and a given sound. For example, if we were discussing a sound that was the same pressure as the referent (i.e., dB = 20 log 0.0002 µPa/0.0002 µ, where the referent is 0.0002 µ), the ratio equals 1, and the log of 1 = 0. Therefore, 20 × 0 = 0 dB, and 0 dB means that there is no difference between the two sounds—our sound and its referent. It is also important to be aware that the decibel represents a logarithmic series, not an interval series. Therefore, in pressure measurements, a 20-dB step represents a 10-fold increase (i.e., a ratio of 10:1); a 40-dB step represents a 100-fold increase; a 60-dB step represents a 1,000-fold increase; and so forth. For example, people attending a rock concert where the level of the sound is 140 dB SPL (2,000 dynes/cm²) are exposed to 1,000 times more pressure than they should be exposed to if the safe level is 80 dB SPL (2.0 dynes/cm²).

The basic acoustical measurement that is used for almost all acoustic measures is the sound pressure level (SPL). This

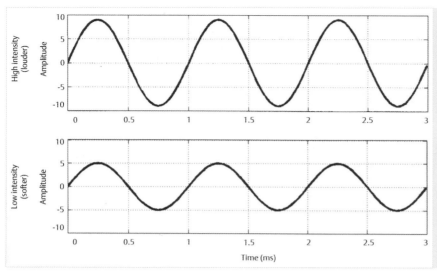

Fig. 2.2 Graphs of two sine waves of the same frequency (1,000 Hz) but different intensities plotted over time. The tones have the same cycles per second but differ in the amplitude of the waves.

Table 2.2 Standard Referenced Sound Pressure Levels (0.0002 dynes/cm²) for 0 dB Hearing Level as Developed for a Standard Audiometer Earphone (TDH 39) (ANSI, 1996)

Frequency (Hz)	Standard Earphore (TDH 39)
125	45.0
250	25.5
500	11.5
750	8.0
1,000	7.0
1,500	6.5
2,000	9.0
3,000	10.0
4,000	9.5
6,000	15.5
8,000	13.0

measure is independent of frequency and has a referent of 0.0002 dyne/cm² (or 0.0002 μ). This referent was determined in the Bell Laboratories many years ago and has stood the test of time. It remains the basic referent for all acoustic measures, but, unfortunately, very few people are able to detect a sound at 0 dB SPL. Therefore, a different system had to be set up using SPL as a referent and criteria ascertained from several studies of auditory sensitivity in humans. The American National Standards Institute (ANSI) in 1969 issued the standard for audiometric zero.

Audiometric zero is frequency-specific and indicates that auditory sensitivity in humans is poorer at lower frequencies (125 Hz) and higher frequencies (8,000 Hz) than it is in the mid-frequency range (500 to 4,000 Hz), as shown in ► Table 2.2. When audiometric zero is the referent, the designation is hearing level (HL); thus, when indicating a decibel measurement, the method of measurement (i.e., SPL or HL) is very important. The use of dB HL instead of dB SPL allows the hearing threshold for normal individuals to be calibrated to audiometric zero across all frequencies (despite normal auditory sensitivity being better for the middle frequencies of the test range).

As previously noted, dB sensation level (SL) refers to any measurement that is above an individual's threshold. This term is both frequency-specific and individual-specific. If patients are tested at 30 dB SL, this means they were tested at 30 dB above their threshold for that particular frequency or for speech. Because the decibel is a measurement based on a referent, it is possible to move back and forth among dB SPL, dB HL, and dB SL. For example, at 250 Hz, a sound is to be presented to a patient at 35 dB SL. The patient's threshold is 40 dB HL. What is the level of presentation in dB SPL? We know from ► Table 2.2 that the 0 dB HL is 25.5 dB SPL; thus, the dB SPL equivalent of 35 dB SL is 100.5. Because all of the units are mathematically related, it is possible to convert from one to another.

2.2.3 Phase

The phase of a sound refers to the relative timing of sound waves. It is simplest to refer to the starting phase of the signal; therefore, at time zero the point of the sine wave where the signal begins will be the starting phase as shown in ► Fig. 2.3. This will act as a referent point for other waves. Two tones of the same frequency that begin 180 degrees out of phase will cancel each other out.

In a complex sound, that is, one that has more than one frequency, the lowest frequency in that sound is called the fundamental. The fundamental frequency of a complex, periodic sound is the frequency at which the source vibrates. All frequencies above that are called overtones. Frequencies that are multiples of the fundamental are called harmonics and those that are not multiples are called aharmonics.

Resonance refers to the phenomenon whereby one body can be set into motion by the vibration of another body. If a given area has a "resonant frequency," then that frequency is amplified when it is presented in that area. In other words, there is an increase in the intensity of that signal because the surface of the area with the resonant frequency vibrates at the particular frequency that has been presented and therefore increases its

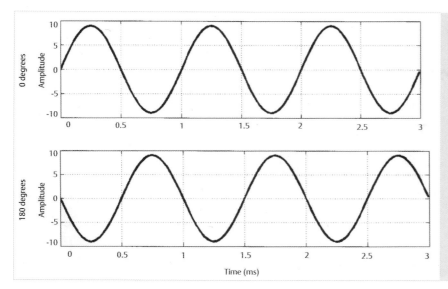

Fig. 2.3 Two tones that are 180 degrees out of phase; note that the starting points for the two waves are the same, creating a mirror image.

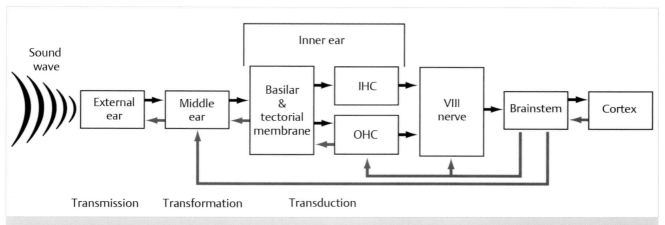

Fig. 2.4 Block diagram of the auditory system. The sound leaves its generator and travels through the external, middle, and inner ear and travels to the auditory cortex. IHC, inner hair cell; OHC, outer hair cell.

intensity. The fundamental frequency of the voice is the slowest rate at which the vocal folds vibrate for a given "voiced" sound. There may be several overtones imposed by the inertial effect of the vibrating vocal folds.

Differences in the sounds that come out of the vocal mechanism are caused by changing the resonating cavities above the vocal folds. Complex sounds may be described in terms of spectra. The spectrum of a sound identifies the frequencies and the relative amplitudes of the various components of a sound.

2.3 Physiology of Hearing

The anatomy of the auditory system is addressed in Chapter 1. This chapter traces the course of the auditory stimulus from its generator to the auditory cortex, as shown in ▶ Fig. 2.4. Although the many relay stations in the auditory system all contribute to signal processing in a unique way, we highlight those areas pertinent to the practicing otologist and to those interested in the complexity of this exciting and mysterious sensory system.

The natural or usual manner by which humans detect sound is via an airborne or acoustic signal. Once the sound is generated, it travels through the air in a disturbance called a sound wave. This sound is slightly modified by the body and head, specifically the head and shoulders, which affect the frequencies below 1,500 Hz by shadowing and reflection.[3] The flange and concha of the pinna collect, amplify, and direct the sound wave to the tympanic membrane by the external auditory meatus. At the tympanic membrane, several transformations of the signal occur: (1) the acoustic signal becomes mechanoacoustic; (2) it is faithfully reproduced; and (3) it is passed along to the ossicular chain, is amplified, or, under certain conditions, is attenuated.

2.4 Transmission and Natural Resonance of the External Ear

Natural resonance refers to inherent anatomic and physiological properties of the external and middle ear that allow certain frequencies to pass more easily to the inner ear.[4] The external ear serves to enhance the sound as it travels to the cochlea and to protect the tympanic membrane.[5] The concha and ear canal increase the intensity of the sound over the frequency range 1,500 to 7,000 Hz by as much as 10 to 20 dB SPL using only simple resonance.[6] The natural resonance of the external auditory canal is 2,700 Hz[6] in the adult, and 5,300 to 7,200 Hz in newborns.[7] This ear canal resonance is dependent on the size and shape of the ear canal and is inversely related to its length.

The natural resonance of the middle ear is 800 Hz. The tympanic membrane is most efficient in transmitting sounds between 800 and 1,600 Hz, whereas the ossicular chain is most efficient in transmitting sounds between 500 and 2,000 Hz. These structures enhance sensitivity to sound between 500 and 3,000 Hz, which are approximately the frequencies that are most important in human speech.[4]

2.4.1 Transformation and the Middle Ear Mechanism

The middle ear system is a mechanical transformer used to help compensate for the impedance mismatch between sound traveling through air and cochlear fluid. This mismatch is caused by the much larger cochlear input impedance, which allows about 3% of the sound energy to be transmitted into the cochlea and reflects 87%.[8] The impedance matching is accomplished by the area effect of the tympanic membrane, the lever ratio of the ossicular chain, the natural resonance and efficiency of the middle ear, and the phase difference between the oval and round windows. Many of these principles were first suggested by Helmholtz,[9] and were later confirmed by Wever and Lawrence.[4]

2.4.2 Area Effect of the Tympanic Membrane

The adult human tympanic membrane measures approximately 90 mm². Of this area, approximately 55 mm² are functional in that primarily the lower two thirds of the membrane vibrates in response to sound. The tympanic membrane in turn is connected to the stapes footplate by way of the ossicular chain. The stapes footplate has an area of 3.2 mm². The hydraulic ratio created by the vibrating area of the tympanic membrane in comparison with that of the stapes footplate produces a 17:1 increase in sound energy transmission across the middle ear.

2.4.3 Lever Ratio of the Ossicular Chain

Tympanic membrane vibrations are transmitted by way of the malleus to the incus. The axis of rotation of the ossicular chain is from the anterior process of the malleus through the posterior (short) process of the incus. The long process of the incus and handle of the malleus move in unison; however, the malleus handle is 1.3 times longer than the long process of the incus. This difference in length produces a 1.3:1 lever ratio of the middle ear ossicles. The overall middle ear transformer ratio is the product of 1.3 × 17, or a transformer ratio of 22:1 due to the combined area effect of the drum and lever ratio of the ossicles.[4] This equates to approximately 27 dB of gain and when combined with the action of the external ear will compensate for the loss of energy due to the impedance mismatch.[10]

2.4.4 Phase Difference Between Oval and Round Windows

As sound energy is transmitted to the stapes footplate, fluid vibrations travel from the scala vestibuli up the cochlear partition to the helicotrema.[8,11] For most frequencies, the helicotrema acts mechanically as though it were closed. Therefore, it is incorrect to assume that displacement of the stapes causes perilymph to flow back and forth through this opening. If this in fact occurred, there would be no displacement of the cochlear partition. The helicotrema is instead involved in the static balance of fluid pressure within the cochlea.[8] The round window membrane is an elastic membrane several cell layers thick that vibrates in response to sound waves traveling through the fluid medium of the inner ear. Because impulses created at the oval window must travel through the vestibule and scala vestibuli before reaching the round window membrane, movements of the stapes footplate precede those of the round window membrane; that is, there is a phase difference between the two windows. Clinically, if the round window niche were sealed by bone or other pathological disease, lack of membrane movements would impede the traveling fluid wave and result in a hearing loss. Similarly, in surgically altered ears where the oval and round windows are "exteriorized" (e.g., a canal wall down, type IV tympanomastoidectomy) and simultaneously exposed to the same acoustic impulse or signal, the concurrent generation of a traveling wave from both the oval and round windows would be anticipated to create a net canceling effect that again would cause a hearing loss.

For the fluid system of the inner ear to transmit sound most efficiently, there must be oval window exposure and round window protection. Oval window exposure permits transmission of tympanic membrane vibrations through the ossicles to the oval window. Round window protection prevents the sound wave from striking the round window simultaneously with the oval window, thus canceling out the vibrations. Phase difference between the oval and round windows produces a minor effect in the normal ear (approximately 4 dB) but a very large effect in the diseased ear.[4]

Middle ear muscles (tensor tympani and stapedius) probably play a role in protecting the inner ear from acoustic trauma.[11] Whether they enhance audition is not known.

2.5 Sound Transmission in the Diseased Ear

Middle ear pathology may alter the normal transformation mechanism by creating stiffness of the eardrum and ossicular chain or by a mass within the middle ear cavity. Both pathological results produce conductive hearing loss, but middle ear stiffness involves primarily low frequencies. Thus, different pathological processes can produce characteristic conductive hearing losses.

Eustachian tube obstruction, negative middle ear pressure, and early effusion produce a stiffening of the middle ear transformation mechanism, causing a low-frequency conductive hearing loss. If effusion becomes secondarily infected and progresses to the stage of suppuration, increased pressure within the middle ear cleft produces a mass effect on the transformation mechanism, resulting in a high-frequency loss in addition to the low-frequency loss. Perforations of the tympanic membrane alter the function of the middle ear transformation mechanism by decreasing the area effect of the drum and by producing abnormal phase on the oval and round windows. Perforation size is more important than its location. For example, a small central perforation may impair the area effect of the drum to produce a relatively small conductive hearing loss (e.g., 15 dB) primarily in the low frequencies, whereas a large central perforation of the tympanic membrane may produce a greater (e.g., 30 dB) conductive hearing loss. This is due not only to further loss of area effect of the drum, but also to passage of sound directly to the round window membrane where the phase effect may be altered.

When the ossicular chain is disrupted, the area effect of the drum and the lever ratio of the ossicles do not contribute to the middle ear transformation mechanism. If a large central perforation of the drum coexists with ossicular discontinuity, at least some sound energy will pass through the perforation to vibrate the stapes, causing a greater conductive hearing loss (e.g., 45 dB). If, however, the tympanic membrane is intact but the ossicular chain is disrupted, sound vibrations from the drum will not be passed to either the oval or round windows, and the result will be a maximal conductive hearing loss of 60 dB.

In the office examination, the clinician should correlate audiometric findings with physical findings. A small attic perforation with cholesteatoma may preserve the larger vibrating portion of the drum, but a coexistent conductive hearing loss of 30 or 40 dB usually implies that ossicular erosion has taken place. Knowledge of the middle ear transformation mechanism often can aid the surgeon in determining the extent of disease preoperatively.

2.6 Clinical Application of the Principles of Middle Ear Mechanics

As described above, the primary role of the middle ear is to bridge the mechanical mismatch between the air-filled outer ear and fluid-filled cochlea. Acoustic immittance tympanometry is used to determine the canal size, pressure, and compliance of the tympanic membrane. In the patient care setting, this allows the clinician to assess the integrity of the tympanic membrane, the presence of effusion, the patency of tympanostomy tube(s), or obstruction by cerumen or debris. For the adult patient who can articulate symptoms or changes in hearing perception, this assessment provides a confirmatory piece of data. However, in very young children, correlation of history and physical exam findings with immittance testing results can enhance the sensitivity and specificity of clinicians' diagnosis of ear pathologies that might impair a child's hearing or vestibular function.

2.6.1 Transduction and the Inner Ear

As the vibrations reach the footplate of the stapes and enter the inner ear (the vestibule) via the oval window, they are transformed into hydroacoustic waves in the perilymph. This disturbance, called a traveling wave, enters the cochlea at its base, via the scala vestibuli, and courses its length, displacing the cochlear partition in a precise fashion. The movement within the inner ear can be described by two components: passive and active cochlear mechanics. Passive linear mechanics consist of the traveling wave and its interactions with the structures of the inner ear. A traveling wave with a certain frequency grows in amplitude as it moves apically up the cochlea until it has reached its maximum displacement at the place where the cochlea is tuned to that frequency and then rapidly dampens out.[12] The tuning of the basilar membrane is such that it vibrates according to its characteristic frequency. Thus the basal end of the basilar membrane is tuned to the high frequencies and the tuning becomes lower in frequency toward the apex. The active cochlear mechanism accounts for the high sensitivity, sharp frequency tuning, and wide dynamic range of the auditory system. This occurs because energy is provided into the system to enhance the vibration of the basilar membrane, resulting in sufficient amplification of the weak vibration to stimulate the inner hair cells (IHCs) and accounting for our ability to hear soft sounds.[13]

The cochlea is a snail-shaped, 32-mm-long structure that makes 2.75 turns in the normal postnatal temporal bone. Delicate membranes divide the cochlea into three fluid-filled chambers. The two outer chambers contain perilymph, which has an ionic composition similar to that of extracellular fluid. These two chambers communicate at the apex of the cochlea where the scala media terminates (helicotrema). The middle cochlear chamber (also called cochlear duct, scala media, and otic duct) contains endolymph, which has an ionic composition similar to that of intracellular fluid. Different ionic compositions of the fluid compartments are ideal for propagation of afferent auditory neural impulses.

With the delivery of an auditory stimulus, transduction of the mechanical traveling wave into neural activity begins with the deflection of the outer hair cells' (OHCs) stereocilia. Each OHC supports three rows of stereocilia, all configured into a W pattern. The actin-filled OHC stereocilia, like the IHCs' stereocilia, are interconnected by cross-links.[14] The OHC stereocilia generally number from 50 to 150 per bundle, with greater numbers appearing toward the cochlear base; they have lengths ranging from 0.5 to 1 μm or greater near the lower frequency cochlear apex. Each stereocilia row is progressively graded in length as a function of its distance from the modiolus.[14] The OHC stereocilia are relatively more rounded at their extremes, compared with the more flattened distal tips of the IHC stereocilia. The OHC stereocilia are also thinner (≈ 0.20 μm) relative to the wider diameters (≈ 0.45 μm) of the IHC stereocilia.[15] The tips of the tallest OHC stereocilia appear to be embedded within the tectorial membrane, whereas by contrast the IHC stereocilia show no evidence of tectorial membrane-embedding.[16] It is therefore likely that the stereocilia of the OHCs are displaced directly by the combined displacement of the tectorial and basilar membranes. The three stereocilia rows, therefore, provide stiffness; the OHC subplasma membrane provides an elastic hair cell attachment (for a restorative force), and the overlying tectorial membrane provides a resonant system.[17] Indeed, the gradient of stiffness along the basilar membrane is the key factor in determining the tonotopic specificity of the basilar membrane.

There are three to five rows of OHCs (approximately 12,000 to 15,000 in humans). The cylindrically shaped mammalian OHCs have lengths ranging from 0.20 µm (near the cochlear base) to 80 µm nearer to the apex of the cochlea.[14] The OHCs are securely attached at their perinuclear region to the Deiters' cells,[15] which are capable of stretching,[18] and to the reticular lamina at the OHC apex. The OHCs exhibit a much poorer afferent innervation compared with the well-innervated IHCs,[19] yet they seem to be capable of both responding to forces, as in detecting and boosting the amplitude of the traveling wave, and generating forces as in the production of otoacoustic emissions (OAEs).[17,20] It is important to note that the existence of OAEs depends largely on the micromechanical integrity of the cochlear OHCs.[21] The current view is that OHCs serve as active, nonlinear force-generating mechanical effectors, providing a threshold boost in basilar membrane mechanics within the initial 40 dB of hearing sensitivity.[20,22]

A depolarizing current applied to the apical region of the OHCs produces a decrease in OHC length and an increase in cell width, whereas hyperpolarizing currents produce increases in cell length and decreases in cell width.[20,22]

These observed contractile properties have never been observed in IHCs or in supporting cells. As effectors, the OHCs are capable of altering the shape of the basilar membrane and reticular lamina independent of the traveling wave, changing their relative position to the tectorial membrane along select frequency regions.[23] Such actions may well serve to facilitate or damp sensitivity at select frequency bands.[24] Therefore, the OHCs are recognized as key elements in the dynamic maintenance of auditory threshold sensitivity and in frequency tuning.[25,26] All available evidence indicates that their dynamic, micromechanical nonlinear properties fall under the modulatory control of the medial efferent olivocochlear (OC) system.[27]

From cochlear base to apex, the flask-shaped mammalian IHCs (which number 3,000 to 3,500) line up in a single row. The IHCs remain constant in morphology, and each supports approximately 60 to 77 stereocilia, having lengths ranging from 1 µm (at the cochlear base) to greater than 8 µm near the cochlear apex. The IHC stereocilia are also interconnected by cross-links and tip-links.[14] Located at or near the distal tips of the stereocilia are the elastically gated, mechanosensitive transduction channels, numbering approximately four per stereocilium.[28–32]

These apical transduction channels prefer cations over anions.[17,20] Stereocilia deflection (1 to 100 nm) in a positive direction, toward the bundle's tall edge, produces IHC depolarization.[33] During the resting state the hair cell is exposed to a constant and random buffeting by surrounding molecules, and each apical transduction channel can randomly fluctuate from an open to a closed state. This permits a small steady flow of positively charged ions to cross into the hair cell. Only approximately 15% of the IHC transducer channels are open during the resting, or inactive state. The two principal cations, K^+ and Ca^{2+}, appear to be the major carriers of the mammalian depolarizing current across the apical IHC membrane.[17,20] At frequencies < 200 Hz, the displacement of the free-standing IHC stereocilia is proportional to basilar membrane velocity, and at frequencies > 200 Hz, to basilar membrane displacement.[34] A positive deflection of the stiff, actin-filled IHC stereocilia is sufficient to gate an inward flow of current through almost

100 mechanosensitive transducer channels associated within each stereocilia bundle.

The IHCs, as shown in ▶ Fig. 2.5, are the primary end-organs for transmitting information to the myelinated type I dendrites of the auditory nerve.[35] The initiation of auditory signaling and hearing within the mammalian periphery is therefore highly dependent on the release of the primary excitatory neurotransmitter from within the IHCs. This afferent neurotransmitter is probably glutamate or a related excitatory amino acid.[36,37]

The central pillar of petrous bone around which the cochlea is wound is the modiolus, and in the cavity (Rosenthal's canal) created within the modiolus are the cell bodies of the neurons that compose the auditory portion of the eighth cranial nerve. Collectively, these cell bodies are called the auditory

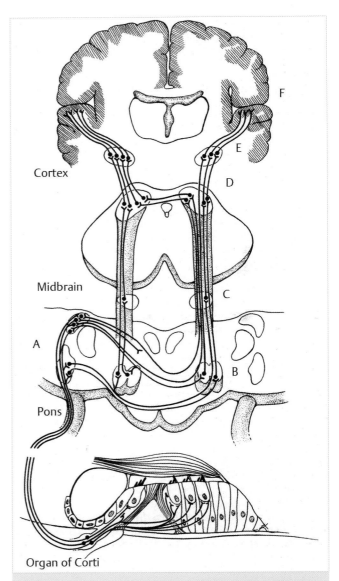

Fig. 2.5 Electrical impulses beginning at the level of the cochlea traverse to the primary auditory cortex through both the ipsilateral and contralateral auditory pathways. A, cochlear nuclei; B, superior olivary complex; C, lateral lemniscus; D, inferior colliculus; E, medial geniculate body; F, auditory cortex.

spiral ganglia. These cell bodies, totaling approximately 30,000 in humans, are of two types, and the dendrites of both types emerge from out of the osseous spiral lamina, and enter the organ of Corti. The myelinated type I neurons make up at least 90 to 95% of the total neurons used in hearing and are therefore responsible for most or all of the auditory input reaching the brain.[19] Type I afferent neurons innervate the IHCs exclusively, with approximately 7 to 10 type I neurons per IHC.

2.7 Auditory Pathways and Cortex

The mammalian auditory system also contains descending neural pathways. Although the efferent system begins at the cortex, we will discuss the system only as it arises from the superior olivocochlear region. These efferent fiber bundles originate from neurons located near the brainstem superior olivary region, and innervate the cochlea via anatomically segregated medial and lateral divisions.[38] Descending lateral efferent axons are distributed primarily within the ipsilateral cochlea and terminate directly upon the dendrites of auditory type I spiral ganglia neurons.[39] The purpose of these unmyelinated lateral efferents is not well defined, although numerous attempts have been made to clarify their role in auditory function.[40,41] Anatomic studies have demonstrated that auditory type I dendrites are segregated with respect to the number of lateral efferent terminations they receive. About 10 to 30% of the total number of type I afferents exhibit relatively high thresholds and relatively low rates of spontaneous discharge. These relatively less responsive afferents receive twice as many lateral efferent terminals, as compared with the remaining afferents that characteristically exhibit lower thresholds and higher rates of spontaneous discharge.[42] This segregated synaptic distribution has suggested that tonic input from the lateral efferents may be required to establish or maintain the distribution of spontaneous activity and sensitivity within primary auditory inputs to the brain.[43]

Centrifugal axons arising from the medial pre- and periolivary efferent nuclei terminate upon the basal and circumnuclear regions of the OHCs, bilaterally.[39] A convincing argument has been made in favor of a medial efferent system that functions to reduce primary afferent neural responses to low levels of "nonessential" auditory stimuli,[44-46] improving the response range ($\approx$ 3 to 8 dB) of individual auditory neurons in backgrounds of noise.[47] The resulting improvement in signal encoding then permits a greater detection of intensity changes in noise backgrounds, at relatively lower signal-to-noise ratios.

A considerable amount of evidence indicates that both efferent divisions utilize several neurotransmitters, including acetylcholine (ACh) and γ-aminobutyric acid (GABA). The lateral efferent system also utilizes neuroactive enkephalin and dynorphin opioid peptides.[36]

At the level of the organ of Corti the stimulus changes from hydroacoustic to synaptic ($\blacktriangleright$ Fig. 2.5). The neural impulses leave the cochlea via the afferent neurons and coalesce to form the acoustic division of the eighth cranial nerve. The nerve enters the brainstem at the level of the pons. Here the fibers bifurcate and send collaterals to the dorsal and ventral cochlear nuclei. The central auditory system (CAS) begins at the cochlear nuclei. It is responsible not only for transferring acoustic information to the brain but also for many subtle but critical functions that afford us the experience of hearing. It plays a critical role in such processes as hearing in noise, localization, temporal judgments, and decoding complex acoustic stimuli.

Approximately 80% of the fibers leave the cochlear nuclei and traverse the brainstem to the contralateral superior olivary nucleus (SON) in a nerve bundle called the trapezoid body. From the SON, fibers travel up the brainstem in another pathway called the lateral lemniscus. At the nucleus of the lateral lemniscus, fibers may synapse, cross to the contralateral nucleus, or may bypass the nucleus on the way to the inferior colliculus, where the same three possibilities may occur. The next stations are the medial geniculates, and from there cortical radiations travel to the surface of the cortex (Brodmann's area 41) located at the superior aspect of the temporal lobe along the floor of the lateral cerebral fissure.

2.8 Conclusion

This chapter has discussed many of the core principles of acoustics; introduced some terms, concepts, and definitions; and described the pathway of a sound from its generator to the brain. Each section in this chapter could have been the subject of a complete text. Therefore, the interested reader should view the information contained within as a threshold and not as an end point.

References

[1] Yost WA. Overview: psychoacoustics. In: Yost WA, Popper AN, Fay RR, eds. Human Psychophysics. New York: Springer-Verlag, 1993:1–12

[2] Martin FN, Clark JG. Introduction to Audiology. Boston: Allyn and Bacon, 2003

[3] Zwicker E, Fastl H. Psychoacoustics: Facts and Models. New York: Springer-Verlag, 1990

[4] Wever EG, Lawrence M. Physiological Acoustics. Princeton, NJ: Princeton University Press, 1954

[5] Peck JE. Development of hearing. Part I: Phylogeny. J Am Acad Audiol 1994; 5: 291–299

[6] Shaw EAG. The external ear. In: Keidel WD, Neff WD, eds. Handbook of Sensory Physiology—Auditory Systems, vol 5. Berlin: Springer-Verlag, 1974:455–490

[7] Kruger B. An update on the external ear resonance in infants and young children. Ear Hear 1987; 8: 333–336

[8] Durrant JD, Lovrinic JH. Bases of Hearing Science, 3rd ed. Owings Mills, MD: William & Wilkins, 1995

[9] Helmholtz H. Die Mechanick der gehorknochelchen und des trommelfells. Pfluegers Arch Ges Physiol 1868

[10] Killion MC, Dallos P. Impedance matching by the combined effects of the outer and middle ear. J Acoust Soc Am 1979; 66: 599–602

[11] Ferraro JA, Melnick W, Gerhardt KR. Effects of prolonged noise exposure in chinchillas with severed middle ear muscles. Am J Otolaryngol 1981; 2: 13–18

[12] Pickles JO. An Introduction to the Physiology of Hearing, 2nd ed. New York: Academic Press, 1988

[13] Ryan A, Dallos P. Effect of absence of cochlear outer hair cells on behavioural auditory threshold. Nature 1975; 253: 44–46

[14] Harrison RV, Hunter-Duvar IM. An anatomical tour of the cochlea. In: Jahn AF, Santos-Sacchi J, eds. Physiology of the Ear. New York: Raven Press, 1988:159–171

[15] Santi PA. Cochlear microanatomy and ultrastructure. In: Jahn AF, Santos-Sacchi J, eds. Physiology of the Ear. New York: Raven Press, 1988:173–199

[16] Lim DJ. Cochlear anatomy related to cochlear micromechanics. A review. J Acoust Soc Am 1980; 67: 1686–1695

[17] Ashmore JF. The electrophysiology of hair cells. Annu Rev Physiol 1991; 53: 465–476

[18] LePage EL. Functional role of the olivo-cochlear bundle: a motor unit control system in the mammalian cochlea. Hear Res 1989; 38: 177–198

[19] Spoendlin HH. Neural anatomy of the inner ear. In: Jahn AF, Santos-Sacchi J, eds. Physiology of the Ear. New York: Raven Press, 1988:201–219

[20] Ashmore JF. Ionic mechanisms in hair cells of the mammalian cochlea. In: Hamann W, Iggo A, eds. Progress in Brain Research, vol 74. New York: Elsevier Science, 1988:3–9

[21] Probst R. Otoacoustic emissions: an overview. Adv Otorhinolaryngol 1990; 44: 1–91

[22] Ashmore JF. A fast motile response in guinea-pig outer hair cells: the cellular basis of the cochlear amplifier. J Physiol 1987; 388: 323–347

[23] Reuter G, Gitter AH, Thurm U, Zenner HP. High frequency radial movements of the reticular lamina induced by outer hair cell motility. Hear Res 1992; 60: 236–246

[24] Patuzzi R, Yates GK, Johnstone BM. Outer hair cell receptor current and its effect on cochlear mechanics. In: Wilson JP, Kemp DT, eds. Cochlear Mechanisms: Structure, Function and Models. New York: Plenum Press, 1989:169–176

[25] Cody AR. Acoustic lesions in the mammalian cochlea: implications for the spatial distribution of the 'active process'. Hear Res 1992; 62: 166–172

[26] Cody AR, Russell LL. Effects of intense acoustic stimulation on the nonlinear properties of mammalian hair cells. In: Dancer AL, Salvi RH, Hamernik RP, eds. Noise-Induced Hearing Loss. St. Louis: Mosby Year Book, 1992:11–27

[27] Brownell WE. Outer hair cell electromotility and otoacoustic emissions. Ear Hear 1990; 11: 82–92

[28] Holton T, Hudspeth AJ. The transduction channel of hair cells from the bull-frog characterized by noise analysis. J Physiol 1986; 375: 195–227

[29] Hudspeth AJ. Extracellular current flow and the site of transduction by vertebrate hair cells. J Neurosci 1982; 2: 1–10

[30] Hudspeth AJ. The hair cells of the inner ear. They are exquisitely sensitive transducers that in human beings mediate the senses of hearing and balance. A tiny force applied to the top of the cell produces an electrical signal at the bottom. Sci Am 1983; 248: 54–64

[31] Hudspeth AJ. The cellular basis of hearing: the biophysics of hair cells. Science 1985; 230: 745–752

[32] Hudspeth AJ, Roberts WM, Howard J. Gating compliance, a reduction in hair-bundle stiffness associated with the gating of transduction channels in hair cells from the bullfrog's sacculus. In: Wilson JP, Kemp DT, eds. Cochlear Mechanisms: Structure, Function and Models. New York: Plenum Press, 1989:117–123

[33] Roberts WM, Jacobs RA, Hudspeth AJ. Colocalization of ion channels involved in frequency selectivity and synaptic transmission at presynaptic active zones of hair cells. J Neurosci 1990; 10: 3664–3684

[34] Russell IJ, Sellick PM. Low-frequency characteristics of intracellularly recorded receptor potentials in guinea-pig cochlear hair cells. J Physiol 1983; 338: 179–206

[35] Santos-Sacchi J. Cochlear Physiology. In: Jahn AF, Santos-Sacchi J, eds. Physiology of the Ear. New York: Raven Press, 1988:271–293

[36] Eybalin M. Neurotransmitters and neuromodulators of the mammalian cochlea. Physiol Rev 1993; 73: 309–373

[37] Guth PS, Aubert A, Ricci AJ, Norris CH. Differential modulation of spontaneous and evoked neurotransmitter release from hair cells: some novel hypotheses. Hear Res 1991; 56: 69–78

[38] Helfert RH, Snead CR, Altschuler RA. The ascending auditory pathways. In: Altschuler RA, Bobbin RP, Clopton BM, Hoffman D, eds. Neurobiology of Hearing: The Central Auditory System. New York: Raven Press, 1991:1–25

[39] Warr WB. Organization of olivocochlear efferent systems in mammals. In: Webster DB, Popper AN, Fay RR, eds. The Mammalian Auditory Pathway: Neuroanatomy. New York: Springer-Verlag, 1992:410–448

[40] Liberman MC. The olivocochlear efferent bundle and susceptibility of the inner ear to acoustic injury. J Neurophysiol 1991; 65: 123–132

[41] Sahley TL, Nodar RH. Improvement in auditory function following pentazocine suggests a role for dynorphins in auditory sensitivity. Ear Hear 1994; 15: 422–431

[42] Liberman MC. Morphological differences among radial afferent fibers in the cat cochlea: an electron-microscopic study of serial sections. Hear Res 1980; 3: 45–63

[43] Liberman MC. Effects of chronic cochlear de-efferentation on auditory-nerve response. Hear Res 1990; 49: 209–223

[44] Guinan JJ, Jr, Gifford ML. Effects of electrical stimulation of efferent olivocochlear neurons on cat auditory-nerve fibers. I. Rate-level functions. Hear Res 1988; 33: 97–113

[45] Guinan JJ, Jr, Gifford ML. Effects of electrical stimulation of efferent olivocochlear neurons on cat auditory-nerve fibers. II. Spontaneous rate. Hear Res 1988; 33: 115–127

[46] Guinan JJ, Jr, Gifford ML. Effects of electrical stimulation of efferent olivocochlear neurons on cat auditory-nerve fibers. III. Tuning curves and thresholds at CF. Hear Res 1988; 37: 29–45

[47] Winslow RL, Sachs MB. Effect of electrical stimulation of the crossed olivocochlear bundle on auditory nerve response to tones in noise. J Neurophysiol 1987; 57: 1002–1021

3 Vestibular Physiology

Maroun T. Semaan, Cameron C. Wick, and Cliff A. Megerian

3.1 Introduction

The vestibular end-organs comprise specialized mechanoreceptors that transduce angular and linear acceleration into afferent neural signals. The vestibular input along with visual and proprioceptive sensory cues allow seamless integration of a complex array of information designed to stabilize gaze during rapid head movements and provide postural control in a gravitational field. Although the sensitivity of the vestibular end-organ spans a wide frequency range of head movements, provision of a unambiguous scheme of the spatial relationship of the body and retinal image requires the integration of multimodal sensory systems.

This chapter explores the basic physiology of the vestibular end-organs and how they are integrated to enable appropriate eye movement, postural control, and fluidity of movement. The anatomy of the semicircular canals, utricle, and saccule are discussed, as are the central neural pathways that facilitate integration and plasticity.

3.2 Vestibular End-Organ Anatomy and Physiology

Encased within the petrous portion of the temporal bone, the membranous vestibular labyrinth includes the paired sensory end-organs of the semicircular canals (SCCs) and the otolithic organs (utricle and saccule).

3.2.1 Mechanoelectric Transduction: The Role of the Hair Cells

Hair cells function as the basic sensory element of the vestibular system that allows mechanoelectric transduction of linear and angular, static and dynamic, head position and velocity. These specialized cells have a characteristic appearance with an apical surface that contains a large, single kinocilium connected via tip-link and side-link proteins to 50 to 100 stereocilia. The kinocilium arises from the basal body, whereas the stereocilia are anchored to the cuticular plate. The apical bundles are embedded in the gelatinous matrix of their respective cupula (SCCs) or macula (utricle, saccule).[1,2] The hair-like stereocilia, for which the cells are named, transduce mechanical energy into electric potential based on the direction of the force applied to them. Hair cells, which are bathed in potassium-rich endolymph, maintain a resting membrane potential of –60 mV. When stereocilia deflect toward the kinocilium, it alters the tip-link tension and opens selectively permeable channels' "gating spring" that allow cations, predominantly potassium, to enter the hair cell (▶ Fig. 3.1). This influx of cations causes hair cell depolarization. When the depolarization reaches –40 mV, voltage-sensitive calcium channels at the basolateral aspect of the cell allow calcium to enter. The influx of calcium causes exocytosis of the excitatory neurotransmitter glutamate. Likewise, stereocilia deflection away from the kinocilium causes hyperpolarization to –64 mV, thus inhibiting glutamate release. The sensory unit returns to its resting potential by allowing efflux of potassium and calcium out of the cytoplasm and neutralization of calcium ions by binding to intracellular proteins.[3–5]

There are two morphologically distinct types of hair cells (▶ Fig. 3.2). Type I hair cell bodies are globular in shape and associated with a calyceal afferent nerve terminal engulfing its base.[6] Type I hair cells are concentrated toward the center of the vestibular end-organs' neuroepithelial structures (i.e., apex of the canal cristae and striola of the otolith maculae). The afferent axons associated with type I hair cells are among the largest axons in the nervous system. They have an irregular baseline firing rate that is modulated by hair cell neurotransmitter release. The ability to increase or decrease the afferent signal based on excitation (depolarization) or inhibition

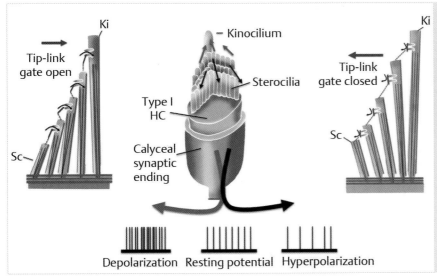

Fig. 3.1 Tip-link mechanotransduction. Stereocilia (Sc) on the apical surface of a hair cell (HC) are oriented adjacent to a single kinocilium (Ki), all of which are connected via extracellular tip-link proteins. At rest, vestibular afferent nerves exhibit a tonic baseline firing rate. Deflection of stereocilia toward the kinocilium opens the ion gate allowing an influx of cations that causes hair cell depolarization and ultimately an increased afferent firing rate. When stereocilia deflect away from the kinocilium, the ion gates close and hyperpolarization occurs.

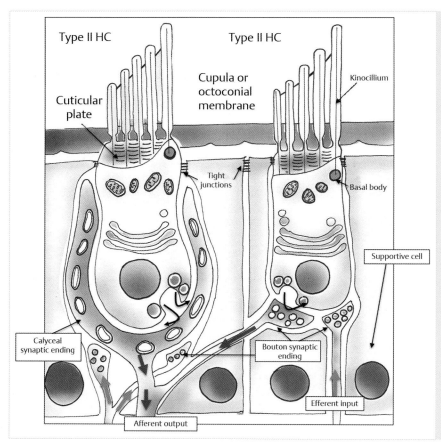

Fig. 3.2 Hair cell morphology. Type I hair cells (HC) have a globular shape and are centrally located on the vestibular neuroepithelium (i.e., apex of the cristae or striola of the maculae). Type I afferents have a large calyceal synapse and irregular baseline firing rate. Type II hair cells are more cylindrical and associated with button afferents that fire at a regular baseline rate.

(hyperpolarization) of the hair cell is an important property termed bidirectional sensitivity.[7] Type II hair cells are more cylindrical and associated with slower conducting axons that fire at regular intervals. Multiple bouton afferent nerve terminals are associated with each type II hair cell. Both hair cell types also receive efferent synaptic contact.[6]

3.2.2 Translation of Head Angular Movement: The Role of the Semicircular Canals

The SCCs [horizontal (hSCC), superior (sSCC), and posterior (pSCC)] respond to angular acceleration and are orthogonal in respect to each other. Each individual canal has a corresponding coplanar SCC. The hSCCs form a coplanar pair and are inclined 30 degrees upward from an axial plane connecting the lateral canthus to the external auditory meatus. The pSCC and contralateral sSCC form a coplanar pair. This peculiar orthogonal orientation of the SCCs allows detection of practically any head position in reference to earth vertical and horizontal planes. Each SCC has one ampullated end that contains the crista ampullaris. Both the sSCC and pSCC share a "common crus" (▶ Fig. 3.3). The crista ampullaris houses the sensory neuroepithelium responsible for transduction of head movement. A gelatinous goblet-shaped structure known as the cupula extends across the lumen of the SCC, filling the full cross section of the ampulla. The cupula has a specific gravity that is equal to that of the endolymph and serves as a mechanical barrier that

separates the endolymph of the SCC from the utricle. As a result, it does not respond to gravitational and static changes in head position but to dynamic head movements that allow a relative movement of the endolymph (and cupula) in the opposite direction of the head movement due to its inertia.

In the ampulla, the hair cells are oriented in a polarized manner, with all of the kinocilia and stereocilia facing the same direction. Therefore, head movements around a canal's axis excite or inhibit all of the hair cells in that particular canal.[2] Because none of the SCCs are perfectly aligned with the earth vertical or horizontal plane, common head movements (i.e., head movement while running) activate concomitantly several SCCs.

Angular head acceleration causes relative endolymph flow in a direction opposite to that of the head movement. The endolymph displaces the cupula, which in turn causes bending of the hair cell bundles and a change in membrane potential. Endolymph that flows toward the ampulla is termed ampullopetal (Latin *petere*, "to seek"), whereas flow away from the ampulla is termed ampullofugal (Latin *fugere*, "to flee"). For the hSCC the kinocilia are arranged closest to the utricle (utriculopetal); thus ampullopetal flow pushes the stereocilia toward the kinocilium, resulting in depolarization. The sSCC and pSCC have reversed hair bundle orientations; therefore, ampullofugal flow of endolymph (utriculofugal movement of the cupula) causes excitation (▶ Fig. 3.4).

For head rotations below 0.1 Hz (low frequency), the vestibular afferent nerves poorly encode head velocity because the rotational stimulus must overcome the elastic restoring force

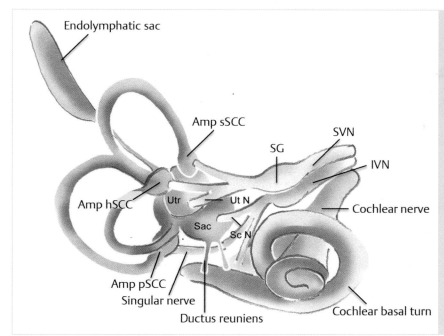

Fig. 3.3 Vestibular end-organs and vestibular nerve: anatomic organization of the peripheral vestibular system. Amp, ampullated; IVN, inferior vestibular nerve; Sac, saccule; SCC, semicircular canal (a, anterior; s, superior; p, posterior); Sc N, saccular nerve; SG, Scarpa's ganglion; SVN, superior vestibular nerve; Ut N, utricular nerve; Utr, utricle.

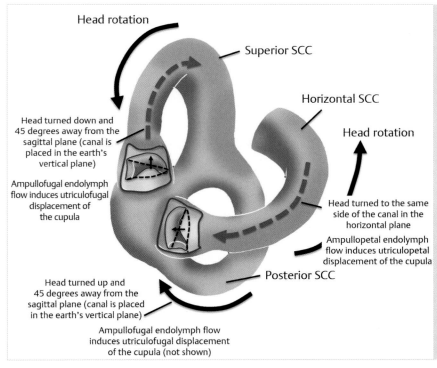

Fig. 3.4 Semicircular canal polarity. Head rotation causes relative endolymph flow in the opposite direction. The cupula, which spans the lumen of the ampulla, is displaced by the endolymph. Based on kinocilium orientation, ampullopetal flow excites the horizontal semicircular canal (SCC) whereas ampullofugal flow excites the superior and posterior SCCs.

of the cupula (i.e., the elastic forces that return the cupula overcome the forces that would deflect the cupula relative to the head [inertia], and the result is absent to minimal afferent stimulation). The weak afferent signals for constant low-frequency head rotation all tend to decay prematurely. To adapt for this decay, the afferent signal is perseverated by the vestibular nuclei and cerebellar feedback loop. This functionality known as velocity storage extends the dynamic range of the vestibular system by allowing for greater overlap between the higher frequency (vestibulo-ocular reflex [VOR]) and lower frequency (smooth pursuit and optokinetic) gaze stabilizing systems.[8–10] Clinically, velocity storage is responsible for the prolonged nystagmus that occurs after termination of a sustained constant rotational velocity in one direction. Lesion studies indicate that velocity storage stems from a feedback loop between the medullary and cerebellar circuits that directly communicate with the vestibular nuclei, particularly the medial vestibular nucleus (MVN) and descending vestibular nucleus (DVN). The clinical correlate is the post-head-shake nystagmus.[11–13]

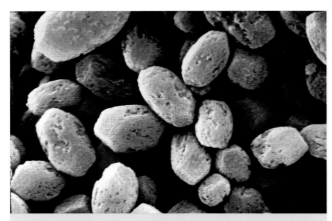

Fig. 3.5 Otoconia. Electron microscopy of otoconia or otolith. Otoconia increased the specific gravity of the maculae utriculi and sacculi relative to the endolymph, allowing detection of gravitational changes by the underlying neuroepithelium. (Courtesy of Dr. M. Bassim.)

3.2.3 Detection of Linear Acceleration, Gravitational Changes and Head-Tilt: The Role of the Otolithic Organs

The saccule and utricle make up the otolithic organs of the membranous labyrinth. The neuroepithelium of the otolithic organ is the macula, on top of which lay the hair cells. The hair cell stereocilia are embedded in a gelatinous matrix analogous to the cupula of the SCCs. This layer is topped with calcium carbonate crystals called otoconia (or otoliths) (▶ Fig. 3.5). The otoconia increase the specific gravity of the gelatinous matrix above that of the endolymph, which unlike the cupula allows the otolithic organ to be responsive both to static and gravitational changes in head position (head tilt and gravity) and dynamic changes in head linear acceleration. In contrast to hair cells on the cristae ampullaris that are polarized in the same direction, otolithic hair cells are oriented in many directions on the macula at right angles to a curvilinear axis called the striola (▶ Fig. 3.6). The striola separates oppositely oriented hair cells, giving the maculae bidirectional sensitivity.[14–16]

There are minimum and maximum stimuli to which the otoliths may respond. The nonlinear macula shape permits the otolithic organs to perceive linear force in a variety of head positions. As with all hair cells, activation occurs with deflection of the stereocilia toward the kinocilium, and compressive forces have no effect. Type I hair cells are mainly found on the central part of the macula (striola), whereas type II cells are on the periphery.[14–17]

Utricle

The utricle is located in the elliptical recess at the superior aspect of the vestibule. It is oriented in a horizontal plane during upright head position (i.e., roughly the same plane as the hSCC). The utricular maculae are C-shaped and tilted upward at a 30-degree angle (▶ Fig. 3.6). This allows sensation of linear acceleration primarily in a horizontal direction (axial plane) relative to gravitational pull.[17,18] Recent studies indicate that ocular vestibular evoked myogenic potentials (oVEMPs) originate

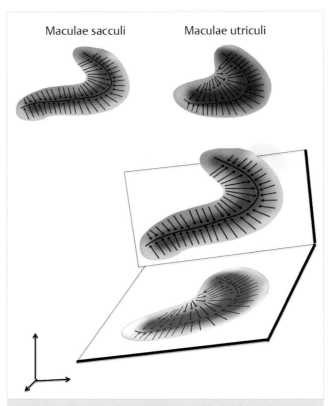

Maculae sacculi   Maculae utriculi

Fig. 3.6 Otolith organ arrangement. The utricle lies roughly in the earth-horizontal plane, is C-shaped, and senses horizontal linear acceleration. The saccule lies in the earth-vertical plane, is J-shaped, and senses vertical linear acceleration. Kinocilia are oriented to the striola, which divides the macula into a bidirectional sensor.

from the utricle and may aid in future diagnosis of utricular dysfunction.[19]

Saccule

The saccule is located in the spherical recess at the inferior aspect of the vestibule. It is oriented parallel to the earth-vertical plane (sagittal plane) during upright head position. The membranous labyrinth of the saccule is connected to the cochlear duct via the ductus reuniens (Hensen's duct). Extensions of the saccular duct and utricular duct form the endolymphatic duct, which leads to the endolymphatic sac. The saccular maculae have an inverted J-shape and sense linear acceleration primarily in a vertical direction (sagittal plane) relative to gravitational pull (▶ Fig. 3.6).[17,18] The utility of cervical vestibular evoked myogenic potentials (cVEMPs) has been appreciated since its first description in 1992 and is a test of saccular function via the vestibulocollic reflex (VCR), which is described below.[20]

3.2.4 Transfer and Regulation of the Vestibular Neural Output: The Role of Neural Pathways

Peripheral Afferent Neurons

Cell bodies of the vestibular nerve form the vestibular (Scarpa's) ganglion (▶ Fig. 3.3). There are approximately 25,000 primary afferent vestibular neurons in each vestibular nerve. These bipolar neurons have one end that synapses at a vestibular end-organ hair cell, whereas the other end synapses at one of the four main vestibular nuclei located in the floor of the medulla. Information from the utricle, sSCC, and hSCC travels along the superior division of the vestibular nerve, whereas information from the saccule and pSCC propagates along the inferior division (► Fig. 3.3). The inferior division is further separated into the saccular nerve that innervates the saccule and the posterior ampullary (singular) nerve that innervates the pSCC.[18,21]

All vestibular afferent neurons have a resting discharge rate of approximately 90 spikes per second (range: 10 to 200 spikes per second). This resting discharge is required for bidirectional sensitivity. Excitatory stimuli cause hair cell depolarization that leads to an increase in the neuronal firing rate, whereas inhibitory stimuli cause hair cell hyperpolarization that leads to a decreased firing rate.

In an intact vestibular system there is constant interplay between ipsilateral and contralateral input. At higher acceleration, the neural discharge rate becomes increasingly asymmetric because excitation and the resultant increase in the neural output is essentially limitless, whereas during inhibition downward modulation cannot go below zero.[22] Otolithic afferent neurons also have baseline activity that is dependent on hair cell orientation to gravitational force. At different states of static head tilt, different hair cells will be polarized to respond to the linear stimulus.[17,23]

Peripheral Efferent Neurons

Efferent neurons also innervate the vestibular end-organs. It is hypothesized that the vestibular efferents may raise baseline afferent firing rates, particularly for irregularly firing afferents, in anticipation of rapid head movement. Still, the full impact of vestibular efferents on everyday movements remains in question.[6,24,25]

3.2.5 The First Docking Station: The Vestibular Nuclei

Primary vestibular afferent neurons enter the brainstem at the pontomedullary junction where they branch into ascending and descending pathways before synapsing with second-order vestibular neurons in one of four vestibular nuclei. The vestibular nuclei are located adjacent to the lateral wall of the fourth ventricle at the floor of the medulla. The four main subnuclei are the superior (Bechterew's) vestibular nucleus (SVN), lateral (Deiters') vestibular nucleus (LVN), medial (Schwalbe's) vestibular nucleus (MVN), and the descending/inferior (spinal) vestibular nucleus (DVN).[22,26]

Each vestibular nucleus has a role in propagating and filtering the afferent vestibular signal as well as early integration of other sensory input. The SVN serves as the primary relay center for conjugate ocular reflexes mediated by the SCC. The LVN enables the "righting-reflex" controlled by the ipsilateral vestibulospinal arc. The MVN connects to the medial longitudinal fasciculus, which allows coordination of eye, head, and neck movements. This function is influenced by many factors including contralateral vestibular input, other sensory input, and cerebral feedback.[26,27]

Although the majority of primary vestibular afferent neurons project to the vestibular nuclei, some primary SCC afferents directly project to the cerebellar flocculus and paraflocculus. These connections permit functional adaptation of the VOR based on visual feedback through the accessory optic tract to cells in the cerebellar cortex.[26]

3.2.6 The Vestibular System at Work: Vestibular Reflexes

The intricate vestibular end-organ and neuronal physiology described above combines with central pathways to provide instantaneous adjustments that allow proper head position, postural control, and visual orientation. Although analogous to three-neuron reflex arcs (i.e., knee-jerk reflex), the vestibular reflex pathways described below are inherently more complex and highlight the brain's ability to seamlessly integrate to the ever-changing external environment.

Vestibulo-Ocular Reflex

The best studied, and arguably most important, vestibular reflex arc is the vestibulo-ocular reflex (VOR). The purpose of the VOR is to stabilize images on the fovea during high-velocity head movements. When head movement occurs at a velocity less than 50 degrees/second (frequency of approximately 1 Hz), the primary visual cortex computes an object's change across the fovea (retinal area of high visual acuity). This computation is passed through the cerebral motor cortex, then back to the brainstem and cerebellum where an oculomotor command is generated to re-center the image on the fovea.[28] In a similar manner, the optokinetic reflex (OKR) also stabilizes low-velocity images. As an image drifts toward the retinal periphery, signals are sent along the accessory optic tract, which then communicates with Purkinje cells in the cerebellum to create compensatory eye movements.[22,29,30] The efficiency of the low-frequency gaze-stabilizing systems (i.e., smooth pursuits, saccades, and optokinetic reflex) decreases with high-velocity head movements. Additional support from the VOR is required to maintain a stable gaze.

Common activities like locomotion even cause visual movements outside the range of the smooth pursuit and OKR systems. The VOR may involve stimulation of any combination of the semicircular canals and otoliths, as head movements rarely occur in one plane.

As originally described by Ewald in 1892, rotational movements that stimulate the SCC cause the eyes to move smoothly in a direction opposite of the head movement but in the same plane as the stimulated SCC.[31] Head rotation in the earth-horizontal plane (yaw plane) primarily involves activation of the hSCCs. Leftward head rotation induces relative endolymph flow to the right due to inertial forces of the fluid. This in turn causes ampullopetal cupular displacement in the left hSCC and ampullofugal displacement in the right hSCC. Hair cells in the crista of the left hSCC are depolarized, and those in the right hSCC are hyperpolarized. This causes an increase in the neuronal firing rate in the left vestibular nerve and a decrease in the neuronal firing in the right.

Central connections for the VOR consist of both excitatory and inhibitory pathways. In the case of the hSCC, primary

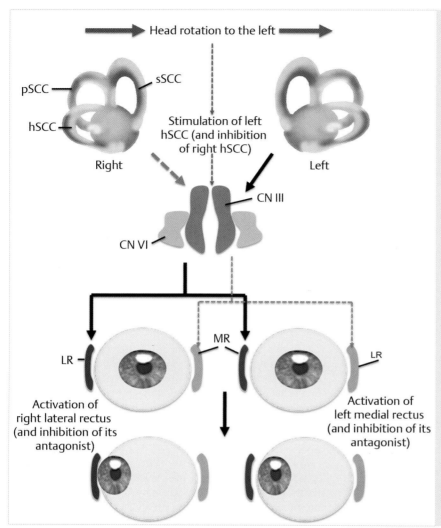

Fig. 3.7 Horizontal semicircular canal activation. Head rotation to the left stimulates the left horizontal semicircular canal (hSCC). Excitatory interneurons from the left vestibular nuclei synapse on the ipsilateral oculomotor nucleus (cranial nerve [CN] III) and contralateral abducens nucleus (CN VI), where their motoneurons excite the medial rectus (MR) and lateral rectus (LR) muscles, respectively (*black arrows*). Inhibitory input from the right hSCC is sent to the antagonistic muscles MR and LR (*gray dashed arrows*). The result is lateral eye deviation opposite that of head rotation.

vestibular afferents from the hSCC synapse in the ipsilateral MVN and LVN. Secondary vestibular neurons synapse in the contralateral abducens nucleus and ipsilateral oculomotor nucleus (the medial rectus subdivision). Finally, motoneurons leaving the contralateral abducens and ipsilateral medial rectus nucleus synapse at the neuromuscular junction of the lateral rectus and medial rectus muscles respectively. Excitation causes deviation of the eyes in a direction counter to the rotational stimulus, thus allowing gaze stabilization (▶ Fig. 3.7). Also, there are inhibitory pathways that exert opposing effects on the antagonist muscle pairs. Meanwhile, in the contralateral vestibular nuclei, the downward modulation of afferent activity leads to concomitant modulation of the neuronal firing rates in the contralateral excitatory and inhibitory pathways, ultimately leading to activation of the same extraocular movements as described above in a compensatory fashion.

When the visual stimulus displacement approaches the limit of normal oculomotor range, the eyes are re-centered in the orbit by the saccadic system, resulting in nystagmus. Nystagmus is a repetitive involuntary eye movement that resets the globe to a more central position within the orbit (fast phase) whereas a reciprocal response directs the eye in accordance to the vestibular input (slow phase). By convention, nystagmus is named for the fast phase, which clinically is often most apparent, but it is the slow phase that is truly driven by the vestibular system.[29,30]

Comprehension of the sSCC and pSCC is more complex. First, activation of these canals is often a sum of vectors or partial activations that get interpreted by the vestibular nuclei and second-order neurons. Second, the kinocilia in the sSCC and pSCC are oriented opposite to the hSCC, which means ampullofugal endolymph flow is excitatory in the sSCC and pSCC (▶ Fig. 3.4). Rotating the head down and rolling it to the left in a 45-degree angle excites the left sSCC, whereas tilting the head up and rolling it to the left excites the left pSCC. In all situations the contralateral coplanar SCC gets inhibited.

Unilateral stimulation of either the sSCC or pSCC results in an unopposed torsional nystagmus around that canal's axis. Stimulation of the sSCC initiates a trisynaptic VOR that ultimately results in activation of the bilateral superior recti muscles (upward globe movement), the ipsilateral superior oblique, and the contralateral inferior oblique (ipsilateral globe intorsion and contralateral extorsion) (▶ Fig. 3.8). Stimulation of the pSCC results in activation of the bilateral inferior recti muscles (downward globe movement), the ipsilateral superior oblique and contralateral inferior oblique (ipsilateral intorsion and

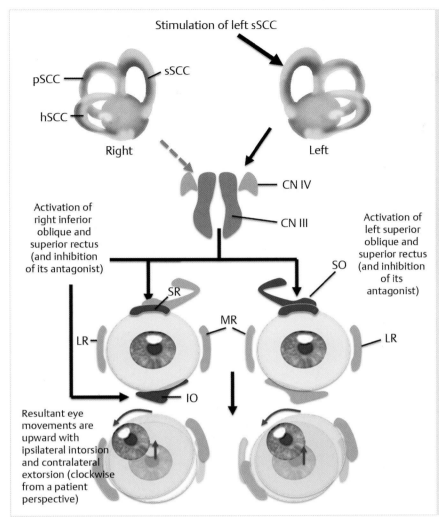

Stimulation of left sSCC

pSCC

sSCC

hSCC

Right

Left

CN IV

CN III

Activation of right inferior oblique and superior rectus (and inhibition of its antagonist)

Activation of left superior oblique and superior rectus (and inhibition of its antagonist)

SO

SR

MR

LR

LR

IO

Resultant eye movements are upward with ipsilateral intorsion and contralateral extorsion (clockwise from a patient perspective)

Fig. 3.8 Superior semicircular canal activation. Head rotation down and 45 degrees to the left activates the left superior semicircular canal (sSCC). Excitatory interneurons from the left vestibular nuclei synapse on the oculomotor nucleus (CN III) and trochlear nucleus (CN IV), which excite the ipsilateral superior oblique (SO) and superior rectus (SR) as well as the contralateral superior rectus and inferior oblique (IO) muscles. The slow phase component is upward/clockwise (from patient's perspective) eye deviation. The corrective nystagmus beats downward and counterclockwise from a patient's perspective. Acoustic energy and positive middle ear pressure excite the sSCC, whereas the Valsalva maneuver and negative middle ear pressure inhibit the sSCC.

contralateral extorsion) (▶ Fig. 3.9). Torsional nystagmus means the upper poles of the globes deviate away from the activated SCC (slow phase), whereas the fast phase beats toward the ipsilateral ear.[30]

The recoil forces applied by the antagonistic muscle groups during reflexive eye movements limit the full range of the VOR. To avoid degradation of the foveal image, a central neural integrator adjusts for the push-pull effect exerted by the recoil force vectors. The horizontal neural integrator is located in the nucleus prepositus hypoglossi (NPH) and the MVN.[32] The vertical and torsional neural integrator is in the interstitial nucleus of Cajal.[33] In peripheral vestibular disorders, the neural integrator becomes leaky and the result is a constant tendency of the eyes to drift to the center.

Vestibulospinal Reflex

The purpose of the vestibulospinal reflex (VSR) is to maintain postural stability. Mediated through the LVN and MVN, the VSR consists of multiple pathways that ultimately provide input to the antigravity muscles of the trunk and extremities. Control of the neck will be discussed separately as part of the VCR. The VSR begins when the otolithic organs, SCCs, and cerebellum sense a head tilt. The saccule is of particular importance in initiating the VSR because of its ability to sense linear acceleration in the earth-vertical plane (i.e., falling down) and its high degree of innervation into the LVN.[34] Neural input from the LVN and MVN is sent to the spinal cord via the lateral vestibulospinal tract (LVST) and medial vestibulospinal tract (MVST).[26,27] The LVST extends down to the lumbosacral region where it excites extensor motoneurons on the same side to which the head is tilted, thus creating the "righting-reflex" and maintaining postural control.

Vestibulocollic Reflex

The VCR controls neck musculature to stabilize the head. A three-neuron arc with second-order vestibular neurons passing through the MVST and LVST before reaching cervical motoneurons has been proposed for the VCR, although lesion studies may indicate that a more complex circuitry exists.[35,36] Although all vestibular end-organs contribute to the VCR, the well-described cVEMP indicates a prominent role for the saccule.[20,37]

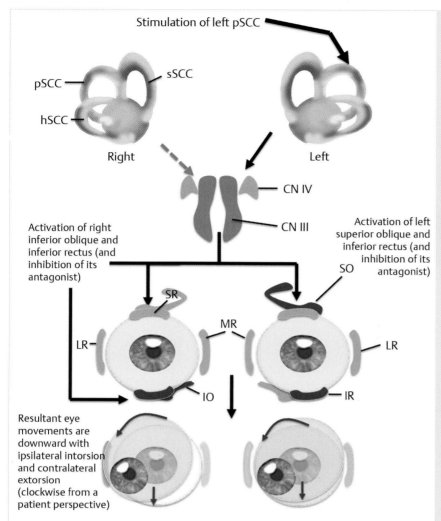

Fig. 3.9 Posterior semicircular canal activation. Head rotation up and 45 degrees to the left activates the left posterior semicircular canal (pSCC). Excitatory interneurons from the left vestibular nuclei synapse on the oculomotor nucleus (CN III) and trochlear nucleus (CN IV), which excite the ipsilateral superior oblique (SO) and inferior rectus (IR) as well as the contralateral inferior rectus and inferior oblique (IO) muscles. The slow phase component is downward/clockwise (from patient's perspective) eye deviation. The corrective nystagmus beats upward and counterclockwise (from patient's perspective). In a patient with left canalolithiasis, excitation of the left posterior SCC with the head down to the left causes a slow phase that takes the meridian to the right and downward. The corrective nystagmus takes the meridian back upward and toward the left ear. When the patient's head is rotated down to the left, the nystagmus appears to beat toward the earth's center of gravity or geotropic.

3.3 Pathophysiological Correlates in Common Vestibulopathies

3.3.1 Posterior Canal Benign Paroxysmal Positional Vertigo

The presence of canalolithiasis in the pSCC increases the specific gravity of the endolymph. Tilting the head up and rolling it to the side (frequently occurs when rolling in bed) causes a relative ampullofugal movement of the endolymph, which stimulates the ipsilateral pSCC (refer to polarization of the SCC). The brainstem interprets that the head rotated in the plane of the ipsilateral pSCC. The reflexive eye movements intended to keep the retinal image result in activation of the bilateral inferior recti muscles (downward globe movement), the ipsilateral superior oblique and contralateral inferior oblique (ipsilateral globe intorsion and contralateral globe extorsion, from a patient's perspective; right pSCC causes a counterclockwise slow phase eye movement and left pSCC causes a clockwise slow phase eye movement). The resultant nystagmus is down-beating (with head down) and geotropic.

3.3.2 Acute Labyrinthine Deafferentiation

Acute deafferentiation of the vestibular end-organ (i.e., after a labyrinthectomy) causes an unopposed activation of the contralateral canal. The brainstem interprets that the head is moving along all the planes that typically activates the three opposing SCCs. Because the effect of the superior and inferior recti muscles are antagonistic and nulled, the resulting activation of the contralateral medial rectus and the superior oblique muscles, and the ipsilateral lateral rectus and the inferior oblique muscles, causes a horizontal and torsional movement of the globe toward the injured labyrinth (slow phase) and a nystagmus beating toward the intact side.[38,39]

In an acute vestibulopathy, the neural integrator becomes "leaky." The result is a constant drift of the eyes to the center of the orbit. This vector force when added to the one resulting from the fast phase of the nystagmus causes an increase in the amplitude and velocity of the nystagmus when looking away from the hypofunctional side. This is also known as Alexander's law and is suggestive of peripheral acute vestibulopathy. Acute end-organ vestibular imbalance resulting from injury is perceived by the brainstem as a rotation/head tilt toward the intact side. This resulting nystagmus disappears within 24 to 48 hours due to vestibular nuclei rebalancing the asymmetry in tonic activity.[38–41]

With total bilateral loss in humans, substitution of pursuit and saccadic eye movements is the primary strategy for gaze fixation. With practice, pursuit efficiency has been shown to increase, and efficient use of "catch-up" saccades helps to stabilize retinal images during head rotation. As previously noted, however, as the frequency or acceleration of head movement increases (> 1–2 Hz, $> 2,000$ degrees/s^2), the efficiency of tracking and preprogrammed saccadic eye movement decreases and oscillopsia occurs.

3.3.3 Superior Canal Dehiscence Syndrome

A dehiscent superior canal creates a "third inner ear window" that decreases the fluid impedances in the vestibular labyrinth. This results in aphysiological stimulation or inhibition of the affected canal when shunted energy causes movement of the endolymphatic fluid.[42] Acoustic energy leaking into the dehiscent SCC enters the ampullated interface and causes an ampullofugal movement of the cupula. This excitation of the ipsilateral sSCC causes a slow phase eye movement upward and torsional (left sSCC stimulation causes clockwise rotation from a patient perspective, whereas right sSCC stimulation causes a counterclockwise rotation from a patient's perspective) that brings the meridian of the globes away from the affected side. The same response occurs with pneumatic otoscopy during positive pressure application. A fast-phase torsional component (nystagmus) brings the globes downward and toward the affected side. Breathing against a closed glottis (Valsalva maneuver) increases intracranial pressure. This leads to an ampullopetal flow of endolymph that results in the opposite cascade of events. The resultant nystagmus has a torsional component that takes the meridian of the globes toward the affected ear.

References

[1] Auer M, Koster AJ, Ziese U et al. Three-dimensional architecture of hair-bundle linkages revealed by electron-microscopic tomography. J Assoc Res Otolaryngol 2008; 9: 215–224

[2] Takumida M. Functional morphology of the crista ampullaris: with special interests in sensory hairs and cupula: a review. Biol Sci Space 2001; 15: 356–358

[3] Hudspeth AJ. Mechanoelectrical transduction by hair cells in the acousticolateralis sensory system. Annu Rev Neurosci 1983; 6: 187–215

[4] Pickles JO, Corey DP. Mechanoelectrical transduction by hair cells. Trends Neurosci 1992; 15: 254–259

[5] Uthaiah RC, Hudspeth AJ. Molecular anatomy of the hair cell's ribbon synapse. J Neurosci 2010; 30: 12387–12399

[6] Jackler RK, Brackman DE. Textbook of Neurobiology. St. Louis: Mosby, 1993

[7] Kalluri R, Xue J, Eatock RA. Ion channels set spike timing regularity of mammalian vestibular afferent neurons. J Neurophysiol 2010; 104: 2034–2051

[8] Wilson VJ, Melvill-Jones G, eds. Mammalian Vestibular Physiology. New York: Plenum Press, 1979

[9] Rabbit RD, Damiano ER, Grant JW. Biomechanics of the semicircular canals and otolith organs. In: Highstein SM, Fay RR, Popper AN, eds. The Vestibular System. New York: Springer, 2004:153–201

[10] Raphan T, Cohen B. Velocity storage and the ocular response to multidimensional vestibular stimuli. Rev Oculomot Res 1985; 1: 123–143

[11] Hain TC, Fetter M, Zee DS. Head-shaking nystagmus in patients with unilateral peripheral vestibular lesions. Am J Otolaryngol 1987; 8: 36–47

[12] Katz E, Vianney de Jong JMB, Buettner-Ennever JA, Cohen B. Effects of midline medullary lesions on velocity storage and the vestibulo-ocular reflex. Exp Brain Res 1991; 87: 505–520

[13] Cohen B, Wearne S, Dai M, Raphan T. Spatial orientation of the angular vestibulo-ocular reflex. J Vestib Res 1999; 9: 163–172

[14] DeVris H. The mechanisms of the labyrinth otoliths. Acta Otolaryngol 1950; 38: 262–273

[15] Lindeman HH. Studies on the morphology of the sensory regions of the vestibular apparatus with 45 figures. Ergeb Anat Entwicklungsgesch 1969; 42: 1–113

[16] Gresty MA, Bronstein AM, Brandt T, Dieterich M. Neurology of otolith function. Peripheral and central disorders. Brain 1992; 115: 647–673

[17] Jaeger R, Takagi A, Haslwanter T. Modeling the relation between head orientations and otolith responses in humans. Hear Res 2002; 173: 29–42

[18] Janfaza P, Nadol JB. Temporal bone and ear. In: Janfaza P, Nadol JB, Galla R, Fabian RL, Montgomery WM, eds. Surgical Anatomy of the Head and Neck. Boston: Harvard University Press, 2011:419–479

[19] Jacobson GP, McCaslin DL, Piker EG, Gruenwald J, Grantham SL, Tegel L. Patterns of abnormality in cVEMP, oVEMP, and caloric tests may provide topological information about vestibular impairment. J Am Acad Audiol 2011; 22: 601–611

[20] Rosengren SM, Welgampola MS, Colebatch JG. Vestibular evoked myogenic potentials: past, present and future. Clin Neurophysiol 2010; 121: 636–651

[21] Park JJ, Tang Y, Lopez I, Ishiyama A. Age-related change in the number of neurons in the human vestibular ganglion. J Comp Neurol 2001; 431: 437–443

[22] Baloh RW, Honrubia V, eds. Clinical Neurophysiology of the Vestibular System, 2nd ed. Philadelphia: FA Davis, 1990

[23] Bush GA, Perachio AA, Angelaki DE. Encoding of head acceleration in vestibular neurons. I. Spatiotemporal response properties to linear acceleration. J Neurophysiol 1993; 69: 2039–2055

[24] Highstein SM. The central nervous system efferent control of the organs of balance and equilibrium. Neurosci Res 1991; 12: 13–30

[25] Sadeghi SG, Goldberg JM, Minor LB, Cullen KE. Efferent-mediated responses in vestibular nerve afferents of the alert macaque. J Neurophysiol 2009; 101: 988–1001

[26] Barmack NH. Central vestibular system: vestibular nuclei and posterior cerebellum. Brain Res Bull 2003; 60: 511–541

[27] Rutka JA. Physiology of the vestibular system. In: Roland PS, Rutka JA, eds. Ototoxicity. Hamilton, Ontario: BC Decker, 2004:20–27

[28] Tychsen L, Lisberger SG. Visual motion processing for the initiation of smooth-pursuit eye movements in humans. J Neurophysiol 1986; 56: 953–968

[29] Schweigart G, Mergner T, Evdokimidis I, Morand S, Becker W. Gaze stabilization by optokinetic reflex (OKR) and vestibulo-ocular reflex (VOR) during active head rotation in man. Vision Res 1997; 37: 1643–1652

[30] Leigh RJ, Zee DS. Contemporary Neurology Series: The Neurology of Eye Movements. New York: Oxford University Press, 2006

[31] Ewald JR. Physiologische Untersuchungen eber das Endorgan des Nervus Octavus. Wiesbaden: Bergman, 1892

[32] Cannon SC, Robinson DA. Loss of the neural integrator of the oculomotor system from brain stem lesions in monkey. J Neurophysiol 1987; 57: 1383–1409

[33] Farshadmanesh F, Klier EM, Chang P, Wang H, Crawford JD. Three-dimensional eye-head coordination after injection of muscimol into the interstitial nucleus of Cajal (INC). J Neurophysiol 2007; 97: 2322–2338

[34] Newlands SD, Vrabec JT, Purcell IM, Stewart CM, Zimmerman BE, Perachio AA. Central projections of the saccular and utricular nerves in macaques. J Comp Neurol 2003; 466: 31–47

[35] Goldberg JM, Cullen KE. Vestibular control of the head: possible functions of the vestibulocollic reflex. Exp Brain Res 2011; 210: 331–345

[36] Wilson VJ, Boyle R, Fukushima K et al. The vestibulocollic reflex. J Vestib Res 1995; 5: 147–170

[37] Colebatch JG, Halmagyi GM. Vestibular evoked potentials in human neck muscles before and after unilateral vestibular deafferentation. Neurology 1992; 42: 1635–1636

[38] Cass SP, Kartush JM, Graham MD. Patterns of vestibular function following vestibular nerve section. Laryngoscope 1992; 102: 388–394

[39] Curthoys IS, Halmagyi GM. Vestibular compensation: a review of the oculomotor, neural, and clinical consequences of unilateral vestibular loss. J Vestib Res 1995; 5: 67–107

[40] Leveque M, Seidermann L, Tran H, Langagne T, Ulmer E, Chays A. Vestibular function outcomes after vestibular neurectomy in Meniere disease: can vestibular neurectomy provide complete vestibular deafferentation? Auris Nasus Larynx 2010; 37: 308–313

[41] Cullen KE, Minor LB, Beraneck M, Sadeghi SG. Neural substrates underlying vestibular compensation: contribution of peripheral versus central processing. J Vestib Res 2009; 19: 171–182

[42] Minor LB, Solomon D, Zinreich JS, Zee DS. Sound- and/or pressure-induced vertigo due to bone dehiscence of the superior semicircular canal. Arch Otolaryngol Head Neck Surg 1998; 124: 249–258

4 The Eustachian Tube

Ilkka Kivekäs and Dennis S. Poe

4.1 Introduction

The eustachian tube forms a dynamic connection between the middle ear and nasopharynx. This link is important for middle ear aeration and drainage and thus for optimal conduction of sound to inner ear. Surgical therapy for eustachian tube disorder has not met long-term success in the past, but recent findings of the anatomy, physiology, and pathophysiology have led to new strategies in surgical intervention.

4.2 History

The first known mention of the eustachian tube was in the writings of Alcmaeon of Sparta circa 400 B.C.[1] The credit for the discovery of the eustachian tube belongs to Bartolomeus Eustachius in 1562, when he published a detailed description of its anatomy and physiological function. In the early 1700s, Antonio Maria Valsalva gave the tube its name, described the eustachian tube as having cartilaginous and osseous parts, and was the first to recognize the importance of the tensor veli palatini muscle in opening the eustachian tube. He also described the Valsalva maneuver, which remains clinically relevant to this day.[2] The 19th-century English otologist Joseph Toynbee furthered our understanding of the eustachian tube through investigations of the peritubal muscles and popularized the Toynbee test to assess tubal dilatory function.[3] At the end of 19th century, Adam Politzer made important contributions in recognizing the role of the eustachian tube in middle ear pathology.[1]

4.3 Anatomy

The eustachian tube measures approximately 31 to 38 mm in overall length in the normal adult and about 21 mm in an infant.[4,5] The eustachian tube reaches its full length at about 7 years of age.[6] The eustachian tube originates from the anterior aspect of the middle ear cavity at its proximal end and extends to the nasopharynx, where it terminates distally.

The eustachian tube is composed of two portions: a proximal osseous one third that is contained within the skull base, and a distal two thirds that is the cartilaginous portion. It has a slightly S-shaped course and passes generally posterosuperiorly and laterally from the nasopharynx. At the nasopharyngeal orifice, its cross section is triangular in shape, measuring 2 to 3 mm vertically and 3 to 4 mm in the horizontal base. The narrowest portion of the eustachian tube, the isthmus, which is located in the cartilaginous portion, is a vertical slit measuring 2 mm in height and 0.6 to 0.9 mm in width. The segment in which the cartilaginous and osseous portions connect has been termed the junctional portion by Sudo et al.[7] The osseous portion opens funnel-like into the middle ear, and it remains fixed and patent under normal circumstances; in contrast, the cartilaginous portion of the eustachian tube is dynamic (particularly the most nasopharyngeal portion), closed at rest and opened when active. Within the cartilaginous superior and middle portion, the mucosal surfaces of the anterolateral and posteromedial walls meet in apposition, closing the lumen in the resting position. This roughly 8- to 15-mm-long section serves as a functional "valve" and is composed of the mucosa, submucosa, lateral cartilaginous lamina, the Ostmann's fat pad, and the relaxed bulk of the tensor veli palatini muscle.

The bony portion is lined by a layer of cuboidal respiratory epithelium[8] and the cartilaginous portion is lined by pseudostratified columnar respiratory epithelium that is taller, more densely ciliated, and abundant in secreting goblet cells.[5,9]

The eustachian tube orifice can be identified just posterior to the inferior turbinate. The fossa of Rosenmüller is located posterior to the torus tubarius and courses laterally toward the internal carotid artery, which lies just deep to the apex of the fossa. The torus tubarius, also known as the posterior cushion, contains the medial cartilaginous lamina, which is the mobile portion of the eustachian tube orifice. The lateral cartilaginous lamina (anterolaterally located) is smaller and immobile. The entire cartilaginous skeleton is shaped like an inverted J in cross section.

4.3.1 Peritubal Muscles

There are four peritubal muscles: the tensor veli palatini, the levator veli palatini, the tensor tympani, and the salpingopharyngeus. The principal dilatator muscle is the tensor veli palatini. It originates from the sphenoid bone and is composed of two bundles of muscle fibers. These two muscle bundles course anteriorly and inferiorly and converge in a tendon that runs under, or at times inserts into, the hamulus of the medial pterygoid processes before inserting into the soft palate. The tubae portion of the tensor veli palatini originates directly along the anterolateral membranous wall of the eustachian tube and is important for active tubal dilation as well as tubal closure.[9]

The levator veli palatini muscle is another important muscle in opening the eustachian tube. Contraction of the levator veli palatini raises and supports the soft palate, affecting the initial phase of dilation of the eustachian tube by medially rotating the medial cartilaginous lamina.[4,10] It originates in the base of the temporal bone, runs along the floor of the eustachian tube, and inserts into the soft palate. The salpingopharyngeus muscle appears to depress the floor of the eustachian tube lumen to facilitate dilation. It originates from the medial and inferior borders of the cartilaginous eustachian tube and inserts into the palatal musculature. The tensor tympani arises from the cartilaginous portion of the eustachian tube and attaches to the medial surface of the malleus in the middle ear cavity. It has no functional purpose for the eustachian tube.

The mandibular division of the trigeminal nerve innervates the tensor veli palatini and the tensor tympani muscles.[11] The pharyngeal branch of the vagus nerve innervates the levator veli palatini and salpingopharyngeus muscles.[12]

There are several anatomic differences between the pediatric and adult eustachian tubes that likely influence the pathogenesis of otitis media. The pediatric eustachian tube is significantly shorter, narrower, more compliant, and more horizontally oriented, and it contains more mucosal folds.[9]

4.4 Physiology

4.4.1 Eustachian Tube Dilation and Closure

The cartilaginous eustachian tube is maintained closed in the resting position by a "valve" that opens intermittently for ventilation of the middle ear. The tube ordinarily opens with swallows and yawns, but not every swallow or yawn is accompanied with opening of the tube. Tubal dilation occurs about 1.4 times per minute in the daytime, lasts approximately 400 to 500 ms, and is substantially decreased during sleep.[13,14]

The dilation of the eustachian tube can be divided into two phases. In the first phase, palatal elevation begins due to the contraction of the levator veli palatini muscle. This phase also includes medial rotation of the torus tubarius and the posteromedial wall of the eustachian tube. The levator veli palatini remains contracted throughout the tubal dilatation phase and serves as a scaffold against which the tensor veli palatini acts. In the second phase the tensor veli palatini contracts and causes active dilation of the eustachian tube's functional valve with a lateral traction force on the anterolateral membranous wall. Full contraction of the tensor veli palatini results in maximal opening of the eustachian tube valve and creates a rounded lumen (► Fig. 4.1). The tubal dilation propagates from the nasopharyngeal opening toward the isthmus of the eustachian tube (distal-to-proximal direction), and closure proceeds in the opposite direction. The mucosal surfaces of the cartilaginous eustachian tube contact one another to create an air- and watertight seal. Dilation of the normal eustachian tube provides adequate ventilation of the middle ear space, and maintains air pressure at near ambient levels.

4.4.2 Middle Ear Gas Exchange

When the eustachian tube is closed, an ongoing exchange of gas occurs between the middle ear and mastoid cavity and the mucosa. This exchange process continually generates a net absorption of gases and it causes an increasingly negative pressure between tubal dilations.[15–18] Exchange of middle ear gases with venous gases results in a slowly decreasing net pressure within the middle ear. The most important and abundant of these middle ear gases is nitrogen, which has a very slow coefficient of diffusion that causes it to pass, in net, from the middle ear space into the venous blood, driven by its partial pressure gradient. The exchange of nitrogen is most likely the principal factor behind the increasingly negative pressure that develops within the middle ear space when the eustachian tube opening process is compromised. The dilation of the eustachian tube is a result of voluntary and involuntary actions such as yawning and swallowing, but the autonomic nervous system may also have a reflex that stimulates dilation via alterations in gas composition and pressure that are detected by baroreceptors and chemoreceptors.[19,20]

4.4.3 Clearance of the Middle Ear

In addition to middle ear aeration, the eustachian tube also serves as a drainage pathway for secretions, fluids, and debris from within the middle ear. The middle ear is cleared by two primary mechanisms. The first mechanism involves mucociliary function within the eustachian tube, which actively transports secretions, fluids, and debris toward the distal nasopharyngeal opening of the tube.[21,22] However, in the presence of extremely viscous secretions, mucociliary clearance may be reduced. Surfactants are also found in eustachian tube and middle ear. Mucosal surfactants help reduce surface tension within the lumen of the eustachian tube and improve mucociliary clearance, tubal dilation, and exchange of gases across the mucosal barrier.[23,24] The second clearance mechanism is the pumping action of the peritubal muscles, which during the tubal closing process serves as an additional and synergistic means of tubal clearance. When the eustachian tube closes in a proximal-to-distal (superior to inferior) direction, it creates an expelling force, generated by the relaxing cartilage and peritubal muscles.[22]

4.4.4 Protection of the Middle Ear

Reflux of nasopharyngeal secretions into the middle ear is limited or prevented by the functional valve of the eustachian tube and by the trapped volume of gas in the middle ear and mastoid bone, which creates a "gas cushion."[14] Reflux of the sounds of breathing and vocalization are similarly blocked by the closed resting position of the pharyngeal eustachian tube.[14]

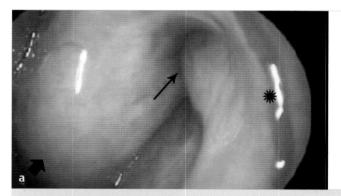
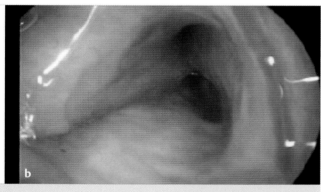

Fig. 4.1 Normal left eustachian tube: posterior cushion (*arrowhead*), orifice (*arrow*), anterolateral wall (*asterisk*). Images have been taken from the ipsilateral nasal cavity with a 30-degree Hopkins rod endoscope. (a) Closed, resting position. (b) Open, dilated position.

4.5 Evaluation of Eustachian Tube Function

4.5.1 History and Physical Examination

Evaluation of patients with eustachian tube problems begins with a comprehensive history and physical examination. Patients should be questioned about inflammatory disorders such as allergies, asthma, laryngopharyngeal reflux, and chronic or recurrent rhinosinusitis. In the pediatric population it is important to additionally inquire about recurrent otitis media, persistent or recurrent respiratory infections, smoke or wood stove exposure, day-care attendance, and immune deficiency.[25] Eustachian tube disorders may also be familial. Ciliary motility disorders such as Kartagener's syndrome are also important to take into account. Nevertheless, cystic fibrosis is not associated with eustachian tube dysfunction.[26] Tobacco use or smoke exposure can reduce mucociliary clearance. Surgical history, with reference, for example, to tympanostomy tube placements or adenoidectomy, is also relevant information. Medications, especially nasal preparations of topical corticosteroids and oxymetazoline, as well as for allergies and reflux disease, oral contraceptives, and any hormonal replacement therapies should also be noted.

Physical examination includes a comprehensive head and neck evaluation with otomicroscopy assessment. The external auditory canal, tympanic membrane, and middle ear pressure status are important to assess and tympanometry may be helpful. Eustachian tube dilatory dysfunction is often, but not always, associated with negative pressure in the middle ear, so it is crucial to look for tympanic membrane retraction, retraction pockets, effusion, perforations, tympanosclerosis, or cholesteatoma. Tympanic membrane movements with normal breathing indicate a patulous eustachian tube. A tympanogram and an audiogram should be obtained to determine the middle ear pressure and hearing.

4.5.2 Endoscopic Examination

The initial examination with a flexible endoscope should assess the nasal mucosa, nasopharynx, pharynx, larynx, hypopharynx, and subglottic space for signs of inflammation or underlying allergy, granulomatous disease, laryngopharyngeal reflux, or other pathology.[27] A rigid 4-mm endoscope with a 30- or 45-degree viewing angle is ideal to see into eustachian tube. The scope should be directed laterally and, upon successful recognition of the orifice, rotated superiorly by 45 degrees.[28] Signs of edema or hypertrophy with diminished tubal dilation are often seen with dilatory dysfunction.[29] The adenoid should be assessed for its size, degree of inflammation, and degree of contact with the posterior cushions of the eustachian tubes.

Evaluation with slow-motion endoscopy helps to differentiate obstructive from dynamic causes of eustachian tube dilatory dysfunction. An assessment of the mostly isolated contraction of the levator veli palatine muscle can be performed by asking the patient to phonate the letter K repeatedly. The tubal orifice will begin to dilate, but the valve should not open. Swallowing provides an assessment of normal tubal dilation, whereas yawning evaluates the maximal dilatory effort. Slow-motion video allows for detailed assessment of the tubal dilatory

phases, and the orifice will be seen to change from its resting S-shaped convexity into a rounded opening.[30]

4.5.3 Imaging

The primary purpose of the imaging is to find other possible pathologies that involve eustachian tube dysfunction. These include nasal and sinus diseases, middle ear diseases, nasopharynx tumors, and the position of the internal carotid canal within the skull base if surgery is contemplated. Exclusion of carotid canal dehiscence by computed tomography (CT) before eustachian tube operation within the bony portion is recommended. In a recent study, the dynamic opening of the eustachian tube was investigated with cine CT.[31] Sequential "peristaltic-like" movement of an air bolus was observed passing through the eustachian tube in normal subjects but not in subjects with eustachian tube dysfunction. These results are preliminary, but sequential peristaltic opening of the eustachian tube may be an important newly recognized mechanism for middle ear ventilation. More data are needed to support these new findings before the clinical value of cine CT will be realized.

4.6 Eustachian Tube Function Tests

The Valsalva and Toynbee tests are traditional, but still usable, tests in clinical practice. In the Valsalva test, the patient performs a forced exhalation against a closed airway, with a closed mouth and pinching of the nose. A positive result indicates that middle ear air pressure equalized with nasopharynx and a "pop" sensation in the ear is usually experienced. In the Toynbee test, the patient swallows while the nose is pinched, creating a change in pressure within the middle ear. Traditionally, in normal subjects, the test has been thought to create a negative pressure with accompanying retraction of the tympanic membrane, but in actual practice it may result in either a positive or negative pressure change.

4.6.1 Nine-Step Inflation-Deflation Test

Charles Bluestone has developed a nine-step inflation-deflation test, in which a series of tympanometric evaluations during inflation and deflation of pressure in the ear canal can be used to assess eustachian tube function with an intact tympanic membrane.[32] In step 1, a tympanogram is obtained to assess the resting middle ear pressure. In step 2, after the ear canal has been properly sealed and pressurized to $+200$ mm H_2O, the patient is instructed to attempt to equilibrate the resultant overpressure within the middle ear cavity with several swallows. In step 3, the external ear canal pressure is released to return to normal and the patient avoids swallowing, leaving a slightly negative pressure in the middle ear. In step 4, the patient tries to equilibrate the middle ear cavity again with several swallows. In step 5, if the eustachian tube function is intact, air should flow from the nasopharynx into the middle ear cavity, equilibration should result, and a tympanogram is then obtained. In step 6, the external ear canal is depressurized to -200 mm H_2O, and the patient is then asked to swallow several times to equilibrate the middle ear pressure. In step 7, the patient avoids swallowing and the external ear canal pressure is returned to normal, which should create a positive pressure environment in the middle ear quantified by tympanogram. In steps 8 and 9, the patient swallows to reduce the positive pressure in the middle ear, and a tympanogram is then obtained to verify the degree of equilibration. This test has been used to assess eustachian tube function in children prior to tympanoplasty and correlates well with favorable outcomes. However, poor tubal function failed to correlate with poor tympanoplasty outcomes.[33]

4.6.2 Tubomanometry

Tubomanometry is based on detecting the movement of gas from the nasopharynx to the middle ear during pressure equilibration. With a pressure transducer fitted into the external auditory canal and a bilateral nasal pressure generator and pressure transducer in place, the patient is instructed to swallow. The pressure transducer senses the initial action and sends a precise amount of positive pressure into the nasopharyngeal space via the nasal pressure generator. The ear canal pressure transducer is sensitive to pressure changes secondary to tympanic membrane displacement, and it can also detect the transmission of pressure from the nasopharynx when a ventilation tube or perforation is present.[34,35] The clinical relevance of the test remains to be demonstrated.

4.6.3 Sonotubometry

In sonotubometry, tubal dilation is evaluated using a speaker in the subjects' nose and a microphone placed within the external auditory canal. The test is based on the principle that the sound amplitude measured in the middle ear will increase during eustachian tube dilation.[36] Confounders for sonotubometry are that the eustachian tube does not open uniformly, or at all, with every swallow, even in normal subjects. Arbitrary testing frequencies and confounding noise further limit its clinical use.[36] Sonotubometry sensitivity and reproducibility may be improved with the use of specific sound frequencies in the range of 5,500 to 8,500 Hz[37] and can detect acute dysfunction as seen by application of histamine onto the nasopharyngeal orifice in healthy individuals.[38] The simultaneous and synchronous use of endoscopy and sonotubometry may improve the assessment of tubal function compared to the use of either test separately.[39] In some cases, eustachian tube dilation was observed to have probably occurred on endoscopy, but not recorded on sonotubometry, despite the middle ear being normally ventilated. In these cases, endoscopy may be judged as a false positive. In contrast, in the cases in which the eustachian tube was thought to open on endoscopy, but an increase in ear canal sound pressure did not reach adequate threshold, the sonotubometry could be judged as a false negative. Sonotubometry testing in children with otitis media with effusion, having undergone tympanostomy tube placement, detected a reduced incidence of tubal opening at 1 week and improvement to normal levels after 3 months.[40]

4.7 Pathology and Treatment of Eustachian Tube Dysfunction

Eustachian tube endoscopy has demonstrated that in most cases, eustachian tube dysfunction has identifiable pathology within the cartilaginous portion.[8,28,41] The problem of inadequate dilation of the eustachian tube (dilatory dysfunction) is the most common type of eustachian tube dysfunction. Failure of tubal closure results in a patulous eustachian tube dysfunction.

When eustachian tube dilatory dysfunction causes prolonged and a severe negative pressure at approximately –400 dPa, transudates may fill the middle ear and mastoid space as a serous effusion.[42] Patients with dilatory dysfunction frequently complain of aural fullness and varying degrees of conductive hearing loss, and they often have an abnormal-appearing tympanic membrane. Less common symptoms are otalgia, otorrhea, and fever.

Isolated chronic aural fullness without tympanic membrane retractions, effusion, or abnormalities are unlikely to have eustachian tube dilatory dysfunction. In these cases other causes should be investigated, such as patulous eustachian tube, musculoskeletal and temporomandibular joint disorders, and "third labyrinthine window" (Minor's syndrome) disorders.

The familial history of dilatory dysfunction is quite common. The etiology of eustachian tube dilatory dysfunction is divided into two categories: obstructive and dynamic. Obstructive dysfunction is more common and usually involves a functional or physiological compromise of dilation rather than true anatomic blockage. Mucosal inflammation with edema is the leading source of the obstruction that may cause reductions in dilation diameter, duration of dilation, frequency of dilation, or a combination of these (▶ Fig. 4.2).

Mucosal inflammation typically appears to involve the lymphoid tissues in the posteromedial wall of the posterior cushion mucosal surfaces at the orifice, but less commonly occurs within the lumen of the valve or more proximally. Adenoid-like lymphoid hyperplasia can be seen as "cobblestone"-appearing mucosa on the posterior cushions and may contribute to mucosal inflammation within the eustachian tube lumen. In a previous study, mucosal edema was found in 83% of subjects with otitis media with effusion or nonadherent tympanic membrane retraction, and 74% had reduced anterolateral wall movement of the eustachian tube compared to 13% of normal subjects who had only mild inflammatory changes.[43] Adjacent inflammation

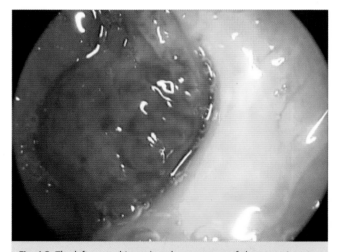

Fig. 4.2 The left eustachian tube where mucosa of the posterior cushion is inflamed and there is also lymphoid hyperplasia. There was otitis media with effusion.

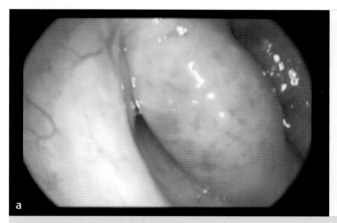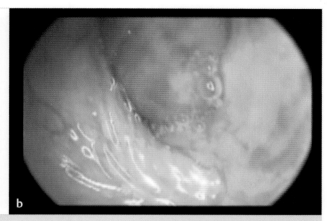

Fig. 4.3 The right eustachian tube with inflamed adenoid (upper right corner) abutting an inflamed posterior cushion. There was otitis media with effusion. (a) Closed resting position. (b) Patient is attempting to open the eustachian tube by swallowing, but a swollen posterior cushion is compressed against the adenoid, thrusting the posterior cushion anteriorly and preventing opening of the orifice.

in the adenoid tissue is common. The presence of chronic inflammation has been correlated significantly with the presence of laryngopharyngeal reflux and allergies in adults, raising suspicions that these factors may be important contributors to dilatory dysfunction.[41,43] Mucosal inflammation in the eustachian tube with dilatory dysfunction can be caused by diseases in the respiratory tract, including those affecting the nasal cavity, sinuses, nasopharynx, and the remainder of the upper and lower airway. Chronic mucosal disorders such as Wegener's disease, Samter's triad (asthma, polyps, and aspirin allergy), and granulomatous diseases are less common etiologies. In children, there is the additional burden of frequent upper respiratory infections that are increased with day care, reflux disease in younger children, and exposure to smoke from tobacco or wood-burning stoves.[25] Additionally, genetic disorders, such as Kartagener's syndrome, can impair mucociliary function. The effect of hormonal disturbances on the eustachian tube can be observed in pregnancy, particularly in the third trimester when progesterone levels are peaking. Progesterone has a direct effect on the mucosa, with ensuing edema and occasional dilatory dysfunction.

Anatomic obstructive causes of dilatory dysfunction are less common, with the exception of adenoid hypertrophy as it commonly impinges on the posterior cushion in children, but seen also in affected adults. Contraction of the pharyngeal constrictors during swallowing can compress a nonobstructive adenoid into the posterior cushions, causing them to be thrust anteriorly, resulting in paradoxical closure of the tubal orifice during the dilatory phase in which it should be opening (► Fig. 4.3).

True anatomic obstructions from benign and malignant lesions are rare. Benign anatomic obstructions include severe adenoid hypertrophy, large Thornwaldt's cysts, mucus retention cysts, teratomas and dermoids, and synechiae after adenoidectomy or other head and neck surgeries. Malignant tumors such as nasopharyngeal carcinoma (the most common malignant lesion), lymphoma, chondrosarcoma, and mucosal melanoma are rare, but important to rule out with contrast-enhanced imaging studies, particularly in unilateral persistent otitis media with effusion cases.[44]

Dynamic causes of eustachian tube dilatory dysfunction can be due to hypoactive, hyperactive, or uncoordinated contraction of tensor or levator veli palatini muscles. Tensor veli palatini muscle weakness or dysfunction is the most common dynamic cause of decrease in anterolateral wall dilatory movement. Weakened or disorganized tensor veli palatini contractions may reduce the lateral excursion of the anterolateral wall in the final step of dilation. Excessive disorganized contractions have been observed in both tensor and levator muscles, causing a bulky mass effect and paradoxical impairment of valve dilation (► Fig. 4.4). Uncoordinated contractions can result in impaired dilation when the levator veli palatini relaxes prematurely before contraction of the tensor veli palatini.

4.8 Treatment of Eustachian Tube Dysfunction

Mucosal disease is the most common cause of dilatory dysfunction. Attempts should be made to identify and minimize the known risk factors of mucosal disorders as discussed above. Conservative medical treatment should be instituted before consideration of surgical therapy.

4.8.1 Medical Therapy

Conservative and medical therapy for allergic disease may include allergen avoidance, oral antihistamine, nasal topical steroid sprays or drops (available in Europe but not in the United States), saline irrigations, nasal antihistamine, mast cell stabilizer sprays, leukotriene inhibitors, combination therapy, and immunotherapy. Chronic rhinosinusitis should be treated as thoroughly as indicated. Laryngopharyngeal reflux disease should be treated with dietary and behavioral modifications as well as antireflux medications and even surgery if appropriate. A recent randomized, placebo-controlled, double-blinded study, in which nasal corticosteroid spray was given for eustachian tube dilatory dysfunction without specified etiologies, found that it provided no benefit.[45] Anatomic obstruction re-

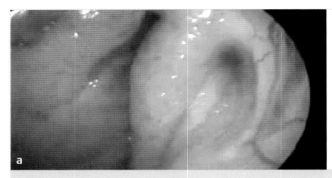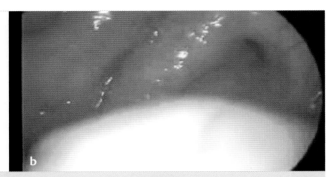

Fig. 4.4 The left eustachian tube with dynamic dysfunction of the levator veli palatini muscle. Excessively high contractions of the levator veli palatini during swallows caused blockage of the lumen during dilatory effort. There was otitis media with effusion. (a) Resting closed position. (b) When the patient swallowed, elevation of the palate and levator veli palatini muscle blocked the tubal lumen.

quires often more than medical management, including excision of benign or malignant lesions.

4.8.2 Surgical Therapy

Chronic dilatory dysfunction despite maximal efforts to control possible underlying etiologies may imply that the mucosa has become irreversibly injured or perhaps involved with biofilm. Surgical treatment may be considered for the disease when medical therapy is inadequate. Tympanostomy tubes may relieve the negative middle ear pressure, tympanic membrane retraction, effusion, or atelectasis. In cases with persistent tubal dilatory dysfunction repeatedly following tympanostomy tube extrusion, the use of larger flanged tubes such as T-tubes or subannular semipermanent tubes may be considered. If the effusion or inflammation continues despite a tube in place, it should raise the suspicion of a primary mucosal disorder or other disorders. Thick proteinaceous "gluelike" effusions that repeatedly occlude the ventilating tube may be due to primary mucosal inflammation where MUC protein production is upregulated and will often respond to oral or topical corticosteroids.[46] Adenoidectomy may provide significant relief for patients with otitis media with effusion and adenoid hypertrophy, especially if the adenoid is in contact with the posterior cushions (torus tubarius).[47,48] Endoscope-assisted adenoidectomy permits more complete removal of the tissue in contact with the posterior cushion and allows for light cauterization of the "cobblestoned" hyperplastic mucosa that also may be involving the posterior cushion.

There are two currently used surgical approaches to restore eustachian tube dilatory function: shaver or laser-assisted tuboplasty and balloon dilation tuboplasty. Eustachian tuboplasty has received increased attention as a safe and effective surgical option for patients with eustachian tube dilatory dysfunction. Patients with chronic tubal dilatory dysfunction, despite receiving maximal medical therapy and multiple tympanostomy tube placements, are potential candidates for eustachian tuboplasty.

Eustachian tuboplasty can be accomplished by the removal of inflamed soft tissue, as indicated by using tools such as a laser or microdebrider, along the luminal side of the posteromedial wall, beginning from the leading edge of the torus tubarius and extending up to the valve. This procedure is based on the hypothesis that dilation of the lumen by surgical debulking may facilitate the dilatory action of the tensor veli palatini muscle,

and removal of irreversibly diseased mucosa may allow it to regrow in a healthier and thinner state. Removal of submucosal tissue and cartilage within the valve region may be done, but the mucosa is preserved to prevent synechiae. Injury to the mucosa of the anterolateral wall should be avoided for the same reason.[49] The internal carotid artery lies in increasingly close proximity to the eustachian tube as it courses superiorly, and care should always be made to protect and avoid the artery. In a previous 2-year follow-up study of eustachian tuboplasty using an argon or potassium titanyl phosphate (KTP) laser for tissue ablation, an overall improvement rate was 68%.[50] Results of eustachian tuboplasty have been studied also in preoperative and postoperative pressure chamber tests demonstrating significant improvement of eustachian tube dilatory function.[51] Failures of laser eustachian tuboplasty correlated with the presence of symptomatic allergic and laryngopharyngeal reflux disease, underscoring the need to continue to treat any underlying conditions postoperatively.[50,52]

Preliminary result from balloon dilation eustachian tuboplasty has been assessed for feasibility, safety, and clinical application.[53–56] In this endoscope-assisted approach, a balloon catheter is inserted into the cartilaginous portion of the eustachian tube and dilated to 12 atmospheres for 2 minutes, after which the balloon is deflated and removed. It is important for the surgeon to recognize that the eustachian tube initially curves slightly posteromedially before coursing anterolaterally toward the ear. The lumen should be opened gently by retracting medially on the posterior cushion with the guiding catheter, allowing for a view deep into the lumen before beginning the insertion. Failure to medially rotate the posterior cushion could result in laceration of the mucosa with bleeding or creation of a false passage into the submucosal tissue as the catheter is advanced. The catheter is passed through the lumen gently and slowly until meeting slight resistance as the catheter engages the isthmus. The catheter should never be inserted forcefully (► Fig. 4.5). Preoperative histology has shown significant lymphocyte infiltration and even follicles within the submucosa and loss of the cilia in areas, whereas postoperatively the lymphocyte infiltration is markedly reduced and replaced in part by thinner fibrotic tissue. There has been regeneration of a healthy pseudocolumnar ciliated epithelium (► Fig. 4.6).

In a recent study of 11 patients with chronic otitis media with effusion (OME) of over 5 years' duration, postoperatively all 11

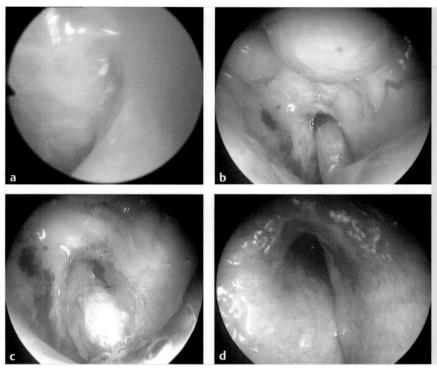

Fig. 4.5 Left eustachian tube balloon dilation in a patient with prolonged otitis media with effusion. (a) Preoperative resting position. There is edema and inflammation on the posterior cushion. (b) A guide catheter is inserted into the lumen of eustachian tube. (c) A 7- × 16-mm balloon catheter has been inserted to 16 mm depth and inflated to 12 atm for 2 minutes. (d) The catheter has been removed. The lumen appears wider and there are some minimal mucosal lacerations.

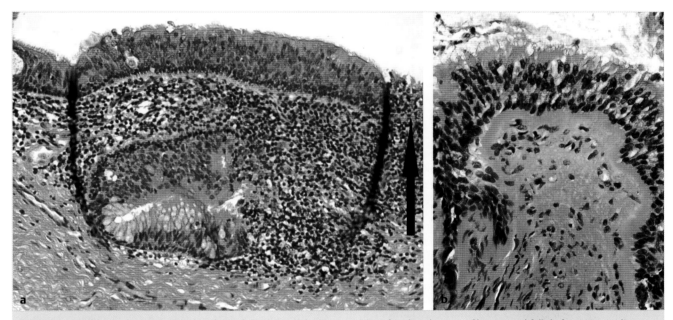

Fig. 4.6 Preoperative and postoperative histology of eustachian tube mucosa. (a) Profuse lymphocytic infiltration and follicle formation in the submucosa indicates chronic inflammation in preoperative eustachian tube mucosa. There is increased lymphocyte infiltration in the mucosa layer. (b) Postoperative histology shows significantly reduced amount of lymphocytes in submucosa, but also some fibrotic tissue.

patients were able to perform a Valsalva maneuver, whereas they had previously been unable to do so, but this declined to seven of 11 patients (63.6%) at the end of the follow-up period from 6 to 14 months.[53] Resolution of OME occurred in the five patients (45.5%) who had an intact tympanic membranes (no perforation or tube); also there was a significant reduction in inflammation of the mucosa of the eustachian tube. Additional clinical studies of balloon dilation eustachian tuboplasty are needed to determine the long-lasting follow-up results of these procedures.

4.9 Patulous Eustachian Tube

The patulous eustachian tube has been defined as a prolonged situation with an abnormal patency in the lumen that results in

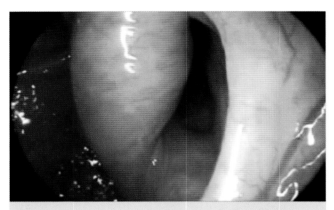

Fig. 4.7 Patulous left eustachian tube demonstrating a marked concave anterolateral wall. There is no visible anterolateral cartilaginous lamina or evidence of a significant Ostmann's fat pad.

free and unrestricted passage of air and sound between the nasopharynx and the middle ear cavity.[57] Patients frequently complain of an amplified perception of their own voice and breathing sounds, called autophony, and an accompanying sensation of aural fullness. Autophony is often described as similar to talking into a wind tunnel or barrel. Patulous dysfunction causes a wide spectrum of symptom severity that can range from mild discomfort to severe impairment. Symptoms are often intermittent, although in severe cases the symptoms may persist for hours. Nasal or oral decongestants are of no benefit and may exacerbate the condition. Symptoms may occur after a dramatic and substantial weight loss such as after pregnancy or with cachectic diseases, dietary weight loss, or bariatric surgery. One third of patients with a patulous eustachian tube have a history of substantial weight loss; one third have an associated systemic disorder, usually rheumatologic; and the remaining third are idiopathic.

Loss of tubal tissue volume (Ostmann's fat pad, mucosal and muscle atrophy) within the valve area is the likely etiology for many patients with patulous eustachian tube dysfunction, with noted longitudinal concavity in the resting position and inadequate closing of the tubal lumen (▶ Fig. 4.7).[58] In one study, CT scans revealed smaller Ostmann's fat pad and glandular tissues in patulous patients compared with normal control subjects, supporting the theory of tissue loss and patulous function.[59] The size of the Ostmann's fat pad in magnetic resonance imaging also diminishes with age even in asymptomatic patients.[60]

The symptoms of a patulous eustachian tube can overlap with many other conditions, such as eustachian tube dilatory dysfunction, temporomandibular joint (TMJ) disorders, superior semicircular canal dehiscence (Minor's) syndrome, and Ménière's disease. Patulous eustachian tube dysfunction can be diagnosed by the history and physical examination, and also with endoscopic-assisted inspection. Audiogram and tympanometry should be normal. Examination with an otoscope or otomicroscope is essential to look for the classic sign of medial and lateral tympanic membrane excursions during nasal breathing with the opposite nostril pinched shut; this only occurs while the patients are actively experiencing their autophony. The examination usually needs to be done with the patient seated upright, because most patulous eustachian tubes will close in the supine

position. If it is not seen, symptoms may be provoked by a few minutes of physical activity prior to otoscopy.

Patients can usually experience relief of symptoms by lying supine, placing their head down in a dependent position, sniffing inward against a closed nostril, or compressing their ipsilateral internal jugular vein. The symptoms usually abate due to venous engorgement and at least temporarily close the patulous eustachian tube. If a tympanostomy tube is placed, ventilatory excursions can be observed by placing a drop of clear topical otologic medication onto the tube and watching for movement of the meniscus.

Vestibular evoked myogenic potential (VEMP) testing can aid in differentiating patulous dysfunction from Minor's syndrome. Minor's syndrome patients generally lack autophony with breathing and have abnormally low thresholds on VEMP. Impedance tympanometry is one of the most sensitive tests for patulous eustachian tube dysfunction, showing ventilatory fluctuations in the compliance of the tympanic membrane while a 10- to 15-second run is performed on the reflex decay mode. Also, sonotubometry research with recent improvements in detecting tubal patency status have demonstrated a correlation between the severity of autophony and the measurement of tubal function.[61]

4.10 Medical Therapy of a Patulous Eustachian Tube

A healthy humidified mucosa and competence of the tubal valve are the primary goals of treatment. Treatment should be started in a stepwise fashion, beginning with reassuring the patient that it is a benign disorder. Discontinuation of medications such as decongestants and topical nasal corticosteroid sprays may result in symptom relief. Patients should be encouraged to increase hydration, particularly during exercise, and nasal saline drops or irrigations may be effective in restoring tubal mucosal volume. Although up to a third of patulous patients have a history of significant weight loss, weight gain is generally not advised unless there is obvious malnutrition. Several medications have been tried with varied results. Saturated solution of potassium iodide (SSKI) enhances viscosity of the mucus. It is taken three times daily, 8 to 10 drops diluted in water or juice. Irritating nasal drops that cause tissue inflammation, increased mucus production, and reduced tubal patency may work, and treatments with boric and salicylic acid powder, silver nitrate, nitrate acid, and phenol have shown temporary benefit. Hydrochloric acid-based nasal drops are available and have some success. The off-label use of Premarin or estradiol estrogens as nasal drops may provide variable lengths of relief in adults by causing localized mucosal hypertrophy. Drops are most effective when applied with the nose pointed straight upward and the head turned 45 degrees to the ipsilateral side as the drops pass through the nasal cavity, and the drops should cause a tickle sensation radiating toward the ear.[62]

4.11 Surgical Therapy of a Patulous Eustachian Tube

When medical treatments afford no relief, surgical options can be considered. The most common intervention is myringotomy

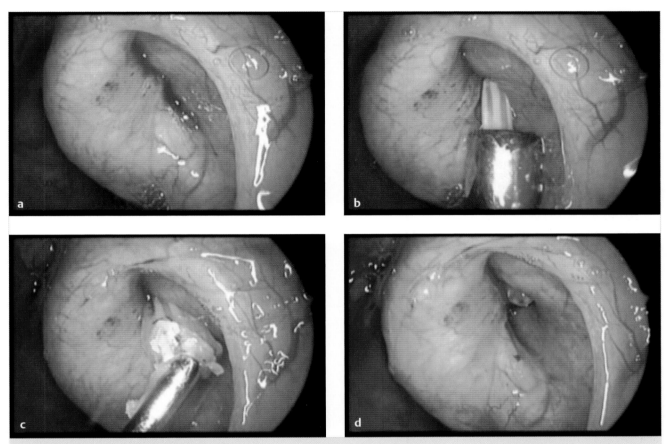

Fig. 4.8 Insertion of an intravenous catheter into the left patulous eustachian tube. The catheter has been filled with bone wax. (a) The left tubal orifice before insertion. (b) The catheter is housed in an introducer tool and is being inserted into the tubal orifice. The posterior cushion is rotated posteromedially to open the lumen and view the direction of the lumen, which usually curves slightly medially before subsequently coursing laterally toward the temporal bone. Failure to recognize this curve can result in mucosal laceration or a false submucosal passage as the catheter is advanced. (c) The catheter is firmly wedged into the bony–cartilaginous junction. (d) The catheter is in the final position at the level of the orifice of posterior cushion.

with tympanostomy tube placement.[63] It may be effective for aural fullness and tympanic membrane excursion, but it is generally not effective for treating autophony. Monopolar cauterization of the nasopharyngeal orifice lumen mucosa with fat graft occlusion or occlusion of the bony eustachian tube lumen with a catheter filled with and surrounded by bone wax has been used. This intervention is effective in alleviating autophony, but it entails the risk of predisposing the patient to OME and the likely need for long-term tympanostomy tubes.[64] Mucoid middle ear effusions have been known to occur after eustachian tube obliteration, creating problems with tympanostomy tube occlusion and the persistence of effusion. Complete obliteration is therefore reserved for a procedure of last resort.

In an effort to correct the patulous symptoms while preserving tubal function, shims may be inserted into the lumen, or autologous cartilage may be placed into submucosal pockets within the lumen. A shim can be inserted into the nasopharyngeal orifice, wedging it into position within the isthmus, and the flexible material lies within the longitudinal concave defect in the valve to effectively relieve the symptoms. A regular intravenous catheter filled with bone wax can be used in this off-label application (▶ Fig. 4.8). If the catheter extrudes prematurely, patulous eustachian tube reconstruction may be done with

cauterization of the tubal lumen and near occlusion with fat graft, leaving a stent in place for 6 weeks to preserve a limited, but functional lumen.

4.12 Conclusion

Proper function of the eustachian tube is essential for aeration, protection, and clearance of the middle ear cavity. Disorders of the eustachian tube commonly have identifiable pathology within the cartilaginous portion seen on endoscope-assisted evaluation. In most cases, conservative management directed at the underlying etiology is adequate therapy. If eustachian tube dilatory dysfunction persists after a trial of a tympanostomy tube, surgical intervention may be considered. Nasal or sinus surgery may be done if indicated. Adenoidectomy with attention to the posterior cushions is often beneficial. Surgical intervention on the eustachian tube itself is now possible for selected cases, although greater experience in controlled clinical trials is needed to determine the long-term effect of these new procedures. Basic science investigations are also needed for a better understanding of the etiology of eustachian tube dysfunction and the mechanisms of action of the surgical therapies.

References

[1] Bluestone CD. Introduction. In: Bluestone MB, ed. Eustachian Tube: Structure, Function, Role in Otitis Media. Hamilton, Ontario; Lewiston, NY: BC Decker, 2005:1–9

[2] Canalis RF. Valsalva's contribution to otology. Am J Otolaryngol 1990; 11: 420–427

[3] Toynbee J. On the muscles that open the eustachian tube. Proc R Soc Lond 1853; 6: 286–287

[4] Proctor B. Anatomy of the eustachian tube. Arch Otolaryngol 1973; 97: 2–8

[5] Sando I, Takahashi H, Matsune S, Aoki H. Localization of function in the eustachian tube: a hypothesis. Ann Otol Rhinol Laryngol 1994; 103: 311–314

[6] Ishijima K, Sando I, Balaban CD, Suzuki C, Takasaki K. Length of the eustachian tube and its postnatal development: computer-aided three-dimensional reconstruction and measurement study. Ann Otol Rhinol Laryngol 2000; 109: 542–548

[7] Sudo M, Sando I, Ikui A, Suzuki C. Narrowest (isthmus) portion of eustachian tube: a computer-aided three-dimensional reconstruction and measurement study. Ann Otol Rhinol Laryngol 1997; 106: 583–588

[8] Hopf J, Linnarz M, Gundlach P et al. [Microendoscopy of the eustachian tube and the middle ear. Indications and clinical application] Laryngorhinootologie 1991; 70: 391–394

[9] Bluestone CD. Anatomy. In: Bluestone MB, ed. Eustachian Tube: Structure, Function, Role in Otitis Media. Hamilton, Ontario; Lewiston, NY: BC Decker, 2005:25–50

[10] Rich A. A physiological study of the eustachian tube and its related muscles. Bull Johns Hopkins Hosp 1920; 31: 3005–3010

[11] Cantekin EI, Doyle WJ, Reichert TJ, Phillips DC, Bluestone CD. Dilation of the eustachian tube by electrical stimulation of the mandibular nerve. Ann Otol Rhinol Laryngol 1979; 88: 40–51

[12] King PF. The eustachian tube and its significance in flight. J Laryngol Otol 1979; 93: 659–678

[13] Mondain M, Vidal D, Bouhanna S, Uziel A. Monitoring eustachian tube opening: preliminary results in normal subjects. Laryngoscope 1997; 107: 1414–1419

[14] Bluestone CD. Physiology. In: Bluestone MB, ed. Eustachian Tube: Structure, Function, Role in Otitis Media. Hamilton, Ontario; Lewiston, NY: BC Decker, 2005:51–63

[15] Felding JU, Rasmussen JB, Lildholdt T. Gas composition of the normal and the ventilated middle ear cavity. Scand J Clin Lab Invest Suppl 1987; 186: 31–41

[16] Ostfeld EJ, Silberberg A. Gas composition and pressure in the middle ear: a model for the physiological steady state. Laryngoscope 1991; 101: 297–304

[17] Ars B, Ars-Piret N. Middle ear pressure balance under normal conditions. Specific role of the middle ear structure. Acta Otorhinolaryngol Belg 1994; 48: 339–342

[18] Doyle WJ, Seroky JT. Middle ear gas exchange in rhesus monkeys. Ann Otol Rhinol Laryngol 1994; 103: 636–645

[19] Rockley TJ, Hawke WM. The middle ear as a baroreceptor. Acta Otolaryngol 1992; 112: 816–823

[20] Sadé J, Ar A. Middle ear and auditory tube: middle ear clearance, gas exchange, and pressure regulation. Otolaryngol Head Neck Surg 1997; 116: 499–524

[21] Nuutinen J, Kärjä J, Karjalainen P. Measurement of mucociliary function of the eustachian tube. Arch Otolaryngol 1983; 109: 669–672

[22] Honjo I, Hayashi M, Ito S, Takahashi H. Pumping and clearance function of the eustachian tube. Am J Otolaryngol 1985; 6: 241–244

[23] McGuire JF. Surfactant in the middle ear and eustachian tube: a review. Int J Pediatr Otorhinolaryngol 2002; 66: 1–15

[24] Grace A, Kwok P, Hawke M. Surfactant in middle ear effusions. Otolaryngol Head Neck Surg 1987; 96: 336–340

[25] Bluestone CD. Epidemiology. In: Bluestone MB, ed. Eustachian Tube: Structure, Function, Role in Otitis Media. Hamilton, Ontario; Lewiston, NY: BC Decker, 2005:11–24

[26] Todd NW, Martin WS. Temporal bone pneumatization in cystic fibrosis patients. Laryngoscope 1988; 98: 1046–1049

[27] Poe DS, Gopen Q. Eustachian tube dysfunction. In: Snow JB, Wackym PA, Ballenger JJ, eds. Ballenger's Otorhinolaryngology: Head and Neck Surgery, 17th ed. Lewiston, NY: BC Decker, 2009:201–208

[28] Poe DS, Pyykkö I, Valtonen H, Silvola J. Analysis of eustachian tube function by video endoscopy. Am J Otol 2000; 21: 602–607

[29] Takahashi H, Honjo I, Fujita A. Endoscopic findings at the pharyngeal orifice of the eustachian tube in otitis media with effusion. Eur Arch Otorhinolaryngol 1996; 253: 42–44

[30] Poe DS, Pyykkö I. Measurements of eustachian tube dilation by video endoscopy. Otol Neurotol 2011; 32: 794–798

[31] McDonald MH, Hoffman MR, Gentry LR, Jiang JJ. New insights into mechanism of eustachian tube ventilation based on cine computed tomography images. Eur Arch Otorhinolaryngol 2012; 269: 1901–1907

[32] Bluestone CD. Diagnosis and tests of function. In: Bluestone MB, ed. Eustachian Tube: Structure, Function, Role in Otitis Media. Hamilton, Ontario; Lewiston, NY: BC Decker, 2005:113–141

[33] Manning SC, Cantekin EI, Kenna MA, Bluestone CD. Prognostic value of eustachian tube function in pediatric tympanoplasty. Laryngoscope 1987; 97: 1012–1016

[34] Ars B, Dirckx J. Tubomanometry. In: Ars B, ed. Fibrocartilaginous Eustachian Tube: Middle Ear Cleft. The Hague: Kugler, 2003:151–158

[35] Esteve D. Tubomanometry and pathology. In: Ars B, ed. Fibrocartilaginous Eustachian Tube: Middle Ear Cleft. The Hague: Kugler, 2003:159–175

[36] van der Avoort SJ, van Heerbeek N, Zielhuis GA, Cremers CW. Sonotubometry: eustachian tube ventilatory function test: a state-of-the-art review. Otol Neurotol 2005; 26: 538–543, discussion 543

[37] Palva T, Marttila T, Jauhiainen T. Comparison of pure tones and noise stimuli in sonotubometry. Acta Otolaryngol 1987; 103: 212–216

[38] van Heerbeek N, van der Avoort SJ, Zielhuis GA, Cremers CW. Sonotubometry: a useful tool to measure intra-individual changes in eustachian tube ventilatory function. Arch Otolaryngol Head Neck Surg 2007; 133: 763–766

[39] Handzel O, Poe D, Marchbanks RJ. Synchronous endoscopy and sonotubometry of the eustachian tube: a pilot study. Otol Neurotol 2012; 33: 184–191

[40] van der Avoort SJ, van Heerbeek N, Zielhuis GA, Cremers CW. Sonotubometry in children with otitis media with effusion before and after insertion of ventilation tubes. Arch Otolaryngol Head Neck Surg 2009; 135: 448–452

[41] Edelstein DR, Magnan J, Parisier SC et al. Microfiberoptic evaluation of the middle ear cavity. Am J Otol 1994; 15: 50–55

[42] Bluestone CD. Pathophysiology. In: Bluestone MB, ed. Eustachian Tube: Structure, Function, Role in Otitis Media. Hamilton, Ontario; Lewiston, NY: BC Decker, 2005:67–91

[43] Poe DS, Abou-Halawa A, Abdel-Razek O. Analysis of the dysfunctional eustachian tube by video endoscopy. Otol Neurotol 2001; 22: 590–595

[44] Muzzi E, Cama E, Boscolo-Rizzo P, Trabalzini F, Arslan E. Primary tumors and tumor-like lesions of the eustachian tube: a systematic review of an emerging entity. Eur Arch Otorhinolaryngol 2012; 269: 1723–1732

[45] Gluth MB, McDonald DR, Weaver AL, Bauch CD, Beatty CW, Orvidas LJ. Management of eustachian tube dysfunction with nasal steroid spray: a prospective, randomized, placebo-controlled trial. Arch Otolaryngol Head Neck Surg 2011; 137: 449–455

[46] Elsheikh MN, Mahfouz ME. Up-regulation of MUC5AC and MUC5B mucin genes in nasopharyngeal respiratory mucosa and selective up-regulation of MUC5B in middle ear in pediatric otitis media with effusion. Laryngoscope 2006; 116: 365–369

[47] Gates GA. Adenoidectomy for otitis media with effusion. Ann Otol Rhinol Laryngol Suppl 1994; 163: 54–58

[48] Nguyen LH, Manoukian JJ, Yoskovitch A, Al-Sebeih KH. Adenoidectomy: selection criteria for surgical cases of otitis media. Laryngoscope 2004; 114: 863–866

[49] Poe DS, Metson RB, Kujawski O. Laser eustachian tuboplasty: a preliminary report. Laryngoscope 2003; 113: 583–591

[50] Poe DS, Grimmer JF, Metson R. Laser eustachian tuboplasty: two-year results. Laryngoscope 2007; 117: 231–237

[51] Jumah MD, Jumah M, Pazen D, Sedlmaier B. Laser eustachian tuboplasty: efficiency evaluation in the pressure chamber. Otol Neurotol 2012; 33: 406–412

[52] Kujawski OB, Poe DS. Laser eustachian tuboplasty. Otol Neurotol 2004; 25: 1–8

[53] Poe DS, Silvola J, Pyykkö I. Balloon dilation of the cartilaginous eustachian tube. Otolaryngol Head Neck Surg 2011; 144: 563–569

[54] Ockermann T, Reineke U, Upile T, Ebmeyer J, Sudhoff HH. Balloon dilatation eustachian tuboplasty: a clinical study. Laryngoscope 2010; 120: 1411–1416

[55] McCoul ED, Anand VK. Eustachian tube balloon dilation surgery. Int Forum Allergy Rhinol 2012; 2: 191–198

[56] Schröder S, Reineke U, Lehmann M, Ebmeyer J, Sudhoff H. Chronic obstructive eustachian tube dysfunction in adults: Long-term results of balloon eustachian tuboplasty. HNO 2012[German].

[57] O'Connor AF, Shea JJ. Autophony and the patulous eustachian tube. Laryngoscope 1981; 91: 1427–1435

[58] Poe DS. Diagnosis and management of the patulous eustachian tube. Otol Neurotol 2007; 28: 668–677

[59] Kikuchi T, Oshima T, Ogura M, Hori Y, Kawase T, Kobayashi T. Three-dimensional computed tomography imaging in the sitting position for the diagnosis of patulous eustachian tube. Otol Neurotol 2007; 28: 199–203

[60] Amoodi H, Bance M, Thamboo A. Magnetic resonance imaging illustrating change in the Ostmann fat pad with age. J Otolaryngol Head Neck Surg 2010; 39: 440–441

[61] Hori Y, Kawase T, Oshima T, Sakamoto S, Kobayashi T. Objective assessment of autophony in patients with patulous eustachian tube. Eur Arch Otorhinolaryngol 2007; 264: 1387–1391

[62] Karagama YG, Rashid M, Lancaster JL, Karkanevatos A, William RS. Intranasal delivery of drugs to eustachian tube orifice. J Laryngol Otol 2011; 125: 934–939

[63] Dyer RK, Jr, McElveen JT, Jr. The patulous eustachian tube: management options. Otolaryngol Head Neck Surg 1991; 105: 832–835

[64] Doherty JK, Slattery WH, III. Autologous fat grafting for the refractory patulous eustachian tube. Otolaryngol Head Neck Surg 2003; 128: 88–91

5 Molecular Biology of the Inner Ear

Elodie M. Richard, Rizwan Yousaf, Zubair M. Ahmed, and Saima Riazuddin

5.1 Introduction

The inner ear is a complex organ responsible for the perception of sounds and head movements. Through studies involving human genetics and animal models, we have improved our understanding of the genes involved in the development of the inner ear structures and their functions. This chapter broadly summarizes these findings.

5.2 Development of the Inner Ear

5.2.1 From the Otic Placode to the Inner Ear

The inner ear derives from the otic placode, an ectodermal thickening adjacent to rhombomeres 5 and 6 of the hindbrain.[1, 2] In mammals, after invagination, the otic placode pinches off from the surface ectoderm to form an epithelial sac known as the otocyst or otic vesicle. Individual neuroblasts from the anteroventral region of the otocyst differentiate to form the statoacoustic ganglion (SAG), which provides sensory innervation for the inner ear. The otocyst then undergoes morphological changes to reshape into a fluid-filled labyrinth, holding the auditory and vestibular sensory structures. At the end of the otic vesicle development, the mammalian adult inner ear is composed of six specialized structures: (1) The cochlea, located along the coil of the cochlear duct, is the primary auditory organ. The (2) saccule and (3) utricle, located in the center of the inner ear, perceive linear and angular accelerations. Finally,

three semicircular canals (4,5,6) together with three cristae ampularis provide perception and maintenance of balance. Next, the SAG segregates to form the spiral ganglion, along the length of the cochlear duct and the vestibular ganglion, which is localized at the surface of the inner ear and innervates the vestibular sensory epithelia.

The six structures of the adult mammalian inner ear exhibit the same basic epithelial-derived components as seen in SAG segregation: a sensory epithelium is flanked by nonsensory cells and innervated by neurons. Indeed, during its development, the otic vesicle is subdivided into sensory, nonsensory, and neurosensory domains (► Fig. 5.1). These domains are further subdivided into hair cells [outer hair cells (OHCs) and inner hair cells (IHCs)], supporting cells (SCs), mesenchymal cells, and auditory and vestibular neurons.

5.2.2 Pathways Involved in the Development and Differentiation of the Inner Ear

The development and patterning of the inner ear are under the control of a very sophisticated network of genes whose expression is temporally and spatially coordinated. These genes orchestrate the cellular proliferation and differentiation, as well as the morphogenesis and maturation that lead to a functional inner ear. A large group of regulatory proteins, including transcription factors, fibroblast growth factors, Sonic-Hedgehog (shh), Wnt and Notch pathways are involved in this process. With a subtle, back-and-forth pattern of inhibition and induc-

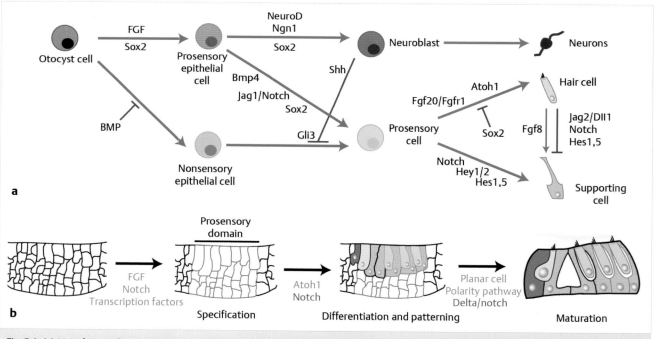

Fig. 5.1 (a) Main factors directing sensory cell fates in the inner ear. (b) Development of the auditory epithelium.

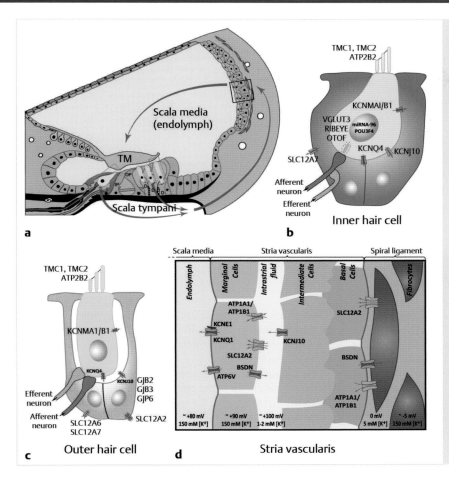

Fig. 5.2 Schematic diagrams illustrating recycling of K + and the generation of the endocochlear potential. (a) Cross section of cochlea indicating the flow of K + recycle path (*red arrows*). (b,c) Cellular structure of the outer and inner hair cells. (d) Cellular structure of the stria vascularis indicating the flow of K + (*red arrows*).

tion signaling, genes generate the specialized substructures described above (▶ Fig. 5.1; ▶ Fig. 5.2).

In the cochlear duct, a converging pathway that includes fibroblast growth factors, Notch signaling, and several other transcription factors leads to the specification of the prosensory domain. This process is coupled with a synchronized cell cycle exit, with a specific role for CDK inhibitors, such as p27Kipl and the Delta/Jagged1/Notch pathway. Upon activation of Atoh1 and inhibition of Notch, differentiation begins at the base of the cochlear duct and progresses through to the apex. Differentiation then occurs along the medial-lateral axis. Although less is known about this process, *Fgf20* was recently identified as an important component of differentiation between the medial (OHCs and SCs) and lateral compartments (IHCs and SCs) of the inner ear.[3] During differentiation and maturation the morphological changes and movements, as well as the convergent extension of the cochlea, are driven by the planar cell polarity signaling pathway and the Delta/Notch signaling pathway.

5.2.3 New Insights from microRNA

MicroRNAs (miRNA) are negative regulators that act at the level of protein translation. Hundreds of different miRNA are involved in regulating gene expression in the inner ear.[4,5] Prominent examples include the miR-183 family, consisting of the miR-96, miR-182, and miR-183 triplet. Mutations in miR-96 in humans[6,7] and in mouse (diminuendo[8]) have been associated with progressive hearing loss. Recent studies show that miR-183 may play a role in the molecular mechanisms involved in the differentiation and patterning of cells in the inner ear[9] and also in hair cell maintenance and survival.[10] Our understanding of the importance of miRNA is strengthened by the study of mouse model: mice that are genetic mutants for Dicer, an enzyme responsible for the maturation of miRNA, fail to develop an inner ear.[11]

5.3 Stereocilium and Hair Bundle Structure

Once matured, the cochlea is a complex structure: a spiral-shaped cavity framed by the bony labyrinth, divided into three fluid-filled compartments. The sensory organ, the organ of Corti, is distributed along the coil of the cochlea and is bathed in the endolymph of scala media (▶ Fig. 5.2). The hair cells are arranged in four rows in the organ of Corti: three rows of OHCs and one row of IHCs. In the vestibular epithelium, hair cells can be classified as type I and II, which correspond to the inner and outer hair cells of the cochlea, respectively. It is through the actin-based structures, known as stereocilia, located on the apical poles of hair cells that the adult inner ear is able to perceive sound and head movements.

In mammals, stereocilia are organized in three or four rows of decreasing height, forming a staircase pattern (▶ Fig. 5.3). A

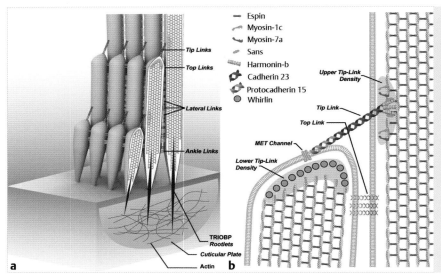

Fig. 5.3 Scheme of stereocilia and molecular components of mechanotransduction channel. (a) Scheme of the apical surface of a hair cell, showing tens to hundreds of stereocilia that compose the hair bundle. (b) Scheme showing putative locations of some of the identified hair-bundle molecular components of the mechano-transduction complex in stereocilia.

single axonemal primary cilium, the kinocilium, composed of a doublet of microtubules, is located at the vertex of the V-shaped stereocilia bundle. Present only in the developing hair bundle of the organ of Corti, the kinocilium degenerates after birth, which suggests a unique role kinocilium might play during development.

Stereocilia are composed of highly cross-linked F-actin filaments, uniformly polarized, with the barbed (plus) ends located at their tips. These microfilaments contain β (beta) and γ (gamma) actin, cross-linked with espin, plastin 1, and T-plastin proteins.[12–15] Mutations in the genes encoding these proteins severely impact the hair bundle structure and function, which points to their important role in stereocilia morphogenesis and stabilization.[16,17] Actin filaments provide a structural stability to the stereocilium and must be replaced if they are damaged. Until recently, it was generally hypothesized that actin filaments were continuously being renewed and remodeled by the incorporation of new actin monomers, resulting in a "treadmilling" action along the stereocilia to maintain their length.[18,19] A recent study, however, showed rapid turnover of the actin filaments only at the tips of stereocilia.[20] Specifically, researchers found no "treadmilling" along the length of stereocilia, but only the tips of stereocilia being continuously renewed.[20]

When deflected, stereocilia pivot at their insertion point, where their diameters taper. Mutations in the deafness genes *Myo6* and *Ptprq* (▶ Table 5.1) result in a loss of this tapering, which suggests that the genes regulate the formation and maintenance of this morphology.[21–23] Mutations in the gene encoding Taperin, a protein named because of its accumulation in the taper region of hair cells, also leads to deafness, emphasizing the important role of this region of hair cells in the hearing process.[24] At the tapered end, the composition of the stereocilia differs and the actin filaments form a rootlet, a dense actin-based structure that penetrates into the hair cell body. Two different roles for the rootlet have been proposed: (1) the rootlet anchors the stereocilia in the actin-rich meshwork of the cuticular plate, or (2) the rootlet allows for elasticity to maintain the pivoting action of the stereocilium at the insertion point. Tropomyosin and spectrin are proteins that are known to accumulate in the cuticular plate.[25] Recently, mutations of *TRIOBP* have

been associated with deafness in humans (DFNB28).[26,27] Based on this and further studies in mice, this actin-bundling protein has been identified as critical for the formation and maintenance of rootlets (▶ Fig. 5.1).[28]

The stereocilia are organized in a bundle that is composed of 20 to 300 stereocilia at the apical surface of a hair cell. To guarantee the structure and the function of the bundle, stereocilia are interconnected by up to five different types of links. These links include the tectorial membrane attachment crown, the tip link, horizontal top connectors, shaft connectors, and the ankle links, seen in that order along the length of the hair bundle, from top to bottom (▶ Fig. 5.1). Tip links have been widely studied because of their predicted implication in the mechanoelectrical transduction (MET) process. Tip links are formed by two members of the cadherin superfamily: protocadherin 15 (Pcdh15) and cadherin 23 (Cdh23). These two proteins interact to form an asymmetric complex and are both present as homodimers. Pcdh15 is located in the lower part of the tip link and Cdh23 is in the upper part (▶ Fig. 5.2).

The lower end of the tip-link is anchored in the stereociliary membrane at the lower tip-link density (LTLD) of the stereocilia, whereas the upper end is inserted in the upper tip-link density (UTLD) of the nearest taller stereocilium.[29] The tip links are oriented along the functional axis of the hair bundle. Mutations in the genes for these proteins lead to Usher syndrome type 1 as well as to nonsyndromic hearing loss in humans.[30–32] The other stereocilia links are not directly involved in the MET process but are supposed to help transmit force across the hair bundle or maintain the integrity of the structure. The lateral links are mainly composed of Cdh23[33] and Pcdh15,[34] whereas the main component of the shaft connectors is PTPRQ.[22] Finally, VLGR1 and Usherin form the ankle links (▶ Fig. 5.1 and ▶ Fig. 5.2).[35,36]

Other proteins, such as Whirlin, Espin, Myo3a, Myo7a, and Myo15, also have been shown to be essential for the development and maintenance of the hair bundle. Mutations of these genes cause deafness in humans, and defects in the hair bundle morphology, particularly the regulation of stereocilia growth, have been described in mice mutants for these genes. In addition to these proteins, three newly identified stereocilia

Table 5.1 Overview of the Genes That Are Frequently Associated with Inherited Hearing Loss

Gene	Protein	Function	Locus Name	Deafness
CDH23	Cadherin 23	Stereocilia organization and hair bundle formation	DFNB12	Progressive prelingual
CLDN14	Claudin 14	Component of tight junction	DFNB29	Profound congenital
COCH	Cochlin	Extracellular matrix	DFNBA9	Progressive
COL11A2	Collagen 12	Component of the tectorial membrane	DFNA13 DFNB53	Progressive
CX26 or GJB2	Connexin 26	Flow of potassiun	DFNB1 DFNA3	Nonprogressive prelingual
CX30 or GJB6	Connexin 30	Flow of potassiun	DFNB1, DFNA3	Nonprogressive prelingual
CX31 or GJB3	Connexin 31	Flow of potassiun	DFNA2i	Progressive
DIAPH1	Diaphanous	Cell polarization and cytokenesis	DFNA1	Progressive postlingual
ESPN	Espin	Microfilament binding protein	DFNB36, DFNAi	Profound sensorineural
EYA4	Eyes absent 4	Transcriptional activator	DFNA10	Progressive postlingual
KCNQ4	Potassium channels	Outflow of potassium	DFNA2	Progressive
MARVELD2	Tricellulin	Component of tight junction	DFNB49	Profound congenital
miR96			DFNA50	Progressive postlingual
MYO15	Myosin XV	Unconventional myosin, intracellular movement	DFNB3	Profound congenital
MYO3A	Myosin IIIa	Unconventional myosin, intracellular movement	DFNB30	Progressive
MYO6	Myosin VI	Unconventional myosin, intracellular movement	DFNA22, DFNB37	Progressive postlingual
MYO7A	Myosin VIIa	Unconventional myosin, intracellular movement	DFNB2 DFNA11	Moderate
OTOA	Otoancorin	Noncollagenous glycoprotein, unique to inner ear	DFNB22	Moderate to severe prelingual
OTOF	Otoferlin	Vesicle membrane fusion	DFNB9	Profound prelingual
PCDH15	Protocadherin-15	Morphogenesis and cohesion of stereocilia bundles	DFNB23	Prelingual
PJVK	Pejvakin	Activity of auditory pathway neurons	DFNB59	Profound prelingual
POU3F4	Transcription factor POU3F4	Potassium ion homeostasis	DFNX2	Profound sensorineural
POU4F3	Transcription factor POU4F3	Maturation and survival of supporting cells	DFNA15	Progressive
PTPRQ	Protein tyrosine phosphatase receptor type Q	Stereociliar membrane protein involved in inter-stereocilia link	DFNB84	Moderate to severe prelingual
SLC17A8	Vglut3	Glutamate vesicle transporter	DFNA25	Progressive sensorineural
SLC26A4	Pendrin	Anion transporter	DFNB4	Progressive congenital
SLC26A5	Prestin	Motor protein involved in electromotility	DFNB61	Moderate to severe
STRC	Stereocilin	Associated with stereocilia	DFNB16	Nonprogressive
TECTA	Alpha-tectorin	Component of the tectorial membrane	DFNA8/12 DFNB21	Nonprogressive prelingual
TMC1	Transmembrane cochlear 1	Suspected to be the mechanoelectrical transduction (MET) channel	DFNB7/11 DFNA36	Profound prelingual, progressive postlingual
TPRN	Taperin	Unknown	DFNB79	Prelingual, severe to profound sensorineural
TRIOBP	Trio- and f-actin-binding protein	Controlling actin cytoskeleton organization, cell motility, and cell growth	DFNB28	Profound prelingual
USH1C	Harmonin	Part of a transmembrane complex that connects stereocilia into a bundle	DFNB18	Severe prelingual
WHRN	Whirlin	Organization and stabilization of stereocilia elongation and actin cystoskeletal assembly	DFNB31	Profound prelingual

proteins—twinfilin2,[37] gelsolin,[38] and Eps8[39,40]—seem to control actin elongation in the stereocilia via their actin capping or bundling activity.

The structure, integrity, and stability of the hair bundle are critical features for the successful transduction of stimuli. Nonetheless, the orientation of the hair bundle is equally important. The hair bundle deflection toward the tallest row of stereocilia can lead to maximal opening of the MET channels. The mechanisms responsible for this polarity of the hair bundle are not fully understood, though planar cell polarity genes are strong candidates, given that mice with mutations in these genes show defects in hair bundle orientation.[41,42] The kinocilium also appears to be involved in the establishment of polarity of the hair bundle; Mice carrying mutations in genes involved in kinocilium development have misoriented bundles and are linked to ciliopathies (Bardet-Biedl syndrome,[43] Ift88[44]). Finally, Usher genes have also been identified as components of the polarization process of the hair bundle.[45,46]

5.4 Mechanotransduction

Auditory and vestibular stimuli are transduced by the mechanoreceptors of the inner ear. Mechanical stimuli are converted by the mechanoreceptors into an electrochemical signal that is then transmitted to the brain through a nerve impulse: this phenomenon is termed mechanoelectrical transduction (MET). After receiving auditory stimuli, the tympanic membrane vibrates and creates a pressure wave in the perilymph. This wave vibrates the basilar membrane and creates a shearing motion in the tectorial membrane. The tips of the tallest row of stereocilia are embedded in the tectorial membrane, whereas the base of a hair cell sits on top of the basilar membrane. Therefore, the vibration due to auditory stimuli causes the deflection, or movement, of the hair bundle. It is at the hair bundle, due to its deflection, where MET occurs. In the vestibular system, stimuli create a displacement of acellular structures, which overlay the hair cells and thus provoke deflection. This deflection is called excitatory when the hair bundle is deflected in the direction of tallest row of stereocilia. The transduction channels then open, allowing cations (mostly K^+ but also Ca^{2+}) to enter the cell, thereby depolarizing the cell. An inhibitory deflection (toward the shortest row of stereocilia) closes the transduction channels, and the hair cells become hyperpolarized. The release of neurotransmitters from synapses at the basolateral surfaces of hair cells increases (excitatory) or decreases (inhibitory) according to these variations of membrane potential. The transduction channel is thought to be opened by "gating springs," elastic elements in the hair bundle that are coupled to the MET channel. Gating springs stretch when a positive deflection occurs. The release of this tension then causes the channel to close. Tip links are the suspected molecular identities for gating springs, due to their orientation and position.[47] However, evidence does not currently exist to support this theory.

5.4.1 Transduction Channels

By studying the flow and entry sites of Ca^{2+} with high-resolution imaging, following the deflection of the hair bundle, the MET channel has been localized in hair cells to the lower tip-link end, at the tips of all but the tallest stereocilia.[48] In zebrafish, TRPN1 has been identified as the primary molecule of the transduction channel.[49] In mammals, however, molecules of the transduction channel remain unknown, though recently, TMC1, TMC2, TRPC3, and TRPC6 were proposed to be part of the mechanotransduction complex.[50,51] Clear identification of these molecules is particularly difficult, as the transduction channel has few properties that distinguish it from other channels. It has a large single-channel conductance of approximately 100 pS and a rapid activation (on the order of microseconds). It is permeable to cations, without any selectivity, and larger molecules. Several pharmaceutical reagents are known to block the transduction channels, but a selective and high-affinity antagonist has not been identified.

5.4.2 Adaptation by Hair Cells

To maintain their sensitivity to stimulation, hair cells have two different forms of adaptation: fast and slow. After stimulation, the fast adaptation leads to a rapid reclosure of the channel through the binding of Ca^{2+} to the MET channel or to elements near the MET channel. Slow adaptation is thought to be mediated by a cluster of myosin motor proteins, located at the tip-link ends, near the stereocilia tips. At rest, the cluster generates a tension in the gating springs to maintain sensitivity of the MET channel. During deflection, tension in the gating springs increases. The myosin motor proteins travel down the stereocilium, leading to a decrease of the tension that closes the channel. The hair cell is again at rest, but the tension is too low and as a result the motor cluster climbs up the stereocilium to reestablish the resting tension in the spring gates. Myosin 1C, an unconventional myosin, is a strong candidate to be the actin-based motor that takes part in the adaptation of the MET channel and the maintenance of a resting tension in the hair bundle.[52] Mutations of myosin 1C affect the adaption process and have been shown to be involved in deafness.[53,54]

5.4.3 Regulation of the Mechanotransduction Process

Proteins associated with tip links have been shown to regulate the MET. Cadherin23 and Pcdh15 are of particular interest as they are the two major components of the tip link itself. Few proteins are known to interact with the tip-link proteins; these include harmonin and myosin VIIa. Present at the upper end of the tip link,[55] harmonin is related to MET channel function and the process of slow adaptation. Myosin VIIa has been shown to impact the resting tension of the tip links[56] and is localized in the UTLD. This protein interacts with harmonin and sans, which are known scaffolding proteins also found in this region[57] (▸ Fig. 5.2).

Furthermore, the mechanical stimulation of hair cells relies on the integrity of the extracellular matrix surrounding the basilar membrane and the tectorial membrane. Temporal and spatial dysregulation of protein expression (α-tectorin, collagen type XI-α2, cochlin, otoancorin, otogelin, and stereocilin) in this matrix leads to various types of hearing impairment (reviewed elsewhere[58]).

5.4.4 Neuronal Transmission Mediated by the OHCs and IHCs

After auditory or vestibular stimulation, the OHCs and IHCs have two distinct roles in neurotransmission of the stimuli. The OHCs are responsible for the local amplification of the auditory stimuli, whereas the IHCs respond to the amplified stimulus and elicit action potentials in the afferent neural fibers that carry the signal to the brain. The cochlea is able to analyze and transduce complex sounds according to a spatial distribution of the frequencies of those sounds along the coil of the organ of Corti (high frequencies at the basal end and low frequencies at the apex), which is referred to as the toponic principle. According to this principle, sound causes the basilar membrane to vibrate, and the amplitude will be maximal at a specific location of the organ of Corti. The change in membrane voltage of the OHCs, due to the hair bundle deflection, leads to a phenomenon termed "electromotility." The lateral walls of the OHCs undergo a contraction/extension cycle that increases the length of the cells, enhancing the vibration of the basilar membrane. Prestin and spectrin, present at the membrane level of the OHCs, have been identified as main proteins participating in the elongation of the cells and thereby enhance the discrimination of frequencies.[59,60] However, whether this dynamic mechanism of amplification is the result of OHC electromotility itself, active movements of the hair bundle,[61] or both, is still undetermined. In addition to their amplifier role, the OHCs also create distortions of the original signal that we can hear, and they generate a suppressive masking effect to weaken competing signals by increasing the contrast between tones. Stereocilin, a protein of the top connectors of the stereocilia, plays a crucial role in these two latter aspects, suggesting that the integrity of the hair bundle is critical for sound.[62]

Unlike the OHCs, the basilar membrane located under the IHCs does not vibrate. After deflection of the hair bundle, depolarization of the membrane leads to a release of neurotransmitters at the basal pole of the IHCs—the synaptic ribbon. This exocytosis of glutamate is triggered by the Ca^{2+} entry in the IHCs. In contrast to conventional synapses, IHC stimulation induces a finely graded depolarization of the plasma membrane and a graded release of neurotransmitters. This gradation allows the IHCs to respond according to the intensity of stimulation. The IHCs lack proteins usually present in conventional synapses and even in photoreceptors synapses (synaptophysin, synapsin, and SNARE proteins). They express a specific ribbon synapse protein RIBEYE[63] but also Otoferlin (reviewed elsewhere[64]) and Vglut3,[65,66] two proteins associated with auditory neuropathies. Pejvakin[67,68] and diaphanous-3[69] have been recently linked to auditory neuropathy too, although their roles are still unclear. Despite a great improvement of the understanding of the neuronal transmission recently, much remains to be uncovered.

5.5 Fluid Homeostasis of the Inner Ear

The membranous labyrinth of the inner ear is surrounded by a fluid termed endolymph, whereas the perilymph is the fluid located between the outer wall of the membranous labyrinth and the wall of the bony labyrinth (▶ Fig. 5.2a). Mechanoelectrical transduction of a signal, as described above, is based on the transduction of the auditory/vestibular stimuli from the middle ear to the inner ear, through these fluids. Stimuli travel through the perilymph and create endolymph waves. Fluid waves (auditory stimulus) or angular acceleration (vestibular stimulus) of the endolymph stimulates hair cells, which leads to the MET process. The homeostasis of the fluids in these two compartments (endolymph and perilymph), therefore, is crucial for sound transduction. Both fluids have unique ionic compositions that directly relate to their activities in the MET process.

To preserve the K^+-rich profile of endolymph and Na^+-rich profile of perilymph, the integrity of the epithelia encasing these compartments is crucial. Tight junction proteins, embedded in the plasma membrane, prevent any molecular leakage by strengthening the contacts between neighboring cells. The claudin family of proteins (in particular Cldn14,[70] Cldn11, and Cldn9[71–73]), the tight junction proteins (TJP/ZO), and Tricellulin[74] are of particular interest because we know that mutations in these genes are associated with deafness. Connexins are the structural components of the gap junctions, which allow the flow of proteins and ions between cells, and more particularly, ions between hair cells. Mutations of Connexin-26, -30, and -31, the main connexins expressed in the cochlea, also lead to deafness.[75]

The transduction of a signal depends also on ionic gradients and the opening of Ca^{2+} and K^+ channels. The high K^+ gradient in the endolymph is generated by the epithelium of the stria vascularis, in the lateral wall of the scala media. After stimulation, K^+ enters the hair cells and is then released into the perilymph. The genes participating in the secretion and recycling of K^+ (e.g., *KCNQ1*, *KCNE1*, *KCNQ4*, *KCNJ10* and *SLC12A2*, *KCC3*, *KCC4*) encode potassium channels and potassium transporters that are crucial for proper sound transduction (see ▶ Fig. 5.2b–d).[76]

Similarly, even if Ca^{2+} contributes only to 0.2% of the ionic current during stimulation, a functional inner ear must maintain a proper Ca^{2+} balance in the endolymph. Recently, some studies have shown that PMCA2 is implicated in deafness through its role in ejection of Ca^{2+} from the stereocilia back into the endolymph after MET stimulation.[77,78] Calcium-binding proteins, therefore, also play an important role by buffering cytoplasmic calcium. In addition to Calbindin-D28k, Calretinin, Parvalbumin-α, and Parvalbumin-β, the four well-known buffering proteins, CIB2 and CABP2 have been described recently as new buffering proteins in the inner ear.[79,80] These two proteins also have been associated with deafness. Mutations in *Pendrin*, a solute carrier transporter gene, leading to hearing loss further validate the need to maintain proper electrolyte levels.[81] Finally, it has been shown that 11 members of the aquaporin family (water channel, AQ1 to AQ11) are expressed in the mammalian inner ear. Their functions in water transport and their localization in the inner ear suggest a fluid regulation role in the hearing process.[82] Their potential role in Ménière's disease is still under investigation.

5.6 Clinical Perspectives

The main cause of hearing loss and balance disorders is the degeneration of hair cells, which can result from many different factors. Electronic devices, such as hearing aids or cochlear implants, help restore hearing loss and allow patients to develop significant hearing and communicative skills. However, the benefits of this technology to patients are limited as the success of electronic devices depends on multiple factors and varies from one patient to another. Moreover, there is no device that is capable of recovering vestibular function. In the 1980s, the discovery of the regenerative ability of avian hair cells gave hope to scientists and clinicians that similar outcomes could be possible in humans as well.[83,84] Research is currently focused on the molecular pathways involved in the development of the mammalian inner ear, with the hope of finding genes that will induce regeneration of hair cells. Based on our knowledge of these pathways, gene therapy centered around virus-mediated delivery of Atoh1 into the inner ear has been developed.[85,86] Numerous studies have shown that Atoh1 is able to promote, in specific conditions, regeneration of hair cells in avian populations[87] as well as in mammals.[88] However, further studies are needed as Atoh1 can itself induce profound hearing loss with the development of supernumerary cells. Moreover, this technique is limited because it does not permit delivery of the virus along the entire cochlea duct.

Another approach is drug delivery, for the modulation of specific genes in the cell-signaling pathways. In this way, if active compounds are found that affect or control cell cycles, these can be injected into the inner ear, thus potentially leading to the generation of new hair cells, or proactively fighting against the degeneration of existing hair cells. A critical, current limitation of drug delivery, however, is that drug therapies cannot access the whole cochlear duct.

Stem cell–based therapies have been another focus of attention in the recent years. The primary challenge for researchers is overcoming the obstacles to utilization of exogenously derived stem cells. Two possible approaches are being considered and tested: (1) finding signaling pathways that are able to reactivate stem cell skills, and (2) the local delivery of autologous stem cells.

5.7 Conclusion

Studies conducted in the last few decades have tremendously increased our knowledge of the development and functions of the inner ear. A better understanding of the genes and molecular pathways involved in the inner ear has allowed scientists to develop therapeutic strategies for dealing with hearing loss, deafness, and balance impairments. More understanding and information is need, however, to fill the gaps in our knowledge. In time, with continued study into the genetics and molecular pathways of the inner ear, we have every reason to believe that real and efficacious treatments will be developed, allowing clinicians to restore or even prevent hearing loss and balance impairments in humans altogether.

References

[1] Noramly S, Grainger RM. Determination of the embryonic inner ear. J Neurobiol 2002; 53: 100–128

[2] Solomon KS, Fritz A. Concerted action of two dlx paralogs in sensory placode formation. Development 2002; 129: 3127–3136

[3] Huh SH, Jones J, Warchol ME, Ornitz DM. Differentiation of the lateral compartment of the cochlea requires a temporally restricted FGF20 signal. PLoS Biol 2012; 10: e1001231

[4] Weston MD, Pierce ML, Rocha-Sanchez S, Beisel KW, Soukup GA. MicroRNA gene expression in the mouse inner ear. Brain Res 2006; 1111: 95–104

[5] Friedman LM, Dror AA, Mor E et al. MicroRNAs are essential for development and function of inner ear hair cells in vertebrates. Proc Natl Acad Sci U S A 2009; 106: 7915–7920

[6] Mencía A, Modamio-Høybjør S, Redshaw N et al. Mutations in the seed region of human miR-96 are responsible for nonsyndromic progressive hearing loss. Nat Genet 2009; 41: 609–613

[7] Soldà G, Robusto M, Primignani P et al. A novel mutation within the MIR96 gene causes non-syndromic inherited hearing loss in an Italian family by altering pre-miRNA processing. Hum Mol Genet 2012; 21: 577–585

[8] Lewis MA, Quint E, Glazier AM et al. An ENU-induced mutation of miR-96 associated with progressive hearing loss in mice. Nat Genet 2009; 41: 614–618

[9] Sacheli R, Nguyen L, Borgs L et al. Expression patterns of miR-96, miR-182 and miR-183 in the development inner ear. Gene Expr Patterns 2009; 9: 364–370

[10] Weston MD, Pierce ML, Jensen-Smith HC et al. MicroRNA-183 family expression in hair cell development and requirement of microRNAs for hair cell maintenance and survival. Dev Dyn 2011; 240: 808–819

[11] Rudnicki A, Avraham KB. microRNAs: the art of silencing in the ear. EMBO Mol Med 2012; 4: 849–859

[12] Zine A, Romand R. Development of the auditory receptors of the rat: a SEM study. Brain Res 1996; 721: 49–58

[13] Zheng L, Sekerková G, Vranich K, Tilney LG, Mugnaini E, Bartles JR. The deaf jerker mouse has a mutation in the gene encoding the espin actin-bundling proteins of hair cell stereocilia and lacks espins. Cell 2000; 102: 377–385

[14] Li H, Liu H, Balt S, Mann S, Corrales CE, Heller S. Correlation of expression of the actin filament-bundling protein espin with stereociliary bundle formation in the developing inner ear. J Comp Neurol 2004; 468: 125–134

[15] Daudet N, Lebart MC. Transient expression of the t-isoform of plastins/fimbrin in the stereocilia of developing auditory hair cells. Cell Motil Cytoskeleton 2002; 53: 326–336

[16] Sekerková G, Zheng L, Mugnaini E, Bartles JR. Differential expression of espin isoforms during epithelial morphogenesis, stereociliogenesis and postnatal maturation in the developing inner ear. Dev Biol 2006; 291: 83–95

[17] Sekerková G, Richter CP, Bartles JR. Roles of the espin actin-bundling proteins in the morphogenesis and stabilization of hair cell stereocilia revealed in CBA/CaJ congenic jerker mice. PLoS Genet 2011; 7: e1002032

[18] Schneider ME, Belyantseva IA, Azevedo RB, Kachar B. Rapid renewal of auditory hair bundles. Nature 2002; 418: 837–838

[19] Rzadzinska AK, Schneider ME, Davies C, Riordan GP, Kachar B. An actin molecular treadmill and myosins maintain stereocilia functional architecture and self-renewal. J Cell Biol 2004; 164: 887–897

[20] Zhang DS, Piazza V, Perrin BJ et al. Multi-isotope imaging mass spectrometry reveals slow protein turnover in hair-cell stereocilia. Nature 2012; 481: 520–524

[21] Hasson T, Gillespie PG, Garcia JA et al. Unconventional myosins in inner-ear sensory epithelia. J Cell Biol 1997; 137: 1287–1307

[22] Goodyear RJ, Legan PK, Wright MB et al. A receptor-like inositol lipid phosphatase is required for the maturation of developing cochlear hair bundles. J Neurosci 2003; 23: 9208–9219

[23] Sakaguchi H, Tokita J, Naoz M, Bowen-Pope D, Gov NS, Kachar B. Dynamic compartmentalization of protein tyrosine phosphatase receptor Q at the proximal end of stereocilia: implication of myosin VI-based transport. Cell Motil Cytoskeleton 2008; 65: 528–538

[24] Rehman AU, Morell RJ, Belyantseva IA et al. Targeted capture and next-generation sequencing identifies C9orf75, encoding taperin, as the mutated gene in nonsyndromic deafness DFNB79. Am J Hum Genet 2010; 86: 378–388

[25] Furness DN, Katori Y, Nirmal Kumar B, Hackney CM. The dimensions and structural attachments of tip links in mammalian cochlear hair cells and the effects of exposure to different levels of extracellular calcium. Neuroscience 2008; 154: 10–21

[26] Riazuddin S, Khan SN, Ahmed ZM et al. Mutations in TRIOBP, which encodes a putative cytoskeletal-organizing protein, are associated with nonsyndromic recessive deafness. Am J Hum Genet 2006; 78: 137–143

[27] Shahin H, Walsh T, Sobe T et al. Mutations in a novel isoform of TRIOBP that encodes a filamentous-actin binding protein are responsible for DFNB28 recessive nonsyndromic hearing loss. Am J Hum Genet 2006; 78: 144–152

[28] Kitajiri S, Sakamoto T, Belyantseva IA et al. Actin-bundling protein TRIOBP forms resilient rootlets of hair cell stereocilia essential for hearing. Cell 2010; 141: 786–798

[29] Furness DN, Hackney CM. Cross-links between stereocilia in the guinea pig cochlea. Hear Res 1985; 18: 177–188

[30] Alagramam KN, Murcia CL, Kwon HY, Pawlowski KS, Wright CG, Woychik RP. The mouse Ames waltzer hearing-loss mutant is caused by mutation of Pcdh15, a novel protocadherin gene. Nat Genet 2001; 27: 99–102

[31] Di Palma F, Holme RH, Bryda EC et al. Mutations in Cdh23, encoding a new type of cadherin, cause stereocilia disorganization in waltzer, the mouse model for Usher syndrome type 1D. Nat Genet 2001; 27: 103–107

[32] Wilson SM, Householder DB, Coppola V et al. Mutations in Cdh23 cause non-syndromic hearing loss in waltzer mice. Genomics 2001; 74: 228–233

[33] Michel V, Goodyear RJ, Weil D et al. Cadherin 23 is a component of the transient lateral links in the developing hair bundles of cochlear sensory cells. Dev Biol 2005; 280: 281–294

[34] Ahmed ZM, Goodyear R, Riazuddin S et al. The tip-link antigen, a protein associated with the transduction complex of sensory hair cells, is protocadherin-15. J Neurosci 2006; 26: 7022–7034

[35] McGee J, Goodyear RJ, McMillan DR et al. The very large G-protein-coupled receptor VLGR1: a component of the ankle link complex required for the normal development of auditory hair bundles. J Neurosci 2006; 26: 6543–6553

[36] Adato A, Lefèvre G, Delprat B et al. Usherin, the defective protein in Usher syndrome type IIA, is likely to be a component of interstereocilia ankle links in the inner ear sensory cells. Hum Mol Genet 2005; 14: 3921–3932

[37] Peng AW, Belyantseva IA, Hsu PD, Friedman TB, Heller S. Twinfilin 2 regulates actin filament lengths in cochlear stereocilia. J Neurosci 2009; 29: 15083–15088

[38] Mburu P, Romero MR, Hilton H et al. Gelsolin plays a role in the actin polymerization complex of hair cell stereocilia. PLoS ONE 2010; 5: e11627

[39] Manor U, Disanza A, Grati M et al. Regulation of stereocilia length by myosin XVa and whirlin depends on the actin-regulatory protein Eps8. Curr Biol 2011; 21: 167–172

[40] Zampini V, Rüttiger L, Johnson SL et al. Eps8 regulates hair bundle length and functional maturation of mammalian auditory hair cells. PLoS Biol 2011; 9: e1001048

[41] Rida PC, Chen P. Line up and listen: Planar cell polarity regulation in the mammalian inner ear. Semin Cell Dev Biol 2009; 20: 978–985

[42] Wansleeben C, Meijlink F. The planar cell polarity pathway in vertebrate development. Dev Dyn 2011; 240: 616–626

[43] Ross AJ, May-Simera H, Eichers ER et al. Disruption of Bardet-Biedl syndrome ciliary proteins perturbs planar cell polarity in vertebrates. Nat Genet 2005; 37: 1135–1140

[44] Jones C, Roper VC, Foucher I et al. Ciliary proteins link basal body polarization to planar cell polarity regulation. Nat Genet 2008; 40: 69–77

[45] Lefèvre G, Michel V, Weil D et al. A core cochlear phenotype in USH1 mouse mutants implicates fibrous links of the hair bundle in its cohesion, orientation and differential growth. Development 2008; 135: 1427–1437

[46] Webb SW, Grillet N, Andrade LR et al. Regulation of PCDH15 function in mechanosensory hair cells by alternative splicing of the cytoplasmic domain. Development 2011; 138: 1607–1617

[47] Pickles JO, Comis SD, Osborne MP. Cross-links between stereocilia in the guinea pig organ of Corti, and their possible relation to sensory transduction. Hear Res 1984; 15: 103–112

[48] Beurg M, Fettiplace R, Nam JH, Ricci AJ. Localization of inner hair cell mechanotransducer channels using high-speed calcium imaging. Nat Neurosci 2009; 12: 553–558

[49] Sidi S, Friedrich RW, Nicolson T. NompC TRP channel required for vertebrate sensory hair cell mechanotransduction. Science 2003; 301: 96–99

[50] Kawashima Y, Géléoc GS, Kurima K et al. Mechanotransduction in mouse inner ear hair cells requires transmembrane channel-like genes. J Clin Invest 2011; 121: 4796–4809

[51] Quick K, Zhao J, Eijkelkamp N et al. TRPC3 and TRPC6 are essential for normal mechanotransduction in subsets of sensory neurons and cochlear hair cells. Open Biol 2012; 2: 120068

[52] Holt JR, Gillespie SK, Provance DW et al. A chemical-genetic strategy implicates myosin-1c in adaptation by hair cells. Cell 2002; 108: 371–381

[53] Zadro C, Alemanno MS, Bellacchio E et al. Are MYO1C and MYO1F associated with hearing loss? Biochim Biophys Acta 2009; 1792: 27–32

[54] Adamek N, Geeves MA, Coluccio LM. Myo1c mutations associated with hearing loss cause defects in the interaction with nucleotide and actin. Cell Mol Life Sci 2011; 68: 139–150

[55] Grillet N, Xiong W, Reynolds A et al. Harmonin mutations cause mechanotransduction defects in cochlear hair cells. Neuron 2009; 62: 375–387

[56] Kros CJ, Marcotti W, van Netten SM et al. Reduced climbing and increased slipping adaptation in cochlear hair cells of mice with Myo7a mutations. Nat Neurosci 2002; 5: 41–47

[57] Grati M, Kachar B. Myosin VIIa and sans localization at stereocilia upper tip-link density implicates these Usher syndrome proteins in mechanotransduction. Proc Natl Acad Sci U S A 2011; 108: 11476–11481

[58] Richardson GP, Lukashkin AN, Russell IJ. The tectorial membrane: one slice of a complex cochlear sandwich. Curr Opin Otolaryngol Head Neck Surg 2008; 16: 458–464

[59] Zheng J, Shen W, He DZ, Long KB, Madison LD, Dallos P. Prestin is the motor protein of cochlear outer hair cells. Nature 2000; 405: 149–155

[60] Legendre K, Safieddine S, Küssel-Andermann P, Petit C, El-Amraoui A. alphaII-betaV spectrin bridges the plasma membrane and cortical lattice in the lateral wall of the auditory outer hair cells. J Cell Sci 2008; 121: 3347–3356

[61] Fettiplace R. Active hair bundle movements in auditory hair cells. J Physiol 2006; 576: 29–36

[62] Verpy E, Leibovici M, Michalski N et al. Stereocilin connects outer hair cell stereocilia to one another and to the tectorial membrane. J Comp Neurol 2011; 519: 194–210

[63] Uthaiah RC, Hudspeth AJ. Molecular anatomy of the hair cell's ribbon synapse. J Neurosci 2010; 30: 12387–12399

[64] Zak M, Pfister M, Blin N. The otoferlin interactome in neurosensory hair cells: significance for synaptic vesicle release and trans-Golgi network.(Review) Int J Mol Med 2011; 28: 311–314

[65] Seal RP, Akil O, Yi E et al. Sensorineural deafness and seizures in mice lacking vesicular glutamate transporter 3. Neuron 2008; 57: 263–275

[66] Ruel J, Emery S, Nouvian R et al. Impairment of SLC17A8 encoding vesicular glutamate transporter-3, VGLUT3, underlies nonsyndromic deafness DFNA25 and inner hair cell dysfunction in null mice. Am J Hum Genet 2008; 83: 278–292

[67] Delmaghani S, del Castillo FJ, Michel V et al. Mutations in the gene encoding pejvakin, a newly identified protein of the afferent auditory pathway, cause DFNB59 auditory neuropathy. Nat Genet 2006; 38: 770–778

[68] Schwander M, Sczaniecka A, Grillet N et al. A forward genetics screen in mice identifies recessive deafness traits and reveals that pejvakin is essential for outer hair cell function. J Neurosci 2007; 27: 2163–2175

[69] Schoen CJ, Emery SB, Thorne MC et al. Increased activity of Diaphanous homolog 3 (DIAPH3)/diaphanous causes hearing defects in humans with auditory neuropathy and in Drosophila. Proc Natl Acad Sci U S A 2010; 107: 13396–13401

[70] Wilcox ER, Burton QL, Naz S et al. Mutations in the gene encoding tight junction claudin-14 cause autosomal recessive deafness DFNB29. Cell 2001; 104: 165–172

[71] Gow A, Davies C, Southwood CM et al. Deafness in Claudin 11-null mice reveals the critical contribution of basal cell tight junctions to stria vascularis function. J Neurosci 2004; 24: 7051–7062

[72] Kitajiri S, Miyamoto T, Mineharu A et al. Compartmentalization established by claudin-11-based tight junctions in stria vascularis is required for hearing through generation of endocochlear potential. J Cell Sci 2004; 117: 5087–5096

[73] Nakano Y, Kim SH, Kim HM et al. A claudin-9-based ion permeability barrier is essential for hearing. PLoS Genet 2009; 5: e1000610

[74] Riazuddin S, Ahmed ZM, Fanning AS et al. Tricellulin is a tight-junction protein necessary for hearing. Am J Hum Genet 2006; 79: 1040–1051

[75] Nickel R, Forge A. Gap junctions and connexins in the inner ear: their roles in homeostasis and deafness. Curr Opin Otolaryngol Head Neck Surg 2008; 16: 452–457

[76] Zdebik AA, Wangemann P, Jentsch TJ. Potassium ion movement in the inner ear: insights from genetic disease and mouse models. Physiology (Bethesda) 2009; 24: 307–316

[77] Giacomello M, De Mario A, Lopreiato R et al. Mutations in PMCA2 and hereditary deafness: a molecular analysis of the pump defect. Cell Calcium 2011; 50: 569–576

[78] Giacomello M, De Mario A, Primerano S, Brini M, Carafoli E. Hair cells, plasma membrane Ca^{2+} ATPase and deafness. Int J Biochem Cell Biol 2012; 44: 679–683

[79] Riazuddin S, Belyantseva IA, Giese AP et al. Alterations of the CIB2 calcium- and integrin-binding protein cause Usher syndrome type 1J and nonsyndromic deafness DFNB48. Nat Genet 2012; 44: 1265–1271

[80] Schrauwen I, Helfmann S, Inagaki A et al. A mutation in CABP2, expressed in cochlear hair cells, causes autosomal-recessive hearing impairment. Am J Hum Genet 2012; 91: 636–645epub ahead

[81] Wangemann P. The role of pendrin in the development of the murine inner ear. Cell Physiol Biochem 2011; 28: 527–534

[82] Ishiyama G, López IA, Ishiyama A. Aquaporins and Meniere's disease. Curr Opin Otolaryngol Head Neck Surg 2006; 14: 332–336

[83] Corwin JT, Cotanche DA. Regeneration of sensory hair cells after acoustic trauma. Science 1988; 240: 1772–1774

[84] Ryals BM, Rubel EW. Hair cell regeneration after acoustic trauma in adult Coturnix quail. Science 1988; 240: 1774–1776

[85] Albu S, Muresanu DF. Vestibular regeneration—experimental models and clinical implications. J Cell Mol Med 2012; 16: 1970–1977

[86] Di Domenico M, Ricciardi C, Martone T et al. Towards gene therapy for deafness. J Cell Physiol 2011; 226: 2494–2499

[87] Lewis RM, Hume CR, Stone JS. Atoh1 expression and function during auditory hair cell regeneration in post-hatch chickens. Hear Res 2012; 289: 74–85

[88] Kelly MC, Chang Q, Pan A, Lin X, Chen P. Atoh1 directs the formation of sensory mosaics and induces cell proliferation in the postnatal mammalian cochlea in vivo. J Neurosci 2012; 32: 6699–6710

6 Pharmacology of Otologic Drugs

Leonard P. Rybak

6.1 Introduction

The therapy of inner ear diseases has undergone an explosion of publications dealing with the use of new and established drugs. Novel methods of drug delivery to the inner ear have been tested in the past several years. This chapter discusses the pharmacology of several agents used to treat sensorineural hearing loss and vertigo, and offers new perspectives for drug delivery to the inner ear.

6.2 Corticosteroids

6.2.1 Indications

Naturally occurring corticosteroids are used to replace deficient hormone levels in patients with adrenocortical insufficiency. Various synthetic corticosteroids are used for pharmacological effects because of their greater potency, longer duration of action, and superior efficacy in the treatment of disease states. Corticosteroids are used to treat a variety of nonotologic diseases, including disorders of the upper and lower respiratory tract, endocrine diseases, collagen diseases, skin disorders, neoplasms, allergic problems, diseases of the eye and blood-forming organs.[1]

Corticosteroids are employed to treat a variety of otologic diseases, ranging from illnesses affecting the pinna and external auditory canal, such as contact dermatitis and eczema, and as an adjunct in combination with topical antibiotic solutions or powders to treat external otitis. These drugs may also be used in combination with antibiotics topically to treat otitis media in patients with an opening into the middle ear, whether it is a ventilation tube or a spontaneous perforation of the tympanic membrane. They are also frequently used to treat a number of inner ear disorders: sudden sensorineural hearing loss, whether idiopathic or of suspected vascular, traumatic or viral etiology; Ménière disease; autoimmune inner ear disease (AIED); and certain vestibular disorders.

6.2.2 Mechanisms of Action

The glucocorticoids are those corticosteroids that are most commonly utilized to treat ear disease. These drugs are derivatives of the naturally occurring hormones in the adrenal cortex. These compounds affect carbohydrate, lipid, and protein metabolism by combining with their receptors in the tissues affected. Interaction with the receptors causes a change in gene expression within the cells. The resulting effects include immune suppression, membrane stabilization, anti-inflammatory effects with a reduction in tissue edema, sodium transport regulation, and increased perfusion of target tissues.[2] Steroids have been shown to prevent hearing loss in patients with bacterial meningitis by inhibiting the actions of cell adhesion molecules, thereby reducing the inflammatory response to molecules released in response to the bacterial injury, such as the arachidonic acid metabolites.[3,4] Nevertheless, the exact molecular mechanisms by which steroids reverse or prevent hearing loss are not yet known.[2]

New mechanisms for the actions of glucocorticoids have been elucidated recently. These drugs clearly act on diverse targets through multiple mechanisms to control inflammation. The glucocorticoid receptor in humans is located on chromosome 5q31–32. The details of its regulation are discussed in a review article.[1] Glucocorticoids interacting with their receptor initiate a complex regulatory network that blocks several inflammatory pathways. The glucocorticoids can block the production of prostaglandins through three independent mechanisms: the induction and activation of annexin I, the induction of mitogen-activated protein kinase (MAPK) phosphatase 1, and the repression of transcription of cyclo-oxygenase 2. The latter step is accomplished by blocking the transcriptional activity of nuclear factor kappa-B (NF-κB). Glucocorticoids and their receptor also modulate the activity of other transcription factors. These include numerous cytokines and chemokines. The expression of interleukin-1 (IL-1), IL-2, IL-3, IL-4, IL-5, IL-6, IL-9, IL-11, IL-13, IL-16, IL-17, IL-18, tumor necrosis factor-alpha (TNF-α), and granulocyte-macrophage stimulating factor (GM-CSF) can be repressed as well as that of regulated and normal T-cell expressed and secreted (RANTES), macrophage inflammatory protein-1-alpha (MIP-1-alpha), and eotaxin.[5] Organ of Corti explants from rats that were exposed to TNF-α underwent hair cell apoptosis. This was prevented by dexamethasone via activation of phosphatidylinositol (PI$_3$)/Akt and NF-κB upregulation.[6] Thus in certain situations NF-κB can be proapoptotic or antiapoptotic, and the effects of glucocorticoids on this transcription factor may vary depending on the tissue and pathological process taking place.

By a nongenomic mechanism, glucocorticoids activate endothelial nitric oxide synthase, thus protecting against ischemia-reperfusion injury. Glucocorticoids can also decrease inflammation by decreasing the stability of messenger RNA (mRNA) for inflammatory proteins, such as vascular endothelial growth factor and cyclo-oxygenase 2.[1]

Glucocorticoid receptors have been demonstrated in various inner ear tissues in experimental animals (rat and mouse).[7,8] In the human temporal bone, the highest concentration of glucocorticoid receptor protein was found in the spiral ligament by enzyme-linked immunosorbent assay, whereas the lowest concentration of glucocorticoid receptors was measured in the macula of the saccule. The presence of glucocorticoid receptors in the human inner ear tissues implies that glucocorticoids may act directly on select inner ear cells, rather than by a broad-systemic anti-inflammatory or immunosuppressive mechanism in patients with inner ear disorders.[9]

6.2.3 Pharmacokinetics

Corticosteroids, such as dexamethasone, are primarily metabolized in the liver and excreted by the kidneys. The most commonly used systemic glucocorticoids are hydrocortisone, prednisolone, methylprednisolone, prednisone, and dexamethasone. These drugs have good oral bioavailability. Plasma concentrations follow a biexponential pattern. Two compartment models are used after intravenous administration, but one-compartment models are sufficient to describe pharmacokinetics after oral administration. Pharmacokinetic parameters such as the elimination half-life, and pharmacodynamic parameters such as the concentration producing the half-maximal effect, determine the duration and intensity of the effects of the glucocorticoids.[10] Measurable concentrations of steroids are reached in inner ear fluids, but the concentrations are much lower than those achieved following intratympanic administration (see below).

A review of reports on the use of corticosteroids for AIED stated that 4 weeks of high-dose corticosteroids consisting of 60 mg or 1 mg/kg prednisone per day may be required in order to elicit a significant response.[11]

6.2.4 Adverse Reactions

A host of adverse reactions have been reported following systemic administration of corticosteroids. These tend to be more frequent and more severe following chronic administration. Adverse events include increased susceptibility to infection; disturbances in fluid and electrolyte balance (hypokalemia, retention of sodium and water); congestive heart failure and myocardial rupture after recent acute myocardial infarction; muscle weakness and wasting; disturbances in bone metabolism (osteoporosis, aseptic necrosis of the heads of the femur or humerus, compression fractures of the vertebrae); and tendon ruptures.

Endocrine problems found with corticosteroid therapy include suppression of growth in children and secondary lack of responsiveness to stress by the adrenal cortex and pituitary gland, such as trauma, illnesses, and surgery. Carbohydrate intolerance may occur, especially in latent or insulin-dependent diabetics, making them relatively resistant to insulin. Hirsutism or cushingoid changes in body habitus, including "buffalo hump," and cushingoid facies, as well as hypertension, may develop.

Gastrointestinal complications may include nausea, perforation of the bowel, peptic ulcers with hemorrhage and possible perforation, pancreatitis, and ulcers of the esophagus. Ophthalmologic complications include posterior subcapsular cataracts, increased intraocular pressure or glaucoma, and exophthalmos. Neurologic side effects include seizures, increased intracranial pressure, headache, and psychological changes, including severe depression. Skin changes include petechiae, increased fragility of the skin and capillaries, with petechiae and ecchymosis, impairment of wound healing, and diaphoresis. Additional side effects such as thromboembolism, weight gain, increased appetite, and malaise may occur.[1,1,2]

However, a prospective study of a large series of patients with AIED treated with high-dose prednisone was reported with relatively few adverse reactions. Of 116 patients, seven had to stop steroid therapy during the 1-month challenge phase due to adverse events. Five of 34 patients were unable to complete the full 22-week course of prednisone because of adverse reactions. The most common side effects were hyperglycemia and weight gain during the 22-week steroid course. No fractures or osteonecrosis were reported. This study suggests that with appropriate patient selection, monitoring, and patient educa-

tion, high-dose corticosteroids can be relatively safe and effective treatment for AIED.[13]

Although particular concerns are raised in the treatment of children with systemic corticosteroids for AIED, a series of seven children was reported. Six of the seven children had significant hearing improvement after treatment with steroids or cytotoxic medication with no serious side effects.[14]

Systemic corticosteroids raise a particular concern for safety in pregnancy. They are classified as category C drugs by the United States Food and Drug Administration (FDA). Systemic corticosteroids have been associated with the development of oral clefts,[15–17] which appears to be of greatest concern during the first trimester.[18] Most experts believe that systemic corticosteroids can be safely administered during the second and third trimester if necessary.[19] Either prednisone or prednisolone is preferred in these cases, because the fetal liver is unable to convert prednisone to its active metabolite and because the placenta can convert prednisolone to prednisone.[17,20,21]

Systemic corticosteroids have been found to increase the risk of preterm delivery independent of other factors in three large-cohort studies.[22–24] The use of intratympanic injection of corticosteroids in pregnant women with sudden sensorineural hearing loss can be considered as an alternative route for administration of corticosteroids in pregnant patients.[25] The systemic administration of corticosteroids to a pregnant patient may result in fetal adrenal suppression. The child may develop early hypoglycemia and late hyponatremia in the neonatal period and requiring extended corticosteroid replacement therapy.[26]

6.2.5 Drug–Drug Interactions

Corticosteroids have a hyperglycemic effect and may increase the requirement for insulin or oral hypoglycemic drugs. The potassium balance needs to be monitored in patients receiving corticosteroids, especially when these patients are receiving concomitant diuretics, such as thiazides or loop diuretics, or when they are being treated concurrently with amphotericin B. Such combinations can cause potassium depletion.[1] The hypokalemia induced by glucocorticoids may enhance the blockade of nondepolarizing neuromuscular blocking agents, which may lead to increased or prolonged respiratory depression or paralysis, resulting in apnea. Prolonged paralysis with cisatracurium for mechanical ventilation in combination with methylprednisolone resulted in acute motor axonal polyneuropathy manifested as flaccid quadriplegia with absent deep tendon reflexes.[27] Patients receiving digitalis glycosides may be more likely to experience arrhythmias or digitalis toxicity associated with hypokalemia.[28] The natriuretic and diuretic effects of diuretics may be decreased by the sodium- and fluid-retaining effects of corticosteroids.[28]

Corticosteroids given in combination with salicylates can result in increased clearance of salicylates. The efficacy of anticoagulants can be diminished by steroid therapy, and the dosage of the former may need to be adjusted when steroid therapy is initiated or discontinued. The risk of gastrointestinal ulceration or hemorrhage may be increased during concurrent use. The induction of hepatic enzymes by corticosteroids may increase the formation of a hepatoxic acetaminophen metabolite, thereby increasing the risk of hepatotoxicity when they are used concurrently with high-dose or chronic acetaminophen therapy.[28]

The metabolism of corticosteroids is increased by drugs that induce drug metabolizing enzymes in the liver. Such drugs include phenobarbital, phenytoin, and rifampin. If one or more of these drugs is administered concurrently with corticosteroids, the maintenance dose of the latter may need to be increased in order to maintain the desired effect.

The simultaneous use of certain antibiotics, such as troleandomycin or erythromycin, may reduce the clearance of corticosteroids, resulting in an exaggerated steroid activity or cushingoid side effects, and the dose of steroid may need to be reduced.[29]

Large doses of intravenous methylprednisolone can increase the plasma concentrations of cyclosporine in renal transplant patients. This may require that the physician reduce the dose of cyclosporine in the face of glucocorticoid therapy.[30]

Estrogens have a dual effect on the pharmacokinetics of corticosteroids. The former hormones increase the levels of corticosteroid-binding globulin, thus increasing the fraction of bound steroid and rendering it less active. In contrast, the metabolism of corticosteroids is decreased, thus prolonging their half-life. Therefore, when estrogen therapy is begun, a reduction in the dose of glucocorticoids may be in order, and when estrogen therapy is discontinued in patients on concomitant corticosteroid therapy, the dose of the latter may need to be increased.[28]

Tricyclic antidepressants do not relieve, but rather may exacerbate, corticosteroid-induced mental disturbances, and they should not be used to treat these adverse effects.[28]

6.3 Aminoglycoside Antibiotics

6.3.1 Indications

Aminoglycosides are polyanionic amino sugars that have been derived from soil bacteria. They were first developed in 1944 to treat gram-negative bacterial infections, such as those occurring in malignant otitis externa and chronic otitis media. The members of this family of drugs are streptomycin, kanamycin, neomycin, gentamicin, amikacin, tobramycin, and netilmicin. Intramuscular streptomycin has been used for vestibular ablation in patients with bilateral Ménière disease, or Ménière disease in an only hearing ear, or in the second ear that is symptomatic after contralateral ablation.[31]

6.3.2 Mechanisms of Action

The aminoglycosides are bactericidal. They are actively transported across the bacterial cell membrane, irreversibly bind to one or more specific receptor proteins on the 30S subunit of bacterial ribosomes, and interfere with an initiation complex between mRNA and the 30S subunit. DNA may be incorrectly read, and this can lead to the formation of nonfunctional proteins. Polyribosomes are split apart, resulting in the inability to synthesize new proteins. This then accelerates uptake of the antibiotic molecules, disrupting the cytoplasmic membrane of the bacteria, leading to leakage of ions and other substances out of the bacterial cell, which in turn leads to cell death.[32]

The mechanisms of action of aminoglycosides in the treatment of Ménière disease are not entirely clear. They are thought to include ablation of type I hair cells of the crista ampullaris of the semicircular canals and damage to the dark cells of the ampulla.[33]

6.3.3 Pharmacokinetics

Aminoglycosides are poorly absorbed after oral administration. They are well absorbed from intramuscular injection sites. These drugs may be absorbed in significant amounts from certain body surfaces, such as from the peritoneal or pleural cavity, following local irrigation of these body cavities.[32] They are absorbed through the round window membrane to a significant degree (see below).

Aminoglycosides are not significantly metabolized following systemic administration. They are not bound to serum proteins to any great extent (usually less than 10%). They are distributed to all body tissues and accumulate within cells. These drugs achieve high concentrations in highly perfused organs like liver, lungs, and kidneys. Lower concentrations are found in muscle, fat and bone. They are excreted by the kidney, and a high concentration is found in the urine. Distribution half-life after systemic administration is quite short, 5 to 15 minutes. Elimination half-life is 2 to 4 hours in adults with normal renal function, but is significantly longer in neonates and in patients with renal insufficiency. The terminal half-life is greater than 100 hours and this is because of slow release from binding to intracellular sites.[32] Animal studies have shown that aminoglycosides may be detected in inner ear tissues up to a year after systemic administration.[34] To avoid systemic toxicity and to achieve selective vestibular ablation, especially in one ear only, aminoglycosides have been applied intratympanically for Ménière disease (see below).

6.3.4 Adverse Reactions

Hypersensitivity reactions to aminoglycosides occasionally occur, and, when they are documented, cross-sensitivity to other members of this class of drugs must be considered. Hearing loss and nephrotoxicity are risks with any of the aminoglycosides. All aminoglycosides cross the placenta and cause nephrotoxicity or total, irreversible congenital deafness in children born to mothers treated with these drugs during pregnancy. All aminoglycosides have the potential to cause neuromuscular blockade. Very young infants have been reported to experience central nervous system depression, with stupor, flaccidity, coma, or deep respiratory depression. Caution needs to be used in the treatment of elderly patients because of an age-related decrease in renal function and perhaps increased susceptibility to toxicity.[32] Systemic aminoglycosides can cause unintended severe bilateral vestibular loss, resulting in clumsiness, ataxia, and oscillopsia. Toxicity to peripheral nerves can also occur. Optic neuritis has only been reported following streptomycin.

6.3.5 Drug–Drug Interactions

Aminoglycoside antibiotics may interact with other nephrotoxic or ototoxic medications to produce a higher incidence or a greater severity of kidney damage or ototoxic injury.

Neuromuscular blocking agents used in patients receiving aminoglycosides may result in respiratory depression or skeletal muscle weakness after surgery.

6.4 Methotrexate

6.4.1 Indications

Methotrexate is widely used to treat rheumatoid arthritis. Several reports have suggested that methotrexate may be useful for the treatment of AIED. Hearing and balance were improved in patients with AIED and Ménière disease treated with oral methotrexate.[35,36] Although open-label studies demonstrate that this drug may be beneficial in some patients with mild AIED, randomized controlled trials do not support its use.[37,38] Methotrexate has been used to try to maintain hearing improvement after steroid therapy in AIED in order to avoid adverse effects associated with long-term use of systemic corticosteroids. To investigate the efficacy of long-term methotrexate in maintaining hearing improvements achieved with prednisone therapy in patients with AIED, a randomized, double-blind, placebo-controlled study of 67 patients with rapidly progressive, steroid-responsive, bilateral sensorineural hearing loss was conducted at 10 tertiary care centers in the United States. Methotrexate was no more effective than placebo in maintaining the hearing improvement achieved with prednisone treatment.[38]

The efficacy of methotrexate may be enhanced by combining it with etanercept, a TNF-α receptor antagonist. This combination has been used to successfully treat rheumatoid arthritis.[39]

Another option may exist for methotrexate-resistant AIED. A 69-year-old man with sensorineural hearing loss and iritis was diagnosed with atypical Cogan's syndrome. He improved initially after receiving high doses of prednisolone. However, his condition relapsed within 1 year. His illness was resistant to several immunosuppressive drugs, including methotrexate, cyclosporine, azathioprine, and adalimumab. Ultimately he responded to treatment with tocilizumab, a humanized anti–interleukin-6 receptor antibody.[40]

6.4.2 Mechanism of Action

Methotrexate is an antimetabolite that is an analogue of folic acid. In the treatment of cancer, it is specific for the S phase of cell division. Methotrexate inhibits the synthesis of DNA, RNA, thymidylate, and protein by binding irreversibility to the enzyme, dihydrofolate reductase. Rapidly dividing cells, including tumor cells and normal cells in the bone marrow, buccal and intestinal mucosa, cells in the urinary bladder, spermatogonia, and cells in the fetus have their growth inhibited by this drug. In nonmalignant conditions, such as AIED, methotrexate has a mild immunosuppressive action.[28]

6.4.3 Pharmacokinetics

Methotrexate is absorbed by the oral route, but the absorption is highly variable. It is moderately (about 50%) bound to serum proteins. It has only limited penetration of the blood–brain barrier. It is metabolized by the liver where metabolites are retained in the hepatocytes. The half-life for low doses is variable —from 3 to 10 hours. The clearance rates vary a great deal for individuals. Peak concentration after oral administration is 1 to 2 hours; 80 to 90% is absorbed primarily by the kidney as the unchanged molecule within 24 hours. Biliary excretion occurs to a slight extent; only 10% or less of methotrexate administered is eliminated in the bile.

6.4.4 Adverse Reactions

Methotrexate crosses the placenta and is teratogenic. It is also a potent abortifacient. It is potentially carcinogenic. Methotrexate can cause ulcerative stomatitis, gingivitis, and pharyngitis. It is also hepatotoxic. Gastrointestinal ulceration, bleeding, or perforation may occur with methotrexate. Bone marrow suppression from methotrexate may result in thrombocytopenia, with easy bruising and bleeding. Leukopenia may also occur, resulting in bacterial infections or septicemia.

6.4.5 Drug Interactions

Methotrexate may increase the risk of hepatotoxicity when used in combination with alcohol or hepatotoxic medications, such as the sulfonamides. Methotrexate may cause an additive effect on the bone marrow when used in combination with bone marrow–suppressant medications.

Oral neomycin may increase the absorption of methotrexate. Probenecid and weak organic acids such as salicylates may inhibit the renal tubular secretion of methotrexate, resulting in higher blood concentrations. Drugs that are highly protein bound, such as sulfonamides and salicylates, may displace bound methotrexate in the blood, resulting in toxic concentrations of unbound methotrexate.

6.5 Etanercept

6.5.1 Indications

Etanercept is a dimeric fusion protein (decoy receptor) consisting of the extracellular ligand-binding protein of the human 75-kd TNF receptor linked to the Fc portion of the human immunoglobulin IgG1. It is a drug that has been approved for the treatment of rheumatic arthritis in adults and children, and for the treatment of psoriatic arthritis, ankylosing spondylitis, and psoriasis.[41,42] Animal studies suggested that prompt intervention with etanercept reduces inflammation and hearing loss in treated ears.[43] It has been used to treat immune-mediated cochleovestibular disorders.[44] It is administered twice weekly by subcutaneous injection of 25 mg per dose. Recent clinical studies suggest that etanercept therapy does not improve hearing loss in AIED compared with placebo,[45] but may stabilize hearing in patients with pretreatment intractable progressive hearing loss.[44] Vertigo and tinnitus may be improved, however.[44]

6.5.2 Mechanism of Action

Etanercept binds to TNF, acting as a "decoy receptor," thereby blocking the interaction of TNF with cell surface receptors and preventing the proinflammatory effects of this cytokine. Tumor necrosis factor has a pivotal role in inflammation, and its crucial role has been demonstrated in a number of autoimmune diseases.[42]

6.5.3 Pharmacokinetics

A single 25-mg dose of etanercept given subcutaneously (SC) to healthy adults is slowly absorbed from the injection site, reaching a peak concentration at 51 hours. Mean bioavailability was 58% following a single SC dose of 10 mg etanercept. It is assumed that the complex of etanercept with TNF is metabolized through peptide and amino acid pathways, with either recycling of amino acids or elimination in bile and urine. Age, body size, gender, and ethnic origin can have an effect on the pharmacokinetics of etanercept.[42]

6.5.4 Adverse Reactions

Etanercept is generally safe and well tolerated. However, because TNF-α may play a role in the host defense against tuberculosis and other infections, there is a risk of infection with the use of drugs like etanercept. Case reports of tuberculosis in patients treated with etanercept have been reported to the FDA.[46] Fulminant pneumonia with adult respiratory distress syndrome can occur, especially in patients receiving both systemic corticosteroids and etanercept.[47]

6.5.5 Drug–Drug Interactions

Drug interactions of etanercept with warfarin, digoxin, and methotrexate were investigated. To date, no clinically relevant drug–drug interactions between etanercept and other commonly prescribed drugs have been detected.[42]

A positive interaction with methotrexate has been reported in the treatment of rheumatoid arthritis. This positive interaction has been exploited to effectively treat hearing loss from AIED.[39]

6.5.6 Intratympanic Therapy

Over the past one or two decades, intratympanic drug therapy has become an increasingly utilized method to deliver drugs to the inner ear in higher concentrations than can be achieved by systemic administration and in order to circumvent systemic toxicity of these agents. The inner ear is isolated from the rest of the body by the blood–labyrinth barrier.[48] This route of drug treatment has been utilized primarily to deliver corticosteroids or aminoglycosides to the inner ear. Other less frequently used medications applied by this route include antioxidants, growth factors, antiviral agents, diuretics, and volume expanders.[2] The drug selected for treatment may be injected through an intact tympanic membrane, through a ventilation tube, or through a myringotomy incision with endoscopic guidance. Also various wicks and catheters have been devised to deliver the drug directly to the round window membrane of the patient to be treated. A recent paper reported the use of endoscope-assisted intratympanic methylprednisolone injection through a laser myringotomy for refractory sensorineural hearing loss; 13 of 38 patients (34.2%) demonstrated an improvement in hearing levels, with complete recovery of hearing in 21% (eight of 38). This method allows direct visualization of the round window membrane, which may provide more effective delivery of the drug to the round window membrane.[25]

6.5.7 Anatomy of the Round Window

The round window membrane is located in the medial wall of the middle ear within the round window niche. This membrane is partially obscured by the bony promontory. The latter may frequently have mucoperiosteal folds that may tend to obstruct access to the round window membrane. Such folds may be known as "false round window membranes."[49] Studies of adult human temporal bones have found that 21% had false round window membranes and 11% had a plug of fat or fibrous tissue obstructing the round window niche. Only 56% had no obstruction, whereas 22% had bilateral obstruction.[50] In 41 living patients undergoing middle ear endoscopy prior to intratympanic therapy, 29 round windows appeared to be unobstructed, seven were partially obstructed, and five were completely obstructed by adhesions.[51]

The round window membrane is thicker around the edges and thinner in the center. The average thickness of the human round window membrane is about 70 μm, but it is much thinner in rodents, ranging from 10 to 14 μm in thickness, and in cats it varies from 20 to 40 μm in average thickness.[52] It consists of three layers: an epithelial layer facing the middle ear, a core of connective tissue, and an inner epithelial layer facing the inner ear.[49] Animal experiments have shown that the round window membrane acts as a semipermeable membrane, allowing the passage of cationic ferritin, horseradish peroxidase, 1-μm latex spheres, and neomycin-gold spheres.[49]

6.6 Principles of Pharmacokinetics of Intratympanic Drug Therapy

The inner ear is a geometrically complex organ containing spaces (scalae) filled with fluid, and each scala has multiple interfaces with other scalae and with other compartments, including the middle ear space and the systemic blood circulation. The scala tympani and scala vestibule contain perilymph, which has characteristics of extracellular fluid, namely low potassium and high sodium concentrations. The scala media contains endolymph, a fluid high in potassium and a relatively high positive charge. Recent studies have revealed that inner ear fluids do not circulate to any significant degree and are not actively stirred. Therefore, drugs applied locally to the round window membrane enter the ear slowly, mainly by passive diffusion. The rate at which drugs spread depends on the physical properties of the diffusing molecules. Their molecular weight appears to have the greatest influence on their diffusion. Animal experiments suggest that the round window acts as a semipermeable membrane. A major process that determines drug concentration in the inner ear is clearance, which expresses the rate of removal of drugs from the inner ear fluids into the circulation. Large gradients of drug concentration can occur with intratympanic application, resulting in higher levels of drug near the round window, with diminishing concentrations at more apical locations in the inner ear.[53] In order to direct drugs to particular parts of the inner ear, various delivery strategies need to be utilized. If the clinician wishes to target the basal turn of the cochlea or the vestibular system, single intratympanic injections may be effective.[53] Fluid sampling in order to determine the kinetics of locally applied drugs from animal cochleae has specific challenges, as discussed in a recent review.[53]

A variety of drug application systems has been employed, varying from intratympanic injections of fluids, to the use of wicks, catheters, implantable pumps, polymers, and gels in animal and human studies. Based on animal studies, it appears that the application protocol is a major factor that determines the drug level achieved in the inner ear. The time that the drug is present in the middle ear plays a primary role.[53]

The use of a poloxamer hydrogel–based dexamethasone formulation may provide a more effective technique for a prolonged delivery of dexamethasone to the inner ear because it provides a more uniform distribution than do single injections. This method may also obviate the need for multiple injections.[54] A study performed using mice compared two gentamicin delivery systems following intratympanic injection. These two methods resulted in different kinetic curves. The hydrogel-loaded gentamicin provided sustained release during a 7-day period. The intratympanic injection of the gentamicin solution without the hydrogel demonstrated a dramatic decline after achieving a peak concentration in perilymph on the first day. Gentamicin was almost completely eliminated by the third day when applied without the hydrogel. The hydrogel system administration provided significant balance dysfunction without any hearing changes. However, the solution of gentamicin had no effect on inner ear function with the dose of 40 mg. Thus, the hydrogel system appears to provide a more sustained, consistent, and efficient drug release to the inner ear than does a traditional intratympanic gentamicin injection. This method may offer a novel way of treating Ménière disease in patients in the future.[55]

The differences in anatomy between animals and humans make it difficult to extrapolate the results from animal studies to clinical intratympanic therapy.[52]

6.7 Intratympanic Corticosteroid Therapy

6.7.1 Indications

Intratympanic administration of corticosteroids has been used to provide high concentrations of these antiinflammatory drugs to the inner ear tissues. Clinical otologic conditions that have been treated with this technique include sudden sensorineural hearing loss, Ménière disease, and tinnitus.

A high rate of improvement in hearing was recently reported following the administration of intratympanic dexamethasone injected through a perforation created by laser-assisted myringotomy. Nineteen patients studied received dexamethasone intratympanic injection as initial treatment. Eighteen of the 19 patients (95%) demonstrated an improvement of more than 10 dB in the pure-tone audiogram, with a mean improvement of 40 dB. Patients who failed systemic steroid therapy were treated with intratympanic dexamethasone. In this group 14 of 24 patients (58%) improved more than 10 dB, with a mean improvement of 16 dB. Two patients showed complete recovery in

this salvage treatment group. There are at least three requirements that need to be met in order to have success with intratympanic steroid treatment: (1) A secure and reliable delivery method is needed, and it is important to replace the air bubbles around the round window membrane with the drug solution. (2) It may be necessary to provide sequential or continuous administration of the drug to achieve sufficient concentration of the drug in the target areas of the cochlea. (3) The method should be simple and painless.[56]

The combined use of an intratympanic dexamethasone/hyaluronic acid mix with intravenous steroid therapy in patients with severe idiopathic senorineural hearing loss was reported because of the suspected need for more aggressive treatment in the presence of severe hearing loss. The use of systemic steroids alone was utilized in patients with less severe disease. In the group with severe hearing loss, hearing improved to a level comparable to that obtained with intravenous therapy alone.[57]

The results of double-blind, placebo-controlled studies of intratympanic steroid therapy for severe to profound sudden sensorineural hearing loss have yielded somewhat modest results. A multicenter study was conducted in Germany on the safety and efficacy of continuous intratympanic dexamethasone-phosphate for severe to profound sudden idiopathic sensorineural hearing loss or sudden idiopathic anacusis after failure of systemic therapy. The average hearing improvement in the treatment group was 13.9 dB (standard deviation [SD]: 21.3), and in the placebo group it was 5.4 dB (SD: 10.4). This difference in hearing improvement between the two groups (mean: 8.4 dB, SD: 17.0, 95% confidence interval [CI]: −7.1 to 24.1) was statistically not significant ($p = 0.26$). Of the secondary outcome parameters, the largest benefit of local salvage therapy was found for maximum speech discrimination, with an improvement of 24.4% (SD: 32.0) in the treatment group and 4.5% (SD: 7.6) in the placebo group ($p = 0.07$). Perhaps the severity of the cochlear damage in these patients was too severe to ameliorate with intratympanic steroid therapy. However, the authors concluded that the tendency to obtain better hearing improvement in the treatment group, the rather conservative inclusion criteria, the limited placebo-controlled observation period, and the absence of serious adverse events support further investigation of local inner ear drug delivery as a first- or second-line treatment option for idiopathic sudden sensorineural hearing loss.[58]

A prospective, double-blind, placebo-controlled study of 60 patients with idiopathic sudden sensorineural hearing loss who did not respond to an initial round of systemic steroid therapy was performed. The subjects were randomized into an intratympanic steroid group and an intratympanic normal saline injection group, which were matched by age and sex. A total of 55 subjects completed the study. Both groups received four injections within a 2-week period. The response rate and the extent of hearing improvement were significantly greater in the intratympanic steroid group than in the intratympanic saline group. The authors concluded that intratympanic steroid injections are useful as a salvage therapy for patients with idiopathic sudden sensorineural hearing loss who do not respond to initial systemic steroid therapy.[59]

A recent review of the literature sought to determine the efficacy of intratympanic steroid treatment for idiopathic sudden sensorineural hearing loss. The authors found 176 relevant publications, 32 of which were studies of initial or salvage intratympanic steroid injections for sudden hearing loss. These included six randomized trials and only two randomized controlled trials. Although there were few well-executed trials, the overwhelming majority of studies of intratympanic steroids for salvage treatment showed that intratympanic steroid therapy was beneficial. A limited meta-analysis of the higher quality studies revealed a mean difference in improvement of 13.3 dB (95% CI: 7.7–18.9; $p < 0.0001$). The authors believe it is still uncertain whether this difference is clinically significant. In the larger literature, including studies of lesser quality, it was apparent that initial intratympanic therapy was equivalent to systemic steroid treatment for this condition.[60]

In another recent review, the authors searched the Cochrane Ear, Nose, and Throat Disorders Group Trials Register, the Cochrane Central Register of Controlled Trials (CENTRAL), PubMed, EMBASE, CINAHL, Web of Science, BIOSIS Previews, Cambridge Scientific Abstracts, ICTRP, and additional sources for published and unpublished trials through January 2011. The criteria used were randomized controlled trials of intratympanic dexamethasone versus placebo in patients with Ménière disease. A single trial containing 22 patients, with a low risk of bias, was found. This trial involved daily intratympanic injections of dexamethasone for 5 consecutive days. After 24 months, the dexamethasone-treated group showed a statistically and clinically significant improvement in vertigo compared with placebo. This positive result was defined as (1) improvement in functional level American Academy of Otolaryngology–Head and Neck Surgery (AAO-HNS) class; (2) improvement in Dizziness Handicap Inventory scores; and (3) subjective improvement of vertigo. Importantly, no complications were reported. The reviewers concluded that there is limited evidence that intratympanic steroids are effective in controlling vertigo in patients with Ménière disease.[61] Future rigorously controlled studies should confirm or refute these findings. If vertiginous symptoms persist after 6 months of medical treatment, intratympanic dexamethasone may be initiated. Satisfactory control of vertigo was 72% among patients receiving intratympanic dexamethasone.[62]

Intratympanic dexamethasone infusion was performed as a treatment for cochlear tinnitus, and its efficacy was investigated. The overall effective rate for the 1,214 patients with 1,466 affected ears was 71%. Cochlear tinnitus was seen frequently in the age group of 50 to 69 years. The results of the treatment for tinnitus in different age groups did not show a correlation between age and efficacy rate of treatment. The efficacy rate was high for tinnitus accompanying chronic otitis media, Ménière disease, and labyrinth syphilis. The efficacy rate tended to decrease with longer disease duration. The efficacy rate was high in tinnitus of low tone pitch and low in tinnitus with high tone pitch.[63]

6.7.2 Adverse Effects

Intratympanic steroid therapy has been associated with tympanic membrane perforation, chronic otitis media, disequilibrium, and dysgeusia[64] exacerbation of hearing loss (▶ Table 6.1).[2,65]

Table 6.1 Adverse Effects of Intratympanic Corticosteroids

Event	Reference
Tympanic membrane perforation:	
Temporary	Parnes et al, 1999[68]
Slow healing	Silverstein et al, 1996[85]
Chronic	Shulman and Goldstein, 2000[86]
	Doyle et al, 2004[12]
Ear blockage	Shulman and Goldstein, 2000[86]
Increased tinnitus intensity	Shulman and Goldstein, 2000[86]
Otitis media:	
Acute	Doyle et al, 2004[12]
Chronic	Herr and Marzo, 2005[64]
Worsening hearing loss	Arriaga and Goldman, 1998[87]
	Chandrasekhar, 2001[88]
Increased insulin requirement	Doyle et al, 2004[12]
Pain:	
Methylprednisolone	Parnes et al, 1999[68]
Dexamethasone	Barrs et al, 2001[89]
Vertigo (temporary)	Doyle et al, 2004[12]
Disequilibrium	Herr and Marzo, 2005[64]
Dysgeusia	Herr and Marzo, 2005[64]

6.7.3 Pharmacokinetics

Intratympanic dexamethasone administration in animals resulted in greater concentrations in perilymph than those resulting from intravenous injection.[66] The perilymph kinetics of methylprednisolone, dexamethasone, and hydrocortisone were compared in the guinea pig after intratympanic administration. Methylprednisolone reached the highest concentration in both perilymph and endolymph. Concentrations in endolymph were greater than in perilymph. The peak perilymph concentrations were attained within the first hour, and then diminished rapidly. Peak endolymph levels occurred at 1 to 2 hours, followed by a rapid decline. Plontke and Salt[67] used computer simulation to determine the pharmacokinetics of steroids in the inner ear using the data published by Parnes et al[68] and Bachmann et al.[69] From these data, Plontke and Salt determined that the clearance half-time of these corticosteroids was 130 minutes. They calculated that continuous delivery resulted in the highest maximum concentration, and a brief single application gave the lowest maximum concentration. Because of the rapid clearance half-time, it was ascertained that although the method of drug delivery and its concentration determined the absolute concentration at any given place in the scala tympani, it did not alter the relative concentration. A steady state is achieved within hours, and this is not significantly affected by additional drug application.[52,67]

6.7.4 Intratympanic Therapy with Tumor Necrosis Factor-α Blockers

A pilot study of patients with AIED utilized transtympanic delivery of the TNF-α blocker infliximab once weekly for 4 weeks using a Silverstein microwick, which allowed patients to be tapered off steroids and resulted in hearing improvement and reduced relapses. Infliximab appeared to be safe and effective following intratympanic delivery for AIED.[70] However, in a series of eight patients resistant to steroid and immunosuppressive drug therapy, no improvements in objective hearing tests were observed after intratympanic administration of infliximab.[71] These results suggest that infliximab may only be effective in steroid-responsive patients with AIED. Further large-scale studies are needed to determine the role of infliximab in AIED.

6.7.5 Growth Factors

Patients with sudden sensorineural hearing loss who showed no recovery to systemic glucocorticoid administration were recruited to test the safety and efficacy of topical insulin-like growth factor-1 (IGF-1) application using gelatin hydrogels as a treatment for sudden sensorineural hearing loss. This study was single arm, nonrandomized, and open. No placebo applications were administered and no blinding was used. At 12 weeks after the test treatment, 48% (95% CI: 28 to 69%; $p = 0.086$) of the patients showed hearing improvement. At 24 weeks after the test treatment, the proportion of patients showing hearing improvement was 56% (95% CI: 35 to 76%; $p = 0.015$), No serious adverse events were recorded.[72]

6.8 Intratympanic Therapy with Aminoglycosides

6.8.1 Indications

The intratympanic use of aminoglycoside antibiotics, primarily gentamicin, has been primarily focused on the treatment of peripheral vertigo associated with unilateral Ménière disease.

6.8.2 Adverse Effects

A major concern with the intratympanic administration of the ototoxic antibiotic gentamicin is hearing loss. However, a meta-analysis was published of articles reporting clinical trials of patients diagnosed as having definitive Ménière disease according to the 1985 or 1995 criteria of the Committee on Hearing and Equilibrium of the AAO-HNS and receiving gentamicin administered into the middle ear by transtympanic injection or using a specially designed catheter. Toxic effects of intratympanic gentamicin on hearing and word recognition were found to be neither statistically significant nor clinically important. However, it was reported that patients treated with a titration regimen experienced a lesser degree of worsening of hearing and word recognition than those receiving the drug on a fixed-dose regimen (0.02 dB and 0.4% in the former group versus 5.4 dB and 6.5% for the latter group).[73] However, another meta-analysis of intratympanic gentamicin for Ménière disease reported an estimated hearing loss of 25.1% from all studies combined. The weekly method of gentamicin dosing was associated with less hearing loss (13.1%) than the multiple daily dosing methods, which resulted in hearing loss in nearly 35% of patients treated in this manner. Other delivery methods, so-called low-dose, titration or continuous administration, displayed similar rates of hearing loss to the group as a whole.[74] The discrepancies between these two meta-analyses published in 2004 likely represent differences in inclusion criteria between the two studies.

A recent study of 393 patients with Ménière disease reported excellent results for hearing preservation and vertigo control after one or more 3-day treatments utilizing a combination of low-dose streptomycin and high-dose dexamethasone injections into the middle ear. Ninety percent of patients indicated improvement in their quality of life, and 88% reported improvement in their vertigo. Clinically significant hearing loss was reported in 19%.[75]

6.8.3 Pharmacokinetics

Gentamicin kinetics in the chinchilla inner ear varied according to whether the drug was administered by bolus intratympanic injection or by round window microcatheter infusion.[76] After transtympanic injection, a peak concentration of gentamicin was found in perilymph at 24 hours, followed by a decline in concentration that followed first-order kinetics. On the other hand, when the drug was applied by round window microcatheter infusion, a small peak was reached at 4 hours, followed by a slight decline. A higher, sustained peak concentration was measured at 24 hours and persisted for 72 hours. This was followed by a gradual decline in spite of continued infusion of gentamicin.[76] Plontke and colleagues[77] combined the data from studies in the chinchilla to create a computer simulation of gentamicin in the chinchilla and human, and determined that the peak concentration of gentamicin after a single application of a 10-mg/mL solution would occur between 600 to 700 minutes after application, followed by a rapid decline. Using this computer simulation and comparing the relative size of the human and chinchilla inner ear, they calculated that the drug levels in the vestibule would be similar for the chinchilla and human. Because of the greater length of the human cochlea, the concentration of gentamicin at the apex would be two orders of magnitude lower than at the base in humans, as opposed to being 10-fold lower in the chinchilla.[52,77] Comparing different protocols of drug administration using computer simulation, Plontke and colleagues found that continuous delivery of gentamicin resulted in the highest maximum concentration. Middle ear volume stabilization with fibrin glue gave intermediate maximum concentrations, and a single application of gentamicin without volume stabilization in the middle ear resulted in the lowest concentrations in perilymph.[52,77]

From animal studies, it appears that there is great variation in the maximum concentration of gentamicin after single-dose intratympanic administration; however, peak concentrations appear to be achieved in 8 to 24 hours. Elimination from perilymph appears to follow first-order kinetics and may be energy dependent. Continuous administration appears to lead to more predictable and stable concentrations.[52]

6.9 The Future of Intratympanic Therapy

The use of the intratympanic route to administer drugs, such as corticosteroids, is a rational approach to the treatment of diseases that may involve the release of inflammatory cytokines into the inner ear in order to reduce the damage caused by the latter molecules. This approach needs further study to define the ideal pharmacological parameters for steroid delivery.[78] The use of computer simulation of concentration time courses can guide the design of preclinical animal experiments and can help to estimate inner ear drug concentrations prior to designing clinical protocols.[53] The use of carrier substances, such as biopolymers to prolong the time that a drug remains in the middle ear and other methods of inner ear delivery, such as nanotechnology and gene therapy, may provide exciting prospects for improving the therapy of inner ear diseases with intratympanic drug administration. Biodegradable carriers offer a promising method to provide controlled local drug delivery to the inner ear. These materials appear to be effective in providing sustained release of active drug without toxic effects of the carriers.[72,79,80]

Intratympanic drug therapy could be replaced by cochleostomy, which is an invasive procedure with risks to hearing. It could be combined with cochlear implants to preserve residual hearing. Experiments in laboratory animals are being carried out to deliver drugs by cochleostomy using devices that pump drugs into the inner ear without causing cochlear damage.[81]

The application of nanotechnology for delivery of drugs to the cochlea appears to be quite promising. The local application of rhodamine nanoparticles to the round window membrane was more effective in targeted delivery to the guinea pig cochlea than was systemic administration of these nanoparticles. After local application of these nanoparticles, strong fluorescence was found in the scala tympani of the basal and middle turns of the cochlea, with the majority of rhodamine particles localized to the basal turn. The number of rhodamine particles in the cochlea was about 10-fold greater after round window application 10 minutes after application compared with systemic administration.[82] Another study examined the properties of lipid-core nanocapsules, which are 50 nm in size and were shown to penetrate through the round window membrane and to reach all other cell types in the inner ear. Round window delivery in rats resulted in no adverse effects after 28 days. No changes in hearing or cochlear morphology were observed. Lipid-core nanocapsules may provide vectors for delivery of drugs to the inner ear.[83] Future studies should provide additional insights into the feasibility of nanotechnology for clinical applications. Numerous clinical trials are in progress to determine the efficacy of various drugs to prevent acquired sensorineural hearing loss from various causes. These trials could produce some exciting and clinically useful drugs.[84]

References

[1] Rhen T, Cidlowski JA. Antiinflammatory actions of glucocorticoids—new mechanism for old drugs. N Engl J Med 2006; 353: 1711–1723

[2] Seidman MD, Vivek P. Intratympanic treatment of hearing loss with novel and traditional agents. Otolaryngol Clin North Am 2004; 37: 973–990

[3] Kaplan SL. Prevention of hearing loss from meningitis. Lancet 1997; 350: 158–159

[4] Coyle PK. Glucocorticoids in central nervous system bacterial infection. Arch Neurol 1999; 56: 796–801

[5] Grzanka A, Misiołek M, Golusiński W, Jarząb J. Molecular mechanisms of glucocorticoids action: implications for treatment of rhinosinusitis and nasal polyposis. Eur Arch Otorhinolaryngol 2011; 268: 247–253

[6] Haake SM, Dinh CT, Chen S, Eshraghi AA, Van De Water TR. Dexamethasone protects auditory hair cells against TNFalpha-initiated apoptosis via activation of PI3K/Akt and NFkappaB signaling. Hear Res 2009; 255: 22–32

[7] Rarey KE, Curtis LM, ten Cate WJ. Tissue specific levels of glucocorticoid receptor within the rat inner ear. Hear Res 1993; 64: 205–210

[8] Shimazaki T, Ichimiya I, Suzuki M, Mogi G. Localization of glucocorticoid receptors in the murine inner ear. Ann Otol Rhinol Laryngol 2002; 111: 1133–1138

[9] Rarey KE, Curtis LM. Receptors for glucocorticoids in the human inner ear. Otolaryngol Head Neck Surg 1996; 115: 38–41

[10] Czock D, Keller F, Rasche FM, Häussler U. Pharmacokinetics and pharmacodynamics of systemically administered glucocorticoids. Clin Pharmacokinet 2005; 44: 61–98

[11] Buniel MC, Geelan-Hansen K, Weber PC, Tuohy VK. Immunosuppressive therapy for autoimmune inner ear disease. Immunotherapy 2009; 1: 425–434

[12] Doyle KJ, Bauch C, Battista R et al. Intratympanic steroid treatment: a review. Otol Neurotol 2004; 25: 1034–1039

[13] Alexander TH, Weisman MH, Derebery JM et al. Safety of high-dose corticosteroids for the treatment of autoimmune inner ear disease. Otol Neurotol 2009; 30: 443–448

[14] Huang NC, Sataloff RT. Autoimmune inner ear disease in children. Otol Neurotol 2011; 32: 213–216

[15] Schatz M. The efficacy and safety of asthma medications during pregnancy. Semin Perinatol 2001; 25: 145–152

[16] Oren D, Nulman I, Makhija M, Ito S, Koren G. Using corticosteroids during pregnancy. Are topical, inhaled, or systemic agents associated with risk? Can Fam Physician 2004; 50: 1083–1085

[17] Vlastarakos PV, Nikolopoulos TP, Manolopoulos L, Ferekidis E, Kreatsas G. Treating common ear problems in pregnancy: what is safe? Eur Arch Otorhinolaryngol 2008; 265: 139–145

[18] Park-Wyllie L, Mazzotta P, Pastuszak A et al. Birth defects after maternal exposure to corticosteroids: prospective cohort study and meta-analysis of epidemiological studies. Teratology 2000; 62: 385–392

[19] Ambro BT, Scheid SC, Pribitkin EA. Prescribing guidelines for ENT medications during pregnancy. Ear Nose Throat J 2003; 82: 565–568

[20] Guillonneau M, Jacqz-Aigrain E. [Maternal corticotherapy. Pharmacology and effect on the fetus](French) J Gynecol Obstet Biol Reprod (Paris) 1996; 25: 160–167

[21] Lockshin MD, Sammaritano LR. Corticosteroids during pregnancy. Scand J Rheumatol Suppl 1998; 107: 136–138

[22] Bracken MB, Triche EW, Belanger K, Saftlas A, Beckett WS, Leaderer BP. Asthma symptoms, severity, and drug therapy: a prospective study of effects on 2205 pregnancies. Obstet Gynecol 2003; 102: 739–752

[23] Schatz M, Dombrowski MP, Wise R et al. Maternal-Fetal Medicine Units Network, The National Institute of Child Health and Development, National Heart, Lung and Blood Institute. The relationship of asthma medication use to perinatal outcomes. J Allergy Clin Immunol 2004; 113: 1040–1045

[24] Bakhireva LN, Jones KL, Schatz M, Johnson D, Chambers CD Organization Of Teratology Information Services Research Group. Asthma medication use in pregnancy and fetal growth. J Allergy Clin Immunol 2005; 116: 503–509

[25] Chen Y, Wen L, Hu P, Qiu J, Lu L, Qiao L. Endoscopic intratympanic methylprednisolone injection for treatment of refractory sudden sensorineural hearing loss and one case in pregnancy. J Otolaryngol Head Neck Surg 2010; 39: 640–645

[26] Kurtoğlu S, Sarıcı D, Akın MA, Daar G, Korkmaz L, Memur Ş. Fetal adrenal suppression due to maternal corticosteroid use: case report. J Clin Res Pediatr Endocrinol 2011; 3: 160–162

[27] Fodale V, Praticò C, Girlanda P et al. Acute motor axonal polyneuropathy after a cisatracurium infusion and concomitant corticosteroid therapy. Br J Anaesth 2004; 92: 289–293

[28] USP DI. Drug Information for the Health Care Professional, Volume I, 19th ed. Englewood, CO: Micromedix, 1999:1000–1001, 1969–1973

[29] Szefler SJ, Rose JQ, Ellis EF, Spector SL, Green AW, Jusko WJ. The effect of troleandomycin on methylprednisolone elimination. J Allergy Clin Immunol 1980; 66: 447–451

[30] Klintmalm G, Säwe J. High dose methylprednisolone increases plasma cyclosporin levels in renal transplant recipients. Lancet 1984; 1: 731

[31] Monsell EM, Cass SP, Rybak LP, et al. Chemical treatment of the labyrinth. In: Brackman DE, Shelton C, Arriaga MA, eds. Otologic Surgery, 2nd ed. Philadelphia: Saunders, 2001:413–421

[32] USP DI. Drug Information for the Health Care Professional, Volume I, 19th ed. Englewood, CO: Micromedix, 1999:70–72 (aminoglycosides)

[33] Monsell EM, Cass SP, Rybak LP. Therapeutic use of aminoglycosides in Ménière's disease. Otolaryngol Clin North Am 1993; 26: 737–746

[34] Aran JM. Current perspectives on inner ear toxicity. Otolaryngol Head Neck Surg 1995; 112: 133–144

[35] Sismanis A, Wise CM, Johnson GD. Methotrexate management of immune-mediated cochleovestibular disorders. Otolaryngol Head Neck Surg 1997; 116: 146–152

[36] Matteson EL, Tirzaman O, Facer GW et al. Use of methotrexate for autoimmune hearing loss. Ann Otol Rhinol Laryngol 2000; 109: 710–714

[37] Matteson EL, Fabry DA, Facer GW et al. Open trial of methotrexate as treatment for autoimmune hearing loss. Arthritis Rheum 2001; 45: 146–150

[38] Harris JP, Weisman MH, Derebery JM et al. Treatment of corticosteroid-responsive autoimmune inner ear disease with methotrexate: a randomized controlled trial. JAMA 2003; 290: 1875–1883

[39] Street I, Jobanputra P, Proops DW. Etanercept, a tumour necrosis factor alpha receptor antagonist, and methotrexate in acute sensorineural hearing loss. J Laryngol Otol 2006; 120: 1064–1066

[40] Shibuya M, Fujio K, Morita K et al. Successful treatment with tocilizumab in a case of Cogan's syndrome complicated with aortitis. Mod Rheumatol 2012 [Epub ahead of print]

[41] Atzeni F, Turiel M, Capsoni F, Doria A, Meroni P, Sarzi-Puttini P. Autoimmunity and anti-TNF-alpha agents. Ann N Y Acad Sci 2005; 1051: 559–569

[42] Zhou H. Clinical pharmacokinetics of etanercept: a fully humanized soluble recombinant tumor necrosis factor receptor fusion protein. J Clin Pharmacol 2005; 45: 490–497

[43] Wang X, Truong T, Billings PB, Harris JP, Keithley EM. Blockage of immune-mediated inner ear damage by etanercept. Otol Neurotol 2003; 24: 52–57

[44] Matteson EL, Choi HK, Poe DS et al. Etanercept therapy for immune-mediated cochleovestibular disorders: a multi-center, open-label, pilot study. Arthritis Rheum 2005; 53: 337–342

[45] Cohen S, Shoup A, Weisman MH, Harris J. Etanercept treatment for autoimmune inner ear disease: results of a pilot placebo-controlled study. Otol Neurotol 2005; 26: 903–907

[46] Rychly DJ, DiPiro JT. Infections associated with tumor necrosis factor-alpha antagonists. Pharmacotherapy 2005; 25: 1181–1192

[47] Zimmer C, Beiderlinden M, Peters J. Lethal acute respiratory distress syndrome during anti-TNF-alpha therapy for rheumatoid arthritis. Clin Rheumatol 2006; 25: 430–432

[48] Juhn SK, Rybak LP, Prado S. Nature of blood-labyrinth barrier in experimental conditions. Ann Otol Rhinol Laryngol 1981; 90: 135–141

[49] Goycoolea MV, Lundman L. Round window membrane. Structure function and permeability: a review. Microsc Res Tech 1997; 36: 201–211

[50] Alzamil KS, Linthicum FH, Jr. Extraneous round window membranes and plugs: possible effect on intratympanic therapy. Ann Otol Rhinol Laryngol 2000; 109: 30–32

[51] Silverstein H, Rowan PT, Olds MJ, Rosenberg SI. Inner ear perfusion and the role of round window patency. Am J Otol 1997; 18: 586–589

[52] Banerjee A, Parnes LS. The biology of intratympanic drug administration and pharmacodynamics of round window drug absorption. Otolaryngol Clin North Am 2004; 37: 1035–1051

[53] Salt AN, Plontke SK. Principles of local drug delivery to the inner ear. Audiol Neurootol 2009; 14: 350–360

[54] Salt AN, Hartsock J, Plontke S, LeBel C, Piu F. Distribution of dexamethasone and preservation of inner ear function following intratympanic delivery of a gel-based formulation. Audiol Neurootol 2011; 16: 323–335

[55] Xu L, Heldrich J, Wang H et al. A controlled and sustained local gentamicin delivery system for inner ear applications. Otol Neurotol 2010; 31: 1115–1121

[56] Kakehata S, Sasaki A, Futai K, Kitani R, Shinkawa H. Daily short-term intratympanic dexamethasone treatment alone as an initial or salvage treatment for idiopathic sudden sensorineural hearing loss. Audiol Neurootol 2011; 16: 191–197

[57] Gouveris H, Schuler-Schmidt W, Mewes T, Mann W. Intratympanic dexamethasone/hyaluronic acid mix as an adjunct to intravenous steroid and vasoactive treatment in patients with severe idiopathic sudden sensorineural hearing loss. Otol Neurotol 2011; 32: 756–760

[58] Plontke SK, Löwenheim H, Mertens J et al. Randomized, double blind, placebo controlled trial on the safety and efficacy of continuous intratympanic dexamethasone delivered via a round window catheter for severe to profound sudden idiopathic sensorineural hearing loss after failure of systemic therapy. Laryngoscope 2009; 119: 359–369

[59] Wu HP, Chou YF, Yu SH, Wang CP, Hsu CJ, Chen PR. Intratympanic steroid injections as a salvage treatment for sudden sensorineural hearing loss: a randomized, double-blind, placebo-controlled study. Otol Neurotol 2011; 32: 774–779

[60] Spear SA, Schwartz SR. Intratympanic steroids for sudden sensorineural hearing loss: a systematic review. Otolaryngol Head Neck Surg 2011; 145: 534–543

[61] Phillips JS, Westerberg B. Intratympanic steroids for Ménière's disease or syndrome. Cochrane Database Syst Rev 2011 Issue 7: CD008514

[62] Sennaroglu L, Sennaroglu G, Gursel B, Dini FM. Intratympanic dexamethasone, intratympanic gentamicin, and endolymphatic sac surgery for intractable vertigo in Meniere's disease. Otolaryngol Head Neck Surg 2001; 125: 537–543

[63] Sakata E, Itoh A, Itoh Y. Treatment of cochlear-tinnitus with dexamethasone infusion into the tympanic cavity. Int Tinnitus J 1996; 2: 12: 9–135

[64] Herr BD, Marzo SJ. Intratympanic steroid perfusion for refractory sudden sensorineural hearing loss. Otolaryngol Head Neck Surg 2005; 132: 527–531

[65] Kopke RD, Hoffer ME, Wester D, O'Leary MJ, Jackson RL. Targeted topical steroid therapy in sudden sensorineural hearing loss. Otol Neurotol 2001; 22: 475–479

[66] Chandrasekhar SS, Rubinstein RY, Kwartler JA et al. Dexamethasone pharmacokinetics in the inner ear: comparison of route of administration and use of facilitating agents. Otolaryngol Head Neck Surg 2000; 122: 521–528

[67] Plontke SK, Salt AN. Quantitative interpretation of corticosteroid pharmacokinetics in inner fluids using computer simulations. Hear Res 2003; 182: 34–42

[68] Parnes LS, Sun AH, Freeman DJ. Corticosteroid pharmacokinetics in the inner ear fluids: an animal study followed by clinical application. Laryngoscope 1999; 109: 1–17

[69] Bachmann G, Su J, Zumegen C et al. Permeabilitat des runden Fenstermembranen fur prednisolon-21-hydrogensuccinat. HNO 2001; 49: 538–541

[70] Van Wijk F, Staecker H, Keithley E, Lefebvre PP. Local perfusion of the tumor necrosis factor alpha blocker infliximab to the inner ear improves autoimmune neurosensory hearing loss. Audiol Neurootol 2006; 11: 357–365

[71] Liu YC, Rubin R, Sataloff RT. Treatment-refractory autoimmune sensorineural hearing loss: response to infliximab. Ear Nose Throat J 2011; 90: 23–28

[72] Nakagawa T, Sakamoto T, Hiraumi H et al. Topical insulin-like growth factor 1 treatment using gelatin hydrogels for glucocorticoid-resistant sudden sensorineural hearing loss: a prospective clinical trial. BMC Med 2010; 8: 76

[73] Cohen-Kerem R, Kisilevsky V, Einarson TR, Kozer E, Koren G, Rutka JA. Intratympanic gentamicin for Ménière's disease: a meta-analysis. Laryngoscope 2004; 114: 2085–2091

[74] Chia SH, Gamst AC, Anderson JP, Harris JP. Intratympanic gentamicin therapy for Ménière's disease: a meta-analysis. Otol Neurotol 2004; 25: 544–552

[75] Shea PF, Richey PA, Wan JY, Stevens SR. Hearing results and quality of life after streptomycin/dexamethasone perfusion for Meniere's disease. Laryngoscope 2012; 122: 204–211

[76] Hoffer ME, Allen K, Kopke RD, Weisskopf P, Gottshall K, Wester D. Transtympanic versus sustained-release administration of gentamicin: kinetics, morphology, and function. Laryngoscope 2001; 111: 1343–1357

[77] Plontke SK, Wood AW, Salt AN. Analysis of gentamicin kinetics in fluids of the inner ear with round window administration. Otol Neurotol 2002; 23: 967–974

[78] Staecker H. Broadening the spectrum of treatment options for SNHL. Arch Otolaryngol Head Neck Surg 2005; 131: 734

[79] Paulson DP, Abuzeid W, Jiang H, Oe T, O'Malley BW, Li D. A novel controlled local drug delivery system for inner ear disease. Laryngoscope 2008; 118: 706–711

[80] Nakagawa T, Ito J. Local drug delivery to the inner ear using biodegradable materials. Ther Deliv 2011; 2: 807–814

[81] Rivera T, Sanz L, Camarero G, Varela-Nieto I. Drug delivery to the inner ear: strategies and their therapeutic implications for sensorineural hearing loss. Curr Drug Deliv 2012; 9: 231–242

[82] Tamura T, Kita T, Nakagawa T et al. Drug delivery to the cochlea using PLGA nanoparticles. Laryngoscope 2005; 115: 2000–2005

[83] Zhang Y, Zhang W, Löbler M et al. Inner ear biocompatibility of lipid nanocapsules after round window membrane application. Int J Pharm 2011; 404: 211–219

[84] Mukherjea D, Rybak LP, Sheehan KE et al. The design and screening of drugs to prevent acquired sensorineural hearing loss. Expert Opin Drug Discov 2011; 6: 491–505

[85] Silverstein H, Choo D, Rosenberg SI, Kuhn J, Seidman M, Stein I. Intratympanic steroid treatment of inner ear disease and tinnitus (preliminary report). Ear Nose Throat J 1996; 75: 468–471, 474, 476 passim

[86] Shulman A, Goldstein B. Intratympanic drug therapy with steroids for tinnitus control: a preliminary report. Int Tinnitus J 2000; 6: 10–20

[87] Arriaga MA, Goldman S. Hearing results of intratympanic steroid treatment of endolymphatic hydrops. Laryngoscope 1998; 108: 1682–1685

[88] Chandrasekhar SS. Intratympanic dexamethasone for sudden sensorineural hearing loss: clinical and laboratory evaluation. Otol Neurotol 2001; 22: 18–23

[89] Barrs DM, Keyser JS, Stallworth C, McElveen JT, Jr. Intratympanic steroid injections for intractable Ménière's disease. Laryngoscope 2001; 111: 2100–2104

Part 2

Evaluation

7 Temporal Bone Imaging

Rebecca S. Cornelius and Humberto Morales

7.1 Introduction

Imaging of temporal bone pathology relies primarily on computed tomography (CT) and magnetic resonance imaging (MRI).[1-3] Other modalities, including angiography and nuclear medicine imaging, have a role limited to specific clinical situations.

Imaging procedures of choice in various clinical situations are discussed in this chapter. In general, MRI offers advantages of multiplanar imaging capability without requiring the patient to lie in uncomfortable positions. Also, MRI provides better detail of soft tissue abnormalities as well as more specific characteristics of mass lesions. However, imaging time is usually considerably longer than with CT and requires a higher level of patient cooperation to achieve high-quality images. Likewise, patients with claustrophobia usually experience greater difficulty with MRI than with CT. Newer generation helical multislice CT technology now allows for rapid scan times and high-quality multiplanar reconstructions, often obviating the need for scanning directly in two planes.[4,5] A high-detail temporal bone CT performed using these techniques requires less than 10 minutes patient time in the CT scanner and actual scan time of under 30 seconds for a single plane study.

Magnetic resonance imaging is contraindicated in patients with implanted metallic devices or foreign bodies, such as pacemakers, certain aneurysm clips, cardiac valves, cochlear and other metallic implants, and metallic foreign bodies in the globe or orbit. MRI centers keep extensive lists of implanted devices that are known to be MRI compatible or incompatible. Radiologists and technologists operating MRI scanners should be able to determine whether a particular device implanted in a patient can be exposed to the magnetic field without risk. There are greater limitations when scanning at 3 Tesla as opposed to 1.5 Tesla.

The cost of CT examination is usually 20 to 40% less than that of MRI; however, in most instances of temporal bone evaluation, one test is clearly the procedure of choice over the other as far as diagnostic value. Thus, the issue of cost differential does not realistically come into play in most situations.

As a general guideline for choosing imaging modalities, CT is helpful as the primary test in cases of conductive hearing loss (CHL), cholesteatoma, otosclerosis, otomastoiditis, trauma, and any time bony detail is required. Magnetic resonance imaging is indicated as the primary test in sensorineural hearing loss (SNHL), tinnitus, vertigo/dizziness (central cause), soft tissue mass/tumors, and cranial nerve involvement. Readers are referred to the introductory chapter of *Imaging of the Temporal Bone* by Swartz and Loevner,[3] which covers in detail the imaging approach based on the patient's clinical presentation.

7.2 External Auditory Canal

Disease processes that affect the external auditory canal (EAC) include congenital dysplasias/branchial cleft abnormalities,

benign and malignant neoplasms, and inflammatory disease. These entities are covered in detail in Chapter 16.

Imaging of EAC disease is best accomplished with CT scanning to ensure that the cortex of the osseous portion of the EAC is fully evaluated (▶ Fig. 7.1).[3,6]

In patients with aggressive malignant neoplasms additional evaluation with MRI with gadolinium contrast enhancement may be warranted if there is evidence of intracranial extension. Extension into adjacent extracranial tissue such as the parotid space usually can be evaluated with either contrast-enhanced CT or MRI.

Likewise, patients with necrotizing external otitis (NEO) with suspicion of intracranial spread may require additional imaging with MRI (▶ Fig. 7.2). Detection of meningeal involvement and complications such as abscess or sinus thrombosis are better detected with MRI than with CT.

Extracranial spread into the temporomandibular joint, parapharyngeal space, and masticator space is usually adequately evaluated with contrast-enhanced CT,[7] but is also well evaluated with MRI, which also detects bony signal changes in osteomyelitis (▶ Fig. 7.2).[8,9]

Some studies advocate the use of radionuclide imaging in the diagnosis and follow-up of NEO. Both technetium (Tc)-99 m and gallium-67 citrate have been used.[9-11] Technetium-99 m is a bone-scanning agent that demonstrates increased uptake in areas of increased osteoblastic activity. It is more sensitive than CT for early changes of osteomyelitis in the skull base,[12] but does not delineate soft tissue changes, which are clearly seen with CT scanning. The bone scan remains abnormal for months even if there is no active infection. Gallium-67 citrate scintigraphy is more specific for active infection, and serial scanning has been used to predict resolution of NEO (▶ Fig. 7.2).[13] However, there are documented cases of patients with recurrent or persistent NEO who have had normal gallium scans.[14]

Indium-111 white blood cell scan in combination with Tc-99 m single photon emission computed tomography (SPECT) scan has also been shown to be useful in the diagnosis and follow-up of skull base osteomyelitis in patients with NEO.[15]

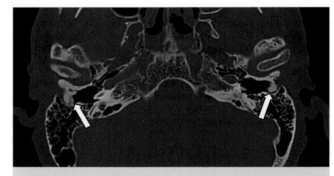

Fig. 7.1 External auditory canal exostosis (surfer's ear). Axial CT image through the level of the external auditory canals shows bilateral exophytic ossific lesions (*arrows*) covering the entry of the bony canal. They have a "pedicle" contiguous with the tympanic bone.

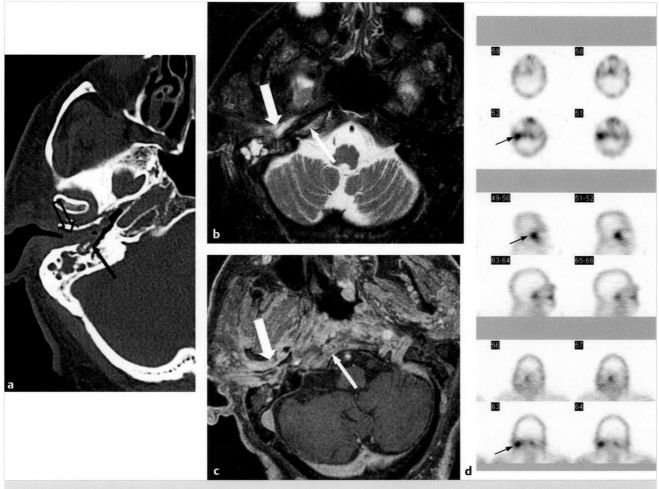

Fig. 7.2 Malignant (necrotizing) external otitis. (a) Axial CT image shows thick soft tissue density within the external auditory canal (*large white arrow*) and associated erosion of the posterior wall of the canal (*small white arrow*). (b,c) Axial T2-weighted and postcontrast MR images through the same level better demonstrate enhancing soft tissue abnormality within the external auditory canal (*large white arrows*). There is also abnormal bone marrow signal and enhancement in the petrous apex and clivus (*small white arrows*) consistent with extensive osteomyelitis. (d) Multiplanar gallium-67 citrate scintigraphy images show abnormal increased uptake in the region of the right temporal bone (*small black arrows*) consistent with osteomyelitis.

7.3 Mastoid and Middle Ear

Diseases of the mastoid and middle ear cavity include congenital anomalies (see Chapter 1), inflammatory disease (Chapters 18 and 19), and neoplasms (Chapters 25 and 27).

The initial imaging evaluation of mastoid and middle ear pathology relies primarily on high-resolution noncontrast CT (▶ Fig. 7.3; ▶ Fig. 7.4).[4,16,17] Magnetic resonance imaging is extremely valuable in the assessment of patients with intracranial complications from otomastoiditis and cholesteatoma. Meningitis, subdural or epidural empyema, and intracranial abscess are much better demonstrated with MRI than with CT.

Sigmoid sinus thrombophlebitis is also better demonstrated with MRI (▶ Fig. 7.5). If findings of venous thrombosis are equivocal on routine spin-echo images, magnetic resonance venography can be utilized for confirmation. Magnetic resonance imaging is also superior in detecting encephaloceles, which may develop at sites of postsurgical or erosive defects in the tegmen.[18]

Recent advances in MRI, particularly improvements on diffusion-weighted images (DWI), have shown promising results in the evaluation of the temporal bone.[19,20] Diffusion-weighted images can be particularly useful in the diagnosis of cholesteatoma,[21–24] which has increased signal intensity on DWI, partially due to restricted water diffusion (oily consistency of the contained fluid) and predominantly to the T2-weighted shine-through effect of the lesion (▶ Fig. 7.6).[21] This characteristic signal can be useful for the evaluation of recurrent/residual cholesteatoma to avoid unnecessary second-look surgeries.[25]

The temporal bone course of the facial nerve can be clearly depicted by CT and is of paramount importance in patients who undergo middle ear surgery. A variety of processes can affect the facial nerve; CT and MRI are complementary techniques in its evaluation.[26]

Paragangliomas including glomus tympanicum and jugulotympanicum involve the middle ear cavity. Their imaging evaluation is discussed later in this chapter.

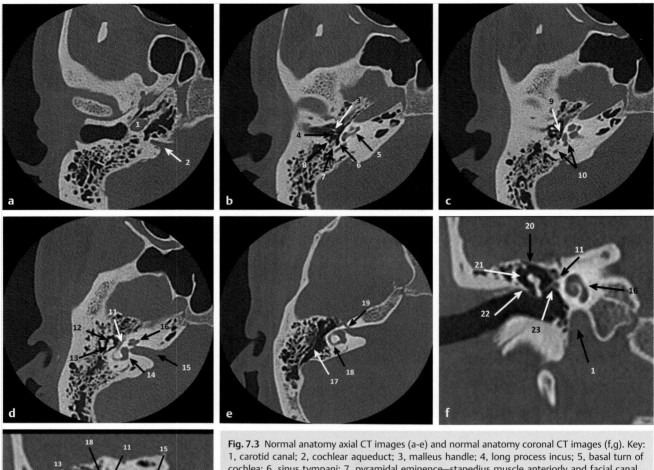

Fig. 7.3 Normal anatomy axial CT images (a-e) and normal anatomy coronal CT images (f,g). Key: 1, carotid canal; 2, cochlear aqueduct; 3, malleus handle; 4, long process incus; 5, basal turn of cochlea; 6, sinus tympani; 7, pyramidal eminence—stapedius muscle anteriorly and facial canal posteriorly; 8, facial recess; 9, stapes crura; 10, posterior semicircular canal; 11, tympanic segment facial nerve canal; 12, malleus head; 13, incus body; 14, vestibule; 15, internal auditory canal; 16, cochlea—second turn and apex; 17, Koerner septum; 18, lateral semicircular canal; 19, labyrinthine segment facial nerve canal; 20, tegmen tympani; 21, Prussak space; 22, scutum; 23, tensor tympani; 24, lenticular process of incus; 25, oval window.

7.4 Inner Ear

Congenital malformations of the inner ear are covered in Chapters 1 and 23. Other processes that may lead to imaging evaluations include inflammatory disease, bony dehiscences, otodystrophies, and neoplasms.

An interesting concept in the evaluation of CHL is the "third-window lesions" of the inner ear. These lesions cause a mobile window on the scala vestibule side of the cochlear partition; thus, CHL results from the dual mechanism of worsening of air conduction thresholds and improvement of bone conduction thresholds.[27,28] Third-window lesions are better evaluated by high-resolution CT and include abnormalities of the semicircular canals (superior, lateral, or posterior canal dehiscence), bony vestibule (vestibular aqueduct enlargement or dehiscence), or the cochlea (carotid-cochlear dehiscence) (▶ Fig. 7.7).

Imaging of patients with suspected otodystrophy also relies heavily on high-resolution CT scanning (▶ Fig. 7.8).[29–32] Otosclerosis is covered in detail in Chapter 21.[33–35] Other otodystrophies including fibrous dysplasia and Paget disease demonstrate classic findings on CT.[3] Extensive areas of bony demineralization are evident with the cotton-wool appearance seen in calvarial bone in Paget disease.[36,37] Patients with fibrous dysplasia demonstrate areas of enlarged dense bone with a ground-glass appearance to the matrix. Although patients with Paget disease and those with fibrous dysplasia have visible abnormalities on MRI, the changes are frequently less diagnostic on MRI than on CT and do not warrant the added expense.

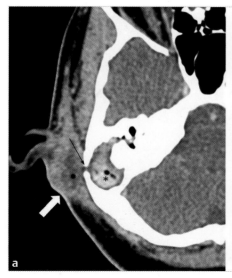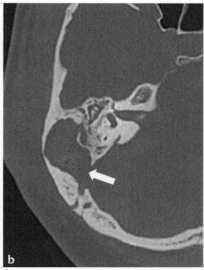

Fig. 7.4 Mastoiditis, subperiosteal abscess, and cholesteatoma. (a) Axial CT image with soft tissue algorithm shows coalescent hyperdensity in the mastoid (*asterisk*) and cortical erosion (*small black arrow*) with associated subperiosteal rim–enhancing fluid collection (*large white arrow*). (b) Axial CT image with bone algorithm shows opacification of the middle ear and dehiscence of the sigmoid plate (*white arrow*). Patient underwent surgery that showed large cholesteatoma within the mastoid cavity (hyperdensity on CT) and associated abscess/osteomyelitis.

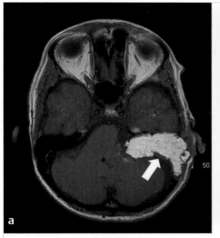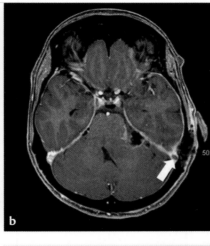

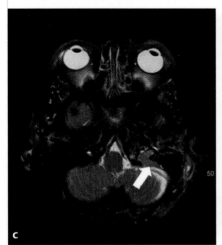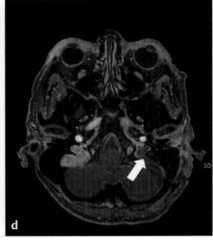

Fig. 7.5 Dural sinus thrombosis post–internal auditory canal (IAC) schwannoma resection. (a) Axial T1-weighted MRI shows postsurgical changes in the left temporal bone with fat packing (*arrow*). (b–d) Images on the same patient. (b) Axial postcontrast MR image shows filling defect within the dural sinus (*arrow*) at the junction of the transverse and sigmoid sinus. (c, d) Axial T2-weighted and postcontrast MR images show abnormal signal within the sigmoid sinus extending into the jugular bulb on the left (c, *arrow*) with associated filling defect (d, *arrow*).

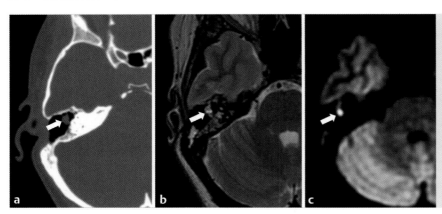

Fig. 7.6 Recurrent cholesteatoma. (a) Axial CT image shows mastoidectomy cavity on the right and small nodular-like soft tissue opacification in the middle ear (*arrow*). It is suspicious but not specific for cholesteatoma. (b,c) Axial T2-weighted and DWI images show hyperintense signal in the area corresponding to soft tissue opacification (*arrow*) on CT. Restricted diffusion has shown high specificity for cholesteatoma in the temporal bone.

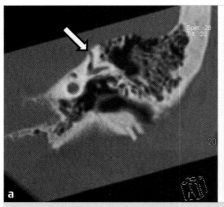
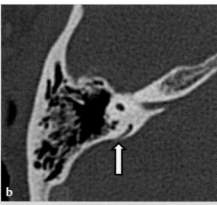
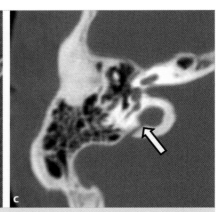

Fig. 7.7 Examples of third-window lesions of the inner ear. (a) Coronal oblique reconstructed CT images of the temporal bone at the level of the superior semicircular canal shows small focal dehiscence (*arrow*) with no bone covering the upper portion of the canal. (b) Axial CT image shows focal dehiscence of the posterior semicircular canal (*arrow*). (c) Axial CT image shows dehiscence of the vestibular aqueduct into a high-riding jugular bulb (*arrow*).

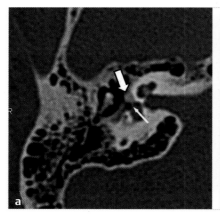
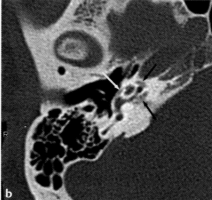

Fig. 7.8 Otosclerosis. (a) Axial CT image through the level of the cochlea and oval window shows subtle area of demineralization/lucency adjacent to the oval window (*small arrow*) in the region of the fissula ante fenestram (*large arrow*) consistent with fenestral otosclerosis. (b) Axial CT image through the level of the cochlea shows extensive areas of demineralization/lucencies surrounding the cochlea (*white and black arrows*), most consistent with severe cochlear otosclerosis.

Imaging of patients with inner ear inflammatory disease is performed to exclude other causes of vertigo. Patients with acute labyrinthitis frequently show abnormal signal or enhancement within the membranous labyrinth on MRI. The findings are a nonspecific indication of inflammation.[38]

Labyrinthitis ossificans can occur as a sequela of labyrinthitis, most frequently following a bacterial infection. Both CT and MRI are useful in the detection of labyrinthitis ossificans.[39,40] On MRI obliteration of the normal fluid signal within the mem-branous labyrinth on high-resolution T2-weighted sequences can be detected. In the early stages, MRI findings may be more obvious than the CT findings of subtle labyrinthine sclerosis.[41] Rare intralabyrinthine schwannomas are easily detected on gadolinium-enhanced MRI.[42]

With the improved visualization of inner ear structures using three-dimensional (3D) and high-resolution techniques, MRI is playing an increasing role in the detection and diagnosis of inner ear pathology.[43–61]

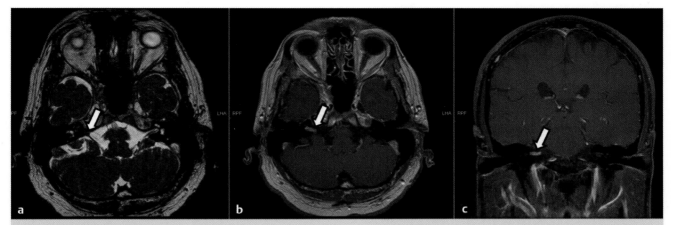

Fig. 7.9 Intracanalicular vestibular schwannoma. (a) Axial high-resolution T2-weighted 3D Fourier transform-constructive interference in steady state (3DFT-CISS) MRI shows small mass within the IAC obliterating the normal cerebrospinal fluid (CSF) signal (*arrow*). (b,c) Axial and coronal postcontrast MR images show small enhancing mass within the IAC (*arrows*).

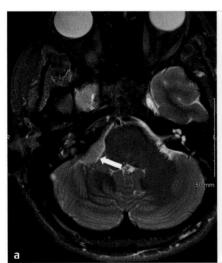
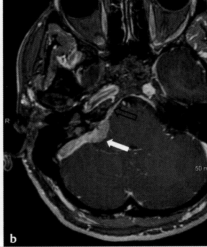

Fig. 7.10 Cerebellopontine angle meningioma. (a) Axial T2-weighted MR image shows an intermediate signal intensity mass in the CPA (*arrow*). (b) Axial postcontrast MR image shows enhancing mass in CPA (*white arrow*) with linear extension of enhancement into the retroclival region (*open black arrow*) consistent with dural tail.

7.5 Skull Base, Internal Auditory Canal, and Cerebellopontine Angle

The main categories of disease to be considered include neoplasms and cysts, inflammatory disease, and vascular lesions including normal vascular variants. Imaging of the skull base, internal auditory canal (IAC), and cerebellopontine angle (CPA) have been greatly improved since the advent of MRI.[62–66] This is the one area of temporal bone imaging where MRI clearly supplants CT as the initial imaging test of choice in most instances. MRI also plays a role in the evaluation of patients with pulsatile tinnitus.[67] Magnetic resonance imaging/magnetic resonance angiography (MRA) can detect petrous carotid aneurysm, glomus tumor, atherosclerotic carotid stenosis, advanced fibromuscular dysplasia (FMD), and high-flow dural arteriovenous malformation/fistula.[68,69] However, many patients with objective pulsatile tinnitus require conventional angiography for more complete evaluation of lesions detected on MRI or for treatment purposes. Low-flow dural fistulas may not be detected with MRI/MRA. Likewise, subtle FMD may be mistaken as an artifactual finding on MRA. Thus, it may be more cost-effective to proceed directly to conventional angiography in patients with objective pulsatile tinnitus. In patients with subjective pulsatile tinnitus, imaging to exclude a number of normal vascular variants is necessary. These are all well demonstrated with CT imaging.[69] Uncommonly subjective tinnitus may be related to kinking or stenosis in the high cervical internal carotid artery, or to venous sinus stenosis. Magnetic resonance angiography and MR venography can be of use in detecting such abnormalities. Pulsatile tinnitus is covered in more detail in Chapter 37.

Magnetic resonance imaging provides excellent delineation of tumors and cysts of the skull base, IAC, and CPA.[70–72]

Schwannomas of the fifth, seventh, and eighth cranial nerves typically demonstrate intermediate signal on T1-weighted images (T1WI) and high signal on T2-weighted images (T2WI).[73] They enhance intensely with gadolinium. Even small intracanalicular acoustic schwannomas are easily detected with MRI with gadolinium and with high-resolution 3D technique (▶ Fig. 7.9).[74–76]

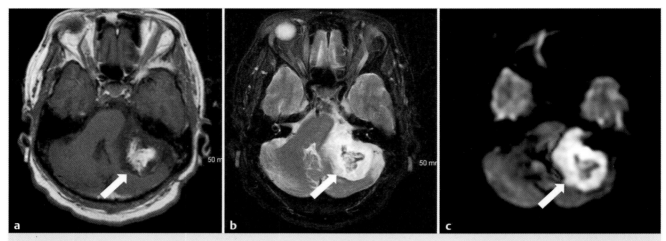

Fig. 7.11 Cerebellopontine angle epidermoid-dermoid. (a) Axial T1-weighted MR image shows large mixed signal mass in the left CPA (*arrow*) with central areas of increased (fat) signal. (b) Axial T2-weighted MR image with fat saturation shows the mass (*arrow*) with predominant increased signal and superimposed areas of decreased signal centrally, related to the saturation of fat signal. It is most consistent with mixed fluid and fatty tumor. (c) Axial DWI MR image shows significant increased signal of the lesion most consistent with restricted water diffusion, which is typical for epidermoid tumors.

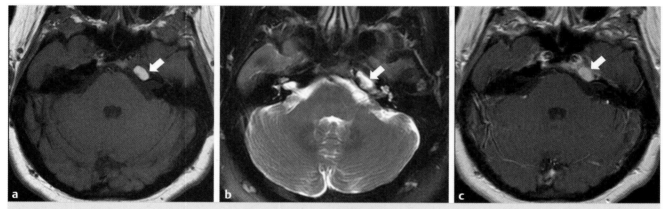

Fig. 7.12 Cholesterol granuloma of the petrous apex. Axial T1-weighted (a), T2-weighted (b), and postcontrast (c) MR images show abnormal signal within the petrous apex (*arrows*) with mild expansion. There is increased signal on T1WI and T2WI and no abnormal enhancement, most consistent with cholesterol granuloma. Increased signal on T1WI is believed to be secondary to hemorrhagic by-products.

Meningiomas typically demonstrate intermediate signal on T1WI and T2WI, usually isointense to gray matter, with intense gadolinium enhancement. The multiplanar imaging capability of MRI allows for easier determination of the dural base of a meningioma (▶ Fig. 7.10). Some meningiomas demonstrate increased signal on T2WI.

Epidermoid tumors, frequently seen in the CPA, have a characteristic appearance on MRI. Signal characteristics parallel cerebrospinal fluid (CSF), but are usually not identical. These lesions demonstrate low signal on T1WI and high signal on T2WI. They do not demonstrate enhancement. They usually have characteristic frond-like borders when occurring in the CPA. Differentiation from arachnoid cyst is sometimes difficult if the lesions have smooth borders. In these cases diffusion weighted imaging is helpful as epidermoid tumors demonstrate restricted diffusion (▶ Fig. 7.11).

Cholesterol granulomas of the petrous apex demonstrate characteristic findings on MRI, with high signal intensity seen on both T1- and T2-weighted images (▶ Fig. 7.12).[77-84] This is in contrast to cholesteatoma, which has low T1-weighted signal intensity.[80,81,85-87] CT findings are less specific, showing expansile smooth erosion of the petrous apex.[78,79,86,87] These are covered in detail in Chapter 26.

Dermoids and lipomas have a characteristic fat signal on MRI. They demonstrate increased signal on T1WI and low signal on T2WI. Fat suppression techniques are also useful showing loss of signal within the tumor (▶ Fig. 7.11).

Tumors of the skull base, including chordoma, chondrosarcoma, and metastatic disease, frequently require both MRI and CT for complete evaluation (▶ Fig. 7.13).[88-93] CT is useful in evaluating subtle foraminal erosion[94-96] and for evaluating the chondroid matrix in chondrosarcoma or chordomas (▶ Fig. 7.14).[97-99]

MRI provides elegant visualization of the skull base and intracranial and extracranial extent of tumor by virtue of its multiplanar imaging capabilities.[100-103] It is virtually the only

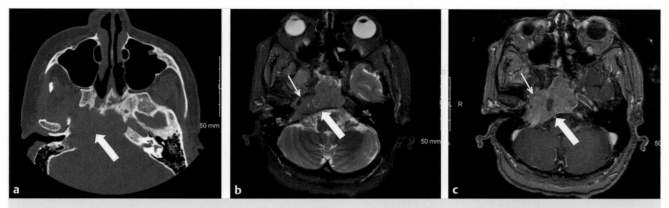

Fig. 7.13 Metastatic squamous cell carcinoma to the skull base. (a) Axial CT image shows complete osseous destruction of the right petrous apex and clivus (*arrow*). (b,c) Axial T2-weighted and postcontrast MR images show isointense T2 and heterogeneously enhancing mass centered in the skull base and right petrous apex (*arrows*). The mass is also encasing the carotid artery in its petrous segment (*small arrows*).

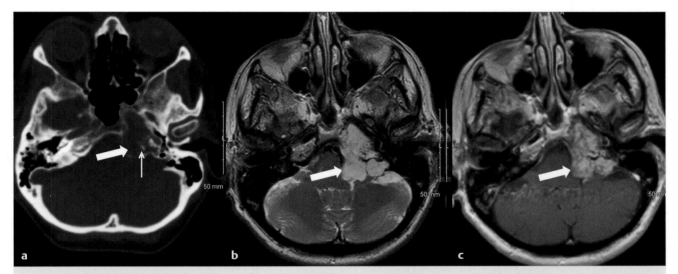

Fig. 7.14 Petrous apex chondrosarcoma. (a) Axial CT image shows destruction and expansion of the petrous apex on the left (*arrow*). There are small areas of increased density (*small arrow*) most consistent with calcific chondroid matrix. (b,c) Axial T2-weighted and postcontrast MR images show the bone destruction secondary to a large enhancing mass with T2 hyperintensity centered in the petrous apex with an exophytic component extending into the CPA.

imaging technique that clearly demonstrates perineural spread of skull base/head and neck tumors (▶ Fig. 7.15). Intrinsic skull base tumors show replacement of normal fatty marrow signal on T1WI by abnormal intermediate signal intensity.[104] T2-weighted images show abnormal increased signal (▶ Fig. 7.14).[97] Chordomas tend to have extremely bright signal on T2WI.[99,102,105–108]

Paragangliomas of the temporal bone may involve the middle ear cavity (glomus tympanicum), jugular foramen (glomus jugulare), or both (glomus jugulotympanicum).[109] High-resolution CT with contrast should be used as the first step in the evaluation of patients with suspected temporal bone glomus tumor.[110,111] Glomus tympanicum can frequently be diagnosed and completely evaluated with CT only.[112,113] If the tumor is large enough to involve the eustachian tube, MRI may be necessary to differentiate fluid within the middle ear cavity from enhancing tumor mass.[114]

High-resolution CT is needed to assess subtle bony erosion of the jugular foramen in small glomus jugulare tumors.[115,116] Erosion of the bony plate between the jugular bulb and hypotympanum may be subtle, but can usually be detected with high-resolution CT in cases of glomus jugulotympanicum. In large glomus jugulare tumors, MRI is useful for evaluation of intracranial extension, inferior extension in the neck, and multicentric tumors. On MRI glomus tumors demonstrate intermediate signal on T1WI. Larger lesions demonstrate an inhomogeneous "salt and pepper" pattern with areas of foci of subacute hemorrhage and areas of low signal representing vascular flow voids. On T2WI the lesion usually has inhomogeneous bright signal with areas of low signal flow voids. The lesions demonstrate significant enhancement with gadolinium.

A radionuclide imaging technique has been described that may be useful in evaluating multicentric glomus tumors.

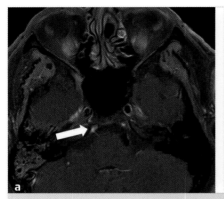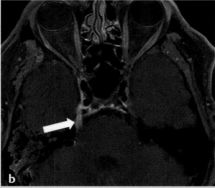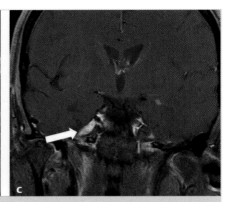

Fig. 7.15 Perineural spread of squamous cell carcinoma of the head and neck. (a) Axial postcontrast MR image shows abnormal enhancement of the right sixth cranial nerve, including the Dorello canal (*arrow*). (b) Axial postcontrast MR image shows abnormal enhancement of the cisternal portion of the fifth cranial nerve (*arrow*). (c) Coronal postcontrast MR image in the same patient shows abnormal enhancement of the Meckel cave on the right (*arrow*).

Indium-111 octreotide, a somatostatin analogue, has been investigated in identifying tumors of neuroendocrine origin. Limitations of the technique include identification of small tumors. It usually identifies tumors larger than 1 cm.[117]

Petrous apicitis may be diagnosed earlier with MRI than with CT. T2-weighted images demonstrate abnormal high signal intensity in the petrous apex.[82,118] Gadolinium-enhanced images demonstrate abnormal enhancement within the petrous apex and adjacent leptomeninges.[3] CT imaging may show fluid-filled pneumatized petrous apex cells or in severe cases bone erosion.

7.6 Trauma

This subject is covered in detail in Chapter 22. Evaluation of temporal bone fractures is best achieved with high-resolution CT scanning in axial projection with coronal reconstructions.[119–125]

If fractures are seen to extend into the carotid canal, further imaging is indicated to assess for vascular injury. Conventional angiography is still considered the gold standard for evaluation, though CT angiography is being increasingly utilized to evaluate dissections.[126,127]

Magnetic imaging angiography is less useful in evaluation of vascular injury at the skull base level due to frequently encountered artifacts in this region.

References

[1] Swartz JD. Current imaging approach to the temporal bone. Radiology 1989; 171: 309–317

[2] Swartz JD. The temporal bone: imaging considerations. Crit Rev Diagn Imaging 1990; 30: 341–417

[3] Swartz JD, Loevner LA. Imaging of the Temporal Bone, 4th ed. New York: Thieme, 2009

[4] Phillips GS, LoGerfo SE, Richardson ML, Anzai Y. Interactive Web-based learning module on CT of the temporal bone: anatomy and pathology. Radiographics 2012; 32: E85–E105

[5] Fujii N, Inui Y, Katada K. Temporal bone anatomy: correlation of multiplanar reconstruction sections and three-dimensional computed tomography images. Jpn J Radiol 2010; 28: 637–648

[6] Gassner EM, Mallouhi A, Jaschke WR. Preoperative evaluation of external auditory canal atresia on high-resolution CT. AJR Am J Roentgenol 2004; 182: 1305–1312

[7] Rubin J, Curtin HD, Yu VL, Kamerer DB. Malignant external otitis: utility of CT in diagnosis and follow-up. Radiology 1990; 174: 391–394

[8] Gherini SG, Brackmann DE, Bradley WG. Magnetic resonance imaging and computerized tomography in malignant external otitis. Laryngoscope 1986; 96: 542–548

[9] Chang PC, Fischbein NJ, Holliday RA. Central skull base osteomyelitis in patients without otitis externa: imaging findings. AJNR Am J Neuroradiol 2003; 24: 1310–1316

[10] Uri N, Gips S, Front A, Meyer SW, Hardoff R. Quantitative bone and 67Ga scintigraphy in the differentiation of necrotizing external otitis from severe external otitis. Arch Otolaryngol Head Neck Surg 1991; 117: 623–626

[11] Parisier SC, Lucente FE, Som PM, Hirschman SZ, Arnold LM, Roffman JD. Nuclear scanning in necrotizing progressive "malignant" external otitis. Laryngoscope 1982; 92: 1016–1019

[12] Ostfeld E, Aviel A, Pelet D. Malignant external otitis: the diagnostic value of bone scintigraphy. Laryngoscope 1981; 91: 960–964

[13] Mendelson DS, Som PM, Mendelson MH, Parisier SC. Malignant external otitis: the role of computed tomography and radionuclides in evaluation. Radiology 1983; 149: 745–749

[14] Kraus DH, Rehm SJ, Kinney SE. The evolving treatment of necrotizing external otitis. Laryngoscope 1988; 98: 934–939

[15] Seabold JE, Simonson TM, Weber PC et al. Cranial osteomyelitis: diagnosis and follow-up with In-111 white blood cell and Tc-99m methylene diphosphonate bone SPECT, CT, and MR imaging. Radiology 1995; 196: 779–788

[16] Silver AJ, Janecka I, Wazen J, Hilal SK, Rutledge JN. Complicated cholesteatomas: CT findings in inner ear complications of middle ear cholesteatomas. Radiology 1987; 164: 47–51

[17] Torizuka T, Hayakawa K, Satoh Y et al. High-resolution CT of the temporal bone: a modified baseline. Radiology 1992; 184: 109–111

[18] Martin N, Sterkers O, Nahum H. Chronic inflammatory disease of the middle ear cavities: Gd-DTPA-enhanced MR imaging. Radiology 1990; 176: 399–405

[19] De Foer B, Vercruysse JP, Spaepen M et al. Diffusion-weighted magnetic resonance imaging of the temporal bone. Neuroradiology 2010; 52: 785–807

[20] De Foer B, Vercruysse JP, Pilet B et al. Single-shot, turbo spin-echo, diffusion-weighted imaging versus spin-echo-planar, diffusion-weighted imaging in the detection of acquired middle ear cholesteatoma. AJNR Am J Neuroradiol 2006; 27: 1480–1482

[21] Vercruysse JP, De Foer B, Pouillon M, Somers T, Casselman J, Offeciers E. The value of diffusion-weighted MR imaging in the diagnosis of primary acquired and residual cholesteatoma: a surgical verified study of 100 patients. Eur Radiol 2006; 16: 1461–1467

[22] Baráth K, Huber AM, Stämpfli P, Varga Z, Kollias S. Neuroradiology of cholesteatomas. AJNR Am J Neuroradiol 2011; 32: 221–229

[23] De Foer B, Vercruysse JP, Bernaerts A et al. Middle ear cholesteatoma: non-echo-planar diffusion-weighted MR imaging versus delayed gadolinium-enhanced T1-weighted MR imaging—value in detection. Radiology 2010; 255: 866–872

[24] Más-Estellés F, Mateos-Fernández M, Carrascosa-Bisquert B, Facal de Castro F, Puchades-Román I, Morera-Pérez C. Contemporary non-echo-planar diffusion-weighted imaging of middle ear cholesteatomas. Radiographics 2012; 32: 1197–1213

[25] Dubrulle F, Souillard R, Chechin D, Vaneecloo FM, Desaulty A, Vincent C. Diffusion-weighted MR imaging sequence in the detection of postoperative recurrent cholesteatoma. Radiology 2006; 238: 604–610

[26] Raghavan P, Mukherjee S, Phillips CD. Imaging of the facial nerve. Neuroimaging Clin N Am 2009; 19: 407–425

[27] St Martin MB, Hirsch BE. Imaging of hearing loss. Otolaryngol Clin North Am 2008; 41: 157–178, vi–viivi–vii.

[28] Merchant SN, Rosowski JJ. Conductive hearing loss caused by third-window lesions of the inner ear. Otol Neurotol 2008; 29: 282–289

[29] Swartz JD. The otodystrophies: diagnosis and differential diagnosis. Semin Ultrasound CT MR 2004; 25: 305–318

[30] Odrezin GT, Krasikov N. CT of the temporal bone in a patient with osteopathia striata and cranial sclerosis. AJNR Am J Neuroradiol 1993; 14: 72–75

[31] d'Archambeau O, Parizel PM, Koekelkoren E, Van de Heyning P, De Schepper AM. CT diagnosis and differential diagnosis of otodystrophic lesions of the temporal bone. Eur J Radiol 1990; 11: 22–30

[32] Shah LM, Wiggins RH, III. Imaging of hearing loss. Neuroimaging Clin N Am 2009; 19: 287–306

[33] Ziyeh S, Berlis A, Ross UH, Reinhardt MJ, Schumacher M. MRI of active otosclerosis. Neuroradiology 1997; 39: 453–457

[34] Saunders JE, Derebery MJ, Lo WW. Magnetic resonance imaging of cochlear otosclerosis. Ann Otol Rhinol Laryngol 1995; 104: 826–829

[35] Goh JP, Chan LL, Tan TY. MRI of cochlear otosclerosis. Br J Radiol 2002; 75: 502–505

[36] Crain MR, Dolan KD. Internal auditory canal enlargement in Paget's disease appearing as bilateral acoustic neuromas. Ann Otol Rhinol Laryngol 1990; 99: 833–834

[37] Alkadhi H, Rissmann D, Kollias SS. Osteogenesis imperfecta of the temporal bone: CT and MR imaging in Van der Hoeve-de Kleyn syndrome. AJNR Am J Neuroradiol 2004; 25: 1106–1109

[38] Lemmerling MM, De Foer B, Verbist BM, VandeVyver V. Imaging of inflammatory and infectious diseases in the temporal bone. Neuroimaging Clin N Am 2009; 19: 321–337

[39] Ball JB, Jr, Miller GW, Hepfner ST. Computed tomography of single-channel cochlear implants. AJNR Am J Neuroradiol 1986; 7: 41–47

[40] Swartz JD, Mandell DM, Faerber EN et al. Labyrinthine ossification: etiologies and CT findings. Radiology 1985; 157: 395–398

[41] Arriaga MA, Carrier D. MRI and clinical decisions in cochlear implantation. Am J Otol 1996; 17: 547–553

[42] Mafee MF, Lachenauer CS, Kumar A, Arnold PM, Buckingham RA, Valvassori GECT. CT and MR imaging of intralabyrinthine schwannoma: report of two cases and review of the literature. Radiology 1990; 174: 395–400

[43] Mark AS, Fitzgerald D. Segmental enhancement of the cochlea on contrast-enhanced MR: correlation with the frequency of hearing loss and possible sign of perilymphatic fistula and autoimmune labyrinthitis. AJNR Am J Neuroradiol 1993; 14: 991–996

[44] Stillman AE, Remley K, Loes DJ, Hu X, Latchaw RE. Steady-state free precession imaging of the inner ear. AJNR Am J Neuroradiol 1994; 15: 348–350

[45] Casselman JW, Kuhweide R, Deimling M, Ampe W, Dehaene I, Meeus L. Constructive interference in steady state-3DFT MR imaging of the inner ear and cerebellopontine angle. AJNR Am J Neuroradiol 1993; 14: 47–57

[46] Casselman JW, Kuhweide R, Ampe W, Meeus L, Steyaert L. Pathology of the membranous labyrinth: comparison of T1- and T2-weighted and gadolinium-enhanced spin-echo and 3DFT-CISS imaging. AJNR Am J Neuroradiol 1993; 14: 59–69

[47] Mark AS, Seltzer S, Harnsberger HR. Sensorineural hearing loss: more than meets the eye? AJNR Am J Neuroradiol 1993; 14: 37–45

[48] Tien RD, Felsberg GJ, Macfall J. Fast spin-echo high-resolution MR imaging of the inner ear. AJR Am J Roentgenol 1992; 159: 395–398

[49] Seltzer S, Mark AS. Contrast enhancement of the labyrinth on MR scans in patients with sudden hearing loss and vertigo: evidence of labyrinthine disease. AJNR Am J Neuroradiol 1991; 12: 13–16

[50] Harnsberger HR, Dart DJ, Parkin JL, Smoker WR, Osborn AG. Cochlear implant candidates: assessment with CT and MR imaging. Radiology 1987; 164: 53–57

[51] Brogan M, Chakeres DW, Schmalbrock P. High-resolution 3DFT MR imaging of the endolymphatic duct and soft tissues of the otic capsule. AJNR Am J Neuroradiol 1991; 12: 1–11

[52] Kim HJ, Song JW, Chon KM, Goh EK. Common crus aplasia: diagnosis by 3D volume rendering imaging using 3DFT-CISS sequence. Clin Radiol 2004; 59: 830–834

[53] Dahlen RT, Harnsberger HR, Gray SD et al. Overlapping thin-section fast spin-echo MR of the large vestibular aqueduct syndrome. AJNR Am J Neuroradiol 1997; 18: 67–75

[54] Fitzgerald DC, Mark AS. Sudden hearing loss: frequency of abnormal findings on contrast-enhanced MR studies. AJNR Am J Neuroradiol 1998; 19: 1433–1436

[55] Lemmerling M, Vanzieleghem B, Dhooge I, Van Cauwenberge P, Kunnen MCT. CT and MRI of the semicircular canals in the normal and diseased temporal bone. Eur Radiol 2001; 11: 1210–1219

[56] Naganawa S, Koshikawa T, Nakamura T, Fukatsu H, Ishigaki T, Aoki I. High-resolution T1-weighted 3D real IR imaging of the temporal bone using triple-dose contrast material. Eur Radiol 2003; 13: 2650–2658

[57] Guirado CR, Martínez P, Roig R et al. Three-dimensional MR of the inner ear with steady-state free precession. AJNR Am J Neuroradiol 1995; 16: 1909–1913

[58] Held P, Fellner C, Fellner F, Seitz J, Strutz J. MRI of inner ear anatomy using 3D MP-RAGE and 3D CISS sequences. Br J Radiol 1997; 70: 465–472

[59] Stone JA, Chakeres DW, Schmalbrock P. High-resolution MR imaging of the auditory pathway. Magn Reson Imaging Clin N Am 1998; 6: 195–217

[60] Naganawa S, Satake H, Iwano S, Fukatsu H, Sone M, Nakashima T. Imaging endolymphatic hydrops at 3 tesla using 3D-FLAIR with intratympanic Gd-DTPA administration. Magn Reson Med Sci 2008; 7: 85–91

[61] Naganawa S, Yamazaki M, Kawai H, Bokura K, Sone M, Nakashima T. Visualization of endolymphatic hydrops in Ménière's disease with single-dose intravenous gadolinium-based contrast media using heavily T-weighted 3D-FLAIR. Magn Reson Med Sci 2010; 9: 237–242

[62] Sartoretti-Schefer S, Wichmann W, Valavanis A. Idiopathic, herpetic, and HIV-associated facial nerve palsies: abnormal MR enhancement patterns. AJNR Am J Neuroradiol 1994; 15: 479–485

[63] Han MH, Jabour BA, Andrews JC et al. Nonneoplastic enhancing lesions mimicking intracanalicular acoustic neuroma on gadolinium-enhanced MR images. Radiology 1991; 179: 795–796

[64] Madden GJ, Sirimanna KS. Cavernous hemangioma of the internal auditory meatus. J Otolaryngol 1990; 19: 288–291

[65] Atlas MD, Fagan PA, Turner J. Calcification of internal auditory canal tumors. Ann Otol Rhinol Laryngol 1992; 101: 620–622

[66] Lakshmi M, Glastonbury CM. Imaging of the cerebellopontine angle. Neuroimaging Clin N Am 2009; 19: 393–406

[67] Kang M, Escott E. Imaging of tinnitus. Otolaryngol Clin North Am 2008; 41: 179–193, viivii.

[68] Remley KB, Coit WE, Harnsberger HR, Smoker WR, Jacobs JM, McIff EB. Pulsatile tinnitus and the vascular tympanic membrane: CT, MR, and angiographic findings. Radiology 1990; 174: 383–389

[69] Lo WW, Solti-Bohman LG. High-resolution CT of the jugular foramen: anatomy and vascular variants and anomalies. Radiology 1984; 150: 743–747

[70] Press GA, Hesselink JR. MR imaging of cerebellopontine angle and internal auditory canal lesions at 1.5 T. AJR Am J Roentgenol 1988; 150: 1371–1381

[71] Julien J, Bismuth P, Martin N, Molas G, Sterkers O. [Hemangioma of the petrous bone. Diagnosis and treatment] Ann Otolaryngol Chir Cervicofac 1992; 109: 335–340

[72] Salzman KL, Davidson HC, Harnsberger HR et al. Dumbbell schwannomas of the internal auditory canal. AJNR Am J Neuroradiol 2001; 22: 1368–1376

[73] Sanna M, Zini C, Gamoletti R, Pasanisi E. Primary intratemporal tumours of the facial nerve: diagnosis and treatment. J Laryngol Otol 1990; 104: 765–771

[74] Linskey ME, Lunsford LD, Flickinger JC. Neuroimaging of acoustic nerve sheath tumors after stereotaxic radiosurgery. AJNR Am J Neuroradiol 1991; 12: 1165–1175

[75] Mueller DP, Gantz BJ, Dolan KD. Gadolinium-enhanced MR of the postoperative internal auditory canal following acoustic neuroma resection via the middle fossa approach. AJNR Am J Neuroradiol 1992; 13: 197–200

[76] Litt AW, Kondo N, Bannon KR, Kricheff II. Role of slice thickness in MR imaging of the internal auditory canal. J Comput Assist Tomogr 1990; 14: 717–720

[77] Greenberg JJ, Oot RF, Wismer GL et al. Cholesterol granuloma of the petrous apex: MR and CT evaluation. AJNR Am J Neuroradiol 1988; 9: 1205–1214

[78] Griffin C, DeLaPaz R, Enzmann DMR. MR and CT correlation of cholesterol cysts of the petrous bone. AJNR Am J Neuroradiol 1987; 8: 825–829

[79] Latack JT, Graham MD, Kemink JL, Knake JE. Giant cholesterol cysts of the petrous apex: radiologic features. AJNR Am J Neuroradiol 1985; 6: 409–413

[80] Goldofsky E, Hoffman RA, Holliday RA, Cohen NL. Cholesterol cysts of the temporal bone: diagnosis and treatment. Ann Otol Rhinol Laryngol 1991; 100: 181–187

[81] Rosenberg RA, Hammerschlag PE, Cohen NL, Bergeron RT, Reede DL. Cholesteatoma vs. cholesterol granuloma of the petrous apex. Otolaryngol Head Neck Surg 1986; 94: 322–327

[82] Chapman PR, Shah R, Curé JK, Bag AK. Petrous apex lesions: pictorial review. AJR Am J Roentgenol 2011; 196 Suppl: WS26–WS37, Quiz S40–S43

[83] Gore MR, Zanation AM, Ebert CS, Senior BA. Cholesterol granuloma of the petrous apex. Otolaryngol Clin North Am 2011; 44: 1043–1058

[84] Connor SE, Leung R, Natas S. Imaging of the petrous apex: a pictorial review. Br J Radiol 2008; 81: 427–435

[85] Morrison GA, Dilkes MG. Cholesterol cyst and cholesterol granuloma of the petrous bone. J Laryngol Otol 1992; 106: 465–467

[86] Latack JT, Kartush JM, Kemink JL, Graham MD, Knake JE. Epidermoidomas of the cerebellopontine angle and temporal bone: CT and MR aspects. Radiology 1985; 157: 361–366

[87] Clifton AG, Phelps PD, Brookes GB. Cholesterol granuloma of the petrous apex. Br J Radiol 1990; 63: 724–726

[88] Horowitz SW, Leonetti JP, Azar-Kia B, Fine M, Izquierdo RCT. CT and MR of temporal bone malignancies primary and secondary to parotid carcinoma. AJNR Am J Neuroradiol 1994; 15: 755–762

[89] Lo WW, Applegate LJ, Carberry JN et al. Endolymphatic sac tumors: radiologic appearance. Radiology 1993; 189: 199–204

[90] Birzgalis AR, Ramsden RT, Lye RH, Richardson PL. Haemangiopericytoma of the temporal bone. J Laryngol Otol 1990; 104: 998–1003

[91] Han JS, Huss RG, Benson JE et al. MR imaging of the skull base. J Comput Assist Tomogr 1984; 8: 944–952

[92] Borges A. Imaging of the central skull base. Neuroimaging Clin N Am 2009; 19: 669–696

[93] De Foer B, Kenis C, Vercruysse JP et al. Imaging of temporal bone tumors. Neuroimaging Clin N Am 2009; 19: 339–366

[94] Ginsberg LE, Pruett SW, Chen MY, Elster AD. Skull-base foramina of the middle cranial fossa: reassessment of normal variation with high-resolution CT. AJNR Am J Neuroradiol 1994; 15: 283–291

[95] Daniels DL, Williams AL, Haughton VM. Jugular foramen: anatomic and computed tomographic study. AJR Am J Roentgenol 1984; 142: 153–158

[96] Lanzieri CF, Duchesneau PM, Rosenbloom SA, Smith AS, Rosenbaum AE. The significance of asymmetry of the foramen of Vesalius. AJNR Am J Neuroradiol 1988; 9: 1201–1204

[97] Ginsberg LE. Neoplastic diseases affecting the central skull base: CT and MR imaging. AJR Am J Roentgenol 1992; 159: 581–589

[98] Meyers SP, Hirsch WL, Jr, Curtin HD, Barnes L, Sekhar LN, Sen C. Chondrosarcomas of the skull base: MR imaging features. Radiology 1992; 184: 103–108

[99] Brown RV, Sage MR, Brophy BPCT. CT and MR findings in patients with chordomas of the petrous apex. AJNR Am J Neuroradiol 1990; 11: 121–124

[100] Daniels DL, Czervionke LF, Pech P et al. Gradient recalled echo MR imaging of the jugular foramen. AJNR Am J Neuroradiol 1988; 9: 675–678

[101] Laine FJ, Braun IF, Jensen ME, Nadel L, Som PM. Perineural tumor extension through the foramen ovale: evaluation with MR imaging. Radiology 1990; 174: 65–71

[102] Oot RF, Melville GE, New PF et al. The role of MR and CT in evaluating clival chordomas and chondrosarcomas. AJR Am J Roentgenol 1988; 151: 567–575

[103] Laine FJ, Nadel L, Braun IFCT. CT and MR imaging of the central skull base. Part 2. Pathologic spectrum. Radiographics 1990; 10: 797–821

[104] West MS, Russell EJ, Breit R, Sze G, Kim KS. Calvarial and skull base metastases: comparison of nonenhanced and Gd-DTPA-enhanced MR images. Radiology 1990; 174: 85–91

[105] Meyers SP, Hirsch WL, Jr, Curtin HD, Barnes L, Sekhar LN, Sen C. Chordomas of the skull base: MR features. AJNR Am J Neuroradiol 1992; 13: 1627–1636

[106] Sze G, Uichanco LS, III, Brant-Zawadzki MN et al. Chordomas: MR imaging. Radiology 1988; 166: 187–191

[107] Lipper MH, Cail WS. Chordoma of the petrous bone. South Med J 1991; 84: 629–631

[108] Koutourousiou M, Snyderman CH, Fernandez-Miranda J, Gardner PA. Skull base chordomas. Otolaryngol Clin North Am 2011; 44: 1155–1171

[109] Duncan AW, Lack EE, Deck MF. Radiological evaluation of paragangliomas of the head and neck. Radiology 1979; 132: 99–105

[110] Chakeres DW, LaMasters DL. Paragangliomas of the temporal bone: high-resolution CT studies. Radiology 1984; 150: 749–753

[111] Lo WW, Solti-Bohman LG, Lambert PR. High-resolution CT in the evaluation of glomus tumors of the temporal bone. Radiology 1984; 150: 737–742

[112] Curtin HD. Radiologic approach to paragangliomas of the temporal bone. Radiology 1984; 150: 837–838

[113] Larson TC, III, Reese DF, Baker HL, Jr, McDonald TJ. Glomus tympanicum chemodectomas: radiographic and clinical characteristics. Radiology 1987; 163: 801–806

[114] Phelps PD, Cheesman AD. Imaging jugulotympanic glomus tumors. Arch Otolaryngol Head Neck Surg 1990; 116: 940–945

[115] Rubinstein D, Burton BS, Walker AL. The anatomy of the inferior petrosal sinus, glossopharyngeal nerve, vagus nerve, and accessory nerve in the jugular foramen. AJNR Am J Neuroradiol 1995; 16: 185–194

[116] Ong CK, Fook-Hin Chong V. Imaging of jugular foramen. Neuroimaging Clin N Am 2009; 19: 469–482

[117] Whiteman ML, Serafini AN, Telischi FF, Civantos FJ, Falcone S. 111 In octreotide scintigraphy in the evaluation of head and neck lesions. AJNR Am J Neuroradiol 1997; 18: 1073–1080

[118] Schmalfuss IM. Petrous apex. Neuroimaging Clin N Am 2009; 19: 367–391

[119] Avrahami E, Chen Z, Solomon A. Modern high resolution computed tomography (CT) diagnosis of longitudinal fractures of the petrous bone. Neuroradiology 1988; 30: 166–168

[120] Zimmerman RA, Bilaniuk LT, Hackney DB, Goldberg HI, Grossman RI. Magnetic resonance imaging in temporal bone fracture. Neuroradiology 1987; 29: 246–251

[121] Swartz JD, Zwillenberg S, Berger AS. Acquired disruptions of the incudostapedial articulation: diagnosis with CT. Radiology 1989; 171: 779–781

[122] Betz BW, Wiener MD. Air in the temporomandibular joint fossa: CT sign of temporal bone fracture. Radiology 1991; 180: 463–466

[123] Saraiya PV, Aygun N. Temporal bone fractures. Emerg Radiol 2009; 16: 255–265

[124] Johnson F, Semaan MT, Megerian CA. Temporal bone fracture: evaluation and management in the modern era. Otolaryngol Clin North Am 2008; 41: 597

[125] Gladwell M, Viozzi C. Temporal bone fractures: a review for the oral and maxillofacial surgeon. J Oral Maxillofac Surg 2008; 66: 513–522

[126] Rogers FB, Baker EF, Osler TM, Shackford SR, Wald SL, Vieco P. Computed tomographic angiography as a screening modality for blunt cervical arterial injuries: preliminary results. J Trauma 1999; 46: 380–385

[127] Munera F, Soto JA, Palacio D, Velez SM, Medina E. Diagnosis of arterial injuries caused by penetrating trauma to the neck: comparison of helical CT angiography and conventional angiography. Radiology 2000; 216: 356–362

8 Diagnostic Audiology

Lisa L. Hunter and David K. Brown

8.1 Introduction

Patients who present with hearing problems are most effectively evaluated with a combined medical-audiological approach. The basic audiological test battery is composed of behavioral techniques that require patients to respond to pure-tone or speech stimuli. Physiological tests are also used that do not require active participation by the patient.

8.2 Pure-Tone Audiometry

Pure-tone audiometry is the most fundamental component of the audiological evaluation. Results from pure-tone testing are used to (1) determine the severity of hearing loss; (2) diagnose the type of hearing loss (i.e., conductive, sensory, neural, or mixed) by comparing air- and bone-conduction thresholds as well as results of physiological tests; (3) describe the configuration of hearing loss (i.e., pattern of pure-tone thresholds from low to high frequencies); (4) determine the intensity levels at which other audiological procedures will be performed; (5) determine the need for rehabilitative treatment; and (6) evaluate effects of surgery or treatment. Pure-tone audiometry is based on obtaining a series of thresholds at various pure-tone frequencies. Threshold is defined as the lowest intensity at which the patient is able to respond to the stimulus 50% of the time (e. g., two out of four trials). Thresholds are routinely assessed at octave frequency intervals, for example, 250, 500, 1,000, 2,000, 4,000, and 8,000 Hz. Pure-tone thresholds are obtained using an audiometer that is calibrated to specifications established by the American National Standards Institute to ensure the validity and reliability of test results.[1] Pure-tone air and bone thresholds are recorded on the audiogram, with frequency displayed on the abscissa and intensity in dB HL (hearing level) on the ordinate. ▶ Fig. 8.1 shows two audiograms with their associated symbol set used to document patient responses.

▶ Fig. 8.1a is used for adults with a normal range of –10 to 25 dB HL, and ▶ Fig. 8.1b is used for children with a lower normative range (–10 to 15 dB HL). Children require better hearing thresholds in order to develop optimal speech, language, and academic skills.[2] Air-conduction thresholds are measured using supra-aural earphones or insert phones that assess the entire peripheral auditory system including the conductive (outer ear and middle ear), cochlear, and neural pathways (eighth cranial nerve, brainstem, and cortical regions). In contrast, bone-conduction thresholds are measured using a vibratory bone oscillator placed on the mastoid or forehead. Comparison of air and bone conduction audiometry provides a measure of cochlear reserve. Extended high-frequency thresholds at frequencies greater than 8,000 Hz may be measured using specialized earphones.[3] Hearing in extended high frequencies is strongly age-related, and this frequency range is sensitive to noise, ototoxicity, and cochlear damage due to chronic otitis media.

8.3 Audiogram Interpretation

Obtaining and interpreting valid and reliable pure-tone thresholds requires a trained and experienced clinician. Automated software has been developed that can aid in obtaining accurate audiometry more efficiently, but it cannot replace the interpretive skill of an experienced, licensed audiologist.[4] Variables such as patient understanding and motivation, false-positive or false-negative responses, cerumen blockages, collapsed ear canals, equipment malfunction, ambient noise in the test environment, and earphone/bone-oscillator placement can influence the results and must be controlled. The degree of hearing loss is expressed using the average of 500, 1,000, and 2,000 Hz, known as the *pure-tone average* (PTA). Alternatively, the two best thresholds of 500, 1,000, and 2,000 Hz are often more consistent with the speech reception threshold (SRT) for sloping hearing losses. ▶ Table 8.1 shows a classification scheme that is appropriate for adults; however, minimal hearing loss between 15 to 25 dB HL can have negative effects on academic performance of children.

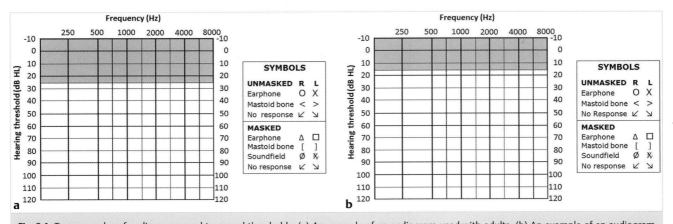

Fig. 8.1 Two examples of audiograms used to record thresholds. (a) An example of an audiogram used with adults. (b) An example of an audiogram used with children. Note the difference in the shaded area, which represents the range of normal hearing.

Table 8.1 Hearing Loss Classification Scheme Based on Pure-Tone Average (PTA; 500, 1,000, 2,000 Hz) and Associated Communication Difficulty

PTA (in dB HL)	Category	Communication Difficulty
0–25	Normal	No significant difficulty
26–40	Mild	Difficulty understanding soft-spoken speech
41–55	Moderate	An understanding of speech at 3 to 5 feet
56–70	Moderately severe	Speech must be loud for auditory reception; significant difficulty in group settings
71–90	Severe	Loud speech may be understood at 1 foot from the ear; may distinguish vowel but not consonant sounds
90 +	Profound	Does not rely on audition as primary mode of communication

Adapted with permission from Roeser RJ, Buckley KA, Stickney GS. Pure tone test. In: Roeser RJ, Valente M, Hosford-Dunn H, eds. Audiology Diagnosis. New York: Thieme, 2000:239.
HL: hearing level (referring to the ANSI-1996 scale).

8.4 Type of Hearing Loss

There are three main types of hearing loss: conductive, sensorineural, and mixed. The type can be determined by comparing air-conduction thresholds to bone-conduction thresholds for each ear, as shown in ▶ Fig. 8.2. The difference between the air- and bone-conduction thresholds or the *air–bone gap* reflects the degree of the conductive component contributing to the overall hearing loss. Conductive hearing loss is caused by disorders of the outer ear and/or middle ear, with normal bone-conduction threshold responses, and air-conduction thresholds falling outside the normal limits. Sensory or cochlear hearing loss involves damage to portions of the cochlea, such as the outer or inner hair cells or stria vascularis. Sensory hearing loss is characterized by relatively equal (i.e., within 10 dB) air- and bone-conduction thresholds, both outside normal limits. Mixed hearing loss is a combination of middle-ear and cochlear hearing loss with elevation of both the air- and bone-conduction thresholds as well as air–bone gaps.

Auditory neuropathy spectrum disorder (ANSD) is a heterogeneous auditory disorder that is characterized by sensorineural hearing loss that is variable in degree and shape, absent or abnormal auditory brainstem responses, and preserved otoacoustic emissions or cochlear microphonics. This combination of test results indicates relatively normal function of cochlear outer hair cells. Thus, the primary lesion might be located in the inner hair cells, in the auditory nerve or in the intervening synapse.[5] A key feature of ANSD is very poor speech intelligibility, poorer than predicted by the PTA, which is postulated to be caused by dyssynchronous neural responses.[6]

8.5 Speech Audiometry

Speech audiometry is useful for cross-checking the validity of pure-tone thresholds, quantifying suprathreshold speech recognition, estimating communication function, and evaluating the benefit of rehabilitative interventions. Speech reception threshold (SRT), speech awareness threshold (SAT), and suprathreshold word recognition testing (WRT) in quiet and noise are the primary tests used routinely. Similar to pure-tone thresholds, the SRT is the lowest hearing level at which the patient can correctly recognize two-syllable words 50% of the time. Young children or others who cannot repeat back the words can respond using pictured items. There is close agreement between the patient's PTA and SRT. Discrepancy in the SRT compared to the PTA may occur due to functional or nonorganic hearing loss, eighth cranial nerve disorders, sloping hearing loss, or cognitive or language disorders. Word recognition testing uses monosyllabic phonetically balanced (PB) words that contain all of the phonetic elements of connected discourse representative of everyday English speech. The most popular 50-item word lists are the Central Institute for the Deaf (CID) Auditory Test W-22 and the Northwestern University Test No. 6.

For standardization purposes, these word lists are presented in quiet conditions using commercially available recordings rather than "live voice" presentations, and using an "open response" format wherein the patient repeats the word verbally. Word recognition scores are expressed as the percentage of words correctly repeated from the 50 (full) or 25 (one-half) word lists and are used to estimate speech understanding ability. For example, word recognition scores of 90 to 100% are classified as excellent, 80 to 88% good, 70 to 78% fair, and below 70% is poor. For patients with normal hearing sensitivity, PB Max occurs at or near 100% when the words are presented at 35 to 40 dB SL. Patients with conductive hearing loss perform similarly to normal individuals once the intensity level of the signal is increased to overcome the reduction in audibility caused by the conductive component. For patients with cochlear disorders, PB Max is generally reduced and is consistent with the severity of hearing loss. Further, no significant decline is expected in the word recognition score as intensity levels are increased. In contrast, patients with eighth cranial nerve disorders may show word recognition scores disproportionately poorer in relationship to the severity of hearing loss.

Speech recognition tests in noise have been developed to better estimate speech understanding using word or sentence materials in the presence of a competing background noise. Tests such as the Bamford-Kawal-Bench Speech in Noise (BKB-SIN) and the Words-in-Noise (WIN) test use an adaptive method of seeking the signal-to-noise ratio for a given percent correct, which has better sensitivity and reliability than a single-intensity level test scored as percent correct.[7]

8.6 Clinical Masking

Masking noise may be required during pure-tone and speech audiometry to eliminate the participation of the nontest ear when evaluating the test ear. Unless the examiner uses

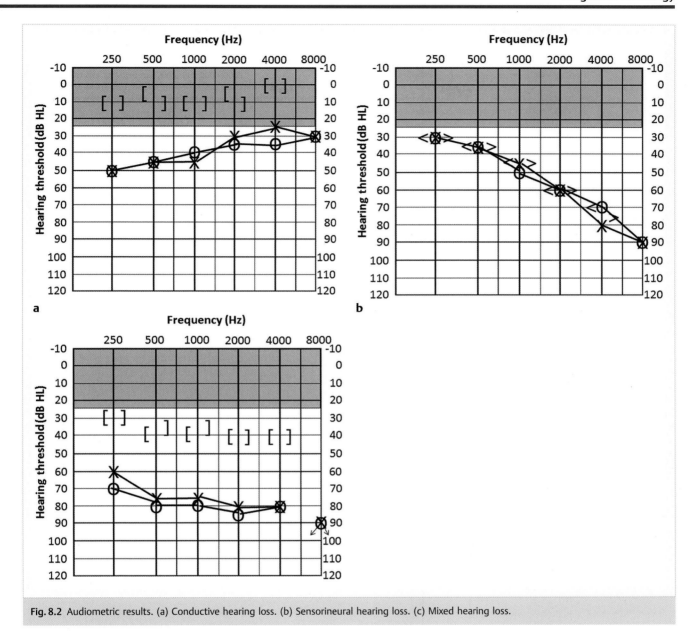

Fig. 8.2 Audiometric results. (a) Conductive hearing loss. (b) Sensorineural hearing loss. (c) Mixed hearing loss.

appropriate masking levels and procedures, serious errors in diagnosing the type and severity of hearing loss may occur. For example, a sensorineural loss may appear as conductive loss, or a profound loss may be viewed as a moderate loss. When a signal is presented to the poorer test ear at a sufficiently loud intensity level, it may cross over to the opposite ear and be perceived by that ear.

8.7 Immittance Measurement

Acoustic immittance measurements are considered a routine component of the audiological test battery, serving at least two primary functions: (1) detecting middle ear disorders, and (2) differentiating cochlear from retrocochlear disorders. *Acoustic immittance* is a general term referring to acoustic impedance, or opposition to energy flow (Za), and acoustic admittance, or

ease of energy flow (Ya). Most commercially available immittance instrumentation measures Ya. Tympanometry is a dynamic measure of immittance in the ear canal as a function of changes in air pressure in the ear canal above and below atmospheric pressure. A tympanogram is a graphical display of acoustic admittance, displayed on the y-axis, relative to ear canal air pressure, displayed on the x-axis. Ear canal pressure is expressed in units called deca-pascals (daPa). The unit of immittance is the millimho (mmho). Tympanometry typically is measured at a single, low-frequency probe tone (e.g., 226 Hz). Higher frequency probe tones have been studied, and better sensitivity and specificity are achieved for detection of middle ear dysfunction using probe tones of 1,000 or higher in newborns.[8]

The peak height of the tympanogram, also known as compensated static acoustic admittance, is sensitive to many

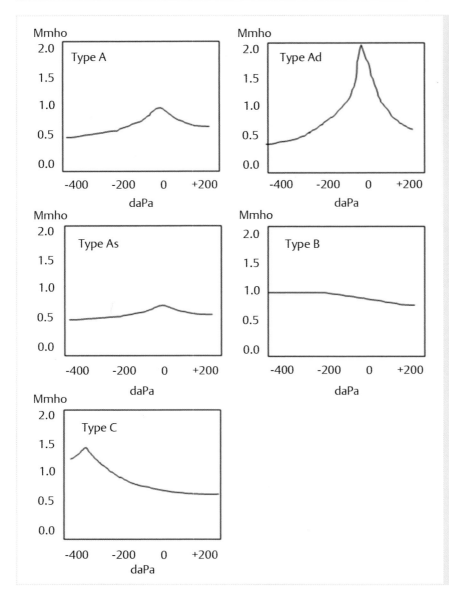

Fig. 8.3 Examples of tympanograms for each of the main types. Type A has normal admittance, width, and peak pressure. Type Ad has abnormally increased admittance. Type As has low peak admittance. Type B is flattened admittance with no peak and broad admittance. Type C has negative pressure and may or may not have normal admittance and width.

different middle ear conditions, including otitis media effusion, chronic otitis media sequelae such as cholesteatoma and ossicular adhesions, and cholesteatoma. Tympanometric width (TW) is the width of the tympanogram (in daPa) measured at half of the height from the peak to the tail. Abnormally wide TW is considered an indication of middle ear dysfunction.[9,10] Equivalent ear canal volume (Vea) is an estimate of the volume air trapped between the probe tip and the tympanic membrane. In the presence of a flat tympanogram, a large Vea is useful for detecting tympanic membrane perforations or patency of tympanostomy tubes. Normative ranges should be used for consistency and reliability in classification.[11] Traditionally, tympanograms have been described using a typing system (▶ Fig. 8.3).

8.8 Acoustic Reflex Testing

Measuring acoustic reflexes for differential diagnosis purposes is especially helpful in (1) confirming middle ear disease; (2) distinguishing between sensory (cochlear) and neural (eighth nerve) disease; (3) identifying lower brainstem pathology; and (4) identifying the site of a facial nerve lesion. The acoustic reflex threshold is defined as the lowest intensity level at which a change in middle ear admittance can be detected in response to sound. Acoustic reflexes are measured by assessing changes in acoustic admittance of the ear caused by a contraction of the stapedius muscle. The reflex is a bilateral phenomenon that occurs when a high-intensity stimulus (i.e., usually 80 dB HL or greater) is presented to either ear of a patient with normal hearing to moderate cochlear hearing loss, causing the stapedius muscle to contract bilaterally. For bilateral middle ear disorders, acoustic reflexes typically are absent when both ipsilateral and contralateral ears are stimulated with the acoustic signal. In cases of a unilateral conductive disorder, stimulation of the unaffected ear elicits an ipsilateral reflex, whereas the occurrence of a reflex caused by stimulating the contralateral affected ear is determined by the severity of the conductive hearing loss in that abnormal ear.

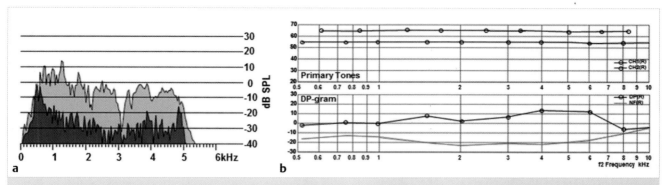

Fig. 8.4 Example of OAEs obtained from adults with normal hearing. (a) Transient evoked otoacoustic emission (TEOAE). The dark response shows the noise floor (NF), and the gray response is the transient evoked (TE) emission. (b) Distortion product otoacoustic emission (DPOAE). The levels (in dB SPL) of the two primary tones (F1 and F2) are shown in the top plot (CH1 and CH2). In the lower plot, O is the distortion-product (DP) response and the line below it is the noise floor (NF).

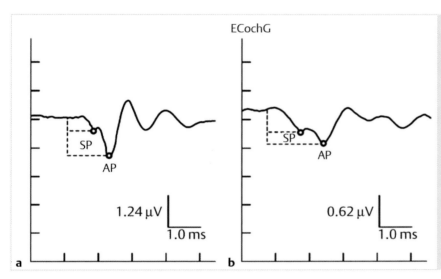

Fig. 8.5 Example of electrocochleography (ECochG) recordings from (a) a normal ear and (b) a patient with Ménière disease showing an enlarged SP/AP ratio. SP, summating potential; AP, whole-nerve action potential.

Acoustic reflex thresholds in ears with cochlear disorders are determined by the degree of sensory hearing loss. For cochlear hearing loss < 80 dB HL, acoustic reflex thresholds may be present but at reduced sensation levels relative to hearing level. In contrast, reflexes are usually absent when audiometric thresholds exceed 80 dB HL. In cranial nerve VII disorders and in particular for auditory neuropathy, acoustic reflexes are generally elevated or absent with stimulation to the affected ear regardless of the degree of loss.[12] In cranial nerve VIII disorders, rapid decay to less than 50% of baseline may be observed if the stimulus is presented for 5 to 10 seconds. In facial nerve disorders, acoustic reflexes are abnormal or absent when the probe is placed in the ear with facial nerve paralysis. Acoustic reflex responses are affected only if the site of the lesion is central to the innervation at the stapedius muscle. Patients with brainstem disorders may demonstrate normal ipsilateral reflexes with abnormalities in contralateral reflex measures. The exact site and size of the brainstem disorder influences the crossed and uncrossed reflex patterns.

8.9 Otoacoustic Emissions

Otoacoustic emissions (OAEs) are low-intensity sounds generated by the cochlea that emanate into the middle ear and are detected in the ear canal by a microphone. They are considered by-products of outer hair cell motility, thereby providing an objective noninvasive technique for assessing preneural cochlear function. Applications of OAE include (1) newborn and infant hearing screening and assessment;[13] (2) cross-checks for behavioral testing in difficult-to-test patients;[13] (3) assessment of cochlear hearing losses;[14] and (4) ototoxicity monitoring.[15] There are two types of evoked OAEs: transient-evoked otoacoustic emissions (TEOAE) and distortion-product otoacoustic emissions (DPOAE). TEOAEs use time-synchronous averaging techniques and are accomplished using an 80- to 85-dB sound pressure level (SPL) click that stimulates a wide range of frequencies, but the response (▶ Fig. 8.4a) can be analyzed to provide frequency-specific information. In response to the presentation of a pair of primary tones (i.e., F1 and F2), the outer hair cells generate a response due to nonlinearities called the distortion product, the most robust of which occurs at a frequency equal to 2f1 – f2. When emissions are present, as illustrated in ▶ Fig. 8.4b, it is likely that outer hair cells are functioning in the frequency region of the F2. In general, OAEs will be absent when cochlear hearing loss exceeds approximately 30 dB HL. A conductive hearing loss may prevent an OAE response, but it may be present with patent tympanostomy tubes. OAEs provide an objective measure of preneural cochlear function, thereby assisting in the differentiation between sensory and neural dysfunction.

8.10 Auditory Evoked Potential Measurement

Auditory evoked potentials (AEPs) are a series of bioelectric responses recorded from the scalp and reflect neural synchrony and transmission in the auditory system. The obtained waveforms consist of a series of peaks and troughs (i.e., wave components) that can be quantified by amplitude and latency measures. The two most clinically used AEPs are electrocochleography (ECochG) and the auditory brainstem response (ABR).

8.11 Electrocochleography

The ECochG response arises in the first 2 or 3 ms following an abrupt signal onset and it is recorded using noninvasive extratympanic or tympanic membrane electrodes. ▶ Fig. 8.5a shows a normal ECochG waveform that consists of two cochlear potentials, the summating potential (SP) and compound action potential (AP) of the eighth cranial nerve. Although the exact source of the SP is unknown, it is attributed to distortion products associated with basilar membrane and hair cell displacement. The AP arises from the distal portion of the eighth cranial nerve. The primary clinical application of ECochG is for the diagnosis and monitoring of Ménière disease/endolymphatic hydrops.[16] This is accomplished by comparing the amplitude relationships between the SP and AP, forming the SP/AP ratio. ▶ Fig. 8.5b illustrates an abnormal ECochG reflected by an abnormally large SP in comparison to the AP (SP/AP ratio). An SP/AP ratio of 0.45 or greater is considered abnormal, suggesting increased labyrinth pressure. In addition, ECochG is used as an enhancement technique for wave I of the ABR when the patient has significant hearing loss or when recording conditions are less than optimal. ECochG recordings have been used intraoperatively, which can be helpful for monitoring cochlear and auditory nerve function during surgical procedures involving the auditory periphery.[17]

8.12 Auditory Brainstem Response

The auditory brainstem response (ABR) occurs during the first 10 ms following a rapid-onset signal, such as a click. As shown in ▶ Fig. 8.6, the response is composed of a series of vertex-positive waves. Waves I and II are generated by the distal and proximal portions of the eighth cranial nerve. It is generally agreed the latter responses have multiple generator sites; however, wave III represents the cochlear nucleus, wave IV the superior

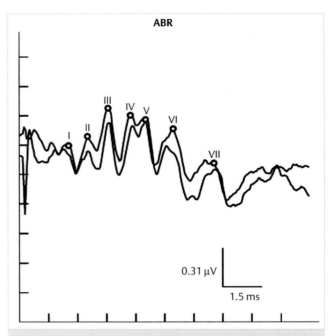

Fig. 8.6 Example of an auditory brainstem response (ABR) recording obtained from a normal ear. The individual waves of the ABR are labeled with roman numerals I to VII.

olivary complex with input from the cochlear nucleus and lateral lemniscus, and wave V is associated with the termination of fibers from the lateral lemniscus into the inferior colliculus. The ABR has two main uses when testing a patient, either threshold estimation or neurologic testing. ABR is used to evaluate the neurologic integrity of the eighth cranial nerve and brainstem pathways,[18] and to estimate peripheral hearing sensitivity of patients who cannot cooperate with behavioral testing, such as children or individuals with developmental delay.[19]

For neurologic applications, ABR interpretation is based on latencies for waves I, III, and V, wherein absolute latency values, interaural differences, interwave differences, and absent waveforms serve as diagnostic indices. However, there is not any one ABR pattern that is diagnostic for a particular disease process. ▶ Fig. 8.6 shows standard ABR latency measures, which are valuable in detecting extracanalicular and intracanalicular tumors larger than 1.0 cm; however, smaller tumors often go undetected using standard clinical techniques. ABR is also useful for neurophysiological monitoring of surgical procedures that place hearing at risk. During the surgical procedure, ABR responses are compared with the baseline recordings. For example, wave V latency shifts of 1 ms or greater and amplitude reduction for wave V of greater than 50% have been considered clinically significant changes from baseline. According to Hall,[20] hearing preservation is best for patients with small tumors (less than 1.5 cm) and intact hearing (PTA of 30 dB or better and word recognition scores better that 70%).[20]

Auditory brainstem response testing is not a true test of hearing, but it is highly correlated with hearing thresholds. With the worldwide acceptance of newborn hearing screening, ABR provides a reliable method of estimating normal hearing for infants at risk for hearing loss. The process of hearing sensitivity

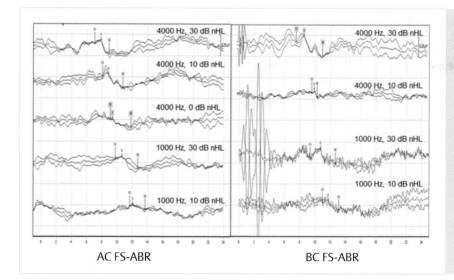

Fig. 8.7 Examples of FS-ABR responses at threshold from an infant showing wave V at 1 and 4 kHz utilizing air- (AC) and bone-conduction (BC) stimuli.

prediction is a determination of the lowest level at which wave V of the ABR can be identified. Frequency-specific ABR (FS-ABR) thresholds utilizing both air- and bone-conduction are determined from 500 to 4,000 Hz using frequency-specific tone bursts (▸ Fig. 8.7). The ABR response is best used as a cross-check principle to verify threshold with other audiological measures such as OAEs, tympanograms, and behavioral audiometry.

8.13 Conclusion

Diagnostic audiology is dependent on examining relationships among the behavioral and physiological measures employed during the test session. Each procedure adds a piece of information to the audiological picture of the patient. Diagnostic procedures, especially those capitalizing on physiological responses to auditory signals, continue to be refined, and new technology and related clinical applications continue to emerge.

References

[1] American National Standards Institute (ANSI). Specifications for threshold pure tone audiometry S 3.36
[2] Northern and Downs textbook
[3] ISO/TR 389–5 (1998). Acoustics—reference zero for the calibration of audiometric equipment. Part 5: Reference equivalent threshold sound pressure levels for pure tones in the frequency range 8 kHz to 16 kHz (Technical Report)
[4] Margolis RH, Morgan DE. Automated pure-tone audiometry: an analysis of capacity, need, and benefit. Am J Audiol 2008; 17: 109–113
[5] Del Castillo FJ, Del Castillo I. Genetics of isolated auditory neuropathies. Front Biosci (Landmark Ed) 2012; 17: 1251–1265
[6] Berlin CI, Hood LJ, Morlet T et al. Multi-site diagnosis and management of 260 patients with auditory neuropathy/dys-synchrony (auditory neuropathy spectrum disorder). Int J Audiol 2010; 49: 30–43
[7] Wilson RH, McArdle RA, Smith SL. An evaluation of the BKB-SIN, HINT, Quick-SIN, and WIN materials on listeners with normal hearing and listeners with hearing loss. J Speech Lang Hear Res 2007; 50: 844–856

[8] Sanford CA, Schooling T, Frymark T. Determining the presence or absence of middle ear disorders: an evidence-based systematic review on the diagnostic accuracy of selected assessment instruments. Am J Audiol 2012; 21: 251–268
[9] Nozza RJ, Bluestone CD, Kardatzke D, Bachman R. Towards the validation of aural acoustic immittance measures for diagnosis of middle ear effusion in children. Ear Hear 1992; 13: 442–453
[10] Nozza RJ, Bluestone CD, Kardatzke D, Bachman R. Identification of middle ear effusion by aural acoustic admittance and otoscopy. Ear Hear 1994; 15: 310–323
[11] Hunter LL, Margolis RH. Middle ear measurement. In: Seewald R, Tharpe AM, eds. Comprehensive Handbook of Pediatric Audiology. San Diego: Plural Publishing, 2011:365–388
[12] Berlin CI, Hood LJ, Morlet T et al. Absent or elevated middle ear muscle reflexes in the presence of normal otoacoustic emissions: a universal finding in 136 cases of auditory neuropathy/dys-synchrony. J Am Acad Audiol 2005; 16: 546–553
[13] Prieve BA, Driesbach L. Otoacoustic emissions. In: Seewald R, Tharpe AM, eds. Comprehensive Handbook of Pediatric Audiology. San Diego: Plural Publishing, 2011:389–408
[14] Gorga MP, Dierking DM, Johnson TA, Beauchaine KL, Garner CA, Neely ST. A validation and potential clinical application of multivariate analyses of distortion-product otoacoustic emission data. Ear Hear 2005; 26: 593–607
[15] Stavroulaki P, Apostolopoulos N, Segas J, Tsakanikos M, Adamopoulos G. Evoked otoacoustic emissions—an approach for monitoring cisplatin induced ototoxicity in children. Int J Pediatr Otorhinolaryngol 2001; 59: 47–57
[16] Hornibrook J, Kalin C, Lin E, O'Beirne GA, Gourley J. Transtympanic electrocochleography for the diagnosis of Ménière's disease. Int J Otolaryngol 2012; 2012: 852714
[17] Cueva RA. Preoperative, intraoperative, and postoperative auditory evaluation of patients with acoustic neuroma. Otolaryngol Clin North Am 2012; 45: 285–290, vii
[18] Stone JL, Calderon-Arnulphi M, Watson KS et al. Brainstem auditory evoked potentials—a review and modified studies in healthy subjects. J Clin Neurophysiol 2009; 26: 167–175
[19] Stapells DR. Frequency-specific threshold assessment in young infants using the transient ABR and the brainstem ASSR. In: Seewald R, Tharpe AM, eds. Comprehensive Handbook of Pediatric Audiology. San Diego: Plural Publishing, 2011:409–448
[20] Hall JW. New Handbook of Auditory Evoked Responses. New York: Pearson Allyn and Bacon, 2007

9 Assessment of Auditory Processing Disorders

Lisa W. Hilbert

9.1 Introduction

As the field of audiology continues to grow, one aspect of this discipline that is developing rapidly in evaluation and treatment is (central) auditory processing. This chapter discusses (central) auditory processing, indications for evaluation, and the importance of a test battery approach in combination with a multidisciplinary evaluation. Case studies are provided in this chapter.

9.2 History of Central Auditory Processing Disorders

The study of (central) auditory processing disorders [(C)APD or APD] emerged from both a medical and an educational perspective. Early research conducted by otolaryngologists provided a medical model for (central) auditory processing. The works of Bocca, Calearo, Antonelli, and their colleagues published in the mid-1950s provided a basis for subsequent development of central auditory testing.[1,2] They identified adults with what they called "cortical or subcortical deafness." These adults were found to have lesions involving the central auditory pathway and auditory centers of the brain.

In the 1950s and 1960s, the emphasis was on the identification of auditory pathway lesions and neurologic disorders in adults. With the development of sophisticated diagnostic imaging techniques (e.g., magnetic resonance imaging), the need for (central) auditory processing testing in this population diminished. However, a second area was emerging in the educational setting. In 1954, Helmer Myklebust,[3] a psychologist with an interest in the evaluation of deaf children, identified a problem in which children with normal hearing presented with a disorder of auditory perception. The 1960s brought increased interest in using adult measures of auditory processing with children. The National Institutes of Health authorized the first formal study of auditory processing in children in the 1960s.[4] Central auditory testing of children with learning disabilities began to gain interest in the 1970s.[5] The Willeford test battery was designed in 1977 to assess central auditory processing skills in children. The goal of these tests was to identify areas of weakness that could account for academic, communicative, or social skills difficulties. The SCAN: A Test for Auditory Processing Disorders, developed by Robert W. Keith in 1968, utilized a battery of tests in one assessment. The current revision, the SCAN 3, is a popular tool used for screening and diagnostic testing of children and adults.

Interest in the area of (C)APD continues to grow among professionals and lay public alike. The Internet has provided a source of information and misinformation on the subject. Some of the confusion may, in part, be due to the lack of agreement on a "gold standard" for diagnosis of (C)APD. Both the American Speech-Language-Hearing Association (ASHA) and the American Academy of Audiology (AAA) have offered guidelines for the diagnosis and management of (central) auditory processing disorders.

9.3 Definition of Auditory Processing Disorder

Before defining a disorder of the central auditory pathway, it is important to understand its normal function. In very simple terms, central auditory processing refers to "what the brain does with what the ears hear." ASHA defines (central) auditory processing as the "perceptual processing of auditory information in the central nervous system (CNS) and the neurobiologic activity that underlies that processing and gives rise to electrophysiologic auditory potentials."[6] In other words, it is the efficiency and effectiveness of the CNS in using auditory information. This includes the auditory mechanisms that underlie the following:

- Sound localization and lateralization
- Auditory discrimination
- Auditory pattern recognition
- Temporal aspects of audition:
  - Temporal integration
  - Temporal discrimination (e.g., temporal gap detection)
  - Temporal ordering
  - Temporal masking
- Auditory performance in competing acoustic signals (including dichotic listening)
- Auditory performance with degraded acoustic signals[7,8]

Difficulty in the processing of auditory information involving the above skills is the basis of central auditory processing disorder.

The prevalence of (C)APD is unknown as there is no gold standard for the disorder. Learning disabilities in children have a prevalence of 7.66 to 9.7%.[9,10] Many of these children may have (C)APD as well,[11] but the occurrence is unknown and estimates reported in the literature are speculative.

9.4 Principles of Central Auditory Dysfunction

Calearo and Antonelli[12] summarized several principles that explain how the normal CNS handles auditory messages:

1. *Channel separation*: A signal delivered to one ear is kept distinct from a different signal in the other ear.
2. *Binaural fusion*: If a single auditory message is divided into two bands by filtering or switching, and these bands are delivered binaurally and simultaneously, fusion will take place (at the brainstem level) and the subject will perceive one message only.
3. *Contralateral pathways*: Auditory messages from one ear cross at the brainstem level and reach the temporal lobe of the opposite side.
4. *Hemispheric dominance for language*: Although one cerebral hemisphere (usually the left) is verbally dominant, the other hemisphere appears to possess limited verbal abilities. Adding to Bocca and Calearo, we now understand that linguistic

information reaching the nondominant hemisphere (the right hemisphere from information presented to the left ear) crosses to the dominant language hemisphere through the densely myelinated fibers in the splenium of the corpus callosum.

Most diseases affecting central auditory pathways do not produce a loss in peripheral threshold sensitivity. Therefore, pure-tone tests do not generally identify (C)APD. Also, undistorted speech audiometry is not sufficiently challenging to the central auditory nervous system (CANS) to identify the presence of a central auditory lesion/disorder.

9.5 Neurophysiological Basis of Central Auditory Disorders

A (central) auditory processing disorder is a deficit in neural processing of auditory stimuli that is not due to higher-order language, cognitive, or related factors. However, (C)APD may lead to or be associated with difficulties in higher-order language, learning cognition, and communication functions.[13]

The auditory nervous system presents a complex interaction of neural signals that integrates acoustic information from both ears at nearly all levels of the CANS from the cochlear nucleus to the auditory cortex. These neural pathways are not simply passive conductors of an electrical signal. Auditory analysis takes place at all levels of the auditory system from the cochlea to the cortex.

The final common pathway is the auditory area of the cerebral cortex that lies in the Heschl gyrus. Anatomically, the brain contains regions that are typically different in size on the two sides. The best-defined asymmetry is in the primary auditory reception area in centers known to be associated with language comprehension. This asymmetry is present in newborns. What we know about auditory processing and the brain is as follows:

1. Language centers are usually situated in the left hemisphere. Ninety-five percent of persons are left-hemisphere dominant for language. Although production of speech is controlled from one hemisphere, there is a continuum of lateralization for speech perception. The right hemisphere is probably capable of processing paralinguistic aspects of language such as emotional tone, context, inference, and connotation. Therefore, motor speech production is a single-hemisphere function, whereas speech perception is a dual-hemisphere function that has implications for interpretation of auditory perceptual test results.
2. Maturation of neural structures, especially association fibers, takes place over many years. Sensory deprivation results in failure of certain neural centers to develop, at least in the brainstem and probably cortically.[14]
3. Dominance for language is present in the left cerebral hemisphere at early ages, but the brain is sufficiently plastic to allow language to be controlled by other areas if early damage occurs.[15] Linguistic processing is more completely centered in the dominant hemisphere in older persons who are less able to recover from damage to language centers.
4. Failure to establish cerebral dominance is associated with problems related to language development, learning to read, and integration of information from the several senses. Causes of brain dysfunction include congenital abnormal-ities, anoxia, maternal virus, other birth injury or illness, head trauma, seizures, genetic factors, and unknown factors.

According to Ferry,[16] delay or deviation in language development is due to disordered brain functioning. Normal speech and language development is a reflection of an intact, functioning brain. A speech or language delay, or auditory processing disorder, may be the only symptom or sign of neurologic impairment.

9.6 Behaviors of Individuals with Central Auditory Processing Disorders

The following observations are characteristic of children with auditory processing problems[7]:
1. Difficulty hearing spoken messages in the presence of other competing speech messages or in noisy or reverberant environments
2. Difficulty localizing the source of a signal
3. Difficulty learning a foreign language or other novel speech materials, such as technical language
4. Frequent requests for repetition
5. Difficulty processing rapid speech
6. Inconsistent or inappropriate responding to verbal stimuli
7. Inability to detect humor or sarcasm that is signaled by subtle changes in prosody
8. Being easily distracted by external stimuli
9. Difficulty maintaining attention
10. Difficulty following directions
11. Poor musical ability
12. Reading, spelling, and learning problems

These characteristics are not unique to those with (C)APD. Many of these behaviors are also seen in individuals with learning disabilities, attention deficit disorder with or without hyperactivity, language disorders, autism spectrum disorder, other cognitive or behavioral issues, and peripheral hearing loss.[7,17,18] Accordingly, the presence of any of these behavioral characteristics is not sufficient for the diagnosis of (C)APD. They are indicators that a diagnostic evaluation is warranted. Testing should be completed and a diagnosis made by an audiologist specializing in the area of (C)APD.[19,20] The audiologist should work as part of a multidisciplinary team for evaluation and developing plans for remediation. The purpose is to ensure that different aspects of the individual's speech, language, auditory, psychological, emotional, and physical function have been evaluated. Only after all these aspects have been examined can (C)APD be diagnosed and appropriate recommendations for treatment made. This is especially true when evaluating children and adolescents with language and learning problems.

Other candidates for (central) auditory processing evaluation are those with a history of hyperbilirubinemia,[21] seizure disorder (e.g., Landau-Kleffner syndrome[22]), multiple sclerosis or other neurodegenerative disease, traumatic brain injury,[23] space-occupying lesions, and other neurologic conditions that may affect the CANS. This includes military personnel exposed to combat-related trauma.

9.7 Test Battery Approach

Because auditory processing disorders can originate from various levels and regions of the CANS, it is important to have a test battery to assess the entire system.[6] Both speech and nonspeech (nonverbal) stimuli should be incorporated into behavioral testing. Most behavioral tests require a minimal developmental age of 7 or 8 years due to the variability of the maturation of the auditory pathways, specifically, the region of interhemispheric transfer at the corpus callosum.[24] Electrophysiological testing can provide objective information to support behavioral testing or offer information unavailable in populations unable to complete behavioral testing. All evaluations should begin with a comprehensive case history to identify any potential etiologic basis for the disorder and determine how it impacts the patient's communication and education/vocation.

The type of measurement used is individualized and dependent on the presenting complaints and case history. The following categories represent the types of measurements that are available for (C)APD assessment:

1. Auditory discrimination tests: assess the ability to differentiate similar acoustic stimuli that differ in frequency, intensity, or temporal parameters.
2. Auditory temporal processing and patterning tests: assess the ability to analyze acoustic events over time.
3. Dichotic speech tests: assess the ability to separate or integrate disparate auditory stimuli presented to each ear simultaneously.
4. Monaural low-redundancy speech tests: assess recognition of degraded speech stimuli presented to one ear at a time.
5. Binaural interaction tests: assess binaural (i.e., diotic) processes dependent on intensity or time differences of acoustic stimuli.
6. Electroacoustic measures: recordings of acoustic signals from within the ear canal that are generated spontaneously or in response to acoustic stimuli.
7. Electrophysiological measures: recording of electrical potentials that reflect synchronous activity generated by the CNS in response to a wide variety of acoustic events.[6]

9.8 Factors Affecting Central Auditory Test Results

Many variables can affect central auditory test results. Peripheral hearing loss, conductive or sensorineural, can result in hearing asymmetry and cochlear distortion.[5] Patients with peripheral hearing loss cannot be tested with most central auditory measures. Therefore, complete assessment of the peripheral auditory system must be completed prior to testing for (C)APD. Mental age and cognitive status can impact the individual's ability to perform the behavioral testing. Results from individuals with low cognition can be difficult to interpret or may be invalid.[24] Children and adults who are nonnative speakers of English typically have difficulty performing on sensitized speech tasks presented in English, even years after being immersed in the language.[25,26] Individuals referred for testing must also have adequate speech production in order for the examiner to accurately interpret their responses.

Some children with attention deficit hyperactive disorder (ADHD) have comorbidity with (C)APD. Research has focused on attempts to differentiate between (C)APD and ADHD, which have similar behavioral patterns. In general, the literature indicates that the presence of ADHD results in a general reduction of performance on tests of auditory processing. When possible, it is important to differentiate between ADHD and (C)APD because the treatments differ. Children who have (C)APD are not treated with medication for this specific diagnosis. If a child takes medication to treat ADHD, it is important that the medication is taken at the time of (C)APD testing.

9.9 Interpretation

Test results can provide a diagnosis of (C)APD as well as information regarding areas of auditory strengths and weaknesses. This information is helpful in developing an individualized plan for remediation. Diagnosis of (C)APD is commonly defined by performance deficits at least two standard deviations below the mean on two or more tests in the battery.[7] Tests of low-redundancy monaural speech identify how a particular child performs under poor acoustic conditions such as listening under degraded conditions or competing conditions. For example, the auditory figure–ground test enables the examiner to assess a child's ability to understand speech in the presence of competing background noise. Difficulty understanding speech in the presence of background noise is a frequent complaint of individuals with auditory processing difficulties. Many children with (C)APD have poor ability to understand speech under noisy situations, in reverberant rooms, and in other unfavorable listening conditions. These children require management of the acoustic environment and occasionally use of an assistive listening device in the classroom.

Tests of dichotic listening ability are used to determine levels of auditory maturation and hemispheric dominance for language and to identify disordered or damaged central auditory pathways.[27] The advantage of testing binaural separation with signals at simple and more complex linguistic levels (e.g., digits, words, and sentences) is that it serves the purpose of test reliability and it examines how performance, including ear advantage, changes with a different hierarchy of signal. Poor overall performance may indicate a developmental delay in maturation or underlying neurologic disorganization or damage to auditory pathways. Ear advantage is a powerful indicator of hemispheric organization. Normal-achieving children typically have a strong right ear advantage at younger ages with equal performance between ears as the child's auditory system matures. Left-ear advantages for all test conditions indicate the possibility of damage to the auditory reception areas of the left hemisphere, or failure to develop left hemisphere dominance for language. Abnormalities shown by dichotic test results correlate with a wide range of specific disabilities, including (C)APD, language disabilities, learning disabilities, and reading disorders.

Tests of temporal processing identify perceptual disorders that lead to phonological problems of reading and spelling. Tests of binaural integration identify brainstem dysfunction. Finally, tests of pattern recognition access nondominant hemisphere function and, if a verbal report is required, transfer of information from the nondominant to the dominant hemisphere.

Low scores across all tests suggest the possibility of confounding factors such as attention, cognition, or language delay.

9.10 Clinical Populations and Rehabilitation

9.10.1 Adults

Research has been conducted in various adult patient populations including persons who are aging[28,29] and those with Parkinson's disease,[30] chronic alcoholism,[31] Alzheimer's disease,[32] multiple sclerosis, head trauma,[23,33] stroke,[34] learning disabilities and reading disorders,[35,36] and AIDS.[37] In all of these patient groups, results of central auditory tests were poorer than predicted on the basis of peripheral hearing levels. There are several purposes for administration of a central auditory test battery to adults[38]:

1. In chronic CNS disease, to assess progression and to describe functional impairment
2. In head injury and stroke, to monitor recovery and provide a framework for counseling families
3. In pre- and postoperative brain surgery patients, to determine functional disorders of communication
4. In learning-disabled adults, to describe auditory processing abilities
5. In persons with neurologic disease, to monitor degenerative cognitive function and to assess the effectiveness of medical treatment
6. In patients with normal hearing who have histories of decreased ability to understand speech, to identify the presence of an APD
7. In aging patients, to study and describe auditory processing abilities related to changes that occur among healthy elderly persons and among those with chronic disease

Identification of central auditory disorders among these patient populations facilitates counseling the affected individuals and their families about their communication abilities, identifying necessary changes in the patient's listening environment (both physical and psychological changes), and determining specific recommendations for rehabilitation.

9.10.2 Children

The literature is full of examples of APDs in children that are related to language, learning, reading, and other developmental disorders. Auditory processing tests in children do the following:

1. Describe the maturation level of the central auditory pathways and, through longitudinal studies on the same child, demonstrate the development of auditory processing abilities
2. Provide data to document the neurologic origin presumed to exist in children with specific learning disabilities
3. Aid in ruling out abnormalities of the central auditory pathways as contributing to a language-learning problem
4. Describe whether language is appropriately located in the left hemisphere or whether there is a mixed or right hemisphere cerebral dominance for language

5. Describe whether the auditory channel is weak or strong and whether the classroom environment should be modified, with tutoring or remedial material initiated or assistive listening devices recommended to aid the child in the learning environment
6. Help assess the effect of medication (e.g., Ritalin) on performance on tests of (central) auditory processing

Thus, the results of the auditory processing test battery are used to develop remedial strategies for auditory processing/language-learning–disordered children.

9.11 Remediation

Diagnostic testing has greater value when used to design a plan for remediation. Many strategies exist for assisting children and adults found to have (C)APD. The type of treatment should be directed by the area of weakness identified in the evaluation. Remediation should begin immediately following diagnosis to exploit the plasticity of the CNS, maximize successful therapeutic outcomes, and minimize residual functional deficits.[6] In general, remediation of central auditory disorders falls into three categories: direct skills remediation, compensatory strategies, and environmental modifications. The following is a brief overview of strategies for management and remediation of auditory processing disorders.

9.11.1 Direct Skills Remediation

Also referred to as "auditory training," this approach uses bottom-up treatments to reduce or resolve (C)APD. Specially trained audiologists and speech-language pathologists regularly work with individuals diagnosed with (C)APD. Treatment options are developing with a focus on brain plasticity. Several auditory training programs utilize this philosophy, including the Auditory Rehabilitation for Interaural Symmetry (ARIA)[39] and the Dichotic Interaural Intensity Difference Training (DIID).[40] Also, interest continues to grow in computer-based auditory training (CBAT) programs such as Fast ForWord and Earobics.[41] These programs are appealing because of their engaging format, which provides reinforcement, thus encouraging their use. However, more research is needed to demonstrate the effectiveness of these programs[42] and to determine what factors contribute to their success (e.g., type of stimuli, hierarchy of tasks, and training environment[41]).

9.11.2 Compensatory Strategies

Compensatory strategies are designed to teach the individual how to minimize the impact of the residual (C)APD and maximize use of auditory information.[43] These techniques focus on improving learning and listening skills and strengthening language, problem solving, memory, attention, and other cognitive skills.[6] For example, children learn to actively monitor and self-regulate their message comprehension skills and develop new problem-solving skills. Compensatory strategies can include language training, vocabulary development, and the teaching of organizational skills. Individuals learn to take responsibility for their own listening success or failure and to be active participants in daily listening activities.

9.11.3 Environmental Modifications

Environmental modifications include such strategies as preferential seating, use of FM and sound field systems, and attention to classroom acoustics. For example, when an auditory figure–ground deficit is identified, recommendations for remediation are directed toward management of the environment to enhance listening opportunities and to improve signal quality. One way to improve speech understanding is to reduce competing acoustic signals in the listening environment by reducing background noise and reverberation time. Other methods include increasing the intensity of the signal through preferential seating and using assistive listening devices such as FM systems or classroom amplification. Classroom amplification has the additional benefit of helping all children including those with APD, mild or fluctuating hearing loss from otitis media, and children with ADHD. The individual's work and home environments can also be modified to produce the best possible listening condition.[44]

9.12 Case Examples of Auditory Processing Disorders

The following two cases exemplify some of the principles discussed in this chapter. The first case demonstrates a neurologic basis for the central auditory processing disorder. The second case demonstrates improvements seen from initial testing to the follow-up after 1 year of maturation and interventions.

9.12.1 Case 1: Child with Epilepsy and Left-Ear Advantage on Dichotic Testing

This 9-year-old girl was referred to our clinic by her neurologist due to concerns about auditory memory and auditory processing. The mother's pregnancy and the child's birth history were unremarkable. Developmental milestones were age-appropriate; however, speech development was delayed. Speech therapy was initiated at 3 years of age. The patient did not have a significant history of ear infections. Her adenoids were removed due to obstructive sleep apnea. She had a history of seizures, which began in association with fevers. As she grew older, she began having additional afebrile seizures. The seizures are presently under good control with medication. Magnetic resonance imaging (MRI) of the brain was completed prior to testing and was unremarkable. The patient is right-handed and uses the left ear when talking on the phone.

Psychological evaluation indicated solidly average intellect and similarly age-appropriate skills across most domains, including memory, visual-spatial, and visual-motor. Language weaknesses were identified, specifically related to auditory working memory, attention to auditory information, and phonological processing. The patient also had difficulty with working memory, organization, planning, and self-monitoring. There was some concern about ADHD, inattentive subtype.

This child was enrolled in the third grade of a Montessori program, in which she had repeated the second grade. Her individualized education program (IEP) provided classroom support for testing and a reduced work load. She also received group speech therapy at school. Reading phonetically was very

difficult. Most of her reading progress had been through memorization of words.

Peripheral hearing testing revealed normal hearing for pure tones and speech. Word recognition in quiet was excellent. Immittance measurements were normal. Ipsilateral acoustic reflexes were present. Contralateral acoustic reflexes were absent or elevated. The child was cooperative and attentive during testing; however, her demeanor changed during dichotic testing. She hid her face in her hands and became upset. She completed testing with encouragement and returned to her previous happy state. Central auditory test results were as follows:

- SCAN-C composite performance was in the 5th percentile. Scores for Filtered Words and Auditory Figure Ground (speech in noise) subtests were within the range of normal, indicating age-appropriate performance for auditory closure and degraded speech. A weakness was seen in dichotic testing for both auditory integration and auditory separation of information (▶ Table 9.1). A significant left ear advantage was revealed for dichotic testing (▶ Table 9.2).
- Performance on the test of phonemic synthesis was very poor. Of the 25 words presented, the patient repeated only one word correctly. These results indicate a significant weakness in the area of phonemic decoding. This deficit is thought to be strongly associated with difficulties in spelling and reading phonetically.
- The Pitch Pattern Sequence Test indicated age-appropriate scores for temporal processing.
- The Dichotic Digits Test confirmed a left-ear advantage with a score of 92% correct for the left ear and 69% correct for the right ear.

The child was referred for a speech and language evaluation following her diagnosis of (C)APD. She was found to have mildly

Table 9.1 Test Results on the SCAN for the Child in Case 1

SCAN-3 Subtest		
	Scaled Score	Percentile
Filtered Words	8	25%
Auditory Figure Ground	8	25%
Competing Words	5	5%
Competing Sentences	5	5%
Composite Score	76	5%

Table 9.2 Ear Advantage and Prevalence of the Test Results for the Child in Case 1

Subtest	Ear Advantage*	Prevalence
Filtered Words	7	15%
Auditory Figure Ground	0	Typical
Competing Words Directed Ear	Right: −3 Left: −6	Typical 2%
Competing Sentences	−33	2%

*Negative values in the Ear Advantage column indicate a left ear advantage.

deficient receptive and expressive language skills. Her phonological awareness and segmentation skills were moderately deficient. Severe deficits were noted in word discrimination and phonological blending skills. She was unable to retain and manipulate simple sentences of auditory information. She was unable to demonstrate understanding and processing of higher-order language such as implication, idioms, and inference.

Recommendations

This child will be enrolled in language therapy with a speech-language pathologist who specializes in (C)APD to increase phonological skills, memory skills, comprehension of more complex language, morphological skills, and formulating complex sentences. She will also begin deficit-specific auditory training with an audiologist to improve her dichotic listening skills.

9.12.2 Case 2: Child with Dichotic Weakness and Poor Auditory Figure–Ground Skills Before and After Remediation

This 8-year-old girl was referred to our clinic due to concerns regarding her hearing at home and at school. The mother's pregnancy and the child's birth history were unremarkable. Her developmental milestones were reported to be age appropriate. She had seasonal allergies but was otherwise healthy. Her adenoids were removed between her first and second central auditory processing evaluations. Her mother's concern was that she did not appear to hear unless she was looking at the speaker.

At the time of her initial evaluation, the patient was enrolled in the second grade at a private school. She was performing well and had no additional supports or services. She reported difficulty hearing spelling words during oral exams as well as difficulty with Spanish class. She read at or above grade level; however, she did not enjoy reading and had no confidence about her reading skills.

Speech and language testing using the Clinical Evaluation of Language Function (CELF-4) indicated a receptive language score in the 47th percentile and an expressive language score in the 39th percentile. This suggests typical receptive language skills and only mildly impaired expressive language skills. It was noted, however, that she had difficulty formulating her thoughts into organized discourse during conversation.

Central Auditory Processing Disorder Testing

The child was found to be socially engaging and cooperative with testing. She had good attention throughout the testing session. Peripheral hearing testing revealed normal hearing for pure tones and speech. Word recognition in quiet was excellent. Immittance measurements were normal. Both ipsilateral and contralateral acoustic reflexes were present. Central auditory test results were as follows:

- SCAN-C composite performance was in the 3rd percentile. Scores for Filtered Words and Competing Words subtests were within the range of normal, indicating age-appropriate

performance for auditory closure and auditory integration of information. A weakness was seen in the area of binaural separation of information. Significantly delayed skills were demonstrated for auditory figure–ground (speech in noise). There was no significant ear advantage.
- The phonemic synthesis test indicated age-appropriate performance for auditory blending of phonemes.
- The Staggered Spondee Word (SSW) test revealed difficulty with competing conditions for both ears. More errors were made for the left competing condition (16 errors, Number of Errors(NOE) ≤ 10) than the right competing condition (eight errors, NOE ≤ 7).
- Pitch Pattern Sequence Test (PPS) indicated age-appropriate performance for temporal processing. She was easily able to identify the changing tonal patterns and provide the appropriate linguistic label for the patterns.

Recommendations

It was recommended that the patient use Earobics, a home-based, computer-assisted program. She followed this recommendation and used the program daily for 4 months. Sporadic use was continued for the following year. She reached a plateau in the recommended version of Earobics.

Classroom modifications were recommended, including pre-teaching, a buddy system for note-taking, and the use of visual aids. Her teachers were also encouraged to modify their speech patterns and use simpler constructions to ensure that she was receiving and understanding the message. Her teachers were very supportive in meeting her auditory needs.

Follow-Up

She returned in 1 year for a follow-up visit to monitor her progress. At the time of her return, her mother reported significant improvement in her auditory skills. Improvement was also seen in her reading ability. Repeat testing of her peripheral hearing continued to show normal hearing for speech and pure tones. Immittance and acoustic reflex testing were normal as well. Central auditory test results were as follows:

- SCAN-3 composite performance was in the 53rd percentile. Scores for all subtests were improved or remained consistent with previous normal performance (▶ Table 9.3).
- The test of phonemic synthesis continued to show age-appropriate performance for auditory blending of phonemes.
- The SSW test revealed scores in the normal range for three of the four listening conditions. Performance on the right competing condition was just outside the normal range (eight errors, NOE ≤ 6) (▶ Table 9.4).

Discussion

Although this child exhibited significant improvement in her auditory development, her family continued to have concerns regarding her language development. There will be a need for continued language intervention throughout her school years. She can continue to strengthen her auditory processing skills using a more developmentally appropriate level of the Earobics program. This case is an excellent example of the effect of auditory-specific training and maturation on the development of the central auditory system.

Table 9.3 Test Results on the SCAN for the Child in Case 2

SCAN-C and SCAN-3 Subtest	Initial Evaluation		Follow-Up Evaluation	
	Scaled Score	Percentile	Scaled Score	Percentile
Filtered Words	8	25%	15	95%
Auditory Figure–Ground	2	0.4%	8	25%
Competing Words	8	25%	10	50%
Competing Sentences	5	5%	8	25%
Composite Score	71	3%	101	53%

Table 9.4 Test Results on the SSW for the Child in Case 2

SSW Test	Initial Evaluation (Number of Errors)		Follow-Up Evaluation (Number of Errors)	
	Right non-competing	0 (NOE ≤ 3)	Right non-competing	0 (NOE ≤ 2)
	Right competing	8 (NOE ≤ 7)	Right competing	8 (NOE ≤ 6)
	Left non-competing	3 (NOE ≤ 4)	Left non-competing	0 (NOE ≤ 3)
	Left Competing	16 (NOE ≤ 10)	Left Competing	8 (NOE ≤ 8)
Total errors		27		16

References

[1] Bocca E, Calearo C, Cassinari V, Migliavacca F. Testing "cortical" hearing in temporal lobe tumours. Acta Otolaryngol 1955; 45: 289–304

[2] Bocca E, Calearo C, Cassinari V. A new method for testing hearing in temporal lobe tumors. Acta Otolaryngol 1954; 44: 219–221

[3] Myklebust H. Auditory Disorders in Children: A Manual for Differential Diagnosis. New York: Grune and Stratton, 1954

[4] Chalfant J, Scheffelin MA. Central processing dysfunctions in children: a review of research. In: National Institute of Neurological Diseases and Stroke Monograph. Bethesda, MD: Department of Health, Education, and Welfare, 1969

[5] Baran J, Musiek F. Behavioral assessment of the central auditory nervous system. In: Contemporary Perspectives in Hearing Assessment. Boston: Allyn & Bacon, 1999:375–414

[6] Bellis TJ, Chermak GD, Ferre JM, et al. (Central) Auditory Processing Disorders. Rockville, MD: American Speech-Language-Hearing Association, 2005

[7] Chermak GD, Musiek FE. Central Auditory Processing Disorder. San Diego: Singular, 1997

[8] Catts HW. Chermak GD, Craig CH, et al. Central auditory processing: current status of research and implications for clinical practice. Am J Audiol 1996; 5: 41–54

[9] Boyle CA, Boulet S, Schieve LA et al. Trends in the prevalence of developmental disabilities in US children, 1997–2008. Pediatrics 2011; 127: 1034–1042

[10] Altarac M, Saroha E. Lifetime prevalence of learning disability among US children. Pediatrics 2007; 119 Suppl 1: S77–S83

[11] Iliadou V, Bamiou DE, Kaprinis S, Kandylis D, Kaprinis G. Auditory processing disorders in children suspected of learning disabilities—a need for screening? Int J Pediatr Otorhinolaryngol 2009; 73: 1029–1034

[12] Calearo C, Antonelli AR. Disorders of the central auditory nervous system. Otolaryngology 1973; 2: 407–425

[13] Musiek F, Chermak G. Handbook of (Central) Auditory Processing Disorder, vol 1. Auditory Neuroscience and Diagnosis. San Diego: Plural Publishing, 2007:128–129

[14] Phillips DP. Central auditory processing: a view from auditory neuroscience. Am J Otol 1995; 16: 338–352

[15] Gelfand SA. Long-term recovery and no recovery from the auditory deprivation effect with binaural amplification: six cases. J Am Acad Audiol 1995; 6: 141–149

[16] Ferry P. Neurological consideration in children with learning disabilites. In: Central Auditory and Language Disorders in Children. Houston: College Hill Press, 1981:1–12

[17] Bellis T. Assessment and Management of Central Auditory Processing Disorders in the Educational Setting: From Science to Practice, 2nd ed. New York: Thomson Learning, 2003

[18] Baran JA, Musiek FE. Central auditory disorders. In: Textbook of Audiolgical Medicine: Clinical Aspects of Hearing and Balance. London: Martin Dunitz, 2003:495–511

[19] American Speech-Language-Hearing Association. Code of Ethics (revised). ASHA Suppl 2003; 23: 13–15

[20] American Speech-Language-Hearing Association. Scope of Practice in Audiology. Rockville, MD: ASHA, 2004

[21] Dublin W. Fundamentals of Sensorineural Auditory Pathology. Springfield, IL: Charles C. Thomas, 1976

[22] Landau WM, Kleffner FR. Syndrome of acquired aphasia with convulsive disorder in children. Neurology 1957; 7: 523–530

[23] Bergemalm PO, Lyxell B. Appearances are deceptive? Long-term cognitive and central auditory sequelae from closed head injury. Int J Audiol 2005; 44: 39–49

[24] American Academy of Audiology. Diagnosis, Treatment and Management of Children and Adults with Central Auditory Processing Disorder. American Academy of Audiology, 2010

[25] Gat IB, Keith RW. An effect of linguistic experience. Auditory word discrimination by native and non-native speakers of English. Audiology 1978; 17: 339–345

[26] Keith RW, Katbamna B, Tawfik S, Smolak LH. The effect of linguistic background on staggered spondaic word and dichotic consonant vowel scores. Br J Audiol 1987; 21: 21–26

[27] Keith R, Novak KK. Relationships between tests of centralauditory function and receptive language. Semin Hear 1984; 5: 243–250

[28] Golding M, Carter N, Mitchell P, Hood LJ. Prevalence of central auditory processing (CAP) abnormality in an older Australian population: the Blue Mountains Hearing Study. J Am Acad Audiol 2004; 15: 633–642

[29] Jerger J, Chmiel R, Allen J, Wilson A. Effects of age and gender on dichotic sentence identification. Ear Hear 1994; 15: 274–286

[30] Jerger JF. Observations on auditory behavior in lesions of the central auditory pathways. AMA Arch Otolaryngol 1960; 71: 797–806

[31] Spitzer JB, Ventry IM. Central auditory dysfunction among chronic alcoholics. Arch Otolaryngol 1980; 106: 224–229

[32] Strouse AL, Hall JW, III, Burger MC. Central auditory processing in Alzheimer's disease. Ear Hear 1995; 16: 230–238

[33] Musiek FE, Baran JA, Shinn J. Assessment and remediation of an auditory processing disorder associated with head trauma. J Am Acad Audiol 2004; 15: 117–132

[34] Baran JA, Bothfeldt RW, Musiek FE. Central auditory deficits associated with compromise of the primary auditory cortex. J Am Acad Audiol 2004; 15: 106–116

[35] Walker MM, Shinn JB, Cranford JL, Givens GD, Holbert D. Auditory temporal processing performance of young adults with reading disorders. J Speech Lang Hear Res 2002; 45: 598–605

[36] King WM, Lombardino LJ, Crandell CC, Leonard CM. Comorbid auditory processing disorder in developmental dyslexia. Ear Hear 2003; 24: 448–456

[37] Bankaitis AE, Keith RW. Audiological changes associated with HIV infection. Ear Nose Throat J 1995; 74: 353–359

[38] Keith RW, Pensak ML. Central auditory function. Otolaryngol Clin North Am 1991; 24: 371–379

[39] Moncrieff DW, Wertz D. Auditory rehabilitation for interaural asymmetry: preliminary evidence of improved dichotic listening performance following intensive training. Int J Audiol 2008; 47: 84–97

[40] Musiek F, Schochat E. Auditory training and centralauditory processing disorders: a case study. Semin Hear 1998; 19: 357–366

[41] Thibodeau L. Computer-based auditory training (CBAT) for (central) auditory procedssing disorders. In: Chermak GD, Musiek FE, eds. Handbook of (Central) Auditory Processing Disorder: Comprehensive Intervention. San Diego: Plural Publishing, 2007:167–206

[42] Musiek F, Shinn J, Hare C. Plasticity, auditory training, andauditory processing disorders. Semin Hear 2002; 23: 263–276

[43] Whitelaw GM. Auditory processing in adults: beyone the audiogram. AudiologyOnline, 2008

[44] Willeford J, Burleigh J. Handbook of Central Auditory Processing Disorders in Chidren. Orlando, FL: Grune and Stratton, 1985

10 Laboratory Tests of Vestibular and Balance Functioning

Dennis I. Bojrab, Danny J. Soares, and Matthew L. Kircher

10.1 Introduction

Laboratory testing of vestibular and balance functioning is an important tool in the evaluation and management of the dizzy patient. This testing is meant to complement a careful history and neurotologic examination in making an accurate clinical diagnosis. Because many patient complaints arise due to an asymmetry in labyrinthine function, clinical vestibular testing allows a quantifiable comparison in the level of function between the two corresponding vestibular sense organs. Although not every patient requires laboratory vestibular testing, the methods described in this chapter enable assessment and documentation of the patient's vestibular function while providing information on prognosis and recovery.

The semicircular canals encode the rotation of the head, and the otolith organs encode linear head acceleration and tilt by changes in baseline vestibular afferent activity between the two labyrinths. The vestibulo-ocular reflex (VOR), a short latency reflex that compensates for head rotations, is meant to stabilize the visual field on the retina during head movements. The VOR is central to laboratory testing of vestibular and balance disorders. Also, using variable vestibular stimulation, the vestibular evoked myogenic potential (VEMP) provides valuable insight into the integrity of dynamic otolith function. This chapter describes electronystagmography and VEMP testing. Posturography and rotational chair testing are also discussed.

10.2 Electronystagmography

Electronystagmography (ENG) entails a battery of tests that evaluate vestibular and nonvestibular systems. Patients with peripheral or central balance disorders may exhibit abnormal eye movements that can be assessed through the ENG. The VOR is a primary reflex tested in the ENG. Vestibular stimulation generates a modulation in vestibular afferent nerve activity, which in turn generates characteristic eye movements through the VOR (▶ Fig. 10.1a). Central or peripheral dysfunction yields characteristic study findings. The resulting eye movements are monitored and recorded relative to the head position using eye movement recording equipment, the most common of which include electro-oculography (EOG) and video-oculography.

Electro-oculography provides a measure of corneoretinal potentials that exist between the positively charged cornea and negatively charged retina. These potentials create an electric field that rotates as the eyes move within the orbits. Electrodes placed along the lateral orbit monitor horizontal eye position, whereas electrodes placed above and below the eyes monitor vertical eye position (▶ Fig. 10.2a,b). Movement of the eyes causes potential changes relative to the skin electrodes. By convention, an upward deflection on the horizontal channel represents movement of the eye to the right, whereas a downward deflection represents movement to the left. Recorded eye movements by the vertical channels correspond directly with upward and downward movements represented as upward and downward deflections. EOG surface electrodes, however, lack the ability to monitor ocular torsion.

Today, many institutions employ videooculography (VOG) or videonystagmography (VNG), which utilizes digital video recording equipment to capture eye movements under certain vestibular test situations (▶ Fig. 10.2c). These computer systems are programmed to document eye position by detecting and tracking pupil movement. With applied vestibular stimulation, pupillary deflections are captured and analyzed, enabling ocular torsion to be evaluated. Advantages of VNG include storage and retrieval of eye movement data with the ability to playback and review eye movements at a later time. This is especially helpful in cases of subtle nystagmus findings or for use in teaching. Blink artifact, however, may obscure VNG findings, and so the patient must keep the eyes open during testing.

10.3 Routine Components of Electronystagmography

The ENG test battery generally consists of seven components: the Dix-Hallpike maneuver, gaze, positional testing, calorics, saccades, smooth pursuit, and optokinetics. Although saccade and pursuit eye movements are of secondary interest to those who evaluate dizziness, they are nevertheless routinely tested because abnormalities may be evident and may affect vestibular test results.

10.3.1 Gaze Test

Patients' eye movements are monitored while they gaze 30 degrees to the right, 30 degrees to the left, 30 degrees up, and 30 degrees down. Spontaneous nystagmus and the effects of fixation suppression can be determined. Individuals without vestibular pathology rarely have nystagmus while fixating at any of these gaze positions; however, many patients, especially the elderly, display endpoint nystagmus. This nystagmus is usually faint with centripetal slow phases of equal intensity on right and left gaze.

The gaze test detects nystagmus from vestibular origin as well as central nervous system origin. An acute unilateral peripheral vestibular lesion may display spontaneous nystagmus exacerbated with certain gaze positions. For example, a person with acute left vestibular ablation may have spontaneous right-beating nystagmus (▶ Fig. 10.1b). This nystagmus is accentuated with gaze to the right and improved with gaze to the left (Alexander's law). Upbeat nystagmus, which occurs most commonly as a result of medullary lesions involving vertical vestibular pathways, is an example of central nystagmus.[1] Hullar et al[2] give a thorough review of different types of nystagmus based on central or peripheral vestibular lesion location.

10.3.2 Dix-Hallpike Positioning Maneuver

The most common maneuver used to test for positioning nystagmus is the Dix-Hallpike maneuver. This test is performed

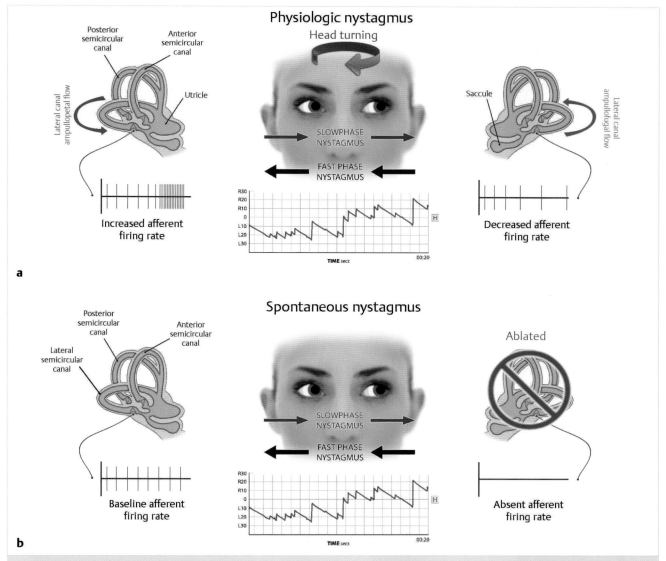

Fig. 10.1 Vestibular afferent firing rate in physiological (a) and spontaneous (b) nystagmus. (a) Head turning to the right stimulates an increase in the afferent firing rate from the right lateral canal and a decreased firing rate from the left lateral canal, resulting in physiological rightward fast-phase nystagmus. (b) Left vestibular ablation (B) results in absent left vestibular afferent firing, and baseline right vestibular afferent activity results in pathological rightward fast-phase spontaneous nystagmus.

first in the battery of positioning and positional testing in order to capture potentially fatigable nystagmus. It is also best performed with the patient wearing Frenzel lenses or video-oculography goggles to suppress visual fixation. With the patient in the sitting position, the head is turned 45 degrees toward one side. The examiner holds the patient's head and then quickly lowers the patient into the supine position, hanging the head over the end of the exam table and keeping the head turned 45 degrees (▶ Fig. 10.3). This position is maintained for at least 30 seconds during which eye movements are monitored or recorded. The examiner then returns the patient to the sitting position. This maneuver may then be repeated with the head turned to the opposite side.

The most common pathology identified with the Dix-Hall-pike positioning maneuver is posterior semicircular canal benign paroxysmal positional vertigo (BPPV), accounting for

approximately 81 to 89% of BPPV cases.[3] Posterior canal BPPV is most commonly a canalithiasis type of BPPV (▶ Fig. 10.3c). (See Chapter 3 for a more detailed discussion of BPPV pathophysiology.) In right posterior canal canalithiasis, placing the patient in the right head-hanging position produces a geotropic up-beating torsional nystagmus (fast-phase up and to the right). These eye movements are in the plane of the undermost posterior canal in accordance with Ewald's first law. Nystagmus is delayed in onset by at least a few seconds, builds in intensity, and then slowly abates over the next 30 seconds as the head remains in the head-hanging position. The nystagmus and associated vertigo also tend to be fatigable in that they progressively diminish in intensity with repetition of the positioning maneuver.

The observed torsional nystagmus in BPPV also changes in character depending on the patient's gaze. In right posterior

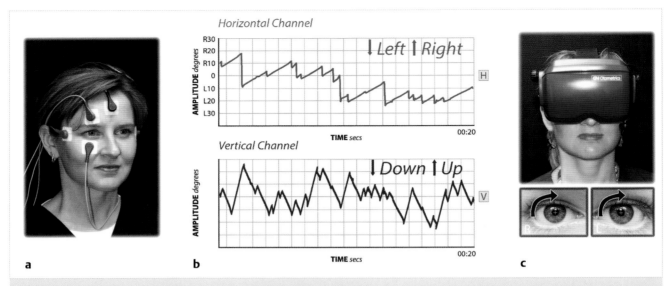

Fig. 10.2 Oculographic electrode placement. (a) Standard lead placement in electro-oculography. (b) Sample horizontal and vertical oculographic tracings describing a left torsional nystagmus. (c) Video-oculography allows for additional verification of the torsional component of nystagmus.

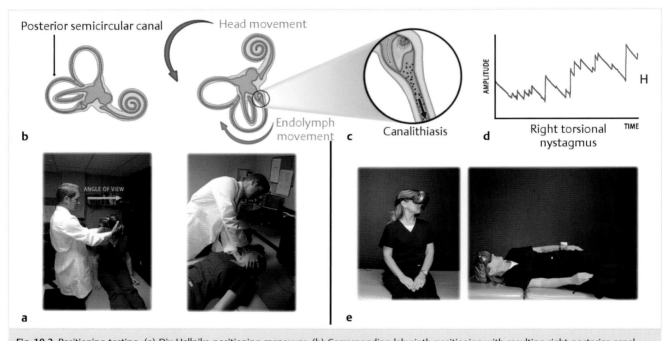

Fig. 10.3 Positioning testing. (a) Dix-Hallpike positioning maneuver. (b) Corresponding labyrinth positioning with resulting right posterior canal ampullofugal endolymphatic flow. (c) Right posterior canalithiasis with stimulatory cupula deflection. (d) Representative horizontal channel electro-oculography showing right torsional (geotropic) nystagmus with right posterior canal benign paroxysmal positional vertigo (BPPV). (e) The Bojrab maneuver is an alternative equivalent posterior canal positioning method.

canal BPPV, the torsional component is most prominent with rightward gaze, and the vertical component is most prominent with leftward gaze. Although less common, the Dix-Hallpike maneuver may also provoke positioning nystagmus responses from the horizontal and superior canal. It is estimated that 8 to 17% of BPPV cases represent horizontal canal responses and 1 to 3% of cases represent superior canal BPPV.[3] The examiner may identify the canal involved by noting the direction of nystag-

mus. Lateral canal BPPV displays horizontal nystagmus, whereas superior canal BPPV displays a down-beating torsional nystagmus. Once again, patient gaze can give valuable information as to the canal from which the nystagmus is generated. For instance, in right superior canal BPPV, the torsional component is most prominent with leftward gaze, and the vertical component is most prominent with rightward gaze (the opposite of right posterior canal BPPV).

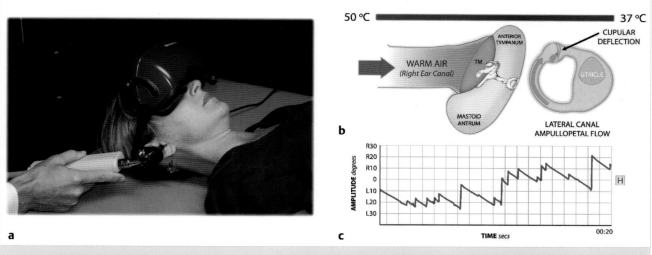

Fig. 10.4 Caloric testing. (a) Right ear warm caloric testing. (b) Warm caloric stimulation results in ampullopetal flow of endolymph within the vertically positioned lateral semicircular canal. (c) Electro-oculography demonstrating rightward horizontal nystagmus.

Horizontal canal BPPV is most effectively identified by placing the patient in the supine position and turning the head quickly to the right (or left) ear-down position for 30 seconds. If nystagmus is provoked, the position is held for several minutes before slowly returning to the neutral position. This maneuver is then repeated to the opposite side. Due to variations in lateral canal cupular deflection and the fact that stimulatory vestibular responses are greater than inhibitory, lateral canal canalithiasis will generate geotropic horizontal nystagmus with the pathologic ear undermost.[4] For lateral canal cupulolithiasis, an ageogropic horizontal nystagmus is generated stronger with the non-pathologic ear undermost.

10.3.3 Positional Test

The positional test determines the ability of different sustained head positions to induce or modify nystagmus. This testing is also best performed with the patient wearing Frenzel lenses or video-oculography goggles. The patient's eye movements are monitored in four head positions: sitting, supine, right ear down, and left ear down. Many protocols monitor eye movements with eyes open in total darkness as an effective means to deny visual fixation and still be able to measure nystagmus. Also, asking the patient to perform mental tasks during testing, such as counting backward or naming common household items, helps to maintain the patient's mental alertness and thus avoid nystagmus suppression.

Patients with central or peripheral vestibular lesions commonly display a sustained, usually horizontal positional nystagmus of low velocity, although this finding may also be present in asymptomatic human subjects.[5] A central lesion may also cause a purely vertical or purely torsional positional nystagmus that typically fails to be suppressed or abolished by visual fixation.[2] It must also be remembered that the positional test may provoke paroxysmal positioning nystagmus if the response has not previously been provoked and fatigued by the Dix-Hallpike maneuver.

10.3.4 Caloric Test

The caloric test is the most widely used test of semicircular canal function. With the patient in the supine position and the head elevated 30 degrees, the lateral semicircular canal assumes a vertical position. The standard caloric stimulus consists of 250 mL of either 30°C or 44°C water irrigated into the external ear canal over 30 seconds. Some examiners use air (8 L at 24°C and 50°C within 60 seconds) instead of water as the caloric stimuli.[1] By introducing cool or warm stimuli into the external auditory canal, a thermal gradient is generated in the most laterally positioned portion of the labyrinth—the lateral semicircular canal. Cool air causes endolymph to fall, whereas warm air causes endolymph to rise. The displacement in endolymph (convective flow) causes cupula deflection away from or toward the utricle, and the horizontal canal afferent pathway is inhibited or stimulated respectively (▶ Fig. 10.4). Slow-phase nystagmus velocity is measured and compared to contralateral cool and warm stimulation. The absolute value of the slow-phase eye velocity to the same thermal stimulus may vary considerably between persons due to differences in size and shape of the external auditory canal and the skull.

The diagnostically valuable measure is the level of slow-phase eye velocity symmetry between labyrinths (▶ Fig. 10.5). This symmetry is calculated by the canal paresis (CP) index. A CP index > 20 to 25% is generally considered to represent significant asymmetric horizontal canal function. Bilateral slow-phase velocity responses below 16 degrees/sec are considered to represent bilateral labyrinthine hypofunction[6] and may result from central or peripheral pathology. In cases of reduced or absent caloric responses, ice water irrigations may be used to attempt to obtain a response. The CP index is calculated as follows:

$$\frac{(RW + RC) - (LW + LC)}{RW + RC + LW + LC} \times 100 = UW\%$$

RW, right warm; RC, right cool; LW, left warm; LC, left cool peak slow-phase velocities; UW, unilateral weakness. Significant unilateral weakness is considered at greater than 20 to 25%.

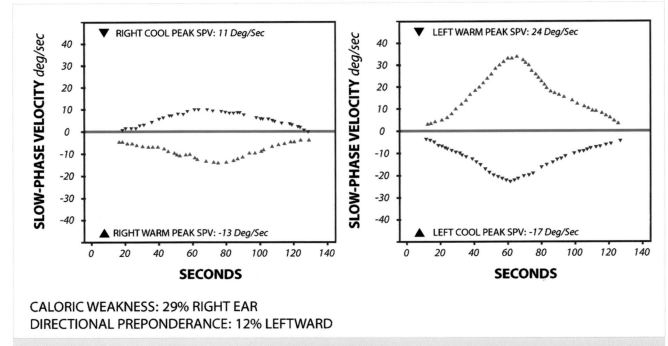

CALORIC WEAKNESS: 29% RIGHT EAR
DIRECTIONAL PREPONDERANCE: 12% LEFTWARD

Fig. 10.5 Caloric response in a patient with a right unilateral weakness. Red and blue arrows represent leftward and rightward slow-phase nystagmus, respectively.

An important advantage of caloric testing is the ability to stimulate each horizontal canal and the associated superior vestibular nerve afferents separately and thereby localize the diseased labyrinth. In this way, calorics are very good in localizing superior vestibular nerve pathology; however, inferior vestibular nerve aferrents will not be well represented. Other vestibular test procedures, such as rotational chair testing and posturography, necessarily involve bilateral labyrinthine stimulation and are therefore nonlocalizing to the diseased labyrinth. In this way, pathology involving inferior vestibular nerve afferents will not be well represented on caloric testing.

10.3.5 Saccade Test

The saccade eye movement functions to cause a rapid change in gaze from one object to another in order to capture peripheral visual field targets onto the fovea. Saccade testing may be performed in both horizontal and vertical eye movement planes. To test horizontal saccades, the patient's head is fixed and he or she is instructed to fixate vision on a series of randomly displayed targets at eccentricities of 5 to 30 degrees in the horizontal plane. The saccade eye movement program consists of recording eye responses to left and right target jumps and computing eye movement latency, amplitude, velocity, and accuracy (▶ Fig. 10.6).

Saccade latency is approximately 180 to 200 ms after presentation of target, although this may be increased in patients with frontal lobe lesions, Alzheimer disease, and Huntington disease. Saccade velocity increases linearly with amplitudes up to 20 degrees but remains relatively constant for higher amplitudes.[2] Abnormalities in saccade velocity are seen in many degenerative and metabolic central nervous system disease processes. Inaccurate saccades, or ocular dysmetria, are classified as hypermetria (overshooting the target) or hypometria (undershooting) and may be seen with cerebellar or brainstem disorders.

10.3.6 Smooth Pursuit Testing

In smooth pursuit or tracking testing, the patient's head is fixed and horizontal eye movements are monitored while the patient follows a visual target moving in the horizontal plane. The target moves smoothly left and right usually following a sinusoidal waveform at frequencies between 0.2 and 0.7 Hz with an amplitude of 15 degrees. The eye velocity gain, defined as the ratio of peak eye velocity to peak target velocity, is calculated and plotted at each target frequency (▶ Fig. 10.7). Individuals with normal functioning pursuit systems are able to follow the target smoothly in both directions at all target frequencies. Patients with impairment in smooth pursuit often display corrective saccades in order to recapture the image on the fovea. Smooth pursuit mechanisms assist visual fixation, suppressing nystagmus from peripheral but not central lesions.[2] Sedating medications and a variety of central neurologic conditions can cause impairment in smooth pursuit. Smooth pursuit is also performed less well by the elderly.

10.3.7 Optokinetic Testing

In optokinetic testing, the physician is trying to capture the patient's ability to track the motion of an entire visual field as opposed to tracking a single object in smooth pursuit. Ideally, this is done in a full field surround test environment; however, not all vestibular laboratories have this capability. Optokinetic responses drive the eyes to follow the visual surround during sustained head movements. Some laboratories test optokinetics

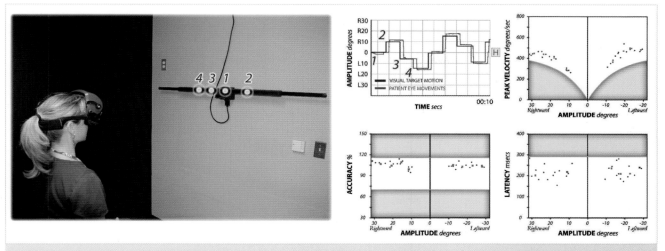

Fig. 10.6 Standard saccade testing setup and tracings. Intermittent light targets are presented sequentially, resulting in a step-configuration on standard horizontal oculography. Peak velocity, accuracy, and latency are plotted (blue-shaded regions denote abnormal response ranges).

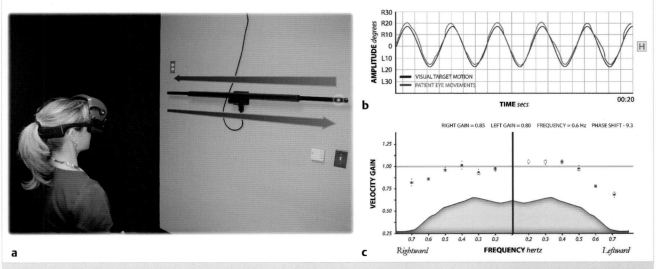

Fig. 10.7 Smooth pursuit testing. (a) Standard setup. (b) Oculographic recording of a normal smooth pursuit response. (c) Velocity gain plotted against moving target frequencies (blue-shaded areas represent abnormal response ranges).

by monitoring eye movements as visual targets provoke slow-phase nystagmus in the direction of target motion, periodically interrupted by fast phases in the opposite direction. In this manner, gain may be computed as in smooth pursuit testing. Also, because smooth pursuit tracking contributes to the generation of optokinetic responses, many of the abnormalities resulting in smooth pursuit deficits also lead to impaired optokinetic nystagmus.

10.3.8 Rotational Chair Testing

Rotational chair testing may be used to assess vestibular function in patients with suspected bilateral vestibular hypofunction, or in children who may not tolerate caloric testing. The rotational chair test monitors eye movements while the patient is rotated horizontally around a vertical axis. The chin is pitched

30 degrees nose down to place the horizontal canal in the plane of rotation. This rotation results in bilateral horizontal canal stimulation. The patient is tested in total darkness with the eyes open while undergoing sinusoidal chair oscillation at different frequencies. The relationship between head and eye movements is measured, and phase, gain, and symmetry parameters are calculated.

Slow-phase eye velocity usually lags behind head velocity by a gain ratio of about 0.6. Phase measures the timing relationship between eye and head velocity; as the head moves to the right, the eyes move to the left and vice versa. Increased phase lead may imply peripheral vestibular system dysfunction, whereas decreased phase lead may suggest a cerebellar lesion. Symmetry, the ratio of rightward and leftward slow-phase eye velocities, gives information as to whether any bias is present in the system, such as a peripheral vestibular weakness.

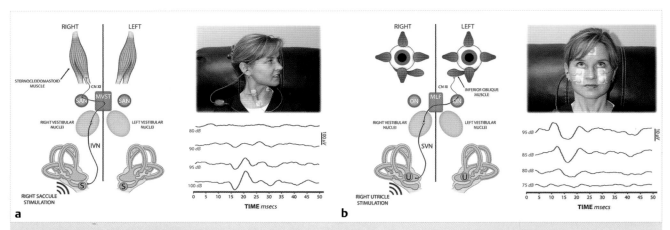

Fig. 10.8 Vestibular-evoked myogenic potential (VEMP) testing. (a) Cervical VEMP pathway, testing setup, and standard ipsilateral sternocleido-mastoid myogenic potential tracings. IVN, inferior vestibular nerve; MVST, medial vestibulospinal tract; S, saccule; SAN, spinal accessory nucleus. (b) Ocular VEMP pathway, testing setup, and standard contralateral extraocular muscle myogenic potential tracings. MLF, medial longitudinal fasciculus; ON, oculomotor nucleus; SVN, superior vestibular nerve; U, utricle.

10.3.9 Dynamic Posturography

Balance is maintained using a combination of vestibular, visual, and proprioceptive cues. Dynamic posturography is a test that in part determines the effects of manipulation of visual and proprioceptive information on standing balance function. A specialized test platform capable of tilting back and forth in a pitch plane about an axis collinear with the patient's ankle joints is used. During testing, the patient wears a harness for safety and faces a visual screen capable of tilting independently or simultaneously about the platform axis. The patient's postural stability as measured by sway angle at the platform is evaluated under the following six conditions:[7]

1. Support fixed, eyes open, visual fixed
2. Support fixed, eyes closed, visual fixed
3. Support fixed, eyes open, visual sway-referenced
4. Support swayed, eyes open, visual fixed
5. Support swayed, eyes closed, visual fixed
6. Support swayed, eyes open, visual sway-referenced

An equilibrium score for each condition is calculated and compared to normal controls. Patients with bilateral vestibular hypofunction or uncompensated unilateral vestibular hypofunction sway excessively under conditions 5 and 6, as these conditions rely on vestibular input to maintain balance.

10.4 Vestibular Evoked Myogenic Potential

10.4.1 A Test of Otolith Function

Animal studies have shown that both air- and bone-conducted sound activates otolith afferents (saccular and utricular) and rarely semicircular canal afferents.[8] The utricular and saccular macula have different neural projections. Uchino et al and other researchers have shown that saccular neurons have strong projections to the neck muscles, whereas utricular afferents project primarily to the eye muscles.[9–12]

Sound evoked potentials recorded from electrodes over the sternocleidomastoid muscle persist in patients with profound sensorineural hearing loss but disappear after vestibular nerve section. There is general consensus that cervical VEMPs (cVEMPs) are saccular and inferior vestibular nerve dependent (▶ Fig. 10.8a).[13–15] VEMPs may also be recorded from periocular electrodes and are called ocular VEMPs (oVEMPs) (▶ Fig. 10.8b). These potentials are thought to arise primarily from inferior oblique and inferior rectus muscles. The majority of the otolith ocular connections originate from the utricle, and oVEMPs are useful for assessing utricular function. Patients with vestibular neuritis, which frequently involves the superior division of the vestibular nerve, were found to often have normal cVEMPs but absent oVEMPS.[16]

10.4.2 Clinical Implications

Because cVEMPS originate in the saccule and are carried in the inferior vestibular nerve, vestibular lesions that damage the saccule or inferior vestibular nerve should cause abnormal cVEMPs. Patients with Ménière disease have a decreased or absent cVEMP on the involved side 50% of the time when tested between attacks.[17,18] With gentamicin intratympanic treatment for Ménière disease, cVEMPs may be used to monitor the effectiveness of treatment.[19] In up to 80% of patients with vestibular schwannomas, cVEMPs are abnormal. Vestibular neuritis typically involves the superior division of the nerve; however, some cases have normal caloric responses with abnormal cVEMPs, suggesting selective involvement of the inferior division of the vestibular nerve. cVEMPs are also helpful in confirming the diagnosis of superior canal dehiscence syndrome (SCDS), displaying a large cVEMP amplitude and low cVEMP threshold. oVEMPs may have an additional advantage in screening for SCDS because they reflect an excitatory response that does not saturate with increasing intensity as the inhibitory cVEMP response. The oVEMP and cVEMP tests are vestibular because patients who are totally deaf show the myogenic potentials to air-conducted sound (ACS) or bone-conducted vibration (BCV), and patients treated with systemic gentamicin with presumed absent vestibular function but residual hearing do not show the myogenic potentials.[20,21] In patients with complete unilateral vestibular loss following vestibular schwannoma removal, there is a reduced or absent oVEMP n10 from beneath the contralateral eye (as the subject looks up) in response to BCV or ACS stimulation of the affected ear[22-24] and reduced or absent cVEMP p13-n23 from over the ipsilateral SCM in response to BCV at the midline forehead at the hairline (Fz).

References

[1] Barber HO, Stockwell CW. Manual of Electronystagmography, 2nd ed. St. Louis: CV Mosby, 1980

[2] Hullar TEZD, Minor LB. Evaluation of the patient with dizziness. In: Flint P, ed. Flint Cummings Otolaryngology: Head and Neck Surgery, 5th ed. Philadelphia: Mosby Elsevier, 2010:2305–2327

[3] Fife TD, Iverson DJ, Lempert T et al. Quality Standards Subcommittee, American Academy of Neurology. Practice parameter: therapies for benign paroxysmal positional vertigo (an evidence-based review): report of the Quality Standards Subcommittee of the American Academy of Neurology. Neurology 2008; 70: 2067–2074

[4] Baloh RW, Kerber KA. Clinical Neurophysiology of the Vestibular System, 4th ed. New York: Oxford University Press, 2011

[5] McAuley JR, Dickman JD, Mustain W, Anand VK. Positional nystagmus in asymptomatic human subjects. Otolaryngol Head Neck Surg 1996; 114: 545–553

[6] Sills AW, Baloh RW, Honrubia V. Caloric testing 2. Results in normal subjects. Ann Otol Rhinol Laryngol Suppl 1977; 86 Suppl 43: 7–23

[7] Nashner L. Computerized dynamic posturography. In: Jacobson G, Newman CW, Kartush JM, eds. Handbook of Balance Function Testing. St. Louis: CV Mosby, 1996:280–307

[8] Curthoys IS, Kim J, McPhedran SK, Camp AJ. Bone conducted vibration selectively activates irregular primary otolithic vestibular neurons in the guinea pig. Exp Brain Res 2006; 175: 256–267

[9] Kushiro K, Zakir M, Ogawa Y, Sato H, Uchino Y. Saccular and utricular inputs to sternocleidomastoid motoneurons of decerebrate cats. Exp Brain Res 1999; 126: 410–416

[10] Goto F, Meng H, Bai R et al. Eye movements evoked by selective saccular nerve stimulation in cats. Auris Nasus Larynx 2004; 31: 220–225

[11] Uchino Y, Sasaki M, Sato H, Imagawa M, Suwa H, Isu N. Utriculoocular reflex arc of the cat. J Neurophysiol 1996; 76: 1896–1903

[12] Goto F, Meng H, Bai R et al. Eye movements evoked by the selective stimulation of the utricular nerve in cats. Auris Nasus Larynx 2003; 30: 341–348

[13] Colebatch JG, Halmagyi GM, Skuse NF. Myogenic potentials generated by a click-evoked vestibulocollic reflex. J Neurol Neurosurg Psychiatry 1994; 57: 190–197

[14] Uchino Y, Sato H, Sasaki M et al. Sacculocollic reflex arcs in cats. J Neurophysiol 1997; 77: 3003–3012

[15] Colebatch JG, Rothwell JC. Motor unit excitability changes mediating vestibulocollic reflexes in the sternocleidomastoid muscle. Clin Neurophysiol 2004; 115: 2567–2573

[16] Iwasaki S, Chihara Y, Smulders YE et al. The role of the superior vestibular nerve in generating ocular vestibular-evoked myogenic potentials to bone conducted vibration at Fz. Clin Neurophysiol 2009; 120: 588–593

[17] de Waele C, Huy PT, Diard JP, Freyss G, Vidal PP. Saccular dysfunction in Ménière's disease. Am J Otol 1999; 20: 223–232

[18] Murofushi T, Shimizu K, Takegoshi H, Cheng PW. Diagnostic value of prolonged latencies in the vestibular evoked myogenic potential. Arch Otolaryngol Head Neck Surg 2001; 127: 1069–1072

[19] Helling K, Schönfeld U, Clarke AH. Treatment of Ménière's disease by low-dosage intratympanic gentamicin application: effect on otolith function. Laryngoscope 2007; 117: 2244–2250

[20] Iwasaki S, Smulders YE, Burgess AM et al. Ocular vestibular evoked myogenic potentials to bone conducted vibration of the midline forehead at Fz in healthy subjects. Clin Neurophysiol 2008; 119: 2135–2147

[21] Rosengren SM, McAngus Todd NP, Colebatch JG. Vestibular-evoked extraocular potentials produced by stimulation with bone-conducted sound. Clin Neurophysiol 2005; 116: 1938–1948

[22] Chiarovano E, Zamith F, Vidal PP, de Waele C. Ocular and cervical VEMPs: a study of 74 patients suffering from peripheral vestibular disorders. Clin Neurophysiol 2011; 122: 1650–1659

[23] Iwasaki S, Smulders YE, Burgess AM et al. Ocular vestibular evoked myogenic potentials in response to bone-conducted vibration of the midline forehead at Fz. A new indicator of unilateral otolithic loss. Audiol Neurootol 2008; 13: 396–404

[24] Manzari L, Burgess AM, Curthoys IS. Effect of bone-conducted vibration of the midline forehead (Fz) in unilateral vestibular loss (uVL). Evidence for a new indicator of unilateral otolithic function. Acta Otorhinolaryngol Ital 2010; 30: 175

11 Clinical Evaluation of the Cranial Nerves

Aaron C. Moberly and D. Bradley Welling

11.1 Introduction

The clinical evaluation of the cranial nerves (CNs) requires a thorough understanding of their anatomy, a detailed patient history, and a complete bedside examination. This chapter reviews the anatomy and clinical assessment of the CNs as they pertain to the otologist or neurotologist, and provides an up-to-date report on the current state of intraoperative neurophysiological CN monitoring. Several excellent texts are recommended for a more comprehensive review of CN anatomy and the clinical evaluation.[1–3]

The 12 pairs of CNs provide motor and sensory function for the head and neck. ▶ Fig. 11.1 illustrates the topographic anatomy of the CNs at the brainstem: CNs I and II are direct extensions of the central nervous system (CNS); CNs III and IV arise from the midbrain; CNs V to VIII originate in the pons; and CN IX to XII arise from the medulla.

11.2 Anatomy and Clinical Evaluation of Cranial Nerves

11.2.1 Cranial Nerve I: Olfactory Nerve

The olfactory pathway begins at the olfactory epithelium, a specialized sensory area of mucosa that is present along the roof of the nasal cavity, including the superior concha and superior nasal septum. This epithelium contains molecular receptors arising from the dendrites of olfactory bipolar neurons, whose axonal processes together form approximately 20 olfactory filaments. These bundles of axons traverse the cribriform plate and synapse with secondary olfactory neurons within the olfactory bulb. From here, axons travel within the olfactory tract to the primary olfactory areas within the uncus, entorhinal area, liman insula, and amygdaloid body. Further central projections travel to the limbic system as secondary olfactory areas.

The bedside evaluation of olfaction begins with a complete (including endoscopic) nasal, sinus, and nasopharyngeal examination. A quick screening test of olfaction can be performed using a series of bottles of nonirritating odorants, such as coffee or chocolate, delivered separately to each nostril with occlusion of the opposite nostril. A variety of more sophisticated commercial tests are reliable and convenient, including the University of Pennsylvania Smell Identification Test (UPSIT), the Smell Identification Test (Sensonics, Inc., Haddon Heights, NJ), the Japanese Odor Stick Identification Test (OSIT), the Scandinavian Odor Identification Test (SOIT), the Smell Diskettes (Novimed, Dietikon, Switzerland), and Sniffin'Sticks.[4] In our clinic we routinely utilize the UPSIT.

11.2.2 Cranial Nerve II: Optic Nerve

Light enters the eye and is transformed at the retina into electrical signals. These signals are transmitted centrally via the optic nerve (▶ Fig. 11.2). This nerve enters the middle cranial fossa through the optic canal, an opening in the lesser wing of the sphenoid bone. The optic chiasm is formed at the junction of the two optic nerves. Here fibers from the medial half of each retina cross into the contralateral optic tract. The majority of fibers from each optic tract terminate in the lateral geniculate nucleus of the thalamus. Optic radiations leave the thalamus, pass through the internal capsule, and terminate in each occipital lobe's primary visual cortex. Further radiations project to adjacent visual association areas.

The clinical evaluation of CN II includes testing basic visual acuity for macular function with a Snellen chart at 20 feet or using a handheld visual acuity card at the bedside. Visual field testing is performed by having the patient cover one eye and focus the other eye on the clinician's nose. The clinician covers his or her opposite eye and brings the index finger from beyond the periphery of vision toward the center of the visual field. The patient responds when the finger is first seen, with testing done in all four quadrants of the visual field. The pupillary constriction response evaluates function of both CN II (sensory) and CN III (motor) and is assessed as both a direct response (constriction of the ipsilateral pupil to light) and an indirect or consensual response (constriction of the contralateral pupil to light). A swinging flashlight test will identify an afferent pupillary defect, in which the light is swung from one eye to the other in a darkened room while the patient's eyes are fixed on a distant object. Stimulation of the normal eye causes constriction of both pupils, but stimulation of the affected eye leads to dilation of both pupils, suggesting pathology of the afferent branch of the pupil light reflex. Finally, an ophthalmoscopic examination should be done to examine the fundus. Dimming the room lights and having the patient focus on a distant object helps maximally dilate the pupils. The optic disk should be examined for sharp margins, as blurred margins may reveal increased intracranial pressure (ICP). Optic cup vessel venous pulsations should be present but may disappear with elevated ICP. A more detailed evaluation of the retina and macula generally requires consultation with the ophthalmology service.

11.2.3 Cranial Nerves III, IV, and VI: Oculomotor, Trochlear, and Abducens Nerves

The oculomotor nerve (CN III) serves a major role in eye movement, innervating four of the extrinsic eye muscles, along with the intrinsic ocular muscles (the constrictor pupillae and ciliary muscles) and the levator palpebrae superioris of the upper eyelid. The oculomotor complex (oculomotor and Edinger-Westphal nuclei) is located in the midbrain ventral to the cerebral aqueduct. The oculomotor nerve emerges ventrally from the caudal midbrain, passes between the posterior cerebral and superior cerebellar arteries, and enters the lateral aspect of the cavernous sinus. It then enters the orbit through the superior orbital fissure. Just inside the orbit, CN III splits into superior and inferior divisions. The superior division supplies motor input to the superior rectus and levator palpebrae muscles, whereas the inferior division innervates the medial rectus,

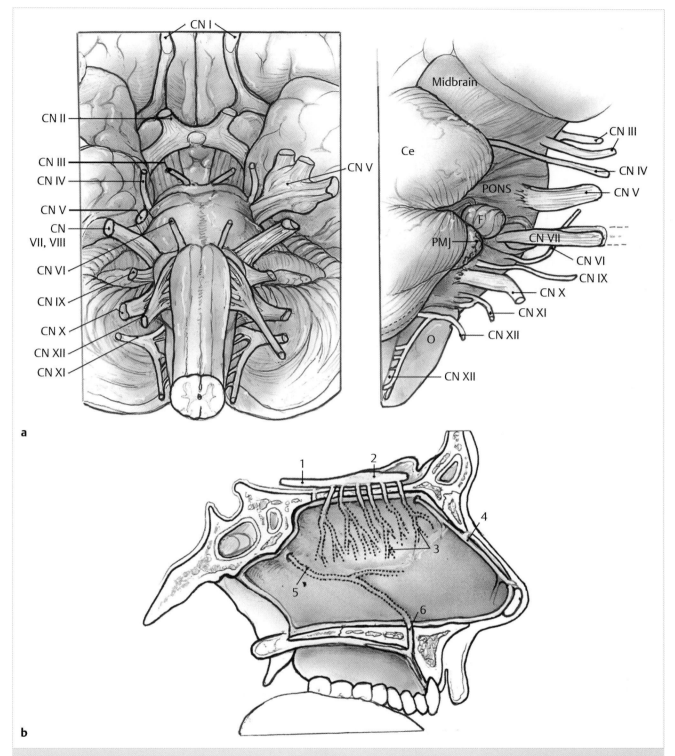

Fig. 11.1 Topographic anatomy of the cranial nerves (CNs) at the brainstem in frontal (a) and lateral (b) views. Ce, cerebellum; F, flocculus; PMJ, pontomedullary junction; O, olive. 1, olfactory tract; 2, olfactory bulb; 3, septal olfactory nerves; 4, branch of anterior ethmoidal nerve; 5, nasopalatine nerve; 6, nasopalatine nerve at incisive foramen.

inferior rectus, and inferior oblique. The inferior division also carries preganglionic parasympathetic fibers from the Edinger-Westphal nucleus to the ciliary ganglion. Postganglionic fibers travel to the ciliary body and constrictor pupillae muscles.

The trochlear nerve (CN IV) is the smallest of the CNs and innervates only the superior oblique muscle. Its fibers originate in the midbrain caudal to the oculomotor complex. Interestingly, this nerve decussates within the brainstem before exiting on

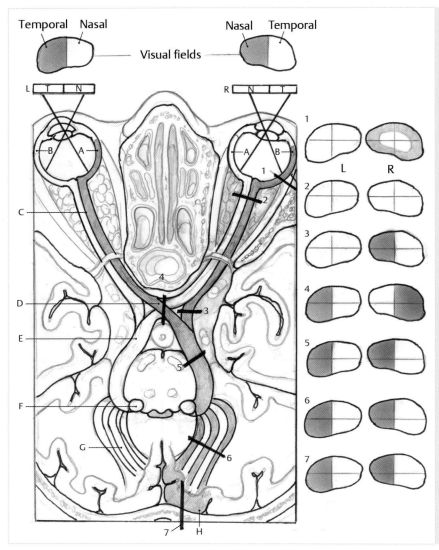

Fig. 11.2 The optic pathway. As shown, injuries at various locations along the pathway result in characteristic visual field defects, noted by the darkened areas. A, nasal retina; B, temporal retina; C, optic nerve; D, optic chiasm; E, optic tract; F, lateral geniculate nucleus; G, optic radiation; H, primary visual cortex.

the dorsal surface of the midbrain. The trochlear nerve travels along the lateral wall of the cavernous sinus just inferior to the oculomotor nerve prior to entering the orbit through the superior orbital fissure. This nerve has the longest intracranial course of any CN.

The abducens nerve (CN VI) provides motor input to the lateral rectus muscle. Its nucleus is located in the pons anterior to the fourth ventricle and adjacent to the facial motor nucleus. CN VI exits the ventral pontomedullary junction, travels rostrally along the clivus, passes through the Dorello canal, and emerges within the cavernous sinus. It enters the orbit through the superior orbital fissure.

The bedside evaluation of CN III starts with evaluation of eyelid position, with ptosis of the upper eyelid suggesting CN III injury from loss of function of the levator palpebrae superioris. With the patient looking directly ahead, the upper eyelid should not fall above the upper limit of the pupil, and the upper eyelids should be symmetrical. If the parasympathetic portion of CN III is damaged, the ipsilateral pupil will not constrict as a response to light presented to that pupil or to the contralateral pupil. Accommodation, the process of focusing on a near object,

can be tested by having the patient follow the clinician's finger from a distance to near the patient's nose. Convergence of the eyes and pupillary constriction suggest a functional CN III.

Cranial nerves III, IV, and VI together move the globe, and their motor functions are tested together. The clinician draws a large "H" in the air with his or her finger a few feet in front of the patient, who follows the movement with the eyes. Horizontal movement tests the medial and lateral rectus muscles. The vertical movements of the "H" test the superior or inferior recti and the superior or inferior obliques. A complete third nerve palsy will present with an ipsilateral eye that is deviated inferiorly and laterally, ipsilateral ptosis, and an ipsilateral enlarged and nonreactive pupil.[5] Trochlear nerve dysfunction results in hypertropia (elevation of the affected eye) and vertical diplopia, worse with downward gaze with the eye adducted, which attempts to isolate the function of the superior oblique. A resting head tilt toward the nonaffected side may result from a chronic trochlear nerve injury. Isolated abducens palsy results in impaired ipsilateral abduction, with worsening diplopia on ipsilateral lateral gaze.[5]

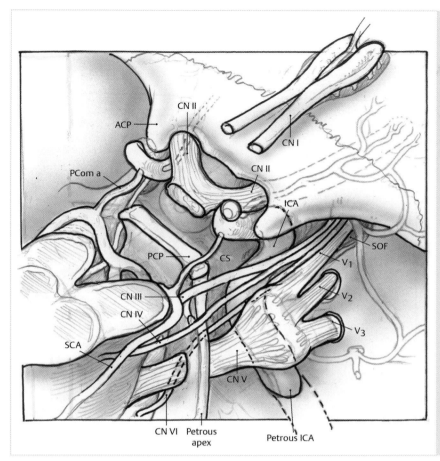

Fig. 11.3 Drawing of the anterior and middle cranial fossae depicting cranial nerves I (olfactory), II (optic), III (oculomotor), IV (trochlear), V (trigeminal), and VI (abducens). Note the dorsal origin of the trochlear nerve as well as the ascent of the abducens nerve along the clivus. ACP, anterior clinoid process; PCP, posterior clinoid process; ICA, internal carotid artery; SOF, superior orbital fissue; CS, clivus; V1, ophthalmic division of trigeminal nerve; V2, maxillary division of trigeminal nerve; V3, mandibular division of trigeminal nerve; PCom a, posterior communicating artery; SCA, superior cerebellar artery.

11.2.4 Cranial Nerve V: Trigeminal Nerve

The principal brainstem nuclei of CN V are the motor (masticator) nucleus and the pontine (sensory) trigeminal nucleus (▶ Fig. 11.3; ▶ Fig. 11.4).

The trigeminal nerve emerges from the mid-lateral pons as a large sensory and smaller motor root. Its principal sensory ganglion, the semilunar or gasserian ganglion, is situated in the Meckel cave along the anteromedial floor of the middle cranial fossa. From the ganglion, three divisions of the nerve (ophthalmic V_1, maxillary V_2, and mandibular V_3) exit the intracranial space through the superior orbital fissure, foramen rotundum, and foramen ovale, respectively. The ophthalmic division divides into its four terminal branches (the frontal nerve, the nasociliary nerve, the lacrimal nerve, and a meningeal branch) within the orbit. The maxillary division splits into a meningeal branch, the zygomatic nerve, the infraorbital nerve, and the superior alveolar nerve within the pterygopalatine fossa. The peripheral ganglion of the maxillary nerve, the pterygopalatine ganglion, is located within the pterygopalatine fossa. The mandibular nerve traverses the foramen ovale and enters the infratemporal fossa. Here it divides into its terminal branches, the auriculotemporal nerve, the buccal nerve, the lingual nerve, and the inferior alveolar nerve. Accompanying V_3 of the trigeminal nerve is the parasympathetic otic ganglion, situated in the infratemporal fossa. The trigeminal nerve provides motor innervation to the muscles of mastication, the mylohyoid, the anterior belly of the digastric muscle, the tensor tympani, and the tensor veli palatini muscles. It also receives general sensory information from the face and scalp (up to the vertex of the head), conjunctiva, paranasal sinuses and nasal cavity, oral cavity (including tongue and dentition), anterior ear canal, lateral surface of the tympanic membrane, and the meninges of the anterior and middle cranial fossa.

Primary bedside evaluation of the trigeminal nerve assesses both sensory and motor functions. The presence and symmetry of sensation over the forehead (V_1), cheeks (V_2), and chin (V_3) are tested. Pain (with a toothpick), temperature (with a warm or cool object), and light touch (with cotton) pathways can be tested more specifically. The sensory portion of the corneal reflex (V_1) can be tested as a blink response to a light touch of a cotton wisp on the cornea.

The motor component of the trigeminal nerve (part of V_3) can be tested by having the patient clench the jaws tightly while the clinician palpates the masseter and temporalis muscles. Examination for jaw deviation to one side on wide mouth opening suggests a lesion of the ipsilateral trigeminal nerve. A mandibular reflex (jaw jerk) can be tested by tapping the middle of the chin with a reflex hammer with the mouth partially open. A normal response is a slight closing of the jaws.

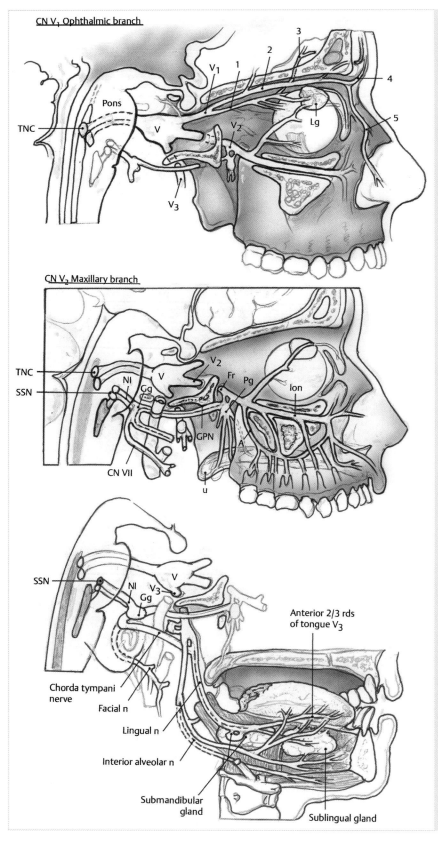

CN V₁ Ophthalmic branch

CN V₂ Maxillary branch

Fig. 11.4 Drawing of the V₁, V₂, and V₃ divisions of the trigeminal nerve. TNC, trigeminal nucleus; V, gasserian ganglion; 1, nasociliary nerve; 2, frontal nerve; 3, intracranial branch; 4, supratrochlear nerve; 5, external branch of anterior ethmoidal nerve; Lg, lacrimal gland; SSN, superior salivary nucleus; NI, nervus intermedius; Gg, geniculate ganglion; GPN, greater petrosal nerve; Fr, foramen rotundum; Pg, pterygopalatine ganglion; Ion, infraorbital nerve; u, uvula.

11.2.5 Cranial Nerve VII: Facial Nerve

Cranial nerve VII emerges from the caudal pons, passes through the cerebellopontine angle (CPA), and enters the internal auditory canal (IAC), where it assumes an anterosuperior position at the fundus (► Fig. 11.5). The helpful phrase "7-Up, Coke down" has been used to remember the arrangement of the seventh and eighth CNs in the lateral IAC fundus. Several named segments characterize the intratemporal course of the facial nerve, including the labyrinthine, geniculate, tympanic (horizontal), and mastoid (vertical) segments. The nerve exits the temporal bone through the stylomastoid foramen and divides at the pes anserinus into temporozygomatic and cervicofacial trunks. These primary branches then split into five terminal branches: frontal (zygomatic), orbital, buccal, marginal mandibular, and cervical nerves.

The facial nerve contains motor fibers from the facial motor nucleus, parasympathetic fibers from the superior salivatory nucleus, taste afferents to the nucleus solitarius, and general sensory afferents to the spinal trigeminal tract. The nerve provides motor innervation to the stapedius, stylohyoid, posterior belly of digastric, auricular muscles, muscles of facial expression, buccinator, and platysma. Parasympathetic innervation of the lacrimal gland occurs via the greater superficial petrosal nerve. The chorda tympani nerve stimulates salivation from the submandibular and sublingual glands. Special sensory fibers within the chorda tympani transmit taste afferents from the anterior two thirds of the tongue, whereas the greater superficial petrosal nerve mediates taste from the posterior soft palate. General sensation from the posterior meatal skin of the ear canal is carried by the facial nerve, along with branches of CN V, IX, and X (► Fig. 11.6).

A full clinical evaluation of the facial nerve examines the motor, parasympathetic, taste, and general sensory functions of the nerve. Topographic testing historically was performed to localize a lesion along CN VII but has not been found to be reliable. The initial clinical examination should classify the extent of motor weakness (using the House-Brackmann scale) and approximate the location of nerve injury. The upper face receives bilateral central motor innervation. As a result, brainstem and peripheral facial nerve injuries cause a paralysis of the entire ipsilateral face, whereas injuries rostral to the facial motor nucleus spare the upper face. The clinician should observe the patient's spontaneous facial movements, followed by examination while the patient raises his or her eyebrows (frontalis), closes the eyes tightly against attempted opening by the clinician (orbicularis oculi), presses the lips together firmly (orbicularis oris), puffs out the cheeks (buccinators), and clinches the jaw to examine for platysma contraction. Asymmetric rapid eye blinking acts as a sensitive measure of slight facial nerve weakness. Function of the stapedius can be evaluated by the stapedial reflex performed by an audiologist.

The parasympathetic function of CN VII can be evaluated with the Schirmer test for tearing. A piece of filter paper 5 mm by 25 mm can be placed into the lower conjunctival sac with the remainder hanging over the edge of the lower lid. After 5 minutes, an individual with parasympathetic dysfunction will have moistened less than 10 mm of the paper. This test is rarely performed as its specificity is low. A patient history of dry eyes may be more useful, as is a history of dry mouth for assessment of salivatory function.

Taste is rarely tested clinically, but it may be evaluated with a cotton swab moistened with a sugary or salty solution with the patient identifying the solution placed on the ipsilateral tongue. Liquid drops and taste strips may also be used with qualitative responses from the patient.[6]

General sensation is tested by evaluating sensation of over the lateral auricular concha or posterior external auditory canal. Loss of sensation here is called "Hitselberger's sign" and suggestive of compression of CN VII by a CPA tumor.

11.2.6 Cranial Nerve VIII: Vestibulocochlear Nerve

The vestibulocochlear nerve (► Fig. 11.5) exits the brainstem as one nerve but separates into the cochlear, superior vestibular, and inferior vestibular nerves as it approaches the IAC. The cochlear nerve is initially inferior to the vestibular nerve within the CPA but rotates into an anteroinferior position by the time it reaches the IAC. The superior and inferior vestibular nerves are situated in the posterosuperior and posteroinferior quadrants, respectively, whereas the facial nerve is located in an anterosuperior position at the fundus. Nerve cell bodies in the spiral ganglion (cochlear) and Scarpa's ganglion (vestibular) transmit information from specialized sensory end-organs within the cochlea (organ of Corti), the utricle and saccule (maculae), and the semicircular canals (cristae ampullaris).

The auditory pathway begins with cochlear hair cells that transduce mechanical energy into electrical impulses. These impulses are transmitted along the auditory nerve to the ipsilateral cochlear nucleus by the neurons of the spiral ganglion. From the cochlear nucleus, ipsilateral and contralateral auditory pathways are generated. The majority of fibers cross the brainstem and synapse in the contralateral superior olivary complex or pass through the lateral lemniscus to the inferior colliculus. Information is then relayed to the medial geniculate body of the thalamus from which it is transmitted to the primary auditory complex of the temporal lobe.

The bedside evaluation begins with a thorough otologic examination of the external and middle ear. A complete evaluation of hearing requires audiological testing. Basic bedside tests of hearing include the whisper test and a tuning fork examination. In the Weber test, a 512-Hz tuning fork lateralizes toward the side with a conductive hearing loss and away from the ear with a sensorineural loss. The Rinne test is positive (normal) if air conduction (tuning fork next to the pinna) is greater than bone conduction (tuning fork placed on the mastoid tip). Bone conduction greater than air conduction typically reflects a 25-dB or greater conductive hearing loss.

Bedside vestibular testing includes evaluating the patient's gait and performing the Romberg and tandem Romberg tests; normal balance requires intact somatosensory, visual, and vestibular input. Spontaneous, gaze, positional, and positioning (including Dix-Hallpike) nystagmus should be sought. A post–head-shake nystagmus will beat away from an ear with unilateral vestibular loss. The presence of a post–head-thrust refixation saccade reflects a vestibular weakness in the ear toward which

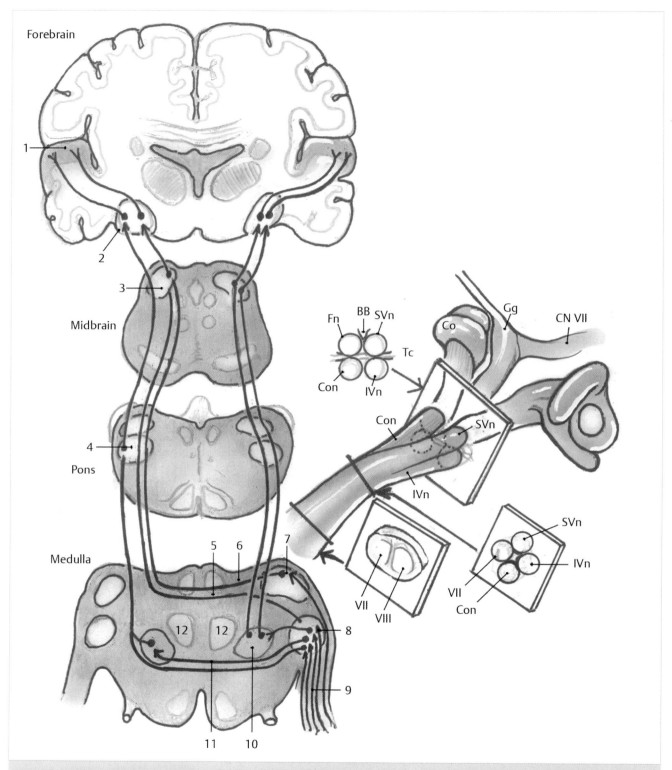

Fig. 11.5 Anatomy of the seventh (facial) and eighth (vestibulocochlear) CNs. At the fundus of internal auditory canal, the facial nerve is in the anterosuperior quadrant, the cochlear nerve is in the anteroinferior quadrant, and the superior and inferior vestibular nerves are in the posterosuperior and posteroinferior quadrants. 1, primary auditory cortex; 2, medial geniculate nucleus; 3, inferior colliculus; 4, lateral lemniscus; 5, intermediate acoustic stria; 6, dorsal acoustic stria; 7, dorsal cochlear nucleus; 8, ventral cochlear nucleus; 9, auditory nerve; 10, superior olivary complex; 11, trapezoid body; 12, reticular formation; Fn, facial nerve; SVn, superior vestibular nerve; Con, cochlear nerve; IVn, inferior vestibular nerve; BB, Bill's bar; Tc, transverse crest; Co, cochlea; Gg, geniculate ganglion.

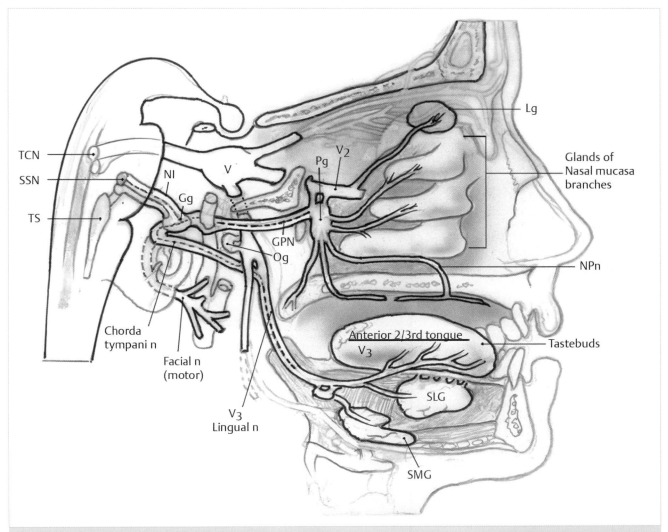

Fig. 11.6 Facial nerve innervation. This nerve stimulates lacrimation and nasal secretions, contributes to taste sensation along the soft palate and anterior tongue, is motor to the mimetic facial musculature, and sensory to the skin of external auditory meatus. TCN, trigeminal nerve; SSN, superior salivary nucleus; TS, tractus solitaries; NI, nervus intermedius; Gg, geniculate ganglion; GPN, greater petrosal nerve; Og, otic ganglion; Pg, pteryngopalatine ganglion; Lg, lacrimal gland; NPn, nasopalatine nerve; SLG, sublingual gland; SMG, submandibular gland.

the head is thrust. Detailed descriptions regarding these and other tests are covered in Chapters 10 and 14.

11.2.7 Cranial Nerve IX: Glossopharyngeal Nerve

The ninth CN provides motor innervation to the stylopharyngeus muscle (arising from the nucleus ambiguus), parasympathetic input to the parotid gland (inferior salivatory nucleus), innervation to the carotid body and carotid sinus (nucleus solitarius), general sensation (trigeminal tract) and taste (nucleus solitarius) to the posterior third of the tongue, and is sensory to a portion of the ear canal and internal surface of the tympanic membrane (trigeminal tract). It exits the medulla as rootlets, which enter the jugular foramen. Superior and inferior glossopharyngeal ganglia are present within the foramen. As the

nerve enters the jugular foramen, the tympanic branch (Jacobson's nerve) separates and enters the middle ear through the inferior (hypotympanic) canaliculus. A plexus is formed on the promontory of the cochlea after which the nerve reconstitutes as the lesser petrosal nerve. This petrosal nerve enters the middle cranial fossa, descends through the foramen ovale, and synapses with the otic ganglion in the infratemporal fossa. Parasympathetic fibers from CN IX eventually join the auriculotemporal nerve (V₃) within the otic ganglion.

Bedside examination of CN IX tests only the sensory component. This involves testing the afferent limb of the oropharyngeal gag reflex by lightly touching the right and left sides of the pharynx with a tongue depressor or cotton swab. Supraglottic sensation may be tested during flexible fiberoptic laryngoscopy. A history of xerostomia, particularly during mastication, may reflect parotid dysfunction secondary to CN IX palsy.

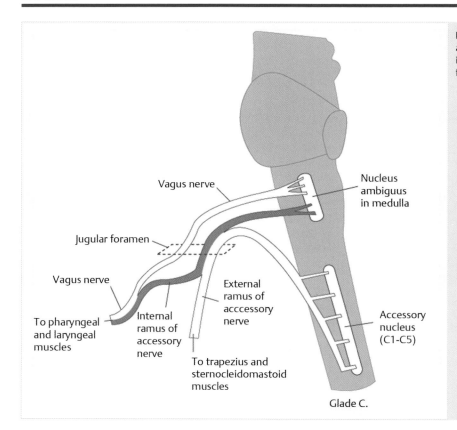

Fig. 11.7 Cranial nerves X (vagus) and XI (spinal accessory). Note that some fibers initially traveling with CN XI join CN X distal to the jugular foramen.

Vagus nerve

Nucleus ambiguus in medulla

Jugular foramen

Vagus nerve

External ramus of acccessory nerve

To pharyngeal and laryngeal muscles

Internal ramus of accessory nerve

To trapezius and sternocleidomastoid muscles

Accessory nucleus (C1-C5)

Glade C.

11.2.8 Cranial Nerve X: Vagus Nerve

Vagal nerve rootlets emerge from the medulla and join as they enter the jugular foramen (▶ Fig. 11.7). The superior (jugular) and inferior (nodose) ganglia of CN X are located within this foramen. Some fibers from the caudal aspect of the nucleus ambiguus exit the brainstem within the spinal accessory nerve (CN XI) but later join CN X after it exits the skull base. Motor branches from the vagus nerve (nucleus ambiguus) include the pharyngeal branch, the superior laryngeal nerve, and the recurrent laryngeal nerve. Parasympathetic fibers (dorsal vagal nucleus) innervate glands within the pharyngeal, laryngeal, gastric, and intestinal mucosa. Visceral sensation from the gut is transmitted to the nucleus solitarius. General sensory afferents from the pharynx, larynx, skin of the external auditory canal (auricular branch), external surface of the tympanic membrane (auricular branch), and meninges of the posterior fossa travel with CN X to the trigeminal tract and nucleus.

Clinical testing of the vagus nerve includes evaluation of the efferent limb of the gag reflex. Inspection of the palate while having the patient say "ahhh" should reveal contraction of the superior pharyngeal constrictor muscle. Unilateral constrictor paresis will result in deviation of the uvula to the normal side with lowering of the palatal arch on the affected side. A bedside swallow evaluation can be performed to rule out aspiration. Appraisal of voice quality for hypernasality, hoarseness, or breathiness may suggest a vagal lesion. Fiberoptic or direct laryngoscopy should be performed to examine vocal cord motion with vocalization.

11.2.9 Cranial Nerve XI: Spinal Accessory Nerve

The accessory nucleus is located within the spinal cord. Axons from lower motor neurons emerge as rootlets that ascend through the foramen magnum into the posterior cranial fossa. These are joined by fibers of the nucleus ambiguus to form CN XI (▶ Fig. 11.7). The spinal accessory nerve exits the posterior fossa through the jugular foramen and provides motor innervation to the sternocleidomastoid (SCM) and trapezius muscles.

Clinical evaluation of CN XI requires testing of both the SCM and trapezius. The muscles should be examined for asymmetry caused by denervation atrophy, and a winged scapula suggests trapezius weakness. The SCM is tested by having the patient tilt the chin toward the opposite side against resistance. The trapezius is tested by having the patient abduct the arm 180 degrees against resistance; failure to abduct more than 100 degrees suggests CN XI weakness. Shrugging the shoulders against resistance can also test trapezius function.

11.2.10 Cranial Nerve XII: Hypoglossal Nerve

The hypoglossal nerve provides motor input to the ipsilateral tongue by innervating all intrinsic and extrinsic tongue musculature except the palatoglossus muscle (CN X). The hypoglossal nucleus is located within the medulla. Nerve rootlets exit between the pyramids and olive to form a common trunk, which then traverses the hypoglossal (anterior condylar) canal.

The hypoglossal nerve is evaluated first by examining the tongue at rest, looking for fasciculation or atrophy. The patient is then asked to protrude the tongue, with weakness manifesting as deviation of the tongue toward the weaker side because of the unopposed action of the contralateral genioglossus.

11.3 Nerve Injury

Seddon's[7] 1943 three-tier classification of neural injury was later expanded in 1951 by Sunderland[8] into a five-tier system (▶ Fig. 11.8).

Sunderland used the terms *first-* and *second-degree injury* in place of Seddon's *neurapraxia* and *axonotmesis,* while subclassifying Seddon's *neurotmesis* into third-, fourth-, and fifth-degree injuries. A first-degree injury (neurapraxia) is a conduction block resulting from edema and compression at the site of injury. Once edema resolves, complete recovery usually occurs within days or weeks, or up to 3 months if demyelination has occurred. Second-degree injury (axonotmesis) results in wallerian degeneration distal to the injured site. Electromyographic (EMG) testing confirms denervation for motor nerves, but reinnervation is expected as axons grow toward their target musculature roughly 1 mm/day. A second-degree injury is more severe than a first-degree conduction block, but endoneurial

tubules remain intact to guide regenerating axons. Complete recovery is expected. Seddon used the term *neurotmesis* to mean complete disruption of the nerve. Sunderland's subclassification divided neurotmesis into third-degree injury (endoneurial disruption without loss of perineurium or epineurium), fourth-degree injury (disruption of endoneurium and perineurium), and fifth-degree injury (transection of endoneurium, perineurium, and epineurium). Third-degree injuries usually recover some function but with varying degrees of synkinesis. Fourth- and fifth-degree injuries do not recover. Unfortunately, electrical tests are unable to differentiate between axonotmesis and neurotmesis because both undergo wallerian degeneration. One should recognize that each nerve trunk (within its epineurial sheath) contains numerous perineurial fascicles, which in turn ensheath large numbers of axon-containing endoneurial tubules. A compound nerve action potential and the resulting muscle twitch it engenders reflect the net effect of the electrical activity within the entire nerve trunk.

11.4 Electrophysiologic Testing of the Facial Nerve

Several electrophysiological tests can be performed to evaluate the function of the facial nerve. Two forms of testing are

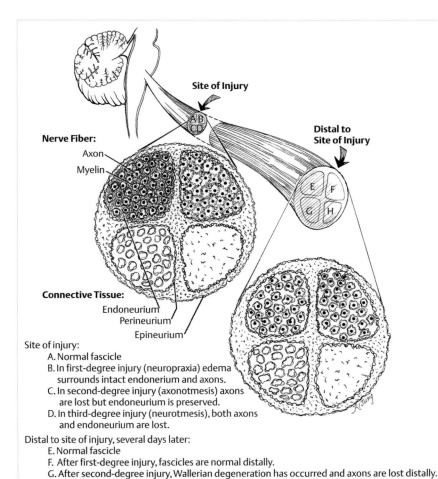

Fig. 11.8 Cross-sectional model of microanatomic changes in mild to moderate CN injury. The effects of neural injury dictate the potential for successful, appropriate patterns of fiber regeneration across the site of nerve injury. (Courtesy of John K. Niparko, MD.)

Nerve Fiber:
Axon
Myelin

Connective Tissue:
Endoneurium
Perineurium
Epineurium

Site of injury:
A. Normal fascicle
B. In first-degree injury (neuropraxia) edema surrounds intact endonerium and axons.
C. In second-degree injury (axonotmesis) axons are lost but endoneurium is preserved.
D. In third-degree injury (neurotmesis), both axons and endoneurium are lost.

Distal to site of injury, several days later:
E. Normal fascicle
F. After first-degree injury, fascicles are normal distally.
G. After second-degree injury, Wallerian degeneration has occurred and axons are lost distally.
H. After third-degree injury, loss of endoneurium at the site of injury prevents guidance of regenerating fibers into distal nerve segment.

Site of Injury

Distal to Site of Injury

qualitative and require a subjective assessment by the observer. The nerve excitability test (NET) uses an electrical current to stimulate the facial nerve at the stylomastoid foramen. A minimum threshold stimulus for initiating perceptible facial motion on the uninjured side is established first. This threshold is then compared with the threshold obtained from the injured side. A 3.5-mA or greater difference in thresholds between the two sides represents a significant difference. The maximal stimulation test (MST) delivers suprathreshold stimuli at the stylomastoid foramen bilaterally while an observer grades the maximal mimetic response obtained from each side.

To improve interobserver reliability, electroneurography (ENoG) was developed. This is a semiquantitative electrical test of facial nerve function. As with MST, suprathreshold electrical stimuli are applied bilaterally at the stylomastoid foramina to elicit a maximal contraction on each side. In its original description, bipolar pads placed along the nasolabial folds recorded the compound action potential from the underlying mimetic musculature. Direct measurement of these potentials using EMG electrodes is now referred to as evoked electromyography (EEMG). The amplitude of these potentials is proportional to the number of functional motor axons present within the facial nerve.[9] Peak-to-peak amplitude differences between the normal and involved sides of the face are expressed as percent degeneration of axons within the injured nerve. ENoG should be performed between 3 and 21 days after neural injury. Wallerian degeneration distal to the site of an intracranial or intratemporal facial nerve injury takes place within 72 hours, and a proximally injured nerve continues to stimulate at the stylomastoid foramen until that time. Therefore, ENoG is unreliable for the first 3 days after the onset of facial paralysis. This test also becomes unreliable after 3 weeks. By this time, axons in varying stages of degeneration and regeneration create asynchronous neural activity.

Spontaneous or voluntary EMG activity can be recorded from mimetic muscles innervated by all five terminal branches of the facial nerve. Spontaneous EMG activity is classified as normal (di- or triphasic), polyphasic, or fibrillation potentials. The presence of fibrillation potentials reflects relatively recent denervation at the motor end plate, whereas long-standing denervation results in electrical silence.[10,11] Testing spontaneous EMG is most useful during nerve regeneration. The presence of polyphasic EMG potentials in a patient with complete clinical facial paralysis reflects active neuronal reinnervation. In fact, these polyphasic potentials can precede functional recovery by several weeks.

Clinically, ENoG has been used to determine when surgical intervention might be appropriate for patients with facial paralysis.[12,13] Fisch[13] suggested that greater than 90% degeneration on ENoG within 3 weeks of facial nerve injury justifies surgical decompression. Gantz and associates,[10] in a multicenter clinical trial of Bell palsy, demonstrated that patients with greater than 90% degeneration on ENoG testing and no evidence of voluntary potentials on EMG within 14 days of facial paralysis had improved outcomes with surgical decompression of the labyrinthine segment. Outcomes in patients electing middle fossa decompression medial to the geniculate ganglion were compared with those patients who refused surgery. Those undergoing surgical decompression exhibited a House-Brackmann

(HB) grade I or II in 91% of cases, whereas the control group had a 58% chance of an unfavorable HB grade III or IV recovery at 7 months. In 1999, Chang and Cass[14] extensively reviewed the literature on facial nerve injury in temporal bone trauma. They suggested that patients with greater than 95% degeneration within 2 weeks of injury may benefit from decompression. In both studies antiviral medications were not used. For children with Bell palsy, the presence of any identifiable ENoG response may indicate a favorable recovery of facial movement.[15] Takemoto et al[16] found that an ENoG response of greater than 85% degeneration has a specificity of 77.8% and sensitivity of 71.4% in predicting nonrecovery of facial movement (with recovery defined as an improvement on the Yanagihara grading system to at least 36 out of 40) in patients with Bell palsy and Ramsay Hunt syndrome.

11.5 Intraoperative Cranial Nerve Monitoring

Intraoperative monitoring of the cranial nerves has become common in skull base operations as the goals of treatment have been refined from reducing mortality to preserving functional integrity of the surrounding anatomy. During the late 19th and early 20th centuries, Krause[17] and Frazier[18] described using monopolar electrical current for stimulating the facial nerve. Responses were evaluated by subjective observation for facial movement. In 1979, Delgado and associates[19] introduced intraoperative, recordable facial EMG. Sugita and Kobayashi[20] then coupled the EMG to a loudspeaker, making muscle activity audible to the surgeon. Neurophysiological monitoring has become a profession in itself with various societies and certifying bodies including the American Board of Registered Electrodiagnostics Technologists (ABRET), the Certification in Neurophysiological Intraoperative Monitoring (CNIM), and the American Board of Neurophysiologic Monitoring (ABNM).

Cranial nerves III to VII and IX to XII are typically monitored using spontaneous or evoked EMG. Multichannel EMG devices are capable of recording electrical activity in several muscle groups simultaneously. Because the operating room is an electrically and acoustically hostile environment, these systems must mute their audible responses upon detecting interference from other equipment. High- and low-pass acoustic filters can help reduce signal artifacts.[21]

Several electrode designs are available. These include monopolar or bipolar surface and needle electrodes. Bipolar needle electrodes inserted directly into the muscles being monitored provide the best signal-to-noise ratio. Insulated needle electrodes or hook-wire electrodes allow for deeper insertions when necessary. Stimulator probes also come in monopolar and bipolar varieties. Insulated monopolar probes are less bulky and provide 1-mm spatial resolution.[22] Equipment manufacturers now make surgical dissection instruments coupled directly to monopolar stimulating probes.

11.5.1 Intraoperative Monitoring of the Facial Nerve

Modern vestibular schwannoma (VS) surgery successfully preserves the anatomic integrity of the facial nerve in more than

90% of cases.[23,24] Acoustically coupled EMG remains the gold standard for intraoperative facial nerve monitoring.[25,26] It has been found to be cost-effective in mastoid surgery in addition to skull base procedures,[27] and it may shorten surgical time.[28] Spontaneous EMG recordings detect direct mechanical stimulation of the nerve but may also represent spontaneous facial nerve activity (if the depth of anesthesia is not adequate) or artifact from instrumentation. Stimulus-evoked EMG at suprathreshold stimulation helps surgeons identify the nerve during difficult dissections, such as during dissection of large or cystic tumors of the CPA. Prass and Luders[29] described two patterns of EMG activity. "Burst" activity refers to short, synchronized motor unit potentials resulting from direct stimulation, whereas "train" activity reflects asynchronous, often prolonged motor unit responses secondary to intraoperative nerve irritation or traction. Trains are more frequently observed from nerves that have sustained preoperative compression, stretch, or ischemic injury.[21] In general, a greater number and higher rate of trains correlates with greater nerve irritation.[30] Irrigating with body temperature saline and reducing nerve traction usually quells a train response.

The optimal type, intensity, and duration of the stimulus applied during intraoperative facial nerve stimulation is debated. Constant-voltage stimulation and constant-current stimulation both have their advocates.[21] Surgeon preference usually dictates the type of stimulus used. Most surgeons use electrical stimuli of between a 50- and 200-μs duration. Some guidelines for facial nerve stimulus intensity during surgery are 0.05 to 0.2 mA for intracranial stimulation, 0.1 to 0.3 mA for intratemporal stimulation, and 0.1 to 0.5 mA for extracranial stimulation.[21]

Although a positive stimulation response may help the operator identify the facial nerve, a negative response can mean anything from the nerve not being present in that location to a monitor malfunction, temporary nerve dysfunction, effects from anesthesia, electrical interference, or probe failure. The 1991 National Institutes of Health (NIH) consensus conference on vestibular schwannoma advocated routine facial nerve monitoring during neurotologic resection.[31] The American Academy of Otolaryngology–Head and Neck Surgery has supported the "proven efficacy" of intraoperative nerve monitoring to minimize the risk of facial nerve injury.[32] Several studies have found a higher rate of HB grade I or II outcomes and fewer HB V or VI in monitored patients.[33–35] A recent meta-analysis of 79 articles showed that the use of EMG facial nerve monitoring was one of three factors (the other two being tumor size and surgical approach) that improved long-term facial nerve function.[36] The monitor, however, is not a substitute for thorough knowledge of anatomy, surgical experience, and good judgment.

Intraoperative facial nerve monitoring can help predict postoperative facial function. Prell et al[37] found EMG train time, a quantitative parameter of time intervals of nerve response trains, to correlate strongly with deterioration of postoperative facial nerve function. Intraoperative monitoring parameters, including proximal stimulation threshold and proximal-to-distal response amplitude ratio, were found to predict risk of long-term facial nerve dysfunction using a logistic regression equation in 60 patients with positive and negative predictive values of 95% and 67%, respectively.[38] Grayeli et al[39] found that a proximal threshold between 0.01 and 0.04 mA with a response greater than 100 μV had a positive predictive value of 94% for a

HB grade I or II outcome using a four-channel EMG device in 89 patients. Electrical silence portends a bad outcome.[40] Thresholds less than 0.05 mA or 0.2 V using monopolar stimulation indicate a good long-term prognosis for facial nerve function.[41] Neff and colleagues[24] found that if the EMG response to facial nerve stimulation was greater than or equal to 240 μV at a stimulus intensity less than or equal to 0.05 mA, this predicted an HB grade I or II outcome in 98% of patients. Mandpe and coworkers[42] reported that only 41% of patients stimulating to less than 200 μV achieved an HB grade I or II recovery. Assessment methods utilizing proximal/distal response ratios for amplitude and latency may be more useful than absolute values.[43]

A specific EMG response has been identified on stimulation of the nervus intermedius.[44] The observed response is low amplitude, is only identified in the orbicularis oris channel, and has a prolonged latency as well as later onset relative to the facial nerve. Knowledge of this response and recognition of the nervus intermedius may prevent inadvertent injury to the facial nerve. Additionally, antidromic (retrograde) stimulation of the greater superficial petrosal nerve during middle fossa surgery may help to identify the facial nerve where the greater superficial petrosal enters at the facial hiatus.[45]

A significant limitation of EMG-based monitoring of the facial nerve is the large electrical artifact induced by electrocautery, which limits the ability to monitor the nerve during the use of instrumentation that may put the nerve at risk. Video-based and webcam video monitoring systems for intraoperative facial nerve monitoring have been developed as an alternative.[46,47] Another limitation of EMG monitoring is the requirement that the surgeon actively stimulate the nerve to obtain a response, which may be difficult in large tumors. A possible solution and a method that is familiar to neurosurgeons is transcranial electrical stimulation, which is widely used for monitoring corticospinal tracts during spinal surgery. Transcranial stimulation of the contralateral motor cortex with measurement of facial nerve motor evoked potentials (FNMEPs) may provide an alternative method of facial nerve monitoring.[48,49] Fukuda et al[50] found that initial postoperative and long-term facial nerve function correlated significantly with FNMEP responses in 35 patients with cranial base tumors. Response amplitude reduction by 30% or more dictates a change in surgical activity to enable rapid nerve recovery.[51] A final limitation of EMG-based facial nerve monitoring techniques is the contraindication to the use of muscle relaxants by the anesthesiologist.

11.5.2 Intraoperative Monitoring of Auditory Function (CN VIII)

Intraoperative auditory brainstem response (ABR), electrocochleography (ECochG), otoacoustic emissions (OAEs), and direct eighth nerve monitoring (DENM) are techniques used to monitor the vestibulocochlear nerve. Intraoperative ABR requires a sound source, surface electroencephalogram (EEG) electrodes and amplifiers, a computer for averaging ABR sweeps, and a monitor for displaying the tracing. The ABR is a set of seven peaks named by consecutive roman numerals. Preoperative presence of an ABR may help prognosticate chances for hearing preservation.[52] Only patients with a discernible wave V on ABR preoperatively can be monitored with intraoperative ABR, Each patient must have a baseline ABR established just prior to the start of the operation. Click stimuli > 70 dB sound level (SL) are typically delivered at 20 to 30 clicks per second.[53] Each ABR sweep is filtered and averaged by a computer, which then provides waveforms. The delay from stimulus to averaged waveform may be up to several minutes. Acoustic interference from instruments such as electrocautery, drills, and the cavitron ultrasonic aspirator (CUSA) is a significant limitation.[54] Cerebellar retraction, dissection, acoustic trauma, temperature changes, and interruptions to cochlear blood flow can also affect the ABR.[53]

Matthies and Samii[55] reported the utility of intraoperative bilateral ABR in more than 200 VS resections. Temporary or permanent losses of waves V, I, and III occurred in 21%, 27%, and 29% of patients, respectively. Wave III disappearance was the earliest and most sensitive sign of trauma to the auditory nerve. Other clinicians prefer to monitor wave V. Bischoff et al[56] posited that reversible intraoperative changes in ABR responses are likely caused by disturbances of microcirculation to the nerve, whereas abrupt or irreversible loss suggested a mechanical nerve injury. Much of the more recent literature on intraoperative ABR monitoring compares this modality to other, newer monitoring techniques.

Electrocochleography also requires a sound source but can utilize a variety of different recording electrodes. Transtympanic electrodes provide the best ECochG tracing but risk tympanic membrane perforation and subsequent cerebrospinal fluid (CSF) leakage. Tympanic membrane electrodes placed in contact with the eardrum generate the next best signal-to-noise ratio. Electrocochleography records the cochlear microphonic (CM), summating potential (SP), and the eighth nerve action potential (AP) in response to sound stimuli. ECochG reflects only the status of the cochlea and distal auditory nerve. However, some reports have shown a good correlation between changes in the AP and postoperative hearing loss, even when the cochlea itself is not directly injured.[57,58]

Direct eight nerve monitoring (DENM) techniques use wire electrodes, wick electrodes, or the Cueva electrode. The Cueva electrode (Ad-Tech, Racine, WI) is a C-shaped monopolar electrode that can be attached directly to the cochlear nerve. The DENM response may be present even when a preoperative ABR is absent.[59] The high-amplitude DENM responses require minimal signal averaging and permit nearly real-time data acquisition, with intraoperative feedback given within 1 to 2 seconds, as compared with 2 to 3 minutes for ABR.[21,60] In general, monopolar electrodes are used more frequently than bipolar electrodes. Rosenberg and colleagues, however, reported a specially designed flush-tipped, bipolar electrode to help define the cochlear-vestibular cleavage plane during vestibular nerve section.[61] Electrodes have been developed that consist of a tuft of cotton against the brain or a malleable wire attached to a retractor with a flexible wire that allows stable positioning of the electrode on the cisternal portion of the nerve.[62,53]

Robust compound nerve action potentials (CNAPs) were found in some cases with unreliable ABRs, and the positive presence of CNAPs was 100% predictive of postoperative serviceable hearing. Most electrode designs are limited because the electrode must be placed on a clear segment of normal cochlear nerve. Møller and coworkers[63] have described placement of a monopolar recording electrode in the lateral recess of the fourth ventricle to record directly from the cochlear nucleus. Roberson et al[64] has described using a plate electrode placed along the floor of the IAC during middle fossa procedures. As with ABR, stretching the nerve increases response latency before affecting amplitude.[65]

Recording OAEs requires a sound source and microphones placed within the ear canal. OAEs reflect intact outer hair cell function within the organ of Corti. Telischi and colleagues[66] reported that changes in distortion-product otoacoustic emissions (DPOAEs) were exquisitely sensitive to interruptions in cochlear blood flow. Recordings could be obtained as frequently as every 2 seconds and provided nearly real-time data. Morawski and associates[67] used DPOAEs monitoring in 20 patients undergoing resection of acoustic tumors using a retrosigmoid approach. They found that DPOAEs from the basal regions of the cochlea were more readily affected by surgical manipulation than those from middle and apical segments. Microcoagulation of small vessels, tumor debulking, and compression or stretch of IAC contents resulted in altered DPOAEs. This group felt that the DPOAEs did not assist the surgeon during tumor dissection, but the presence of DPOAEs at the end of the procedure correlated with postoperative hearing outcomes.

Several studies have compared or examined combinations of ABR, ECochG, and DENM for intraoperative monitoring. Tucker and coworkers[68] found that the presence of both ABR and CNAP at the end of resection was associated with successful hearing preservation, whereas their absence was associated with loss of hearing in 75.5% of cases. No association was found between ABR, CNAP, and hearing preservation in nearly 25% of cases. Yamakami and coworkers[69] found DENM to be more useful than ABR in 10 patients undergoing CPA tumor surgery. Hearing was preserved in eight of the 10 patients postoperatively. ABR was useless in six of the 10 patients due to severe artifacts. This group found that DENM more accurately predicted postoperative hearing outcome. Battista and colleagues[70] compared ABR, ECochG, and DENM retrospectively in 66 patients. Overall, 24% of patients retained useful hearing. Forty percent of DENM patients retained their hearing, whereas only 18% of ABR and 17% of ECochG patients retained theirs. Jackson and Roberson[71] compared CNAP with ABR in 25 patients undergoing hearing preservation acoustic tumor surgery. Pure-tone average < 50 dB and word recognition > 50% were used to define successful hearing preservation. CNAPs were obtained in 92% of patients, whereas ABR was recordable in only 48%. For tumors less than or equal to 2 cm, hearing was preserved in 67% of those monitored with CNAPs; ABR monitoring did not significantly alter hearing preservation rates.

Danner and associates[72] retrospectively compared use of DENM using the Cueva electrode in one group of patients with intraoperative ABR in another cohort. A total of 77 patients undergoing retrosigmoid resection of vestibular schwannomas were included in the study. In the DENM group, hearing was preserved in 71% of patients with tumors 1 cm or less and 32% with tumors between 1 and 2.5 cm. Hearing preservation using ABR was 41% and 10%, respectively. These authors concluded that DENM was superior to ABR in preserving hearing. In comparing ABR, CNAP, and ECochG, Colletti and associates[73] found that CNAPs were most predictive of hearing preservation. In fact, irreversible loss of CNAPs was 100% predictive of poor postoperative hearing.

11.5.3 Intraoperative Monitoring of Other Cranial Nerves

Although not routinely performed for neurotologic procedures, progress has been made for monitoring the remaining cranial nerves. Intraoperative olfactory evoked potentials have been measured in animal and clinical studies during the removal of brain tumors and aneurysm clippings during frontotemporal operations.[74] Stimulating electrodes were affixed to the olfactory mucosa, and recording electrodes were placed on the exposed olfactory tract after craniotomy with frontal lobe retraction. A 50% decrease in response amplitude or 10% increase in response latency is used as a standard to alert the surgeon to impending nerve injury,[75] although these criteria have not been tested in detail.

Visual-evoked potentials for monitoring of CN II have been done during anterior skull base procedures and endoscopic sinus surgery but were initially unreliable in the operating room.[76] Newer stimulus delivery techniques have improved the validity of CN II monitoring. These potentials can be measured by scalp recordings over the visual cortex as a response to fiber-optic light flashes delivered through closed eyelids. Reversible changes in the responses and loss of responses were associated with postoperative vision loss.[77]

Cranial nerves III, IV, and VI may be monitored directly by inserting long, insulated needle or hookwire electrodes into the extraocular muscles. Ultrasound guidance may be used to improve accuracy and safety of electrode placement.[78] Conventional neuronavigation systems may be used with placement of a skin fiducial marker near the orbit prior to brain imaging.[79] Another option is the use of shorter bipolar electrodes placed in proximity to the extraocular muscles to obtain electrical signals by volume conduction. Noninvasive monitoring using electrooculography, which measures the electrical potential difference between the retina and cornea, has also been used to monitor the eyes for movement.[80]

The motor division of the mandibular nerve (V_3) can be monitored using fine hookwire EMG electrodes placed in either the temporalis or masseter muscles. Because of interference from overlying mimetic muscles, surface electrodes are discouraged.[81] Monitoring the temporalis muscle is ideal but may be limited during neurotologic cases. More recently, trigeminal somatosensory evoked potentials have been evaluated as a potential method for intraoperative monitoring of CN V with stimulating needle electrodes placed in the lower and upper lips and recording electrodes from the contralateral scalp overlying the sensory cortex.[82]

Monitoring of CN IX should always be performed in conjunction with CN X, because the majority of the pharyngeal musculature is innervated by CN X. EMG responses from stylopharyngeus activity without concurrent activity of the laryngeal musculature suggests a true CN IX response. Hookwire electrodes are placed into the ipsilateral lateral pharyngeal wall under direct observation. Alternatively, surface electrodes can be mounted on a laryngeal mask airway (LMA) placed against the lateral pharyngeal wall with the patient intubated through the LMA.[83] CN X can be monitored by recording from an endotracheal tube with affixed or built-in electrodes. Medtronic-Xomed (Jacksonville, FL) offers a commercially available tube with integrated EMG electrodes. Needle or hookwire electrodes may be placed under laryngoscopic guidance or percutaneously, and these electrodes provide a better signal-to-noise ratio than surface electrodes on an endotracheal tube.[84] It is worth noting that monitoring of CN IX and X may evoke bradycardia or hypotension because these nerves innervate the carotid body baroreceptors and the heart, respectively; these responses should be treated intraoperatively with atropine.

Monitoring of CN XI requires EMG monitoring of the trapezius or SCM muscle. The upper trapezius can be conveniently needled along the medial half of the top ridge of the shoulder.[85] The SCM may be used, but the wire electrode must be placed well within the SCM deep to the platysma (innervated by CN VII) with care to avoid the great vessels. CN XII can be monitored with electrodes placed directly into the tongue or into the genioglossus muscle through a percutaneous submandibular approach.

11.6 Conclusion

Accurate assessment of CN function begins with a thorough anatomic and functional understanding. Supplemental electrical testing is now part of the surgeon's technological armamentarium for diagnostic purposes, as well as in helping the surgeon preserve neurologic function while removing disease. Minimizing patient morbidity with respect to CN function has now become a primary objective in the practice of otology and neurotology.

References

[1] Wilson-Pauwels L, Stewart PA, Akesson EJ, Spacey SD. Cranial Nerves: Function and Dysfunction. Shelton, CT: People's Medical Publishing House, 2010

[2] Brazis PW, Masdeu JC, Biller J. Localization in Clinical Neurology. Philadelphia: Lippincott Williams & Wilkins, 2011

[3] Snell RS. Clinical Neuroanatomy. Philadelphia: 2010

[4] Simmen D, Briner HR. Olfaction in rhinology—methods of assessing the sense of smell. Rhinology 2006; 44: 98–101

[5] Rucker JC. Cranial neuropathies. In: Daroff RB, ed. Bradley's Neurology in Clinical Practice. Philadelphia: Elsevier, 2012:1745–1761

[6] Mueller C, Kallert S, Renner B et al. Quantitative assessment of gustatory function in a clinical context using impregnated "taste strips." Rhinology 2003; 41: 2–6

[7] Seddon HJ. Three types of nerve injury. Brain 1943; 66: 237–288

[8] Sunderland S. Nerve and Nerve Injuries, 2nd ed. New York: Churchill Livingstone, 1978

[9] Esslen E. The Acute Facial Palsies. Berlin: Springer-Verlag, 1977

[10] Gantz BJ, Rubinstein JT, Gidley P, Woodworth GG. Surgical management of Bell's palsy. Laryngoscope 1999; 109: 1177–1188

[11] Dumitru D, Walsh NE, Porter LD. Electrophysiologic evaluation of the facial nerve in Bell's palsy. A review. Am J Phys Med Rehabil 1988; 67: 137–144

[12] Esslen E. The Acute Facial Palsies. Berlin: Springer-Verlag, 1977

[13] Fisch U. Prognostic value of electrical tests in acute facial paralysis. Am J Otol 1984; 5: 494–498

[14] Chang CY, Cass SP. Management of facial nerve injury due to temporal bone trauma. Am J Otol 1999; 20: 96–114

[15] Baba S, Kondo K, Kanaya K, Ushio M, Tojima H, Yamasoba T. Bell's palsy in children: relationship between electroneurography findings and prognosis in comparison with adults. Otol Neurotol 2011; 32: 1554–1558

[16] Takemoto N, Horii A, Sakata Y, Inohara H. Prognostic factors of peripheral facial palsy: multivariate analysis followed by receiver operating characteristic and Kaplan-Meier analyses. Otol Neurotol 2011; 32: 1031–1036

[17] Krause F. Surgery of the Brain and Spinal Cord, vol 2. New York: Rebman, 1912

[18] Frazier CH. Intracranial division of the auditory nerve for persistent aural vertigo. Surg Gynecol Obstet 1912; 15: 524–529

[19] Delgado TE, Bucheit WA, Rosenholtz HR, Chrissian S. Intraoperative monitoring of facila muscle evoked responses obtained by intracranial stimulation of the facila nerve: a more accurate technique for facila nerve dissection. Neurosurgery 1979; 4: 418–421

[20] Sugita K, Kobayashi S. Technical and instrumental improvements in the surgical treatment of acoustic neurinomas. J Neurosurg 1982; 57: 747–752

[21] Martin WH, Mishler ET. Intraoperative monitoring of auditory evoked potentials and facial nerve electromyography. In: Katz ed. Handbook of Clinical Audiology, 5th ed. Philadelphia: Lippincott Williams & Wilkins, 2002:323–348

[22] Kartush JM, Niparko JK, Bledsoe SC, Graham MD, Kemink JL. Intraoperative facial nerve monitoring: a comparison of stimulating electrodes. Laryngoscope 1985; 95: 1536–1540

[23] Kartush JM, Lundy LB. Facial nerve outcome in acoustic neuroma surgery. Otolaryngol Clin North Am 1992; 25: 623–647

[24] Neff BA, Ting J, Dickinson SL, Welling DB. Facial nerve monitoring parameters as a predictor of postoperative facial nerve outcomes after vestibular schwannoma resection. Otol Neurotol 2005; 26: 728–732

[25] Nadol JB, Jr, Chiong CM, Ojemann RG et al. Preservation of hearing and facial nerve function in resection of acoustic neuroma. Laryngoscope 1992; 102: 1153–1158

[26] Beck DL, Benecke JE, Jr. Intraoperative facial nerve monitoring. Technical aspects. Otolaryngol Head Neck Surg 1990; 102: 270–272

[27] Wilson L, Lin E, Lalwani A. Cost-effectiveness of intraoperative facial nerve monitoring in middle ear or mastoid surgery. Laryngoscope 2003; 113: 1736–1745

[28] Grosheva M, Klussmann JP, Grimminger C et al. Electromyographic facial nerve monitoring during parotidectomy for benign lesions does not improve the outcome of postoperative facial nerve function: a prospective two-center trial. Laryngoscope 2009; 119: 2299–2305

[29] Prass RL, Lüders H. Acoustic (loudspeaker) facial electromyographic monitoring: Part 1. Evoked electromyographic activity during acoustic neuroma resection. Neurosurgery 1986; 19: 392–400

[30] Minahan RE, Mandir AS. Neurophysiologic intraoperative monitoring of trigeminal and facial nerves. J Clin Neurophysiol 2011; 28: 551–565

[31] National Institutes of Health Consensus Statement. Acoustic neuromas. NIH Consensus Development Conference, Bethesda MD, December 11–13, 1991

[32] American Academy of Otolaryngology. Facial Nerve Monitoring Policy of the American Academy of Otolaryngology–Head Neck Surg, 2006. http://www.entlink.net/practice/rules/facial_nerve_monitoring.cfm

[33] Kwartler JA, Luxford WM, Atkins J, Shelton C. Facial nerve monitoring in acoustic tumor surgery. Otolaryngol Head Neck Surg 1991; 104: 814–817

[34] Kartush JM. Electroneurography and intraoperative facial monitoring in contemporary neurotology. Otolaryngol Head Neck Surg 1989; 101: 496–503

[35] Hammerschlag PE, Cohen NL. Intraoperative monitoring of facial nerve function in cerebellopontine angle surgery. Otolaryngol Head Neck Surg 1990; 103: 681–684

[36] Sughrue ME, Yang I, Rutkowski MJ, Aranda D, Parsa AT. Preservation of facial nerve function after resection of vestibular schwannoma. Br J Neurosurg 2010; 24: 666–671

[37] Prell J, Rampp S, Romstöck J, Fahlbusch R, Strauss C. Train time as a quantitative electromyographic parameter for facial nerve function in patients undergoing surgery for vestibular schwannoma. J Neurosurg 2007; 106: 826–832

[38] Isaacson B, Kileny PR, El-Kashlan HK. Prediction of long-term facial nerve outcomes with intraoperative nerve monitoring. Otol Neurotol 2005; 26: 270–273

[39] Grayeli AB, Guindi S, Kalamarides M et al. Four-channel electromyography of the facial nerve in vestibular schwannoma surgery: sensitivity and prognostic value for short-term facial function outcome. Otol Neurotol 2005; 26: 114–120

[40] Nakao Y, Piccirillo E, Falcioni M et al. Prediction of facial nerve outcome using electromyographic responses in acoustic neuroma surgery. Otol Neurotol 2002; 23: 93–95

[41] Bernat I, Grayeli AB, Esquia G, Zhang Z, Kalamarides M, Sterkers O. Intraoperative electromyography and surgical observations as predictive factors of facial nerve outcome in vestibular schwannoma surgery. Otol Neurotol 2010; 31: 306–312

[42] Mandpe AH, Mikulec A, Jackler RK, Pitts LH, Yingling CD. Comparison of response amplitude versus stimulation threshold in predicting early postoperative facial nerve function after acoustic neuroma resection. Am J Otol 1998; 19: 112–117

[43] Goldbrunner RH, Schlake HP, Milewski C, Tonn JC, Helms J, Roosen K. Quantitative parameters of intraoperative electromyography predict facial nerve

[44] Ashram YA, Jackler RK, Pitts LH, Yingling CD. Intraoperative electrophysiologic identification of the nervus intermedius. Otol Neurotol 2005; 26: 274–279

[45] Arriaga M, Haid R, Masel D. Antidromic stimulation of the greater superficial petrosal nerve in middle fossa surgery. Laryngoscope 1995; 105: 102–105

[46] Filipo R, Pichi B, Bertoli GA, De Seta E. Video-based system for intraoperative facial nerve monitoring: comparison with electromyography. Otol Neurotol 2002; 23: 594–597

[47] De Seta E, Bertoli GA, De Seta D, Covelli E, Filipo R. New development in intraoperative video monitoring of facial nerve: a pilot study. Otol Neurotol 2010; 31: 1498–1502

[48] Yingling CD, Gardi JN. Intraoperative monitoring of facial and cochlear nerves during acoustic neuroma surgery. 1992. Neurosurg Clin N Am 2008; 19: 289–315, vii

[49] Dong CC, Macdonald DB, Akagami R et al. Intraoperative facial motor evoked potential monitoring with transcranial electrical stimulation during skull base surgery. Clin Neurophysiol 2005; 116: 588–596

[50] Fukuda M, Oishi M, Hiraishi T, Saito A, Fujii Y. Intraoperative facial nerve motor evoked potential monitoring during skull base surgery predicts long-term facial nerve function outcomes. Neurol Res 2011; 33: 578–582

[51] Matthies C, Raslan F, Schweitzer T, Hagen R, Roosen K, Reiners K. Facial motor evoked potentials in cerebellopontine angle surgery: technique, pitfalls and predictive value. Clin Neurol Neurosurg 2011; 113: 872–879

[52] Brackmann DE, Owens RM, Friedman RA et al. Prognostic factors for hearing preservation in vestibular schwannoma surgery. Am J Otol 2000; 21: 417–424

[53] Yingling CD, Ashram YA. Intraoperative monitoring of cranial nerves in skull base surgery. In: Jackler RK, Brackmann DE eds. Neurotology, 2nd ed. Philadelphia: Elsevier Mosby, 2005:958–994

[54] Simon MV. Neurophysiologic intraoperative monitoring of the vestibulocochlear nerve. J Clin Neurophysiol 2011; 28: 566–581

[55] Matthies C, Samii M. Management of vestibular schwannomas (acoustic neuromas): the value of neurophysiology for intraoperative monitoring of auditory function in 200 cases. Neurosurgery 1997; 40: 459–466, discussion 466–468

[56] Bischoff B, Romstöck J, Fahlbusch R, Buchfelder M, Strauss C. Intraoperative brainstem auditory evoked potential pattern and perioperative vasoactive treatment for hearing preservation in vestibular schwannoma surgery. J Neurol Neurosurg Psychiatry 2008; 79: 170–175

[57] Attias J, Nageris B, Ralph J, Vajda J, Rappaport ZH. Hearing preservation using combined monitoring of extra-tympanic electrocochleography and auditory brainstem responses during acoustic neuroma surgery. Int J Audiol 2008; 47: 178–184

[58] Battista RA, Wiet RJ, Paauwe L. Evaluation of three intraoperative auditory monitoring techniques in acoustic neuroma surgery. Am J Otol 2000; 21: 244–248

[59] Jackson LE, Roberson JB, Jr. Acoustic neuroma surgery: use of cochlear nerve action potential monitoring for hearing preservation. Am J Otol 2000; 21: 249–259

[60] Cueva RA. Preoperative, intraoperative, and postoperative auditory evaluation of patients with acoustic neuroma. Otolaryngol Clin North Am 2012; 45: 285–290, vii

[61] Rosenberg SI, Martin WH, Pratt H, Schwegler JW, Silverstein H. Bipolar cochlear nerve recording technique: a preliminary report. Am J Otol 1993; 14: 362–368

[62] Yamakami I, Yoshinori H, Saeki N, Wada M, Oka N. Hearing preservation and intraoperative auditory brainstem response and cochlear nerve compound action potential monitoring in the removal of small acoustic neurinoma via the retrosigmoid approach. J Neurol Neurosurg Psychiatry 2009; 80: 218–227

[63] Møller AR, Jho HD, Jannetta PJ. Preservation of hearing in operations on acoustic tumors: an alternative to recording brain stem auditory evoked potentials. Neurosurgery 1994; 34: 688–692, discussion 692–693

[64] Roberson J, Senne A, Brackmann D, Hitselberger WE, Saunders J. Direct cochlear nerve action potentials as an aid to hearing preservation in middle fossa acoustic neuroma resection. Am J Otol 1996; 17: 653–657

[65] Moller AR. Evoked Potentials in Intraoperative Monitoring. Baltimore: Williams & Wilkins, 1988

[66] Telischi FF, Widick MP, Lonsbury-Martin BL, McCoy MJ. Monitoring cochlear function intraoperatively using distortion product otoacoustic emissions. Am J Otol 1995; 16: 597–608

[67] Morawski K, Namyslowski G, Lisowska G, Bazowski P, Kwiek S, Telischi FF. Intraoperative monitoring of cochlear function using distortion product otoacoustic emissions (DPOAEs) in patients with cerebellopontine angle tumors. Otol Neurotol 2004; 25: 818–825

[68] Tucker A, Slattery WH, III, Solcyk L, Brackmann DE. Intraoperative auditory assessments as predictors of hearing preservation after vestibular schwannoma surgery. J Am Acad Audiol 2001; 12: 471–477

[69] Yamakami I, Oka N, Yamaura A. Intraoperative monitoring of cochlear nerve compound action potential in cerebellopontine angle tumour removal. J Clin Neurosci 2003; 10: 567–570

[70] Battista RA, Wiet RJ, Paauwe L. Evaluation of three intraoperative auditory monitoring techniques in acoustic neuroma surgery. Am J Otol 2000; 21: 244–248

[71] Jackson LE, Roberson JB, Jr. Acoustic neuroma surgery: use of cochlear nerve action potential monitoring for hearing preservation. Am J Otol 2000; 21: 249–259

[72] Danner C, Mastrodimos B, Cueva RA. A comparison of direct eighth nerve monitoring and auditory brainstem response in hearing preservation surgery for vestibular schwannoma. Otol Neurotol 2004; 25: 826–832

[73] Colletti V, Fiorino FG, Mocella S, Policante Z. ECochG, CNAP and ABR monitoring during vestibular Schwannoma surgery. Audiology 1998; 37: 27–37

[74] Sato M, Kodama N, Sasaki T, Ohta M. Olfactory evoked potentials: experimental and clinical studies. J Neurosurg 1996; 85: 1122–1126

[75] Balzer JR, Rose RD, Welch WC, Sclabassi RJ. Simultaneous somatosensory evoked potential and electromyographic recordings during lumbosacral decompression and instrumentation. Neurosurgery 1998; 42: 1318–1324, discussion 1324–1325

[76] Cedzich C, Schramm J. Monitoring of flash visual evoked potentials during neurosurgical operations. Int Anesthesiol Clin 1990; 28: 165–169

[77] Kodama K, Goto T, Sato A, Sakai K, Tanaka Y, Hongo K. Standard and limitation of intraoperative monitoring of the visual evoked potential. Acta Neurochir (Wien) 2010; 152: 643–648

[78] Schlake HP, Goldbrunner R, Siebert M, Behr R, Roosen K. Intra-Operative electromyographic monitoring of extra-ocular motor nerves (Nn. III, VI) in skull base surgery. Acta Neurochir (Wien) 2001; 143: 251–261

[79] Alberti O, Sure U, Riegel T, Bertalanffy H. Image-guided placement of eye muscle electrodes for intraoperative cranial nerve monitoring. Neurosurgery 2001; 49: 660–663, discussion 663–664

[80] Fukaya C, Katayama Y, Kasai M, Kurihara J, Yamamoto T. Intraoperative electrooculographic monitoring of oculomotor nerve function during skull base surgery. Technical note. J Neurosurg 1999; 91: 157–159

[81] Harper CM. Intraoperative cranial nerve monitoring. Muscle Nerve 2004; 29: 339–351

[82] Malcharek MJ, Landgraf J, Hennig G, Sorge O, Aschermann J, Sablotzki A. Recordings of long-latency trigeminal somatosensory-evoked potentials in patients under general anaesthesia. Clin Neurophysiol 2011; 122: 1048–1054

[83] Husain AM, Wright DR, Stolp BW, Friedman AH, Keifer JC. Neurophysiological intraoperative monitoring of the glossopharyngeal nerve: technical case report. Neurosurgery 2008; 63 Suppl 2: 277–278, discussion 278

[84] Bigelow DC, Patterson T, Weber R, Stecker MM, Judy K. Comparison of endotracheal tube and hookwire electrodes for monitoring the vagus nerve. J Clin Monit Comput 2002; 17: 217–220

[85] Skinner SA. Neurophysiologic monitoring of the spinal accessory nerve, hypoglossal nerve, and the spinomedullary region. J Clin Neurophysiol 2011; 28: 587–598

12 Otologic Photography and Videography

Ken Yanagisawa and Eiji Yanagisawa

12.1 Introduction

The first American photographic documentation of the tympanic membrane[1] occurred in 1887 when Randall and Morse[2] published a series of normal and pathological images of the tympanic membrane. Since that time, many different methods of tympanic membrane photography have evolved.[3–16] Open-tube photography was popularized using a variety of different cameras including the Cameron, Brubaker-Holinger, and Kowa.[3–6] Buckingham[3] first adapted the Brubaker-Holinger camera to ear photography in the mid-1950s, and produced beautiful, high-quality images of the tympanic membrane and middle ear. Smith et al[6] described an inexpensive method of producing high-resolution images of the tympanic membrane using a Kowa Fundus camera. Both of these methods produced small images that required editing and enlargement to be appreciated when projected. The introduction of the Carl Zeiss operating microscope in the late 1950s permitted large images of the tympanic membrane. Attachments to the microscope were developed that utilized photo adapters to capture 35-mm and video images.[8,9] An alternative, less expensive method of photographing the tympanic membrane through the eyepiece of the microscope with a 35-mm single lens reflex (SLR) camera was described by Hughes et al[7] and Yanagisawa.[8]

The development of the Hopkins telescope was a significant advancement in endoscopic technology.[8–15] Rather than air-containing spaces between conventional lenses, glass rods with polished ends separated by small air lenses were used, greatly improving image quality, brightness, and magnification. Many clinicians including Konrad et al,[10] Chen et al,[11] Chole,[12] Nomura,[13] Yanagisawa,[8] and Hawke[14] have refined the techniques for improving the quality of images captured with the telescope. Several excellent textbooks of telescopic tympanic membrane photography have been published.[17–21] Selkin[16] recommended fiberscopic photography as an alternative means to capture images of the tympanic membrane. Transtympanic endoscopy of the middle ear was pioneered by Nomura[13] in 1982 and advocated by Poe et al[22] as an office procedure to precede middle ear exploration using a 2-mm or smaller telescope, which yielded acceptable pictures of middle ear structures.

With the advent of video cameras, Yanagisawa[23–26] promoted videography as an ideal method for endoscopic documentation; it provided a real-time record of anatomic structures and their associated movements, and allowed instantaneous review, confirming adequate image capture. Retakes, if necessary, could be immediately recorded. He advocated the wider use of videography and video printers in all branches of otolaryngology.[23–27] Excellent still images could be produced from selected videotape images using an analog video printer.[23–28]

The era of widespread digital imaging has arrived.[29–32] Newer digital image capture systems such as the Stryker Digital Capture System (SDCS; Kalamazoo, MI) allow rapid image transport to a high-density computer disk. Image capture time takes 1 second. Stored images can be viewed, selected, and easily retrieved.[30]

The D-scope system (Medical Digital Developers, New York, NY) allows image transfer from the endoscope to the video capture and control unit.[33] Digital still images and videos can be viewed on the monitor screen individually, or played back next to previously stored images or videos, for comparison or surveillance. Files are saved by patient name and date of examination and are readily accessible.

With the widespread use of still digital cameras, their use in otorhinolaryngological endoscopy has been recommended.[30–37] Melder and Mair[34] compared an off-the-shelf digital camera with a standard 35-mm SLR endoscopic camera and introduced a simple, inexpensive, and easily available endoscopic digital photography system. They stated that digital photography offered numerous advantages over analog photography, predicting that digital imaging would soon replace 35-mm camera photography. This time has come.

Haynes et al[37] described the microscopic photographic technique with a handheld digital camera placed in contact with one of the microscope ocular lenses and discussed the merits of digital photography. Using this practical and inexpensive technique, well-taken pictures of a variety of microsurgical procedures through the eyepiece of the microscope could be obtained.

With new technologies come new challenges such as equipment size and data archiving. Much of the equipment available for high-quality image and video recording is costly and often bulky in size. Harris and Goyal[38] reported on the use of a portable media device that offers an affordable and small video capture device with reasonable resolution and clarity. Image and video files can be simply transferred to a computer using a universal serial bus (USB) connected drive. The issues of database management and retrieval of images and videos are real and valid problems, especially as image libraries continually enlarge. Calhoun and Decherd[39] discussed various options for setting up an effective and efficient digital image archiving system that could retrieve appropriate images based on, for example, disease categories or chronological timing after surgery.

Telemedicine (the use of electronic communications to exchange medical information) represents a potential future direction in health care, especially as the quality of digital images continues to improve.[40–42] Aronzon et al[41] reported that the accuracy of otologic diagnosis from digital images approached the accuracy of a live physical examination, particularly when the evaluation was performed by an experienced otolaryngologist. Kokesh et al[42] reported on the successful use of digital images for otoscopic diagnosis, and supported the use of these images in telemedicine applications to help providers in rural, underserved, or remote locations such as theirs in Alaska. The key to the success of telemedical diagnoses is the assurance that digital images for review are of acceptable quality, and adequately visualize the structures of interest (e.g., the entire tympanic membrane free of obstructing cerumen).

This chapter discusses traditional (film) photography, digital (i.e., filmless) photography, and videography of the ear.

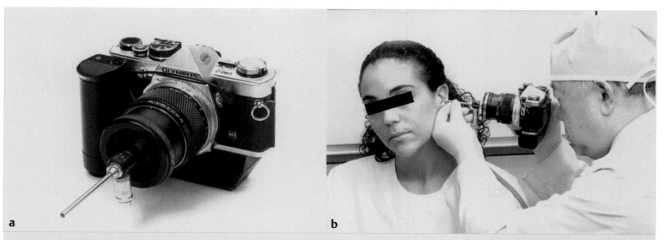

Fig. 12.1 Telescopic film photography of the ear. (a) Equipment used for telescopic film photography included the Olympus OM2 35-mm SLR camera with autowinder, a 100-mm macrolens, the Karl Storz quick-connect adapter, and the Hopkins 4-mm, 0-degree 1215A ototelescope. (b) The technique of telescopic film photography. An Olympus OM-2 SLR camera with a Hopkins 4-mm, 0-degree 1215A ototelescope is held in one hand while the tip of the telescope and the head of the patient are supported by the other hand to prevent injury to the ear canal.

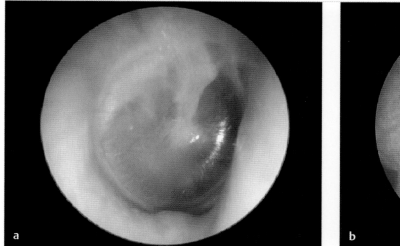
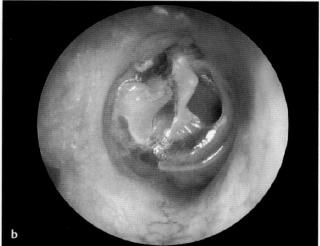

Fig. 12.2 Telescopic film photography of the ear using a 35-mm SLR camera and Hopkins 4-mm, 0-degree 1215A ototelescope. (a) Normal right tympanic membrane. (b) Right postoperative tympanoplasty with incus repositioning.

12.2 Traditional (Film) Photography

Silver-based photography has now been firmly eclipsed by digital photography and technology. History will remember traditional film photography as the initial method of "permanent" and accurate image recording; previously, the recall capabilities of human memory, or the notations of hand-drawn sketches, were the only methods of documentation. For medical conditions, silver photography was transformational in allowing comparisons of pre- and post- interventions and treatments, seeing the progression of diseases over time, and serving as a teaching tool to educate patients and students of medicine about disease processes.

The drawbacks of traditional film photography include (1) the time required for film/slide processing (causing a delay in seeing the final image); (2) image degradation over time; (3) the need for different films with different film speeds (ASAs) and different lighting characteristics (e.g., tungsten versus daylight); and (4) storage issues that have been overcome by the digital technologies now available.

Previous versions of this chapter have clearly documented the techniques for traditional film photography (► Fig. 12.1; ► Fig. 12.2; ► Fig. 12.3; ► Fig. 12.4). Much of the equipment, the techniques, and the setups are identical for film versus digital cameras, the main difference being the recording medium. Tips for successful image capture are discussed in detail below (see Digital Photography).

12.3 Digital Photography

Digital imaging has arrived as the newest, and now widely accepted, technology for permanently recording images. An

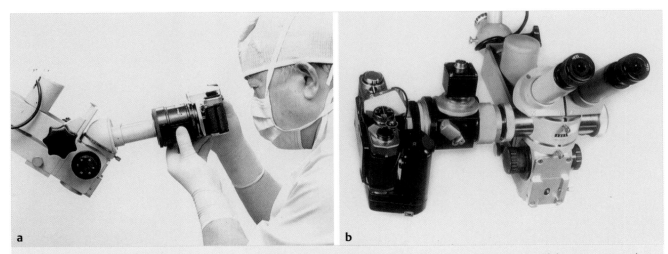

Fig. 12.3 Microscopic film photography of the ear. (a) Technique of microscopic film photography through the eyepiece of the microscope without photoadapter. Recessed housing of the macrolens of an SLR camera is held against the eyepiece of the microscope. Make sure the optical line of the microscope and the camera is straight. The tympanic membrane is focused through the camera viewfinder and photographs are taken. (b) Technique of microscopic film photography with a photoadapter. The SLR camera is attached to the operating microscope using the photoadapter and the beam splitter. The subject is focused through the camera viewfinder and photographs are taken.

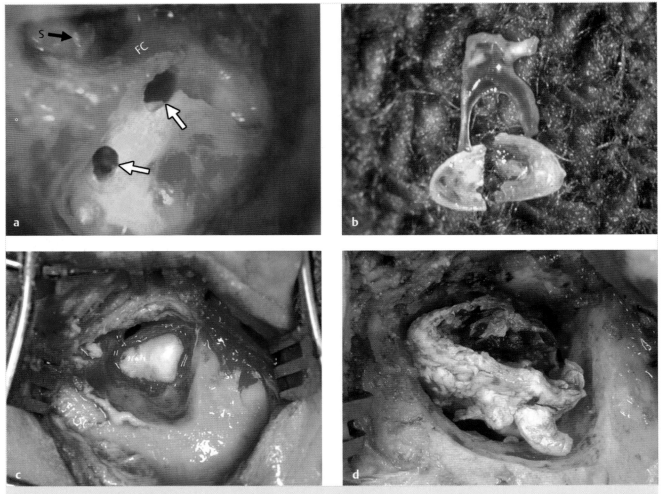

Fig. 12.4 Microscopic film photography through the eyepiece of the microscope without a photoadapter. (a) Left mastoid cavity with opened horizontal semicircular canal (*white arrows*) during labyrinthectomy. S, stapes; FC, facial canal. (b) Otosclerotic stapes removed during total stapedectomy. Microscopic film photography with a photoadapter. (c) Cholesteatoma filling the medial portion of the left mastoid cavity. (d) Large cholesteatoma filling the left mastoid cavity.

image obtained via a video camera is converted to an electronic signal that a computer can read, record, and store in a digital fashion.[30] There are three primary approaches to creating digital images:

1. Convert a photograph or slide into a still digital image using a scanner connected to a computer.
2. Convert an analog signal from a video camera or videotape into streaming digital video with an image capture board installed in a computer. Such hardware is universally compatible with either a Macintosh- or a PC-based system. Using this method, excellent images have been produced for publications by one of us (E.Y.).[23–27] E.Y. used ¾-inch prerecorded videotapes, a Macintosh computer, Avid Media Suite Pro video editing software, Adobe Photoshop, and a Sony digital dye-sublimation printer. Several easy and useful video editing applications are commercially available such as that by Pinnacle Studio (Mountain View, CA).
3. Capture the image directly with a charge-coupled device (CCD) digital camera. This method bypasses conversion and starts with a digital image at the time of capture. Components of a digital imaging system include a digital camera, computer, removable memory storage, digital image capture device, and color digital printer. Direct digital image capture is the simplest and most common method to obtain digital images.

Digital still cameras, like conventional film-based cameras, are available in point-and-shoot and SLR models (DSLR). Utilizing non-interchangeable lenses, point-and-shoot cameras are inexpensive, easy to use, and generally smaller and lighter than SLR cameras. The disadvantages of point-and-shoot models include less flexibility in controlling the features of the camera, lower resolution, and restriction to the built-in lens. In contrast, DSLR cameras have modified the typical film-based 35-mm camera by replacing film with a CCD and processing hardware, and a liquid crystal diode (LCD) screen. DSLR cameras are usually larger and more expensive than point-and-shoot digital cameras, produce superior quality images, permit advanced controls over numerous features, and allow for changing to different lenses.

The choices for digital still cameras available that can be used for endoscopy are numerous and continually improving, but include the following: (1) Nikon CoolPix 5000,[35] (2) Olympus C-4040, (3) Canon Power Shot G12,[34] (4) Canon EOS 6D,[36] and (5) Nikon D90 and D7000. Specific digital camera adapters are available for the Nikon CoolPix 5000 and Olympus C4040. Step-up or step-down rings may be necessary to couple the camera lens to the endoscopic adapter (if the lens and adapter diameters are slightly different). Rapid technological advances lead to constant improvements in the features and size of the camera, and to reduced prices. For medical use, one should choose a 3.1 or greater megapixel digital camera, which produces high-quality images.[35] It should also be lightweight, compact, convenient, affordable, and easy to handle.

Digital imaging allows instantaneous confirmation of appropriate and acceptable quality images. Areas of particular interest can be closely scrutinized by scrolling or magnifying within the LCD display. Furthermore, digital images are easily annotated or edited utilizing commercially available applications such as Adobe Photoshop. Digital imaging is an effective and convenient method for storing, delivering, and archiving multiple images.

The camera the authors use is the Nikon CoolPix 5000 with an endoscopic adapter designed for the camera (▶ Fig. 12.5). It is a 5.0-megapixel CCD camera with a 3X zoom lens, with a focal range of 7.1 to 21.4 mm (equivalent to 28 to 85 mm in 35-mm format) producing high-resolution images (2560 × 1920 pixels). Its small size and compact design are advantages. The Nikon CoolPix 5000 has a liquid crystal display (LCD) that allows for better visualization before image capture as well as immediate review. The camera can also be connected to an external monitor or television through the audiovisual output cable. The Nikon CoolPix 5000 allows image transfer to a computer hard drive via a USB cable.

The endoscopic adapter was designed specifically for the Coolpix 5000, but unfortunately there are no longer any companies (that the authors are aware of) that design adapters for specific cameras, due to the constant changes in camera models and designs. Endoscopic adapters, however, are available for digital SLR cameras. These adapters thread onto the end of a lens, and are available from Precision Optics Corporation (Gardner, MA) in 28-, 37-, and 49-mm diameters. Stepping rings are available to connect the adapters to different-sized (diameter) lenses.

12.3.1 Telescopic Digital Photography

Telescopic digital photography requires (1) a Hopkins 4-mm, 0-degree telescope (Karl Storz 1215A, Culver City, CA) (▶ Fig. 12.5a); (2) a light source (Karl Storz 615, 610, 481C, Xenon Nova) and light cable; (3) a digital camera (e.g., Nikon CoolPix 5000); (4) an endoscopic digital camera mounting adapter; and (5) a computer.

With the patient in a sitting position, the 4-mm telescope is carefully inserted into the ear canal. The camera is held in one hand. The other hand grasps the telescope several centimeters away from the tip, and is stabilized against the patient's head to prevent excessive length from sliding into the ear canal, thus avoiding injury to the ear canal and the tympanic membrane (▶ Fig. 12.5b).

Select the size of the images by controlling the zoom button. When the desired image is visualized, gently press the shutter release button on the camera halfway for focus, and all the way down to take the picture. Digital imaging allows immediate observation of the image on the LCD monitor; if it is unsatisfactory, simply reshoot (▶ Fig. 12.6).

The advantages of the telescopic technique include the following: (1) unlike the microscopic technique, the entire tympanic membrane can be visualized, because the tip of the telescope can be passed through the narrow isthmus of the ear canal (▶ Fig. 12.2); and (2) the wide-angle view of the telescope allows an almost infinite depth of field, so that all areas of the tympanic membrane are typically in focus.

The disadvantages of the telescopic technique include the following: (1) lens fogging can be annoying, and frequent dips into warm water or anti-fog solution are needed; and (2) care must be taken not to touch the ear canal or the tympanic membrane, which can potentially cause discomfort or injury. Be sure to position the patient with the head held steady by an assistant, or in the case of pediatric patients, by a parent (or assistant).

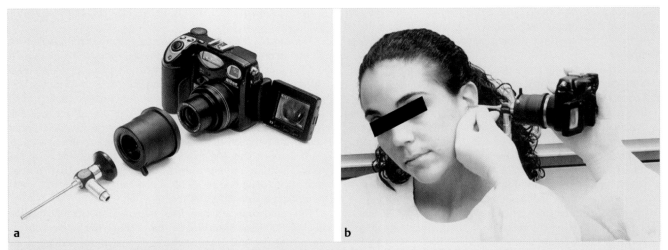

Fig. 12.5 Telescopic digital photography of the ear. (a) Equipment recommended for telescopic digital photography of the ear includes a digital camera (e.g., Nikon CoolPix 5000), an endoscopic digital camera mounting adapter, and a Hopkins 4-mm ototelescope. The Nikon CoolPix 5000 has an LCD monitor that flips and twists. (b) Technique of telescopic digital photography. A Hopkins telescope attached to a Nikon CoolPix 5000 is carefully inserted into the ear canal. When the desired image is visualized, gently press the shutter release button on the camera halfway down for focus, then press the shutter release button all the way to capture the image.

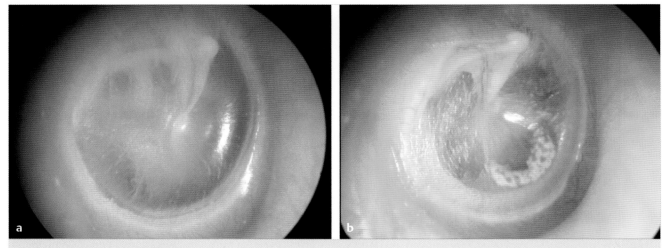

Fig. 12.6 Telescopic digital photography of the ear. (a) Right normal tympanic membrane. (b) Right atrophic tympanic membrane with healed perforation.

12.3.2 Microscopic Digital Photography

Microscopic Digital Photography Through the Eyepiece of the Microscope (Without a Photoadapter)[37]

Microscopic photography through the eyepiece of the microscope using a digital SLR camera without a photoadapter requires the following equipment: (1) a digital SLR camera, and (2) a 50-mm macrolens (with the glass surface of the lens recessed into the barrel of the lens).

Ensure that the microscope is stable and fixed. The subject is centered and focused through the microscope first. The front end of the digital camera is placed gently but snugly against the eyepiece of the microscope (▸ Fig. 12.7a) or the assistant's observation eyepiece (▸ Fig. 12.7b). Make sure that the optical line of the long axis of the microscope eyepiece is aligned with the axis of the digital camera. When the image is confirmed, depress the shutter release button halfway. Auto-focus should show a clear, focused image. If not, switch the camera to manual focus mode, and manually focus the desired image. Depress the shutter release button all the way. The picture is immediately reviewed in the LCD monitor of the digital camera (▸ Fig. 12.8). If the captured image is unsatisfactory, repeat this procedure until the desired image is obtained.

The advantages of this technique include the following: (1) the technique is easy and simple to perform, and (2) magnification changes can be made through the microscope or using the camera zoom control. Surprisingly good pictures can be taken using this inexpensive technique using a 35-mm film SLR camera (▸ Fig. 12.4) or a digital SLR camera (▸ Fig. 12.8).

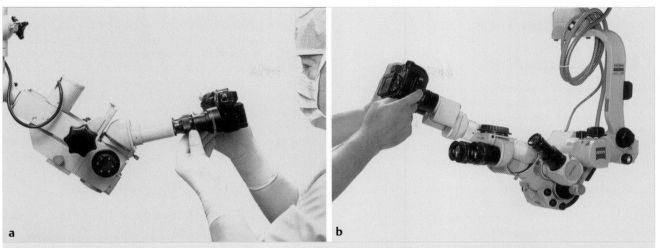

Fig. 12.7 Microscopic digital photography of the ear. (a) Microscopic digital photography through the eyepiece of the microscope. The camera is handheld and the tip of the camera is held against the eyepiece of the microscope. Ensure that the axis of the camera aligns with the axis of the microscope eyepiece. The subject is centered and focused. To capture the image, depress the shutter release button all the way. (b) Microscopic digital photography through the eyepiece using the assistant observation tube. When the pictures are taken in this way, the operation is not interrupted.

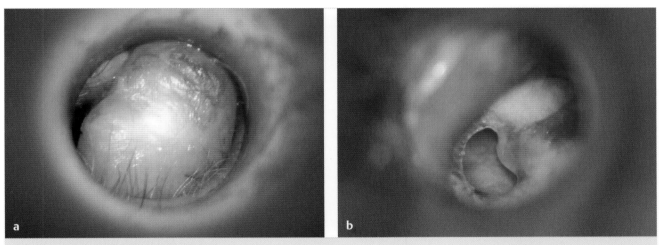

Fig. 12.8 Microscopic digital photography through the eyepiece of the microscope. (a) A large osteoma nearly completely occluding the left external auditory canal. (b) A large left inferior tympanic membrane perforation.

The disadvantages of this technique include the following: (1) it may be difficult to hold the camera perfectly still on the microscope eyepiece, and proper long axis orientation must be maintained for a successful image; and (2) sterile operative procedures must be interrupted—the assistant has to take the picture or the surgeon has to change gloves to take the picture.

Microscopic Digital Photography with a Photoadapter

This is a more expensive but more desirable method of digital photography because the digital camera is fixed, and the surgeon can easily be the photographer. This technique requires (1) a Zeiss operating microscope; (2) a Zeiss beam splitter; (3) a photo adapter, such as Zeiss digital photoadapter, which fits into the SLR digital camera body, Zeiss-Urban dual adapter, or De-

sign for Vision; (4) a digital camera (e.g., Nikon CoolPix 5000, Nikon D7000, Nikon D90); and (5) a SanDisk (SD) memory card.

The image is identified, centered, and focused through the operating microscope. Magnification is selected to best demonstrate the otologic findings. The camera is attached to a side arm via the beam splitter and photoadapter (▶ Fig. 12.3b). It is set on automatic mode, and selected photographs are taken by depressing the shutter release button. Inspect the images for proper focus and exposure. If not in focus, switch to manual focus. If exposures are incorrect, bracketing of exposures both under and over by one and two stops can help determine the optimal exposure.

The advantages of this technique include the following: (1) the camera is steady and properly aligned, (2) the picture shooting is not as disruptive, and (3) different magnifications of the microscope are readily available.

The disadvantage of this technique is that the photo-adapter and beam splitter may be expensive.

12.4 Videography

With the technical improvements in video documentation devices, including video cameras, high-intensity lighting, high-quality endoscopes, and video printers, video imaging is our recommended procedure of choice for otologic documentation. Like digital photography, video documentation permits instantaneous imaging and verification of successful image capture. Nearly instantaneous video printouts of outstanding quality can be obtained using video printers, even at the time of the otologic examination. Equipment required for videography includes a video camera, a light source, an image capture device, a video monitor, and a video printer:

- *Video cameras:* The best resolution and brightness of images are obtained with compact three-chip CCD video cameras such as the Karl Storz Tricam, Stryker 782, or Karl Storz Image 1 HD. These cameras are expensive, but produce superior images with outstanding color and clarity. Less expensive single lens chip cameras, such as the Karl Storz Telecam, are producing increasingly improved images.
- *Light sources:* Xenon light sources such as the Karl Storz 487C, 610, or 615C Xenon Nova are recommended. Other satisfactory light sources are also available.
- *Image capture devices:* Replacing the videotape recorders of the past, digital image capture devices are the current preferred method of video capture. These devices permit image transport to a computer for print generation and image storage. These systems allow for safe, degradation-free storage of video clips with easy retrieval and manipulation through computer software. The primary disadvantages are the high cost and the need to create a user-friendly archiving system for retrieval. Devices that are available include the Stryker SDC system and the D-scope system. The D-scope system digitally stores video clips based on patient name and date of examination. Multiple images can be retrieved for simultaneous monitor display making comparisons and patient education seamless and fast. The authors use the D-scope system.
- *Video printers:* We use the Sony UP5600, which produces the best images, but it is costly. The Sony CVP M3 is more affordable and produces acceptable images. The videoprints are sharp and clear and can be used for journal and textbook publications as well as in poster presentations. Videoprints can be scanned, or pictures of the video monitor image can be photographed with a digital camera, for digital presentations. We currently capture images from the D-scope image capture system, and create video printouts.
- *Video monitors:* Any Sony or Panasonic monitor is adequate. Innovations in display design (e.g., high-definition televisions, plasma screen displays, or LCD monitors) may take full advantage of the superior image quality afforded by newer digital capture devices.

The advantages of video imaging are the following: (1) reliable images of high color and resolution quality; (2) immediate images that can be easily captured and played back at a later time for more careful analysis; and (3) nearly instantaneous video printouts can be produced for patient charts, teaching, publication, and effective communication with referring physicians.

The disadvantages of video imaging are the following: (1) the equipment is costly, (2) the equipment can become outdated quickly due to rapid technological advances, and (3) video printouts fade with time. We have seen significant fading over 10 to 20 years, with high humidity, high temperatures, and light exposure hastening the degradation. We recommend storing images digitally, whenever possible, because the images should show no degradation over time. Backups of stored images are also a must.

12.4.1 Telescopic Videography

Telescopic Video-Otoscopy in the Office

Video-otoscopy may be performed with the 4-mm, 0-degree (adult and older children) or 2.7-mm, 0-degree (younger children) rigid telescopes. A light-sensitive and lightweight CCD video camera (single-chip or three-chip CCD camera) is used for video recording (▶ Fig. 12.9a).

With the patient in the sitting position, the telescope, which is attached to the video camera, is dipped into warm water to prevent fogging and passed into the ear canal. The video camera should be held in one hand while the other hand holds the distal tip of the telescope to prevent it from injuring the ear canal or the tympanic membrane (▶ Fig. 12.9a). When the desired image is seen on the video monitor, focus is confirmed, and video recording is begun. Hardcopies of the selected video image can be easily obtained using a color video printer (▶ Fig. 12.9b). These can be used for medical records, teaching, patient education, and physician referrals. Mastoidectomy cavities can be thoroughly examined by angling the tip of the telescope. A retrograde telescope (30, 70, or 120 degrees) may be helpful to visualize hidden areas of the mastoidectomy cavity in some cases.

The advantages of this technique include the following: (1) it is a simple and safe technique that permits excellent visualization of the entire ear canal and tympanic membrane (▶ Fig. 12.10); (2) it is a fast technique, with the entire procedure taking less than 3 minutes to perform; (3) video images can be immediately confirmed, and video prints can be nearly instantaneously made using a color video printer; and (4) the video camera can be connected to one of the digital capture systems, resulting in prompt digital image storage. This is the most useful technique of imaging of the tympanic membrane.

The disadvantages of this technique include the following: (1) the equipment is expensive; (2) lens fogging can be annoying, so frequent dips into warm water or anti-fog solution are needed; (3) some image distortion occurs due to the wide-angle effect of the telescope lens; and (4) care must be taken not to touch the ear canal skin or the tympanic membrane.

Telescopic Pneumatic Video-Otoscopy

The mobility of the tympanic membrane can best be documented by pneumatic video-otoscopy. Although there are several excellent commercially available video-pneumatic otoscopes, video-pneumatic otoscopy can be simply accomplished by the Welch-Allen (Skaneateles Falls, NY) otoscope technique.

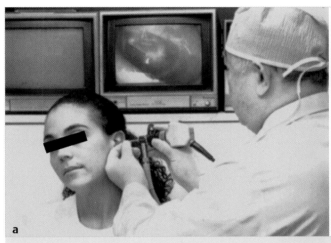
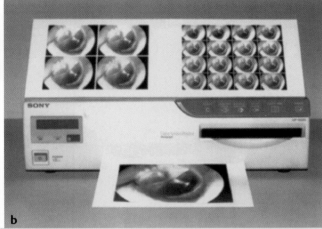

Fig. 12.9 Telescopic video-otoscopy. (a) Technique of telescopic video-otoscopy. A Hopkins 4-mm, 0-degree ototelescope is attached to the Stryker 3-chip CCD camera and used to examine the left ear canal. (b) Color video printers. Color video images obtained from the video camera can be printed almost simultaneously with a Sony UP5000 Mavigraph color video printer. Note that single- or multiple-image printouts can be produced.

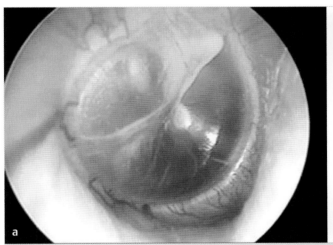
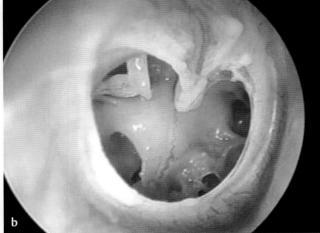

Fig. 12.10 Telescopic video-otoscopy. (a) Glomus jugulare tumor of the right ear. (b) Subtotal tympanic membrane perforation of the right ear.

A simple and effective method of documenting pneumatic otoscopy has been described using an adapted Welch-Allen otoscope head.[23] The open end of the otoscope head with the pneumatic bulb attached is filled with Mack's ear plug molds, and a 4-mm central opening through the ear plug mold is made with a hemostat. The telescope is then passed through the hole so that the telescope tip extends just beyond the tip of the speculum. To produce a better seal within the ear canal, a rubber tourniquet may be wrapped around the tip of the speculum. Video adapters are then attached to the eyepiece of the telescope and video recordings with pneumatic insufflation documented.

The normal tympanic membrane moves readily with pneumatic otoscopy. Decreased mobility may be observed in patients with serous otitis media and tympanosclerosis. Excessive mobility may be noted with an atrophic tympanic membrane or ossicular discontinuity.

Telescopic Transtympanic Middle Ear Videography

Transtympanic middle ear endoscopy has been described as an office procedure using a small-diameter telescope such as the 1.9-mm, 0- or 30-degree telescope attached to a video camera.[22,27] The telescope is introduced into the middle ear cavity through a small myringotomy, a tympanomeatal flap, or an existing perforation. Structures that can be well visualized and documented include the promontory, round window, oval window, stapes suprastructure, long process of the incus, and, with the 30-degree telescope, the sinus tympani, facial nerve, pyramidal eminence, cochleariform process, and eustachian tube orifice. Poe et al[22] described the diagnosis of a labyrinthine fistula using this technique through a myringotomy.

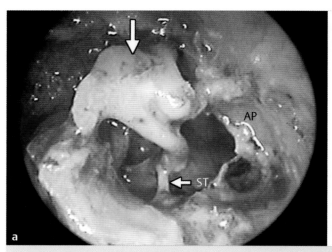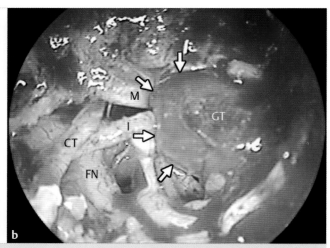

Fig. 12.11 Telescopic videography of the ear in the operating room. (a) Fused malleus and incus (*large arrow*) found in a patient with right congenital atresia of the ear canal. AP, atresia plate; ST, stapedial tendon (*small arrow*). (b) Intraoperative view of right middle ear showing glomus tumor (GT), malleus (M), incus (I), chorda tympani (CT), and facial nerve (FN).

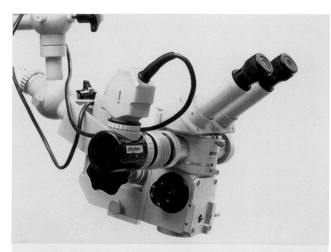

Fig. 12.12 The technique of microscopic videography of the ear. Stryker 782 3-chip CCD video camera (other cameras such as the Tricam 3-chip CCD, Sony DXC-C33 3-chip CCD, Image-1 3-chip CCD, and Telecam 1-chip CCD can be used) attached to the Zeiss TV adapter and beam splitter of the microscope with an appropriate adapter. Make sure that the proper connection between the video camera and the photoadapter is chosen.

Telescopic Videography of the Ear in the Operating Room

The main advantage of performing telescopic videography of the ear in the operating room is that the patient remains immobile during the procedure while under general anesthesia. Clear images for permanent records and teaching can be obtained with this method (▶ Fig. 12.11). Also, intraoperative documentation during middle ear surgery can be performed with the telescope, allowing excellent depth of field, color reproduction, and clear images. Nearly instantaneous video printouts can be produced using the color video printer.

12.4.2 Microscopic Videography

Microscopic videography of the ear is the most convenient and useful method of documenting and teaching of otologic surgery (▶ Fig. 12.12 and ▶ Fig. 12.13). Videomicroscopic documentation requires (1) a Zeiss operating microscope; (2) a Zeiss beam splitter; (3) a photoadapter (Design for Vision, Ronkonkoma, NY; Zeiss; or Zeiss-Urban dual adapter); and (4) a video camera including a single-chip CCD camera such as Telecam (Chatham, MA) microscopic camera head (20210136U) or three-chip cameras such as the Tricam, Stryker, or Karl Storz Image 1 HD camera. A camera can also be attached to the C-mount of a photoadapter of the Zeiss microscope utilizing a special endo-camera adapter (Karl Storz). With their small size and weight, the miniature CCD cameras interfere minimally with the operative procedure.

With the patient lying supine, an ear speculum is used to expose the tympanic membrane or ear canal lesion. The microscope is positioned to visualize the lesion, and appropriate magnification is selected. The video camera is white-balanced. The image is centered and focused on the video monitor and video recording is begun.

The advantages of this technique include the following: (1) it is an easy and effective technique that requires no interruption of surgery; (2) different magnifications are readily available using the magnification dial of the microscope (▶ Fig. 12.13); and (3) digital images can be obtained in real time if the video camera is connected to the digital capture system, thus obviating the need for analog-to-digital conversion later.

The disadvantages of this technique include the following: (1) the photoadapter and beam splitter are expensive; (2) the depth of field is shallow; and (3) it is difficult to photograph the entire tympanic membrane through the transcanal approach.

The authors believe microscopic videography of the ear is the single best method of documenting and teaching otologic surgery. Live images of the procedure can be observed on video monitors placed in the operating room, permitting ear, nose, and throat residents and all operating room personnel to learn

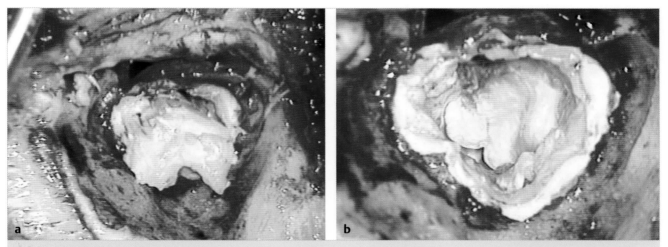

Fig. 12.13 Microscopic videography of the ear. (a) Cholesteatoma filling the right mastoid cavity. (b) Closer view of cholesteatoma contents.

and understand the fundamentals of otologic surgery. The images obtained with a single-chip CCD (Telecam DX camera) are usually adequate, as the quality of the single-chip cameras continues to improve. Images of the highest quality can be obtained with a three-chip CCD video camera such as the Tricam, Stryker, or Karl Storz Image 1 HD camera. Nearly instantaneous video printouts of surgical anatomy and pathology can be made using the color video printers, which can be placed in the patient's chart or sent to the referring physician. If the video camera is attached to a digital capture system, almost simultaneous digital image captures are possible.

12.5 Conclusion

Over the past four decades, photographic techniques for the tympanic membrane have changed dramatically from the open tube (speculum) photography of Buckingham to microscopic photography with a photoadapter or through the eyepiece of the microscope, to telescopic film photography, to digital filmless telescopic and microscopic photography. Today, many options are available. In the office, telescopic video otoscopy with a video camera is the most useful procedure. This technique permits immediate exact diagnosis, patient counseling, and adequate treatment. The quality of the images is outstanding, and high-resolution images can be obtained nearly instantaneously using the video printer. The image from the videoprint can be digitized. Telescopic digital photography of the ear in the office using a digital camera is a very economical method to obtain high-quality images.

In the operating room, microscopic videography is the most useful and convenient method of otologic teaching and documentation. Microscopic digital photography through the eyepiece of the microscope remains a simple and inexpensive method for documenting the surgical procedures of the ear. Microscopic digital photography using a photoadapter is more costly but may be the ideal method for capturing digital microscopic images.

With the continued advances in computer technology and the ability to digitize video images, image storage will continue

primarily in digitized formats. Digital images are predicted to last nearly indefinitely compared with other formats such as 35-mm slides and videotape, where image distortion or degradation occurs. Appealing features of digital technology includes immediate image review, ease of storage of digital images and videos into computer files and folders, and ability to insert into presentation software programs for lectures, or into publications for figures. Sequential comparisons of disease state and progression over time are made easier with rapid and simple image retrieval, and the ability to view images or videos side by side on the computer monitor.

Expanded applications now include remote diagnosis confirmation based on a digital image. The need to store and retrieve images in digital format is reinforced with the escalating presence of the electronic health record, which in the near future will be utilized by most, if not all, medical practices. Additional innovations will emerge for cost-effective and efficient data storage and archiving. Digital imaging has evolved into the ideal modality for otologic photography, videography, and documentation.

References

[1] Pensak ML, Yanagisawa E. Tympanic membrane photography: historical perspective. Am J Otol 1984; 5: 324–332
[2] Randall BA, Morse HL. Photographic Illustrations of the Anatomy of the Human Ear, Together with Pathological Conditions of the Drum Membrane. Philadelphia: P. Blakiston's, 1887
[3] Buckingham RA. Endoscopic otophotography. Laryngoscope 1963; 73: 71–84
[4] Brubaker JD, Holinger PH. Recent progress in open tube endoscopic and cavity still and motion picture photography. J Biol Photogr Assoc 1957; 24: 104–113
[5] Holinger PH, Tardy ME Jr. Photography in otorhinolaryngology and bronchoesophagology. In: English GM, ed. Otolaryngology, vol 5, rev. ed. Philadelphia: Lippincott, 1988:1–21
[6] Smith HW, Rosnagle RS, Yanagisawa E. Tympanic membrane photography. Arch Otolaryngol 1974; 99: 125–127
[7] Hughes GB, Yanagisawa E, Dickins JRE, Jackson CG, Sismanis A. Microscopic otologic photography using a standard 35-mm camera. Am J Otol 1981; 2: 243–247
[8] Yanagisawa E. Effective photography in otolaryngology-head and neck surgery: tympanic membrane photography. Otolaryngol Head Neck Surg 1982; 90: 399–407

[9] Yanagisawa E. Documentation of otologic surgery. In: Yanagisawa E, Gardner G, eds. The Surgical Atlas of Otology and Neuro-Otology. New York: Grune & Stratton, 1983

[10] Konrad HR, Berci G, Ward P. Pediatric otoscopy and photography of the tympanic membrane. Arch Otolaryngol 1979; 105: 431–433

[11] Chen B, Fry TL, Fischer ND. Otoscopy and photography: a new method. Ann Otol Rhinol Laryngol 1979; 88: 771–773

[12] Chole RA. Photography of the tympanic membrane. A new method. Arch Otolaryngol 1980; 106: 230–231

[13] Nomura Y. Effective photography in otolaryngology-head and neck surgery: endoscopic photography of the middle ear. Otolaryngol Head Neck Surg 1982; 90: 395–398

[14] Hawke M. Telescopic otoscopy and photography of the tympanic membrane. J Otolaryngol 1982; 11: 35–39

[15] Gonzalez C, Bluestone CD. Visualization of a retraction pocket/cholesteatoma: indications for use of the middle ear telescope in children. Laryngoscope 1986; 96: 109–110

[16] Selkin SG. Endoscopic photography of the ear, nose, and throat. Laryngoscope 1984; 94: 336–339

[17] Chole RA. Color Atlas of Ear Disease. New York: Appleton-Century-Crofts, 1982

[18] Hawke M, Keene M, Alberti PW. Clinical Otoscopy—A Text and Colour Atlas. Edinburgh: Churchill Livingstone, 1984

[19] Hawke M. Clinical Pocket Guide to Ear Disease. Philadelphia: Lea & Febiger, 1987

[20] Owens TW. Ear Disease—A School Nurse Manual of Common Ear Problems. Houston: Peanut, 1992

[21] Wormald PJ, Browning GG. Otoscopy—A Structural Approach. San Diego: Singular, 1996

[22] Poe DS, Rebeiz EE, Pankratov MM, Shapshay SM. Transtympanic endoscopy of the middle ear. Laryngoscope 1992; 102: 993–996

[23] Yanagisawa E, Carlson RD. Telescopic video-otoscopy using a compact home video color camera. Laryngoscope 1987; 97: 1350–1355

[24] Yanagisawa E. The use of video in ENT endoscopy: its value in teaching. Ear Nose Throat J 1994; 73: 754–763

[25] Mambrino L, Yanagisawa E, Yanagisawa K, Gallo O. Endoscopic ENT photography: a comparison of pictures by standard color films and newer color video printers. Laryngoscope 1991; 101: 1229–1232

[26] Yanagisawa K, Shi JM, Yanagisawa E. Color photography of video images of otolaryngological structures using a 35 mm SLR camera. Laryngoscope 1987; 97: 992–993

[27] Yanagisawa E. Color Atlas of Diagnostic Endoscopy in Otorhinolaryngology. New York: Igaku Shoin, 1997

[28] Silverstein H, Seidman M, Rosenberg S. Documentation is a snap. Laryngoscope 1992; 102: 1395–1398

[29] Spiegel JH, Singer MI. Practical approach to digital photography and its applications. Otolaryngol Head Neck Surg 2000; 123: 152–156

[30] Yanagisawa E, Joe JK, Yanagisawa R. Digital imaging in otolaryngology-head and neck surgery. In: Citardi MJ, ed. Computer-Aided Otorhinolaryngology—Head and Neck Surgery. New York: Marcel Dekker, 2002:117–134

[31] Blevins NH, Lustig LR. Current digital imaging for the otolaryngologist. Curr Opin Otolaryngol Head Neck Surg 2003; 11: 166–172

[32] Spiegel JH, Singer MI. Practical approach to digital photography and its applications. Otolaryngol Head Neck Surg 2000; 123: 152–156

[33] Tabaee A, Johnson PE, Anand VK. Office-based digital video endoscopy in otolaryngology. Laryngoscope 2006; 116: 1523–1525

[34] Melder PC, Mair EA. Endoscopic photography: digital or 35 mm? Arch Otolaryngol Head Neck Surg 2003; 129: 570–575

[35] Manarey CRA, Anand VK. Office-based digital photography in rhinology. Laryngoscope 2004; 114: 593–595

[36] Benjamin B. Digital photography of the larynx. Ann Otol Rhinol Laryngol 2002; 111: 603–608

[37] Haynes DS, Moore BA, Roland P, Olson GT. Digital microphotography: a simple solution. Laryngoscope 2003; 113: 915–919

[38] Harris TM, Goyal P. Recording video endoscopy using a portable media device: a novel solution in the age of digital media. Laryngoscope 2009; 119: 500–501

[39] Calhoun KH, Decherd ME. Digital image archiving. Otolaryngol Clin North Am 2002; 35: 1191–1202, vi

[40] Bashshur RL, Shannon G, Krupinski EA, Grigsby J. Sustaining and realizing the promise of telemedicine. Telemed J E Health 2013; 19: 339–345

[41] Aronzon A, Ross AT, Kazahaya K, Ishii M. Diagnosis of middle ear disease using tympanograms and digital imaging. Otolaryngol Head Neck Surg 2004; 131: 917–920

[42] Kokesh J, Ferguson AS, Patricoski C et al. Digital images for postsurgical follow-up of tympanostomy tubes in remote Alaska. Otolaryngol Head Neck Surg 2008; 139: 87–93

13 Clinical Evaluation of Hearing Loss

Lesley A. Rabach and John F. Kveton

13.1 Introduction

Hearing loss is prevalent in nearly two thirds of adults aged 70 years and older in the United States population.[1] According to the National Institute on Deafness and Other Communication Disorders (NIDCD), approximately 36 million (17%) of American adults have reported having hearing loss.[2,3] The number of people with severe to profound hearing impairment or deafness ranges from 500,000 to 750,000.[4] The Centers for Disease Control and Prevention (CDC) estimates that > 12,000 infants are born with hearing impairment and that 45% of infants do not pass newborn screening tests.[5] The average lifetime cost for one person with hearing loss is approximately $420,000 (in 2003 dollars); this includes household and workplace productivity loss.[6]

Given the prevalence of hearing loss, a cost-effective and accurate diagnostic approach is essential for assessing the degree and nature of hearing loss and to arrive at the underlying cause. Patients may undergo hearing loss assessment because of subjective complaints or because of risk factors for hearing loss, such as low birth weight or ototoxicity chemotherapy. It is imperative to understand the differential diagnosis of hearing loss to help guide clinical evaluation.

13.2 Differential Diagnosis of Hearing Loss

A critical step in establishing a differential diagnosis is to determine whether the hearing loss is conductive, sensorineural, or mixed. Sensorineural hearing loss (SNHL) is caused by a cochlea or auditory nerve lesion. Conductive hearing loss (CHL) is caused by a transmission mechanism lesion of sound energy from the external environment to the cochlea and may involve external ear, tympanic membrane, or middle ear contents. Some patients have both SNHL and CHL simultaneously; in this situation, hearing loss is categorized as mixed. Conditions associated with mixed hearing loss include chronic otitis media, cholesteatoma, temporal bone trauma, certain hereditary syndromes, and otosclerosis. Central hearing loss is caused by a lesion along the neural pathway, either from the inner ear to the auditory region of the brain or in the brain itself. Auditory neuropathy, a recently defined spectrum of disorders, is a hearing impairment in which outer hair cell function is normal but afferent neural conduction in the auditory pathway is disordered. This is another consideration in the differential of central hearing loss.[7,8]

History and physical examination findings are extremely important in narrowing the list of clinical possibilities. To refine the differential diagnosis, data from the audiogram, impedance testing, brainstem evoked response testing, vestibular-evoked myopotentials, and otoacoustic emissions may be analyzed. Additional examinations such as laboratory testing and diagnostic imaging can serve as an adjunct to further narrow the diagnosis.

The differential diagnosis for a patient with unilateral SNHL varies considerably from that for a patient with bilateral SNHL. However, for the purposes of giving a broad overview, the differential diagnoses for sensorineural and CHL are discussed in this chapter. See the boxed text below.

Differential Diagnosis of Sensorineural Hearing Loss

- Congenital
- Genetic disorders
  - Dominant: Waardenburg, Stickler
  - Recessive: Usher, Jervell and Lange-Nielsen, Pendred, branchio-oto-renal
- TORCH infections (toxoplasmosis, rubella, cytomegalovirus, and herpes simplex virus), syphilis
- Teratogens: thalidomide, aminoglycosides, diuretics, quinine
- Perinatal hypoxia-anoxia/prematurity/low birth weight
- Hyperbilirubinemia
- Inner ear malformations
  - Michel aplasia, Mondini aplasia, Scheibe aplasia, Alexander aplasia, enlarged vestibular aqueduct
- Hereditary: delayed onset
- Dominant: neurofibromatosis, Paget
- Recessive: *DFNB1*, connexin 26/30
- X-linked: Norrie, otopalatodigital, Alport
- Mitochondrial: maternally inherited deafness and diabetes MIDD
- Infectious
- Postmeningitis
- Chronic otitis media
- Viral: cytomegalovirus (CMV), herpes simplex virus (HSV), human immunodeficiency virus (HIV)
- Lyme disease
- Tuberculosis
- Inflammatory
- Primary vs. systemic autoimmune
- Neoplastic
- Primary vs. metastatic tumors: schwannomas, paragangliomas, small-cell carcinoma (SCC)
- Metabolic
- Diabetes
- Hypothyroidism
- Hyperlipidemia
- Traumatic
- Temporal bone fractures: transverse > longitudinal
- Perilymphatic fistula
- Barotrauma
- Noise exposure
- Postsurgical
- Traumatic brain injury/auditory concussion
- Vascular-hematologic
- Vascular occlusion/emboli
- Inner ear hemorrhage
- Miscellaneous
- Auditory neuropathy
  - Cochlear otosclerosis
  - Ménière disease
- Multiple sclerosis
- Ototoxicity
- Presbycusis
- Superior semicircular canal dehiscence
- Radiation injury

Differential Diagnosis of Conductive Hearing Loss

- Congenital
- Ossicular fusion/malformation/fixation
- Ear canal atresia
- Congenital cholesteatoma
- Hereditary
- Otosclerosis
- Osteogenesis imperfecta
- Paget disease
- Osteopetrositis (Albers-Schönberg disease)
- Crouzon disease
- Marfan disease
- Turner syndrome
- Goldenhar syndrome
- Down syndrome
- Treacher Collins syndrome
- Infectious-inflammatory
- Otitis media
- Otitis externa
- Cholesteatoma
- Neoplastic
- Ear canal masses
  - Benign: osteoma, exostoses, sebaceous adenoma, ceruminoma
  - Malignant: small-cell carcinoma (SCC), basal cell carcinoma (BCC), adenoid cystic carcinoma, rhabdomyosarcoma, lymphoma, metastatic carcinoma, osteosarcoma, chondrosarcoma
- Glomus tumor
- Histiocytosis
- Fibrous dysplasia
- Traumatic
- Tympanic membrane perforation
- Ossicular discontinuity
- Mechanical
- Cerumen
- Ear canal foreign body
- Superior semicircular canal dehiscence syndrome

13.3 Sensorineural Hearing Loss

Sensorineural hearing loss can be categorized in several ways. One scheme uses age of onset. Congenital hearing loss is defined as that which is present from birth. This can occur from hereditary factors, prenatal exposure or infection, or perinatal events. In contrast, hereditary hearing loss may not be present at birth. Fifty percent of congenital hearing loss is due to genetic factors, 25% is acquired, and 25% is unknown etiology. Causes of congenital SNHL include various genetic disorders, intrauterine infections, teratogenic agent exposure, prematurity, perinatal anoxia, and hyperbilirubinemia. Congenital infections, known as the TORCH infections, can cause hearing loss. Some of these factors may result in inner ear aplasia; however, such deformities may also exist without identifiable cause. Severe low-birth-weight infants (< 1.5 kg) are also at increased risk for permanent SNHL; in fact, rates of permanent hearing loss among extremely preterm survivors range from 0.8 to 8.0%.[9,10]

Delayed-onset hearing loss can be caused by a variety of factors, including genetic factors, infection, trauma, and ototoxic medications. Hereditary hearing loss may be dominant, recessive, X-linked, or mitochondrially inherited, and may exist in a syndromic or nonsyndromic entity.

Of the 50 to 60% of congenital hearing loss that is hereditary, approximately 70% is nonsyndromic. Eighty percent of nonsyndromic congenital hearing loss is inherited in an autosomal recessive fashion.[11] Several loci have been mapped, including autosomal recessive, autosomal dominant, and X-linked loci. The gene coding for connexin 26 is located at locus *DFNB1* on human chromosome 13q12; the most common mutation of which is 35delG. Both connexin 26 and connexin 30 compose gap junctions that are expressed in the cochlea, where they aid in returning potassium ions to the endolymph following hair cell stimulation. The connexin gene codes a protein called gap junction protein B2 (GJB2).[12] More than 100 GJB2 mutations have now been discovered and are located in the human gene mutation database (HGMD); they are responsible for mild to profound hearing loss with both syndromic and nonsyndromic hearing loss and cases of both incomplete penetrance and delayed disease onset.[13]

Infectious agents and inflammatory processes can lead to SNHL. The infectious agents include both bacteria and viruses. Although there is no consensus on the pathogenesis of SNHL due to otitis media, the most likely etiology is the passage of toxins across the round window membrane.[14] Tuberculosis is a rare cause of otitis media and is diagnostic challenge; furthermore, it may be associated with SNHL.[15]

Cytomegalovirus, HSV, and human immunodeficiency virus (HIV) can lead to SNHL. In HIV/AIDs, hearing loss may result from opportunistic infections or ototoxic medications used to treat infections, or may possibly be due to the direct effects of the virus on the cochlea.[16] Between 20 and 40% of HIV patients present with some type of auditory or vestibular manifestation as a result of the infection by the AIDs virus.[17]

Sensorineural hearing loss occurs in 7 to 36% of patients following bacterial meningitis.[18,19] Since the introduction of the *Haemophilus influenzae* type B vaccine, most cases of bacterial meningitis are caused by *Streptococcus pneumoniae*. Bacterial meningitis is the most common cause of acquired SNHL in children (85%).[20,21] Systemic inflammatory processes such as Cogan's syndrome, relapsing polychondritis, Wegener's granulomatosis, lupus erythematosus, Takayasu's disease, and giant cell arteritis can be associated with SHNL. In addition, primary autoimmune hearing loss may present without systemic manifestations, though 15 to 30% have coexistent systemic manifestations.[22,23]

Sensorineural hearing loss may result from primary tumors arising within the temporal bone as well as from metastatic lesions. The most common neoplasm causing SNHL is vestibular schwannoma. Squamous cell carcinoma and paragangliomas arising within the temporal bone may also cause SNHL, though they are more commonly associated with CHL.[24] Metastatic lesions to the temporal bone, most commonly breast, lung, and prostrate carcinoma, are associated with SNHL.[25]

There are many associations between SNHL and metabolic disorders. Importantly, diabetes mellitus has been postulated to result in auditory damage secondary to microangiopathy. Additionally, hypothyroidism, hyperlipoproteinemia, hypertension, and other vascular and hematologic diseases have also been implicated in SNHL. Decreased blood flow to the inner ear may result from narrowed blood vessels, as in atherosclerosis or diabetes mellitus, or secondary to abnormal flow or hypercoagulability, as in sickle cell and other hypercoagulable disorders. Platelet dysfunction, thrombocytopenia, and hypocoagulable states can also lead to hemorrhage within the inner ear, thus causing hearing loss.[26] A rare maternally inherited form of deafness and diabetes (MIDD) has also recently been discovered, in which a mitochondrial gene defect results in type 2 diabetes and bilateral SNHL presenting at an average age of 35 years.[27]

Trauma causes SNHL in a variety of ways. Disruption of the labyrinth can occur with longitudinal and transverse fractures of the temporal bone, though more commonly with transverse fractures. Perilymph fistula can result from both blunt injuries to the head as well as barotrauma. Concussive injuries and traumatic brain injuries can also damage the inner ear or cause central hearing loss. Surgical trauma is always a possible cause of SNHL. Noise exposure damages the outer hair cells, causing hearing loss with a characteristic pattern on audiogram. Other conditions known to lead to SNHL include Ménière's disease, cochlear otosclerosis, multiple sclerosis, ototoxic drugs, radiation injury, and aging (presbycusis).

13.4 Conductive Hearing Loss

Congenital causes of CHL include ossicular fixation and ossicular malformations, as well as atresia or stenosis of the external auditory canal. These anomalies may exist in conjunction with other craniofacial abnormalities as well as with SNHL.

Hereditary delayed-onset CHL can be caused by otosclerosis, which is thought to be an autosomal dominant disease with incomplete penetrance.[28,29]

Osteogenesis imperfecta tarda, another autosomal dominant disorder, leads to delayed-onset CHL by causing stapes footplate fixation or ossicular fracture. Other hereditary causes of CHL include osteopetrosis, Marfan syndrome, Paget disease, and Crouzon syndrome. The presence of congenital cholesteatoma in the middle ear can also cause CHL.

The most common cause of CHL is otitis media with effusion, which can be either acute or chronic. Cholesteatoma or granulation tissue caused by chronic otitis media can interfere with sound transmission to the oval window; it can even cause ossicular erosion. Other infectious sequelae include tympanosclerosis, middle ear atelectasis, and severe otitis externa in which edema of the ear canal interferes with hearing. Trauma may also lead to CHL, caused by tympanic membrane perforation, hemotympanum, or ossicular discontinuity. Lastly, mechanical

occlusion of the external auditory canal from cerumen, foreign bodies, or large exostoses or osteomas can cause CHL.

Rarer causes of CHL include neoplasms involving the external auditory canal or middle ear. These may be benign or malignant. Superior semicircular canal dehiscence syndrome was first described in 1998 by Minor et al[30–32] and can be a cause of CHL even with normal middle ear function and stapedial reflexes.[33]

13.5 History

The history is the first and most important step in the clinical evaluation of hearing loss. The history may identify individuals with hearing loss and can direct the clinician to the appropriate diagnosis.

13.5.1 History in Infants and Children

Family history, the mother's pregnancy history, and the patient's birth history are particularly important in the clinical evaluation of infants and children because they can identify factors that may increase the risk of hearing loss. The incidence of severe permanent bilateral congenital hearing loss is approximately 1 to 3 per 1,000 live births.[33] Hearing loss occurs more frequently than other newborn conditions for which newborns are routinely screened.[34] In 2001 the Joint Committee on Infant Hearing (JCIF) mandated that hearing screening should identify infants at risk for specifically defined hearing loss that interferes with development.[35] Together with the federal government, universal newborn hearing screening measures include testing of all newborns with either auditory brainstem response (ABR) or otoacoustic emissions (OAEs), or both. In 2007, an update for the U.S. Preventive Services Task Force (USPSTF) on universal newborn hearing screening (UNHS) was undertaken to detect moderate to severe permanent, bilateral congenital hearing loss. The review focused on three key questions regarding the effectiveness of universal screening and early interventions in improving language and other outcomes in childhood, the effectiveness of universal screening in identifying infants with hearing loss and leading them to early interventions, and adverse effects of screening and early interventions. Results of this review indicate that infants identified with post-natal CHL through UNHS have significantly earlier referral, diagnosis, and treatment than those identified in other ways.[35,36]

Further issues that are important in the history of the child with hearing loss include a history of bacterial meningitis or other infections associated with hearing loss, a history of head trauma associated with loss of consciousness or skull fracture, the use of ototoxic medications including intravenous (IV) antibiotics, recurrent or persistent otitis media with effusion for more than 3 months, and parental concern about hearing, speech, language, or development.

Parental concerns regarding hearing loss have often been found to be correct. Delays in speech development can be assessed based on the lack of age-appropriate milestones as noted by Matkin and Wilcox:[37]

1. Absence of differentiated babbling or vocal imitation by 12 months
2. Failure to use single words by 18 months
3. A single-word vocabulary of 10 words or less by 24 months
4. A vocabulary of < 100 words, failure to use two-word combinations, and unintelligible speech at 30 months
5. A vocabulary of < 200 words, no use of telegraphic sentences, and clarity less than 50% at 36 months
6. A vocabulary of < 600 words, no use of simple sentences, and clarity of less than 80% at 48 months

Developmental milestones have been established for receptive abilities. From birth to 4 months, infants should startle to loud sounds, quiet to their mother's voice, and cease activity when sound is presented at a conversational level. From 5 to 6 months, infants should be able to localize to sound in the horizontal plane, imitate sounds in their own speech repertoire, and vocalize reciprocally with an adult. Between 7 to 12 months, infants should localize to sound in any plane and respond to their name. By 13 to 15 months, children should be able to point in the direction of an unexpected sound as well as familiar objects or people when asked. Between 16 to 18 months, children should begin to follow simple directions without cues and should be able to be trained to reach toward a midline toy when a sound is presented. Finally, by 19 to 24 months, children should be able to point to parts of the body when named.[38]

13.5.2 History in General

The history should include the patient's age and the duration and progression of symptoms. It is important to establish whether the hearing loss is unilateral or bilateral, sudden in onset or gradual, stable or fluctuating. Associated otologic symptoms such as tinnitus, otalgia, aural fullness, and otorrhea should be inquired about, as well as any vertigo or instability suggestive of vestibular dysfunction. Most patients report noise- or pressure-related vertigo only on direct questioning, highlighting the importance of good history-taking in diagnosing superior semicircular canal dehiscence syndrome.[39] After the otologic history has been taken, further questioning should establish the existence of other systemic illnesses, symptoms of those illnesses, history of infections, and history of head trauma. Particular attention should be paid to both current and prior medications for ototoxic potential, taking care to include over-the-counter and homeopathic drugs (see boxed text below).[40] Any allergies should be noted, and a complete 12-point review of systems should be obtained. Family history of hearing loss or anomalies associated with syndromic hearing loss should be reviewed. The occupational history should be obtained with careful questioning about noise exposure, not only in the workplace but also in leisure activities such as firing ranges and concerts. History of prior otologic and neurologic surgery should be reviewed as well.

Ototoxic Drugs

- Antibiotics:
  - Aminoglycoside
    - Streptomycin, gentamicin, neomycin, tobramycin, amikacin, netilmicin, dihydrostreptomycin, kanamycin
  - Erythromycin
  - Vancomycin
- Chemotherapeutic agents
- Cisplatin
- Bleomycin
- Nitrogen mustard
- Chemicals
- Carbon monoxide
- Alcohol
- Nicotine
- Arsenic
- Potassium bromide
- Heavy metals
- Lead
- Tin
- Gold
- Mercury
- Loop diuretics
- Furosemide
- Ethacrynic acid
- Miscellaneous
- Pentobarbital
- Hexadine
- Salicylates/nonsteroidal antiinflammatory drugs (NSAIDs)
- Quinine

13.6 Physical Examination

The physical examination begins with examination of the external ear. The size, shape, and position of the pinna should be noted. In cases of microtia, the degree of external malformation can be correlated to developmental abnormalities of the middle and possibly the inner ear.[41] The preauricular area should be examined carefully for pits or skin tags, whereas postauricular inspection should make note of tenderness, erythema, swelling, or evidence of previous surgery. Even before the external auditory canal is inspected visually, pain may be elicited by traction on the pinna, which can suggest otitis externa.

Visual inspection of the external auditory canal and tympanic membrane (TM) can be performed with the handheld otoscope, which enables pneumatic otoscopy, or the otomicroscope, which provides improved visualization and ability to use instruments. Cerumen, foreign bodies, pus, fungal infection, keratinaceous debris, and granulation tissue may be noted; the canal itself may be erythematous and edematous or dry and flaky. Sagging of the posterosuperior canal wall is suggestive of mastoid disease. Step-offs of the superior canal may signify a temporal bone fracture. For optimal visualization, the canal should be carefully and thoroughly cleaned, and, if indicated, material from the canal may be sent for culture. Polyps, osteomas, or exostoses may partially or completely occlude the ear canal, making visualization of the TM difficult. However, under optimal circumstances, the entire TM should be inspected, making note of perforations, sclerotic areas, and retraction pockets.

The color of the TM provides additional clinical information. The normal TM is pearly gray. However, serous fluid may make it appear amber, whereas hemotympanum appears bluish. Masses may appear behind the TM and may be white (cholesteatoma), blue (dehiscent jugular bulb), or red (glomus tumor or more rarely aberrant carotid artery). Pneumatic otoscopy should be performed to assess drum mobility. Poor mobility suggests middle ear space fluid, whereas a healed perforation may be flaccid and hypermobile. Pneumatic otoscopy can also be used to perform the fistula test by applying positive and negative pressure and observing the patient for nystagmus. Dehiscence of bone overlying the superior semicircular canal can cause a syndrome of vertigo and oscillopsia induced by loud sounds (Tullio phenomenon),[42] by changes in pressure in the external canal that are transmitted to the middle ear (Hennebert sign),[43] or by Valsalva maneuvers.[44] These patients may have hyperacusis to bone-conducted sounds, with symptoms such as hearing their eye movements or pulse.[45,46]

A thorough head and neck examination can also provide important information. Initial examination may reveal physical findings suggestive of syndromic hearing loss, such as white forelock or facial asymmetry. Examination of the eyes should include assessment of pupillary function, evaluation of extraocular movements, and inspection for spontaneous or gaze nystagmus. Eye examination may also reveal abnormalities such as blue sclerae and heterochromia iridis that can be associated with hearing loss. In addition to the nasal examination, either mirror or fiberoptic examination of the nasopharynx may be performed, especially if the presence of a unilateral serous effusion in an adult is noted.[48]

The oral cavity should be examined for abnormalities such as submucous cleft or palatal malformation. The presence of a neck mass found during the neck examination can alert the examiner to a temporal bone malignancy. Cranial nerve examination is an invaluable part of the physical in that it can provide information about cerebellopontine angle tumors, SNHL, and various otologic systemic diseases. In a patient who presents with vestibular complaints in addition to hearing loss, assessment should also include observation of the patient's gait, a Romberg test, and tests of position sense such as the finger-nose and heel-shin tests.

Tuning fork examination should be performed as a method to confirm formal audiometric testing results. In situations where formal audiometric testing is not possible, such as the bedside,

tuning fork testing is the only means to assess hearing loss. The Rinne and Weber tests are standardly performed with a 512-Hz tuning fork. In the Rinne test, the tuning fork is held first against the mastoid bone and then in front of the ear canal. In CHL, sound is heard better over the mastoid. In the Weber test, the tuning fork is placed in the midline against a solid structure such as the nasal bone, forehead or maxillary incisor. In CHL, the sound is heard better in the involved ear, whereas in SNHL the sound is heard better in the better hearing hear.

Lastly, the physician may acquire additional information that may be pertinent by performing a more generalized physical examination where appropriate. For example, pigmentation abnormalities such as café-au-lait spots and vitiligo may suggest congenital disorders associated with hearing loss. Similarly, limb, stature, or phalangeal abnormalities may be associated with syndromic hearing loss. Cardiovascular examination may reveal bruits or murmurs that point to the possibility of vascular or embolic disease. Stigmata such as rheumatoid nodules, skin rashes, or neuromuscular abnormalities may identify systemic diseases with otologic manifestations.

13.6.1 Audiological Testing

All patients suspected of having hearing loss should undergo formal audiological examination, including pure-tone threshold testing for air and bone as well as assessment of speech threshold and discrimination. Subjective assessment tests rely on the participation of the patient, whereas physiological tests do not rely on the patient's interaction with the audiologist. (See also Chapter 8.)

13.6.2 Subjective Hearing Assessment

For children under 3 years of age or those with developmental delay, visual reinforcement audiometry (VRA) or conditioned play audiometry (CPA) replaces conventional audiological examination.[48] VRA is commonly used in children between the ages of 6 and 24 months. A signal is presented in the sound field, and the child is conditioned to turn toward the sound by the activity of a toy that is located close to the sound source. At 6 months old, a normal response occurs to sound stimuli of 20 dB or higher.[49]

For children 2 to 6 years old, CPA is commonly used. In this technique, the child is taught to perform a simple task, such as dropping a toy into a bucket or stacking a ring on a pole, in response to auditory signals. In CPA, the child wears headphones and pure-tone thresholds for both air and bone can be obtained. In small children, speech reception testing is best performed by allowing the child to point to a picture rather than repeating the word.

For children younger than 6 months, physiological tests of the auditory system provide greater accuracy than behavioral observation audiometry techniques. For children older than 6 years and for adults, a pure-tone audiogram is used to assess hearing in cooperative patients. Both air conduction and bone conduction thresholds are obtained across the frequency range from 250 to 8,000 Hz.[50] The span between 500 and 3,000 Hz is the most significant, as this range includes the majority of human speech sounds. In pure-tone testing, the authors define normal hearing as less than or equal to 25 dB, mild hearing loss as 26 to 40 dB, moderate hearing loss as 41 to 60 dB, severe hearing loss as 61 to 90 dB, and profound as greater than 90 dB.

13.6.3 Immittance Measures

In addition to basic audiometry, tests that may aid in identifying the cause of hearing loss include tympanometry and acoustic reflex testing. Tympanometry provides information about the compliance of the tympanic membrane and can be used to assess middle ear pathology as a cause of hearing loss. Tympanometry in infants younger than 4 months old should be obtained by using a probe frequency of 600 to 1,000 Hz because when tested with a standard probe tone frequency of 226 Hz infants with otitis media with effusion can have a normal-appearing tympanogram due to extensibility of skin in the ear canal.

Acoustic reflex testing assesses a reflex arc that involves the eighth cranial nerve, the brainstem, the facial nerve, and the stapedius muscle. An acoustic signal presented to one ear can produce bilateral reflex contraction of the stapedius muscle, producing a change in impedance. The threshold of the acoustic reflex can be measured as well as the duration of the response to a sustained signal. Although both middle ear and retrocochlear pathology may result in absent or abnormal reflexes, they are usually present in mild to moderate cochlear disorders. Abnormal decay of acoustic reflexes is suggestive of retrocochlear pathology. In otosclerosis, the tympanogram can be normal but reflexes are absent. In superior canal dehiscence, the tympanogram is normal and reflexes are present.[32]

Lastly, in cases where pseudohypoacusis is suspected, either because of the clinical scenario or because of inconsistent responses on basic audiological testing, additional tests can be used. The presence of normal acoustic reflexes with responses characteristic of a profound SNHL on pure-tone testing suggests a functional problem. The Stenger test can be used to test asymmetrical hearing loss, whereas the Doerfler-Stewart test is used in cases of bilateral hearing loss that are thought to be nonorganic. Other tests monitor the patient's spoken responses in the presence of masking noise or with delayed auditory feedback of his or her own voice.

13.6.4 Physiological Hearing Assessment

Physiological tests of the auditory system that may provide clinical information in cases of hearing loss include ABR, OAEs, and electrocochleography (ECochG). These tests may provide information about auditory thresholds in infants or in patients who are unwilling or unable to cooperate with basic audiological testing. In addition, these tests may identify the site of the lesion in cases of SNHL.

13.6.5 Auditory Brainstem Response

The ABR tests the auditory pathway from the eighth cranial nerve to the midbrain. Surface electrodes are used to measure evoked electrical responses to an acoustic signal, commonly a wideband click. The ABR is a noninvasive test that does not depend on the patient's level of consciousness or cooperation, and it has been widely used as a screening test for hearing loss in newborn infants.[36] It also is useful to determine functional hearing loss. Identification of threshold hearing levels is thought to be most accurate in cases of flat hearing loss because the wideband click includes a range of frequencies that stimulate the entire cochlea. To elicit more frequency specific threshold sensitivity, a stimulus with a narrower frequency band can be used, such as a tone pip. In addition, in cases of asymmetric hearing loss, it has been used to detect acoustic neuromas because of the delay in response latency produced by these tumors. Because the ABR can be normal in small (< 1 cm) vestibular schwannomas, magnetic resonance imaging (MRI) with gadolinium contrast enhancement remains the gold standard for diagnosis of suspected tumor. This may be useful in cases where hearing loss is too profound to permit ABR testing on the ipsilateral side. Aside from cerebellopontine angle tumors, diseases known to cause abnormal ABR results include vertebrobasilar vascular disease, central nervous system infections, demyelinating diseases, and polyneuropathies.[51,52] In infants, the auditory nerve and brainstem structures continue to develop from 18 to 24 months of age as reflected in decreasing interpeak latencies in the ABR.[36]

13.6.6 Otoacoustic Emissions

Otoacoustic emissions, discovered in 1978 by Kemp, are produced by the cochlea. These signals may be spontaneous (SOAEs), or may be produced in response to external stimulation. Different patterns of OAEs are produced by different stimuli. The most commonly used in clinical practice are transient-evoked OAEs (TEOAEs) and distortion-product OAEs (DPOAEs). The former are produced by a broadband tone click similar to that used for the ABR. DPOAEs are produced by using two tones of different frequency simultaneously. Less commonly used are stimulus-frequency OAEs (SFOAEs), which are evoked by pure-tone stimuli and provide frequency-specific responses. For all types, testing is noninvasive; a probe in the ear canal is used to produce the stimulus and record the response.

The presence of OAEs generally indicates that hearing is present because positive OAEs indicate functioning outer hair cells. OAEs are affected by outer and middle ear pathology, so that the absence of OAEs does not necessarily indicate hearing loss. Berlin et al[53] first recognized the presence of OAEs with absent ABR waveforms as an unusual type of hearing loss known as auditory dyssynchrony (auditory neuropathy spectrum disorder). Auditory neuropathy spectrum disorder (ANSD) is a recently defined entity that is thought to be a hearing impairment in which outer hair cell function is normal but afferent neural conduction in the auditory pathway is disordered. Characteristics of ANSD have been reported in patients with histories of prematurity, neonatal insult, hyperbilirubinemia, perinatal asphyxia, artificial ventilation, and various infectious processes.[7] A diagnosis of ANSD is made if the ABR conducted in this manner shows an absent or grossly abnormal ABR with only the presence of a cochlear microphonic. OAEs may be present initially but disappear over time; thus, absence of emissions does not preclude the diagnosis of ANSD. Stapedial reflexes are almost always absent.[53] Although approximately 7 to 10% of these patients have no observable symptoms other than an absent ABR, most others show minimal benefit from hearing aids trials based on behavioral audiograms, and some respond extremely well to cochlear implants even when the audiogram is not consistent with severe-to-profound hearing loss because cochlear implants bypass the site of neuropathy, which is thought to be at or near the spiral ganglion.[54]

13.6.7 Electrocochleography

Electrocochleography (ECochG) measures evoked potentials arising from the cochlea and the auditory nerve, usually using a broadband click stimulus. The responses that provide the most clinical information are the summating potential and the compound action potential of the eighth cranial nerve. ECochG can provide information about auditory thresholds. However, because a transtympanic needle electrode has produced the most accurate data, ECochG has not found widespread clinical use.

13.6.8 Vestibular Testing

The need for formal vestibular testing is determined primarily by the patient's history and physical examination. In children, vestibular screening tests should be performed when the hearing impairment is caused by a factor that also causes vestibular systems; examples include Pendred and Usher syndromes, aminoglycoside toxicity, bacterial meningitis, perilymphatic fistula, inner ear dysplasia, CHARGE syndrome (coloboma, heart anomaly, choanal atresia, retardation, and genital and ear anomalies), and a balance or motor delay.[55] In adults, there is a battery of testing available to help delineate vestibular symptoms. Vestibular evoked myogenic potentials (VEMPs) is a test that assesses vestibular function through the vestibulocollic reflex.[56] Clicks or tones presented to the ear stimulate the saccule, inferior vestibular nerve, vestibular nucleus, medial vestibulospinal tract, accessory nucleus, and cranial nerve XI. An electromyograph (EMG) of the sternocleidomastoid (SCM) records output after click stimulation of the ear being tested.[57] This test may be absent in patients with vestibular neuritis, in bilateral vestibular loss in aminoglycoside toxicity, and in acoustic neuromas. If there is a lower threshold associated with CHL on the same side, one must consider a diagnosis of superior semicircular canal dehiscence syndrome. If VEMPs show higher thresholds and are absent, one must consider Ménière's disease.[57]

13.6.9 Laboratory Testing

Testing is usually directed at uncovering underlying systemic diseases that may result in hearing loss, and the need for a specific test can be determined by the history and physical examination. Basic hematologic evaluation should include a complete blood count, platelet count, and sedimentation rate. Coagulation studies may include prothrombin and partial thromboplastin time. Blood chemistries include serum electrolytes, BUN,

creatinine, and urinalysis. Metabolic abnormalities may be identified by thyroid function tests, fasting blood sugar or glucose tolerance, adrenocorticotropic hormone (ACTH)-cortisol stimulation tests, and determination of serum cholesterol and triglycerides.

When the differential diagnosis includes immune-mediated hearing loss, the laboratory evaluation may include both nonspecific and specific tests. Most common testing includes antinuclear antibodies (ANAs) and rheumatroid factor (RF). Additional testing includes Western blot for 68-kd antibody, 31-kd antibody (thought to induce autoimmune hearing loss), and antibodies for heat shock protein 70 (HSP-70) (linked to Ménière disease with an autoimmune basis).

When indicated, laboratory tests for infectious diseases should be performed. Testing for syphilis should be performed by the fluorescent treponemal antibody absorption (FTA-ab) test. In suspected cases of neurosyphilis a lumbar puncture should be done. Cerebrospinal fluid studies should include opening pressure, cell count with differential, protein, glucose, Venereal Disease Research Laboratory (VDRL) test, culture, and Gram stain. Other serum tests include Lyme titers and tests for viral illnesses such as CMV. Specific immunoglobulin M (IgM) antibody assays should be performed if intrauterine infection is suspected, as IgM does not cross the placenta.[58]

Because Jervell and Lange-Nielsen syndrome with prolonged Q-T interval on electrocardiography (ECG) may be the only hereditary ear disease, which can lead to sudden death, some clinicians routinely obtain ECG in children with congenital profound hearing loss, especially if there is a history of syncopal episodes.

13.6.10 Genetic Testing

Given the rising prevalence of hearing loss, our knowledge of genetic testing has also rapidly expanded. With more than 150 loci for deafness genes and over 70 of them being identified (see the website http://hereditaryhearingloss.org/), it is also known that hereditary hearing loss is a very heterogeneous condition.[59] Genetic testing and genetic counseling play an important role in caring for patients with SNHL, as early intervention programs can significantly improve development and quality of life.[60] Autosomal recessive nonsyndromic hearing loss caused by mutations in connexin 26 is known as *DFNB1*, which is characterized by a prelingual, nonprogressive bilateral loss. It has been shown in multiple studies that the most common *DFNB1* mutation is 35delG, and this has a carrier frequency of 1.3 to 4.0%.[61] Testing for mitochondrial DNA inheritance associated with aminoglycoside ototoxicity can be linked to A1555G mutation and the A7445G mutation.[62] For patients with progressive SNHL, if inner ear malformations are detected by routine inner ear imaging, screening for SLC26A4 mutations for Pendred syndrome/*DFNB4* should be undertaken.[62] Similarly, several genetic abnormalities related to auditory neuropathy have also been identified; these include *OTOF, PMP22, MPZ,* and *NDRGI.*[63]

13.6.11 Radiological Evaluation

In the evaluation of temporal bone pathology, high-definition computed tomography (CT) with fine cuts of the temporal bone and MRI provide excellent information. High-definition CT with fine cuts in the axial, coronal, and oblique planes provides information about the bony anatomy of the temporal bone. This study should be performed in all children and should be considered in older patients with progressive hearing loss and craniofacial anomalies. The reported incidence of CT anomalies is 6.8 to 31%, with the most common abnormality being the enlarged vestibular aqueduct.[64] Other abnormalities diagnosed include Mondini dysplasia, common cavity deformity of the cochlea, and abnormalities of semicircular canals including superior semicircular canal dehiscence syndrome. For imaging pathology of the cerebellopontine angle and central nervous system, MRI with gadolinium contrast is superior. Additional imaging beyond the head and neck may be indicated in patients who are suspected of having syndromic hearing loss with pathology involving other systems.

13.7 Conclusion

Clinical evaluation of the patient with hearing loss requires an understanding of the differential diagnosis of conductive and SNHL. Patients may require evaluation because of their subjective complaints or because of identifiable risk factors for hearing loss, particularly of children. A complete history and physical examination provides important information about the nature, degree, and symmetry of hearing loss. Additional testing to identify the site of lesion and underlying pathological process may include more extensive audiological testing, physiological assessment of the auditory system, vestibular testing, laboratory tests, genetic testing, and radiological studies. On the basis of this evaluation, the physician can determine the appropriate diagnosis so that treatment and rehabilitation can be undertaken.

References

[1] Lin FR, Thorpe R, Gordon-Salant S, Ferrucci L. Hearing loss prevalence and risk factors among older adults in the United States. J Gerontol A Biol Sci Med Sci 2011; 66: 582–590

[2] Sataloff RT. Hearing loss: economic impact. Ear Nose Throat J 2012; 91: 10–12

[3] National Institute on Deafness and Other Communication Disorders. Statistics about hearing, balance, ear infections, and deafness: quick statistics. www.nidcd.nih.gov/health/statistics/Pages

[4] Mohr PE, Feldman JJ, Dunbar JL et al. The societal costs of severe to profound hearing loss in the United States. Int J Technol Assess Health Care 2000; 16: 1120–1135

[5] Centers for Disease Control and Prevention (CDC) http://www.cdc.gov/ncbddd/AboutUs/human-development-hearingloss.html

[6] Centers for Disease Control and Prevention (CDC). Economic costs associated with mental retardation, cerebral palsy, hearing loss, and vision impairment —United States, 2003. MMWR Morb Mortal Wkly Rep 2004; 53: 57–59

[7] Starr A, Picton TW, Sininger Y, Hood LJ, Berlin CI. Auditory neuropathy. Brain 1996; 119: 741–753

[8] Roush P. Auditory neuropathy spectrum disorder: evaluation and management. The Hearing Journal. 2008; 61: 36–41

[9] Robertson CM, Howarth TM, Dietlind LR, Dinu IA. Permanent bilateral sensory and neural hearing loss of children after neonatal intensive care because of extreme prematurity: a thirty-year study. Pediatrics 2009; 123: 797–807

[10] Fawke J. Neurological outcomes following preterm birth. Semin Fetal Neonatal Med 2007; 12: 374–382

[11] Erbe CB, Harris KC, Runge-Samuelson CL, Flanary VA, Wackym PA. Connexin 26 and connexin 30 mutations in children with nonsyndromic hearing loss. Laryngoscope 2004; 114: 607–611

[12] Snoeckx RL, Huygen PL, Feldmann D et al. GJB2 mutations and degree of hearing loss: a multicenter study. Am J Hum Genet 2005; 77: 945–957

[13] Battelino S, Repič Lampret B, Zargi M, Podkrajšek KT. Novel connexin 30 and connexin 26 mutational spectrum in patients with progressive sensorineural hearing loss. J Laryngol Otol 2012; 126: 763–769

[14] da Costa SS, Rosito LP, Dornelles C. Sensorineural hearing loss in patients with chronic otitis media. Eur Arch Otorhinolaryngol 2009; 266: 221–224

[15] Vaamonde P, Castro C, García-Soto N, Labella T, Lozano A. Tuberculous otitis media: a significant diagnostic challenge. Otolaryngol Head Neck Surg 2004; 130: 759–766

[16] Araújo EdaS, Zucki F, Corteletti LC, Lopes AC, Feniman MR, Alvarenga KdeF. Hearing loss and acquired immune deficiency syndrome: systematic review. J Soc Bras Fonoaudiol 2012; 24: 188–192

[17] Mata Castro N, Yebra Bango M, Tutor de Ureta P, Villarreal García-Lomas M, García López F. [Hearing loss and human immunodeficiency virus infection. Study of 30 patients] Rev Clin Esp 2000; 200: 271–274

[18] Worsøe L, Cayé-Thomasen P, Brandt CT, Thomsen J, Østergaard C. Factors associated with the occurrence of hearing loss after pneumococcal meningitis. Clin Infect Dis 2010; 51: 917–924

[19] Kutz JW, Simon LM, Chennupati SK, Giannoni CM, Manolidis S. Clinical predictors for hearing loss in children with bacterial meningitis. Arch Otolaryngol Head Neck Surg 2006; 132: 941–945

[20] Wellman MB, Sommer DD, McKenna J. Sensorineural hearing loss in postmeningitic children. Otol Neurotol 2003; 24: 907–912

[21] Külahli I, Oztürk M, Bilen C, Cüreoglu S, Merhametsiz A, Cağil N. Evaluation of hearing loss with auditory brainstem responses in the early and late period of bacterial meningitis in children. J Laryngol Otol 1997; 111: 223–227

[22] Bovo R, Ciorba A, Martini A. The diagnosis of autoimmune inner ear disease: evidence and critical pitfalls. Eur Arch Otorhinolaryngol 2009; 266: 37–40

[23] Huang NC, Sataloff RT. Autoimmune inner ear disease in children. Otol Neurotol 2011; 32: 213–216

[24] Swartz JD. Lesions of the cerebellopontine angle and internal auditory canal: diagnosis and differential diagnosis. Semin Ultrasound CT MR 2004; 25: 332–352

[25] Gloria-Cruz TI, Schachern PA, Paparella MM, Adams GL, Fulton SE. Metastases to temporal bones from primary nonsystemic malignant neoplasms. Arch Otolaryngol Head Neck Surg 2000; 126: 209–214

[26] Kaźmierczak H, Doroszewska G. Metabolic disorders in vertigo, tinnitus, and hearing loss. Int Tinnitus J 2001; 7: 54–58

[27] Masindova I, Varga L, Stanik J et al. Molecular and hereditary mechanisms of sensorineural hearing loss with focus on selected endocrinopathies. Endocr Regul 2012; 46: 167–186

[28] Ealy M, Smith RJ. Otosclerosis. Adv Otorhinolaryngol 2011; 70: 122–129

[29] Schrauwen I, Van Camp G. The etiology of otosclerosis: a combination of genes and environment. Laryngoscope 2010; 120: 1195–1202

[30] Minor LB, Solomon D, Zinreich JS, Zee DS. Sound- and/or pressure-induced vertigo due to bone dehiscence of the superior semicircular canal. Arch Otolaryngol Head Neck Surg 1998; 124: 249–258

[31] Puwanarajah P, Pretorius P, Bottrill I. Superior semicircular canal dehiscence syndrome: a new aetiology. J Laryngol Otol 2008; 122: 741–744

[32] Thabet EM, Abdelkhalek A, Zaghloul H. Superior semicircular canal dehiscence syndrome as assessed by oVEMP and temporal bone computed tomography imaging. Eur Arch Otorhinolaryngol 2012; 269: 1545–1549

[33] Barsky-Firkser L, Sun S. Universal newborn hearing screenings: a three-year experience. Pediatrics 1997; 99: E4

[34] Mehl AL, Thomson V. The Colorado newborn hearing screening project, 1992–1999: on the threshold of effective population-based universal newborn hearing screening. Pediatrics 2002; 109: E7

[35] Nelson HD, Bougatsos C, Nygren P. Universal Newborn Hearing Screening: Systematic Review to Update the 2001 U.S. Preventive Services Task Force Recommendation. Oregon Evidence-based Practice Center. Agency for Healthcare Research and Quality (US), 2008

[36] American Academy of Pediatrics, Joint Committee on Infant Hearing. Year 2007 position statement: Principles and guidelines for early hearing detection and intervention programs. Pediatrics 2007; 120: 898–921

[37] Matkin ND, Wilcox AM. Considerations in the education of children with hearing loss. Pediatr Clin North Am 1999; 46: 143–152

[38] Swartz JD. Lesions of the cerebellopontine angle and internal auditory canal: diagnosis and differential diagnosis. Semin Ultrasound CT MR 2004; 25: 332–352

[39] Suzane da Cunha F. Lima Marco Antonio de Melo Tavares de. Superior Canal Dehiscence Syndrome. Rev Bras Otorrinolaringol (Engl Ed) 2006; 72: 414–418

[40] Mukherjea D, Rybak LP, Sheehan KE et al. The design and screening of drugs to prevent acquired sensorineural hearing loss. Expert Opin Drug Discov 2011; 6: 491–505

[41] Ishimoto S, Ito K, Karino S, Takegoshi H, Kaga K, Yamasoba T. Hearing levels in patients with microtia: correlation with temporal bone malformation. Laryngoscope 2007; 117: 461–465

[42] Minor LB, Carey JP, Cremer PD, Lustig LR, Streubel SO, Ruckenstein MJ. Dehiscence of bone overlying the superior canal as a cause of apparent conductive hearing loss. Otol Neurotol 2003; 24: 270–278

[43] Minor LB. Superior canal dehiscence syndrome. Am J Otol 2000; 21: 9–19

[44] Minor LB, Cremer PD, Carey JP, Della Santina CC, Streubel SO, Weg N. Symptoms and signs in superior canal dehiscence syndrome. Ann N Y Acad Sci 2001; 942: 259–273

[45] Ostrowski VB, Byskosh A, Hain TC. Tullio phenomenon with dehiscence of the superior semicircular canal. Otol Neurotol 2001; 22: 61–65

[46] Watson SRD, Halmagyi GM, Colebatch JG. Vestibular hypersensitivity to sound (Tullio phenomenon): structural and functional assessment. Neurology 2000; 54: 722–728

[47] Sham JS, Wei WI, Lau SK, Yau CC, Choy D. Serous otitis media. An opportunity for early recognition of nasopharyngeal carcinoma. Arch Otolaryngol Head Neck Surg 1992; 118: 794–797

[48] Johnson KC. Audiologic assessment of children with suspected hearing loss. Otolaryngol Clin North Am 2002; 35: 711–732

[49] Kumar A, Maudelonde C, Mafee M. Unilateral sensorineural hearing loss: analysis of 200 consecutive cases. Laryngoscope 1986; 96: 14–18

[50] Schulman-Galambos C, Galambos R. Brain stem evoked response audiometry in newborn hearing screening. Arch Otolaryngol 1979; 105: 86–90

[51] Burkey JM, Rizer FM, Schuring AG, Fucci MJ, Lippy WH. Acoustic reflexes, auditory brainstem response, and MRI in the evaluation of acoustic neuromas. Laryngoscope 1996; 106: 839–841

[52] Telian SA, Kileny PR, Niparko JK, Kemink JL, Graham MD. Normal auditory brainstem response in patients with acoustic neuroma. Laryngoscope 1989; 99: 10–14

[53] Berlin CI, Morlet T, Hood LJ. Auditory neuropathy/dyssynchrony: its diagnosis and management. Pediatr Clin North Am 2003; 50: 331–340, vii–viii

[54] Rapin I, Gravel J. "Auditory neuropathy": physiologic and pathologic evidence calls for more diagnostic specificity. Int J Pediatr Otorhinolaryngol 2003; 67: 707–728

[55] Angeli S. Value of vestibular testing in young children with sensorineural hearing loss. Arch Otolaryngol Head Neck Surg 2003; 129: 478–482

[56] Zhou G, Cox LC. Vestibular evoked myogenic potentials: history and overview. Am J Audiol 2004; 13: 135–143

[57] Isaradisaikul S, Navacharoen N, Hanprasertpong C, Kangsanarak J. Cervical vestibular-evoked myogenic potentials: norms and protocols. Int J Otolaryngol 2012; 2012: 913515

[58] Mathews J, Kumar BN. Autoimmune sensorineural hearing loss. Clin Otolaryngol Allied Sci 2003; 28: 479–488

[59] King PJ, Xiaomei O, Lilin D, Yan D. Etiologic diagnosis of nonsyndromic genetic hearing loss in adult vs pediatric populations. Otolaryngol Head Neck Surg 2012; 5: 932–936

[60] Kochhar A, Hildebrand MS, Smith RJ. Clinical aspects of hereditary hearing loss. Genet Med 2007; 9: 393–408

[61] Lipan M, Ouyang XM, Yan D, Angeli S, Du LL, Liu XZ. Clinical comparison of hearing-impaired patients with DFNB1 against heterozygote carriers of connexin 26 mutations. Laryngoscope 2011; 121: 811–814

[62] Estivill X, Govea N, Barceló E et al. Familial progressive sensorineural deafness is mainly due to the mtDNA A1555G mutation and is enhanced by treatment of aminoglycosides. Am J Hum Genet 1998; 62: 27–35

[63] Madden C, Rutter M, Hilbert L, Greinwald JH, Jr, Choo DI. Clinical and audiological features in auditory neuropathy. Arch Otolaryngol Head Neck Surg 2002; 128: 1026–1030

[64] Mafong DD, Shin EJ, Lalwani AK. Use of laboratory evaluation and radiologic imaging in the diagnostic evaluation of children with sensorineural hearing loss. Laryngoscope 2002; 112: 1–7

14 Evaluation of the Dizzy Patient

Joel A. Goebel and Eric L. Slattery

14.1 Introduction

Dizziness is a commonly seen complaint by both primary care physicians and specialists, such as otolaryngologists or neurologists. Dizziness can refer to symptomatology from derangements of the central and peripheral nervous systems, vestibular system, vision, and cardiovascular system.[1] Given this varied pathophysiology, a systematic approach is necessary to diagnose and manage patients effectively. Often a well-performed history and physical examination can identify or greatly narrow the differential diagnosis in the majority of patients. This chapter discusses maximizing both the history and physical examination in evaluating the dizzy patient, with an emphasis on vestibular causes of dizziness.

14.2 History

The history is critical in understanding the patient describing dizziness. Time spent precisely defining the "dizzy" symptom in the history allows for the narrowing of etiologic causes, and has been shown to have a high degree of predictive ability in diagnosing dizziness.[2] Written questionnaires completed by the patient prior to the interview can greatly increase the efficiency of the encounter. Encouraging patients to describe the sensation in an open-ended manner will greatly help the clinician better understand their condition. Vertigo, light-headedness, presyncope, visual disturbances, imbalance, and dissociated feelings have very different presenting symptoms that can usually be ascertained from the patient's history. Sometimes more directed questioning is needed to help patients describe their sensation.

The term *vertigo* implies an illusion of movement between the patient and the environment. Patients usually report the environment is moving, although sometimes they feel as if they are moving. Most commonly the sensation is rotary and is described as spinning.[3] Although vertigo is a common complaint with otologic causes of dizziness, suggesting a peripheral vestibular dysfunction, vertigo can occur in diseases of the central nervous system as well.

The sensations of light-headedness, nearly losing consciousness (presyncope), or loss of consciousness (syncope) most likely do not have a vestibular origin. These symptoms suggest a cardiovascular or occasionally a psychiatric etiology. Eliciting a history of cardiac or peripheral vascular disease, usage of antihypertensive medication, chest palpitations, or increased symptoms when standing (orthostatic hypotension) suggest a cardiovascular component and warrant further investigation. Psychiatric disease should be entertained after other causes for symptoms have been eliminated in patients having other symptoms or triggers consistent with mood and anxiety disorders.

Patients often report symptoms of general imbalance rather than attacks of dizziness. Often they describe a feeling of unsteadiness when standing or walking. Some patients describe a sensation of falling, swaying, or listing to one side, whereas other patients have no side predominance. Disorders of the somatosensory, proprioceptive, vestibular, and visual systems can contribute to imbalance. Ataxia, having a lack of coordi-

nated movements, is usually caused by lesions of the cerebellum. Patients may describe oscillopsia, that is, bobbing or blurring of the visual field. Oscillopsia with head movement commonly occurs after bilateral or uncompensated unilateral impairment of the vestibular system, causing an inability of the ocular system to maintain gaze during head movement.

After obtaining a better understanding of the dizzy sensation, the following questions should be addressed: (1) Is the sensation episodic? (2) What is the duration of episodes? (3) Are the symptoms brought on by position changes? (4) What other otologic or nonotologic symptoms are associated with the dizzy sensation? Deciding whether the symptoms are periodic, and if so, the duration of symptoms is crucial in narrowing the differential diagnosis. Otologic causes of dizziness usually manifest with episodic vertigo or imbalance. Ménière disease, vestibular neuritis, and benign paroxysmal positional vertigo (BPPV) are the three most prevalent inner ear disorders causing discrete episodes of vertigo. These disorders can readily be distinguished by the duration of symptoms. Ménière disease often manifests as severe recurrent vertigo that abruptly occurs, lasting minutes to hours. Vertigo from vestibular neuritis is often severe, abrupt in onset, and sustained for typically hours to even days. It should be noted that acute ischemia of the cerebellum can give signs and symptoms similar to vestibular neuritis and should be excluded. BPPV occurs for less than a minute and is induced with head movements. A fourth common entity that can cause episodic vertigo or imbalance, which is nonotologic in etiology, is vestibular migraine.[4] The time course of vestibular migraine overlaps with Ménière disease, although symptoms of vestibular migraine can last for days. However, associated symptoms of fluctuating hearing loss with Ménière disease versus photophobia with vestibular migraine help in making the diagnosis, although distinguishing between the two can be difficult.

Discovering if symptoms are brought on by position changes is useful in making a diagnosis. Symptoms of light-headedness or presyncope with standing strongly suggests a cardiovascular etiology. Brief vertigo with head movements implies BPPV. Position changes that induce symptoms depend both on the side and semicircular canal affected. Movements that are within the plane of the affected canal will cause the most vigorous vertigo. Most commonly the posterior canal is involved, with patients reporting that symptoms occur while looking up and rolling over in bed. Vertigo brought on by neck movements associated with other neurologic or visual symptoms lasting up to 15 minutes may be a sign of vertebrobasilar insufficiency.

Associated symptoms experienced by the patient is another very important aspect of the history and can often guide the clinician to the source of the dizziness. Hearing loss, aural fullness, or tinnitus not only helps suggest an otologic origin, but also can help lateralize which ear is involved. Classically, symptoms of Ménière disease include fluctuating low-frequency sensorineural hearing loss, aural fullness, and tinnitus that accompanies attacks of vertigo as set forth by the American Academy of Otolaryngology Committee on Hearing and Equilibrium.[5]

Possible Ménière disease:
- Episodic vertigo of the Ménière type without documented hearing loss or sensorineural hearing loss
- Fluctuating or fixed, with disequilibrium but without definitive episodes
- Other causes excluded

Probable Ménière disease:
- One definitive episode of vertigo
- Audiometrically documented hearing loss on at least one occasion
- Tinnitus or aural fullness in the treated ear
- Other causes excluded

Definitive Ménière disease:
- Two or more definitive spontaneous episodes of vertigo 20 minutes or longer
- Audiometrically documented hearing loss on at least one occasion
- Tinnitus or aural fullness in the treated ear
- Other causes excluded

Certain Ménière disease:
- Definitive Ménière disease, plus histopathological confirmation

Diplacusis (perception of two separate tones from a single auditory stimulus) and hyperacusis (increased sensitivity to sound) also are well-known symptoms in Ménière disease. Many patients suffering from autoimmune hearing loss have complaints of imbalance and progressive hearing loss. Herpes zoster oticus (Ramsay-Hunt syndrome) presents with facial palsy, vesicles of the concha, sensorineural hearing loss, and severe vertigo. Fluctuating hearing loss and sound or pressure-induced vertigo can be seen in perilymph fistulas, although sound-induced vertigo or imbalance (Tullio phenomenon) is also a common symptom of superior semicircular canal dehiscence. Otalgia and otorrhea suggest an infectious etiology. Symptoms suggesting a cardiovascular origin include chest pain or palpitations and shortness of breath with episodes. Many neurologic symptoms can also occur, alerting the clinician to a neurologic origin. Headaches, focal signs such as motor weakness or sensation changes, tremors, visual or olfactory auras, neck stiffness, photophobia and other visual complaints, other cranial neuropathies, and incontinence are all neurologic symptoms. A history of chronic anxiety and a persistent sensation of imbalance may suggest a psychiatric etiology.

Special attention should be made toward the symptomatology of dizziness associated with migraine, as the diagnosis is usually made based on the history and confirmed with treatment. Although vertigo and imbalance is currently recognized only as an aura in basilar migraine by the International Classification of Headache Disorders, imbalance and vertigo have recently been described as a common sensation in patients with migraine.[6]

Diagnostic criteria for both "definite" and "probable" vestibular migraine have been proposed by Neuhauser (see box below) and shown to have a high degree of reliability.[7] Patients are often primarily diagnosed in early or middle age and rarely after 60 years of age. Although patients have been diagnosed with current or prior migraine headaches, often the symptoms of vertigo or imbalance occur during headache-free intervals or with no temporal association to the cephalgia. Symptoms of photophobia or phonophobia during the dizzy attacks have a high concordance with vestibular migraine.[2]

A thorough history also involves past medical and surgical history, which can give clues to why patients are experiencing dizziness. Prior cardiovascular and neurologic history should be obtained. Reviewing any previous imaging of the head and brain can sometimes suggest causes (e.g., multiple sclerosis, tumors, or Arnold-Chiari malformations). An investigation of current medications is necessary as many can causes dizziness. Prior exposure to known ototoxic medications such as aminoglycosides, platinum-based antineoplastic agents, and loop diuretics should be explored.

14.3 Physical Examination

Although diagnosis of many types of dizziness can be made based on the history, a structured thorough physical examination is essential in deriving the etiology. As with the history, conducting the examination systematically increases its efficiency and yield in these patients. The examination begins with a thorough head and neck examination. Testing for orthostatic hypotension is performed by taking a resting blood pressure while the patient is lying down and then after the patient is standing. A drop in the systolic blood pressure by 20 mm Hg or the diastolic blood pressure by 10 mm Hg while standing is considered orthostatic hypotension, although symptoms can occur with little or no change in pressure. The patient should be asked if presyncopal symptoms are occurring as well. A negative test does not rule out cardiac or autonomic nervous system etiologies of dizziness. Careful attention should be given to the otologic examination including visualization of the tympanic membrane during pneumatic otoscopy. A fistula test can be performed by placing positive pressure in the ear canal with a pneumatic otoscope, with a positive test constituting pressure-induced vertigo or nystagmus. Tuning fork exams, including the Weber and Rinne tests, should be undertaken with a 512-Hz tuning fork. Cranial nerves II to XII should also be evaluated.

The neurotologic examination for dizziness entails (1) evaluation for nystagmus; (2) tests of ocular function; (3) tests of the vestibulo-ocular reflex (VOR); (4) positioning/positional tests; (5) limb tests; and (6) tests of gait and posture.

Migraine without aura:

a) At least five attacks fulfilling criteria b to d
b) Headache attacks lasting 4 to 72 hours (untreated or unsuccessfully treated)
c) Headache has at least two of the following characteristics:
- Unilateral location
- Pulsating quality
- Moderate or severe pain intensity
- Aggravation by or causing avoidance of routine physical activity (e.g., walking or climbing stairs)
d) During headache at least one of the following:
- Nausea or vomiting
- Photophobia and phonophobia
- Not attributed to another disorder

Migraine with aura:

a) At least two attacks fulfilling criteria b to d
b) Aura consisting of at least one of the following, but no motor weakness:
- Fully reversible visual symptoms including positive features (e.g., flickering lights, spots, or lines) or negative features (i.e., loss of vision)
- Fully reversible sensory symptoms including positive features (i.e., pins and needles) or negative features (i.e., numbness)
- Fully reversible dysphasic speech disturbance
c) At least two of the following:
- Homonymous visual symptoms[1] or unilateral sensory symptoms
- At least one aura symptom develops gradually over ≥ 5 minutes or different aura symptoms occur in succession over ≥ 5 minutes
- Each symptom lasts ≥ 5 and ≤ 60 minutes
d) Headache fulfilling criteria b to d for migraine without aura that begins during the aura or follows the aura within 60 minutes
e) Not attributed to another disorder

Basilar migraine:

a) At least two attacks fulfilling criteria b to d
b) Aura consisting of at least two of the following fully reversible symptoms, but no motor weakness:
- Dysarthria
- Vertigo
- Tinnitus
- Hyperacusia
- Diplopia
- Visual symptoms simultaneously in both temporal and nasal fields of both eyes
- Ataxia
- Decreased level of consciousness
- Simultaneously bilateral paraesthesias
c) At least one of the following:
- At least one aura symptom develops gradually over ≥ 5 minutes or different aura symptoms occur in succession over ≥ 5 minutes
- Each aura symptom lasts ≥ 5 and ≤ 60 minutes

d) Headache fulfilling criteria b to d for migraine without aura that begins during the aura or follows aura within 60 minutes
e) Not attributed to another disorder

Definite:
- Recurrent episodic vestibular symptoms of moderate severity
- Current or previous history of migraine headaches meeting International Headache Society criteria
- At least one of the following migrainous symptoms during at least two of these attacks:
  - Migraine-type headache
  - Visual or other auras
  - Photophobia
  - Phonophobia
- Other causes ruled out by appropriate investigations

Probable:
- Recurrent episodic vestibular symptoms of moderate severity
- One of the following:
  - Current or previous history of migraine headaches meeting International Headache Society criteria
  - Migrainous symptoms during attacks of vertigo
  - Migraine-precipitants before vertigo in more than 50% of attacks: food triggers, sleep irregularities, hormonal changes
  - Response to migraine medications in more than 50% of attacks
- Other causes ruled out by appropriate investigations

- Nystagmus
  - Spontaneous
  - Gaze-evoked
- Tests of ocular motor function
  - Smooth pursuit
  - Saccades
  - Fixation suppression of rotary nystagmus
- Tests of the VOR
  - Head impulse test
  - Dynamic visual acuity test
  - Post–head-shake test
  - Vibration test
  - Hyperventilation test
- Positioning/positional tests
  - Dynamic positioning tests
  - Static positional tests
- Limb tests
  - Coordination
  - Vibrotactile testing with 128-kHz tuning fork
- Tests of posture and gait

14.3.1 Evaluation for Nystagmus

Nystagmus is an involuntary rhythmic movement of the eyes that can be physiological (optokinetic or rotation-induced) or pathological (central or peripheral vestibular or oculomotor pathway dysfunction). Maintaining visual fixation on a target during rapid impulsive head movement occurs via the VOR, which consists of a vestibular afferent neuron, an interneuron, and an ocular motor neuron. This reflex is fast and accurate, as visual acuity degrades with as little as 2 to 3 degrees/second of retinal slippage. Linear motion is detected by the otolithic organs and angular motion by the semicircular canals. Ewald's laws refer to examination of eye movements in relationship to vestibular input.[8] Ewald's first law states that eye motion in relation to angular movement occurs in the plane of the stimulated semicircular canal(s) in the direction of endolymph flow. The second law states that ampullopetal endolymph flow in the horizontal canal produces a stronger response than ampullofugal movement. The third law states the opposite is true for the vertical canals: ampullofugal flow is more stimulating than ampullopetal flow. Knowing these principles help clinicians understand findings associated with vestibular lesions.

Spontaneous Nystagmus

Spontaneous nystagmus refers to an involuntary rhythmic eye movement seen in the seated position without stimuli. Testing for spontaneous nystagmus is performed with the patient sitting upright and with a neutral gaze with and without visual fixation. Spontaneous nystagmus from a peripheral vestibular injury that affects the whole labyrinth creates a mixed horizontal-torsional nystagmus. In the case of a vestibular deficit, the contralateral labyrinth causes the eyes to drift toward the injured ear with a compensatory fast eye movement toward the uninvolved ear. By convention, nystagmus is usually defined by the direction of the fast phase. Other features of nystagmus resulting from peripheral vestibular disease include nystagmus that is direction fixed and decreased with visual fixation. Removal of fixation is possible with the use of Frenzel lenses, which aid in documenting the presence of spontaneous nystagmus. Most nystagmus caused by the peripheral vestibular system intensifies with gaze toward the fast phase. Alexander's law states that nystagmus that is present with gaze away from the fast phase, gaze neutral, and gaze toward the fast phase is termed third-degree nystagmus and is commonly seen in acute peripheral vestibular dysfunction.[9] As compensation occurs, the nystagmus decreases in severity, and second degree (nystagmus only with gaze neutral and toward the fast phase) and then first degree (nystagmus only toward the fast phase) is noted. Components of spontaneous nystagmus that suggest a central origin include nystagmus that increases or does not decrease with fixation, direction-changing nystagmus, and purely vertical nystagmus. Many types of central nystagmus have been described, including downbeat, upbeat, seesaw, convergence-retraction, square wave, ocular flutter, and opsoclonus. Often cerebellar or medullary lesions, multiple sclerosis, or medication effects have been described with central nystagmus.

Gaze-Evoked Nystagmus

Gaze-evoked nystagmus refers to nystagmus that occurs with attempted eccentric gaze. Clinical testing for gaze-evoked nystagmus is performed by asking the patient to look at the examiner's finger held 20 to 30 degrees to the right, left, up, and down from center for 10 to 20 seconds. As the patient tries to look at an eccentric position, the eyes slowly drift back to a neutral position and a corrective refixation saccade places the eyes back to the eccentric position. This usually results from disorders of the cerebellum or brainstem, which acts as a central integrator of ocular movements. Medication and drug effect also can induce gaze-evoked nystagmus. This should be differentiated from spontaneous nystagmus, which follows Alexander's law and is accentuated by eye movements in the direction of the fast phase. Gaze-evoked nystagmus is also distinct from physiological end-gaze nystagmus that can be induced in normal patients by looking beyond 30 degrees from the neutral position.

14.4 Tests of Ocular Function

14.4.1 Ocular Alignment and Movement

Alignment of the eyes should be inspected with both eyes open while the patient fixates on a target in neutral and eccentric gaze in the horizontal and vertical planes. The patient should be asked if diplopia was experienced with any motion. Misalignment that happens only in certain gazes is termed noncomitant and suggests restriction or weakness of the extraocular muscles. The "cover/uncover test" can reveal less apparent misalignment. The patient fixates on a target with one eye being covered, and then refixates with the opposite eye, and any refixation ocular movement is noted. Vertical misalignment is termed skew deviation and is often thought to be associated with brainstem or cerebellum injury, especially of the supranuclear lesions; however, acute otolithic damage of the peripheral vestibular system can also produce transient vertical misalignment.

Saccades

Saccades are movements of the eye used to redirect the retina's fovea to new targets. The hallmarks of a saccade are that it is a conjugate movement that is highly accurate and fast, and that it entails minimal delay. Testing of saccades involves having a patient look rapidly and repeatedly at a raised finger 15 degrees left from neutral position and then look at a second finger 15 degrees right from neutral position. Saccadic testing should also be evaluated in both the superior and inferior directions as well. Accuracy, velocity, and initiation time should be noted for all saccades. Lesions of the frontal lobe, midbrain, pons, and cerebellum can cause abnormal saccades. Internuclear ophthalmoplegia, commonly seen in multiple sclerosis, displays slowing of saccades in the adducting eye coupled with nystagmus in the abducting eye due to lesions of the medial longitudinal fasciculus. Cerebellar disease can manifest as inaccurate saccadic movement, resulting in either ocular overshoot or undershoot of the visual target.

Smooth Pursuit

Smooth pursuit eye movements produce a continuous view of a moving target on the fovea, such that the eyes "track" with the movement of the target. Examination of smooth pursuit occurs by having an individual follow a moving finger that is positioned about 3 feet from the patient's head. Impairment of smooth pursuit can happen with brainstem and cerebellar lesions as well as with medication effects. It should be noted that smooth pursuit is not developed well in small children, and that there is deterioration with age and reduced visual acuity, often with older patients displaying "catch-up" saccades to make up for this deterioration; thus, a mild impairment of smooth pursuit is not specific in elderly patients.

Fixation Suppression of Per-Rotational Nystagmus

The flocculus of the cerebellum allows for suppression of rotation-induced nystagmus while viewing an object rotating with the subject. The patient is asked to keep his or her eyes gazing straight ahead while the exam chair is rotated and the nystagmus is noted. Visual fixation is induced with the patient maintaining gaze on his or her outstretched thumb during chair rotation. There should be minimal or no nystagmus during fixation. If nystagmus is not suppressed and visual acuity is intact, this is a strong sign of flocculo-cerebellar dysfunction.

14.4.2 Tests of the Vestibulo-Ocular Reflex

The VOR is a three-neuron brainstem reflex that maintains visual clarity during rapid impulsive movements of the head. Loss of the VOR can cause symptoms of oscillopsia, as slippage of the visual field occurs with head movements. This is most pronounced in bilateral weakness of the vestibular system but can be seen in poorly compensated unilateral lesions. Clinical tests of VOR function include the head impulse test, the post–head-shake test, the vibration test, the hyperventilation test, and the dynamic visual acuity test.

Head Impulse Test

The head impulse test was first described by Halmagyi and Curthoys[10] in 1988. This test examines the integrity of the high-frequency VOR and is considered a direct test of the peripheral vestibular system. To perform the test, the patient's head is turned rapidly 30 degrees (either from midline to right and left or from right and left to midline) while the patient attempts to maintain eye fixation on a target (▶ Fig. 14.1).

Although the lateral canal is commonly tested by movements in the horizontal plane, utilizing Ewald's first law (which states that eye movements from activation of the semicircular canals occur in the plane of the semicircular canal), the test can be done in the vertical planes of the superior and posterior canals as well. In the injured vestibular system, the patient's eyes do not remain on the target. Instead, a compensatory or "catch-up" saccade is employed to bring the eyes back to the target. In unilateral vestibular weakness, eye lag occurs with head movement in the direction that causes excitation. In the case of the lateral canal, lag would occur with the head thrust toward the lesioned side. In bilateral vestibular damage, the head thrust may be positive in both directions. Similar to the head thrust test is the head heave test, in which a linear (usually horizontal) movement instead of an angular thrust has also been described and is thought to test the linear VOR generated by the otolithic organs.

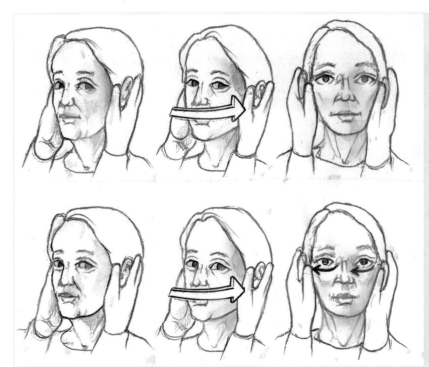

Fig. 14.1 The head impulse test. Patient keeps her gaze fixed forward with the head turned 30 degrees to the right and then rapidly turned to the midline, testing the left horizontal canal function. The top row demonstrates the normal response, with the ability to maintain gaze on target after rapid head turn. The bottom row displays an abnormal test of the right horizontal canal with initial slippage of gaze with the head turn to the left, and then late refixation back to the initial target gaze.

Dynamic Visual Acuity Test

The dynamic visual acuity test assesses degradation of the VOR by examining the change in visual acuity with head movement. The acuity of the patient is first tested with the head still using a Snellen eye chart. Then the head is moved back and forth in the horizontal plane at 90 to 120 degrees per second at 2 Hz. The frequency must be greater than 1 cycle/second, as the smooth pursuit system can maintain fixation up to this frequency. In normal individuals visual acuity usually remains within two lines on the Snellen chart. Unilateral vestibular loss that is poorly compensated or bilateral dysfunction may cause three or more lines of loss.

Post–Head-Shake Nystagmus

Velocity storage refers to "charging" of the central vestibular system during a period of vestibular activation. Once the activation ceases, the central vestibular system then discharges over 5 to 20 seconds. In the case of unilateral vestibular loss, following symmetric stimuli to the peripheral vestibular system, increased peripheral input occurs on the side with the stronger vestibular system compared to the lesioned side, and then subsequently asymmetric discharge of this velocity storage ensues, which results in nystagmus toward the intact side.[11]

Post–head-shake nystagmus tests this phenomenon by having the examiner shake the patient's head in the horizontal plane at 2 Hz for 20 to 30 seconds. The head is then abruptly stopped. If asymmetry is present in the system, nystagmus will occur with the fast phase beating toward the intact ear. Symmetric function, whether it is normal or bilaterally reduced, will not display nystagmus. Frenzel lenses increase the sensitivity of the exam by inhibiting the patient's ability to fixate to suppress the nystagmus.

Vibration-Induced Nystagmus

Vibration of both the neck and skull has been shown to cause nystagmus in cases of unilateral vestibular loss. A high-frequency vibrator (50–100 Hz) is placed over either the mastoid or the sternocleidomastoid muscle. A positive response typically beats in the same direction regardless of whether the stimulus is on the right or left, with the fast phase directed toward the intact ear. Torsional/vertical nystagmus in the direction of the superior semicircular canal has been described in cases of superior semicircular canal dehiscence.[12] Frenzel lenses should be worn during this test.

Hyperventilation-Induced Nystagmus

Dizziness associated with hyperventilation was historically only associated with psychogenic causes. However, deep and vigorous breathing that produces transient hypocarbia has been shown to cause nystagmus in patients with multiple sclerosis and lesions of cranial nerve VIII. Nystagmus has recently been described following stereotactic radiosurgery of an acoustic neuroma.[13] Frenzel lenses should be worn while the patient vigorously breathes in for 20 to 30 seconds. The nystagmus may be "irritative" (fast phase toward the diseased ear) or destructive (fast phase toward the intact ear).

14.4.3 Positioning/Positional Tests

Dynamic Positioning Tests

The Dix-Hallpike test is the most commonly employed positioning test for nystagmus.[14] Posterior canal BPPV, which accounts for 90% of BPPV, and likely most horizontal BPPV, results from canalithiasis, where free-floating otolithic debris exists in a semicircular canal. Maneuvering of the head in the plane of the posterior semicircular canal in this test triggers nystagmus and vertigo in patients by inducing movement of the debris. To examine the right ear (▶ Fig. 14.2), the test is performed by having the patient sit with his or her head turned 45 degrees to the right. The patient is rapidly brought down into the supine position with the head to the right and slight extension of the neck. A positive test for posterior BPPV is indicated by upbeat torsional geotropic nystagmus with the affected ear down. Positioning nystagmus usually has a latency of 10 to 15 seconds, a short duration of less than a minute, and fatigues with repeated maneuvers. The patient often will have symptoms when he or she is brought back to a sitting position, and a reversal of the nystagmus is sometimes seen. The same maneuvering is then performed for the left side. Often the nystagmus is brisk and detectable without Frenzel lenses. If a purely horizontal nystagmus is seen during this maneuver, horizontal canal BPPV is suspected and a supine roll test can be performed by placing the patient in the supine position and turning the head 90 degrees to the right.

Two different variants of nystagmus have been described for horizontal canal BPPV.[15] The first is geotropic horizontal nystagmus, which appears stronger with the affected ear down and is thought to be caused by otoconial movement in the non-ampullated side of the canal moving toward the ampulla. The second variant is ageotropic horizontal nystagmus, which is thought to be triggered by debris in the ampullated end of the canal moving away from the ampulla. In such cases, the nystagmus is weaker with the involved ear down. It should be noted that during liberation maneuvers for the treatment of BPPV, a "canal switch" can occur as debris settles unintentionally in another semicircular canal, leading to symptoms and nystagmus suggestive of BPPV in the new canal. Canal switch most commonly occurs with debris moving from the posterior canal to the horizontal canal.

Static Positional Testing

Nystagmus should be evaluated during various static head positions. This is commonly performed by having the patient lie supine with Frenzel lenses. The head starts in a neutral position. The head then is turned laterally to the right for 10 to 30 seconds and the eyes are observed for nystagmus. The head is returned to the midline and then tested on the left. Both central and peripheral causes for vertigo may trigger static positional nystagmus. Central nystagmus often will have very short or no latency, will be persistent in duration, will be direction changing, and vertical.

14.4.4 Limb Tests

Limb tests are designed to examine the function of the peripheral and central nervous system. Some of these tests specifically

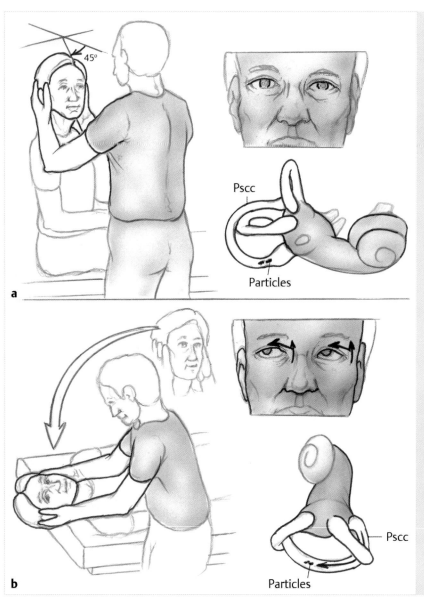

Fig. 14.2 The Dix-Hallpike test. To test for right posterior benign paroxysmal positional vertigo, the patient is placed in a sitting position with the head turned 45 degrees to the right (a). The patient is then rapidly placed in a supine position (b). This positioning allows for alignment of the posterior canal such that debris within the canal moves in an ampullopetal direction, causing geotropic eye movement toward the down (right) ear.

examine the cerebellum, which acts to integrate and modulate both afferent and efferent systems. The flocculonodular lobe within the cerebellum interacts and regulates the vestibular system. Disorders arising in the cerebellum often cause inaccurate function. Motor function manifests with dysmetria and ataxic gait, and speech loses fluidity. Upper extremity cerebellar testing can be examined by having the patient touch an examiner's finger placed several feet away. Over- or undershoot may be seen and is a form of dysmetria. An intention tremor, which is increased jerky movements with intended motion, may also be seen. A similar test asks a patient to touch an examiner's finger that is several feet away with his or her eyes open. Then the task is repeated with the patient's eyes closed. Significant drift can be seen with cerebellar or brainstem lesions. Rapid alternating motion can also be disturbed by cerebellar injury, and is termed dysdiadochokinesia. Foot tapping and rapid alternation of outstretched hands from prone to supine tests rapid alternating movement. Lower extremity movements can be tested as well, most commonly by having the heel of one foot slide along the shin of the opposite leg. Excessive to-and-fro motion suggests a positive test. Limb strength and motion should be examined. The somatosensory system can be assessed by applying a 128-kHz tuning fork on the limbs and having the patient report whether or not he or she feels the vibration.

14.4.5 Tests of Posture and Gait

Posture Tests

The Romberg test is the most commonly examined posture test. It tests primarily the effect of proprioception on static posture control. The patient is asked to stand with his or her eyes open and feet together with arms either folded or at the side. Balance is assessed first with eyes open and then closed. The sharpened or tandem Romberg is performed with feet in the tandem position, and may be more sensitive for detection of patients with vestibular dysfunction. The Quix test operates on a similar principle, only the arms are outstretched anteriorly during the test.

These postural tests can also be tested on 4-inch foam, which decreases somatosensory feedback from the support surface and prompts the patient to rely more on vestibular input for balance. Patients with uncompensated vestibular injury will sway more with the addition of foam. Fall strategies should be examined as the patient sways. Ankle strategies are appropriate on hard surfaces, but hip strategies are often needed on foam. Usage of an ankle strategy on foam suggests incorrect usage of strategy and can be seen in vestibular loss or dysfunction. The Fukuda step is a specialized posture exam that has the patient march in place with eyes closed and arms extended anteriorly for 30 seconds. In patients with vestibular loss, the patient may deviate toward the side of the loss.[16]

Gait Tests

Simple gait can be examined by watching the patient walk. This can often be observed as the patient moves to the examination room. Gait should be assessed if generally appearing normal or not. Abnormal gait can be wide based and ataxic, suggesting cerebellar dysfunction or shuffling and hesitant as seen in Parkinson disease. Patients may list to one side, which suggests vestibular imbalance. Musculoskeletal abnormalities are ubiquitous and can change gait and should be considered in patients in whom abnormal gait is a confounding factor. Tandem stance and gait (walking heel to toe) should also be examined. Inability to perform this task with eyes open may suggest vestibular, cerebellar, or musculoskeletal dysfunction. Failure to maintain tandem stance with eyes closed may indicate a vestibular problem.

14.5 Central versus Peripheral Findings on Physical Exam

▶ Table 14.1 outlines the typical examination findings that distinguish peripheral from central causes of dizziness and imbalance. In general, patients with peripheral vestibular disease describe stereotypical vertigo attacks of a certain character and duration consistent with the disease process. Signs of peripheral disease include direction-fixed spontaneous nystagmus, which suppresses with fixation; a positive head impulse sign; post–head-shake nystagmus; and a positive Dix-Hallpike test with normal ocular motility and central oculomotor function. Conversely, central disease may include impaired ocular alignment and motility, direction-changing nystagmus, and atypical responses to position testing.

Table 14.1 Central Versus Peripheral Findings of the Physical Exam

	Peripheral Vestibular Disease	Central Nervous System Disease
Spontaneous nystagmus	Horizontal/rotary	Vertical or horizontal
	Direction-fixed	Direction-changing
	Fixation suppression	No fixation suppression
Gaze nystagmus	Horizontal/rotary	Vertical or horizontal
	Direction fixed	Direction-changing
Smooth pursuit	No abnormalities	Saccadic pursuit
Saccades	No abnormalities	Disconjugate: medial longitudinal fasciculus (MLF) lesion
		Inaccurate: cerebellar lesion
		Slow: brainstem lesion
Fixation suppression of rotary nystagmus	No nystagmus with fixation	Nystagmus despite attempted fixation
Head impulse test	Saccadic refixation with movement toward lesioned side	No abnormalities
		Variable
Post–head-shake nystagmus	Horizontal/rotary nystagmus toward intact side (most common)	Variable
Dynamic visual acuity	>3 line reduction in acuity	Variable
Hyperventilation	Horizontal/rotary nystagmus	Pure horizontal, vertical or torsional nystagmus
Positional testing	No nystagmus	Pure horizontal, vertical or torsional nystagmus
Positioning testing	Upbeat geotropic torsional posterior semicircular canal (SCC) or horizontal (lateral SCC) nystagmus	Incoordination, dysmetria
Limb coordination	No abnormalities	Severe increase in sway with eyes closed
Romberg	Slight increase sway with eyes closed	Variable
4"-foam test	Increased sway, falls eyes closed	Ataxic, incoordinated gait
Gait	Deviation toward lesioned side	Delayed initiation of movement

14.6 Conclusion

Thorough evaluation of the dizzy patient requires a detailed gathering of the history and a systematic examination. The nature and timing of the dizziness are often the most important factors in deciding the cause and designing an effective treatment plan. In similar fashion, the presence of signs of peripheral dysfunction in the absence of brainstem symptoms and signs guides the examiner with regard to treatment or further audiovestibular or radiological testing prior to therapy.

References

[1] Tusa RJ. Dizziness. Med Clin North Am 2009; 93: 263–271, viivii.

[2] Zhao JG, Piccirillo JF, Spitznagel EL, Jr, Kallogjeri D, Goebel JA. Predictive capability of historical data for diagnosis of dizziness. Otol Neurotol 2011; 32: 284–290

[3] Baloh RW. Approach to the evaluation of the dizzy patient. Otolaryngol Head Neck Surg 1995; 112: 3–7

[4] Neuhauser H, Lempert T. Vestibular migraine. Neurol Clin 2009; 27: 379–391

[5] Committee on Hearing and Equilibrium guidelines for the diagnosis and evaluation of therapy in Menière's disease. American Academy of Otolaryngology-Head and Neck Foundation, Inc. Otolaryngol Head Neck Surg 1995; 113: 181–185

[6] Lempert T, Neuhauser H, Daroff RB. Vertigo as a symptom of migraine. Ann N Y Acad Sci 2009; 1164: 242–251

[7] Lempert T, Neuhauser H. Migrainous vertigo. Neurol Clin 2005; 23: 715–730, vivi.

[8] Ewald JR. Physiologische Untersuchungen uber das Endorgan des Nervus Octavus. Wiesbaden, Germany: Bergmann, 1982

[9] Jeffcoat B, Shelukhin A, Fong A, Mustain W, Zhou W. Alexander's law revisited. J Neurophysiol 2008; 100: 154–159

[10] Halmagyi GM, Curthoys IS. A clinical sign of canal paresis. Arch Neurol 1988; 45: 737–739

[11] Hain TC, Fetter M, Zee DS. Head-shaking nystagmus in patients with unilateral peripheral vestibular lesions. Am J Otolaryngol 1987; 8: 36–47

[12] White JA, Hughes GB, Ruggieri PN. Vibration-induced nystagmus as an office procedure for the diagnosis of superior semicircular canal dehiscence. Otol Neurotol 2007; 28: 911–916

[13] Bradley JP, Hullar TE, Neely JG, Goebel JA. Hyperventilation-induced nystagmus and vertigo after stereotactic radiotherapy for vestibular schwannoma. Otol Neurotol 2011; 32: 1336–1338

[14] Dix MR, Hallpike CS. The pathology, symptomatology and diagnosis of certain common disorders of the vestibular system. Ann Otol Rhinol Laryngol 1952; 61: 987–1016

[15] Steddin S, Ing D, Brandt T. Horizontal canal benign paroxysmal positioning vertigo (h-BPPV): transition of canalolithiasis to cupulolithiasis. Ann Neurol 1996; 40: 918–922

[16] Fukuda T. The stepping test: two phases of the labyrinthine reflex. Acta Otolaryngol 1959; 50: 95–108

[17] The International Classification of Headache Disorders, 2nd ed. Cephalalgia 2004;24(Suppl 1):9–160

Part 3

Management

15 Disorders of the Auricle

Nael M. Shoman

15.1 Introduction

Clinical disorders involving the auricle span a broad spectrum of congenital and acquired conditions, and may be isolated to the external ear or part of a generalized condition involving other organ systems. The embryology of the external ear development is a fascinating journey of complex interactions, and can result in a myriad of clinical presentations including preauricular pits and tags, as well as the spectrum of microtia with or without aural atresia. These congenital conditions may have various implications, including functional and cosmetic sequelae. Many infectious disorders may involve the auricle, either primarily, for example following ear piercing, or secondarily, from adjacent infections of the external auditory canal. The unique structure and location of the auricle expose it to various etiologic risk factors not commonly encountered in other body organs. Its prominence increases the relative sun exposure it receives, and the ear is one of the most common sites of skin cancer. This prominent location and physiology also makes the ear susceptible to traumatic and thermal pathologies. The ears can also be part of various systemic manifestations of underlying autoimmune and metabolic conditions.

15.2 Bacterial Infections

The auricle may be subject to the same skin and soft tissue infectious pathologies encountered elsewhere in the body. Furthermore, its cartilaginous framework, and tightly adherent overlying thin skin facilitates the extension of infection to the perichondrial layer and underlying cartilage.

Impetigo is the most common skin infection in children throughout the world. It presents as superficial, nonfollicular pustules that are mostly caused by *Staphylococcus aureus* or β-hemolytic streptococci. Folliculitis is an infection of the hair follicle, frequently caused by *S. aureus*, whereby inflammation is limited to the superficial layer with suppuration present in the epidermis. Furuncles are deeper follicular infections extending to the deep dermis, where a small abscess develops. The term *cellulitis* is often used to encompass a spectrum of soft tissue infections, from erysipelas to the more severe infectious forms including tissue necrosis. Erysipelas is an acute, superficial, nonnecrotizing infection involving the dermis and hypodermis. It is often of sudden onset, and is sharply demarcated by a shiny erythematous plaque. Cellulitis, on the other hand, is often defined as a deeper infection that involves the subcutaneous tissues.

15.2.1 Impetigo

Impetigo is a common skin infection, accounting for 50 to 60% of all bacterial skin infections.[1] It is a superficial vesiculopustular skin infection occurring mostly on exposed areas of the face and extremities, and usually arises at the site of a minor skin break such as a skin bite or abrasion. Patients typically have no associated systemic symptoms.

Impetigo is a common skin infection throughout the world and occurs most frequently among economically disadvantaged children in tropical or subtropical regions, but it is also quite frequent in northern climates during the summer months.[2] The annular incidence of impetigo is reported at around 0.01 events per person-year.[3-5] The incidence is highest in children under 5 years, followed by that for children 5 to 14 years, affecting boys and girls equally. The incidence drops thereafter and is least common in the elderly (65 years and older).[4] Epidemics have been identified that always started during summer.[5]

Impetigo is nearly always caused by β-hemolytic streptococci or *S. aureus*. The lesions can be bullous or nonbullous. Whereas, in the past, nonbullous lesions were usually caused by streptococci, most cases are now caused by staphylococci, either alone or in combination with streptococci.[2] *S. aureus* accounts for about 80% of cultured swabs,[5] and streptococci isolated from lesions are primarily group A organisms. Bullous impetigo is caused by strains of *S. aureus* that produce exfoliative toxins that cause the loss of keratinocyte cell-to-cell adhesion, resulting in cleavage in the superficial epidermis. Methicillin-resistant *S. aureus* (MRSA) is a major nosocomial pathogen that may also cause impetigo, and its incidence may be on the rise.

Impetigo involving the auricle typically arises as an extension from an ear canal infection. The organisms are usually carried there by instruments or fingers to relieve an itch or clean the ear canal of wax, and enter through small abrasions. Impetigo can also result as a secondary infection associated with a primary skin condition, such as atopic dermatitis, with staphylococcal colonization. The lesions develop into small vesicles or pustules that expand into thin walled blisters, which often erupt to express straw colored fluid, and leave honey or brown-sugar colored crusts. Although the crusts are friable, they have an adherent quality that gives them the appearance of "stuck on cornflakes."[6] The crusts eventually exfoliate and leave an erythematous base behind. Although hyperpigmentation can occur following an infection on pigmented skin, this is usually self-limited and resolves over time. The blisters are rarely painful, although they can be sore and itchy. The episode usually lasts between 2 and 4 weeks.

Systemic antibiotics do not appear to be helpful in treating local impetigo. In 2004, a Cochrane review of interventions for impetigo concluded that topical antibiotics showed better cure rates than placebo, and that topical and oral antibiotics did not show different cure rates, nor did most trials comparing oral antibiotics. Although there is no consensus on the best management approach for auricular impetigo, topical mupirocin and fusidic acid are considerably better than other agents such as bacitracin and neomycin. Patients who have numerous lesions or who are not responding to topical agents should receive oral antimicrobials effective against both *S. aureus* and *S. pyogenes*, such as cephalexin, newer macrolides (instead of erythromycin), and amoxicillin/clavulanic acid. It has been demonstrated that simple local care (including cleansing with soap and water, and removal of crusts and wet dressings) is useful for treating impetigo,[7] and that handwashing with daily bathing also prevents impetigo in children.[8]

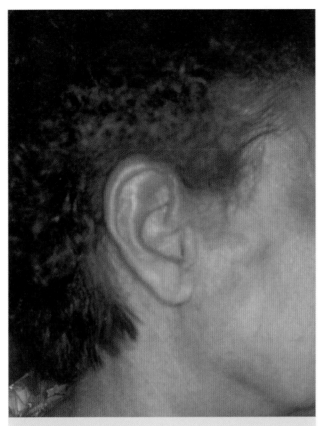

Fig. 15.1 Erysipelas auricle.

Glomerulonephritis following streptococcal infection may be a complication of impetigo caused by certain strains of *S. pyogenes*, but is quite rare in developed countries (less than one case per 1,000,000 population per year); to date, there are no data demonstrating that treatment of impetigo prevents this severe complication.[9,10]

15.2.2 Erysipelas

Erysipelas is a characteristic form of cellulitis that affects the superficial epidermis, producing marked swelling. The erysipelas skin lesion has a raised border, which is sharply demarcated from normal skin, differentiating that from cellulitis (▶ Fig. 15.1).

Erysipelas affects predominantly adult patients in the sixth or seventh decade. It uncommonly involves the auricle, with lower limb involvement in 80% of the cases.[2] Predisposing factors for auricular involvement are extrapolated from data of erysipelas and cellulitis of the lower limb, which mostly include locoregional factors (disruption of the cutaneous barrier, such as local wound and ulceration), as well as local surgical procedures. Edema is a risk factor for cellulitis/erysipelas,[11] as well as a consequence of the disease.[12]

Erysipelas is most commonly caused by β-hemolytic streptococci of group A, less so by group B, C, or G streptococci, and rarely by staphylococci.[10,13,14] Bulla formation is a frequent late local complication of the disease. Although most cases of erysipelas are caused by β-hemolytic streptococci, many other bacteria can produce nonnecrotizing cellulitis. For example, a cat bite or dog bite to the auricle can result in erysipelas secondary to *Pasteurella*. Likewise, *Aeromonas* hydrophila may follow exposure to freshwater, and *Vibrio* species after saltwater exposure.[2]

The infection typically follows a break in the auricular skin, as with trauma, lacerations, bites, or rarely following surgery. The onset is abrupt, and the skin is painful, edematous, intensely erythematous, and indurated. There is usually accompanying fever, systemic toxicity, and chills. The infection may then spread anteriorly from the auricle to involve the face with no specific progression pattern, disrespecting boundaries. Preexisting skin ulcers or eczematous lesions may predispose to this infection.

Erysipelas is treated with an antibiotic active against streptococci. Penicillin, given either parenterally or orally depending on clinical severity, is the treatment of choice.[10,13] Patients with mild to moderate erysipelas without severe systemic signs can be treated orally by amoxicillin (3.0 to 4.5 g daily) for 10 to 14 days, usually as outpatients.[13] Clindamycin (300 mg t.i.d.) may also be used orally in penicillin-allergic patients.[10] Patients with more severe infections usually require hospital admission and intravenous antibiotics, including parenteral penicillin G, amoxicillin, or cefazolin. Patients can then be switched to oral amoxicillin once the infection is better controlled.

15.2.3 Perichondritis

Generally speaking, inflammation of the auricular perichondrial and cartilaginous layers may be categorized as infectious, or suppurative perichondritis, and noninfectious, termed relapsing polychondritis (discussed in the next section). Suppurative perichondritis of the auricle is a complication of the traumatized ear, whether blunt or penetrating (▶ Fig. 15.2). Although the term *perichondritis* implies involvement of only the perichondrial layer, this is a misnomer as the cartilage is almost always involved to a variable extent. This involvement can be limited to a small area in uncomplicated cases, or the entire cartilaginous framework may be involved in more significant injuries, such as with burns (▶ Fig. 15.3).[15,16]

Common traumatic etiologies can be penetrating or nonpenetrating. Penetrating etiologies include ear scratching, insect bites, and piercings. Perichondritis may also arise subsequent to zoster infection of the auricle, and has also been described following ear surgery.[17–20] Nonpenetrating etiologies usually result in a hematoma formation between the cartilage and perichondrial layer, which may then secondarily become infected. This is the commonest form of perichondritis. This blunt trauma may be localized, as with an ill-fitting hearing device, or more generalized, as with a punch to the ear. These observations suggest that direct damage to the cartilage is not likely mandatory for the initiation of perichondritis. The tight adhesion of the perichondrial layer to the underlying cartilage suggests that minimal trauma or inflammation to the auricular skin may cause the cartilage to secondarily become infected.

As with otitis externa, the most common microbiological agent implicated in perichondritis is thought to be *Pseudomonas aeruginosa*.[15] This organism is ubiquitous, with an affinity for moist environments. It may thus be found in the eternal auditory canal and then be introduced through a break in the skin to subsequently involve the cartilaginous layer. The organ-

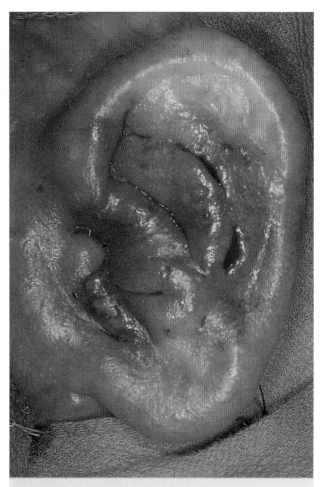

Fig. 15.2 Perichondritis auricle.

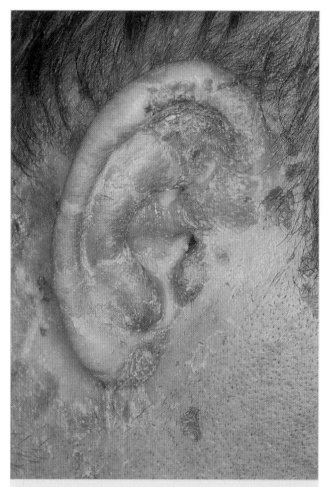

Fig. 15.3 Burn pinna.

ism may be introduced following exposure to lakes or swimming pools, moisturized solid soap, and contaminated disinfectants.[21,22] The organism possesses high invasive capacity and virulence factors.[23] The infection may start with superficial skin colonization before quick progression to deeper layers. This organism appears to have a special affinity for traumatized cartilage.[24] It may subsequently extend beyond the cartilage to involve the soft tissues surrounding the auricle and external auditory canal, the condition clinically termed malignant external otitis. Other organisms commonly implicated in perichondritis include *Proteus* species,[18] *S. aureus*,[15] and *Escherichia coli*.[25]

Perichondritis has an insidious onset. It initially presents as a dull ache that progressively worsens over the course of days, with an average time from symptoms to treatment of 3 days.[22] With disease progression, there is usually associated erythema, edema, and warmth. Cutaneous involvement typically may start in the ear canal if the primary infection is that of otitis externa, with subsequent spread to the auricle. Alternatively, the infection may start in the skin of the auricle, typically first involving the helix and antihelix. Cutaneous extension may then spread beyond the ear to involve the pre- or postauricular regions. As the auricular infection progresses, an abscess may develop between the perichondrial layer and the underlying cartilage. This may result in cartilaginous necrosis and secondary deformity with irreversible sequelae if the abscess is not quickly drained.

In reviewing 61 patients with perichondritis, Prasad et al[24] proposed a two-group clinical classification system based on disease severity, and they have found that this system correlated with patient prognosis. Group A comprised patients with perichondritis of the auricle without malignant otitis externa. Within this group, stage one denoted early perichondritis without an abscess; stage two, perichondritis with an abscess but no cartilage destruction; and stage three, perichondritis with an abscess and cartilage destruction. Group B comprised patients with perichondritis secondary to malignant otitis externa, with or without osteomyelitis of the temporal bone.

It is debatable whether patients with perichondritis should be treated as outpatients or admitted for intravenous antibiotics. If the disease presents in its early stages, with mild erythema and tenderness only, then initiation of an antibiotic with antipseudomonal properties, such as an oral fluoroquinolone, with close clinical follow-up, is reasonable. The concern with this management approach is the possibility of development of resistance of *Pseudomonas* to fluoroquinolones, which are currently the only oral antibiotics with antipseudomonal coverage. In certain clinical setting, such as perichondritis secondary to an animal or human bite, antibiotic choice must include coverage for likely causative organisms, such as *Pasteurella*, with consideration of rabies or tetanus coverage. More severe clinical signs at presentation, such as an elevated white cell count, fever,

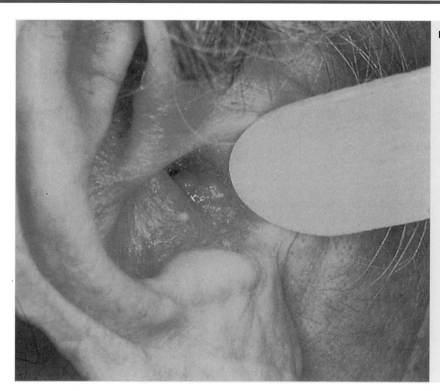

Fig. 15.4 Herpes zoster.

or the presence of an immunosuppressed state or diabetes, warrant intravenous treatment, and this can be undertaken in an outpatient setting or through hospital admission. If an abscess is present, then incision and drainage is undertaken, typically under local anesthetic and using aseptic technique. A swab is taken for culture and sensitivity. The cartilage is then inspected and, if not involved, then the wound is left open and a pressure dressing is applied. In cases of cartilage necrosis, devitalized cartilage is debrided back to healthy tissue. The wound is then left open and a firm pressure dressing applied. If the abscess recurs, then the procedure is repeated. Management of perichondritis secondary to malignant otitis externa follows a similar approach, with the treatment algorithm focused on wound debridement as well as possibly more extensive surgical intervention, as discussed in Chapter 16.

15.3 Viral Infection: Herpes Zoster Oticus (Ramsay Hunt Syndrome)

In 1907 James Ramsay Hunt postulated that the combination of herpes zoster oticus and facial paralysis results from the reactivation of latent varicella zoster virus (VZV) in the geniculate ganglion. Recent evidence adds merit to this hypothesis. Using polymerase chain reaction (PCR), VZV DNA was found in the ipsilateral geniculate ganglion,[26] facial nerve sheath,[27] and in the spiral and vestibular ganglion[28] of patients with facial paralysis associated with herpes zoster oticus.

It is postulated that in the acute infectious stage of VZV, the virus localizes in the skin, resulting in a vesicular eruption. Viral multiplication is profuse in the epithelial stage. This primary infection is varicella (chickenpox), which is common and extremely contagious. Viral multiplication extends to the free nerve endings in the deeper layers of the stratum basale.

Subsequently, the viral particles travel in a retrograde fashion to the neuronal cell bodies of the sensory ganglion. Within this structure, nonneuronal cells are infected and viral reproduction then halts, transforming the viral particles into a state of latency.[29] The latent presence of VZV in sensory ganglia has been demonstrated by the use of PCR, and the reactivation of the virus in herpes zoster oticus (HZO) is suggested by multiple factors, including the simultaneous cutaneous eruption, intense contrast enhancement on magnetic resonance imaging (MRI) in the area of the geniculate ganglion during the acute phase,[30] histopathological studies demonstrating an inflammatory infiltrate around the involved geniculate ganglion,[31] and by seroconversion.[32]

The annual incidence of HZO is estimated to be 1.5 to 4 cases per 1,000 persons,[33,34] and the estimated incidence of HZO is 5 cases per 100,000.[35] HZO is the second most common cause of atraumatic peripheral facial paralysis, with an estimated incidence of about 3 to 20%.[32,36,37] This variable range is reflective of a few factors, including the clinical definition of HZO (for example, with or without vesicles), patients' age distribution, and the presence or absence of vestibulocochlear dysfunction. The condition appears to be more common in women,[32] although this finding was not consistent.[37] It is also more common in those over the age of 60 years. The incidence is higher in children 6 years of age or older than in children younger than 6. In one study, the appearance of vesicles was delayed in children compared with adults.[37]

Herpes zoster oticus is commonly characterized by a viral prodrome, such as an upper respiratory tract infection, followed by ipsilateral otalgia, which can be severe. Facial nerve paralysis may then ensue, and vesicles over the external ear canal, auricle, preauricular skin, or face may subsequently develop up to 2 weeks after the onset of facial palsy (▶ Fig. 15.4).[38] The distribution of vesicles follows a dermatomal pattern that depends on the sensory afferent fibers involved, and may extend to the face and neck down as far as the shoulder and also may appear on the tongue, palate, or buccal mucosa. In a study of the first presenting symptoms in 101 patients with HZO, 54.5% had pain, 22.8% had facial paralysis, and 2% had vesicles.[39] The degree of facial nerve paralysis is variable, with approximately half of the patients having complete paralysis on presentation.[39] In a study of 102 patients with untreated HZO, investigators found that maximal loss of facial function was complete within 1 week, and that complete paralysis occurred more often in patients older than 50.[36] Patients may also have unilateral sensorineural hearing loss, evident in about 50% of patients with HZO.[36,37] Other clinical symptoms include tinnitus in about 25%, and vertigo with nausea and vomiting in about 30%. About 3% of adult patients also show glossopharyngeal and vagal symptoms.

Multiple reports have studied the utility of MRI scan in the early evaluation of patients with HZO. Enhancement of the facial nerve on MRI scanning was found in the majority of patients with facial palsy (57 to 100%).[40] A few of these studies suggested that the degree or the anatomic level of the facial nerve enhancement had prognostic significance,[41–43] but this has not been consistently observed. None of the studies found any significant differences between Bell's palsy and HZO in the degree of facial nerve enhancement. It has also been noted that in patients with HZO with accompanying cochleovestibular symptoms such as vertigo and tinnitus, enhancement was also seen in the vestibular and cochlear nerves.[44] A lag between resolution of facial nerve enhancement on MRI and recovery of facial nerve function has been observed,[40,45] and the significance of this with regard to prognosis is unclear.

Lack of nerve excitability, complete paralysis, and age over 50 were found to be statistically significant factors for a poor prognosis of facial nerve recovery.[36] In patients with partial clinical or electrophysiological function at onset, about 66% show complete facial nerve recovery, compared to about only 10% of patients with complete loss at onset. Increasing clinical severity predicts the development of synkinesis; this occurs in 60 to 70% of patients with complete facial paralysis, and in 10 to 15% of patients with incomplete paralysis. Overall, complete recovery occurs in about 50% of adults and in about 75% of children younger than 16. In a large series of patients with HZO retrospectively reviewed, serial audiograms showed complete recovery in 66% of children and in 37.7% of adults.

Uscategui et al[46] published a Cochrane review of randomized controlled trials in which antiviral agents alone or in combination with other therapies were given in HZO. Based on only one identified prospective study using steroids and antiviral drugs, the authors concluded that antiviral agents had no beneficial effect on outcomes in HZO. This negative result was nevertheless based on one small, statistically underpowered study, and as such does not necessarily indicate that antivirals are ineffective. There are numerous recommendations in the literature regarding the use of steroids and antivirals, but none of these have been tested by randomized placebo-controlled trials. In a recent retrospective study of 101 patients with HZO, those who received a combination of antivirals and steroids recovered significantly more than those who had only one or no pharmacological treatment.[39] In a retrospective review of 80 patients with HZO, there was a statistically significant improvement in facial nerve recovery in patients treated with

prednisone and acyclovir within 3 days of onset. All patients were treated with oral prednisone (1 mg/kg/day for 5 days followed by a 10-day taper), as well as with intravenous acyclovir (250 mg t.i.d.), or oral acyclovir (800 mg five times daily). Complete recovery was seen in 21 patients (75%) treated within the first 3 days ($p < 0.05$), 14 patients (48%) treated at 4 to 7 days, and seven patients (30%) treated after 7 days. Moreover, 26 patients (50%) who were not treated in the first 3 days progressed to a complete loss of response to facial nerve stimulation.

Facial nerve decompression surgery for facial palsy in patients with Bell's palsy and HZO remains controversial. The surgical premise is that axonal ischemia follows as an inflamed facial nerve expands in narrow portions of its intraosseous route, although this has been challenged by some histopathological studies.[47] Most surgical series have been small and retrospective, with a selection bias toward patients with complete palsies and severely deficient axonal function on electrophysiological testing, and none have been randomized. Although some studies showed no benefit,[48–50] Gantz and colleagues[51] employed a middle fossa approach, reporting positive outcomes with complete or almost complete recovery in 91% of patients if operated on within 21 days of onset, compared to only 42% of a similar, medically treated group.

In all patients, eye protection from corneal abrasion and drying is essential during periods of moderate to severe facial paresis with incomplete eye closure. These measures include eye moistening during the day with artificial tears, and the use of an eye lubricant with the eye taped shut overnight. In severe facial palsy, lubrication and occlusion may not be sufficient to protect the cornea, and tarsorrhaphy may then be undertaken to narrow the palpebral fissure. Implanting a gold weight in the upper lid to help with ptosis may augment lid suturing. In cases of incomplete facial nerve recovery, various static and dynamic facial reanimation procedures have been employed.[52] These include grafting an area of damaged nerve with a transposed nerve, bridging fibers from the contralateral facial nerve across the midline to innervate the paralyzed side, and anastomosing the ipsilateral hypoglossal nerve with the damaged nerve. Nerve grafting often involves a muscle transfer procedures, as the ipsilateral paralyzed muscles may atrophy and thus not respond to reinnervation. In cases of partial recover with hemifacial spasm, tonic facial contraction, synkinesis, or "crocodile tear" syndrome, a series of subcutaneous or intramuscular botulinum toxin injections can induce temporary paresis with an improvement of these symptoms.[53–55]

15.4 Inflammatory Conditions

15.4.1 Keloids

Keloids are dermal fibrotic lesions, included in the spectrum of fibroproliferative disorders (▶ Fig. 15.5). The lesions are considered as manifestations of aberrant wound healing resulting in excessive disorganized collagen deposition, forming persistent firm nodules and plaques. Unlike hyperplastic scars, keloids extend beyond the margin of the initiating trauma. The cytokine profile of keloidal fibroblasts differs from normal fibroblasts, with high levels of transforming growth factor-β_1 and -β_2, vascular endothelial growth factor, connective tissue growth factor,

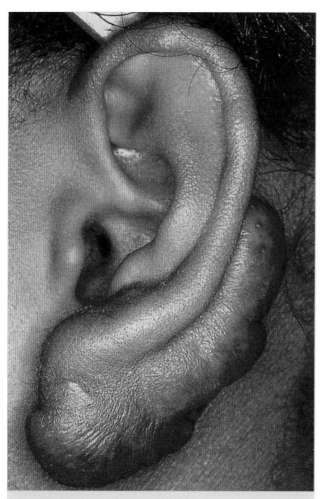

Fig. 15.5 Keloid.

no single established treatment protocol. High recurrence rates have plagued keloid management, and this has been frustrating for patients and treating physicians alike. In general, surgical excision followed by adjuvant therapy is considered the optimal treatment regimen. Surgical excision alone results in recurrence rates of nearly 80%.[63] Various treatment options, either as single modality or in combination, have been described in the literature. These include intralesional corticosteroids injections,[64,65] intralesional 5-fluorouracil (5-FU),[66,67] topical mitomycin-C,[68] bleomycin,[69] silicone compressive therapy,[70] skin grafting,[71] radiotherapy,[72,73] laser therapy,[74–76] cryotherapy,[77] and banding.[78] Variable recurrence rates have been reported with these modalities, but most studies have been limited by smaller numbers, or variable follow-up periods. It is also important to counsel patients regarding potential side effects with these modalities. Radiation may result in hyperpigmentation and telangiectasia. There are also potential side effects from irradiated tissue in the field, including the ear canal, middle and inner ear, and parotid gland. The risk of malignancy is difficult to substantiate in the long term. Local 5-FU or bleomycin injections may also carry a theoretical malignancy transformation risk. In 2007, Mofikoya and colleagues[79] reviewed management modalities published at the time, and concluded that there is no single, reliable, and effective treatment protocol. Instead, they recommended surgical excision followed by postoperative intralesional steroid injection as a reasonable approach with low recurrence rates. The surgical approach is dictated by the size and shape of the keloid. Park and colleagues[80] classified earlobe keloids into five groups, broadly based on whether they are sessile or pedunculated. The proposed surgical approaches followed this classification, spanning from simple core extirpation, to keloidectomy with an elliptical incision, to wedge resection.

15.4.2 Relapsing Polychondritis

Relapsing polychondritis is a rare multisystemic inflammatory disease of unknown etiology. It is presumed to be of autoimmune origin targeting hyaline and elastic cartilage, including the nose, ears, joints, and respiratory tract. It can also affect other proteoglycan-rich structures, such as the eyes, heart, blood vessels, and inner ear (▶ Fig. 15.6).[81]

Relapsing polychondritis usually manifests between the ages of 40 and 60 years, with the average age between 44 and 51 years,[82] but children can also be affected.[83] There does not appear to be a gender predilection.[81,84–86] Relapsing polychondritis can occur in all racial and ethnic groups, with whites being affected predominantly.[82]

Although the etiology of relapsing polychondritis remains unknown, culminating evidence points toward an immunologically mediated pathogenesis. Serum taken from patients with relapsing polychondritis during an acute exacerbation was found to have antibodies against collagen II, IX, and XI.[87,88] In animal models, immunization with type II collagen antibodies induced the development of arthritis and chondritis that is histologically similar to relapsing polychondritis in humans.[89] Cell-mediated immune response was documented in patients with relapsing polychondritis.[90] Likewise, other studies have demonstrated immune responses in affected cartilage, including infiltration by plasma cells, lymphocytes

platelet-derived growth factor-α, and interleukin-6 and -8.[56–58] Keloidal fibroblasts have been shown to have abnormal levels of matrix metalloproteinases and collagen, resulting in an imbalance of normal wound healing.[58] Recent studies have shown that overlying epidermal keratinocytes interact with dermal keloidal fibroblasts, and this may subsequently result in keloid formation.[57]

Keloids commonly affect the ears. They are thought to be a product of an inflammatory response that ensues from infection, excessive wound tension, or foreign material. They may thus follow small skin excisions, drainage of auricular hematomas, repair of auricular traumas, viral infection such as herpes varicella zoster, or as secondary keloid formation after prior keloid excision. They have been frequently associated with ear piercings, possibly resulting from a contact allergy to nickel or other impurities in earrings.[59] In a review of 1,200 pierced ears, Simplot and Hoffman[60] reported keloid formation in 2.5%. Keloids can be found in all skin types and in both genders, but the risk of keloid formation is higher in patients with darker skin pigmentation.[61] In a survey of 32 patients with keloids resulting from ear piercing, Lane et al[62] found that keloids were more likely to form if the piercing occurs after the age of 11.

Despite a sound understanding of the histomorphological structure of keloids, multiple treatment modalities exist with

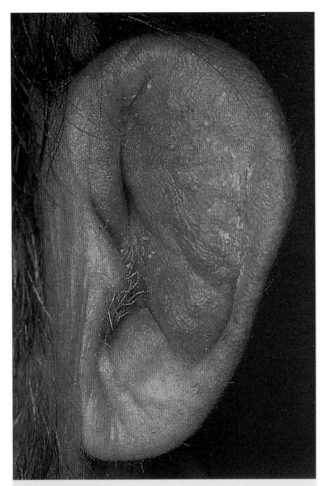

Fig. 15.6 Relapsing polychondritis.

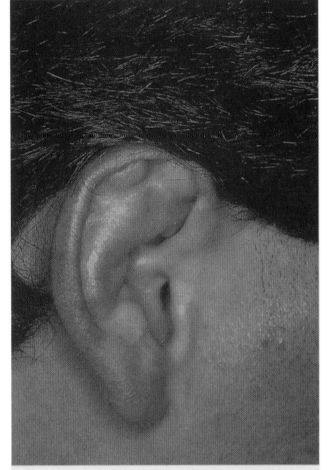

Fig. 15.7 Cauliflower ear.

and polymorphonuclear leukocytes,[91] and deposition of granular immunoglobulin G (IgG), IgA, IgM, and C3 deposits at the junction of membranous and cartilaginous tissues.[92] Further, the association of relapsing polychondritis with other autoimmune disorders and the response of the disease to immunosuppressive agents support the notion that it is probably immunologically mediated.

Over 30% of patients with relapsing polychondritis have a secondary autoimmune or hematologic disease, with systemic vasculitis being the most commonly associated condition.[82,84,85,93] This vasculitis may range from isolated cutaneous leukocytoclastic vasculitis to systemic polyarteritis-type vasculitis such as Wegener granulomatosis and polyarteritis nodosa. Relapsing polychondritis is also associated with other connective tissue disease such as rheumatoid arthritis, systemic lupus erythematosus, Sjögren's syndrome, and hematologic malignancies such as myelodysplastic syndromes, Hodgkin's disease, and acute leukemia.[81] Relapsing polychondritis usually follows the onset of the other condition.

Relapsing polychondritis is generally considered a progressive disease, with most patients experiencing intermittent inflammatory exacerbations. Acute unilateral or bilateral auricular chondritis is the most common clinical finding in relapsing polychondritis, being the presenting complaint in 40% of patients, and occurring in up to 85% of patients over the course of the disease.[82,84,85] The auricular involvement is usually sudden, and is characterized by erythema, warmth, swelling, and pain involving the cartilaginous part of the ear while sparing the lobules. There is absence of infectious symptoms, although this presentation is often misdiagnosed as infectious perichondritis. The episode may last days to weeks, and resolves with or without treatment. Following recurrent attacks, the auricle may start to lose its shape and contour ("cauliflower ear") (▶ Fig. 15.7). There may also be associated hearing loss, which is often conductive, secondary to edema of the external auditory canal. Sudden or gradual sensorineural hearing loss, presumably resulting from vasculitis of the internal auditory artery, or its branches, may occur in up to 40% of patients.

Approximately 50% of patients have involvement of the nasal cartilage during the course of their disease. Nasal symptoms on acute exacerbation include severe pain, epistaxis, congestion, and facial fullness. Recurrent nasal inflammation may result in cartilage damage, with a saddle-nose deformity.

Approximately 50% of patients with relapsing polychondritis have involvement of the cartilage of the larynx or tracheobronchial tree during the course of their disease.[94,95] Respiratory involvement is evident in 25% of patients at initial presentation. Associated symptomatology can be variable, and includes hoarseness, coughing, swallowing difficulties, and respiratory distress either at rest or on exertion. There may be tenderness on laryngeal palpation during an acute exacerbation. Inflammation of the tracheobronchial tree can result in acute respiratory distress, necessitating intubation or tracheostomy placement. The reported mortality from respiratory complications varies from 10 to 50%,[82,94,95] and is the most common cause of death in relapsing polychondritis. Patients with lower airway involvement may remain asymptomatic for quite some time, with this involvement only evident on endoscopic or radiographic evaluation, and may be limited to focal airways or extent over the entire airway.

Episodic polyarthritis or oligoarthritis affecting small or large joints may be the presenting symptom in 30% of cases, and develop in 75% over the course of the disease. The cardiovascular system is involved in 15 to 30% of cases and constitutes the second most frequent cause of death after pulmonary and infectious problems; cardiovascular complications accounted for about 40% of the mortality during a 10-year follow-up.[85] Ocular involvement is common, affecting approximately 20 to 30% of patients at the onset of disease, with about 50% affected during follow-up. Most patients with ocular inflammatory involvement tend to develop multiple systemic manifestations.[81] A variable degree of renal, dermatologic, and hematologic involvement may also be present.[96,97]

McAdam et al[84] proposed clinical diagnostic criteria for relapsing polyarthritis, requiring three or more of the clinical features to confirm the diagnosis:

1. Bilateral auricular chondritis
2. Nasal chondritis
3. Nonerosive, seronegative inflammatory polyarthritis
4. Ocular inflammation (conjunctivitis, keratitis, scleritis and/or episcleritis, uveitis)
5. Respiratory tract chondritis (laryngeal and/or tracheal cartilage)
6. Cochlear and/or vestibular dysfunction (neurosensory hearing loss, tinnitus and/or vertigo)
7. Cartilage biopsy confirmation of a compatible histological picture

In patients where the presentation is characteristic, such as bilateral auricles involvement, or chondritis in multiple sites, a diagnosis is usually reached clinically. However, in some cases, such as early disease, or when other secondary diagnoses exist, a biopsy of the involved ear may be necessary. Once a diagnosis is made, then all patients should undergo upper and lower airway evaluation using pulmonary function tests as well as radiological assessment by computed tomography (CT) scanning.[94]

There are no specific immunologic parameters for relapsing polychondritis. Patients are generally negative for antinuclear antibodies and rheumatoid factor, unless they also have an underlying connective tissue disorder. During acute episodes, patients may have nonspecific inflammatory parameters including an elevated erythrocyte sedimentation rate (ESR), leukocytosis, thrombocytosis, and hypergammaglobulinemia.

As with other immunologic-mediated diseases, corticosteroids remain the cornerstone of treatment. Although they often decrease the frequency, duration, and severity of acute exacerbations, they do not ultimately affect disease progression or alter the natural history of the disease. Most patients with relapsing polychondritis require long-term steroid therapy. Short

courses of high-dose steroids may be administered for exacerbations such as ocular involvement, severe auricular or nasal chondritis, or sudden sensorineural hearing loss. Immunosuppressive steroid sparing drugs, including dapsone,[98] and several cytotoxic agents such as azathioprine,[99] cyclophosphamide,[100] cyclosporine,[101] methotrexate,[102] plasma exchange,[103] and anti-CD4 monoclonal antibody,[104] have been given in an attempt to spare patients the long-term sequelae of steroids. Many of these drugs, as well as intravenous pulse steroids, have been given in cases of severe exacerbations or in acute airway compromise. The latter may also entail surgical intervention. Tracheostomy may be required for significant airway involvement confined to the subglottis. Stenting of the respiratory tree can alleviate more extensive tracheobronchial disease.[105,106]

15.4.3 Chondrodermatitis Nodularis Chronica Helicis

Chondrodermatitis nodularis chronica helicis (CNCH) is a relatively uncommon inflammatory condition of the ear that presents as a painful papule or nodule on the helix or antihelix (▶ Fig. 15.8). In early reports, the majority of affected individuals were middle-aged to elderly men with a smaller prevalence in women.[107,108] More recent studies have found an equal

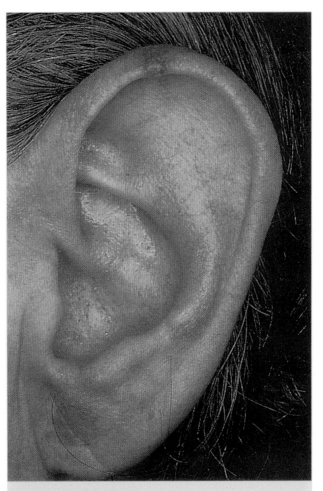

Fig. 15.8 Chondrodermatitis.

gender prevalence with similar age distribution.[109,110] CNCH commonly involves the right ear, but bilateral distribution has also been reported.[109,111–113]

The etiology of this condition remains unknown. Several theories have been proposed, including cold injuries or frostbite, actinic damage, or prolonged focal pressure.[114–116] The latter is substantiated by the observation that these lesions tend to mainly occur on the side the patient sleeps on most, and on the point of maximal pressure on the cartilage, typically the apex of the helix, but can vary in location according to the shape of the pinna.[108,114,116] These factors may act as triggers that set a cascade of events culminating in the formation of these lesions. This notion is supported by the observation of spontaneous regression following avoidance of local pressure from hearing aids, head dressings and hats, and telephonic earpieces.[108,114,117] The lack of a thick subcutaneous layer in the auricle may expose the underlying cartilage and perichondrium to ischemia following prolonged periods of sustained pressure.

It has been found that CNCH primarily presents in adults in their sixth decade of life. It has rarely been reported in children.[118,119] The lesion usually begins as a papule that progresses into a nodule, which is the characteristic clinical finding. It is an oval or round lesion with rolled-out margins. The center of the nodule may have an active sinus tract or a crust from a previous ulcer. There could be a single or multiple lesions, typically on the helix, and less commonly on the antihelix or tragus. The lesions are invariably painful, and patients may wake up at night with pain, having slept on the affected side. The lesions are tender on palpation. There is usually a history of preceding mechanical trauma, and this should be sought on patient questioning. There usually has been no recent change in the appearance of the nodule, which helps in excluding cutaneous malignancy.

If a lesion is not consistent with CNCH on clinical assessment, then histopathological examination is insufficient to make this diagnosis. Nevertheless, in the setting of a painful ulcerating nodule of the helix typical of this lesion, histopathological examination is still important to confirm the diagnosis of CNCH and exclude malignancy and other lesions in the differential. Clinically, the differential diagnosis includes basal cell carcinoma, squamous cell carcinoma, keratoacanthoma, elastotic nodule, and actinic keratosis.[117] Histologically, CNCH demonstrates an epidermal defect similar to that seen in other perforating dermatoses.[120] There is epidermal hyperplasia, parakeratosis, degeneration of elastic tissue, fibrosis, and possible cartilage degeneration.[117]

It should be noted that CNCH is a benign lesion with a favorable natural history that may respond to conservative management approaches.[121] Most authors recommend minimizing mechanical injury, pressure, and actinic exposure. Some authors advise the use of foam padding with a hole cut in it to accommodate the affected ear to relieve any pressure on the ear while the patient is lying on that side, and to wear a headband to keep it applied to the head at night.[122] In cases where conservative management is undertaken, it is important to schedule follow-up for a month later to exclude malignancy if the lesion does not heal.

Steroids, used topically or intralesionally, have been used successfully to treat CNCH.[123–125] Other treatment options described include collagen injections,[126] carbon dioxide laser,[127,128] and curettage[114,129] with variable degrees of success. Surgical excision remains the most commonly described treatment modality in the literature.[110,122,129,130] Surgery usually involves wide excision of the underlying cartilage[131,132] and possibly the skin directly overlying the nodule.[109,130,133] These lesions have been associated with a variable risk of recurrence and may thus require repeat excision.[114,122,123]

15.5 Auricular Trauma

15.5.1 Blunt Trauma

The auricle's prominent position predisposes it to accidental trauma. This conspicuous location also makes deviations in appearance a potential for significant physical and psychological morbidity in both children and adults. The intricate and delicate surface auricular topography makes reconstruction a difficult task for beginning as well as experienced surgeons.

The average adult ear is approximately 6 cm long, with its long axis about 15 to 20 degrees posterior to the vertical, and the top of the ear aligning vertically with the lateral eyebrow, when the head is in the Frankfort horizontal position. The average ear width is about half the length. Normal ear protrusion from the skull is an incline of 20 to 30 degrees from the central plane of the skull, approximately 1.5 to 2 cm from the skull to the tip of the helix. The auricle is supplied by branches of the external carotid artery. Anteriorly, the superficial temporal artery gives off three branches to supply the lobule, tragus, and helix. Posteriorly, the postauricular artery supplies the rest of the ear. An extensive network of anastomoses exists between these two major vessels. Venous drainage ends in the external and internal jugular veins. Ear sensation is supplied by various cranial and cervical nerves. The superolateral surface is supplied by the auriculotemporal nerve (V), the inferior aspect by the anterior branch of the greater auricular (C2–3) nerve, and the posteromedial surface mainly by the posterior branch of the greater auricular nerve, with a small contribution from the lesser occipital (C2). The concha receives a sensory contribution from the Arnold nerve, a branch of the vagus nerve.

The pliable elastic nature of auricular cartilage confers some protection and resiliency to minor trauma. Nevertheless, its anatomic position renders it exposed to avulsion or sharp amputation by a variety of traumatic insults including human and animal bites, falls, and automobile accidents.[134] In minor cases, trauma may result only in simple lacerations. More significant injuries may partially involve the skin or extend to the underlying cartilage, or span the entire thickness of the auricle. Yet more severe traumas may result in complete auricular avulsion. The intricate and delicate soft tissue and neurovascular anatomy are significantly disrupted in traumatic events, making reconstruction and microvascular repair challenging.

Management of auricular trauma is in the context of the underlying etiology. Trauma may solely involve the auricle, or the ear may be a component of a multifacial or even multisystem trauma. When all life-threatening injuries have been addressed, the approach to management of the auricular trauma is systematic. The importance of the external ear is both cosmetic and functional. The functional impairment, such as the inability to wear glasses, may be of more significance to the patient than the cosmetic defect. In cases of surgical auricular defects secondary to malignancy resection, delayed reconstruction may be warranted for tumors with a high recurrence risk, because flap reconstruction may mask recurrence, alter lymphatic disease spread, and facilitate tumor spread along violated tissue planes.[135]

Initial management of the traumatized wound includes copious irrigation and debridement of necrotic tissue. Tetanus and rabies prophylaxis must be addressed. Broad-spectrum antibiotic coverage should be initiated if appropriate.

Auricular hematoma is often observed in contact sports, such as boxing and wrestling (▶ Fig. 15.9). A direct blow to the auricle can result in entrapment of blood or serum in the plane between the perichondrium and cartilage. This may result in dissection of the perichondrial blood supply from the underlying cartilage, causing its devitalization and subsequent fibrosis, distorting its anatomy (cauliflower ear). It is thus important that auricular hematomas are promptly addressed. Needle aspiration is typically ineffective. Most often, incision and suction of the hematoma is advocated, and many authors have recommended tie-through, or compression, sutures, through dental rolls, to obliterate the fluid space following hematoma evacuation. Other pressure dressings have been described, including silicone and thermoplastic splints. In hematomas older than a few days, hyperplastic fibrocartilaginous tissue can develop. In these cases, this fibroneocartilaginous layer is carefully dissected and removed before the placement of a pressure dressing to prevent a cauliflower deformity lower ear.

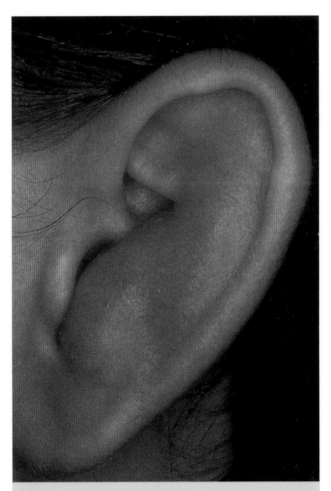

Fig. 15.9 Auricular hematoma.

In the case of exposed cartilage, healing by secondary intention is typically not recommended because of the risk of chondritis development, as well as scar contracture, which can result in variable auricular deformity. Simple auricular lacerations can be approximated by meticulous primary closure of all involved tissue layers. For larger defects, and if perichondrium is present, skin grafting can be appropriate, usually as a full-thickness skin graft. This has some advantages over a split-thickness graft, including potentially good texture, color, and thickness match. It also has a lesser incidence of contracture, and is associated with lower donor-site morbidity. Donor sites that provide a close color match include pre- and postauricular skin, the melolabial fold, submental areas, and the eyelid.[135] If perichondrium is missing, then a skin graft is likely to fail. Options at that point include removal of cartilage if necessary for support (as in concha for example), and supporting the skin graft on the opposing perichondrium. If cartilage support is necessary, then perforations in the cartilage can be made to allow for granulation tissue to grow through, followed by skin graft in a secondary delayed fashion.[135] Whenever cartilage is left exposed, antibiotics with good cartilage penetration, such as the fluoroquinolones, should be administered. Direct reattachment of amputated partial segments has been shown to be unpredictable, with varying degrees of success.[134] Mladick and colleagues[136] described a pocket principle technique for partial composite tissue loss, in which the avulsed ear part is available.

Repair of more extensive auricular trauma is beyond the scope of this chapter. Generally, though, management of subtotal avulsions with any remaining cutaneous attachment is with primary closure, because the extensive auricular blood supply allows for adequate perfusion and healing. In cases of total auricular avulsion, many authors have reported successful microvascular replantation.[137-139] This can be challenging because in many cases anastomotic vessels may be severely injured in trauma. Many supportive measures, including hyperbaric oxygen, anticoagulation, and medicinal leeches, are necessary in these cases.[139-141]

Partial or total auricular prostheses, either via adhesives or osseointegrated titanium implants, present a suitable option for patients who are not surgical candidates, not interested in repair, or require ongoing tumor surveillance.[142] The advantages of these prostheses include good compliance and satisfaction rates, and low rate of complications.[143,144] Disadvantages include cost and prosthetic discoloration over time.[145]

15.5.2 Frostbite

Although more commonly encountered in military environments, there is a rising incidence of cold-induced injuries in the general population (▶ Fig. 15.10).[146,147] Particular settings increase the risk of development of thermal injuries in the civilian population, including exposure to extreme outdoor conditions, immersion, snow, and high altitudes.[146,148-151] Personal factors and individual behavior also play an important role in the risk of cold injuries, including homelessness, smoking, dehydration, old age, ethnic origin, peripheral vascular disease, diabetes, psychiatric illness, drugs (e.g., β-blockers, sedatives), and alcohol and illicit drug intoxication. Ethnic origin also seems to play a role; a large cross-sectional study over 19 years by the United States Army found that men of Afro-Caribbean descent were

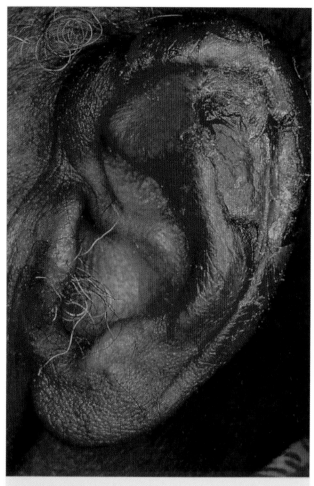

Fig. 15.10 Frostbite pinna.

four times more likely than Caucasian men to sustain cold injuries.[152]

The hands and feet account for 90% of cold injuries reported.[147,153] The ear follows the fingers, toes, noses, and cheeks in order of the sites most commonly affected by frostbite.[154] Although the elderly and young children may be at higher risk of sustaining frostbite injury, studies shows that frostbite tends to mostly affect adults between the ages of 30 and 49 years.[155]

The pathophysiology of frostbite remains poorly understood. Recent work, mainly derived from animal models, describes a series of overlapping events.[147,156] Skin sensation is lost at around 10°C. With further cooling, tissue injury occurs either directly through the formation of intracellular and extracellular ice crystals, or indirectly through the release of proinflammatory cytokines.[156,157] After exposure to temperatures below freezing, the affected extremity exhibits localized vasoconstriction, reducing blood flow, exacerbating cooling, and resulting in more transendothelial leakage of plasma. Microthrombi may also form from endothelial damage, which can occlude capillaries and cause ischemia. Vasoconstriction may be followed by vasodilatation through the so-called hunting response, a normal physiological response thought to protect the extremities from freezing at the expense of heat loss. Tissue ischemia may result in significant tissue loss.

From a clinical standpoint, auricular cold trauma may present on a spectrum from mild to severe injury. Frostnip is the earliest manifestation of significant cold injury, and generally responds well to tissue warming with reversal of the condition. Frostbite, on the other hand, is the most severe form and results in a variable degree of tissue destruction. Initially, most frostbite injuries appear clinically similar. As such, assessment of the degree of injury is best determined after rewarming, and has been categorized into four degrees of severity:

- First-degree frostbite is characterized by an anesthetic central white plaque with peripheral erythema.
- Second-degree injury reveals blisters filled with clear or milky fluid surrounded by erythema and edema, which appears in the first 24 hours.
- Third-degree injury is associated with hemorrhagic blisters that result in a hard black eschar seen over the course of 2 weeks.
- Fourth-degree injury produces complete necrosis and tissue loss.

There are three phases of frostbite treatment.[150] Pre-thaw field care takes place in the field prior to hospital arrival, and involves protecting the auricle from any mechanical trauma that can macerate the skin. Thawing is avoided at this phase until consistent rewarming can be undertaken. The second phase involves immediate rewarming once the patient is in the hospital. Rewarming should be done for 15 to 30 minutes or until thawing is complete, typically demarcated by the red or purple appearance of the auricle. Rewarming is performed within a narrow temperature range, because rewarming at too low a temperature reduces tissue survival, and rewarming at high temperatures increases the thermal damage. White blisters are debrided while hemorrhagic blisters are best left intact to prevent desiccation by exposure if debrided. Aloe vera or Silvadene ointment is used every 6 hours as a thromboxane inhibitor to reduce tissue necrosis. Daily wound care and debridement is important. In the early phase, surgical care consists of limited debridement of blisters and necrotic tissue. More aggressive debridement or amputation is best delayed until the progressive ischemia is complete, usually over 1 to 3 months. Some alterative modalities to rapid rewarming have been studies, including infusion of low molecular weight Dextran, heparin anticoagulation, thrombolysis, and hyperbaric oxygen. However, the efficacy of these modalities has not been substantiated.

15.6 Cutaneous Lesions

15.6.1 Seborrhoic Keratosis

Seborrhoic keratosis (SK) is one of the most common nonmalignant epithelial tumors of the external ear. It initially presents in middle age and often increases in number over time. Most elderly patients will have several SKs, frequently on the head and neck.

Despite their prevalence, the etiology of SK remains unknown. Age is an associated risk factor,[158] as SKs usually appear after the third decade of life. Increased sun exposure is thought to be an independent risk factor, as SKs have been noted to arise in sun-exposed areas of the body.[159] Investigations of the presence of human papillomavirus (HPV) DNA in nongenital SKs have been reported,[160,161] with a prevalence of HPV DNA as high as 76% in SK biopsies. Nevertheless, it is unlikely that the presence of HPV is a causative factor in the development of SKs.

The diagnosis of SK is usually made clinically. The lesions have a typical appearance, commonly presenting as sharply demarcated, brown, "stuck on" papules with granular surfaces. The color is typically dark blue, but may also be other colors including blue-gray, yellow, or black.[162] Although SKs may initially appear flat, they eventually evolve into their verrucous appearance. SKs may spread with time and can potentially affect the whole auricle, and even extend to the external auditory canal.[163] Biopsy is rarely necessary, but may be needed if an SK is difficult to distinguish from a melanoma.[164] In general, histological examination is recommended for any atypical-appearing SKs or for those that have undergone recent inflammation or acute changes.

Seborrhoic keratoses are generally asymptomatic. Some patients may note that they "crumble off" with accidental or intentional trauma.[165] Occasionally they are tender or itchy in light of mild irritation.

No treatment is necessary for SKs, unless sought for cosmetic reasons. Surgical options include cryotherapy, electrodesiccation, CO_2 laser surgery, curettage, and excision.[166,167] Several topical treatments have also been reported, most notable of which is imiquimod (5%) cream,[168] an immune response mediator used in the treatment of external genital warts and common warts, although this will likely prove beneficial only in those SKs possessing HPV DNA.

15.6.2 Actinic Keratosis

Actinic keratosis (AK) is a common lesion that is often located on the auricle, especially on the helix. Its pathogenesis is considered to be a direct result of the photoaging process of the skin from sun exposure.[169] Its frequency increases with age, with an incidence of approximately 10 to 15% in the United States and Europe.[169] Aside from age and ultraviolet (UV) radiation exposure, other risk factors for developing AKs include fair skin pigmentation and immunosuppression.[170] There is a small male predilection. These lesions are considered premalignant, with an approximately 15% malignant transformation rate to squamous cell carcinoma.[169–171]

Actinic keratosis typically presents as an ill-defined 2- to 8-mm lesion with a rough texture. There is a visible erythematous base, and the lesion may grow to a much larger hyperkeratotic plaque. The clinical diagnosis is more of a tactile than visual one. There may be associated signs of inflammation. Although the diagnosis is often made clinically, a biopsy is often recommended if the lesion is recurrent, isolated, or has an atypical appearance.

Actinic keratosis can be managed by close follow-up, with strict sun and ultraviolet radiation exposure. Common treatment modalities include curettage,[172] photodynamic therapy,[173] laser therapy,[174] topical 5-FU, diclofenac, colchicine, imiquimod, and retinoid application.[175]

15.6.3 Seborrheic Dermatitis

Seborrheic dermatitis (SD) is a chronic, relapsing inflammatory skin condition. It has a predilection for areas rich in sebaceous

glands, and the auricle is not an uncommon location, commonly presenting as an itchy ear. SD is considered one of the most frequent skin disorders. A survey of a representative sample of the United States population between 1 and 74 years of age showed that the prevalence of SD, as assessed by a dermatologist, was 11.6% overall and 2.8% among persons with cases considered by the examiner to be clinically significant.[176] The prevalence of SD appears to be lowest among persons younger than 12 years of age, and highest among persons 35 to 44 years old. SD is more prevalent and clinically more severe in persons infected with the human immunodeficiency virus (HIV), particularly in those with CD4 counts below 400 cells per millimeter,[177] and in afflicted individuals the condition may respond to antiretroviral treatment.[178] The etiology of SD remains poorly understood. Although the condition does not primarily involve sebaceous glands or cause excessive secretion of sebum, functioning sebaceous glands may be a permissive factor because SD occurs most often in areas of the skin where sebum is produced. Fungi of the genus *Malassezia,* which are lipid-dependent, ubiquitous normal skin flora, have been considered potentially pathogenic, because they are present on affected skin, and antifungal agents are useful in treatment.[179] It is interesting to note, however, that there is no correlation between the number of *Malassezia* organisms and the severity of disease manifestations. It has been proposed that the inflammatory process may be mediated, in susceptible individuals, by fungal metabolites.[179]

The diagnosis of SD is often made based on history and clinical assessment. The disorder presents as poorly defined erythematous patches, covered by large yellow greasy scales that can be easily scraped. In the ear, it typically involves the concha or the retroauricular area. The lesions are painless, but may present with itchiness, particularly of the external auditory canal, where they may predispose to canal impaction and otitis externa.

Topical agents are used in the management of most cases of SD. The most common of topical agents utilized are the antifungals. These include ketoconazole, bifonazole, and ciclopirox, which are available in various formulations including creams, gels, and foams. Double-blind randomized trials have shown the efficacy of topical ketoconazole in clearing or almost clearing the SD lesions at about 4 weeks.[180,181] Intermittent use of ketoconazole can maintain remission, although this has not been specifically studied in auricular SD. There are only limited data comparing the efficacy of the different antifungal agents. Overall, there are no major side effects reported with topical antifungals, although contact sensitivity has been reported in rare cases or long-term use.[182] There are no case reports of antifungal ototopical medications causing ototoxicity with an intact tympanic membrane, although their use in the setting of a tympanic membrane perforation has not been well studied.[183]

Topical corticosteroids have also been used in the management of SD. Although most studies on their short-term use have been underpowered, they did demonstrate either no difference or only a small difference favoring the topical antifungal agents.[184,185] They are particularly helpful for the short-term control of erythema and itchiness. Topical lithium succinate and lithium gluconate are effective agents in the management of SD.[186] Twice-daily lithium gluconate was shown to be more effective than 2% ketoconazole in an 8-week noninferiority trial involving 288 patients with facial lesions.[187]

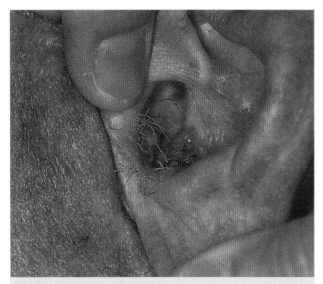

Fig. 15.11 Basal cell carcinoma.

15.7 Cutaneous Malignancies

15.7.1 Nonmelanoma Skin Cancers

Nonmelanoma skin cancers (NMSCs), mainly basal cell carcinomas (BCCs) (▶ Fig. 15.11) and squamous cell carcinomas (SCCs) (▶ Fig. 15.12), represent the most commonly diagnosed cancer in the United States, with more than 2 million new cases each year.[188] UV radiation has been well established as the greatest risk factor for the development of NMSCs. This is supported by epidemiological studies showing that there is a higher predisposition of these cancers on sun-exposed areas of the body.[189] Furthermore, the incidence of NMSCs is higher in lighter-skinned populations, those closer to the equator, in patients in occupations with greater outdoor exposure,[190,191] and in patients with genetic disorders or mutations that compromise the skin's protection from UV radiation such as xeroderma pigmentosum.[192,193] Other possible risk factors for carcinoma of the outer ear include cold injury, radiation exposure, and chronic infection. There is also an association with HPV-induced viral carcinogenesis.[194]

The most recent estimates of NMSC incidence in the United States are 2,152,500 treated persons and 3,507,693 total NMSCs in 2006 based on two Medicare databases.[195] The overall lifetime risk for developing NMSC is 1 in 5.[196,197] The lifetime risk of developing BCC is approximately 30%, and that of developing SCC is 7 to 11%.[198] BCCs account for approximately 80% of NMSCs, but the relative incidence of SCC rises in populations closer to the equator and with increasing age.[199,200] SCC is also more common in males, with a male-to-female ratio of 2.8, compared to about 1.5 for BCC.[196,197] The lower incidence in women may be reflective of the sun protection afforded by longer hair.

Approximately 70 to 80% of NMSCs are found on the head and neck in the United States,[196,197,200,201] and the auricle represents 5 to 10% of new cases of malignant cutaneous neoplasm diagnosed annually.[202,203] Most patients with SCC of the external ear have previously had a skin cancer elsewhere. In a

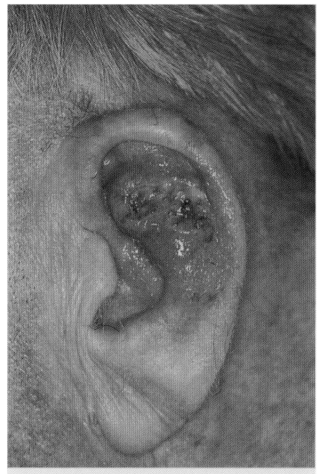

Fig. 15.12 Squamous cell carcinoma.

retrospective review of 167 cases of SCC, 65% of patients had a previous diagnosis of skin SCC elsewhere.[204] The average age of NMSC diagnosis ranges from about 60 to 65 years, peaking in the seventh and eighth decade of life.[191] Rates of SCCs generally increase rapidly with age compared with BCCs. In a retrospective review of 391 auricular and periauricular NMSCs, Niparko and colleagues[205] found a female-to-male ratio of 1:6.6, with an average patient age at presentation of 64.4 years. Similarly, in a retrospective review of 144 patients with SCC of the auricle, Silapunt and colleagues[204] found a dramatic female-to-male ratio of 1:22, with a mean age at presentation of 71 years.

Clinically, BCC may present early as a small, translucent, light-colored skin eminence, completely covered by a thin epidermal layer through which telangiectases can be seen. The tumor is slow growing, but with increased size it becomes nodular in appearance. The nodule has a typical pearly aspect with telangiectasis, and, with ongoing growth, ulceration appears. As with BCC, SCC can present variably with ulceration or frank growth and adjacent soft tissue destruction. SCC typically presents as a scaly, indurated, irregular lesion that shows an exo- or endophytic growth pattern and sometimes accompanied by serosanguinous exudates. A distinguishing feature with BCC is hyperkeratosis, which is usually present in SCC. There may also be associated bloody discharge. In most series of

NMSCs of the ear, the helix is the most commonly involved auricular site.[202,204,205] This is followed by the concha[205] or the antihelix and triangular fossa,[202] depending on the study. Although metastases are extremely rare with NMSCs of the auricle, the indolent invasive nature of these tumors can result in extensive local destruction. The embryonic development of the auricle and temporal bone results in pre- and postauricular fusion planes, which can provide avenues of spread of ear malignancies. The close proximity of various periosteal, perichondrial, fascial, and neurovascular tissue planes can distort tumor extension boundaries and margins of resection.

A complete skin examination is part of the assessment of any auricular lesion suspicious for NMSC. Regional lymph node examination, including the pre- and postauricular regions, parotid, and neck, is important. Suspicious lesions should be biopsied, including the deep dermis if an infiltrating or deeper process is suspected.[191] If palpable lymph nodes are evident, then fine-needle aspiration (FNA) also should be done, and if positive, then additional imaging studies may be necessary. If the FNA is negative, then it can be repeated, or an open biopsy is considered.

Therapy for NMSCs can be categorized into surgical treatments, radiation therapy, and superficial therapy. The choice of treatment is guided by the lesion size, location, histological features, and clinical assessment of recurrence or metastatic risk. Many high-risk factors influence the choice of management approach. The auricles fall in the so-called H-zone of the face, which is a site of high recurrence. Other high-risk factors include larger tumors, ill-defined tumor margins, recurrent disease, immunosuppression status, occurrence at a site of prior radiotherapy or burn, perineural or perivascular invasion, rapid growth, poor histological differentiation, histological subtype, and invasion of surrounding structures (e.g., neurologic symptoms).

Although electrodesiccation and curettage (ED&C) is widely used in the treatment of NMSCs, the auricle is not a favorable site because of the risk of recurrence with this method in H-zone lesions, as well as the possible inferior cosmetic result.[206] Likewise, cryotherapy is not advocated as it can result in cartilage damage, with secondary notching and poor cosmesis. Various topical treatments have been used as both monotherapy or as adjuvant therapy. These are generally used in premalignant lesions (e.g., actinic keratosis), in BCC and SCC in situ, and in other immunocompetent patients without high-risk factors. Their advantages include excellent cosmesis and convenience. Potential disadvantages include cost, patient compliance, and possible delay in definitive management if the therapy fails.[206] Some of the topical agents include imiquimod 5% cream, 5-FU, diclofenac, and retinoids. Newer topical agents include ingenol mebutate[207,208] and resiquimod.[209] Laser ablation with either CO_2 or erbium:yttrium-aluminum-garnet (YAG) has been shown to significantly reduce the number of AKs,[210] and to be effective in the treatment of NMSCs.[211,212] However, laser treatment of NMSCs is limited by the inability to deliver deeper treatments, which carry the risk of scarring.[206]

Radiation can be an effective therapeutic modality, particularly in patients over the age of 60; for younger patients there are concerns about the long-term effects of radiation. Radiation can also be considered as adjuvant treatment in high-risk tumors following surgical excision. It is important to note, however, that radiation side effects in the area of the temporal bone include possible osteitic and non-osteitic complications. The former includes osteoradionecrosis as the end-stage complication of radiation to the temporal bone. The latter includes damage to the ear canal, middle ear, and membranous labyrinth. Clinically, this can present as external canal stenosis, otitis media with effusion, chronic suppurative otitis media with or without cholesteatoma, sensorineural hearing loss, and vestibular dysfunction.[213] Radiation therapy is contraindicated in patients with genetic disorders that predispose them to skin cancers.

Surgical treatments include surgical excision with postoperative margin control, surgical excision with intraoperative frozen section assessment, and Mohs' surgery. National Comprehensive Cancer Network (NCCN) guidelines state that Mohs' surgery is the preferred method of treatment of all high-risk tumors.[214,215] For low-risk tumors (<2 cm and well circumscribed), surgical excision with postoperative margin control can be alternatively used. Inadequate control of surgical margins with primary excision of NMSCs of the external ear carries a high risk of clinical recurrence. Pascal and colleagues[216] found a 33% recurrence rate with BCC of the ear following excision when the surgical margin came within one high-power field of the tumor. Other studies have likewise demonstrated recurrence rates between about 14 and 16% following simple surgical excision.[203,217,218] In contrast, Bumsted et al[219] demonstrated a 4.2% recurrence rate in a series of 71 malignant auricular neoplasms. In Niparko and colleagues'[205] series of 231 auricular malignancies, a recurrence rate of 6.9% was reported following Mohs' excision. It is notable that in this series, preauricular lesions were included. It has been previously reported that the periauricular area has the highest recurrence rate following Mohs' excision compared to all other anatomic sites.[220]

15.7.2 Malignant Melanoma

Cutaneous malignant melanoma is an aggressive malignancy, ranking as the sixth most common cancer in the United States. The incidence of malignant melanoma has steadily increased over the last 40 years at a rate of approximately 5% annually. Among Americans, the current lifetime risk of developing melanoma is 1 in 75.[221] Approximately 25 to 30% of all primary melanomas are located in the head and neck.[222] The predilection for the head and neck region is thought to be attributable to the increased sun exposure, as well as the high melanocytic content in the head and neck, which is two- to threefold higher than in other body regions.[223] Melanoma of the external ear represents 7 to 20% of all melanomas of the head and neck and only 1 to 4% of all cutaneous melanomas.[224-228]

There is a male predilection of approximately 60 to 90% reported in the literature.[224,229-232] As with NMSCs, there is a predilection for fair-skinned individuals, especially redheads.[224,229,232] The average age at presentation is about 50 to 60 years, although all age groups can be affected, with the exception of young children.[233] Peripheral parts of the ear are more frequently affected, and the left ear is more commonly affected, which is thought to be related to the increased exposure of motor vehicle drivers' left ear to UV radiation.[234] The helix is the most commonly affected auricular location.[224,233,235,236]

The characteristic presentation of malignant melanoma is a pigmented lesion that displays the often-quoted ABCDE of melanoma: A, asymmetry of the lesion; B, border irregularity; C, variegated color; D, diameter greater than 6 mm; and E, elevation. The lesion can be flat or may be raised and nodular. There may be surrounding erythema, and the lesion may be associated with pain and itchiness, although these symptoms do not necessarily have to be present. Up to 10% of melanoma lacks melanin, so a high index of suspicion is necessary when clinically warranted. The three most described subtypes are the superficial spreading melanoma (SSM), the nodular melanoma (NM), and the lentigo maligna melanoma (LMM). In the largest literature series of malignant melanoma of the external ear, Jahn et al[233] reported that SSM represented the largest group of histological types, followed by LMM and NM. SSM shows an intermediate radial growth phase before starting to invade the dermis. In contradistinction, the nodular variant is the most aggressive, which is rapidly growing and has a predisposition for dermal invasion early on in its course. The external ear has a thin subcutaneous layer, offering no significant barrier to vertical invasion, and this likely contributes to the poor prognosis attributable to melanoma in this region. Jahn et al found that age, tumor thickness, histological type, level of invasion, and excision margins are significant risk factors for local recurrence. However, overall survival depended only on the tumor thickness and Clark level of invasion. Patients with melanoma of the external ear presented with invasion levels II and III in 36 to 53% of cases, and invasion levels IV and V in 40 to 67% of cases.[225,229,233,237,238]

The current standard management approach is that of surgery with or without adjuvant therapy. Surgical management has evolved over the past two decades. In 1970, Pack et al[228] stated that "the amputation of the ear with total parotidectomy and radical neck dissection is the most effective plan in every case of melanoma of the ear." This recommendation was echoed by other authors as well.[230,239] A decade later, Byers et al[224] proposed less radical management, with 30 of 102 patients managed with partial resection. Yet another decade later, Hudson et al[225] recommended partial resection with wide resection margins. This view has persisted, with many authors proposing controlled resection and subsequent reconstruction with chondrocutaneous or fasciocutaneous flaps, extended locoregional[240,241] advancement flaps, or skin grafts, to afford a good and functional cosmetic outcome.[145,232,233] Recommended excision margins are 10 to 20 mm for primary NM or SSM, and 5 mm with complete three-dimensional (3D) histology of excision margins for LMM.[234] Studies have shown that margins > 10 mm have the lowest risk of recurrence.[233] In recent decades the more aggressive surgical approach has changed toward narrower excision margins, with median excision margins of 13.1 mm and a mean of 10 mm.[236,240] This follows the observation that wider margins only affect the incidence of local recurrence, with little impact on disease specific survival.[233]

Current modalities for evaluation of regional nodal metastases include CT, MRI, positron emission tomography, and lymphoscintigraphy. Formal cervical lymphadenectomy is recommended in patients with a clinically positive neck or in those with a positive sentinel node biopsy. The management of the clinically negative neck in melanoma patients has been controversial. Some studies have demonstrated a benefit to elective

neck dissection in reducing the incidence of local recurrence in patients undergoing resection of head and neck melanoma.[238] Balch et al[242] showed that the presence or absence of nodal metastases is the single most important prognostic factor in the survival of melanoma patients. The current recommendations favor observation in those with primary lesions less than 1 mm in thickness, Clark's level less than IV, and without palpable cervical lymphadenopathy.[221] In a 2002 meta-analysis, however, Lens et al[243] reviewed the three largest prospective trials on the topic and found no survival benefit in those with intermediate-thickness lesions. With regard to sentinel node sapling, most current studies have unfortunately involved small patient numbers,[231,244] precluding any definitive conclusions on the prognostic or therapeutic impact on the management of patients with malignant melanoma of the external ear.

Melanoma is traditionally considered a radioresistant tumor. Radiation has recently seen a promisingly increasing role as an adjuvant treatment modality following definitive surgical treatment, and as a primary treatment in those who are poor surgical candidates, with extensive LMM, neurotropic lesions, extracapsular spread, multiple node involvement (> 4), or recurrence.[245,246] Systemic chemotherapy or immunotherapy plays a principally palliative role in the treatment of malignant melanoma, although recent work has raised hopes that novel chemotherapeutic agents may have a role in the adjuvant setting.[247] Currently chemotherapy is reserved for those who have completed locoregional therapy and are at high risk for recurrence.

15.8 Congenital Anomalies

15.8.1 Microtia

Microtia describes a spectrum of malformations that span a wide range of clinical presentations that can affect the size, orientation, position, and morphology of the auricle. Complete absence of the auricle can also occur (anotia). Using data from birth defects surveillance programs around the world, a systematic review of the prevalence per 10,000 has found the frequency of microtia-anotia 2.06, microtia 1.55, and anotia 0.36.[248]

The etiology of microtia is often multifactorial. Only 15% of patients have a positive family history.[249,250] In a minority of patients, a genetic or environmental cause can be found; in these cases, microtia is usually part of a specific pattern of multiple congenital anomalies. Microtia occurs in association with several single gene disorders, such as Treacher Collins syndrome, as well chromosomal syndromes, such as trisomy 18. It is frequently associated with the oculoauriculovertebral dysplasia spectrum of congenital anomalies, including Goldenhar-Gorlin syndrome.[251] Furthermore, microtia is a component of isotretinoin and thalidomide teratogenicity, and can be part of fetal alcohol syndrome and maternal diabetes embryopathy.[252] The occurrence of microtia is more common in Japanese, Hispanic, and Native American populations but less common in the black and Caucasian populations.[252]

Many classification systems have been proposed and modified over the years. Altmann's classification system is a purely descriptive grouping of clinical features in order of severity (▶ Table 15.1). The De la Cruz classification involves only advanced Altmann groups 2 and 3. It divides malformations into minor and major categories (▶ Table 15.2).

In 1988, Weerda compiled all the classification systems into one scheme that is useful for clinical grading as well as basic management principles:

Weerda's Combined Classification of Auricular Defects, Including Surgical Recommendations

First-degree dysplasia:

- Average definition: most structures of a normal auricle are recognizable (minor deformities).
- Surgical definition: reconstruction does not require the use of additional skin or cartilage.
  a) Microtia
  b) Protruding ear (synonyms: prominent ear, bat ear) (▶ Fig. 15.13)
  c) Cryptotia (synonyms: pocket ear, group IV B [Tanzer])
  d) Absence of upper helix
  e) Small deformities: absence of the tragus, satyr ear, Darwinian tubercle, additional folds (Stahl ear) (▶ Fig. 15.14)
  f) Colobomata (synonyms: clefts, transverse coloboma)
  g) Lobule deformities (pixed lobule, macrolobule, absence of lobule, lobule colobamata [bifid lobule])
  h) Cup ear deformities (▶ Fig. 15.15)
    ○ Type I: cupped upper portion of the helix, hypertrophic concha, reduced height (synonyms: lidding helix, constricted helix, group IV A (Tanzer), lop ear (▶ Fig. 15.16)
    ○ Type II: more severe lopping of the upper pole of the ear; rib cartilage is used as support when a short ear must be expanded or the auricular cartilage is limp

Second-degree dysplasia:

- Average definition: some structures of a normal auricle are recognizable.
- Surgical definition: partial reconstruction requires the use of some additional skin and cartilage.
- Synonym: second-degree microtia (Marx)
  a) Cup ear deformity, type III: the severe cup ear deformity is malformed in all dimensions (synonyms: cockleshell ear, constricted helix, group IV [Tanzer], snail-shell ear)
  b) Mini-ear

Third-degree dysplasia:

- Average definition: none of the structures of a normal ear is recognizable (▶ Fig. 15.17).
- Surgical definition: total reconstruction requires the use of skin and large amounts of cartilage. Synonyms: complete hypoplasia group II, peanut ear, third-degree microtia (Marx); normally concomitant congenital atresia is found.
  a) Unilateral: one ear is normal; no middle ear reconstruction is performed on any child; auricle reconstruction is begun at age 5 or 6 years
  b) Bilateral: bone-conduction hearing aid before the first birthday; middle ear surgery at age 4 years without transposition of the vestige; bilateral reconstruction of the auricle at age 5 or 6 years
- *Anotia:* Complete absence of any recognizable external ear structures. Management is similar to that of third-degree dysplasia.

Table 15.1 Altmann Classification of Congenital Aural Atresia

Group 1 (mild)	Some part of the external auditory canal (EAC), although hypoplastic, is present. The tympanic membrane is hypoplastic and the eardrum is small. The tympanic cavity is either normal in size or hypoplastic.
Group 2 (moderate)	The EAC is completely absent, the tympanic cavity is small and its contents deformed, and the "atresia plate" is partially or completely osseous.
Group 3 (severe)	The EAC is absent and the tympanic cavity is markedly hypoplastic or missing.

Table 15.2 De la Cruz Classification of Congenital Aural Atresia

Minor Malformations	Major Malformations
Normal mastoid pneumatization	Poor pneumatization
Normal oval window/footplate	Abnormal or absent oval window/footplate
Reasonable facial nerve–footplate relationship	Abnormal course of the facial nerve
Normal inner ear	Abnormalities of the inner ear

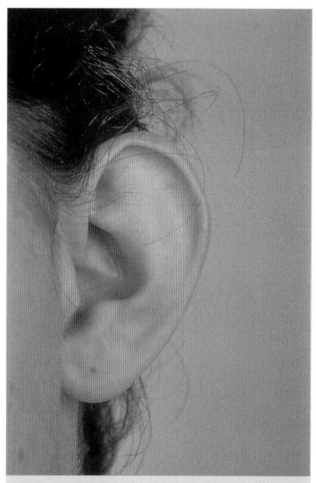

Fig. 15.13 Prominent ear.

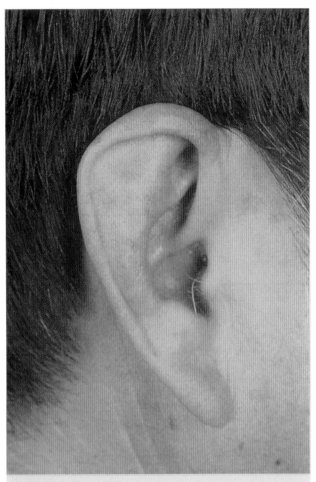

Fig. 15.14 Stahl ear.

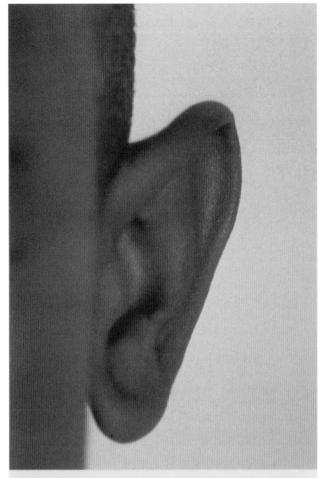

Fig. 15.15 Cup ear.

A thorough physical examination is important to accurately describe the auricular deformity, determine the status of the ear canal, and search for any associated malformations (preauricular pits/sinuses, cervical cysts or sinuses), craniofacial malformations, and other organ systems. This information is helpful in determining a possible syndromic etiology. Microtia, as with congenital aural atresia, is recognized by the American Academy of Pediatrics as a high risk factor for congenital hearing loss. It is paramount that the hearing status of a neonate with a diagnosis of microtia be determined early on. With bilateral microtia, early referral for audiological evaluation is critical so that proper bone conduction hearing aid use can be implemented. With unilateral microtia, a diagnostic auditory brainstem response (ABR) test is typically recommended to ensure that the child has at least one normal hearing ear.

Management of microtia is commonly a multidisciplinary approach. From an otologic perspective, one must initially determine what type of auditory rehabilitation is required and feasible. Patients with microtia associated with congenital aural atresia follow an algorithm to rehabilitate the associated conductive hearing loss (CHL). If surgery is contemplated, microtia repair is undertaken at approximately 5 to 6 years of age with atresia repair following at approximately 6 to 7 years, as atresia repair may disrupt the vascular supply necessary for optimum microtia repair.

Using the Weerda classification, first-degree dysplasia encompasses many common and frequently isolated auricular malformations, including macrotia, protruding ears, and the cup ear deformity. Reconstruction normally does not require the use of additional skin or cartilage. Instead, many otoplastic techniques have been described that attempt to achieve some auricular reduction. These techniques for the most part involve manipulation of the cartilage framework by using sutures or by cutting, abrading, or scoring. Examples of the former include the Mustarde and the Furnas techniques. Examples of the cartilage-cutting techniques include the Converse, Farrior, and Pitanguy techniques.

Second-degree dysplasia has most of the auricular structural components recognizable; there is, however, distinct tissue deficiency that necessitates the transposition of skin and cartilage. The main deficiency often lies in the vertical height of the affected ear. Augmenting this deficiency can be achieved by various techniques depending on the difference in height between the two ears. Donor sites include the contralateral conchal bowl or a rib graft for large deficiencies. A staged skin graft in these instances is often required and may be advanced from a postauricular donor site.

Reconstruction for third-degree dysplasia or anotia requires the use of skin and large amounts of cartilage. This is best initiated when the patient is about 6 years of age, especially for

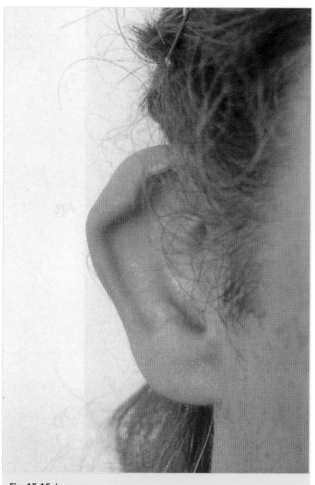

Fig. 15.16 Lop ear.

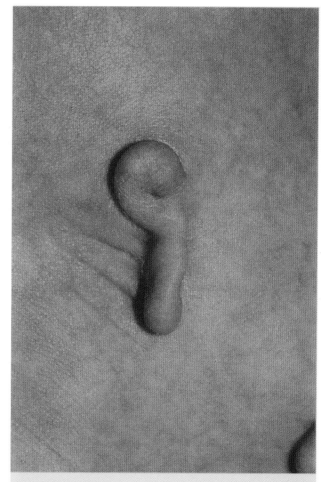

Fig. 15.17 Peanut ear.

unilateral cases, and the best donor tissue is autogenous costal cartilage. By this age, sufficient cartilage is present for the auricular reconstruction, and the patient is more able to cooperate with the necessary postoperative care. The reconstruction is multistaged and incorporates aural atresia repair.

15.8.2 Preauricular Sinus

The preauricular sinus is a benign congenital malformation, also termed preauricular pit, preauricular fistula, and preauricular cyst. It has an estimated incidence of 0.1 to 0.9% in the United States, 2.5% in Taiwan, and 4 to 10% in some areas of Africa.[253] The most accepted theory attributes the development of a preauricular sinus to incomplete fusion of the six auditory hillocks.[254] Unlike branchial cleft anomalies, a preauricular sinus is not associated with the external auditory canal or the facial nerve, although the latter can be at risk during surgical management.

Over 50% of preauricular sinus cases are unilateral, and most often sporadic. They occur more commonly on the right. Bilateral cases are more likely to be inherited. When inherited, the pattern is of incomplete autosomal dominance with reduced penetrance (approximately 85%). The preauricular sinus has been described as part of a number of syndromes, including branchio-otorenal syndrome, branchio-otocostal syndrome, cat eye syndrome, Waardenburg's syndrome, and trisomy 22.

On clinical assessment, a small pit is often incidentally noted adjacent to the external ear. Although the location is variable, and can be along the posterosuperior margin of the helix, the tragus, or the lobule, a preauricular sinus is most commonly found at the anterior margin of the ascending limb of the helix (▶ Fig. 15.18). The opening of the preauricular sinus may be a shallow pit, or may have a variable length with a tortuous course. There may also be an involved cyst intimately associated with the cartilage of the tragus or anterior crus of the helix. The sinus tract is lateral, superior, and posterior to the facial nerve. In some patients, an infected discharging sinus may be the initial presentation. The most common inciting pathogens are *Staphylococcus* species. Less commonly, *Proteus, Streptococcus,* and *Peptococcus* species may be involved.[254]

The majority of children with a preauricular sinus are asymptomatic, and as an isolated finding it requires no treatment. There is a slightly increased risk (odds ratio 1.3) of renal anomalies in children with ear anomalies.[255] Although not commonly agreed upon, many authors suggest that renal ultrasonography be performed on all patients with a preauricular sinus. The risk of associated congenital hearing loss has also been raised, but studies are of small sample size, precluding adequate

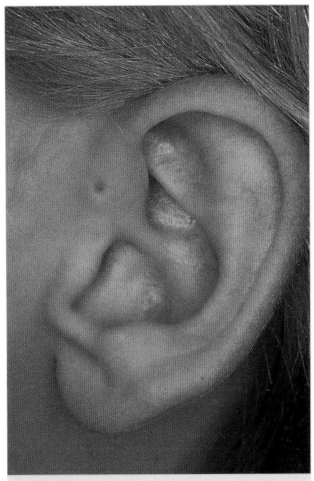

Fig. 15.18 Preauricular sinus.

recommendations. In many centers, newborn screening assessments are in place; however, there has been no evidence to support hearing assessments in the routine evaluation of a newborn with an isolated preauricular pit.

Management of an acutely infected preauricular sinus involves administration of an appropriate antibiotic active against the causative organism. If an abscess is present, then incision and drainage is recommended. Recurrent or persistent preauricular sinus infection is an indication for surgical excision of the sinus and its tract, typically delayed until the infection has resolved and inflammation has settled. There is a risk of recurrence following surgery, reflective of incomplete excision. The reported risk of recurrence has been as high as 42%.[256] As such, complete excision, typically through an elliptical skin incision surrounding the preauricular sinus opening with subsequent meticulous dissection of the entire tract, is important. A portion of the cartilage or perichondrium of the helix at the base of the sinus should be excised to ensure complete removal of the epithelial lining.

References

[1] Dillon HC Jr. Impetigo contagiosa: suppurative and non-suppurative complications. I. Clinical, bacteriologic, and epidemiologic characteristics of impetigo. Am J Dis Child 1968; 115: 530–541

[2] Bernard P. Management of common bacterial infections of the skin. Curr Opin Infect Dis 2008; 21: 122–128

[3] Koning S, Mohammedamin RS, van der Wouden JC, van Suijlekom-Smit LW, Schellevis FG, Thomas S. Impetigo: incidence and treatment in Dutch general practice in 1987 and 2001—results from two national surveys. Br J Dermatol 2006; 154: 239–243

[4] Elliot AJ, Cross KW, Smith GE, Burgess IF, Fleming DM. The association between impetigo, insect bites and air temperature: a retrospective 5-year study (1999–2003) using morbidity data collected from a sentinel general practice network database. Fam Pract 2006; 23: 490–496

[5] Rørtveit S, Rortveit G. Impetigo in epidemic and nonepidemic phases: an incidence study over 4(1/2) years in a general population. Br J Dermatol 2007; 157: 100–105

[6] Watkins P. Impetigo: aetiology, complications and treatment options. Nurs Stand 2005; 19: 50–54

[7] Koning S, van Suijlekom-Smit LW, Nouwen JL et al. Fusidic acid cream in the treatment of impetigo in general practice: double blind randomised placebo controlled trial. BMJ 2002; 324: 203–206

[8] Luby SP, Agboatwalla M, Feikin DR et al. Effect of handwashing on child health: a randomised controlled trial. Lancet 2005; 366: 225–233

[9] Koning S, Verhagen AP, van Suijlekom-Smit LW, Morris A, Butler CC, van der Wouden JC. Interventions for impetigo. Cochrane Database Syst Rev 2004: CD003261

[10] Stevens DL, Bisno AL, Chambers HF et al. Infectious Diseases Society of America. Practice guidelines for the diagnosis and management of skin and soft-tissue infections. Clin Infect Dis 2005; 41: 1373–1406

[11] Dupuy A, Benchikhi H, Roujeau JC et al. Risk factors for erysipelas of the leg (cellulitis): case-control study. BMJ 1999; 318: 1591–1594

[12] Cox NH. Oedema as a risk factor for multiple episodes of cellulitis/erysipelas of the lower leg: a series with community follow-up. Br J Dermatol 2006; 155: 947–950

[13] Article in French. [Management of erysipelas and necrotizing fasciitis] Ann Dermatol Venereol 2001; 128: 463–482

[14] Bernard P, Bedane C, Mounier M, Denis F, Catanzano G, Bonnetblanc JM. Streptococcal cause of erysipelas and cellulitis in adults. A microbiologic study using a direct immunofluorescence technique. Arch Dermatol 1989; 125: 779–782

[15] Martin R, Yonkers AJ, Yarington CT, Jr. Perichondritis of the ear. Laryngoscope 1976; 86: 664–673

[16] Dowling JA, Foley FD, Moncrief JA. Chondritis in the burned ear. Plast Reconstr Surg 1968; 42: 115–122

[17] Tseng CC, Shiao AS. Postoperative auricular perichondritis after an endaural approach tympanoplasty. J Chin Med Assoc 2006; 69: 423–427

[18] Stroud MH. A simple treatment for suppurative perichondritis. Laryngoscope 1963; 73: 556–563

[19] Stevenson EW. Bacillus pyocyaneus perichondritis of the ear. An effective method of treatment. Laryngoscope 1964; 74: 255–259

[20] Wanamaker HH. Suppurative perichondritis of the auricle. Trans Am Acad Ophthalmol Otolaryngol 1972; 76: 1289–1291

[21] Keys TF, Melton LJ III Maker MD, Ilstrup DM. A suspected hospital outbreak of pseudobacteremia due to Pseudomonas stutzeri. J Infect Dis 1983; 147: 489–493

[22] Davidi E, Paz A, Duchman H, Luntz M, Potasman I. Perichondritis of the auricle: analysis of 114 cases. Isr Med Assoc J 2011; 13: 21–24

[23] Veesenmeyer JL, Hauser AR, Lisboa T, Rello J. Pseudomonas aeruginosa virulence and therapy: evolving translational strategies. Crit Care Med 2009; 37: 1777–1786

[24] Prasad HK, Sreedharan S, Prasad HS, Meyyappan MH, Harsha KS. Perichondritis of the auricle and its management. J Laryngol Otol 2007; 121: 530–534

[25] Bassiouny A. Perichondritis of the auricle. Laryngoscope 1981; 91: 422–431

[26] Furuta Y, Takasu T, Fukuda S et al. Detection of varicella-zoster virus DNA in human geniculate ganglia by polymerase chain reaction. J Infect Dis 1992; 166: 1157–1159

[27] Murakami S, Nakashiro Y, Mizobuchi M, Hato N, Honda N, Gyo K. Varicella-zoster virus distribution in Ramsay Hunt syndrome revealed by polymerase chain reaction. Acta Otolaryngol 1998; 118: 145–149

[28] Furuta Y, Takasu T, Suzuki S, Fukuda S, Inuyama Y, Nagashima K. Detection of latent varicella-zoster virus infection in human vestibular and spiral ganglia. J Med Virol 1997; 51: 214–216

[29] Kuhweide R, Van de Steene V, Vlaminck S, Casselman JW. Ramsay Hunt syndrome: pathophysiology of cochleovestibular symptoms. J Laryngol Otol 2002; 116: 844–848

[30] Korzec K, Sobol SM, Kubal W, Mester SJ, Winzelberg G, May M. Gadolinium-enhanced magnetic resonance imaging of the facial nerve in herpes zoster oticus and Bell's palsy: clinical implications. Am J Otol 1991; 12: 163–168

[31] Wackym PA. Molecular temporal bone pathology: II. Ramsay Hunt syndrome (herpes zoster oticus). Laryngoscope 1997; 107: 1165–1175

[32] Robillard RB, Hilsinger RL Jr Adour KK. Ramsay Hunt facial paralysis: clinical analyses of 185 patients. Otolaryngol Head Neck Surg 1986; 95: 292–297

[33] Donahue JG, Choo PW, Manson JE, Platt R. The incidence of herpes zoster. Arch Intern Med 1995; 155: 1605–1609

[34] Ragozzino MW, Melton LJ III Kurland LT, Chu CP, Perry HO. Population-based study of herpes zoster and its sequelae. Medicine (Baltimore) 1982; 61: 310–316

[35] Murakami S, Hato N, Horiuchi J, Honda N, Gyo K, Yanagihara N. Treatment of Ramsay Hunt syndrome with acyclovir-prednisone: significance of early diagnosis and treatment. Ann Neurol 1997; 41: 353–357

[36] Devriese PP, Moesker WH. The natural history of facial paralysis in herpes zoster. Clin Otolaryngol Allied Sci 1988; 13: 289–298

[37] Hato N, Kisaki H, Honda N, Gyo K, Murakami S, Yanagihara N. Ramsay Hunt syndrome in children. Ann Neurol 2000; 48: 254–256

[38] Murakami S, Honda N, Mizobuchi M, Nakashiro Y, Hato N, Gyo K. Rapid diagnosis of varicella zoster virus infection in acute facial palsy. Neurology 1998; 51: 1202–1205

[39] Coulson S, Croxson GR, Adams R, Oey V. Prognostic factors in herpes zoster oticus (Ramsay Hunt syndrome). Otol Neurotol 2011; 32: 1025–1030

[40] Kuo MJ, Drago PC, Proops DW, Chavda SV. Early diagnosis and treatment of Ramsay Hunt syndrome: the role of magnetic resonance imaging. J Laryngol Otol 1995; 109: 777–780

[41] Brügel FJ, Grevers G, Vogl T, Jürgens M. [Reliability of diagnostic procedures in facial paralysis with special reference to magnetic resonance tomography] Laryngorhinootologie 1993; 72: 506–510

[42] Girard N, Poncet M, Chays A et al. MRI exploration of the intrapetrous facial nerve. J Neuroradiol 1993; 20: 226–238

[43] Murphy TP. MRI of the facial nerve during paralysis. Otolaryngol Head Neck Surg 1991; 104: 47–51

[44] Yanagida M, Ushiro K, Yamashita T, Kumazawa T, Katoh T. Enhanced MRI in patients with Ramsay-Hunt's syndrome. Acta Otolaryngol Suppl 1993; 500: 58–61

[45] Tien R, Dillon WP, Jackler RK. Contrast-enhanced MR imaging of the facial nerve in 11 patients with Bell's palsy. AJR Am J Roentgenol 1990; 155: 573–579

[46] Uscategui T, Dorée C, Chamberlain IJ, Burton MJ. Antiviral therapy for Ramsay Hunt syndrome (herpes zoster oticus with facial palsy) in adults. Cochrane Database Syst Rev 2008: CD006851

[47] Liston SL, Kleid MS. Histopathology of Bell's palsy. Laryngoscope 1989; 99: 23–26

[48] Mechelse K, Goor G, Huizing EH et al. Bell's palsy: prognostic criteria and evaluation of surgical decompression. Lancet 1971; 2: 57–59

[49] May M, Klein SR, Taylor FH. Idiopathic (Bell's) facial palsy: natural history defies steroid or surgical treatment. Laryngoscope 1985; 95: 406–409

[50] Aoyagi M, Koike Y, Ichige A. Results of facial nerve decompression. Acta Otolaryngol Suppl 1988; 446: 101–105

[51] Gantz BJ, Rubinstein JT, Gidley P, Woodworth GG. Surgical management of Bell's palsy. Laryngoscope 1999; 109: 1177–1188

[52] Chan JY, Byrne PJ. Management of facial paralysis in the 21st century. Facial Plast Surg 2011; 27: 346–357

[53] May M, Croxson GR, Klein SR. Bell's palsy: management of sequelae using EMG rehabilitation, botulinum toxin, and surgery. Am J Otol 1989; 10: 220–229

[54] Toffola ED, Furini F, Redaelli C, Prestifilippo E, Bejor M. Evaluation and treatment of synkinesis with botulinum toxin following facial nerve palsy. Disabil Rehabil 2010; 32: 1414–1418

[55] Montoya FJ, Riddell CE, Caesar R, Hague S. Treatment of gustatory hyperlacrimation (crocodile tears) with injection of botulinum toxin into the lacrimal gland. Eye (Lond) 2002; 16: 705–709

[56] Music EN, Engel G. Earlobe keloids: a novel and elegant surgical approach. Dermatol Surg 2010; 36: 395–400

[57] Lim CP, Phan TT, Lim IJ, Cao X. Cytokine profiling and Stat3 phosphorylation in epithelial-mesenchymal interactions between keloid keratinocytes and fibroblasts. J Invest Dermatol 2009; 129: 851–861

[58] Fujiwara M, Muragaki Y, Ooshima A. Keloid-derived fibroblasts show increased secretion of factors involved in collagen turnover and depend on matrix metalloproteinase for migration. Br J Dermatol 2005; 153: 295–300

[59] Tian J, Li B, Zhou C, Liu D. [Prevention of keloids of the earlobes] Lin Chuang Er Bi Yan Hou Ke Za Zhi 1999; 13: 157–158

[60] Simplot TC, Hoffman HT. Comparison between cartilage and soft tissue ear piercing complications. Am J Otolaryngol 1998; 19: 305–310

[61] Kelly AP. Keloids. Dermatol Clin 1988; 6: 413–424

[62] Lane JE, Waller JL, Davis LS. Relationship between age of ear piercing and keloid formation. Pediatrics 2005; 115: 1312–1314

[63] Sclafani AP, Gordon L, Chadha M, Romo T III. Prevention of earlobe keloid recurrence with postoperative corticosteroid injections versus radiation therapy: a randomized, prospective study and review of the literature. Dermatol Surg 1996; 22: 569–574

[64] Donkor P. Head and neck keloid: treatment by core excision and delayed intralesional injection of steroid. J Oral Maxillofac Surg 2007; 65: 1292–1296

[65] Chowdri NA, Masarat M, Mattoo A, Darzi MA. Keloids and hypertrophic scars: results with intraoperative and serial postoperative corticosteroid injection therapy. Aust N Z J Surg 1999; 69: 655–659

[66] Apikian M, Goodman G. Intralesional 5-fluorouracil in the treatment of keloid scars. Australas J Dermatol 2004; 45: 140–143

[67] Gupta S, Kalra A. Efficacy and safety of intralesional 5-fluorouracil in the treatment of keloids. Dermatology 2002; 204: 130–132

[68] Stewart CE IV Kim JY. Application of mitomycin-C for head and neck keloids. Otolaryngol Head Neck Surg 2006; 135: 946–950

[69] Naeini FF, Najafian J, Ahmadpour K. Bleomycin tattooing as a promising therapeutic modality in large keloids and hypertrophic scars. Dermatol Surg 2006; 32: 1023–1029, discussion 1029–1030

[70] Savion Y, Sela M. Prefabricated pressure earring for earlobe keloids. J Prosthet Dent 2008; 99: 406–407

[71] Saha SS, Kumar V, Khazanchi RK, Aggarwal A, Garg S. Primary skin grafting in ear lobule keloid. Plast Reconstr Surg 2004; 114: 1204–1207

[72] Eaton DJ, Barber E, Ferguson L, Mark Simpson G, Collis CH. Radiotherapy treatment of keloid scars with a kilovoltage X-ray parallel pair. Radiother Oncol 2012; 102: 421–423

[73] Scrimali L, Lomeo G, Tamburino S, Catalani A, Perrotta R. Laser CO2 versus radiotherapy in treatment of keloid scars. J Cosmet Laser Ther 2012; 14: 94–97

[74] Shih PY, Chen HH, Chen CH, Hong HS, Yang CH. Rapid recurrence of keloid after pulse dye laser treatment. Dermatol Surg 2008; 34: 1124–1127

[75] Nicoletti G et al. Clinical and histologic effects from CO laser treatment of keloids. Lasers Med Sci 2012

[76] Kassab AN, El Kharbotly A. Management of ear lobule keloids using 980-nm diode laser. Eur Arch Otorhinolaryngol 2012; 269: 419–423

[77] Rusciani L, Paradisi A, Alfano C, Chiummariello S, Rusciani A. Cryotherapy in the treatment of keloids. J Drugs Dermatol 2006; 5: 591–595

[78] Parikh DA, Ridgway JM, Ge NN. Keloid banding using suture ligature: a novel technique and review of literature. Laryngoscope 2008; 118: 1960–1965

[79] Mofikoya BO, Adeyemo WL, Abdus-salam AA. Keloid and hypertrophic scars: a review of recent developments in pathogenesis and management. Nig Q J Hosp Med 2007; 17: 134–139

[80] Park TH, Seo SW, Kim JK, Chang CH. Earlobe keloids: classification according to gross morphology determines proper surgical approach. Dermatol Surg 2012; 38: 406–412

[81] Molina JF, Espinoza LR. Relapsing polychondritis. Best Pract Res Clin Rheumatol 2000; 14: 97–109

[82] Trentham DE, Le CH. Relapsing polychondritis. Ann Intern Med 1998; 129: 114–122

[83] Knipp S, Bier H, Horneff G et al. Relapsing polychondritis in childhood—case report and short review. Rheumatol Int 2000; 19: 231–234

[84] McAdam LP, O'Hanlan MA, Bluestone R, Pearson CM. Relapsing polychondritis: prospective study of 23 patients and a review of the literature. Medicine (Baltimore) 1976; 55: 193–215

[85] Michet CJ Jr McKenna CH, Luthra HS, O'Fallon WM. Relapsing polychondritis. Survival and predictive role of early disease manifestations. Ann Intern Med 1986; 104: 74–78

[86] Zeuner M, Straub RH, Rauh G, Albert ED, Schölmerich J, Lang B. Relapsing polychondritis: clinical and immunogenetic analysis of 62 patients. J Rheumatol 1997; 24: 96–101

[87] Foidart JM, Abe S, Martin GR et al. Antibodies to type II collagen in relapsing polychondritis. N Engl J Med 1978; 299: 1203–1207

[88] Yang CL, Brinckmann J, Rui HF et al. Autoantibodies to cartilage collagens in relapsing polychondritis. Arch Dermatol Res 1993; 285: 245–249

[89] Cremer MA, Pitcock JA, Stuart JM, Kang AH, Townes AS. Auricular chondritis in rats. An experimental model of relapsing polychondritis induced with type II collagen. J Exp Med 1981; 154: 535–540

[90] Rajapakse DA, Bywaters EG. Cell-mediated immunity to cartilage proteogly-can in relapsing polychondritis. Clin Exp Immunol 1974; 16: 497–502

[91] Homma S, Matsumoto T, Abe H, Fukuda Y, Nagano M, Suzuki M. Relapsing polychondritis. Pathological and immunological findings in an autopsy case. Acta Pathol Jpn 1984; 34: 1137–1146

[92] Valenzuela R, Cooperrider PA, Gogate P, Deodhar SD, Bergfeld WF. Relapsing polychondritis. Immunomicroscopic findings in cartilage of ear biopsy speci-mens. Hum Pathol 1980; 11: 19–22

[93] Michet CJ. Vasculitis and relapsing polychondritis. Rheum Dis Clin North Am 1990; 16: 441–444

[94] Tillie-Leblond I, Wallaert B, Leblond D et al. Respiratory involvement in re-lapsing polychondritis. Clinical, functional, endoscopic, and radiographic evaluations. Medicine (Baltimore) 1998; 77: 168–176

[95] Lee-Chiong TL, Jr. Pulmonary manifestations of ankylosing spondylitis and re-lapsing polychondritis. Clin Chest Med 1998; 19: 747–757, ixix.

[96] Hebbar M, Brouillard M, Wattel E et al. Association of myelodysplastic syn-drome and relapsing polychondritis: further evidence. Leukemia 1995; 9: 731–733

[97] Diebold L, Rauh G, Jäger K, Löhrs U. Bone marrow pathology in relapsing pol-ychondritis: high frequency of myelodysplastic syndromes. Br J Haematol 1995; 89: 820–830

[98] Barranco VP, Minor DB, Soloman H. Treatment of relapsing polychondritis with dapsone. Arch Dermatol 1976; 112: 1286–1288

[99] Hoang-Xaun T, Foster CS, Rice BA. Scleritis in relapsing polychondritis. Res-ponse to therapy. Ophthalmology 1990; 97: 892–898

[100] Ruhlen JL, Huston KA, Wood WG. Relapsing polychondritis with glomerulo-nephritis. Improvement with prednisone and cyclophosphamide. JAMA 1981; 245: 847–848

[101] Svenson KL, Holmdahl R, Klareskog L et al. Cyclosporin A treatment in a case of relapsing polychondritis. Scand J Rheumatol 1984; 13: 329–333

[102] Park J, Gowin KM, Schumacher HR, Jr. Steroid sparing effect of methotrexate in relapsing polychondritis. J Rheumatol 1996; 23: 937–938

[103] Neilly JB, Winter JH, Stevenson RD. Progressive tracheobronchial polychon-dritis: need for early diagnosis. Thorax 1985; 40: 78–79

[104] Choy EH, Schantz A, Pitzalis C, Kingsley GH, Panayi GS. The pharmacokinetics and human anti-mouse antibody response in rheumatoid arthritis patients treated with a chimeric anti-CD4 monoclonal antibody. Br J Rheumatol 1998; 37: 801–802

[105] Spraggs PD, Tostevin PM, Howard DJ. Management of laryngotracheobron-chial sequelae and complications of relapsing polychondritis. Laryngoscope 1997; 107: 936–941

[106] Dunne JA, Sabanathan S. Use of metallic stents in relapsing polychondritis. Chest 1994; 105: 864–867

[107] Hand EA. Chondrodermatitis nodularis chronica helicis in a woman. Arch Derm Syphilol 1950; 61: 862–863

[108] Shuman R, Helwig EB. Chondrodermatitis helicis: chondrodermatitis nodula-ris chronica helicis. Am J Clin Pathol 1954; 24: 126–144

[109] Munnoch DA, Herbert KJ, Morris AM. Chondrodermatitis nodularis chronica helicis et antihelicis. Br J Plast Surg 1996; 49: 473–476

[110] Hudson-Peacock MJ, Cox NH, Lawrence CM. The long-term results of cartilage removal alone for the treatment of chondrodermatitis nodularis. Br J Derma-tol 1999; 141: 703–705

[111] Bard JW. Chondrodermatitis nodularis chronica helicis. Dermatologica 1981; 163: 376–384

[112] Oelzner S, Elsner P. Bilateral chondrodermatitis nodularis chronica helicis on the free border of the helix in a woman. J Am Acad Dermatol 2003; 49: 720–722

[113] Kaur RR, Lee AD, Feldman SR. Bilateral chondrodermatitis nodularis chronica helicis on the antihelix in an elderly woman. Int J Dermatol 2010; 49: 472–474

[114] Kromann N, Høyer H, Reymann F. Chondrodermatitis nodularis chronica heli-cis treated with curettage and electrocauterization: follow-up of a 15-year material. Acta Derm Venereol 1983; 63: 85–87

[115] Goette DK. Chondrodermatitis nodularis chronica helicis: a perforating nec-robiotic granuloma. J Am Acad Dermatol 1980; 2: 148–154

[116] Newcomer VD, Steffen CG, Sternberg TH, Lichtenstein L. Chondrodermatitis nodularis chronica helicis; report of ninety-four cases and survey of litera-ture, with emphasis upon pathogenesis and treatment. AMA Arch Derm Syphilol 1953; 68: 241–255

[117] Sehgal VN, Singh N. Chondrodermatitis nodularis. Am J Otolaryngol 2009; 30: 331–336

[118] Rogers NE, Farris PK, Wang AR. Juvenile chondrodermatitis nodularis helicis: a case report and literature review. Pediatr Dermatol 2003; 20: 488–490

[119] Grigoryants V, Qureshi H, Patterson JW, Lin KY. Pediatric chondrodermatitis nodularis helicis. J Craniofac Surg 2007; 18: 228–231

[120] Sehgal VN, Jain S, Thappa DM, Bhattacharya SN, Logani K. Perforating dermatoses: a review and report of four cases. J Dermatol 1993; 20: 329–340

[121] Timoney N, Davison PM. Management of chondrodermatitis helicis by protec-tive padding: a series of 12 cases and a review of the literature. Br J Plast Surg 2002; 55: 387–389

[122] Moncrieff M, Sassoon EM. Effective treatment of chondrodermatitis nodularis chronica helicis using a conservative approach. Br J Dermatol 2004; 150: 892–894

[123] Lawrence CM. The treatment of chondrodermatitis nodularis with cartilage removal alone. Arch Dermatol 1991; 127: 530–535

[124] Beck MH. Treatment of chondrodermatitis nodularis helicis and conventional wisdom? Br J Dermatol 1985; 113: 504–505

[125] Cox NH, Denham PF. Intralesional triamcinolone for chondrodermatitis nodu-laris: a follow-up study of 60 patients. Br J Dermatol 2002; 146: 712–713

[126] Greenbaum SS. The treatment of chondrodermatitis nodularis chronica heli-cis with injectable collagen. Int J Dermatol 1991; 30: 291–294

[127] Taylor MB. Chondrodermatitis nodularis chronica helicis. Successful treatment with the carbon dioxide laser. J Dermatol Surg Oncol 1991; 17: 862–864

[128] Karam F, Bauman T. Carbon dioxide laser treatment for chondroderma-titis nodularis chronica helicis. Ear Nose Throat J 1988; 67: 757–758, 762–763

[129] Coldiron BM. The surgical management of chondrodermatitis nodularis chronica helicis. J Dermatol Surg Oncol 1991; 17: 902–904

[130] Sinclair P. Excision technique for chondrodermatitis nodularis helicis. Aus-tralas J Dermatol 1996; 37: 61

[131] Ormond P, Collins P. Modified surgical excision for the treatment of chondro-dermatitis nodularis. Dermatol Surg 2004; 30: 208–210

[132] Hussain W, Chalmers RJ. Simplified surgical treatment of chondrodermatitis nodularis by cartilage trimming and sutureless skin closure. Br J Dermatol 2009; 160: 116–118

[133] Metzger SA, Goodman ML. Chondrodermatitis helicis: a clinical re-evaluation and pathological review. Laryngoscope 1976; 86: 1402–1412

[134] Bardsley AF, Mercer DM. The injured ear: a review of 50 cases. Br J Plast Surg 1983; 36: 466–469

[135] Calhoun KH, Chase SP. Reconstruction of the auricle. Facial Plast Surg Clin North Am 2005; 13: 231–241, vivi.

[136] Mladick RA, Horton CE, Adamson JE, Cohen BI. The pocket principle: a new technique for the reattachment of a severed ear part. Plast Reconstr Surg 1971; 48: 219–223

[137] Mutimer KL, Banis JC, Upton J. Microsurgical reattachment of totally ampu-tated ears. Plast Reconstr Surg 1987; 79: 535–541

[138] Talbi M, Stussi JD, Meley M. Microsurgical replantation of a totally amputated ear without venous repair. J Reconstr Microsurg 2001; 17: 417–420

[139] O'Toole G, Bhatti K, Masood S. Replantation of an avulsed ear, using a single arterial anastamosis. J Plast Reconstr Aesthet Surg 2008; 61: 326–329

[140] Katsaros J, Tan E, Sheen R. Microvascular ear replantation. Br J Plast Surg 1988; 41: 496–499

[141] Lewis D, Goldztein H, Deschler D. Use of hyperbaric oxygen to enhance auric-ular composite graft survival in the rabbit model. Arch Facial Plast Surg 2006; 8: 310–313

[142] Sclafani AP, Mashkevich G. Aesthetic reconstruction of the auricle. Facial Plast Surg Clin North Am 2006; 14: 103–116, vivi.

[143] Thorne CH, Brecht LE, Bradley JP, Levine JP, Hammerschlag P, Longaker MT. Auricular reconstruction: indications for autogenous and prosthetic techni-ques. Plast Reconstr Surg 2001; 107: 1241–1252

[144] Westin T, Tjellström A, Hammerlid E, Bergström K, Rangert B. Long-term study of quality and safety of osseointegration for the retention of auricular prostheses. Otolaryngol Head Neck Surg 1999; 121: 133–143

[145] Butler DF, Gion GG, Rapini RP. Silicone auricular prosthesis. J Am Acad Derma-tol 2000; 43: 687–690

[146] Murphy JV, Banwell PE, Roberts AH, McGrouther DA. Frostbite: pathogenesis and treatment. J Trauma 2000; 48: 171–178

[147] Imray C, Grieve A, Dhillon S Caudwell Xtreme Everest Research Group. Cold damage to the extremities: frostbite and non-freezing cold injuries. Postgrad Med J 2009; 85: 481–488

[148] Harirchi I, Arvin A, Vash JH, Zafarmand V. Frostbite: incidence and predispos-ing factors in mountaineers. Br J Sports Med 2005; 39: 898–901, discussion 901

[149] Roche-Nagle G, Murphy D, Collins A, Sheehan S. Frostbite: management op-tions. Eur J Emerg Med 2008; 15: 173–175

[150] Petrone P, Kuncir EJ, Asensio JA. Surgical management and strategies in the treatment of hypothermia and cold injury. Emerg Med Clin North Am 2003; 21: 1165–1178

[151] Rintamäki H. Predisposing factors and prevention of frostbite. Int J Circumpolar Health 2000; 59: 114–121

[152] DeGroot DW, Castellani JW, Williams JO, Amoroso PJ. Epidemiology of U.S. Army cold weather injuries, 1980–1999. Aviat Space Environ Med 2003; 74: 564–570

[153] Reamy BV. Frostbite: review and current concepts. J Am Board Fam Pract 1998; 11: 34–40

[154] Hallam MJ, Cubison T, Dheansa B, Imray C. Managing frostbite. BMJ 2010; 341: c5864

[155] Valnicek SM, Chasmar LR, Clapson JB. Frostbite in the prairies: a 12-year review. Plast Reconstr Surg 1993; 92: 633–641

[156] Goertz O, Baerreiter S, Ring A et al. Determination of microcirculatory changes and angiogenesis in a model of frostbite injury in vivo. J Surg Res 2011; 168: 155–161

[157] Zook N, Hussmann J, Brown R et al. Microcirculatory studies of frostbite injury. Ann Plast Surg 1998; 40: 246–253, discussion 254–255

[158] Gill D, Dorevitch A, Marks R. The prevalence of seborrheic keratoses in people aged 15 to 30 years: is the term senile keratosis redundant? Arch Dermatol 2000; 136: 759–762

[159] Kwon OS, Hwang EJ, Bae JH et al. Seborrheic keratosis in the Korean males: causative role of sunlight. Photodermatol Photoimmunol Photomed 2003; 19: 73–80

[160] Gushi A, Kanekura T, Kanzaki T, Eizuru Y. Detection and sequences of human papillomavirus DNA in nongenital seborrhoeic keratosis of immunopotent individuals. J Dermatol Sci 2003; 31: 143–149

[161] Li YH, Chen G, Dong XP, Chen HD. Detection of epidermodysplasia verruciformis-associated human papillomavirus DNA in nongenital seborrhoeic keratosis. Br J Dermatol 2004; 151: 1060–1065

[162] Braun RP, Rabinovitz HS, Krischer J et al. Dermoscopy of pigmented seborrheic keratosis: a morphological study. Arch Dermatol 2002; 138: 1556–1560

[163] Konishi E, Nakashima Y, Manabe T, Mazaki T, Wada Y. Irritated seborrheic keratosis of the external ear canal. Pathol Int 2003; 53: 622–626

[164] Hafner C, Vogt T. Seborrheic keratosis. J Dtsch Dermatol Ges 2008; 6: 664–677

[165] Garvey C, Garvey K, Hendi A. A review of common dermatologic disorders of the external ear. J Am Acad Audiol 2008; 19: 226–232

[166] Sowden JM, Lewis-Jones MS, Williams RB. The management of seborrhoeic keratoses by general practitioners, surgeons and dermatologists. Br J Dermatol 1998; 139: 348–349

[167] Noiles K, Vender R. Are all seborrheic keratoses benign? Review of the typical lesion and its variants. J Cutan Med Surg 2008; 12: 203–210

[168] Stockfleth E, Röwert J, Arndt R, Christophers E, Meyer T. Detection of human papillomavirus and response to topical 5% imiquimod in a case of stucco keratosis. Br J Dermatol 2000; 143: 846–850

[169] Oppel T, Korting HC. Actinic keratosis: the key event in the evolution from photoaged skin to squamous cell carcinoma. Therapy based on pathogenetic and clinical aspects. Skin Pharmacol Physiol 2004; 17: 67–76

[170] Rossi R, Mori M, Lotti T. Actinic keratosis. Int J Dermatol 2007; 46: 895–904

[171] Schwartz RA, Bridges TM, Butani AK, Ehrlich A. Actinic keratosis: an occupational and environmental disorder. J Eur Acad Dermatol Venereol 2008; 22: 606–615

[172] Freeman RG, Knox JM, Heaton CL. The Treatment of Skin Cancer. A Statistical Study of 1,341 Skin Tumors Comparing Results Obtained with Irradiation, Surgery, and Curettage Followed by Electrodesiccation. Cancer 1964; 17: 535–538

[173] Szeimies RM, Karrer S, Radakovic-Fijan S et al. Photodynamic therapy using topical methyl 5-aminolevulinate compared with cryotherapy for actinic keratosis: A prospective, randomized study. J Am Acad Dermatol 2002; 47: 258–262

[174] Alexiades-Armenakas MR, Geronemus RG. Laser-mediated photodynamic therapy of actinic keratoses. Arch Dermatol 2003; 139: 1313–1320

[175] Berman B, Amini S. Pharmacotherapy of actinic keratosis: an update. Expert Opin Pharmacother 2012; 13: 1847–1871

[176] Johnson MT, Roberts J. Skin conditions and related need for medical care among persons 1–74 years. United States, 1971–1974. Vital Health Stat 11 1978: i–v, 1–72

[177] Coopman SA, Johnson RA, Platt R, Stern RS. Cutaneous disease and drug reactions in HIV infection. N Engl J Med 1993; 328: 1670–1674

[178] Dunic I, Vesic S, Jevtovic DJ. Oral candidiasis and seborrheic dermatitis in HIV-infected patients on highly active antiretroviral therapy. HIV Med 2004; 5: 50–54

[179] Naldi L, Rebora A. Clinical practice. Seborrheic dermatitis. N Engl J Med 2009; 360: 387–396

[180] Elewski BE, Abramovits W, Kempers S et al. A novel foam formulation of ketoconazole 2% for the treatment of seborrheic dermatitis on multiple body regions. J Drugs Dermatol 2007; 6: 1001–1008

[181] Elewski B, Ling MR, Phillips TJ. Efficacy and safety of a new once-daily topical ketoconazole 2% gel in the treatment of seborrheic dermatitis: a phase III trial. J Drugs Dermatol 2006; 5: 646–650

[182] de Pádua CA, Uter W, Geier J, Schnuch A, Effendy I German Contact Dermatitis Research Group (DKG). Information Network of Departments of Dermatology (IVDK). Contact allergy to topical antifungal agents. Allergy 2008; 63: 946–947

[183] Munguia R, Daniel SJ. Ototopical antifungals and otomycosis: a review. Int J Pediatr Otorhinolaryngol 2008; 72: 453–459

[184] Faergemann J. Seborrhoeic dermatitis and Pityrosporum orbiculare: treatment of seborrhoeic dermatitis of the scalp with miconazole-hydrocortisone (Daktacort), miconazole and hydrocortisone. Br J Dermatol 1986; 114: 695–700

[185] Stratigos JD, Antoniou C, Katsambas A et al. Ketoconazole 2% cream versus hydrocortisone 1% cream in the treatment of seborrheic dermatitis. A double-blind comparative study. J Am Acad Dermatol 1988; 19: 850–853

[186] Efalith Multicenter Trial Group. A double-blind, placebo-controlled, multicenter trial of lithium succinate ointment in the treatment of seborrheic dermatitis. J Am Acad Dermatol 1992; 26: 452–457

[187] Dreno B, Chosidow O, Revuz J, Moyse D STUDY INVESTIGATOR GROUP. Lithium gluconate 8% vs ketoconazole 2% in the treatment of seborrhoeic dermatitis: a multicentre, randomized study. Br J Dermatol 2003; 148: 1230–1236

[188] Siegel R, Naishadham D, Jemal A. Cancer statistics, 2012. CA Cancer J Clin 2012; 62: 10–29

[189] Fears TR, Scotto J. Estimating increases in skin cancer morbidity due to increases in ultraviolet radiation exposure. Cancer Invest 1983; 1: 119–126

[190] Gloster HM Jr Brodland DG. The epidemiology of skin cancer. Dermatol Surg 1996; 22: 217–226

[191] Kim RH, Armstrong AW. Nonmelanoma skin cancer. Dermatol Clin 2012; 30: 125–139, ix

[192] Lynch HT, Fusaro R, Edlund J, Albano W, Lynch J. Skin cancer developing in xeroderma pigmentosum patient relaxing sunlight avoidance. Lancet 1981; 2: 1230

[193] Brash DE, Rudolph JA, Simon JA et al. A role for sunlight in skin cancer: UV-induced p53 mutations in squamous cell carcinoma. Proc Natl Acad Sci U S A 1991; 88: 10124–10128

[194] Molho-Pessach V, Lotem M. Viral carcinogenesis in skin cancer. Curr Probl Dermatol 2007; 35: 39–51

[195] Rogers HW, Weinstock MA, Harris AR et al. Incidence estimate of nonmelanoma skin cancer in the United States, 2006. Arch Dermatol 2010; 146: 283–287

[196] Chuang TY, Popescu NA, Su WP, Chute CG. Squamous cell carcinoma. A population-based incidence study in Rochester, Minn. Arch Dermatol 1990; 126: 185–188

[197] Chuang TY, Popescu A, Su WP, Chute CG. Basal cell carcinoma. A population-based incidence study in Rochester, Minnesota. J Am Acad Dermatol 1990; 22: 413–417

[198] Miller DL, Weinstock MA. Nonmelanoma skin cancer in the United States: incidence. J Am Acad Dermatol 1994; 30: 774–778

[199] Diepgen TL, Mahler V. The epidemiology of skin cancer. Br J Dermatol 2002; 146 Suppl 61: 1–6

[200] Serrano H, Scotto J, Shornick G, Fears TR, Greenberg ER. Incidence of nonmelanoma skin cancer in New Hampshire and Vermont. J Am Acad Dermatol 1991; 24: 574–579

[201] Karagas MR, Greenberg ER, Spencer SK, Stukel TA, Mott LA New Hampshire Skin Cancer Study Group. Increase in incidence rates of basal cell and squamous cell skin cancer in New Hampshire, USA. Int J Cancer 1999; 81: 555–559

[202] Lee D, Nash M, Har-El G. Regional spread of auricular and periauricular cutaneous malignancies. Laryngoscope 1996; 106: 998–1001

[203] Pless J. Carcinoma of the external ear. Scand J Plast Reconstr Surg 1976; 10: 147–151

[204] Silapunt S, Peterson SR, Goldberg LH. Squamous cell carcinoma of the auricle and Mohs micrographic surgery. Dermatol Surg 2005; 31: 1423–1427

[205] Niparko JK, Swanson NA, Baker SR, Telian SA, Sullivan MJ, Kemink JL. Local control of auricular, periauricular, and external canal cutaneous malignancies with Mohs surgery. Laryngoscope 1990; 100: 1047–1051

[206] Galiczynski EM, Vidimos AT. Nonsurgical treatment of nonmelanoma skin cancer. Dermatol Clin 2011; 29: 297–309, xx.

[207] Siller G, Gebauer K, Welburn P, Katsamas J, Ogbourne SM. PEP005 (ingenol mebutate) gel, a novel agent for the treatment of actinic keratosis: results of a randomized, double-blind, vehicle-controlled, multicentre, phase IIa study. Australas J Dermatol 2009; 50: 16–22

[208] Siller G, Rosen R, Freeman M, Welburn P, Katsamas J, Ogbourne SM. PEP005 (ingenol mebutate) gel for the topical treatment of superficial basal cell carcinoma: results of a randomized phase IIa trial. Australas J Dermatol 2010; 51: 99–105

[209] Szeimies RM, Bichel J, Ortonne JP, Stockfleth E, Lee J, Meng TC. A phase II dose-ranging study of topical resiquimod to treat actinic keratosis. Br J Dermatol 2008; 159: 205–210

[210] Jiang SB, Levine VJ, Nehal KS, Baldassano M, Kamino H, Ashinoff RA. Er: YAG laser for the treatment of actinic keratoses. Dermatol Surg 2000; 26: 437–440

[211] Humphreys TR, Malhotra R, Scharf MJ, Marcus SM, Starkus L, Calegari K. Treatment of superficial basal cell carcinoma and squamous cell carcinoma in situ with a high-energy pulsed carbon dioxide laser. Arch Dermatol 1998; 134: 1247–1252

[212] Iyer S, Bowes L, Kricorian G, Friedli A, Fitzpatrick RE. Treatment of basal cell carcinoma with the pulsed carbon dioxide laser: a retrospective analysis. Dermatol Surg 2004; 30: 1214–1218

[213] Smouha EE, Karmody CS. Non-osteitic complications of therapeutic radiation to the temporal bone. Am J Otol 1995; 16: 83–87

[214] Rowe DE, Carroll RJ, Day CL, Jr. Prognostic factors for local recurrence, metastasis, and survival rates in squamous cell carcinoma of the skin, ear, and lip. Implications for treatment modality selection. J Am Acad Dermatol 1992; 26: 976–990

[215] Rowe DE, Carroll RJ, Day CL, Jr. Mohs surgery is the treatment of choice for recurrent (previously treated) basal cell carcinoma. J Dermatol Surg Oncol 1989; 15: 424–431

[216] Pascal RR, Hobby LW, Lattes R, Crikelair GF. Prognosis of "incompletely excised" versus "completely excised" basal cell carcinoma. Plast Reconstr Surg 1968; 41: 328–332

[217] Byers R, Kesler K, Redmon B, Medina J, Schwarz B. Squamous carcinoma of the external ear. Am J Surg 1983; 146: 447–450

[218] Blake GB, Wilson JS. Malignant tumours of the ear and their treatment. I. Tumours of the auricle. Br J Plast Surg 1974; 27: 67–76

[219] Bumsted RM, Ceilley RI, Panje WR, Crumley RL. Auricular malignant neoplasms. When is chemotherapy (Mohs' technique) necessary? Arch Otolaryngol 1981; 107: 721–724

[220] Robins P. Chemosurgery: my 15 years of experience. J Dermatol Surg Oncol 1981; 7: 779–789

[221] Hasney C, Butcher RB II Amedee RG. Malignant melanoma of the head and neck: a brief review of pathophysiology, current staging, and management. Ochsner J 2008; 8: 181–185

[222] Jemal A, Siegel R, Xu J, Ward E. Cancer statistics, 2010. CA Cancer J Clin 2010; 60: 277–300

[223] Jaber JJ, Clark JI, Muzaffar K et al. Evolving treatment strategies in thin cutaneous head and neck melanoma: one institution's experience. Head Neck 2011; 33: 7–12

[224] Byers RM, Smith JL, Russell N, Rosenberg V. Malignant melanoma of the external ear. Review of 102 cases. Am J Surg 1980; 140: 518–521

[225] Hudson DA, Krige JE, Strover RM, King HS. Malignant melanoma of the external ear. Br J Plast Surg 1990; 43: 608–611

[226] Möhrle M, Schippert W, Garbe C, Rassner G, Röcken M, Breuninger H. [Prognostic parameters and surgical strategies for facial melanomas] J Dtsch Dermatol Ges 2003; 1: 457–463

[227] O'Brien CJ, Coates AS, Petersen-Schaefer K et al. Experience with 998 cutaneous melanomas of the head and neck over 30 years. Am J Surg 1991; 162: 310–314

[228] Pack GT, Conley J, Oropeza R. Melanoma of the external ear. Arch Otolaryngol 1970; 92: 106–113

[229] Davidsson A, Hellquist HB, Villman K, Westman G. Malignant melanoma of the ear. J Laryngol Otol 1993; 107: 798–802

[230] Arons MS, Savin RC. Auricular cancer. Some surgical and pathologic considerations. Am J Surg 1971; 122: 770–776

[231] Pockaj BA, Jaroszewski DE, DiCaudo DJ et al. Changing surgical therapy for melanoma of the external ear. Ann Surg Oncol 2003; 10: 689–696

[232] Narayan D, Ariyan S. Surgical considerations in the management of malignant melanoma of the ear. Plast Reconstr Surg 2001; 107: 20–24

[233] Jahn V, Breuninger H, Garbe C, Moehrle M. Melanoma of the ear: prognostic factors and surgical strategies. Br J Dermatol 2006; 154: 310–318

[234] Sand M, Sand D, Brors D, Altmeyer P, Mann B, Bechara FG. Cutaneous lesions of the external ear. Head Face Med 2008; 4: 2

[235] Benmeir P, Baruchin A, Weinberg A, Nahlieli O, Neuman A, Wexler MR. Rare sites of melanoma: melanoma of the external ear. J Craniomaxillofac Surg 1995; 23: 50–53

[236] Bono A, Bartoli C, Maurichi A, Moglia D, Tragni G. Melanoma of the external ear. Tumori 1997; 83: 814–817

[237] Wanebo HJ, Cooper PH, Young DV, Harpole DH, Kaiser DL. Prognostic factors in head and neck melanoma. Effect of lesion location. Cancer 1988; 62: 831–837

[238] Fisher SR. Cutaneous malignant melanoma of the head and neck. Laryngoscope 1989; 99: 822–836

[239] Ward NO, Acquarelli MJ. Malignant melanoma of the external ear. Cancer 1968; 21: 226–233

[240] Cole MD, Jakowatz J, Evans GR. Evaluation of nodal patterns for melanoma of the ear. Plast Reconstr Surg 2003; 112: 50–56

[241] Ollila DW, Foshag LJ, Essner R, Stern SL, Morton DL. Parotid region lymphatic mapping and sentinel lymphadenectomy for cutaneous melanoma. Ann Surg Oncol 1999; 6: 150–154

[242] Balch CM, Soong SJ, Gershenwald JE et al. Prognostic factors analysis of 17,600 melanoma patients: validation of the American Joint Committee on Cancer melanoma staging system. J Clin Oncol 2001; 19: 3622–3634

[243] Lens MB, Dawes M, Goodacre T, Newton-Bishop JA. Elective lymph node dissection in patients with melanoma: systematic review and meta-analysis of randomized controlled trials. Arch Surg 2002; 137: 458–461

[244] Cordova A, Moschella F. Evaluation of nodal patterns for melanoma of the ear. Plast Reconstr Surg 2004; 113: 1528–, author reply 1529

[245] Hong A, Fogarty G. Role of radiation therapy in cutaneous melanoma. Cancer J 2012; 18: 203–207

[246] Burmeister BH, Henderson MA, Ainslie J et al. Adjuvant radiotherapy versus observation alone for patients at risk of lymph-node field relapse after therapeutic lymphadenectomy for melanoma: a randomised trial. Lancet Oncol 2012; 13: 589–597

[247] Davar D, Tarhini AA, Kirkwood JM. Adjuvant therapy for melanoma. Cancer J 2012; 18: 192–202

[248] Luquetti DV, Leoncini E, Mastroiacovo P. Microtia-anotia: a global review of prevalence rates. Birth Defects Res A Clin Mol Teratol 2011; 91: 813–822

[249] Beahm EK, Walton RL. Auricular reconstruction for microtia: part I. Anatomy, embryology, and clinical evaluation. Plast Reconstr Surg 2002; 109: 2473–2482, quiz 2482

[250] Weerda H. Classification of congenital deformities of the auricle. Facial Plast Surg 1988; 5: 385–388

[251] Mastroiacovo P, Corchia C, Botto LD, Lanni R, Zampino G, Fusco D. Epidemiology and genetics of microtia-anotia: a registry based study on over one million births. J Med Genet 1995; 32: 453–457

[252] Luquetti DV, Heike CL, Hing AV, Cunningham ML, Cox TC. Microtia: epidemiology and genetics. Am J Med Genet A 2012; 158A: 124–139

[253] Tan T, Constantinides H, Mitchell TE. The preauricular sinus: a review of its aetiology, clinical presentation and management. Int J Pediatr Otorhinolaryngol 2005; 69: 1469–1474

[254] Ellies M, Laskawi R, Arglebe C, Altrogge C. Clinical evaluation and surgical management of congenital preauricular fistulas. J Oral Maxillofac Surg 1998; 56: 827–830, discussion 831

[255] Wang RY, Earl DL, Ruder RO, Graham JM Jr. Syndromic ear anomalies and renal ultrasounds. Pediatrics 2001; 108: E32

[256] Prasad S, Grundfast K, Milmoe G. Management of congenital preauricular pit and sinus tract in children. Laryngoscope 1990; 100: 320–321

16 Diseases of the External Auditory Canal

John P. Leonetti and Sam J. Marzo

16.1 Introduction

The external auditory canal (EAC) is a bony and cartilaginous tube lined by a thin layer of stratified squamous epithelium. The main function of the EAC is to transmit sound from the pinna to the middle ear. The EAC also has a self-cleaning mechanism. Namely, desquamated skin from the tympanic membrane (TM) migrates out of the canal shaft toward the external meatus. Secretions from ear canal glands lubricate the canal, repel water, and are bacteriostatic. The proper function of the ear canal is necessary for optimal hearing. The various tissues in the EAC can be involved in multiple pathological processes including bacterial infections, inflammatory disorders, traumatic conditions, developmental anomalies, and benign and malignant lesions. This chapter provides an overview of EAC diseases and their management.

16.2 Embryology

An understanding of the developmental anatomy of the EAC is important for physicians treating diseases in this area. The EAC develops primarily from the first branchial cleft. This cleft eventually develops into the fibrocartilaginous EAC. Several medial ossification centers later develop into the bony EAC. Between the eighth and 20th gestational week, a solid core of epithelium grows medially toward the middle ear. By the 21st week, this core begins to resorb, and the innermost layer of ectoderm remains, forming the lining of the bony external canal and the lateral aspect of the TM.[1] Embryological malformations such as congenital aural canal atresia can occur if the reabsorption process does not occur or is incomplete. This process is generally completed by 28 weeks. Development of the middle ear and inner ear occurs earlier in fetal life, with formation of the cochlea, membranous labyrinth, and ossicular chain by 16 weeks. These distinctions are important because patients with congenital aural atresia might have well-developed middle and inner ears, thus allowing the potential for favorable surgical intervention.

16.3 Anatomy

The lateral third of the EAC is fibrocartilaginous, and is composed of an epithelial lining, subcutaneous soft tissue, and cartilage. The cartilaginous portion frequently has several gaps known as the fissures of Santorini, which may allow for the anterior spread of malignant neoplasms of the EAC into the parotid gland. The medial two thirds of the canal is bony and has a thin layer of periosteum and a thin epithelial lining, but lacks substantial subcutaneous soft tissue. This latter characteristic makes it very sensitive to manipulation and prone to trauma. The loss of hair in the ear canal signifies the transition from the cartilaginous portion of the canal to the bony portion, which lacks hair follicles. The examiner must be extremely gentle when cleaning and working in this portion of the ear canal. The epithelial lining of the ear has both apocrine and sebaceous glands that are responsible for producing cerumen. Cerumen is thought to have protective properties, acidifying the ear and creating an environment that is less conducive to infectious overgrowth.[2] The cerumen along with the desquamated epithelial lining has a lateral migratory pattern that allows the ear to self-clean.

The innervation of the EAC is via the fifth, seventh, and tenth cranial nerves and the greater auricular nerve. The tenth nerve contribution, known as the Arnold nerve, is responsible for the cough reflex that can be elicited by touching or irritating the inferior portion of the EAC. The blood supply to the EAC is via the superficial temporal artery and the posterior auricular artery.[3]

16.4 Physiology

Cerumen is a naturally occurring substance of the EAC. It is composed of a combination of sebaceous and apocrine gland secretions in addition to desquamated squamous epithelium.[3] Cerumen is thought to be a bacteriostatic/fungistatic substance whose function is to waterproof the canal. Its components make it extremely hydrophobic and it has an acidic pH, both of which are important in preventing infection.

Constant epithelial proliferation occurs in the EAC and on the lateral surface of the TM. These epithelial proliferation centers have varying locations throughout the TM and EAC.[4] The EAC has an inherent ability for the lateral migration of cerumen and desquamated epithelium. Some cytokeratins are seen specifically in hyperproliferative cells. Studies looking at the cytokeratin content of keratinocytes of the EAC have found some areas to be populated with both normal and hyperproliferative cells. The hyperproliferative subtypes are believed to be important for the lateral epithelial migratory pattern, which is necessary for the EAC to remain free of desquamated epithelium.[5]

16.5 Pathology

16.5.1 Obstructive Masses

Cerumen Impaction

Impaction of cerumen is one of the most common causes of conductive hearing loss (▶ Fig. 16.1). It classically presents with muffled or decreased hearing, but it may be accompanied by other symptoms like fullness, pruritus, or even pain. This is a frequent problem in the elderly, especially in the face of contributing factors such as increased ear canal hair, hearing aids, medications, or use of Q-tips. Primary care doctors frequently see these patients before an otolaryngologist, and are sometimes unable to adequately cleanse the canal. Repeated unsuccessful attempts can result in trauma to the canal, with swelling and inflammation. Treatment with a topical antibiotic-steroid mixture can decrease ear canal edema. Topical softening agents such as carbamide peroxide or mineral oil for several days may also make debridement of cerumen impactions easier.

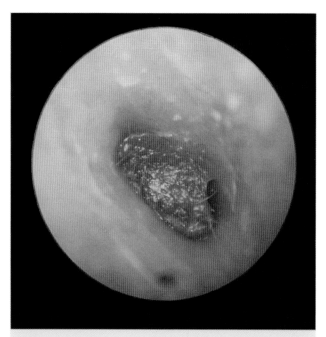

Fig. 16.1 Cerumen.

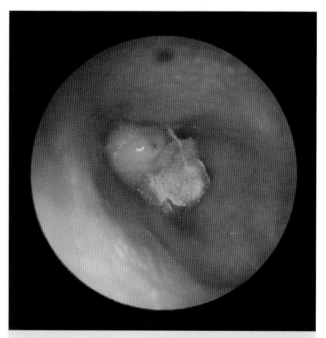

Fig. 16.2 Cotton ball.

There are several methods available to the physician for cerumen removal. Irrigation with a white vinegar (acetic acid) and water mixture often is utilized. The mixture should be kept near body temperature (98°F) to prevent vertigo from horizontal semicircular canal stimulation. This method has its limitations, and may induce damage to the canal, TM, or even the middle/inner ear.[6] It can be useful as first-line treatment of impacted cerumen by primary care personnel. Softening agents like carbamide peroxide (Debrox), hydrogen peroxide, and mineral oil may also be utilized. They can be used alone or as an adjunct to office debridement. Some agents (e.g., triethanolamine polypeptide oleate), if used for long periods of time, can cause inflammation of the EAC and a chemically induced otitis externa.

Perhaps the safest way to remove cerumen is by using binocular microscopic otoscopy. This method allows direct binocular visualization with depth perception and the use of two hands. Small loops, right-angle hooks, suction aspirators, and forceps can safely be used to remove cerumen, hairs, and other debris. If a severe impaction precludes complete removal of the cerumen, the patient may be prescribed softening drops and told to return in several days for completion of the procedure. If the canal has been traumatized, especially in the diabetic patient, the use of antibiotic drops for several days is advisable to prevent infection.

Foreign Bodies

Foreign bodies in the EAC are another frequently encountered problem (▶ Fig. 16.2; ▶ Fig. 16.3; ▶ Fig. 16.4). Common objects include beads, crayons, rocks, food matter, and insects. Small alkali batteries can cause chemical burns, and removal should be performed as soon as possible, followed by topical treatment with antibiotic/steroid drops.[7] Other small objects such are rocks can frequently be removed in the office under binocular

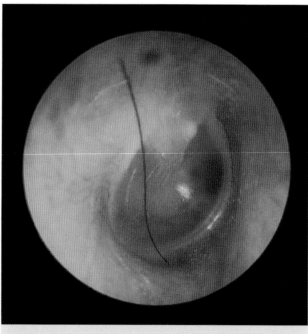

Fig. 16.3 Hair.

vision. A right-angle hook can often be positioned medial to the object and used to pull it laterally, facilitating removal. Small beads and other spherical objects can sometimes be removed with suction. Local ear canal injection with lidocaine can allow office removal of impacted objects.

Young children with foreign bodies in their ears can sometimes be restrained. However, in the uncooperative child, a general anesthetic might be necessary. Food matter like popcorn or beans may also be encountered, and irrigation should be avoided because of the propensity for these foods to swell.

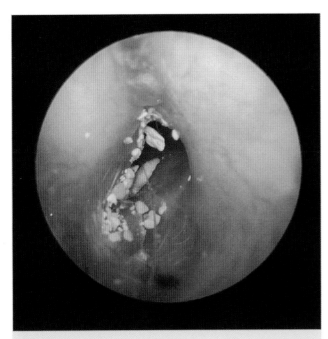

Fig. 16.4 Sand pebbles.

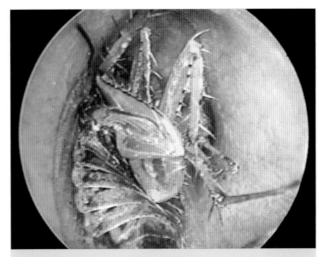

Fig. 16.5 Insect.

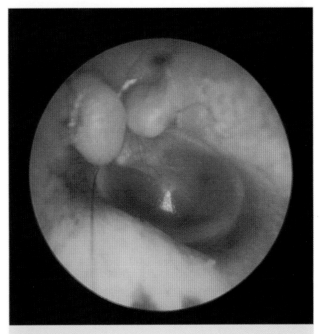

Fig. 16.6 Exostosis.

Insects enter the ear canal at night while the patient is sleeping, but because of their inability for retrograde mobility, and not enough room to turn around, they cannot exit the canal (▶ Fig. 16.5). Patients will often complain of an itching or tickling sensation in the ear and "hear" something in the affected ear if the insect is still alive. In such cases, an insecticidal liquid (alcohol or lidocaine) can be placed in the ear canal for several minutes.[8] Once the insect has died, it can then be removed safely. Except for batteries, which require prompt removal, foreign bodies in the ear canal can usually be removed safely within several days of onset.

Exostosis and Osteomas

Exostoses are bony outgrowths of the EAC (▶ Fig. 16.6). They are frequently multiple and bilateral, and are associated with swimming and water sports. However, their exact pathophysiology is not completely understood.[9,10] Van Gilse[11] proposed that exposure to cold water for long periods of time produces erythema of the canal and a periosteal reaction that induces exostosis formation. More recent research shows that these lesions are not unique to humans, and are found in other mammals that spend considerable amounts of time in the water.[12] These benign growths usually do not involve the suture lines and consist of broad-based lamellar bone.[13] Usually these lesions are asymptomatic, but with excessive growth they can impair water and cerumen drainage from the EAC, resulting in otitis externa and hearing loss. The vast majority of these lesions are asymptomatic and require no treatment. Patients with recurring cerumen impactions medial to the exostoses might require frequent office debridement or use of softening agents such as mineral oil. Patients with obstructing exostoses and conductive hearing losses might benefit from surgical correction via canaloplasty. This is generally performed through an endaural or postauricular approach. It is important to preserve

as much canal skin as possible to prevent potential EAC stenosis. As these lesions are broad-based, removal is best performed using high-speed cutting and diamond burs. Small canal skin defects can be covered with a fascia graft and allowed to heal, in which case the graft acts as a scaffold and the epithelium migrates across during the healing process. Larger defects might require a small skin graft, which can usually be obtained from the postauricular area. Recurrent disease is not uncommon.[14]

Osteomas are bony lesions that are usually unilateral, and almost always found attached to the tympanosquamous or tympanomastoid suture (▶ Fig. 16.7). These lesions differ from exostosis in that they are less common and solitary.[13] The typical location also differs in that these lesions are usually more laterally based. These neoplasms are less likely to be symptomatic, but when they obstruct the canal or impede cerumen

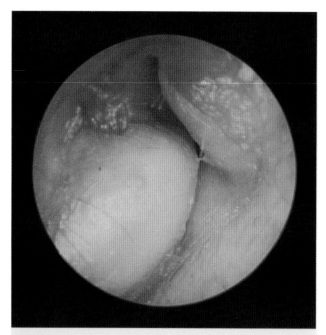

Fig. 16.7 Osteomas.

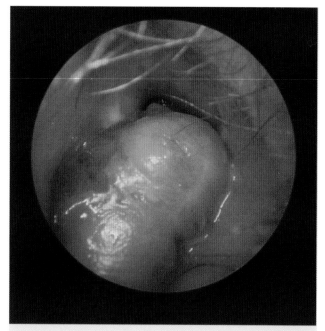

Fig. 16.8 Large obstructing polyp.

migration, they should be removed, usually through an endaural or postauricular approach.

Keratosis Obturans and Canal Cholesteatoma

These two diseases initially were considered to be the same entity, but insight generated by Piepergerdes et al[15] helped to elucidate key differences. Keratosis obturans usually is circumferential in its bony destruction, affects a younger age group, and usually is bilateral. It also has an affiliation for younger patients with bronchiectasis and chronic sinusitis. Its exact etiology is unknown, but it is thought to result from abnormal epithelial kinetics and loss of the lateral migration pattern of the squamous epithelium. Canal cholesteatoma is different in that it usually affects an older age group, is unilateral, and frequently is associated with a dull-aching, chronically draining ear.[16] These lesions are not circumferential in their destruction pattern. They typically result from trauma to the EAC, either postsurgical or self-inflicted. Nontraumatic EAC cholesteatomas are a much rarer entity.

The treatment of keratosis obturans is conservative. These patients generally require serial office debridements under the microscope. Topical therapy with antibiotic or steroid drops is reserved for disease that has a corresponding inflammatory or infectious component. Surgical therapy is generally not indicated.

Canal cholesteatomas usually can initially be managed conservatively, especially in the elderly or debilitated patient.[17] Such patients are typically seen on a regular basis for office debridement. A softening agent, such as mineral oil, can be used by the patient several days prior to the visit to facilitate cleaning under the microscope. In younger patients or in those with progressive, symptomatic disease, surgical intervention may be necessary. This usually requires an endaural or postauricular approach. Normal-appearing ear canal skin should be preserved. The TM and ossicular chain are usually not involved

with EAC cholesteatomas, and should be preserved. Next, a canaloplasty is performed, with removal of disease until healthy appearing bone is identified. Small canal skin defects can be covered with a fascia graft, whereas larger defects might require a small skin graft from the postauricular area.

Inflammatory Polyp

Inflammatory polyps of the middle ear can present as masses in the EAC (▶ Fig. 16.8). These lesions typically are seen with chronic otitis media with or without cholesteatoma.

Other causes include foreign bodies in the EAC or TM, such as retained pressure-equalizing tubes; canal cholesteatoma; osteoradionecrosis; necrotizing otitis externa; benign tumors such as ceruminomas, cystadenomas, and pleomorphic adenomas; and malignant tumors, such as squamous cell carcinomas. Most benign inflammatory polyps are not painful, and will respond to office debridement and topical therapy with steroid-antibiotic drops. Polyps that persist despite conservative treatment for several weeks indicate an underlying disease process. The most common causes are chronic otitis media and cholesteatoma. Perforations and retractions of the TM are usually seen. Temporal bone computed tomography (CT) can help determine the extent of disease. Pain is always worrisome, and is common with necrotizing otitis externa and squamous cell carcinoma. Suspicious lesions should be biopsied. A negative biopsy may indicate no cancer or a nonrepresentative sample. It may be necessary to perform deeper biopsies under local or even general anesthesia to make sure they are representative of the disease process. All polyps should be treated until resolved.

16.5.2 Ear Canal Infections

Otitis Externa

Bacterial otitis externa is a common problem for the otologist as well as the general practitioner (▶ Fig. 16.9). Infections can

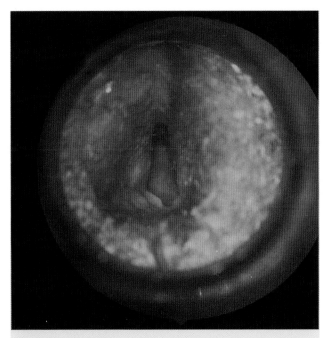

Fig. 16.9 External otitis.

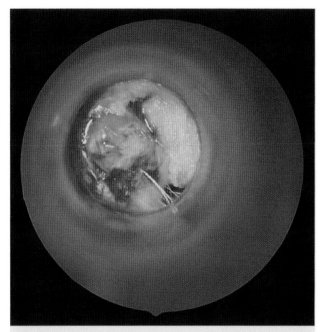

Fig. 16.10 Necrotizing otitis.

range from a brief problem in an immunocompetent individual to a devastating life-threatening infection in the immunocompromised individual. Individuals who are at risk for necrotizing otitis externa are discussed below.

Acute otitis externa is a common problem in swimmers. Swimming in contaminated water (lakes and rivers) increases the risk of pseudomonas otitis externa.[18] The increase in moisture in the EAC causes edema and a more favorable environment for bacterial overgrowth. Cerumen has an acidic pH, and helps prevent bacterial growth in the EAC. A lack of cerumen and exposure to moisture predisposes to infection. Cleaning with cotton applicators can traumatize the thin epithelial lining of the bony EAC, which then predisposes to infection. Patients who wear hearing aids also are at increased risk of otitis externa because of the moist environment that is created in the ear canal and because of occasional EAC trauma. All of the above factors can create an environment that is optimal for bacterial growth, particularly pseudomonas and to a lesser degree staphylococcal species.[19]

Patients with acute otitis externa typically present with unilateral pain and tenderness of the external ear. The pain often is quite severe, and significantly increases with manipulation of the pinna. There is usually some edema of the EAC, and less often some erythema and tenderness in the preauricular soft tissue. Patients may complain of drainage, but typically not as much as patients with chronic otitis media. Binocular microscopy shows an edematous canal, occasionally so severe that the speculum cannot be inserted. It is extremely important to remove as much EAC discharge and debris as can be performed safely. Properly cleaning the ear canal helps topical medications to resolve edematous and inflamed tissue. Occasionally the infection swells the external canal to the point that it is completely closed, and in these cases it is necessary to place a small wick for 4 or 5 days to allow the antibiotic drops to penetrate

the EAC. Forceps are used to place a 1.5-cm piece of absorbable sponge or longer gauze strip, which is able to "wick" the topical antibiotic drops into the inflamed canal.

In patients with disease involving the preauricular soft tissue and in recalcitrant cases that have failed a course of topical antibiotics, systemic antibiotic therapy may be necessary. Because ciprofloxacin has the greatest pseudomonas coverage of the quinolones, it is frequently the oral antibiotic of choice for severe acute otitis externa. Oral quinolones should be reserved for adult patients because of possible effects on cartilage growth plates in the pediatric population. With the increasing use of antibiotics, bacterial sensitivities have changed, as have recommendations for the treatment of acute otitis externa.[19] Aminoglycosides (gentamicin/tobramycin) along with neomycin and polymyxin are available as otic solutions and have proven efficacy against external otitis. However, concerns about ototoxicity have limited their use to ears in which the TM is intact.[20]

Newer antibiotics like Floxin (ofloxacin) (Janssen Pharmaceuticals Inc., Titusville, NJ) and Ciprodex (ciprofloxacin/dexamethasone) (Bayer AG, Leverkusen, Germany) have a safer therapeutic profile and are preferred for external otitis with tympanostomy tubes, or in association with otitis media. Treatment duration varies, but typically lasts 7 to 10 days. A pediatric study investigated a regimen of ofloxacin once daily for 7 days and found that it was effective in eradicating 96% of the organisms.[21]

Necrotizing External Otitis

In the immunocompromised patient otitis externa can be a much more aggressive infection, seen most frequently in the poorly controlled diabetic patients (▶ Fig. 16.10). It is also more frequent in patients with HIV and AIDS. AIDS patients are typically younger and may not have EAC granulation tissue, which is common in patients with diabetes.[22,23]

Necrotizing external otitis (NEO) is a progression of acute otitis externa in the immunocompromised host. Historically termed "malignant otitis externa," the disease can involve the temporal bone and skull base, and is essentially osteomyelitis. It usually begins as an episode of acute otitis externa, but because of the host's compromised immune status, the infection is able to spread beyond the epithelium and soft tissue of the ear canal, and penetrate the periosteum, involving the underlying temporal bone. A chronic infection then occurs, manifesting with granulation tissue formation in the EAC. Granulation and reactive inflammatory tissue replace a significant portion of the bony EAC and can mimic malignant disease. A high index of suspicion should exist in immunocompromised patients with otitis externa. Biopsies should be performed to rule out malignant disease and to obtain tissue necessary for bacterial and fungal cultures. It may be necessary to anesthetize the EAC with injected lidocaine or even perform deep biopsies under general anesthesia to obtain representative tissues samples. The disease can be fatal if not aggressively treated. The infectious organism is typically pseudomonas, but other organisms have been implicated.[24,25]

Disease extension can produce intratemporal and intracranial complications through involvement of neurovascular pathways. Inferior extension into the mastoid portion of the temporal bone can produce facial paresis and paralysis. Medial extension into the petrous apex can produce fifth and sixth nerve signs. Inferomedial extension can involve the jugular foramen, with resulting paralysis of the lower cranial nerves (IX, X, and XI), resulting in hoarseness, dysphonia, and aspiration. Extension of disease to the dura lining the medial and superior surface of the temporal bone can result in vascular (sigmoid sinus thrombosis), and intracranial complications (otitic hydrocephalus, meningitis).

These patients typically present to the otolaryngologist and otologist because they have failed topical therapy provided by their primary care physician or internist. Success in treating this disease is dependent on its early diagnosis and treatment. Any immunocompromised individual with ear pain needs to be evaluated in a timely manner, and NEO should always be suspected in this patient population. Usually the otalgia is severe, despite analgesics, and may prevent the patient from sleeping. Some patients may be febrile and can appear toxic. Frequently the diabetic patient has difficulty with glycemic control, likely secondary to the inflammatory process. Binocular examination usually shows edema and drainage in the EAC, and the pathognomonic finding is granulation tissue at the bony–cartilaginous junction. The granulation tissue should be biopsied as discussed above. The ear should be cleaned to allow topical antibiotic medications to reach the diseased tissues. Laboratory studies including a complete blood count (CBC), metabolic profile, and erythrocyte sedimentation rate (ESR) should be obtained. The patient should be started empirically on oral ciprofloxacin 750 mg p.o. b.i.d. and topical Ciprodex. A CT scan of the temporal bones, bone scan, and gallium scan should be ordered. The CT scan shows the extent of bony erosion and the extension of the disease. Both the bone scan and gallium scan show areas of increased uptake in the affected temporal bone and skull base. However, the bone scan remains positive indefinitely, and

the gallium scan no longer enhances this area once the disease process has resolved.[26]

Infectious disease consultation can be helpful to titrate antibiotics once the culture results are known and to decide the length of therapy. Because infections may be polymicrobial, an antipseudomonal cephalosporin or penicillin might be necessary in addition to oral ciprofloxacin.[27] It is also important to optimize the immune status in the immunocompromised individual, and the patient's internist or family practitioner can be helpful in this regard. Diabetic patients require tight control of blood glucose levels. Neutropenic patients also need to have their immune status optimized. These patients should be seen on a regular basis, and emergently if intratemporal or intracranial complications are suspected. Magnetic resonance imaging (MRI) can be helpful in the diagnosis of suspected intracranial extension.

Hyperbaric oxygen (HBO) therapy may have a role in treating patients with NEO, although there is generally no consensus. HBO increases the wound levels of oxygen, enhancing the abilities of phagocytes, promotes wound healing, and increases vascularization.[28] Treatment consists of 20 dives, administered once a day, 5 days a week, for 4 weeks.[29] HBO may be helpful in patients with disease not responding to conventional antibiotic therapy, in patients with recurrent disease, and in patients with intratemporal or intracranial complications.

The role of surgical therapy in NEO is also not well defined. Surgery in not indicated in patients with disease that is responding to parenteral and topical antibiotics. Aside from biopsy, patients with persistent granulation tissue, necrotic cartilage, bony sequestra, and abscesses can benefit from surgical debridement.[30] Most cranial nerve palsies that occur in NEO are not from compression, but from extension of the disease process, so it is unclear if nerve decompression is helpful.

With appropriate antimicrobial therapy, approximately 80 to 100% of patients can be cured.[31] Patients should be treated until the granulation tissue and pain resolve, and this may require 6 months of treatment. The ESR and gallium scan can be helpful in that therapy should generally be continued until these studies have normalized. Patients should be followed closely for recurrent disease, which can manifest with a recurrence of otalgia.

Furuncle

A furuncle is an abscess that typically arises from a hair follicle in the EAC (▶ Fig. 16.11). It usually presents with a localized swelling in the lateral hair-bearing portion of the ear canal. The infection usually begins as a phlegmon and can proceed to an abscess. It is usually caused by *Staphylococcus aureus*. Treatment of the phlegmon consists of topical antibiotic drops or ointment, warm compresses, and oral antibiotics. Incision and drainage under local anesthesia is performed when the phlegmon progresses to an abscess.

Otomycosis

External otitis due to fungal overgrowth is a common problem especially in patients with hearing aids (▶ Fig. 16.12; ▶ Fig. 16.13), which create a moist environment. *Aspergillus* is the most common fungus isolated from patients with otomyco-

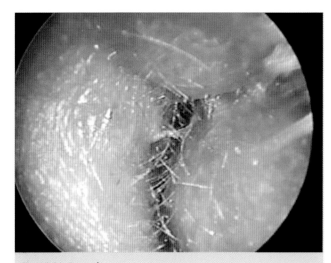

Fig. 16.11 Furuncle.

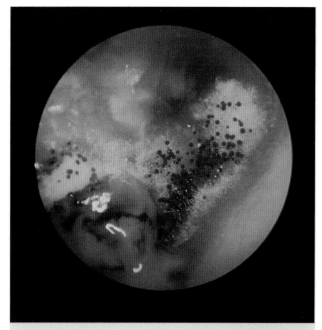

Fig. 16.12 Otomycosis.

sis, but other fungi have also been implicated.[32] The patient frequently presents with pruritus, drainage, and decreased hearing. Pain also can be a symptom, but it is usually not as severe as in bacterial otitis externa. Binocular microscopy typically reveals an edematous ear canal, sometimes with granulation, and frequently the fungal hyphae can be visualized. Usually black granular debris or soft tan discharge appearing like "wet newspaper" will be seen.

This diagnosis is best made by the physical examination, and it should also be suspected in patients treated for bacterial otitis externa that is persistent or not responding to treatment. Several options are available for treatment. Meticulous cleaning is critically important. Empiric treatment with acetic acid mixtures can begin soon after diagnosis and often are indicated for 10 to 14 days. Patients should follow water precautions during treatment. Some refractory cases require specific antifungals, but these often are off-label. Clotrimazole is an effective antifungal with activity against *Aspergillus*, but must be used with caution in patients with perforations of the TM, due to potential ototoxicity. In difficult cases with extensive disease that do not respond to topical antifungals, cultures may be helpful. Rarely are intravenous antifungals indicated in immunocompetent patients. Infectious disease consultation may be beneficial in such cases.

Viral Infections

Viral infections involving the EAC are much less common than bacterial or fungal infections, but can be quite severe. Varicella-zoster virus can manifest as Ramsay Hunt syndrome, characterized by severe ear pain usually preceding vesicular eruptions on the pinna and EAC. Varicella zoster results from reactivation of latent virus usually in the geniculate ganglion, less often in the spiral or vestibular ganglion.[33] It may cause seventh nerve paralysis, hearing loss, and vertigo. This infection is quite painful, and should be treated aggressively with acyclovir or one of the other viral DNA polymerase inhibitors. If a seventh nerve paralysis is found in a patient with a normal immune system, systemic steroids may be prescribed to speed recovery. The role of facial nerve decompression in these cases is unclear.

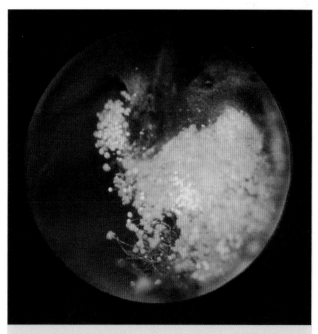

Fig. 16.13 Otomycosis.

Bullous Myringitis

Bullous myringitis is believed secondary to viral or mycoplasmal infection of the tympanic membrane and medial portion of the ear canal. It can be associated with upper respiratory infection and is more common in the winter months. Patients typically present with severe otalgia, serosanguineous otorrhea, and hearing loss. Approximately one third of patients also have serous otitis media.[34] The hearing loss can be conductive, mixed, or sensorineural, with the sensorineural component completely recovering in approximately 60% of patients.[35]

Treatment consists of topical antibiotic/steroid drops, analgesics, oral quinolone, or macrolide antibiotics for 7 to 10 days (for mycoplasma involvement), and occasional myringotomy.

16.5.3 Dermatologic Disease

Dermatitis

Dermatitis of the EAC (also known as chronic external otitis or seborrheic external otitis) may be the result of several irritants. Chemical irritants and allergens affecting the EAC may manifest as intense itching of the canal. Patients frequently complain of itching and dry flaky skin. There may be a history of eczema involving other sites, but it may only be limited to the EAC. Patients frequently report using cotton swabs or other instruments such as toothpicks or bobby pins to scratch the canal in an attempt to relieve itching. These instruments can cause lacerations of the canal, leading to a secondary bacterial infection.

Allergic dermatitis is best treated by avoidance. Hairsprays, perfumes, cosmetics, and hearing aid mold material can all be EAC irritants. Careful elimination helps resolve symptoms. Once resolution has occurred, the patient may start to reuse such items one at a time, watching for a return of symptoms to identify the offending agent. If the agent can be identified, a more hypoallergenic material should be used if the device is necessary (such as hearing aids). In patients whose symptoms persist or are severe, a topical steroid cream or even systemic steroids may be used for a short period of time to expedite resolution of symptoms.

Patients with chronic otitis media may develop dermatitis as a result of chronic drainage from a chronically infected middle ear. The infectious drainage irritates the canal causing itching and edema. Treatment involves cleaning of the ear and removing any drainage or crusts to allow topical medications to reach the middle ear and thus treat the source of the infection. Topical antibiotic drops containing a quinolone antibiotic along with steroid are effective in treating the infection, and also help decrease any secondary inflammation of the EAC.

Most patients with chronic external otitis/dermatitis have no topical allergy, no microbial infection, and no chronic otitis media. They may or may not have a more generalized dermatologic condition. Treatment has both an acute phase and a maintenance phase to prevent recurrence. If the canal is swollen shut, a steroid-impregnated gauze wick is inserted for 2 or 3 days. The patient returns, the wick is removed, and the ear canal is carefully cleaned. If the dermatitis produces copious canal debris, the patient should irrigate the canal with 2 to 3 ounces (or more) of dilute white vinegar (50% white vinegar and 50% water boiled 5 minutes then cooled to body/room temperature) prior to instilling drops. Then four drops of otic solution are placed in the canal for 5 minutes. One particularly effective solution is Locoid (hydrocortisone butyrate) 0.1% topical solution, which also contains alcohol, mineral oil, and other soothing ingredients. After 5 minutes the drops are removed from the canal. This flush-and-drop treatment is repeated at least three times daily for the first week. The patient can return to the physician for cleaning and a progress report if necessary. In the second week, this flush/drop combination is continued twice a day, in the third week once a day, then every other day until the patient titrates the treatment to prevent itching and other symptoms. As water aggravates the condition, the patient should remain on dry ear precautions indefinitely.

16.5.4 Canal Atresia

As discussed in the beginning of this chapter, failure of the canalization of EAC can result in various degrees of canal (and auricular) atresia. This occurs more commonly unilaterally, but may also occur bilaterally. The incidence of canal atresia is 1 in 10,000 to 1 in 20,000 births.[36] Canal atresia can be isolated, or associated with various syndromes. It may be accompanied by microtia or several middle ear anomalies. All of these factors play a role in selecting patients who are amenable to surgical correction. In patients with canal atresia in association with microtia, it is preferable to repair the microtia first, and this is generally performed when the patient is 6 to 8 years old. The reasons for this are several. At age 8, the pinna is almost adult size. Also, most microtia reconstructions are staged and utilize the skin in the pre- and postauricular area. If the canal atresia is repaired first (usually through a postauricular approach), then this skin can no longer be used.

Preoperative Evaluation

Proper patient selection is important when considering congenital canal atresia repair. The surgical procedure can be difficult secondary to the lack of normal landmarks and the potential for an aberrant facial nerve. The facial nerve may also have a more lateral course. Absence of a tympanic membrane and an abnormal ossicular chain may make location of the horizontal semicircular canal difficult. Grading systems have been developed to help decide which candidates may best benefit from surgical repair.

Jahrsdoerfer et al[37] developed a preoperative grading system that utilized temporal bone CT scanning and clinical evaluation of the external ear (▶ Table 16.1). Based on their system, a patient with at least a 60% chance (six out of 10 possible points) of having a 15- to 25-dB speech reception threshold (SRT) postoperatively would be a good surgical candidate. A CT scan is pivotal in the preoperative evaluation of these patients. CT scanning is useful in identifying potential anomalies in the cochlea, vestibule, semicircular canals, endolymphatic duct, internal auditory canal, and course of the facial nerve. Finally, it is important to obtain a preoperative audiogram to document a functioning cochlea. The vast majority of these patients have a 50- to 60-dB conductive hearing loss from loss of function of the EAC and middle ear structures.

Nonsurgical modalities of treatment should also be discussed with the patient and family members. Hearing aids can be beneficial. Patients with unilateral atresia may not desire or want to wear hearing devices even though the benefits of binaural hearing are significant. Patients with bilateral atresia should be aided early to optimize speech development. Previously if the atresia was severe and bilateral, it was not possible for patients to use even small traditional hearing devices. Now with development of bone-anchored hearing aids (BAHAs), even patients with severe microtia and atresia can be aided early without the bulky external devices that were required in the past. Some studies support the use of bilateral BAHAs to improve localization of sound and speech perception.[38] This allows patients to

Table 16.1 Jahrsdoerfer Grading System of Candidacy for Atresia Repair

Parameter	Points
Stapes present	2
Oval window open	1
Normal facial nerve	1
Malleus-incus complex present	1
Appearance of external ear	1
Middle ear space	1
Normal round window	1
Well-pneumatized mastoid	1
Incus-stapes connection	1
Total Points	**Type of Candidate**
10	Excellent
9	Very good
8	Good
7	Fair
6	Marginal
5 or less	Poor

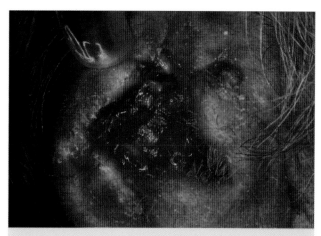

Fig. 16.14 Invasive squamous cell carcinoma.

have excellent hearing during their lengthy staged surgical correction. These devices utilize a titanium implant placed directly into the bone just above the postauricular area. The implant becomes osseointegrated several months after implantation. The patient is then fitted with a sound processor that snaps onto the titanium abutment, which vibrates the temporal bone and cochlea, bypassing the EAC and middle ear structures.

Surgical Treatment

Surgical correction of the atretic ear canal most commonly is performed in a single stage. Occasionally a second stage is required. The first stage addresses the external ear with canaloplasty, tympanoplasty, and meatoplasty. Two surgical approaches are possible: a direct approach using the root of the zygoma and the glenoid fossa as primary landmarks, or a posterior approach utilizing a mastoidectomy and early identification of the facial nerve. In either approach one must be very cognizant of the facial nerve, and in all cases facial nerve monitoring is used. The middle ear structures are identified, the stapes is checked for mobility, and a decision is made about the malleus/incus complex. It may be necessary to remove the malleus/incus complex, especially if it is fixed. An ossiculoplasty can be performed if necessary. Another option is to use a laser to mobilize the malleus/incus complex. If the stapes is fixed, a stapedectomy should be performed at a second stage. A canaloplasty and meatoplasty are performed. A bony trough for the location of the tympanic annulus is created. A fascia graft is used to construct a new TM. This graft is placed over the malleus/incus complex, or on top of the ossiculoplasty.

A split-thickness skin graft is harvested from the ipsilateral thigh and used to line the new ear canal. Laterally, this graft is sutured to the meatoplasty. The meatoplasty should be large enough to allow for routine examination and good visualization of the TM and middle ear. Because the skin graft does not have the same migration kinetics as a normal ear, regular visits are necessary and frequent cleaning is required. Current advances in atresia repair utilizing lasers, thinner split-thickness skin grafts, Silastic sheets, and wicks in the EAC have improved outcomes.[39]

16.5.5 Neoplasms

Benign Neoplasms

Benign neoplasms of the EAC are rare, and usually arise from ceruminous glands. These tumors usually present as a painless mass in the cartilaginous portion of the ear canal. As the tumors enlarge, patients can develop pain, aural fullness, hearing loss, and otorrhea. The two most common types of benign EAC neoplasms are ceruminous adenoma and pleomorphic adenoma. Biopsies should be obtained with a margin of normal tissue to rule out invasion and to help distinguish these benign tumors from adenoid cystic carcinoma and ceruminous adenocarcinoma. The treatment of benign tumors of the EAC is wide local excision with negative margins.[40]

Malignant Neoplasms

Malignancies of the temporal bone are fortunately rare, with an estimated incidence of 1 to 6 per 1,000,000, and malignancies of the EAC comprise approximately 25% of those cases (▶ Fig. 16.14; ▶ Fig. 16.15; ▶ Fig. 16.16).[41] Squamous cell carcinoma is the most common malignancy of the EAC in adults. In children sarcomas are the most frequent malignancy of the temporal bone. Other malignancies seen in the EAC include adenoid cystic carcinoma and acinic cell carcinoma.[42] The presentation of these lesions varies significantly. They may present with pain, drainage, and hearing loss mimicking benign disease, or they may be completely asymptomatic. Because symptoms can imitate benign diseases like chronic otitis externa, the diagnosis can be delayed, and therefore all patients with nonresolving "granulation tissue" should be biopsied to confirm the diagnosis. A negative biopsy may not be diagnostic.

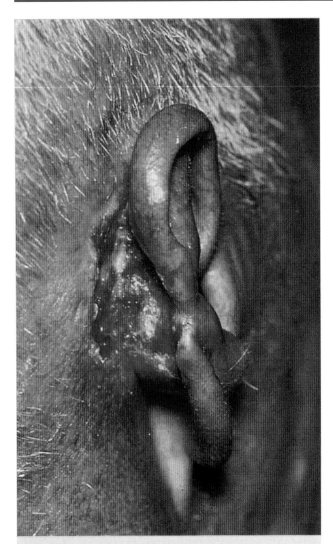

Fig. 16.15 Basal cell carcinoma.

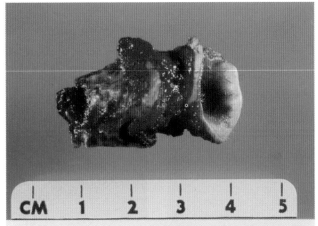

Fig. 16.16 External canal resection specimen.

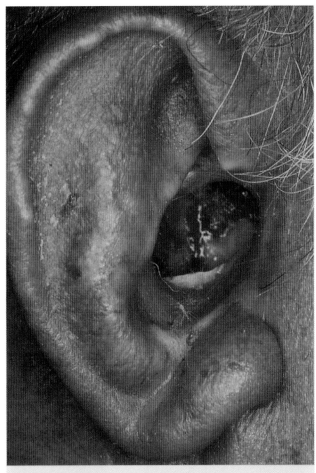

Fig. 16.17 Postoperative osteoradionecrosis.

Multiple biopsies may be necessary, sometimes even under general anesthesia if necessary.

Preoperative imaging should include a CT scan of the temporal bone to assess bony destruction. MRI gives superior detail in assessing local soft tissue invasion. Staging is based on clinical and radiographic findings. Most centers treating malignant disease of the temporal bone utilize a multidisciplinary team including an otologist, head and neck surgical oncologist, reconstructive surgeon, medical oncologist, and radiation therapist. Many patients present with advanced disease, and a combination of surgery and radiation is often required. The surgical procedure required is usually a form of lateral temporal bone resection, with the extent of surgery based on staging. Chapter 27 further discusses this disorder.

16.5.6 Osteoradionecrosis

Osteoradionecrosis (ORN) of the temporal bone is a complication occurring from radiation treatment of skull base malignancies (▶ Fig. 16.17), but idiopathic variants exist.[43]

Patient presentation varies, and symptoms include ear fullness, hearing loss, pain, discharge, tinnitus, and bloody otorrhea. On binocular microscopy there is often debris in the canal, with occasional granulation tissue. There may be single or multiple areas of exposed EAC bone. The devascularized bone is often yellowish in color, spiculated, and soft. Neighboring granulation tissue should be biopsied if persistent. ORN may be localized or diffuse,[44] with localized disease occurring because the EAC is in the radiation portal (as in nasopharyngeal carcinoma), and diffuse disease occurring from direct high-dose radiation therapy to the temporal bone. Localized ORN usually is a less aggressive form of disease and often responds to serial office debridements and topical antibiotic therapy. Diffuse ORN is more lethal, and the necrotic temporal bone is at risk for intratemporal and intracranial neurovascular complications. In such cases, the management is very like the treatment of NEO. Surgical debridement, intravenous antibiotics, and HBO therapy may all be required.

References

[1] Gulya AJ. Developmental anatomy of the temporal bone and skull base. In: Glasscock ME III, Gulya AJ, eds. Surgery of the Ear, 5th ed. Lewiston, NY: BC Decker, 2002:3–8

[2] Okuda I, Bingham B, Stoney P, Hawke M. The organic composition of earwax. J Otolaryngol 1991; 20: 212–215

[3] Gray H. Anatomy of the Human Body. Philadelphia: Lea & Febiger, 1918; www.bartleby.com/107/, 2000

[4] Kakoi H, Anniko M, Kinnefors A, Rask-Andersen H. Auditory epidermal cell migration. VII. Antigen expression of proliferating cell nuclear antigens, PCNA and Ki-67 in human tympanic membrane and external auditory canal. Acta Otolaryngol 1997; 117: 100–108

[5] Vennix PP, Kuijpers W, Peters TA, Tonnaer EL, Ramaekers FC. Epidermal differentiation in the human external auditory meatus. Laryngoscope 1996; 106: 470–475

[6] Bapat U, Nia J, Bance M. Severe audiovestibular loss following ear syringing for wax removal. J Laryngol Otol 2001; 115: 410–411

[7] Capo JM, Lucente FE. Alkaline battery foreign bodies of the ear and nose. Arch Otolaryngol Head Neck Surg 1986; 112: 562–563

[8] Antonelli PJ, Ahmadi A, Prevatt A. Insecticidal activity of common reagents for insect foreign bodies of the ear. Laryngoscope 2001; 111: 15–20

[9] Hurst W, Bailey M, Hurst B. Prevalence of external auditory canal exostoses in Australian surfboard riders. J Laryngol Otol 2004; 118: 348–351

[10] Kroon DF, Lawson ML, Derkay CS, Hoffmann K, McCook J. Surfer's ear: external auditory exostoses are more prevalent in cold water surfers. Otolaryngol Head Neck Surg 2002; 126: 499–504

[11] Van Gilse PHG. Des observations ulterieures sur la genes des exostoses du conduit externe par l'irriations d'eau froide. Acta Otolaryngol 1938; 26: 343

[12] Stenfors LE, Sade J, Hellström S, Anniko M, Folkow L. Exostoses and cavernous venous formation in the external auditory canal of the hooded seal as a functional physiological organ. Acta Otolaryngol 2000; 120: 940–943

[13] Graham MD. Osteomas and exostoses of the external auditory canal. A clinical, histopathologic and scanning electron microscopic study. Ann Otol Rhinol Laryngol 1979; 88: 566–572

[14] Timofeev I, Notkina N, Smith IM. Exostoses of the external auditory canal: a long-term follow-up study of surgical treatment. Clin Otolaryngol Allied Sci 2004; 29: 588–594

[15] Piepergerdes MC, Kramer BM, Behnke EE. Keratosis obturans and external auditory canal cholesteatoma. Laryngoscope 1980; 90: 383–391

[16] Persaud RA, Hajioff D, Thevasagayam MS, Wareing MJ, Wright A. Keratosis obturans and external ear canal cholesteatoma: how and why we should distinguish between these conditions. Clin Otolaryngol Allied Sci 2004; 29: 577–581

[17] Garin P, Degols JC, Delos M. External auditory canal cholesteatoma. Arch Otolaryngol Head Neck Surg 1997; 123: 62–65

[18] Hajjartabar M. Poor-quality water in swimming pools associated with a substantial risk of otitis externa due to Pseudomonas aeruginosa. Water Sci Technol 2004; 50: 63–67

[19] Roland PS, Stroman DW. Microbiology of acute otitis externa. Laryngoscope 2002; 112: 1166–1177

[20] Bath AP, Walsh RM, Bance ML, Rutka JA. Ototoxicity of topical gentamicin preparations. Laryngoscope 1999; 109: 1088–1093

[21] Torum B, Block SL, Avila H et al. Efficacy of ofloxacin otic solution once daily for 7 days in the treatment of otitis externa: a multicenter, open-label, phase III trial. Clin Ther 2004; 26: 1046–1054

[22] Weinroth SE, Schessel D, Tuazon CU. Malignant otitis externa in AIDS patients: case report and review of the literature. Ear Nose Throat J 1994; 73: 772–774, 777–778

[23] Ress BD, Luntz M, Telischi FF, Balkany TJ, Whiteman ML. Necrotizing external otitis in patients with AIDS. Laryngoscope 1997; 107: 456–460

[24] Muñoz A, Martínez-Chamorro E. Necrotizing external otitis caused by Aspergillus fumigatus: computed tomography and high resolution magnetic resonance imaging in an AIDS patient. J Laryngol Otol 1998; 112: 98–102

[25] Soldati D, Mudry A, Monnier P. Necrotizing otitis externa caused by Staphylococcus epidermidis. Eur Arch Otorhinolaryngol 1999; 256: 439–441

[26] Parisier SC, Lucente FE, Som PM, Hirschman SZ, Arnold LM, Roffman JD. Nuclear scanning in necrotizing progressive "malignant" external otitis. Laryngoscope 1982; 92: 1016–1019

[27] Gehanno P. Ciprofloxacin in the treatment of malignant external otitis. Chemotherapy 1994; 40 Suppl 1: 35–40

[28] Davis JC, Gates GA, Lerner C, Davis MG, Jr, Mader JT, Dinesman A. Adjuvant hyperbaric oxygen in malignant external otitis. Arch Otolaryngol Head Neck Surg 1992; 118: 89–93

[29] Mader JT, Love JT. Malignant external otitis. Cure with adjunctive hyperbaric oxygen therapy. Arch Otolaryngol 1982; 108: 38–40

[30] Babiatzki A, Sadé J. Malignant external otitis. J Laryngol Otol 1987; 101: 205–210

[31] Johnson MP, Ramphal R. Malignant external otitis: report on therapy with ceftazidime and review of therapy and prognosis. Rev Infect Dis 1990; 12: 173–180

[32] Kaur R, Mittal N, Kakkar M, Aggarwal AK, Mathur MD. Otomycosis: a clinicomycologic study. Ear Nose Throat J 2000; 79: 606–609

[33] Kuhweide R, Van de Steene V, Vlaminck S, Casselman JW. Ramsay Hunt syndrome: pathophysiology of cochleovestibular symptoms. J Laryngol Otol 2002; 116: 844–848Review.

[34] Marais J, Dale BA. Bullous myringitis: a review. Clin Otolaryngol Allied Sci 1997; 22: 497–499

[35] Hariri MA. Sensorineural hearing loss in bullous myringitis. A prospective study of eighteen patients. Clin Otolaryngol Allied Sci 1990; 15: 351–353

[36] De La Cruz A, Chandrasekhar SS. Congenital malformation of the temporal bone. In: Brackmann DE, Shelton C, Arriaga M, eds. Otologic Surgery. Philadelphia: WB Saunders, 2001:54–67

[37] Jahrsdoerfer RA, Yeakley JW, Aguilar EA, Cole RR, Gray LC. Grading system for the selection of patients with congenital aural atresia. Am J Otol 1992; 13: 6–12

[38] van der Pouw KT, Snik AF, Cremers CW. Audiometric results of bilateral bone-anchored hearing aid application in patients with bilateral congenital aural atresia. Laryngoscope 1998; 108: 548–553

[39] Teufert KB, De la Cruz A. Advances in congenital aural atresia surgery: effects on outcome. Otolaryngol Head Neck Surg 2004; 131: 263–270

[40] Hicks GW. Tumors arising from the glandular structures of the external auditory canal. Laryngoscope 1983; 93: 326–340

[41] Morton RP, Stell PM, Derrick PPO. Epidemiology of cancer of the middle ear cleft. Cancer 1984; 53: 1612–1617

[42] Kinney SE, Wood BG. Malignancies of the external ear canal and temporal bone: surgical techniques and results. Laryngoscope 1987; 97: 158–164

[43] Goufas G. [Diagnosis and pathogenesis of benign necrotic osteitis of the external ear canal] Ann Otolaryngol 1954; 71: 390–396

[44] Ramsden RT, Bulman CH, Lorigan BP. Osteoradionecrosis of the temporal bone. J Laryngol Otol 1975; 89: 941–955

17 Aural Atresia and Unilateral Hearing Loss

Bradley W. Kesser and Daniel I. Choo

17.1 Introduction

Management of unilateral hearing loss in children remains in a state of flux. On the one hand, with normal hearing in one ear and no other cognitive issues, children will develop normal receptive and expressive speech and language skills. In 1978, leaders in audiology issued the following position statement on unilateral hearing loss, "Audiologists and otolaryngologists are not usually concerned over such [unilateral] deafness, other than to identify its etiology and assure the parents that there will be no handicap."[1]

On the other hand, the pioneering work of Bess and Tharpe in the middle to late 1980s clearly demonstrated that a subset of children with unilateral sensorineural hearing loss (USNHL) is at great risk for grade retention and academic difficulty. Otolaryngologists, audiologists, and other hearing health care professionals were awakened to the disabilities associated with unilateral hearing loss in children and have now recommended amplification or other resources for children with USNHL. Despite intervention, however, a more recent review has shown that children with USNHL continue to experience significant rates of grade retention and need for resources and additional educational assistance.[2] Children with USNHL also demonstrate worse language skills than their siblings on the oral portion of the Oral and Written Language Scales (OWLS); these children were more likely to have an individualized education program and to have received speech therapy.[3]

What then, are the current recommendations for children with unilateral hearing loss? This chapter reviews basic information on unilateral hearing loss in children, both sensorineural hearing loss (SNHL) and conductive hearing loss (CHL), and provides a rational algorithm to help otolaryngologists ensure that these children have the optimal resources to succeed in the academic setting.

17.2 Demographics

Older estimates of the prevalence of unilateral hearing loss (UHL) in children range from 3 to 13 (depending on audiometric criteria) per 1,000.[4] In a 1988 review of the second National Health and Nutrition Examination Survey (NHANES-II; 1976–1980), Lee et al[5] found that 6 to 12 per 1,000 school-aged children (6 to 19 years) had some form of UHL, and 0 to 5 per 1,000 had moderate to profound UHL; it was estimated that some 391,000 school-aged children in the United States had UHL. In a more recent review of studies reporting prevalence rates of hearing loss in children and adolescents, the average prevalence of mild (or worse) unilateral or bilateral hearing impairment (pure tone average [PTA]$_{0.5 \text{ to } 2.0 \text{ kHz}}$ > 25 dB) was 3.1% (range, 1.7–5.0%).[6] Another recent study reviewing the third National Health and Nutrition Examination Survey (NHANES-III; 1988–1994) showed that prevalence estimates for UHL varied from 3.0 to 6.3% depending on the case definition of unilateral hearing loss.[7] The 2001–2006 NHANES survey shows an overall prevalence rate of bilateral and unilateral hearing loss

(≥ 25 dB) in adolescents (ages 12 to 19) of 2.3% (range, 1.5–3.1%), an estimated 760,000 adolescents.[8]

By contrast, estimates of the prevalence of congenital aural atresia (in the setting of microtia) range from 0.83 to 17.4 per 10,000 depending on the population studied, with high rates of microtia in Quito, Ecuador; Chile; and the Navajo Indian population; and low rates in Malta, Ireland, and Belgium.[9] In the United States, rates of 2.0 and 2.8 per 10,000 were seen in California and Texas, with a high of 3.8 in Hawaii.[9] Interestingly, in the California population, race was a covariate in prevalence rates of aural atresia, with Hispanics having higher rates (3.23 per 10,000) than Asians (2.18 per 10,000), African Americans (1.22 per 10,000), and whites (1.17 per 10,000).[10] Right ears are more commonly affected than left (57–67%),[9] males more often affected than females,[11] and unilateral atresia far more prevalent than bilateral (75–90%).

17.3 Disability Associated with Unilateral Hearing Loss

From a purely physiological standpoint, the binaural advantage, the advantage gained by having two functioning ears, improves hearing in background noise, enables the listener to pick out the signal from the noise, and facilitates sound localization. Implications and effects of the loss of the binaural advantage have been the focus of major research in corrected bilateral CHL secondary to otitis media with effusion,[12] corrected unilateral CHL after stapedectomy,[13] bilateral cochlear implantation,[14–18] bone-anchored hearing systems,[19–21] corrected USNHL with amplification,[1,22] and the academic success of school-aged children.[2,23–25] In the mid-1980s, Bess and Tharpe[24] reported on a cohort of 60 children with USNHL: 35% of these children failed a grade, and another 13% required some type of resource assistance, such as conventional hearing aid or frequency modulated (FM) system. The authors found that children with more severe hearing loss were at greater risk for academic problems. Other investigators in the 1980s, 1990s, and 2000s confirmed the Bess and Tharpe findings,[1,2,25–28] but what is surprising is that more recent studies show that despite better resource utilization, children with USNHL continue to have academic and language difficulty,[2] as demonstrated by scores on the Oral and Written Language Scales as compared to their normal-hearing siblings,[3] and need a greater signal-to-noise ratio in adverse listening conditions,[29] and as compared to their peers with unilateral aural atresia.[30]

Because of its relative rarity, less is known about the disabilities associated with unilateral congenital aural atresia (CAA). CAA is generally associated with a moderate or moderate to severe CHL with normal bone conduction thresholds. Speech testing generally shows speech reception thresholds that correlate with the PTA, in the 45- to 65-dB HL range. Speech discrimination scores are often very good.[30] Evidence suggests that children with unilateral aural atresia, compared with a matched control group of children with USNHL, have a far lower grade-retention rate (0% vs. 18%) with similar rates of resource utilization (65% vs. 63%).[30] Why these children with a degree of hearing loss that is similar to that of their USNHL peers do better in school is the subject of ongoing research and has implications for the optimal resources needed for these children.

Evidence does not yet exist, however, to determine which children with mild bilateral or unilateral hearing loss will experience difficulties, and consequently which children will benefit from early intervention and early amplification.[1] Identifying that subset and providing the resources they need (and specifically, what exactly those resources are) to succeed in school continues to be a source of research and practical interest.

17.4 Congenital Aural Atresia

Children with bilateral CAA need comprehensive audiological evaluation shortly after birth. Most patients with atresia of the ear canal have associated microtia, so both the cosmetic and functional disabilities are easily recognized. Bone conducted auditory brainstem response testing by a skilled audiologist establishes cochlear function in infants with aural atresia. In general, cochlear function is normal in children with aural atresia because the cochlea and inner ear structures develop from a separate embryological anlage (otocyst and neural tube) than the outer and middle ear (branchial apparatus). Nevertheless, the incidence of inner ear malformations is higher in the atresia population (as high as 22%) than in the general population, although many of the inner ear variants in this study were not associated with SNHL.[32]

These bilateral CAA children are then fitted with bone conducting hearing devices, a hard or soft headband coupled to a bone oscillator, or a power hearing aid. Children with these devices who are given speech therapy have an excellent chance to develop normal speech and language skills. When the child is older, a surgically implanted bone-anchored hearing device (Cochlear BAHA [bone-anchored hearing aid] System, Cochlear Corp., Sydney, Australia; Ponto Pro, Oticon Medical, Somerset, NJ) can be placed as a more comfortable and more efficient sound transducing system; the Food and Drug Administration (FDA) has approved these devices for children 5 years of age and older. Alternatively, when the child is older, a decision can also be made to proceed with atresia surgery if the child is a candidate.

Unlike their peers with unilateral SNHL, children with unilateral CAA are less likely to repeat a grade in elementary school. A large proportion of these children (65%) utilize some resource in the academic setting, such as an individualized education program (IEP), speech therapy, or some form of amplification (including an FM system).[30] One possible explanation for this disparity is that a CHL may not be truly as debilitating as an equivalent degree of SNHL. Given the different embryological derivation of the cochlea and central auditory pathways from the outer and middle ear, theoretically, the cochlea and central pathways should be intact and functioning in patients with aural atresia. As a result, in CHL associated with aural atresia, the cochlea and central auditory pathways are being stimulated when the child speaks or even chews. If ambient sound is loud enough, the atretic ear will also be stimulated. In unpublished data, crossed acoustic reflexes, when the atretic ear is stimulated by sound after surgical repair, can be recorded from the normal hearing ear. The ability to record a crossed acoustic reflex after the atretic ear has been surgically opened offers proof of principle of functional integrity of the acoustic reflex arc despite years of some degree of sensory deprivation to the ear.

Children with unilateral atresia may also fare better in the school setting because of the early identification of the hearing loss with early intervention due to the cosmetic deformity (i.e., microtia) usually accompanying the atresia. The hearing deficit is identified from the day of birth, so children can receive a thorough evaluation and resources early in life. The cosmetic deformity is a constant reminder of the functional deficit, so parents are motivated to continue to use resources to help their child.

The decision to aid a child with unilateral aural atresia with a bone conducting hearing device is a complex one with physiological, psychosocial, and possibly academic ramifications. Because the population of unilateral atresia children is relatively small, large-cohort studies have not systematically examined this question. Randomized trials are not ethical; parents must decide what is best for their child. Some families choose to aid their children with unilateral atresia early on, even from the first months of life; some choose to use other resources, such as speech therapy, IEPs, or FM systems; and some choose simply to monitor their child's academic progress and intervene if necessary. As noted, the cosmetic deformity (microtia) may be a constant reminder of the associated functional disability, so parents and teachers are motivated to pursue resources and to use them consistently to help children succeed in the classroom. Unilateral SNHL is a "silent" disability, so parents, teachers, and children may not be as compulsive about resource use.

One resource potentially available to parents of children with aural atresia not available to children with USNHL is surgery to open the canal and restore the natural sound conducting mechanism of the outer and middle ear. Recent evidence supports a child's improved ability to hear in background noise after atresia repair,[33] but there are no data at this time to suggest that surgery improves a child's academic performance, although such a study is in progress.

17.5 Surgery for Aural Atresia

Significant hearing improvement through a clean, dry, well-epithelialized ear canal and widely patent meatus can be achieved in many patients with aural atresia. Not all children with aural atresia are candidates for surgical repair. Candidacy for surgery rests on audiological and radiological evaluations. Normal bone conduction thresholds for the atretic ear are absolute; surgery is not recommended for patients with SNHL. High-resolution, thin-section (≤ 1 mm) computed tomography (CT) imaging of the temporal bone remains the study of choice to evaluate the bony anatomy of the inner ear, middle ear, mastoid, and atretic plate. The Jahrsdoerfer grading scale focuses the clinician on the critical anatomic aspects of the temporal bone and even has some prognostic significance: Patients with scores of 7 or greater have far better hearing outcomes than do patients scoring 6 or below.[34,35] Surgery for patients with unilateral atresia is not recommended for patients with scores of 6 or below, or scores of 5 or below in patients with bilateral atresia.

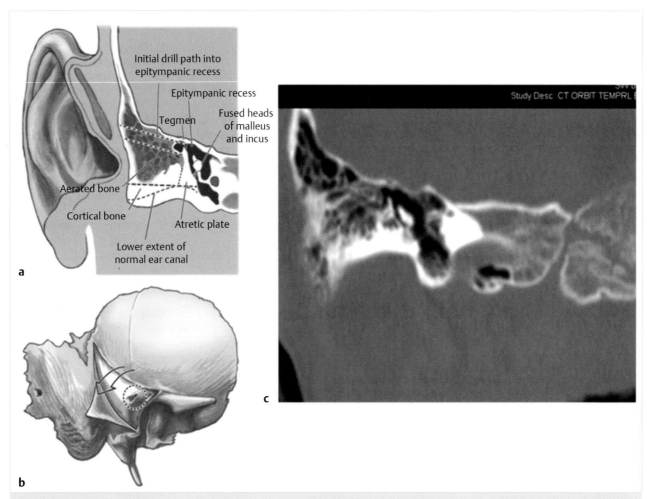

Fig. 17.1 (a) Path of drilling for canaloplasty in repair of aural atresia. Drilling follows the tegmen into the epitympanum, where the fused malleus–incus complex can be identified [correlate with (c), coronal computed tomography image at the level of the fused malleus–incus complex. Drilling follows the tegmen into the epitympanum). (b) Posteriorly based periosteal flap used for exposure of the bony cortex in preparation for canaloplasty drilling. (Used with permission from Kesser BW. Surgery for congenital aural atresia. In: McKinnon BJ, ed. Operative Techniques in Otolaryngology–Head and Neck Surgery: Techniques for the Ear (Part II), vol. 21, issue 4. New York: Elsevier, 2010:278-286.)

Most recent studies analyzing surgery for aural atresia attempt to define preoperative prognostic factors for hearing improvement, including middle ear volume,[35-37] preoperative hearing,[30] and the angulation of the incudostapedial joint.[38] A patient with a well-aerated middle ear has a greater chance of achieving normal hearing with surgery than the patient with a poorly aerated middle ear. Better hearing preoperatively predicts better hearing postoperatively.[32] Wide (> 120°) incudostapedial joint angle predicts worse outcome after atresia surgery.[38] These studies, however, lack long-term follow-up. The long-term complications of atresia surgery, including meatal stenosis (most common) and loss of early preoperative gains, remain a significant problem.[39,40]

The technique of aural atresia repair is well described elsewhere,[41] but a few technical modifications to the anterior approach first described by Jahrsdoerfer[42] merit discussion. The tegmen is identified early in the canaloplasty and followed medially into the epitympanum (▶ Fig. 17.1). The fused malleus–incus complex is identified, and atretic bone is removed 360 degrees around the ossicles, with care taken not to transmit the high energy of the drill to the ossicular chain. The final ligamentous attachments between the neck of the malleus and the atretic plate are incised with a sharp No. 59 beaver blade or laser (▶ Fig. 17.2).

Temporalis fascia is placed in an overlay fashion, draped over the fused malleus–incus complex and extended 1 to 2 mm up onto the canal wall in all directions. The skin graft is taken with a 2-inch guard at 0.006 inches and notched along the medial edge so that the notches align over the temporalis fascia, and all fascia is covered by the skin graft which is meticulously placed up onto the bony canal wall with all skin edges unfurled (▶ Fig. 17.3).

The soft tissue meatus is often low because the bony canal is centered over the epitympanum and not the mesotympanum. As such, the reconstructed auricle occasionally must be elevated to align the meatus with the bony canal. An important note: if the family has chosen Medpor for microtia reconstruction, the atresia surgery must precede Medpor repair so as not to risk exposing the polyethylene implant. For autologous rib cartilage microtia repair, atresia surgery follows the rib graft reconstruction.

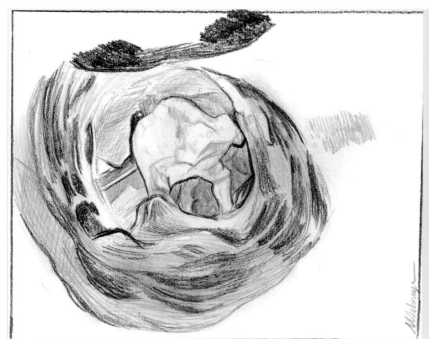

Fig. 17.2 The freed malleus–incus complex after completing the drilling and incising the final ligamentous attachments between the neck of the malleus and the atretic plate.

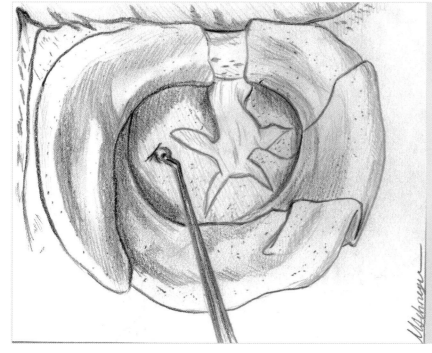

Fig. 17.3 Notches are made along the medial edge of the split-thickness skin graft. These notches are aligned over the temporalis fascia eardrum graft, and the skin graft is delivered up onto the bony canal wall with all skin edges unfurled.

For prevention of postoperative meatal stenosis, a depot steroid (triamcinolone) is injected into the perimeatal skin. Stenting has also been found helpful postoperatively to prevent meatal stenosis.[43] This is instituted after the 1-month postoperative visit and continued for at least 3 to 6 months if the meatus appears to be narrowing. Despite best efforts, meatal stenosis is the most common postoperative complication, and the meatus will occasionally stenose to the point of needing revision surgery. Revision meatoplasty with skin grafting is generally recommended with aggressive postoperative measures of triamcinolone injection and use of a foam earplug coated in water soluble lubricant at night.[40]

Functionally, 1 month after atresia surgery, patients hear better in background noise and perform better than their preoperative performance on a virtual sound localization task. These patients enjoy binaural summation and head shadow effects, but do not reliably exhibit binaural release from masking (squelch).[44] There was an age effect in this study: teenagers perform better than young children and older adults on tests of binaural processing. Perhaps, too, there is a learning curve, in that patients must learn how to "use" their new ear in tasks of true binaural processing; these tests of the binaural advantage are being repeated to gather long-term data.

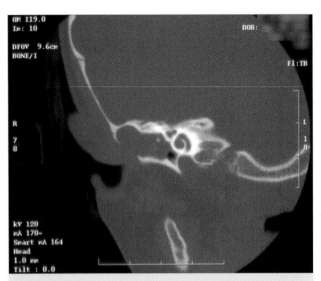

Fig. 17.4 Coronal computed tomography (CT) image of a rounded, soft tissue density filling the external auditory canal and extending into the middle ear space of a patient with an acquired ear canal cholesteatoma in the setting of congenital aural stenosis. Note the rounded smooth bony erosion pattern.

17.6 Other Congenital Unilateral Hearing Losses

17.6.1 Conductive Hearing Loss

Bellucci categorized congenital CHLs as major (aural atresia, absence of the ear canal) or minor malformations. Minor malformations are those characterized by an intact tympanic membrane and patent ear canal, and include congenital stapes fixation or ankylosis (the most common),[45,46] malleus bar,[47] absent oval window,[48] persistent stapedial artery,[49] single stapes crus,[50] shortened or "spindle" malleus,[47] disarticulation of the incudostapedial joint,[50] and other rare configurations. Temporal bone CT imaging is the standard of care prior to surgical intervention in a child with a CHL, normal ear canal, and tympanic membrane, and a clear middle ear space on exam.

Conductive hearing loss in a child can also be caused by congenital cholesteatoma, typically seen as a white mass behind an intact tympanic membrane, often located in the anterosuperior quadrant of the mesotympanum. Congenital cholesteatomas arising posteriorly may not be visible through the tympanic membrane and can achieve large size before abutting the incus and causing CHL. Delay in diagnosis can result in ossicular erosion and overall poor hearing outcomes,[51] prompting many otologists to recommend a CT evaluation for any child with an unexplained CHL.

Acquired ear canal cholesteatoma can develop as a result of congenital aural stenosis. Skin becomes trapped in the stenotic ear canal and develops into cholesteatoma as it erodes surrounding bone (▶ Fig. 17.4). Stenotic canals 2 mm or narrower are at risk.[52] Many patients with aural stenosis have concomitant ossicular hypoplasia/atresia. Preoperative imaging is a necessity. The first priority is to give the child a safe ear, removing the cholesteatoma, performing a canaloplasty to ensure all disease has been removed, and staging the operation by oversewing the lateral ear canal. The ear can be revisited at a later date to complete the formal atresia operation by freeing the ossicular chain and performing tympanoplasty, skin grafting, and wide meatoplasty.

Although not congenital, neoplastic processes causing CHL in a child are rare and include middle ear adenoma, facial nerve hemangioma, rhabdomyosarcoma, paraganglioma, eosinophilic granuloma, schwannoma, choristoma, and others. Any mass behind an intact tympanic membrane must have a radiological evaluation, often with both high-resolution CT and magnetic resonance imaging (MRI), prior to biopsy or surgical intervention.

When sound energy transmitted to the vestibule through the stapes footplate is lost through a third window, the patient can have a sensorineural, conductive, or mixed hearing loss. Audiometric third-window findings include low-frequency CHL (although the hearing loss may be mid-range or high frequency), suprathreshold bone conduction thresholds, and intact acoustic reflexes (as compared to ossicular fixation [e.g., otosclerosis], where acoustic reflexes may be absent or an A_s pattern). An enlarged vestibular aqueduct is one such example of a third window; the condition may be unilateral or bilateral, and the hearing loss can be conductive, sensorineural, or mixed,[53] and stable or progressive.[54] The conductive component is thought to arise from these third-window lesions as sound energy is dissipated through the third window and lost, decreasing the energy available to the cochlea.[55] Dehiscence of the superior semicircular canal also acts as a third window, but reports of this anomaly in children are rare.[56]

The practitioner should be wary about scheduling a child with a CHL for middle ear exploration; the surgeon may encounter a mobile stapes bone if a CT of the temporal bone is not reviewed for the presence of a third window, especially an enlarged vestibular aqueduct.[57,58] If found, treatment is simply supportive, monitoring the hearing over time, and advising the patient to avoid contact sports, as a head injury or blow to the head could transmit high cerebrospinal fluid (CSF) pressures to the inner ear, causing further hearing loss.

17.6.2 Sensorineural Hearing Loss

Sensorineural hearing loss in children, affecting 1 to 3 per 1,000, can be congenital (i.e., present at birth) or acquired, and genetic or nongenetic. Current estimates of the etiology of prelingual SNHL place genetic causes at approximately 50%, idiopathic at 25%, and acquired at 25%. As our understanding of genetic hearing loss deepens, genetic hearing loss will occupy a greater proportion of the etiology. There have been approximately 80 genetic loci linked to hearing loss through family linkage analysis, and about 50 genes identified whose mutations cause hearing loss (see the hereditary hearing loss homepage at http://hereditaryhearingloss.org), the most common of which is *DFNB2*, the genetic locus for the gene *GJB2*, which codes for the protein connexin 26, a gap junction protein responsible for the recirculation of potassium through a syncytium of intercellular junctions in the basal area of the organ of Corti after hair cell depolarization. Carrier rate for *GJB2* mutations is 30%; as an autosomal recessively inherited mutation, two carriers have a 25% chance of having a child with the full mutation and hearing loss.

Loci along the DNA genome associated with hearing loss carry the DFN terminology; DFNA refers to autosomal dominant inheritance, DFNB to autosomal recessive, DFNX to X-linked inheritance. With further research, additional loci will be mapped, and the genetic mutations responsible for those loci will be discovered, furthering our understanding of the genetics of hearing loss, the pathophysiology of genetic hearing loss, and the physiology of the cochlea.

Regarding the genetic causes of hearing loss, the hearing loss is associated with a named syndrome in about one fourth to one third of cases, making nonsyndromic hereditary hearing loss twice as common as syndromic. Evaluation of the child with suspected hearing loss should at least include questions for the parents regarding birth history (especially whether the child passed the newborn hearing screening exam; prematurity, low birth weight, time in the neonatal intensive care unit and medications, especially aminoglycoside antibiotics), jaundice/kernicterus, and a history of kidney (Alport or branchial-oto-renal [BOR]) or heart (Jervell and Lange-Nielson) disease. Physical exam should screen for pigmentation changes including white forelock or heterochromia irides (Waardenburg), branchial cleft cysts or ear pits (BOR), goiter (Pendred), visual loss (Usher), joint laxity (Ehlers-Danlos), syndactyly or polydactyly (Apert), Down syndrome features, palmar crease, "gargoylism" (mucopolysaccharidoses), midface hypoplasia (Crouzon and Treacher Collins, usually associated with aural atresia and CHL), and other syndromic features. Laboratory evaluation may include thyroid stimulating hormone, electrocardiogram, or urinalysis, with possible referral to an ophthalmologist for vision screening and electroretinography. Genetic counseling and testing should be offered with a frank discussion about the costs, benefits, and predictive ability for future children. Temporal bone CT imaging may be more cost-effective than genetic testing for connexin 26 or laboratory testing for other causes of SNHL in an algorithm proposed for the diagnostic management of the child with SNHL.[59]

Structural abnormalities of the cochlea provide a timeline of inner ear embryogenesis, as these anomalies stem from an arrest in the normal embryological development of the cochlea and inner ear.[60] The most common structure affected is the horizontal semicircular canal, the last inner ear structure to complete its development. Structural anomalies can usually be identified on high-resolution CT scanning. The decision to pursue CT scanning in the very young child with SNHL must be made between the physician and the family, weighing the benefits and the yield of the CT scan and the possibility that it would change the management of the child, with the very low but real risk of radiation exposure in the young child.[61] MRI is a nonradiation modality, but it may not be able to detect more subtle inner ear structural findings, although it is the study of choice in cochlear nerve aplasia.[62,63]

The TORCH infections (toxoplasmosis, other agents [syphilis, coxsackievirus, HIV], rubella, cytomegalovirus (CMV), and herpes simplex virus) remain one of the most common acquired causes of hearing loss in children, and CMV is the most common among them. Diagnosis of congenital CMV infection is made by the detection of virus (not antibodies to the virus) in the infant's blood, saliva, or urine. At-risk infants are those whose mothers contracted CMV during pregnancy. Healthy mothers and infants are not routinely screened for CMV. With widespread vaccination, measles, mumps, and meningitis have decreased in frequency, but they should still be screened as some parents elect not to vaccinate their children.

17.7 Treatment Options

What is to be done with children with unilateral hearing loss? Newborn hearing screening now identifies children with hearing loss at birth or shortly thereafter so intervention can be made early in life. One approach is to aid *all* children with unilateral hearing loss because clinicians, audiologists, educators, and parents cannot predict before entry into the school system which child with unilateral hearing loss will fall behind. For children with unilateral mild, moderate, and even severe SNHL, audiologists currently recommend at least a trial of amplification. Some families elect not to get a hearing aid for their child, preferring instead to monitor the hearing on a yearly basis and closely monitor their child's academic progress and possibly utilize other strategies to help their child in school.

Behavioral strategies include preferential seating in class, an IEP, and speech therapy when indicated. Parents may also take advantage of an FM system, in which the teacher wears a microphone and the child either has a speaker at his/her desk or an earbud or hearing aid that transmits the teacher's voice directly to the child's ear. If the hearing loss is mild to moderate, the child may be advised to wear the hearing device in the ear with hearing loss. Alternatively, if the hearing loss in the bad ear is severe to profound, the child may be advised to wear the aid in the good ear, to improve the overall signal-to-noise ratio.

There is evidence that conventional amplification does indeed improve outcomes for children with unilateral hearing loss,[1] with improvement in subjective assessments and quality of life.[22] Hearing aids are preferentially fit by a pediatric audiologist who knows the landscape of available devices on the market and can comfortably make a mold for the child. At times, molds can be made while the child is under anesthesia for a sedated auditory brainstem response test or other exam.

Cochlear implantation (CI) for unilateral profound SNHL is not approved for adults or children in the United States, but there is a preliminary European study in adults assessing CI in unilateral profound SNHL with disabling tinnitus.[64,65]

For children with unilateral CHL, similar strategies of preferential seating in class, an FM system, an IEP, or a trial of conventional amplification may be instituted. Other options for hearing habilitation in children with unilateral CHL include delivering sound energy to the healthy, functioning cochlea through bone conduction. Most children with CHL have normal cochlear function, for the embryological reasons noted earlier. Bone conducting hearing systems capitalize on the intact cochlea and deliver sound to the cochlea through bone vibration. Such systems include a conventional bone oscillator or power hearing aid mounted to a metal headband—the BAHA Softband and BAHA System (Cochlear Corp., Sydney, Australia), Oticon Ponto Pro (Oticon Corp., Somerset, NJ), Sophono (Sophono, Inc., Boulder, CO), and SoundBite (Sonitus Medical, San Mateo, CA) devices. These bone conducting devices provide various ways of delivering sound energy through bone conduction to the cochlea, including (1) a headband worn around the head with the processor tightly applied to

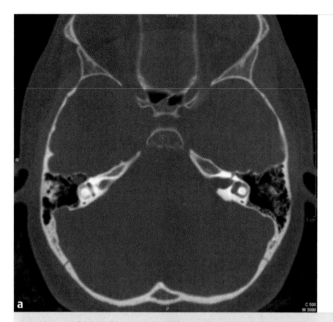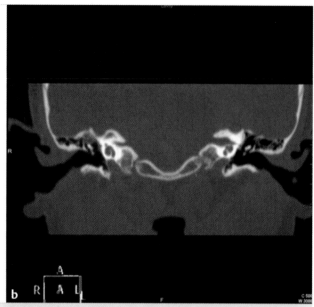

Fig. 17.5 Axial (a) and coronal (b) CT scan of a congenital cholesteatoma located in the posterosuperior epitympanum in a 9-year-old girl with a normal otoscopic exam and CHL.

the mastoid bone (conventional bone conductor, BAHA Softband, Ponto Pro on a softband); (2) a titanium post that is surgically implanted and osseointegrated into the bone of the skull to which the speech processor is "snapped" (BAHA System, Ponto Pro); (3) a magnetic plate surgically placed into the cortical bone of the skull with the bone oscillator applied to the intact skin over the magnet (Sophono); and (4) a microphone worn in the ear that transmits sound energy to a dental appliance that vibrates the bone of the teeth, sending sound energy to the cochlea (SoundBite). Surgically implantable devices (BAHA System, Ponto Pro) are not FDA approved for children under 5 years of age, and the SoundBite is not FDA approved for patients under 18.

The child with unilateral CHL may be a candidate for surgical exploration. As noted, any child with an unexplained CHL should undergo temporal bone CT imaging to investigate the etiology of the hearing loss. An enlarged vestibular aqueduct may cause a CHL not amenable to surgical intervention. A posterior superior congenital cholesteatoma, not visible through the tympanic membrane (▶ Fig. 17.5), needs a far different approach from that for a child with CHL and a clear middle ear and mastoid. Middle ear anatomy and the point of fixation dictate the surgical intervention necessary to restore sound conduction to the middle ear. Congenital stapes fixation is the most common cause of ossicular fixation in the child with congenital CHL ("minor" malformation).

Stapedectomy for congenital stapes ankylosis in children is well established with excellent reported hearing outcomes mirroring the adult stapedectomy results.[45,46,66] There is no ideal age for undergoing a stapedectomy; the timing must be determined individually for each child. Surgery must occur after any eustachian tube issues have resolved. Prior to surgical intervention, imaging is again necessary to investigate the possibility of X-linked progressive hearing loss/mixed hearing loss leading to

a stapes gusher at the time of the stapedectomy, evidenced by bulbous dilatation of the fundus of the internal auditory canal, absence of the bony plates separating the canal from the base of the cochlea, and a large cochlear aperture (▶ Fig. 17.6).[67]

Malleus or incus fixation may be addressed by separating the incudostapedial joint, removing the anomalous or fixed ossicle, and reconstructing with an ossicular replacement prosthesis.[50,68]

If we are to aid all children with unilateral hearing loss, children with unilateral CAA would be fitted with a bone conducting device (not implanted) in infancy. The disadvantages of this approach include the requirement for patient compliance, cosmetic issues, the lack of insurance reimbursement for these devices in unilateral patients, and, above all, the uncertainty of whether this approach truly offers any advantage to the child: Do children with unilateral CAA or even minor middle ear malformations with associated CHL need this technology? Do bone anchored hearing devices make a difference in speech and language development and in the classroom setting for children with unilateral CHL? Can children hear better in background noise and localize speech, the two classic disabilities associated with unilateral hearing loss, with these devices? Do these devices make surgery for aural atresia obsolete?

Studies have shown some improvement in horizontal sound localization in patients with unilateral CHL undergoing bone-anchored hearing aid (BAHA) insertion.[21,69] Interestingly, in the latter study, adult BAHA patients with unilateral CHL fared better than adult BAHA patients with USNHL but never fared as well as normal-hearing controls.[69] Although the bone conducting devices may confer a head shadow advantage, there is no clear evidence that patients are able to locate sound in space on a par with normal-hearing listeners, and no evidence that true binaural processing tasks, such as binaural release from masking, can be achieved with a bone conductor.[20]

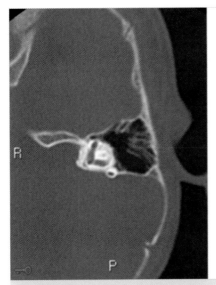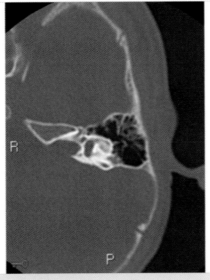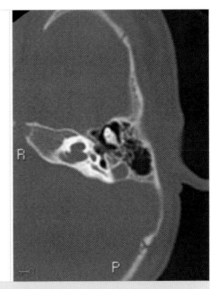

Fig. 17.6 X-linked progressive hearing loss/mixed hearing loss evidenced by bulbous dilatation of the fundus of the internal auditory canal (IAC), absence of the bony plates separating the IAC from the base of the cochlea, and a large cochlear aperture. (Courtesy of Sugoto Mukherjee, MD, Department of Radiology, University of Virginia Health System.)

In background noise, BAHA patients report improved speech understanding, and they score better on some standardized hearing in noise testing.[70] The critical factor is whether these devices overcome the disadvantage of a unilateral CHL in the classroom. In a survey of unilateral CAA families, only six of 40 families polled used some sort of amplification device for their child. As noted previously, in this group of 40 children, no child required repeating a grade in elementary education. Sixty-five percent of this group did use some resource, including speech therapy, an IEP, or an FM system.

As posited earlier, congenital UCHL may not confer as great a functional disability as a similar level of congenital SNHL. In longitudinal studies of young children with chronic otitis media with effusion (COME), binaural auditory processing skills and auditory temporal resolution may be delayed early in development, but do improve as the child grows older and the middle ear disease is corrected.[12,71,72] The fluctuating, milder nature of the hearing loss associated with COME is not equivalent to the unchanging, constant, moderate to severe loss associated with CAA, so the comparison may not be equal. Nevertheless, a unilateral CHL may not be as functionally debilitating as a USNHL. Future studies are warranted to test and examine this hypothesis. If true, these children may need simple monitoring of their hearing with some resource utilization, short of a bone conducting device or a BAHA.

17.8 Conclusion

What has emerged from research involving school-age children with unilateral hearing loss is that some of these children do need help, and, in the case of USNHL, early amplification of all children with mild to moderate and even severe losses appears to be the recommended standard of care, although not all families elect amplification for their child. Children with unilateral

CHL fare a bit better academically than their peers with USNHL, with significant utilization of resources such as speech therapy, IEPs, and FM systems—short of bone conducted amplification—to help in the academic setting. Future research should update, in a multiinstitutional way, how children with UHL do now in school, tracking grade retention rates and use of resources over time to ensure we are making a difference in helping these children succeed and to identify other potential strategies to help them succeed. All families of children with unilateral hearing loss, conductive or sensorineural, must be made aware of the potential disabilities associated with their child's hearing loss and the many options for hearing habilitation so that they can make intelligent, informed decisions about how best to prepare their child for academic success.

References

[1] Tharpe AM. Unilateral and mild bilateral hearing loss in children: past and current perspectives. Trends Amplif 2008; 12: 7–15

[2] Lieu JE. Speech-language and educational consequences of unilateral hearing loss in children. Arch Otolaryngol Head Neck Surg 2004; 130: 524–530

[3] Lieu JE, Tye-Murray N, Karzon RK, Piccirillo JF. Unilateral hearing loss is associated with worse speech-language scores in children. Pediatrics 2010; 125: e1348–e1355

[4] Berg F. Educational Audiology: Hearing and Speech Management. New York: Grune and Stratton, 1972:2

[5] Lee DJ, Gómez-Marín O, Lee HM. Prevalence of unilateral hearing loss in children: the National Health and Nutrition Examination Survey II and the Hispanic Health and Nutrition Examination Survey. Ear Hear 1998; 19: 329–332

[6] Mehra S, Eavey RD, Keamy DG, Jr. The epidemiology of hearing impairment in the United States: newborns, children, and adolescents. Otolaryngol Head Neck Surg 2009; 140: 461–472

[7] Ross DS, Visser SN, Holstrum WJ, Qin T, Kenneson A. Highly variable population-based prevalence rates of unilateral hearing loss after the application of common case definitions. Ear Hear 2010; 31: 126–133

[8] Lin FR, Niparko JK, Ferrucci L. Hearing loss prevalence in the United States. Arch Intern Med 2011; 171: 1851–1852

[9] Klockars T, Rautio J. Embryology and epidemiology of microtia. Facial Plast Surg 2009; 25: 145–148

[10] Harris J, Källén B, Robert E. The epidemiology of anotia and microtia. J Med Genet 1996; 33: 809–813

[11] Suutarla S, Rautio J, Ritvanen A, Ala-Mello S, Jero J, Klockars T. Microtia in Finland: comparison of characteristics in different populations. Int J Pediatr Otorhinolaryngol 2007; 71: 1211–1217

[12] Hall JW III, Grose JH, Pillsbury HC. Long-term effects of chronic otitis media on binaural hearing in children. Arch Otolaryngol Head Neck Surg 1995; 121: 847–852

[13] Hall JW III, Grose JH. Short-term and long-term effects on the masking level difference following middle ear surgery. J Am Acad Audiol 1993; 4: 307–312

[14] Eapen RJ, Buss E, Adunka MC, Pillsbury HC, III, Buchman CA. Hearing-in-noise benefits after bilateral simultaneous cochlear implantation continue to improve 4 years after implantation. Otol Neurotol 2009; 30: 153–159

[15] Aronoff JM, Yoon YS, Freed DJ, Vermiglio AJ, Pal I, Soli SD. The use of interaural time and level difference cues by bilateral cochlear implant users. J Acoust Soc Am 2010; 127: EL87–EL92

[16] Chan JC, Freed DJ, Vermiglio AJ, Soli SD. Evaluation of binaural functions in bilateral cochlear implant users. Int J Audiol 2008; 47: 296–310

[17] Litovsky R, Parkinson A, Arcaroli J, Sammeth C. Simultaneous bilateral cochlear implantation in adults: a multicenter clinical study. Ear Hear 2006; 27: 714–731

[18] Murphy J, O'Donoghue G. Bilateral cochlear implantation: an evidence-based medicine evaluation. Laryngoscope 2007; 117: 1412–1418

[19] Wazen JJ, Spitzer J, Ghossaini SN, Kacker A, Zschommler A. Results of the bone-anchored hearing aid in unilateral hearing loss. Laryngoscope 2001; 111: 955–958

[20] Agterberg MJ, Hol MK, Cremers CW, Mylanus EA, van Opstal J, Snik AF. Conductive hearing loss and bone conduction devices: restored binaural hearing? Adv Otorhinolaryngol 2011; 71: 84–91

[21] Agterberg MJ, Snik AF, Hol MK et al. Improved horizontal directional hearing in bone conduction device users with acquired unilateral conductive hearing loss. J Assoc Res Otolaryngol 2011; 12: 1–11

[22] Briggs L, Davidson L, Lieu JE. Outcomes of conventional amplification for pediatric unilateral hearing loss. Ann Otol Rhinol Laryngol 2011; 120: 448–454

[23] Bess FH, Tharpe AM. Performance and management of children with unilateral sensorineural hearing loss. Scand Audiol 1988 Suppl 30: 75–79

[24] Bess FH, Tharpe AM. Case history data on unilaterally hearing-impaired children. Ear Hear 1986; 7: 14–19

[25] Culbertson JL, Gilbert LE. Children with unilateral sensorineural hearing loss: cognitive, academic, and social development. Ear Hear 1986; 7: 38–42

[26] Bovo R, Martini A, Agnoletto M et al. Auditory and academic performance of children with unilateral hearing loss. Scand Audiol Suppl 1988; 30 Suppl 30: 71–74

[27] Brookhouser PE, Worthington DW, Kelly WJ. Unilateral hearing loss in children. Laryngoscope 1991; 101: 1264–1272

[28] Hartvig Jensen J, Børre S, Johansen PA. Unilateral sensorineural hearing loss in children: cognitive abilities with respect to right/left ear differences. Br J Audiol 1989; 23: 215–220

[29] Ruscetta MN, Arjmand EM, Pratt SR. Speech recognition abilities in noise for children with severe-to-profound unilateral hearing impairment. Int J Pediatr Otorhinolaryngol 2005; 69: 771–779

[30] Kesser BW, Krook K, Gray LC. Impact of unilateral conductive hearing loss secondary to aural atresia on academic performance in children. Laryngoscope. 2013;123(9):2270–2275

[31] Nicholas BD, Krook KA, Gray LC, Kesser BW. Does preoperative hearing predict postoperative hearing in patients undergoing primary aural atresia repair? Otol Neurotol 2012; 33: 1002–1006

[32] Vrabec JT, Lin JW. Inner ear anomalies in congenital aural atresia. Otol Neurotol 2010; 31: 1421–1426

[33] Gray L, Kesser B, Cole E. Understanding speech in noise after correction of congenital unilateral aural atresia: effects of age in the emergence of binaural squelch but not in use of head-shadow. Int J Pediatr Otorhinolaryngol 2009; 73: 1281–1287

[34] Jahrsdoerfer RA, Yeakley JW, Aguilar EA, Cole RR, Gray LC. Grading system for the selection of patients with congenital aural atresia. Am J Otol 1992; 13: 6–12

[35] Shonka DC, Jr, Livingston WJ, III, Kesser BW. The Jahrsdoerfer grading scale in surgery to repair congenital aural atresia. Arch Otolaryngol Head Neck Surg 2008; 134: 873–877

[36] Osborn AJ, Oghalai JS, Vrabec JT. Middle ear volume as an adjunct measure in congenital aural atresia. Int J Pediatr Otorhinolaryngol 2011; 75: 910–914

[37] Oliver ER, Lambert PR, Rumboldt Z, Lee FS, Agarwal A. Middle ear dimensions in congenital aural atresia and hearing outcomes after atresiaplasty. Otol Neurotol 2010; 31: 946–953

[38] Kim DW, Lee JH, Song JJ et al. Continuity of the incudostapedial joint: a novel prognostic factor in postoperative hearing outcomes in congenital aural atresia. Acta Otolaryngol 2011; 131: 701–707

[39] Lambert PR. Congenital aural atresia: stability of surgical results. Laryngoscope 1998; 108: 1801–1805

[40] Oliver ER, Hughley BB, Shonka DC, Kesser BW. Revision aural atresia surgery: indications and outcomes. Otol Neurotol 2011; 32: 252–258

[41] Kesser BW. Repair of congenital aural atresia. In: McKinnon BJ, ed. Operative Techniques in Otolaryngology-Head and Neck Surgery, vol. 21, issue 4. New York: Elsevier, 2010:278–286

[42] Jahrsdoerfer RA. Congenital atresia of the ear. Laryngoscope 1978; 88 Suppl 13: 1–48

[43] Moon IJ, Cho YS, Park J, Chung WH, Hong SH, Chang SO. Long-term stent use can prevent postoperative canal stenosis in patients with congenital aural atresia. Otolaryngol Head Neck Surg 2012; 146: 614–620

[44] Gray L, Kesser B, Cole E. Understanding speech in noise after correction of congenital unilateral aural atresia: effects of age in the emergence of binaural squelch but not in use of head-shadow. Int J Pediatr Otorhinolaryngol 2009; 73: 1281–1287

[45] Thomeer HG, Kunst HP, Cremers CW. Isolated congenital stapes ankylosis: surgical results in a consecutive series of 39 ears. Ann Otol Rhinol Laryngol 2010; 119: 761–766

[46] Teunissen EB, Cremers WR. Classification of congenital middle ear anomalies. Report on 144 ears. Ann Otol Rhinol Laryngol 1993; 102: 606–612

[47] Nomura Y, Nagao Y, Fukaya T. Anomalies of the middle ear. Laryngoscope 1988; 98: 390–393

[48] de Alarcon A, Jahrsdoerfer RA, Kesser BW. Congenital absence of the oval window: diagnosis, surgery, and audiometric outcomes. Otol Neurotol 2008; 29: 23–28

[49] Lau CC, Oghalai JS, Jackler RK. Combination of aberrant internal carotid artery and persistent stapedial artery. Otol Neurotol 2004; 25: 850–851

[50] Kuhn JJ, Lassen LF. Congenital incudostapedial anomalies in adult stapes surgery: a case-series review. Am J Otolaryngol 2011; 32: 477–484

[51] Stapleton AL, Egloff AM, Yellon RF. Congenital cholesteatoma: predictors for residual disease and hearing outcomes. Arch Otolaryngol Head Neck Surg 2012; 138: 280–285

[52] Cole RR, Jahrsdoerfer RA. The risk of cholesteatoma in congenital aural stenosis. Laryngoscope 1990; 100: 576–578

[53] Zhou G, Gopen Q, Kenna MA. Delineating the hearing loss in children with enlarged vestibular aqueduct. Laryngoscope 2008; 118: 2062–2066

[54] Mori T, Westerberg BD, Atashband S, Kozak FK. Natural history of hearing loss in children with enlarged vestibular aqueduct syndrome. J Otolaryngol Head Neck Surg 2008; 37: 112–118

[55] Merchant SN, Rosowski JJ. Conductive hearing loss caused by third-window lesions of the inner ear. Otol Neurotol 2008; 29: 282–289

[56] Hegemann SC, Carey JP. Is superior canal dehiscence congenital or acquired? A case report and review of the literature. Otolaryngol Clin North Am 2011; 44: 377–382, ix

[57] Cama E, Inches I, Muzzi E et al. Temporal bone high-resolution computed tomography in non-syndromic unilateral hearing loss in children. ORL J Otorhinolaryngol Relat Spec 2012; 74: 70–77

[58] Song JJ, Choi HG, Oh SH, Chang SO, Kim CS, Lee JH. Unilateral sensorineural hearing loss in children: the importance of temporal bone computed tomography and audiometric follow-up. Otol Neurotol 2009; 30: 604–608

[59] Preciado DA, Lawson L, Madden C et al. Improved diagnostic effectiveness with a sequential diagnostic paradigm in idiopathic pediatric sensorineural hearing loss. Otol Neurotol 2005; 26: 610–615

[60] Jackler RK, Luxford WM, House WF. Congenital malformations of the inner ear: a classification based on embryogenesis. Laryngoscope 1987; 97 Suppl 40: 2–14

[61] Brenner DJ, Hall EJ. Computed tomography—an increasing source of radiation exposure. N Engl J Med 2007; 357: 2277–2284

[62] Licameli G, Kenna MA. Is computed tomography (CT) or magnetic resonance imaging (MRI) more useful in the evaluation of pediatric sensorineural hearing loss? Laryngoscope 2010; 120: 2358–2359

[63] Mukerji SS, Parmar HA, Ibrahim M, Mukherji SK. Congenital malformations of the temporal bone. Neuroimaging Clin N Am 2011; 21: 603–619, viii

[64] Van de Heyning P, Vermeire K, Diebl M, Nopp P, Anderson I, De Ridder D. Incapacitating unilateral tinnitus in single-sided deafness treated by cochlear implantation. Ann Otol Rhinol Laryngol 2008; 117: 645–652

[65] Punte AK, Vermeire K, Hofkens A, De Bodt M, De Ridder D, Van de Heyning P. Cochlear implantation as a durable tinnitus treatment in single-sided deafness. Cochlear Implants Int 2011; 12 Suppl 1: S26–S29

[66] Welling DB, Merrell JA, Merz M, Dodson EE. Predictive factors in pediatric stapedectomy. Laryngoscope 2003; 113: 1515–1519

[67] Kumar G, Castillo M, Buchman CA. X-linked stapes gusher: CT findings in one patient. AJNR Am J Neuroradiol 2003; 24: 1130–1132

[68] Briggs RJ, Luxford WM. Correction of conductive hearing loss in children. Otolaryngol Clin North Am 1994; 27: 607–620

[69] Grantham DW, Ashmead DH, Haynes DS, Hornsby BWY, Labadie RF, Ricketts TA. Horizontal plane localization in single-sided deaf adults fitted with a bone-anchored hearing aid (Baha). Ear Hear 2012; 33: 595–603

[70] Pfiffner F, Caversaccio MD, Kompis M. Audiological results with Baha in conductive and mixed hearing loss. Adv Otorhinolaryngol 2011; 71: 73–83

[71] Gravel JS, Roberts JE, Roush J et al. Early otitis media with effusion, hearing loss, and auditory processes at school age. Ear Hear 2006; 27: 353–368

[72] Hartley DE, Moore DR. Effects of otitis media with effusion on auditory temporal resolution. Int J Pediatr Otorhinolaryngol 2005; 69: 757–769

18 Otitis Media

Daniel Jensen and Keiko Hirose

18.1 Introduction

Treatment of children and adults with otitis media (OM) is a substantial component of the practice of otolaryngology. Otitis media is second only to viral upper respiratory tract infection (URI) as the most common reason for visits to pediatricians. Epidemiological studies at the University of Pittsburgh found a 90% incidence of OM in urban children within the first 2 years of life.[1,2] The vast majority of OM occurs in children, and although the greater part of these cases resolves by adolescence, the disease may also occur in adults. Tympanostomy with tube placement is the primary surgical treatment for OM and remains the most common surgical procedure performed under general anesthesia in the United States.

In spite of substantial research, discussion continues regarding the role and timing of medical and surgical treatments, which vary across the United States and in other nations. The large annual health care expenditure in the United States for treatment of OM, estimated at more than $5 billion, has caused health care providers and payers to adopt several tactics aimed at reducing costs. The first attempt at development of an evidence-based and cost-effective clinical treatment guideline for OM was introduced by the Agency for Health Care Policy and Research (AHCPR) in 1994.[3] These recommendations were updated in 2004 by the Subcommittee on Management of Acute Otitis Media,[4] composed of experts selected by the American Academy of Pediatrics and the American Academy of Family Physicians, and by the Subcommittee on Otitis Media with Effusion,[5] which included the participation of the American Academy of Otolaryngology—Head and Neck Surgery (AAO-HNS). In 2013, the AAO-HNS issued updated guidance regarding appropriate use of tympanostomy tubes in children, with several important changes to the previous standard of care.[8] These recommendations are intended as guiding principles and allow for adjustments according to the needs of individual patients according to the clinician's judgment.

18.2 Terminology

Otitis media is an infectious and inflammatory condition of the middle ear associated with an effusion behind an intact tympanic membrane. It may be associated with several inciting factors, most commonly URI and eustachian tube dysfunction. OM may be classified according to the composition of the effusion: a serous effusion is characterized by thin, nonpurulent, transparent fluid; a mucoid effusion is thicker, but not infected; and mucopurulent fluid is characteristic of an acutely infected middle ear. This designation encompasses a spectrum of disease, and each classification represents a point along that spectrum rather than a distinct entity. For example, a serous effusion may progress to a mucoid effusion, and an acute otitis media (AOM) characterized by a mucopurulent effusion typically progresses to serous OM during the course of resolution.

Otitis media is also characterized by its chronicity. Acute otitis media is typically characterized by rapid onset of otalgia and erythema of the tympanic membrane in the presence of middle ear effusion (MEE). Otalgia and fever are more evident in younger children and may be absent in older children. Erythema of the tympanic membrane without MEE is called acute myringitis and may be mistaken for AOM. *Recurrent acute otitis media* (RAOM) is a term commonly assigned to patients with multiple self-limited episodes of AOM punctuated by periods of time in which the patient is symptom-free, either with or without a persistent MEE. Current practice guidelines define RAOM as three or more episodes of AOM within 6 months, or four or more episodes within a year.

Chronic otitis media with effusion (COME) refers to an accumulation of liquid in the middle ear cleft without other signs of inflammation or infection (e.g., fever, otalgia, erythema). Alternative names assigned to COME in the literature include glue ear, chronic secretory OM, serous OM, persistent OM, and silent OM. Effusions resulting from barotrauma, skull fracture, or leakage of cerebrospinal fluid are not included in this category. Many, perhaps most, chronic effusions result from resolving AOM. As previously stated, it is appropriate to think of AOM and COME as two points along a continuum of the same disease process. An antecedent history of AOM, however, is not necessary for diagnosis of COME. Chronic effusions of unknown duration as well as all cases of OM persisting for more than 30 days are classified as COME. Chronic otorrhea through a perforated tympanic membrane is termed chronic suppurative otitis media (CSOM) and may be associated with cholesteatoma.

18.3 Risk Factors

Epidemiological factors associated with recurrent OM include male gender, greater number of siblings in the home, day-care attendance, family history of recurrent OM, absence of breast feeding, and cigarette smoke exposure in the home.[7] Susceptibility to OM may result from anomalies of the palate resulting in dysfunction of the tensor veli palatini and eustachian tube or from immunodeficiency, either inherited or acquired. Inherited disorders of mucociliary clearance such as Kartagener syndrome or primary ciliary dyskinesias can predispose children to chronic OM with effusion, although cystic fibrosis classically is not associated with chronic eustachian tube disease. Socioeconomic factors that may contribute to the prevalence of OM include increased exposures, poor nutrition, and lack of access to health care. Certain ethnic groups, notably Native Americans and the Inuit population, have a high incidence of OM presumably due to differences in the anatomy of the eustachian tube and skull base.[8] Infants and toddlers attending day care have a greater incidence of OM than those who receive their care at home with few or no siblings mostly due to infectious exposures. Similarly, children in early grade school who have not had day care or preschool exposures experience an increased incidence of OM. Some authors have also suggested that environmental allergy, food allergy, and gastroesophageal reflux disease contribute to the development of OM, although a definite link between any of these conditions and OM has yet to be established.[9,10]

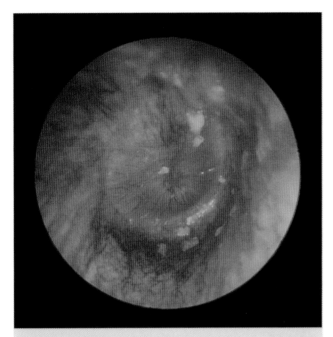

Fig. 18.1 Acute otitis media.

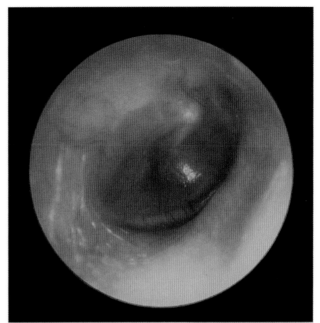

Fig. 18.2 Acute otitis media with effusion.

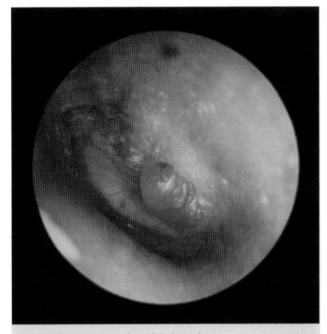

Fig. 18.3 Acute otitis media with bulging drum.

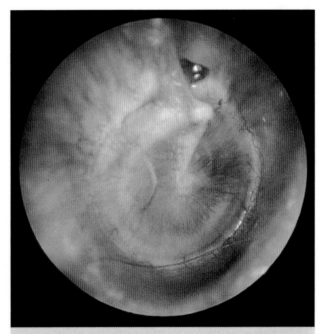

Fig. 18.4 Acute otitis media, exudative stage.

18.4 Pathophysiology

18.4.1 Acute Otitis Media

Acute otitis media (AOM) is an infection of the middle ear space induced by bacteria (▶ Fig. 18.1; ▶ Fig. 18.2; ▶ Fig. 18.3; ▶ Fig. 18.4; ▶ Fig. 18.5; ▶ Fig. 18.6), characterized by the presence of an effusion, usually composed of mucopurulent fluid, and frequently associated with otalgia and fever, particularly in younger children. The most likely route of bacterial entry into the middle ear is from infected secretions from the nasophar-ynx through the eustachian tube. Three factors appear to facilitate bacterial migration into the middle ear: bacterial colonization of the nasopharynx, incompetence of the eustachian tube, and negative pressure in the middle ear space.

Acute otitis media is frequently a sequela of viral URI.[11,12] Viral rhinitis breaks down mucosal barriers and mechanisms of mucociliary clearance that prevent bacterial adherence and growth in both the nose and nasopharynx. In addition, swelling of the nasal mucosa alters the aerodynamics of the upper airway and contributes to eustachian tube dysfunction.

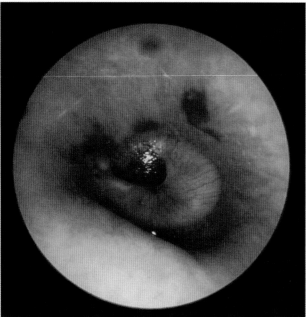

Fig. 18.5 Acute otitis media with bleb.

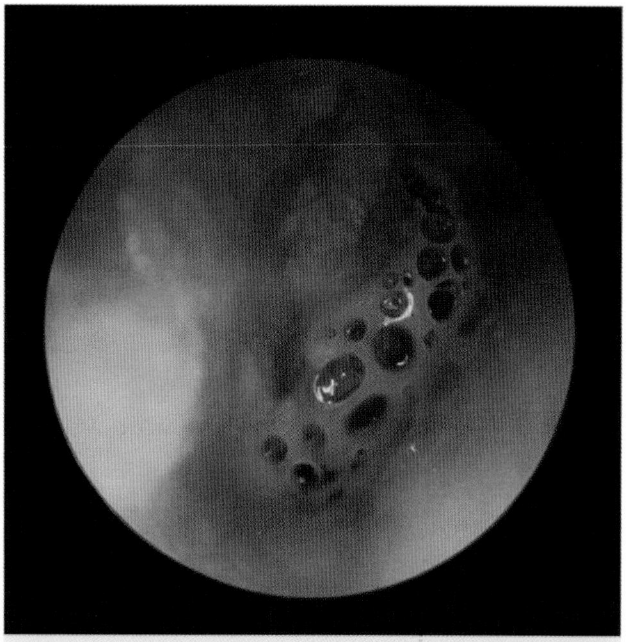

Fig. 18.6 Acute otitis media, suppurative stage.

The bacteriology of AOM has been studied extensively. In a large study at the University of Pittsburgh, the most predominant bacteria cultured from acute MEEs were *Streptococcus pneumoniae* (35%), *Haemophilus influenzae* (23%), and *Moraxella catarrhalis* (14%).[13] These same three pathogenic bacteria appear in the nasopharynx following URI.[14,15] Pillsbury et al[16] demonstrated higher bacterial colony counts in the adenoids of children with recurrent OM than in those undergoing adenoidectomy for adenoid hypertrophy without OM. Bernstein et al[17] have identified the alterations in the microbiology of the nasopharynx in children with RAOM. Normalization of the nasopharyngeal flora in conjunction with a marked decrease in the colonization of pathogenic bacteria has been demonstrated following adenoidectomy in otitis-prone children.[15]

Although eustachian tube dysfunction is generally held to be an underlying cause of OM, controversy remains about whether eustachian tube dysfunction truly causes OM. The eustachian tube has three functions: equalization of pressure between the nose and middle ear, clearance of middle ear secretions, and protection of the middle ear. The child's eustachian tube is short, horizontal, and composed of relatively flaccid cartilage. The protective function of the tube is less effective, and retrograde reflux of nasopharyngeal secretions may occur more readily than in the mature eustachian tube.[18]

Clearance of secretions results mainly from ciliary action. Viral upper respiratory infection is known to cause transient ciliary dysfunction; it is presumed that ciliary function of the middle ear and eustachian tube mucosa is also impaired during AOM. Fluid accumulates as a consequence of ciliary paralysis, and clearance of fluid follows recovery of ciliary function. However, thick viscous fluid may occlude the tube secondarily because of its rheological properties. Pressure equalization is normally mediated by tubal opening from contraction of the tensor veli palatini muscle in response to stimuli mediated by the tympanic plexus.[19] Normal function of the tensor veli

palatini muscle is impaired in patients with submucous or overt cleft palate and is thought to be the main reason for the resultant eustachian tube dysfunction.

The pressure differential that provides the driving pressure for reflux into the middle ear may result from either excessive negative pressure in the middle ear or positive pressure in the nasopharynx. Obstruction of the nose secondary to viral rhinitis may result in increased nasopharyngeal pressure during swallowing, analogous to the Toynbee maneuver, which entails holding the nostrils closed during swallowing. Nose blowing also increases nasopharyngeal pressures that could affect bacterial migration to the middle ear cleft.

18.4.2 Chronic Otitis Media with Effusion

Chronic otitis media with effusion was virtually unknown before antimicrobial therapy began in the 1940s (▶ Fig. 18.7; ▶ Fig. 18.8; ▶ Fig. 18.9; ▶ Fig. 18.10). Whether this is the result of widespread use of antibiotics or better diagnostic methods is unclear. However, perforations of the tympanic membrane are less prevalent after antimicrobial therapy than in the preantibiotic era. It is likely that antibiotics tend to prevent progression of infection to the point of perforation, but that instead these infections develop into quiescent effusions, which otherwise would have drained via perforation of the tympanic membrane.

Early researchers postulated that COME was a primary disorder of multiple causes resulting from the hydrops ex vacuo theory; that is, eustachian tube obstruction resulted in, sequentially, under-aeration of the middle ear, negative middle ear pressure, and fluid transudation.[20] When the drop in pressure is acute, as in barotrauma, these observations adequately explain the development of effusion.[21] However, applying this concept to the pathogenesis of COME does not fully explain

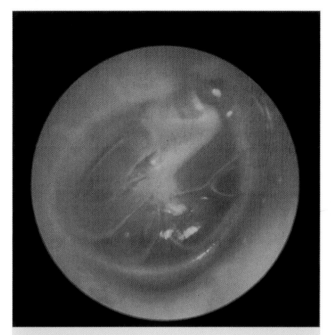

Fig. 18.7 Serous otitis media.

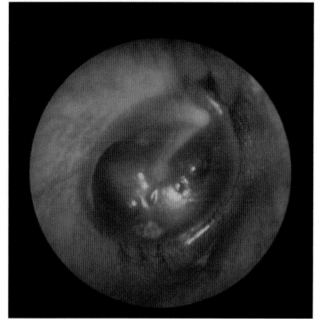

Fig. 18.8 Serous otitis media with retracted drum.

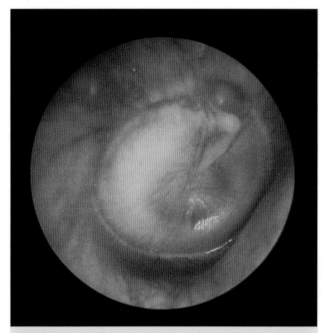

Fig. 18.9 Serous otitis media, advanced.

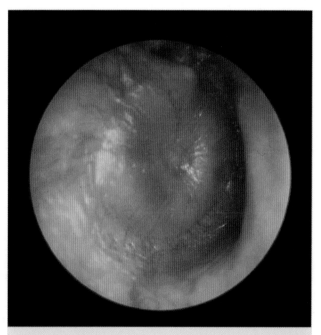

Fig. 18.10 Mucoid otitis media.

more recent observations about the disorder. Normal middle ear gas is now known to be hypoxic and hypercapnic in relation to inspired air,[22] and chronic eustachian tube obstruction per se does not result in severe negative middle ear pressure.[23] Studies in experimental OM[24] have demonstrated that eustachian tube obstruction does not result in mucoid effusion in the absence of bacterial infection.

The Greater Boston Collaborative Otitis Media Study found persistent effusion following AOM for 1 month in 40%, for 2 months in 20%, and for 3 months or longer in 10% of cases.[25] Rosenfeld and Kay[26] performed a search and meta-analysis of

the literature to estimate the natural history of untreated OM. In patients with MEE following an untreated episode of AOM, 59% resolved within 1 month and 74% resolved within 3 months. Patients with chronic MEEs (observed to be present for longer than 3 months) exhibited 26% resolution within 6 months and 33% resolution by 1 year. Many investigators have demonstrated pathogenic bacteria in the fluid obtained from the middle ears of children with COME.[27] The Pittsburgh Otitis Media Research Center study confirmed similar bacteriology in cultured effusions from children with AOM and COME. Children with chronic effusion had a positive culture 70% of the time.[2] In one study, reverse-transcriptase polymerase chain reaction (RT-PCR) analysis of culture-negative chronic effusions in children revealed the presence of bacterial messenger RNA (mRNA) (hence, viable and metabolically active bacteria) in a significant proportion of effusions.[28] It is possible that, in many chronic effusions, bacteria may be present in an attenuated form, existing as biofilms on the mucosal surface. This was demonstrated by Ehrlich et al[29] in a chinchilla model of OM using *H. influenzae*. Thus, the preponderance of available evidence supports the theory that (1) secretory changes in the middle ear in COME are histological sequelae of chronic infection, rather than a separate pathologic disorder; (2) the majority of cases of COME begin as acute infection of the middle ear; (3) postinflammatory alterations in the middle ear mucosa and eustachian tube (e.g., goblet cell metaplasia and hypersecretion) lead to persistence of effusion; and (4) dysfunction of the eustachian tube is an important part of the process.

18.5 Diagnosis

Otitis media is a clinical diagnosis dependent on careful otoscopy by an experienced observer. The guidelines published by the Subcommittee on Management of Otitis Media in 2004 state that the diagnosis of AOM requires "(1) a history of acute onset of signs and symptoms, (2) the presence of MEE, and (3) signs and symptoms of middle ear inflammation."[4] Symptoms such as fever, otalgia, otorrhea, irritability, and decreased hearing should raise suspicion for the presence of OM. In patients with a previous history of OM or with a given history of a preceding URI, the likelihood of MEE is even greater. Direct visualization of the tympanic membrane with an otoscope is required for confirmation of the diagnosis. An erythematous, opaque, and bulging tympanic membrane is consistent with AOM. Bubbles or an air-fluid level may also be visible behind the tympanic membrane and may be associated with an evolving or a resolving OM. COME may be asymptomatic and often is detected incidentally during well-child visits to the pediatrician. Straw or amber-colored fluid may be seen with COME. It is important to document the side and duration of the effusion to follow recommendations for intervention.

Pneumatic otoscopy is useful if the diagnosis is in doubt; on pneumatic otoscopy, we observe reduced mobility of the tympanic membrane when there is fluid in the middle ear. Tympanometry, acoustic reflectometry, and ultrasonography may be useful adjuncts in the diagnosis of OM.[30,31] Tympanometry combined with otoscopy has been demonstrated to raise the sensitivity and specificity of the diagnosis of OM to greater than 90%,[32] whereas pneumatic otoscopy alone has been shown to have 85% sensitivity and 75% specificity in the diagnosis of OM, although this may vary based on the individual clinician's training and experience.[33] Accordingly, the official recommendation of the Subcommittee on Otitis Media with Effusion is to use pneumatic otoscopy as the primary diagnostic method for OM, with tympanometry reserved as a confirmatory test when the diagnosis is in doubt.[5] In the absence of other otologic abnormalities, audiometry may demonstrate a mild or moderate (20–40 dB) conductive hearing loss but is not useful for the initial diagnosis of OM. The history should also include questions regarding the risk factors for learning and speech disabilities, duration of symptoms, sleep quality and irritability, and the presence of environmental risk factors such as exposure to cigarette smoke, participation in day care, breast feeding history, and pacifier use.

Otitis media is much less common in adults than in children. In the absence of an obvious inciting factor (e.g., viral URI, barotrauma) a careful search for the underlying etiology should be undertaken. An adult with unilateral MEE should undergo evaluation for a nasopharyngeal mass, including nasopharyngoscopy.

18.6 Medical Management
18.6.1 Acute Otitis Media

The majority of cases of AOM are due to aerobic organisms, with *S. pneumoniae, H. influenzae*, and *M. catarrhalis* representing the three most commonly isolated organisms in acute MEEs. Historically *S. pneumoniae* has been considered the most common causative organism; however, recent studies have shown a moderate decrease in the proportion of AOM related to *S. pneumoniae*, with a concomitant increase in *H. influenzae*–related cases.[34] Host defenses are usually sufficient on their own to clear an acute episode of OM. There is ongoing debate, however, regarding the role and timing of antibiotics in the treatment of AOM. Tympanocentesis may provide some diagnostic information, but it is not routinely performed and is not considered a therapeutic procedure for OM. In current practice, tympanocentesis is typically reserved for cases in which the clinician suspects a rare or resistant bacterial etiology, or in newborns or immunocompromised patients with OM. Negative cultures in AOM suggest the possibility of a causative agent other than aerobic bacteria (viruses, anaerobes), though cultures can also be spuriously negative, particularly if the patient has already received antibiotic therapy.

Since 2004, the first-line medical therapy for AOM is amoxicillin 80 to 90 mg/kg/day for 7 to 10 days.[4] In cases of severe symptoms, or failure to respond to initial therapy, or if broader coverage is desired, amoxicillin-clavulanate is recommended with weight-based dosing based on the amoxicillin component. In recent years amoxicillin-clavulanate has been used more commonly because of high frequencies of β-lactamase activity in *H. influenza* and *M. catarrhalis* isolates, though high-dose amoxicillin is still commonly prescribed to address the high prevalence of resistant *S. pneumoniae*. Alternative agents include the second- and third-generation cephalosporins such as cefaclor, cefuroxime, and cefpodoxime; macrolide antibiotics such as erythromycin or azithromycin; the combination of sulfisoxazole and erythromycin (Pediazole); or trimethoprim/sulfamethoxazole (Bactrim).

There have been numerous studies investigating the role of antibiotics in treating uncomplicated AOM, and this remains a controversial topic. Many have advocated an initial strategy of observation with symptomatic treatment in children over the age of 24 months with uncomplicated AOM, a practice that has been widely practiced in Europe for years. In a double-blinded, randomized, controlled trial, Tähtinen et al[35] demonstrated clinical improvement in children aged 6 to 35 months who received amoxicillin-clavulanate versus placebo, as evidenced by lower rates of "treatment failure" (19% vs. 45%, with number needed to treat, 3.8), assessed based on signs and symptoms.

They also found in the amoxicillin-clavulanate group significant reductions in day-care absenteeism for patients and work absenteeism for the parents. These effects were tempered by higher rates of diarrhea (48% vs. 27%) and eczema (9% vs. 3%) in the amoxicillin-clavulanate group. Hoberman et al[36] performed a similar, simultaneously published trial in children aged 6 to 23 months, and found significant reductions in overall symptom burden and time to resolution of symptoms among children treated with amoxicillin-clavulanate versus placebo. These two papers would support the use of antibiotics for AOM and support the current thinking for treatment.

Nevertheless, many children who do not receive antibiotic therapy for AOM resolve their infections.[26,37,38] Antibiotic resistance is a public health concern fueled by excessive use of antibiotics, and antibiotic therapy for any individual patient is not without side effects. To balance these considerations, many clinicians opt for initial observation with rescue therapy at 48 to 72 hours (safety net antibiotic prescription) if indicated based on symptoms. This requires either close follow-up or up-front provision of a "safety net" prescription, which the child's parents are instructed to fill only if the child remains febrile or in pain after 48 hours of observation.[39] Guidelines from the 2004 Subcommittee on Management of Acute Otitis Media allow for initial observation with symptomatic treatment for pain and fever in children with uncomplicated AOM depending on age, level of diagnostic certainty, and severity of symptoms.[4] In children over 2 years of age, observation may be considered if the diagnosis is uncertain or symptoms are not severe. In children 6 to 24 months of age, observation is recommended only in cases where there is no fever *and* the diagnosis is uncertain. These guidelines recommend against observation for children under 6 months of age, regardless of other considerations. Treatment decisions should always be made on an individual basis, with consideration for the child's condition, reliability of follow-up, and ability of the family to manage caring for a child who may have a prolonged period of symptoms if antibiotic therapy is deferred.

There are no proven preventive measures for AOM other than avoidance of risk factors. A Finnish study of the efficacy of pneumococcal conjugate vaccine (PCV7) in prevention of AOM in children showed only a modest benefit of 6% reduction in the total number of episodes.[40] Numerous other studies have shown similar small reductions; however, episodes of AOM were known to be declining prior to the advent of pneumococcal conjugate vaccines, suggesting the possibility that these effects may be simply a continuation of a preexisting trend rather than a true effect of the vaccine.[34] Although pneumococcal vaccines are effective in preventing invasive pneumococcal infections, their efficacy in prevention of mucosal disease, such as OM, is equivocal.

18.6.2 Recurrent Acute Otitis Media

Elimination of environmental factors for OM such as smoke exposure and day-care attendance would appear to be an effective first-line intervention against RAOM, but often these factors prove to be difficult to change in the lives of most children. Other interventions are often needed, and escalation of treatment is appropriate in most cases. Prophylactic antibiotic therapy for RAOM was initially popular in the 1980s and 1990s, but

with the emergence of resistant *S. pneumonia* and other resistant bacterial strains, the use of prophylactic antibiotics is no longer recommended.[41] It was estimated as early as 1995 that approximately 25% of pneumococcus strains were penicillin-resistant, and approximately 25% of *H. influenzae* isolates and 90% of *M. catarrhalis* isolates produced β-lactamase.[42]

18.6.3 Chronic Otitis Media with Effusion

As with AOM, the role of antibiotics in the treatment of COME has evolved over time, with gradual reduction in the use of antibiotics in recent years. Nevertheless, it is not uncommon to see children with persistent COME who have received four or more courses of antimicrobials in a 3-month period. Rosenfeld and Post[43] found in a meta-analysis of existing studies that the benefit of antimicrobial therapy in COME is minor. Because most effusions resolve spontaneously after treating AOM, withholding additional treatment in favor of watchful waiting for 3 months is recommended. The 2004 AHCPR guidelines recommend observation of nonacute OM for 3 months in children who are not otherwise at risk for speech, language, or hearing issues. At-risk children may undergo expedited treatment, such as referral to an otolaryngologist, at the discretion of the clinician. If resolution does not occur after 3 months, an audiogram is indicated. After three months of observation, myringotomy and tube placement are indicated if there is a demonstrated conductive hearing loss, and may be considered for other symptoms believed to be attributable to the persistent effusions, such as vestibular dysfunction, social or behavioral problems, ear discomfort, etc.[8] If significant retraction of the tympanic membrane is noted, proceeding with ear tubes without waiting for the presence of hearing loss is considered appropriate.[5]

Certain non-antimicrobial medical therapies have been used as alternatives or adjuncts to antibiotics. Studies of short-term corticosteroid therapy have had conflicting results. Schwartz et al[44] found otoscopic improvement in the treated subjects, whereas Lambert[45] found no difference in outcomes between the corticosteroid group and the control group. Rosenfeld et al[46] performed a meta-analysis of the published studies and found that the odds ratio for clearance was 3.6 in steroid-treated children. A later meta-analysis failed to show any benefit of oral steroids over placebo as treatment for OM.[47] It has not been shown that the long-term benefits of corticosteroid therapy outweigh the risks when used as treatment for OM. Accordingly, the AHCPR does not recommend the use of corticosteroids as treatment of OM, citing lack of proof of long-term efficacy.[5] Antihistamines and decongestants are ineffective treatments for OM.

18.7 Surgical Management

Recurrent AOM is the most common indication for a surgical procedure in children. Over the past two decades, several prospective randomized clinical trials have validated the efficacy of surgical therapy of OM. The goal of surgical therapy is to simplify the care of the child with OM by demystifying the diagnosis, allowing access to the middle ear space with ototopical treatment, to allow for equalization of middle ear pressures, and to

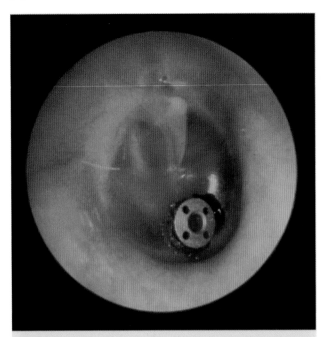

Fig. 18.11 Reuter Bobbin tympanostomy tube.

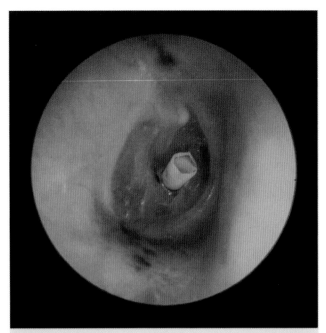

Fig. 18.12 Long-shaft tympanostomy tube.

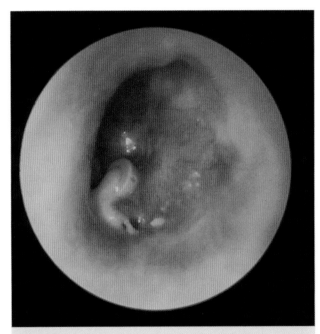

Fig. 18.13 Purulent otitis following tympanostomy tube.

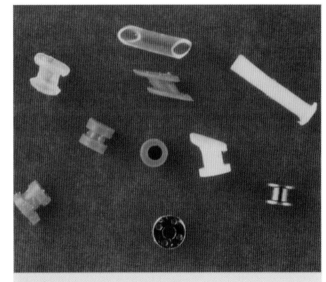

Fig. 18.14 Various tympanostomy tubes.

ameliorate symptoms, primarily pain, fever, and conductive hearing loss, especially during the key periods for development of speech and language. Where persistent eustachian tube dysfunction is present and in cases where obstructive airway symptoms or chronic rhinorrhea are present, adenoidectomy is an important adjunct to ear tubes in the treatment of recurrent AOM. In many cases of COME, both conditions exist concurrently, and thus ear tubes combined with adenoidectomy are often indicated.

Therapy for OM varies with the age of the patient and with whether the process is acute or chronic. Because antimicrobial therapy or watchful waiting represent the standard of care for AOM in the United States, patients with occasional, isolated episodes of AOM do not generally come to the attention of the otolaryngologist.[48] Therefore, only recurrent or chronic cases are considered here.

18.7.1 Tympanostomy Tubes

Tympanostomy tubes were popularized by Armstrong,[49] and insertion of myringotomy tubes is the most common operation performed in children (▶ Fig. 18.11; ▶ Fig. 18.12; ▶ Fig. 18.13; ▶ Fig. 18.14). The myringotomy tube serves as an artificial eustachian tube to ventilate the middle ear and equalize the middle ear pressure to atmospheric pressure. The myringotomy tube also serves as a portal for topical delivery of medications to the middle ear space. Middle ear clearance also is aided because negative pressure cannot occur from the piston effect as a bolus of thick fluid is moved into the eustachian tube by ciliary action. The greater efficacy of myringotomy tubes in OM as opposed to simple drainage by myringotomy has been established.[50]

The finding that the time to recurrence of OM after myringotomy is the same as after extrusion of myringotomy tubes[51] suggests that ventilation of the middle ear provides palliation of the symptoms of OM rather than correcting the underlying pathophysiology. Permanent cure of OM is accomplished only with time, allowing for maturation of the immune system and eustachian tube. Therefore, using myringotomy tubes that remain in place and ventilate the ear for a longer duration compared with myringotomy alone is a logical choice, though not without potential complications.

The major differences among the multitude of available tubes relate to lumen size, length, and retention time. In general, the short grommet tubes extrude sooner than the long, T-shaped tubes. The larger the bore of the tube and the longer it stays in place, the more likely is a persistent perforation of the tympanic membrane. A similar rate of perforations is seen after myringotomy tube insertion using short-term grommets as compared with myringotomy alone.[51] Long-term tubes have a greater perforation rate but greater freedom from OM while in place. Closure of such persistent perforations can usually be easily accomplished with myringoplasty using either fat or cartilage butterfly grafts as an outpatient procedure.[52,53]

An alternative to traditional tympanostomy tubes is placement of a subannular tube. This technique involves elevation of a short flap of external canal skin down to the annulus of the tympanic membrane, and entry into the middle ear around the annulus, analogous to a tympanomeatal flap. The tube is then placed through this tunnel into the middle ear, to function in the same manner as traditional tympanostomy tubes. Although extensive research on this technique is lacking, retrospective reports have generally reported a roughly 7 to 10% rate of tympanic membrane perforation, and duration of tube placement similar to T-tubes.[54] This technique may be attractive in cases of adhesive OM or tympanic membrane retractions.

Patients with myringotomy tubes need periodic monitoring. The modified T-tubes, which are slightly shorter than the original Goode T-tubes,[55] will remain in situ for 2 to 5 years. Patients are examined at 6-month intervals to ensure tubal patency, freedom from infection, and proper position of the tube. These tubes are generally well tolerated, but occasionally granulation tissue will form around the base of the tube, which usually responds well to topical steroid/antibiotic preparations.

Children who receive myringotomy tubes because of hearing loss believed to be attributable to persistent effusion must receive a follow-up audiogram after tube placement to ensure resolution of the hearing loss, as in some cases (particularly in young children), additional pathology will be unmasked after resolution of the effusion. In a case series of children referred for evaluation of persistent hearing loss after myringotomy tube placement, Whittemore et al[56] found a high proportion of other causes, including genetic syndromes, middle or inner ear anomalies, and cholesteatoma. Only a small proportion of these cases were attributable to the tubes themselves, and uniformly

demonstrated mild conductive hearing loss at low frequencies only. The authors recommended further investigation for all children with continued hearing loss after myringotomy tube placement except children with mild low-frequency conductive loss, who should be monitored to ensure correction after tube removal or extrusion.

18.7.2 Adenoidectomy

Adenoidectomy was once the primary surgical treatment offered to children with OM. During the 1960s and 1970s, adenoidectomy was used less often because of the popularity of T-tubes and because several studies, which would be considered flawed by today's standards, failed to show a significant effect of adenoidectomy on outcome. Three separate, prospective, randomized clinical trials have shown that adenoidectomy significantly reduces morbidity from COME.[51,57,58] These studies have demonstrated that (1) adenoidectomy is an effective treatment for patients with OM, and (2) the effect is independent of the size of the adenoid.

Given the following: (1) children in the San Antonio study[51] receiving adenoidectomy had a significant reduction in morbidity as compared with those who did not have their adenoids removed; (2) if adenoidectomy was performed, the outcome in hearing and time with effusion was similar irrespective of myringotomy tubes use; and (3) the complication rate for adenoidectomy was low; then an argument can be made to perform adenoidectomy and myringotomy with or without myringotomy tube insertion as the primary procedure for COME in children 4 years of age and older.[59] Paradise and Bluestone[59] have argued that adenoidectomy, being slightly riskier and more expensive than myringotomy tube insertion, should be reserved for recurrent cases.

The study of Paradise et al[58] showed that the adenoidectomy effect did not differ by age (about one third of the children were under 4 years of age). Clinical experience indicates that there is little physiological difference between a 3-year-old and a 4-year-old. The effect of adenoidectomy was greater for the younger children in the San Antonio study.[51] Therefore, one could make the case that high-risk children should have adenoidectomy at a younger age to accrue the greatest benefit. Adenoidectomy in children over 18 months has been shown to be a safe procedure.[60] When recurrence rate is factored into the initial cost of adenoidectomy versus myringotomy tubes, the cost per quality-adjusted life-year is unchanged.[48]

The preceding arguments are certainly logical, but they are not validated; therefore, clinicians must decide this matter in their own practice according to individual patient needs and practice guidelines. Two important, parallel misconceptions by some physicians still influence clinical decisions about adenoidectomy: first, that adenoidectomy is indicated for OM if the adenoid is enlarged; and second, that the small adenoid is normal. The three clinical trials on adenoidectomy[51,57,58] have all shown that the size of the adenoid is not relevant to outcome. Adenoid hyperplasia is a reaction of the healthy adenoid to antigenic stimulation, whereas the chronically infected adenoid, which is associated with OM,[60] may be small. The decision to do an adenoidectomy, therefore, should be based on the severity and persistence of the middle ear disease, not on the size of the adenoid. As a general rule, most surgeons reserve adenoidectomy in combination with a second set of tympanostomy tubes for children with ongoing OME or recurrent AOM after extrusion of a first set of tubes.

Children being considered for adenoidectomy should be free of defects of the soft palate. The most insidious problem is submucous cleft of the soft palate, which can be suspected by a bifid uvula, a bluish-white band (zona pellucida) in the midline of the palate (where the muscles are absent), absence of a spine on the posterior edge of the hard palate, and a groove in the posterior surface of the soft palate seen on fiberoptic nasopharyngoscopy.

18.7.3 Surgical Treatment of Recurrent Acute Otitis Media

Many children with RAOM have normal otoscopy between episodes, but some retain MEEs. Although antimicrobial prophylaxis was commonly used in the past,[61] overreliance on long-term treatment with low-dose antimicrobial therapy appears to be a contributing factor to the emergence of resistant strains of *S. pneumoniae*. Therefore, surgical treatment is being considered more frequently.[62] Depending on the child's age, myringotomy tubes, adenoidectomy, or both should be considered.

Gebhart[63] was the first to demonstrate a reduction in the number of new episodes of AOM following the insertion of myringotomy tubes. Subsequently, myringotomy tube placement has become the primary surgical prophylaxis against RAOM. Previous guidelines from the AAO-HNS recommended placement of myringotomy tubes in otherwise healthy children with three or more episodes of AOM in 6 months, or four of more episodes within a year.[64] The 2013 AAO-HNS guidelines for tympanostomy tubes in children added the additional stipulation that tympanostomy tubes only be recommended if middle ear effusions were apparent on exam, based on evidence suggesting favorable outcomes with observation in children presenting without middle ear effusions.[8] It is also felt that the presence of middle ear effusion at the time of otolaryngologist examination provides evidence of the reliability of the previously diagnosed episodes of AOM.

In otitis-prone children 18 months and older, adenoidectomy with myringotomy tube placement is the preferred second procedure if the child fails after extrusion of an initial set of myringotomy tubes. If the child is in the older range of the AOM group (i.e., 4 years or older) and the middle ears are well aerated, adenoidectomy and myringotomy *without* myringotomy tubes may be performed in selected cases. Paradise et al,[58] in studying children with recurrent OM despite myringotomy tube placement, found a significant reduction in the incidence of AOM in the first year following adenoidectomy but not in the second year. A study of adenoidectomy in the management of RAOM has demonstrated that although adenoidectomy and adenotonsillectomy may be effective in treating COME, the results when compared with tympanostomy tubes alone were not favorable for RAOM.[65] The efficacy of controlling RAOM with ear tubes alone did not warrant the added risk of the additional procedures of adenoidectomy or adenotonsillectomy as first-line therapy. Nonetheless, adenoidectomy is an effective method for surgical prophylaxis against RAOM and should be employed in the treatment of patients with failure to resolve infections after ear tubes alone. In summary, the AHCPR currently recommends myringotomy tube placement as the preferred initial procedure for surgical treatment of OM. In recurrent or refractory cases, adenoidectomy plus myringotomy (with or without tube placement) is recommended as the second surgical procedure.[5]

18.7.4 Surgical Treatment of Chronic Otitis Media with Effusion

The indication for surgery for COME is failure of medical therapy to clear the MEE and restore hearing to normal levels within a reasonable time. Current AHCPR guidelines recommend surgical treatment (consisting of myringotomy tubes, adenoidectomy, or both) for persistent effusion with documented hearing loss (20 dB or more in the better ear) for bilateral effusions that have not cleared in 3 months, and for a unilateral effusion that persists for 6 months.[5]

In children with documented learning difficulties and bilateral conductive hearing loss, a case can be made to proceed with surgery after 60 days. It is helpful to note that the time criterion is used as an index of the likelihood of spontaneous resolution; many effusions clear within 30 to 60 days, and surgery should not be performed in such self-limited cases. Once an effusion has persisted for 90 days it is possible that it may persist for months or even years. Maw[66] noted an average duration of effusion in the untreated ear of 7.8 years. In such a circumstance there is little doubt that correction of the hearing loss should be done to avoid speech delays. Although the evidence that mild to moderate conductive hearing loss causes speech delay is inconsistent, it is clear that this does occur in many cases and it seems prudent, therefore, to prevent the problem rather than to seek remedial education after the fact.

Early treatment principles for COME were based on the theory that secretory OM was primarily due to eustachian tube obstruction and that ventilation of the middle ear was both necessary and sufficient treatment. It now appears that ventilation of the middle ear via myringotomy tubes bypasses the problem but does not correct the underlying disorder, whereas adenoidectomy appears to modify the underlying pathophysiology. Gates et al[51] compared adenoidectomy (and myringotomy) with tubes and found no significant differences in the outcome variables, including hearing. Further, it was demonstrated that outcome after adenoidectomy did not vary with the size of the adenoid. A multicenter randomized controlled trial conducted in Scotland compared myringotomy tubes alone versus myringotomy tubes with adenoidectomy versus watchful waiting for initial treatment of children with COME with hearing loss (HL) meeting criteria for myringotomy tubes.[67] The study demonstrated a significant benefit to adjuvant adenoidectomy in the form of a reduced rate of eligibility for repeat myringotomy tubes and improved audiometric outcomes during the second year after surgery, with equivalent results during the first year. These results were reasoned to be due to improved physiology in the myringotomy tubes with adenoidectomy group versus the myringotomy tubes alone group after tube extrusion.

It appears clear that although the addition of adjuvant adenoidectomy adds expense and a small amount of risk to the surgical treatment of COME, it does convey some benefit. On the other hand, it would be logistically impractical to perform adenoidectomy as part of initial surgical therapy for every child needing surgical intervention for COME. With these considerations in mind, the 2004 AHCPR guidelines,[5] which recommend reserving adenoidectomy for revision surgery unless a separate indication for adenoidectomy exists, seem appropriate. The 2013 AAO-HNS guidelines on tympanostomy tube placement do not comment on the role of adenoidectomy in management of otitis media.[5] Whenever adenoidectomy is performed for COME, bilateral myringotomy (with or without tube placement) and suction evacuation of the middle ear is always done simultaneously.

18.7.5 Benefits and Limitations of Surgical Treatment

Recurrent AOM often is associated with considerable morbidity from fever, malaise, pain, anorexia, and inadequate sleep. These associated symptoms may produce behavioral changes in children, such as poor attention span and irritability, and lead to social isolation. In addition to the disruptive effects upon the child's behavior, OM produces a mild to moderate conductive hearing loss due to MEE. Because the hearing level fluctuates, the child has difficulty in developing a consistent hearing strategy. Such hearing losses may impair communication and create additional difficulties in interpersonal relations, affect the development of speech and language skills, and, perhaps, retard intellectual achievement.[68,69] A further problem is the impact of sickness upon family dynamics. Time lost from work or social activities due to illness of a child may impose additional hardships upon family relationships. In addition, otitis-prone children are often perceived as being unhealthy, which affects their relations within the family. These considerations contribute substantially to the negative impact of OM on quality of life in affected families.

Patients and parents are advised that surgical therapy for OM is generally not curative, but it does correct the hearing loss and generally reduces the number and severity of subsequent episodes. Pain associated with episodes of AOM is reduced with myringotomy tubes because the tympanic membrane is not under pressure. Further, myringotomy tubes facilitate topical treatment with antibiotic drops. Myringotomy tubes correct the conductive hearing loss as long as they remain open and in place. However, when the tube extrudes, many patients experience recurrent OM. Adenoidectomy removes a source of infection from the nasopharynx and is associated with a reduction in the number of new episodes. Removal of the adenoid often improves sleep and decreases mouth breathing. Surgical therapy for COME has been shown to be highly cost-effective.[48]

18.7.6 Technical Considerations

Myringotomy and Tube Insertion

Sterilization of the external auditory canal is not routinely performed because of the low rate of infection and the lack of efficacy. Thorough cleaning of the canal is important for seeing the tympanic membrane and for postoperative care. In most cases, the incision is made parallel to the annulus fibrosis in the

anteroinferior quadrant of the tympanic membrane. Care is taken to avoid separating the epithelium from the fibrous layer as this predisposes to tympanosclerosis. The fluid is removed with a 5-French (F) cannula, or if very mucoid, a 7F cannula. Gentle flushing of sterile normal saline into the middle ear can facilitate evacuation of tenacious mucus. It is important to position the tube so that the lumen is directly in the line of sight so that it may be inspected postoperatively and suctioned as needed.

Topical antimicrobial drops are often used postoperatively, particularly in younger children and in cases of purulent or mucoid effusion, both to treat infection and in an attempt to maintain patency of the tube during the postoperative period. The ototoxicity of some of these preparations precludes their use in situations where absorption through the round window membrane is possible, such as in ears with normal middle ear mucosa. In cases of thickened mucosa the risk of absorption appears to be low, but there have been few documented episodes of sensorineural loss and vestibular loss in humans from this use. Quinolone antibiotics, which are noncochleotoxic, are now available in a topical otic solution and an ophthalmic solution. Topical quinolone solutions are approved and used quite commonly for both routine postoperative prophylaxis and treatment of ears draining from AOM.[70-72]

The choice of myringotomy tube is dictated by the surgeon's experience and the treatment goals. The choice of tubes available is staggering in number and variety. However, direct comparison of tubes using a prospective randomized study design with stratification by important risk factors has not been done. Three considerations influence the choice of tube: duration of intubation, risk of water contamination, and ease of removal. For short-term intubation (as with placement for a severe AOM), a short grommet is a logical choice. For long-term intubation (e.g., for an 11-month-old boy in day care with eight documented episodes of AOM, persistent effusion, a strong family history of OM, and smoking in the family, or in a child with a history of multiple prior sets of myringotomy tubes) a long-stemmed myringotomy tube may be a better choice. The short, wide-bore tubes offer little resistance to water entry into the middle ear, compared with the long-shafted myringotomy tubes. Finally, the long tubes can be easily removed in the office, whereas removal of the short grommet tubes with rigid flanges may require a general anesthetic. The risk of otorrhea and permanent perforation increases with the duration of the intubation. However, the risk of recurrent effusion appears to lessen as the duration of intubation increases. Thus, there is a trade-off between effectiveness and complications. It is necessary to discuss with the parents the possibility of a permanent perforation rate of 15% that might be expected with a long-stemmed tube staying for 5 years, in light of 5 years' freedom from effusion, and the 90% closure rates of such perforations with an outpatient myringoplasty. It may be argued that the 15% perforation rate, which is lower than the 34% reoperation rate with grommets, is acceptable. However, it is important to involve the parents in such discussions so that they understand the implications of the choices available to them.

Adenoidectomy

General anesthesia is used, and the airway is ensured by endotracheal intubation. The middle ears are aspirated through a myringotomy incision (see above). The patient is placed supine with the neck extended over a roll. A mouth gag is inserted and the soft palate is retracted with a catheter. The adenoid is excised with curved curettes of various sizes and shapes using a large mirror and either a headlight or the operating microscope to inspect the nasopharynx to ensure complete removal. Adenoid curettes are available in several sizes and configurations. Those with an angulated handle are easier to use than those with a straight handle. A malleable suction cautery may be used to control bleeding.

Careful instrumentation minimizes injury to the prevertebral fascia and muscles, which might otherwise result in excessive bleeding. Curved biting forceps are useful to remove tissue not accessible by the curette. The basket adenotome is seldom used because its curved shape may promote incomplete removal. Adenoidectomy is also performed with cautery or the microdebrider by some surgeons.

Bleeding after adenoidectomy usually stops promptly; pressure applied for a few minutes via sponges in the nasopharynx appears to assist the process, as does irrigation with saline at room temperature. Suction electrocautery permits precise coagulation of bleeding vessels and limits the risk of stenosis from indiscriminate field cauterization.

The goal of the surgery is complete removal of the midline adenoid pad to achieve smooth reepithelialization of the nasopharynx. Curettage of the tissue in the fossa of Rosenmüller is not done to avoid scar tissue formation and contracture that might contribute to eustachian tube reflux. Care must be taken to avoid direct injury to the eustachian tube that might result in stenosis. Inadequate removal of adenoid tissue may be avoided by careful inspection of the nasopharynx with a mirror.

Following adenoidectomy, mild ear pain is common. Acetaminophen is prescribed for pain control. The child is able to eat normally as soon as nausea from the anesthetic has subsided. Transient hypernasal speech may occur in a small percentage of cases, but generally resolves within a few weeks. Frank regurgitation of liquids through the nose is rare. These transient sequelae may occur after removal of a large adenoid mass. Palatal and pharyngeal wall compensation occurs quickly, and permanent voice change is highly unusual in patients with normal palate anatomy. Children with submucous cleft of the soft palate are at higher risk.

18.8 Documentation

Current cost-containment strategies by third-party payers have led to increasing scrutiny of the indications for surgical treatment of OM. A variety of schemes has been developed to verify the history, physical findings, and prior treatment. Criteria for precertification vary among the payers in spite of widely circulated indications used by otolaryngologists. As a result, an increasing burden is often placed upon the staff of the surgeon's office to collect the additional information over and above that needed for patient care. A written summary from the referring pediatrician should fulfill the documentation requirements of most payers.

Demonstration of an enlarged adenoid classically has been required to justify adenoidectomy. Now that it is known that the size of the adenoid is not related to outcome, basing the decision on adenoid size is no longer justified, and this is now generally understood by most payers.

18.9 Complications and Sequelae

The complications of untreated AOM are well known, despite being relatively rare (see Chapter 19). OM may progress to mastoiditis, which if also untreated, may lead to life-threatening intracranial complications such as meningitis and brain abscess. Untreated mastoiditis may also result in a Bezold abscess, subperiosteal abscess, and permanent hearing loss.

A well-studied and long-debated topic is the effect of OM-associated conductive hearing loss on speech and language development in children. Over 100 clinical studies have sought to determine if speech and language development is delayed or impaired in children with OM, but most are flawed due to intrinsic study design difficulties. Paradise et al[73] reported the results of a prospective, randomized clinical trial evaluating the difference between time-appropriate and delayed (after 9 months) myringotomy tube insertion on speech and language development in children 3 years of age. Various indicators of developmental outcomes then were measured, which did not differ significantly between early and late treatment groups. Roberts et al[74] performed a meta-analysis of similar prospective trials evaluating speech and language development in children with OM between 1 and 5 years of age. A very small negative association was seen with OM early in life and later speech and language development. The general consensus among many clinicians is that any impairment suffered as a result of OM early in life is temporary, and speech and language skills return to normal with time.[68]

Intraoperative complications following myringotomy tubes placement are few and rarely severe. Accidental displacement of the tube into the middle ear may rarely require elevation of a tympanomeatal flap for recovery. Persistent perforation of the TM following myringotomy tubes removal or extrusion occurs in 1 to 15% of cases depending on the size of the tube, the number of intercurrent infections, and the duration of intubation. If the child is older, it may be possible to close the perforation with cautery to the edges with trichloroacetic acid and application of a paper patch. More often, however, the standard treatment, after it is seen that the ear is dry, is to perform a myringoplasty, usually with fat graft or cartilage button. This offers an effective remedy that can be performed on an outpatient basis. Recurrence of effusion is not uncommon after extrusion or removal of myringotomy tubes.

An expected outcome after myringotomy tube placement is intermittent purulent otorrhea. In young children the organisms recovered are often the same as with AOM. In the past, water precautions with the use of waterproof ear plugs were universally recommended for patients with ear tubes, and many clinicians continue to recommend water precautions. In our experience, however, only a small percentage of patients develop purulent otorrhea following submersion in clean water. These patients are recommended to follow water precautions to prevent future episodes of otorrhea. Most children are able to continue normal activities such as swimming in pool water without problems following myringotomy tube placement. Some physicians recommend the use of ear plugs if the child swims in untreated water, such as ponds or lakes, because of the higher microbial load. The 2013 AAO-HNS guidelines on tympanostomy tubes recommend against routine instructions for water precautions, however, because of a lack of demonstrated benefit and the social burden of consistent plug use. Initial treatment of otorrhea in children with myringotomy tubes is topical antibiotic drops. The topical quinolone preparations (ciprofloxacin, ofloxacin) have been shown to be effective, better tolerated, and without risk of ototoxicity or selecting for resistant organisms outside of the ear.[70,75] If discharge continues for more than 7 days despite topical treatment, additional use of an oral antibiotic is considered. Most cases of myringotomy tube otorrhea are self-limited and resolve with minimal intervention.

If the discharge fails to resolve promptly with ear drops, then office cleaning of the canal, softening any debris in the tube with hydrogen peroxide and opening by gentle suctioning, and culture for identification of the organisms and antimicrobial sensitivity are performed. Office cleaning and use of topical drops are usually effective. If not, the tube may need to be removed and the middle ear inspected and cultured. Rarely, a resistant organism may require intravenous antimicrobial therapy depending on the sensitivity of the isolate. Biofilm formation on the myringotomy tube or chronic granuloma formation around the ear tube may result in persistent otorrhea and removal of the tube is curative in those cases. If otorrhea continues despite appropriate antibiotic management based on cultures from middle ear fluid, tube removal, and, in some cases, adenoidectomy, further anatomic concerns should be considered. Imaging studies may prove to be helpful, to rule out cholesteatoma.

Biofilms are now recognized as a potential cause of chronic myringotomy tube otorrhea. With the aid of electron microscopy, biofilms were visualized on the surface of T-tubes removed from children with refractory posttympanostomy otorrhea.[76] New strategies such as tubes impregnated with silver, phosphorylcholine, or various antibiotics may help combat biofilms as a potential cause of chronic ear tube otorrhea.

The most common complication of adenoidectomy is postoperative bleeding. However, the incidence is low; in one series of 250 cases operated on by 13 surgeons, only one child required operative treatment for bleeding and none needed blood transfusion.[51] Helmus et al[9,8] noted that only four patients in 1,000 (0.4%) bled after outpatient adenoidectomy and that all instances occurred in the first 6 postoperative hours and were managed without transfusion. Other less common complications include nasopharyngeal stenosis and velopharyngeal incompetence (VPI). Stenosis results from excessive tissue destruction such as might occur from excessive use of the electrocautery, excessive curettage of the fossa of Rosenmüller, and removal of the lateral pharyngeal bands. Transient VPI may occur after removal of a large adenoid but resolves spontaneously in the majority of cases. Persistent VPI is a significant concern to both surgeons and parents, as impaired speech can be devastating. The majority of such cases are due to an undetected submucous cleft palate. Preoperative evaluation with fiberoptic nasopharyngoscopy or careful inspection of the palate at the time of surgery is useful in detecting an occult posterior submucous cleft. In patients with a known history of cleft palate or submucous cleft palate, adenoidectomy is contraindicated. In cases of severe nasal airway obstruction, an inferior adenoidectomy may be performed with great caution.

References

[1] Teele DW, Klein JO, Rosner B. Epidemiology of otitis media during the first seven years of life in children in greater Boston: a prospective, cohort study. J Infect Dis 1989; 160: 83–94

[2] Bluestone CD. Studies in otitis media: Children's Hospital of Pittsburgh-University of Pittsburgh progress report—2004. Laryngoscope 2004; 114 Suppl 105: 1–26

[3] Stool SE, and Otitis Media Guideline Panel. Otitis media with effusion in young children. Clinical practice guideline no. 12. Rockville, MD: Department of Health and Human Services, Public Health Service, Agency for Health Care Policy and Research, 1994

[4] Lieberthal A, Ganiats T et al. American Academy of Pediatrics Subcommittee on Management of Acute Otitis Media. Diagnosis and management of acute otitis media. Pediatrics 2004; 113: 1451–1465

[5] Rosenfeld RM, Culpepper L, Doyle KJ et al. American Academy of Pediatrics Subcommittee on Otitis Media with Effusion. American Academy of Family Physicians. American Academy of Otolaryngology–Head and Neck Surgery. Clinical practice guideline: otitis media with effusion. Otolaryngol Head Neck Surg 2004; 130 Suppl: S95–S118

[6] Rosenfeld RM, Schwartz SR, Pynnonen MA, et al. Clinical practice guideline: tympanostomy tubes in children. Otolaryngology-Head and Neck Surgery 149 Suppl: S1-S35.

[7] Bluestone CD, Klein JO. Otitis Media in Infants and Children, 2nd ed. Philadelphia: WB Saunders, 1995

[8] Doyle WJ. A functiono-anatomic description of Eustachian tube vector relations in four ethnic populations: an osteology study. Pittsburgh: University of Pittsburgh, 1977

[9] Aydoğan B, Kiroğlu M, Altintas D, Yilmaz M, Yorgancilar E, Tuncer U. The role of food allergy in otitis media with effusion. Otolaryngol Head Neck Surg 2004; 130: 747–750

[10] White DR, Heavner SB, Hardy SM, Prazma J. Gastroesophageal reflux and eustachian tube dysfunction in an animal model. Laryngoscope 2002; 112: 955–961

[11] Henderson FW, Collier AM, Sanyal MA et al. A longitudinal study of respiratory viruses and bacteria in the etiology of acute otitis media with effusion. N Engl J Med 1982; 306: 1377–1383

[12] Giebink GS, Payne EE, Mills EL, Juhn SK, Quie PG. Experimental otitis media due to Streptococcus pneumoniae: immunopathogenic response in the chinchilla. J Infect Dis 1976; 134: 595–604

[13] Bluestone CD, Stephenson JS, Martin LM. Ten-year review of otitis media pathogens. Pediatr Infect Dis J 1992; 11 Suppl: S7–S11

[14] Howie VM, Ploussard JH. Simultaneous nasopharyngeal and middle ear exudates in otitis media. Pediatrics Digest 1971; 13: 31–35

[15] Dhooge I, Van Damme D, Vaneechoutte M, Claeys G, Verschraegen G, Van Cauwenberge P. Role of nasopharyngeal bacterial flora in the evaluation of recurrent middle ear infections in children. Clin Microbiol Infect 1999; 5: 530–534

[16] Pillsbury HC, III, Kveton JF, Sasaki CT, Frazier W. Quantitative bacteriology in adenoid tissue. Otolaryngol Head Neck Surg 1981; 89: 355–363

[17] Bernstein JM, Faden HF, Dryja DM, Wactawski-Wende J. Micro-ecology of the nasopharyngeal bacterial flora in otitis-prone and non-otitis-prone children. Acta Otolaryngol 1993; 113: 88–92

[18] Bluestone CD, Paradise JL, Beery QC. Physiology of the eustachian tube in the pathogenesis and management of middle ear effusions. Laryngoscope 1972; 82: 1654–1670

[19] Eden AR, Laitman JT, Gannon PJ. Mechanisms of middle ear aeration: anatomic and physiologic evidence in primates. Laryngoscope 1990; 100: 67–75

[20] Politzer A. A Textbook of Diseases of the Ear. Philadelphia: Henry C. Lea's Son, 1883:107

[21] Swarts JD, Alper CM, Seroky JT, Chan KH, Doyle WJ. In vivo observation with magnetic resonance imaging of middle ear effusion in response to experimental underpressures. Ann Otol Rhinol Laryngol 1995; 104: 522–528

[22] Segal J, Ostfeld E, Yinon J, et al. Mass spectometric analysis of gas composition in the guinea pig middle ear-mastoid system. In: Lim DJ, Bluestone CD, eds. Recent Advances in Otitis Media with Effusion, Philadelphia: BC Decker, 1983:68–70

[23] Cantekin EI, Doyle WJ, Phillips DC, Bluestone CD. Gas absorption in the middle ear. Ann Otol Rhinol Laryngol Suppl 1980; 89: 71–75

[24] Goldie P, Hellström S, Johansson U. Vascular events in experimental otitis media models: a comparative study. ORL J Otorhinolaryngol Relat Spec 1990; 52: 104–112

[25] Teele DW, Klein JO, Rosner BA. Epidemiology of otitis media in children. Ann Otol Rhinol Laryngol Suppl 1980; 89: 5–6

[26] Rosenfeld RM, Kay D. Natural history of untreated otitis media. Laryngoscope 2003; 113: 1645–1657

[27] Giebink GS, Mills EL, Huff JS et al. The microbiology of serous and mucoid otitis media. Pediatrics 1979; 63: 915–919

[28] Rayner MG, Zhang Y, Gorry MC, Chen Y, Post JC, Ehrlich GD. Evidence of bacterial metabolic activity in culture-negative otitis media with effusion. JAMA 1998; 279: 296–299

[29] Ehrlich GD, Veeh R, Wang X et al. Mucosal biofilm formation on middle-ear mucosa in the chinchilla model of otitis media. JAMA 2002; 287: 1710–1715

[30] Discolo CM, Byrd MC, Bates T, Hazony D, Lewandowski J, Koltai PJ. Ultrasonic detection of middle ear effusion: a preliminary study. Arch Otolaryngol Head Neck Surg 2004; 130: 1407–1410

[31] Babb MJ, Hilsinger RL, Jr, Korol HW, Wilcox RD. Modern acoustic reflectometry: accuracy in diagnosing otitis media with effusion. Ear Nose Throat J 2004; 83: 622–624

[32] Finitzo T, Friel-Patti S, Chinn K, Brown O. Tympanometry and otoscopy prior to myringotomy: issues in diagnosis of otitis media. Int J Pediatr Otorhinolaryngol 1992; 24: 101–110

[33] Kaleida PH, Stool SE. Assessment of otoscopists' accuracy regarding middle-ear effusion. Otoscopic validation. Am J Dis Child 1992; 146: 433–435

[34] Coker TR, Chan LS, Newberry SJ et al. Diagnosis, microbial epidemiology, and antibiotic treatment of acute otitis media in children: a systematic review. JAMA 2010; 304: 2161–2169

[35] Tähtinen PA, Laine MK, Huovinen P, Jalava J, Ruuskanen O, Ruohola A. A placebo-controlled trial of antimicrobial treatment for acute otitis media. N Engl J Med 2011; 364: 116–126

[36] Hoberman A, Paradise JL, Rockette HE et al. Treatment of acute otitis media in children under 2 years of age. N Engl J Med 2011; 364: 105–115

[37] Rosenfeld RM, Vertrees JE, Carr J et al. Clinical efficacy of antimicrobial drugs for acute otitis media: metaanalysis of 5400 children from thirty-three randomized trials. J Pediatr 1994; 124: 355–367

[38] Glasziou PP, Del Mar CB, Sanders SL, Hayem M. Antibiotics for acute otitis media in children. Cochrane Database Syst Rev 2004; 1: CD000219

[39] Siegel RM, Kiely M, Bien JP et al. Treatment of otitis media with observation and a safety-net antibiotic prescription. Pediatrics 2003; 112: 527–531

[40] Eskola J, Kilpi T, Palmu A et al. Finnish Otitis Media Study Group. Efficacy of a pneumococcal conjugate vaccine against acute otitis media. N Engl J Med 2001; 344: 403–409

[41] Paradise JL. Managing otitis media: a time for change. Pediatrics 1995; 96: 712–715

[42] Barnett ED, Klein JO. The problem of resistant bacteria for the management of acute otitis media. Pediatr Clin North Am 1995; 42: 509–517

[43] Rosenfeld RM, Post JC. Meta-analysis of antibiotics for the treatment of otitis media with effusion. Otolaryngol Head Neck Surg 1992; 106: 378–386

[44] Schwartz RH, Puglese J, Schwartz DM. Use of a short course of prednisone for treating middle ear effusion. A double-blind crossover study. Ann Otol Rhinol Laryngol Suppl 1980; 89: 296–300

[45] Lambert PR. Oral steroid therapy for chronic middle ear perfusion: a double-blind crossover study. Otolaryngol Head Neck Surg 1986; 95: 193–199

[46] Rosenfeld RM, Mandel EM, Bluestone CD. Systemic steroids for otitis media with effusion in children. Arch Otolaryngol Head Neck Surg 1991; 117: 984–989

[47] Butler CC, Van Der Voort JH. Oral or topical nasal steroids for hearing loss associated with otitis media with effusion in children. Cochrane Database Syst Rev 2002; 4: CD001935

[48] Gates GA. Cost-effectiveness considerations in otitis media treatment. Otolaryngol Head Neck Surg 1996; 114: 525–530

[49] Armstrong BW. A new treatment for chronic secretory otitis media. AMA Arch Otolaryngol 1954; 59: 653–654

[50] Mandel EM, Rockette HE, Bluestone CD, Paradise JL, Nozza RJ. Myringotomy with and without tympanostomy tubes for chronic otitis media with effusion. Arch Otolaryngol Head Neck Surg 1989; 115: 1217–1224

[51] Gates GA, Avery CA, Prihoda TJ, Cooper JC, Jr. Effectiveness of adenoidectomy and tympanostomy tubes in the treatment of chronic otitis media with effusion. N Engl J Med 1987; 317: 1444–1451

[52] Gross CW, Bassila M, Lazar RH, Long TE, Stagner S. Adipose plug myringoplasty: an alternative to formal myringoplasty techniques in children. Otolaryngol Head Neck Surg 1989; 101: 617–620

[53] Eavey RD. Inlay tympanoplasty: cartilage butterfly technique. Laryngoscope 1998; 108: 657–661

[54] Daudia A, Yelavich S, Dawes PJ. Long-term middle-ear ventilation with subannular tubes. J Laryngol Otol 2010; 124: 945–949

[55] Goode RL. T-tube for middle ear ventilation. Arch Otolaryngol 1973; 97: 402–403

[56] Whittemore K, Dornan B, Lally T, et al. Persistent conductive or mixed hearing loss after the placement of tympanostomy tubes. Int J Pediatr Otorhinolaryngol 2012;76:1465–1470

[57] Maw AR. Chronic otitis media with effusion (glue ear) and adenotonsillectomy: prospective randomised controlled study. Br Med J (Clin Res Ed) 1983; 287: 1586–1588

[58] Paradise JL, Bluestone CD, Rogers KD et al. Efficacy of adenoidectomy for recurrent otitis media in children previously treated with tympanostomy-tube placement. Results of parallel randomized and nonrandomized trials. JAMA 1990; 263: 2066–2073

[59] Paradise JL, Bluestone CD. Adenoidectomy and chronic otitis media(letter) N Engl J Med 1988; 318: 1470–1471

[60] Brodsky L, Koch RJ. Bacteriology and immunology of normal and diseased adenoids in children. Arch Otolaryngol Head Neck Surg 1993; 119: 821–829

[61] Maynard JE, Fleshman JK, Tschopp CF. Otitis media in Alaskan Eskimo children. Prospective evaluation of chemoprophylaxis. JAMA 1972; 219: 597–599

[62] Bluestone CD, Klein JO. Clinical practice guideline on otitis media with effusion in young children: strengths and weaknesses. Otolaryngol Head Neck Surg 1995; 112: 507–511

[63] Gebhart DE. Tympanostomy tubes in the otitis media prone child. Laryngoscope 1981; 91: 849–866

[64] American Academy of Otolaryngology—Head and Neck Surgery. 2000 Clinical Indicators Compendium. Alexandria, VA: AAO-HNS, 2000

[65] Paradise JL, Bluestone CD, Colborn DK et al. Adenoidectomy and adenotonsillectomy for recurrent acute otitis media: parallel randomized clinical trials in children not previously treated with tympanostomy tubes. JAMA 1999; 282: 945–953

[66] Maw R. Glue Ear in Childhood. Cambridge, England: Cambridge University Press, 1995

[67] Haggard M, Gannon M et al. MRC Multicentre Otitis Media Study Group. Adjuvant adenoidectomy in persistent bilateral otitis media with effusion: hearing and revision surgery outcomes through 2 years in the TARGET randomised trial. Clin Otolaryngol 2012; 37: 107–116

[68] Klein JO, Teele DW, Rosner BA, et al. Otitis media with effusion during the first three years of life and development of speech and language. In: Lim DJ, Bluestone CD, eds. Recent Advances in Otitis Media with Effusion. Philadelphia: BC Decker, 1984:332–335

[69] Hubbard TW, Paradise JL, McWilliams BJ, Elster BA, Taylor FH. Consequences of unremitting middle-ear disease in early life. Otologic, audiologic, and developmental findings in children with cleft palate. N Engl J Med 1985; 312: 1529–1534

[70] Barlow DW, Duckert LG, Kreig CS, Gates GA. Ototoxicity of topical otomicrobial agents. Acta Otolaryngol 1995; 115: 231–235

[71] Dohar JE, Garner ET, Nielsen RW, Biel MA, Seidlin M. Topical ofloxacin treatment of otorrhea in children with tympanostomy tubes. Arch Otolaryngol Head Neck Surg 1999; 125: 537–545

[72] Goldblatt EL. Efficacy of ofloxacin and other otic preparations for acute otitis media in patients with tympanostomy tubes. Pediatr Infect Dis J 2001; 20: 116–119, discussion 120–122

[73] Paradise JL, Feldman HM, Campbell TF et al. Effect of early or delayed insertion of tympanostomy tubes for persistent otitis media on developmental outcomes at the age of three years. N Engl J Med 2001; 344: 1179–1187

[74] Roberts JE, Rosenfeld RM, Zeisel SA. Otitis media and speech and language: a meta-analysis of prospective studies. Pediatrics 2004; 113: e238–e248

[75] Goldblatt EL, Dohar J, Nozza RJ et al. Topical ofloxacin versus systemic amoxicillin/clavulanate in purulent otorrhea in children with tympanostomy tubes. Int J Pediatr Otorhinolaryngol 1998; 46: 91–101

[76] Post JC. Direct evidence of bacterial biofilms in otitis media. Laryngoscope 2001; 111: 2083–2094

[77] Helmus C, Grin M, Westfall R. Same-day-stay adenotonsillectomy. Laryngoscope 1990; 100: 593–596

19 Chronic Otitis Media

Peter C. Weber

19.1 Introduction

This chapter discusses the medical and surgical management of chronic otitis media (COM), including dry tympanic membrane (TM) perforation, mucosal disease, cholesteatoma, draining ear with TM perforation, surgical techniques and surgical complications. Acute otitis media (AOM) and meningeal complications of disease are covered in Chapters 18 and 20, respectively.

19.2 Office Management

19.2.1 Chronic Otitis Media Without Cholesteatoma

In 1965, Thorburn[1] delineated tubotympanic disease into two separate types.[2] Type I is a chronic perforation that may occasionally drain due to colds, weather changes, or water getting into the ear. However, this rarely has significant negative impact on the patient. These dry ears are typically associated with pink middle ear mucosa that is normal and healthy (▶ Fig. 19.1). In contrast, type II is a persistent mucosal infection. Typically the patient presents with a 3- to 6-month history of chronic discharge from the ear, which may or may not have been associated with a respiratory infection and hearing loss (▶ Fig. 19.2).

More than likely, the type II patient has already been treated for several months with multiple courses of systemic and topical antibiotics. Cultures have usually been obtained, which can be helpful. However, the sensitivities are not usually helpful because they do not reflect that topical therapy results in concentrations much greater than those that can be achieved by systemic antibiotics.[3] The typical bacteria are well known.[4–9] *Pseudomonas aeruginosa* and *Staphylococcus aureus* are the most common, whereas *Corynebacterium, Escherichia coli,* and *Streptococcus pneumoniae* are less so. Occasionally a methicillin resistant *S. aureus* may be seen. Foul-smelling drainage also suggests anaerobic *Streptococcus* or *Bacteroides.*[10,11] *Bacteroides* will often respond to chloramphenicol in drop or powder form. Persistent drainage despite antibiotics may indicate *Mycobacterium,* methicillin-resistant *S. aureus* (MRSA), or even cerebrospinal fluid (CSF) leak.[12,13] Cultures and β_2-transferrin testing may be helpful in those cases.

Physical examination of the ear may demonstrate a perforation with significant granulation tissue and purulent discharge (▶ Fig. 19.3). A high-resolution computed tomography (CT) scan typically reveals a middle ear filled with soft tissue extending into the attic and mastoid air cells filled with fluid.[14] Although many clinicians might not obtain a CT scan, even before surgery, I usually obtain a CT scan preoperatively to assess any abnormalities ahead of time and to aid in counseling patients preoperatively.[15]

Chronic otitis media without cholesteatoma is distinctly different from persistent middle ear effusion requiring myringotomy and tube insertion, and from a chronic draining tube requiring tube removal and antibiotics. Such treatment almost always results in a dry ear, although persistent perforation may sometimes occur. Instead, COM describes an ear that drains fluid time and again after a tube is placed and then removed. The patient may have chronic eustachian tube dysfunction, chronic mucosal disease with attic block, or chronic serous mastoiditis.

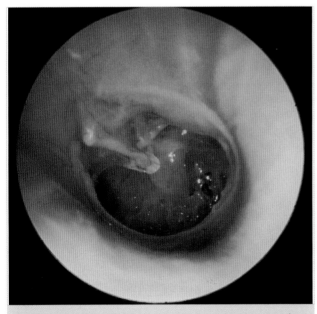

Fig. 19.1 Near-total perforation caused by "necrotizing otitis media" from β-hemolytic streptococcus.

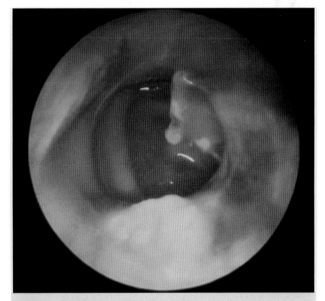

Fig. 19.2 Chronic suppurative otitis media.

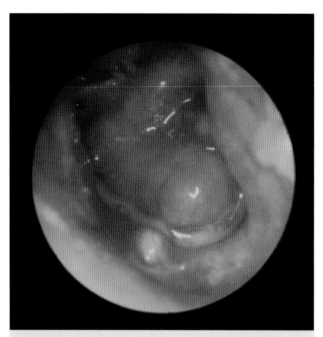

Fig. 19.3 Chronic suppurative otitis media with granuloma.

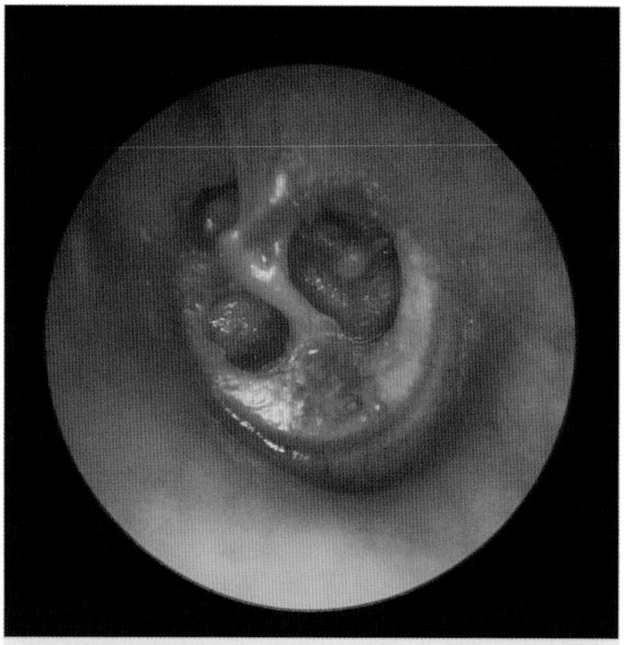

Fig. 19.4 Serous otitis media with retraction.

Many cases of COM can be traced back to an underperforming eustachian tube with effusion and drum retraction (▶ Fig. 19.4).

Many patients with COM without cholesteatoma will eventually need surgery; however, medical therapy should be tried first. The ear should be cleaned thoroughly so that topical drops can reach the middle ear. Cleaning begins in the office under the microscope and then at home with irrigations of 1:1 alcohol/vinegar (essentially acetic acid). The patient repeats the washings several times daily with the ear turned up as described by Sheehy[7] or turned down as preferred by others. The dropper and rubber bulb are filled with solution, the tip of the dropper is placed in the ear opening, and the bulb is compressed and decompressed gently, swishing the solution back and forth to clear the canal. The solution should be near body temperature to avoid dizziness. If acetic acid solution causes pain, then Sheehy also has described using one-half strength Betadine (povidone-iodine). Washings are continued for about 1 week. Steroid antibiotic drops are also used either immediately after each washing or added after the 1 week of washings. An alternative to antibiotic drops is powder combinations.

The preferred medicated drop is a fluoroquinolone with steroid[16] because it is not ototoxic and because corticosteroids can help reduce granulation tissue and edema in the middle ear as well as scaling and itching of the external canal (dexamethasone is even better than hydrocortisone in this regard[17]). Rarely, a fungal infection can occur with fluoroquinolone drops. Potentially ototoxic drops, such as tobramycin, Cortisporin (Epocrates Inc., San Mateo, CA), and Colimycin (Shangqiu Kangmeida Bio-Technology Company Ltd., Henan, China), have been used quite safely for decades, probably because a barrier over the round window membrane is formed by chronic disease. However, if the middle ear mucosa heals with treatment but the patient continues to use ototoxic drops, the drops could penetrate into the inner ear and cause vestibulopathy or hearing loss. Thus, the clinician should inform the patient if a potentially ototoxic

drop is used. However, risks are rare and if fluoroquinolones fail, it may be necessary to use these types of drops. I generally avoid Cortisporin because some patients have an allergy to topical neomycin, which can make the ear worse or make it difficult to tell if the chronic drainage is now due to the ear disease or the allergy.

A recent study demonstrates equivalency between fluoroquinolones with dexamethasone versus powder combinations. In addition, both were significantly better than acetic acid drops. The most common powder mixture that the author uses is composed of chloramphenicol, amphotericin, and boric acid, which creates an environment that is very resistant to bacterial and fungal growth.[18] If the patient has not had any oral antibiotic treatment prior to the first visit, I usually treat with one course. However, the topical drop is more important. If drops or powders fail, the same report demonstrates an 85% salvage rate when Quadriderm is used. IV antibiotics are almost never needed unless there are complications such as petrositis, labyrinthitis, or meningitis. Surgery for COM without cholesteatoma usually is withheld until the ear is dry or maximum improvement is reached.

19.3 Cholesteatoma

Cholesteatomas grow by forming a keratinizing stratified epithelial layer and fibrous subepithelial layer called the matrix. The matrix is constantly desquamating sheets of keratin into the cholesteatoma sac. This keratin or dead skin accumulates in concentric layers. As the sac expands it erodes surrounding bone, even the hard bone of the labyrinth. This generally occurs because of the various aggressive enzymes that the cholesteatoma generates.[19]

Cholesteatoma can be congenital or acquired. Congenital cholesteatomas almost always are seen in children, although adults may present with petrous apex or intracranial epidermoids. By

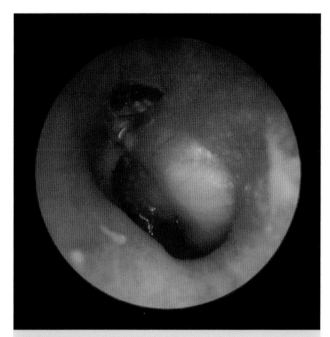

Fig. 19.5 Cholesteatoma behind the posterior drum.

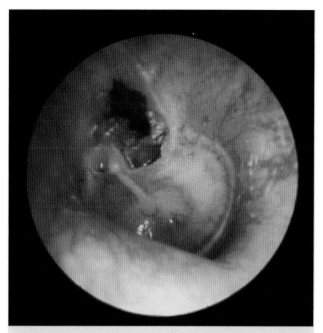

Fig. 19.6 Chronic otitis media with pars flaccida defect.

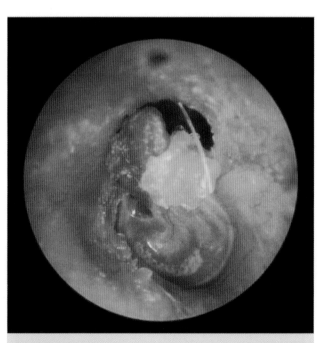

Fig. 19.7 Attic erosion.

definition, congenital cholesteatomas have no history of perforation, myringotomy, or otorrhea and have a normal TM.[20–24] The vast majority of congenital cholesteatomas are found in the anterosuperior quadrant, although at times they may be found in the posterosuperior quadrant, within the TM itself, or in the petrous apex. The pathogenesis of congenital cholesteatoma is controversial, although the following theories have some merit: fetal epithelial cells are trapped in the middle ear; inflamed TM cells invaginate into the middle ear; or squamous metaplasia transforms middle ear mucosa into keratinizing epithelium.[22]

Acquired cholesteatoma is far more common and usually results from retraction of the TM in the pars flaccida or posterosuperior quadrant (► Fig. 19.5; ► Fig. 19.6; ► Fig. 19.7). This retraction and subsequently the cholesteatoma slowly develop and may not be detected until the patient complains of drainage or hearing loss. Previous ear surgery or drum perforation may also be a site for acquired cholesteatoma as keratin can invaginate and proliferate on the undersurface of the perforation. However, the epithelium from the lateral TM usually goes around the edge of a perforation, but then stops growing 1 or 2 mm on the medial surface of the TM where it abuts the mucosal layer.

The diagnosis of cholesteatoma is usually not difficult, as both congenital and acquired types can be seen on microscopic examination in the office. Patients with acquired disease usually complain of foul-smelling discharge and often bleeding. Normally, hearing is impaired to some degree, and this is verified with audiometric testing. Patients may have slight otalgia or headache and occasionally mild dizziness. Diseased mucosa, granulation tissue, and keratin debris may be confined to the epitympanum. Occasionally, drainage and granulation tissue can make it difficult to see the keratin sac (► Fig. 19.3; ► Fig. 19.8).

Cholesteatoma is a disease that requires surgery, but again, antibiotic-steroid drops should be started prior to surgery in order to help decrease the amount of inflammation and granulation tissue. Although this treatment does not cure cholesteatoma, it can decrease the amount of bleeding during surgery. In order to obtain a safe, dry ear, the cholesteatoma must be removed.

Culture and sensitivity studies can be obtained but we know the most common organisms are pseudomonas or bacillus and the results do not alter the treatment, which remains surgery. Culture and sensitivity studies are helpful if the patient is suspected of having a complication from the cholesteatoma.

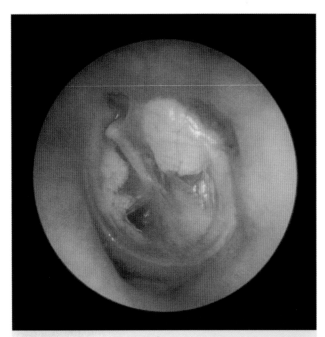

Fig. 19.8 Cartilage is evident in the posterosuperior quadrant after tympanoplasty.

Computed tomography (CT) scanning can be quite useful preoperatively, as it identifies potential abnormalities ahead of time (tegmen erosion, facial nerve dehiscence, and labyrinth fistula) and can lead to better counseling of the patient, but many otologists do not obtain CT scans because it does not change the management. The patient should also be informed that the cholesteatoma can cause hearing loss, facial paralysis, meningitis, dizziness, tinnitus, and other intracranial complications.

19.4 Surgical Management

Whether treating chronic mucosal disease, cholesteatoma, or benign perforation, the surgeon's primary goal is to obtain a safe, dry ear. The approach and technique vary depending on training and experience. However, basic principles apply to all procedures to achieve a good result. These principles and my own preferences are presented.

19.4.1 Preoperative Counseling

Patients should understand that a safe, dry ear is the primary goal of any surgery, so that they do not have unrealistic expectations, such as achieving normal hearing. To this end, the treatment plan may typically require a two-stage procedure, where after the first stage the hearing, by design, is actually worse than it was preoperatively because the ossicular reconstruction occurs at the second surgery/stage. Even without cholesteatoma, attic mucosal disease often necessitates the removal of the incus; failure to do so may not completely eradicate the disease or restore ventilation. Free flow of irrigant from the mastoid into the middle ear is a good indication that disease has been removed and aeration is adequate. I perform second-look surgery

with ossicular reconstruction 6 to 12 months after the first stage. The patient is counseled that even after the ossicular reconstruction the hearing will not be normal and may require amplification or even an implantable device such as a bone-anchored hearing aid.

Indications, risks, benefits, alternatives, and the personnel involved in the surgery are discussed with the patient. The success rate for a safe, dry ear is roughly 90%.[25-27] Risks include but are not limited to partial or total hearing loss (can occur 1 to 2% of the time) vertigo, disequilibrium, facial nerve paralysis, CSF leak, tinnitus, infection, bleeding, meningitis, perilymph fistula, otorrhea, stenosis/fistulization of the external auditory canal, pain, headaches, cosmetic deformities, loss of taste, and visual changes, all of which occur very infrequently.

Underlying sinonasal disease should be treated prior to ear surgery to improve postoperative eustachian tube function. Even if the eustachian tube is not blocked by sinonasal disease, its function is improved anyway by removing disease from the protympanum.

19.5 Terminology

The history of ear surgery has been well described by Glasscock's group.[25,28-30] In chronic ear surgery, residual cholesteatoma refers to disease that is intentionally or unintentionally left behind after the initial surgical procedure; sometimes this is referred to as recidivism. Recurrent cholesteatoma refers to cholesteatoma that forms after the initial surgery, typically in a postoperative retraction pocket.

Although many surgeons define tympanoplasty as closure of a TM perforation, it technically refers to any operation that lifts the TM and removes middle ear disease or reconstructs hearing with or without TM grafting. Tympanoplasty may be performed with or without mastoidectomy. Repair of the TM perforation may be done via a medial (underlay) technique or a lateral (overlay technique). Storrs[31] performed the first medial graft tympanoplasty using temporalis fascia in the United States in 1961. Prior to this, early techniques employed a small rubber disk attached to a silver wire by Toynbee[32] in 1853, skin grafts by Berthold[33] in 1878, and paper patch 10 years later.[34] In the 1950s, Wullstein[35] and Zollner[36] used split- and full-thickness skin grafts to repair chronically diseased ears, not just drum perforations, for better healing and hearing. In 1967, Goodhill[37] first described using tragal cartilage attic reconstruction to minimize recurrent cholesteatoma formation. The approaches used include transcanal, Lempert incision, and postauricular procedures.[38]

Atticotomy is appropriate for disease lateral to the incus body and malleus head that does not extend anterior to the head of the malleus or posterior or medial to the short process of the incus. It involves removal of the scutum to expose the attic tympanum. This approach enables preservation of the posterior external auditory canal while at the same time facilitating removal of cholesteatoma confined to the epitympanum, repair of an attic retraction pocket, and gaining exposure to lateral chain fixation or otosclerosis cases. The scutal wall defect that was made should be reconstructed to prevent recurrence of cholesteatoma.[39] Cartilage obtained from the tragus or cymba can be used for this reconstruction (▶ Fig. 19.8).

Cortical (simple) mastoidectomy removes the lateral aspect of the mastoid bone with exposure of the middle fossa tegmen, sigmoid sinus, and antrum. The facial recess is opened as needed. This procedure is the workhorse for many ear surgeries. It provides ventilation from the middle ear to the mastoid, eradicates disease, and provides exposure for many procedures including endolymphatic sac surgery, cochlear implantation, and labyrinthectomy. Intact canal wall tympanoplasty with mastoidectomy was first described by Jansen[40] in the 1950s. This was a dramatic improvement over the previous techniques,[41–44] first recorded by Jean Louis Petit[45] in Paris.

Modified radical mastoidectomy (MRM) differs from intact canal wall mastoidectomy in that the posterior external auditory canal (EAC) is removed. A meatoplasty is commonly performed to better ventilate the mastoid and facilitate postoperative care. MRM, by definition, includes grafting the TM to cover the mesotympanum or protympanum. The MRM is also commonly referred to as the canal-wall-down (CWD) mastoidectomy.

Although most surgeons strive to not remove the posterior EAC, removal is indicated for extensive disease (in order to see to be able to remove it all), residual epithelium over a labyrinthine fistula, recurrent attic cholesteatoma, the patient's inability to come back for follow-up care, or the patient's unwillingness to undergo a two-staged procedure. Removing the posterior EAC minimizes the chance of recurrent attic disease.[46] Gantz et al[47] described a procedure to remove the posterior EAC and then to put it back after eradication of the disease.

The Bondy MRM, first performed in 1910, is rarely used today.[48] In this procedure the medial wall of the cholesteatoma sac is preserved over the intact TM and ossicular chain. Nowadays most surgeons prefer to remove the entire disease and then return for a second-stage ossicular reconstruction.

Radical mastoidectomy differs from MRM in that the TM is not grafted, the middle ear is not reconstructed, and the eustachian tube is obliterated. It is typically reserved for those situations where the cholesteatoma is so extensive on a revision case that it cannot be completely removed.

19.6 Preoperative Preparation, Anesthesia, and Incisions

The operating room is set up with the anesthesiologist at the foot of the patient and the scrub nurse directly opposite the surgeon so that instruments can be passed back and forth easily while the surgeon continues to work under the microscope. General anesthesia is the mainstay for most patients, typically with a laryngeal mask airway rather than an endotracheal tube. Alternatively, transcanal surgery can be done under local anesthesia or monitored anesthesia care (MAC). The postauricular incision site is injected with 1% lidocaine–1/100,000 epinephrine, although other concentrations can be used. I do not shave any of the patient's hair for any otologic or neurotologic procedure, as studies have indicated that the rate of infection is certainly no worse and may indeed be less than if one does shave the patient.[49] Under microscopic visualization, the EAC is injected with 1% lidocaine–1/40,000 epinephrine (these concentrations vary per surgeon). To facilitate monitoring the facial nerve, the patient should not be paralyzed, although a short-acting paralytic can be used for intubation. In addition, if a medial graft tympanoplasty is performed and the middle ear is packed with Gelfoam, nitrous oxide can be used because it may push the medial graft laterally onto the undersurface of the TM, helping keeping it in place. However, for a lateral graft, nitrous oxide should not be used because of an increase in blunting or lateralization of the graft. Extubation while the patient is "deep" may avoid an increase in middle ear pressure as well. Postoperatively, an antinauseant can be used to minimize straining.

After prepping with iodinated solution (Betadine), or another suitable alternative, a vascular strip incision is made under the microscope for those patients undergoing a postauricular incision (▶ Fig. 19.9). Alternatively, if a transcanal approach is being utilized, a tympanomeatal flap incision is made (▶ Fig. 19.10). The postauricular incision is made a few millimeters behind the postauricular ear crease (▶ Fig. 19.11).

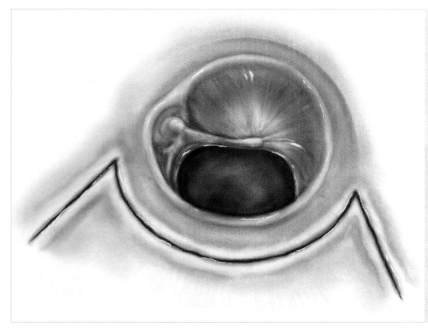

Fig. 19.9 The use of the tympanomeatal and vascular strip incisions for postauricular approach. The horizontal incision parallels and is close to the annulus in this particular incision. The incision at the 6 o'clock position actually starts at 6 o'clock but comes out more at the 7 to 8 o'clock position, as this makes it easier to identify the incision on a postauricular approach. The incision at the 12 o'clock position is angled upward into the incisura of the avascular plane between the helical and antihelical cartilage. Other canal incisions can be used, as the surgeon prefers.

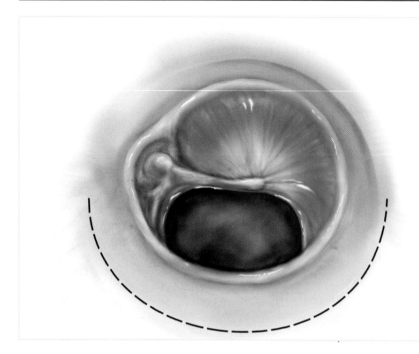

Fig. 19.10 The tympanomeatal incision for transcanal work demonstrates a slightly larger distance between the annulus (about 8 mm) and the horizontal cut. Thus, if the scutum needs to be curetted, it will facilitate closure. If the flap does not lie forward easily, the superior radial incision should be extended beyond 12 o'clock.

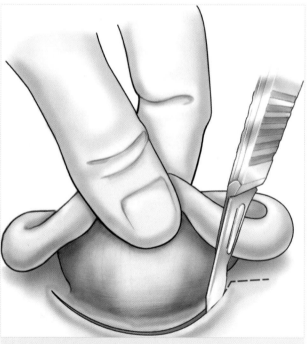

Fig. 19.11 The postauricular incision.

A temporalis areolar tissue or fascia graft is harvested (if needed) to repair the TM. A Palva flap is then raised (▶ Fig. 19.12) by making cuts along the temporal line and mastoid tip, then connecting them posteriorly to create a rectangular flap based anteriorly. Many surgeons use a T-incision to raise the periosteum, but I find the Palva flap helps cover or fill in a mastoid defect, especially in CWD surgery. Alternatively, if a tympanoplasty without mastoidectomy is being performed, then a small curved periosteal incision just posterior to the EAC may be made because no mastoid drilling is done.

19.7 Surgical Technique

19.7.1 Tympanoplasty

Tympanoplasty can be divided into medial or lateral techniques. In the medial graft technique, the perforation edges are "freshened" in order to remove any underlying epithelium. I typically use a microcup forceps to grasp the anterior edge of the perforation and then gently pull posteriorly to remove a circumferentially small rim of tissue. The tympanomeatal flap is elevated, the annulus dissected out of the annular ring, the middle ear entered, and the flap reflected anteriorly. Any disease is removed; then a small piece of Gelfilm is placed onto the floor of the middle ear. This helps prevent adhesions and facilitates filling the mesotympanum with Gelfoam, because the Gelfoam slides across the Gelfilm. The graft is placed medially to cover the perforation and then the middle ear is filled with Gelfoam (▶ Fig. 19.13). Gelfoam facilitates graft placement to cover the defect. For anterosuperior perforations that are not marginal, an anterior wall tympanomeatal flap can be raised in much the same fashion. If the bony overhang prevents adequate visualization, then after windowshading the skin off of the overhang, the overhang is drilled away to facilitate the needed exposure.

The lateral graft technique is typically used for total or near-total perforations, marginal perforations, or revision cases of failed medial grafts. The lateral graft technique differs in that the entire epithelial layer over the TM must be removed to prevent intratympanic cholesteatoma formation (▶ Fig. 19.14). The posterior canal incision is extended circumferentially around the medial aspect of the EAC. The skin is then elevated 360 degrees down to the annulus. Starting inferiorly, the epithelial layer of the TM is then dissected off in continuity with the EAC skin. The TM epithelial layer is typically elevated to the malleus and then gently grabbed superiorly over the short process and gently pulled superior to inferior, removing all the skin in one

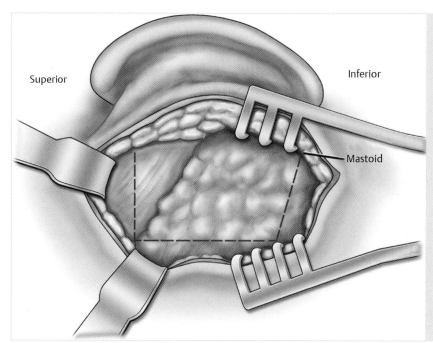

Fig. 19.12 A large Palva flap (dashed line). The superior incision is usually made several millimeters above the actual temporal line, and the inferior incision angles slightly toward the mastoid tip. A T-incision also can be used.

Superior

Inferior

Mastoid

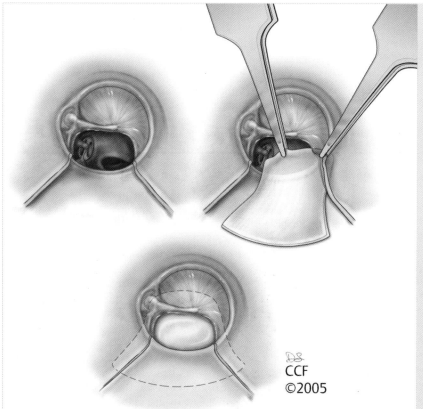

Fig. 19.13 In the medial (underlay) graft technique, the graft is placed medial to the malleus and drum remnant.

piece. This skin is then saved in a moistened fashion for use at the end of the procedure to graft on top of the newly reconstructed TM. If needed, the annulus can be dissected out of the annular ring so that the middle ear can be examined and worked on if needed.

To place a lateral graft so as to avoid blunting or lateralization, the following steps may help. A 1-mm trough can be drilled just lateral to the annulus anteriorly. The anterosuperior

and anteroinferior regions of the EAC are enlarged and squared off. Care is taken not to expose the temporomandibular joint (TMJ). The graft is placed to fit into that trough and then packed tightly down. I find that the size of the fascial graft is typically the size of the nail of my index finger. A small slit is cut into the superior aspect of the graft before placement so that, as the graft is placed under the malleus, the slit yields pieces to wrap around the malleus handle to prevent lateralization

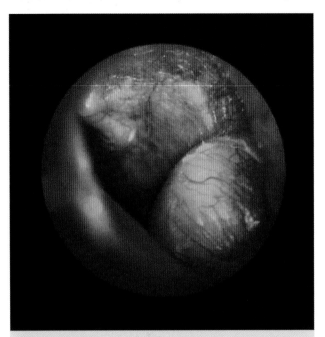

Fig. 19.14 Intratympanic and canal cholesteatoma after a lateral graft technique.

(▶ Fig. 19.15). The posterior portion comes up the posterior EAC slightly. Next, the harvested skin is placed on top of the graft. The skin is typically cut into small pieces or strips. It is placed with the intent of keeping the anterior sulcus on the posterior aspect of the graft. A piece of rolled Gelfoam is placed to help keep the anterior sulcus in place and then the canal is filled with Gelfoam. Postoperatively, the patient is started on antibiotic/steroid eardrops to help dissolve packing and prevent infection and granulation. After 2 weeks, one half to two thirds of the packing is removed, with the patient returning 6 weeks later.

Another option to pack the canal is to use a Rosebud pack. Parachute silk is used to line the medial EAC and new TM. Small cotton pledgets dipped in antibiotic ointment are placed on the silk-lined drum. A second Rosebud packing is placed on top of the first packing to keep the lateral aspect of the EAC open. This is left in place 10 to 14 days before removal and then the patient is started on the same drops. Again, I avoid using neomycin-containing drops.

Cartilage tympanoplasty is indicated when the scutum has been eroded by disease or drilled away in order to facilitate removal of disease. Reconstruction of this area with cartilage is the preferred method of repair. Cartilage may be obtained from either the tragus or the cymba region of the auricle (▶ Fig. 19.16). Perichondrium is left on both sides and then raised on one side to create a cartilage flap. This flap is placed so that the TM is still mobile. It can be extended to cover the head of a partial or total ossicular prosthesis as well. This may be accomplished by scoring a cut in the cartilage or pieces of cartilage can be placed and then covered by a fascial graft (▶ Fig. 19.17). Long-term follow-up is needed because recurrence rates over 20 years are quite high.

19.8 Second-Look Surgery and Ossicular Reconstruction

Occasionally the cholesteatoma is small and easily removed in one piece. The surgeon should be confident that no residual remains, and in these cases ossicular reconstruction can be done immediately, thus precluding a second-look procedure. But second-look surgery is needed when the disease is more extensive. The second look typically occurs 6 to 12 months after the initial surgery. Cartilage graft is typically placed at the initial surgery because that is when a need for ossicular reconstruction is identified, but sometimes there is a need to place a graft of cartilage during the second look for the TORP or PORP.

The published rates of residual cholesteatoma is as high as 30%,[27] with most (85%) occurring in the epitympanum. Fortunately, the residual cholesteatoma is quite small at the second look, resembling a small pearl, and is easily removed. The TORP or PORP is placed (usually made of titanium, hydroxyapatite, or porous polyethylene).

19.9 Mastoidectomy

Prior to performing the mastoidectomy, disease is usually removed in the mesotympanum to facilitate the identification of landmarks. This helps ascertain how deep one is in the mastoid (especially if it is sclerotic). The area may be packed with adrenalin-soaked Gelfoam to improve hemostasis. Two basic rules for mastoidectomy are then followed: (1) "As you go deep, go wide"; that is, the mastoid bowl should be saucerized to improve and minimize the risk from drilling in a confined space (▶ Fig. 19.18). (2) "The tegmen is your friend"; that is, drilling high along the tegmen minimizes risk to the lateral canal and facial nerve as you approach the antrum. This is especially important in sclerotic mastoids.[3]

If possible, some bone should be left over the tegmen and sigmoid sinus to protect the dura, minimize the risk of CSF leak, meningocele formation, and bleeding.[50,51] The posterior EAC should be thinned so as not to drill under a ledge. Drill from one safe area to another. All disease from affected air cells should be removed to prevent the recurrence of infection.

Some surgeons always identify the facial nerve, but others do so only if it is involved with disease. Regardless, the facial nerve landmarks must be kept in mind. In the mesotympanum the tensor tympani (cochleariform process), lateral semicircular canal, and stapedial tendon are good landmarks to identify the geniculate ganglion and tympanic (horizontal) segment. The facial nerve lies superior to the cochleariform process and oval window. In some patients there is a small dehiscence in this segment normally, without disease. The second genu is just anterior/inferior and slightly medial to the lateral semicircular canal as it enters the vertical (mastoid) segment. From the genu to the stylomastoid foramen the nerve courses slightly from medial to lateral. The digastric ridge is the best landmark for the stylomastoid foramen.

The facial recess should be opened if disease fills the posterior epitympanum or posterosuperior mesotympanum. The facial recess is bounded medially by the facial nerve, laterally by

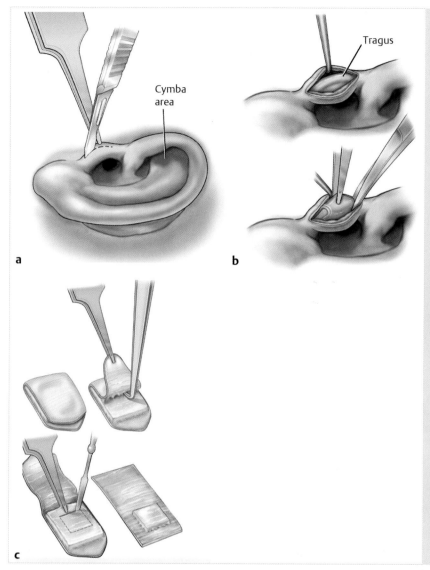

Fig. 19.15 The lateral graft has been put back into the trough with the skin graft and then placed back over the anteroinferior-superior region to help keep the graft from blunting anteriorly. The graft also shows the slit in the middle, which is then wrapped around the malleus to help keep it from lateralizing. The tympanomeatal flap and further skin grafts are being put back down over the fascia graft.

the chorda tympani, and superiorly by the incus buttress (▶ Fig. 19.19). To open the facial recess it helps to have a thin EAC, and the mastoid bone is taken down to the level of the lateral canal to identify the facial nerve. This step should typically allow a 2-mm burr to enter the middle ear via the mastoid. This is then enlarged or narrowed as needed. The sinus tympani is the most difficult area to clean, as it is medial to the facial nerve in the middle ear.[51]

If possible, small cholesteatoma sacs are removed in total, whereas the larger sacs are removed piecemeal.

19.9.1 Canal-Wall-Down Mastoidectomy

The reasons for performing a CWD mastoidectomy have been previously discussed, but the surgeon must also consider the disadvantages of this procedure. Hearing results may be slightly worse because the eardrum is located at a lower level and may vibrate less well. The cavity tends to collect wax and other debris and must be cleaned on a periodic basis, for example, every 6 months. Larger cavities may not tolerate water exposure, which results in infections and dizziness. Custom-fitted ear

molds may help prevent these complications. The surgeon must adhere to the time-honored techniques to maintain a safe, dry ear that can be easily cleaned in the office. The surgeon must avoid a high facial ridge, a dependent mastoid tip, and a small meatus.

The incus and malleus are typically removed. The facial nerve is identified and the posterior canal wall is lowered down to it and the lateral canal. The chorda tympani is sacrificed. Superiorly the tegmen is identified and the zygomatic root is drilled away to facilitate disease removal. The same is accomplished inferiorly. The overhang between the eustachian tube opening and the anterior epitympanum is removed. All disease is removed. Large mastoid tips may be obliterated by drilling the tip off and allowing the soft tissue to fill in. The tympanoplasty technique is exactly the same, although the graft comes up and over the facial nerve.

19.9.2 Meatoplasty

Meatoplasty is often performed before drilling a CWD mastoidectomy so that soft tissue hemostasis is obtained before the

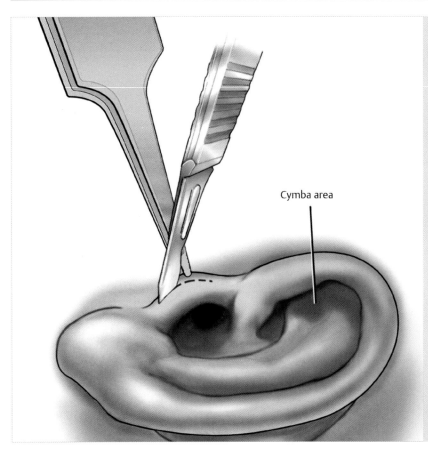

Cymba area

Fig. 19.16 Perichondrium is stripped off of one side of the tragal cartilage graft, and then enough cartilage is removed as needed to fit into the defect. The location for the cymba of cartilage can be obtained underneath the antihelix and the tragus, where cartilage is routinely harvested as well.

delicate middle ear work is begun. A large meatoplasty facilitates office examination and cleaning while maintaining good aeration to the mastoid bowl, thus preventing chronic drainage. Many surgeons advocate removal of 1 cm or 40% of the conchal cartilage to create this opening and prevent cupping of the ear from tension during closure. Such a large piece is removed because the meatus will contract by about 25% over time. This large meatoplasty may be cosmetically unappealing. Thus, I create an incisural meatoplasty. An incision at the 12 o'clock position between the tragal and conchal cartilages is made, similar to an endaural incision. However, this incision stops just at the top of the meatus and forms an opening that the surgeon can place his/her thumb through. To prevent constriction, a suture is placed posteriorly from the vascular strip area to the temporalis fascia posteriorly to keep the meatus open. The mastoid bowl and canal is then packed open. Typically, the bowl and TM are lined with Gelfoam for a few layers, and then are packed open with ¼-inch gauze soaked in bacitracin. I use two pieces, as the lateral piece may be inadvertently removed by the patient.

19.10 Postoperative Care

The gauze packing is removed in 7 to 10 days because after that it becomes malodorous with purulent drainage. Antibiotic/steroid drops are then used to promote healing and dissolve the Gelfoam. Six to 8 weeks are typically required for mastoid epithelization to occur. During this time patients may develop areas with granulation tissue that can be treated locally with silver nitrate, powder, or different drops.

Long-term follow-up for recurrence of cholesteatoma in all patients can involve non–echo planar diffusion-weighted magnetic resonance imaging (MRI), which is far superior to CT scans.[52]

19.11 Complications

Complications from chronic ear surgery are many and varied but fortunately quite rare, occurring in fewer than 1% of patients.[52-54] In contrast, complications can be relatively frequent if disease is left untreated.[54] This section discusses facial nerve injuries, tegmen dehiscence with or without CSF leak, hemorrhage from sigmoid sinus or carotid artery, semicircular canal fistula, and stapes dislocation. Infectious complications are not addressed, but the use of prophylactic antibiotics, which are on call to the operating room and postoperatively, and not shaving the patient minimize this complication.[55]

19.11.1 Facial Paralysis

Facial paralysis is one of the most dreaded complications because of the significant impact it has on a patient's life. The best way to avoid injury to the facial nerve is to thoroughly understand its anatomy.[56-58] The risk of injury to the facial nerve is quite low, less than 1% for primary cases. However, for revision cases it can be as high as 4 to 10%.[59]

Computed tomography scanning may help determine if the nerve is dehiscent or traveling in an anomalous path, but CT of the temporal bone preoperatively is not performed by many ear surgeons. Use of the facial nerve monitor is helpful but not required.[60,61] Even if the CT demonstrates no dehiscence, there

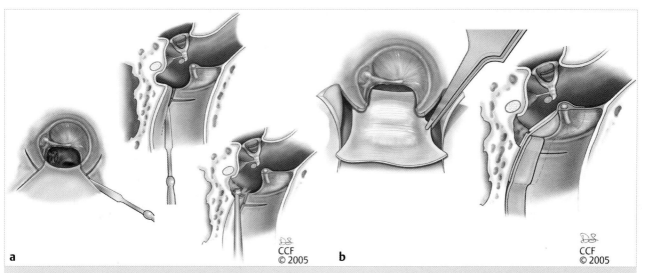

Fig. 19.17 (a) The placement of a medial graft to repair a TM perforation; this can be used with cartilage, especially if a total ossicular reconstruction prosthesis (TORP) or a partial ossicular reconstruction prosthesis (PORP) will be needed. (b) The piece of cartilage sliding medially.

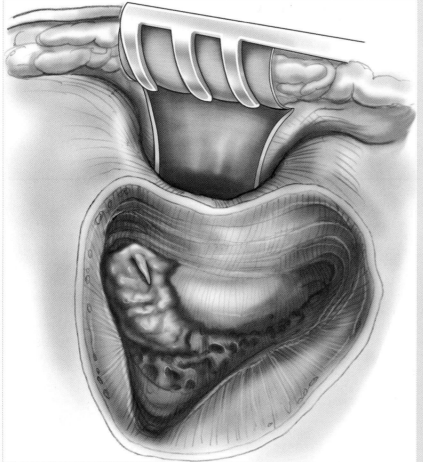

Fig. 19.18 The saucerization of a mastoid bowl identifying the tegmen.

is evidence that up to 50% of patients still have a small, 0.4-mm dehiscence in the tympanic segment.[62] Other areas of dehiscence can involve the geniculate ganglion, facial recess, and mastoid area (where it runs through an air cell).[63] In these cases the stimulator and nerve monitor can be very helpful in identifying the nerve.

If the facial nerve is injured iatrogenically, it is always preferable to identify this occurrence while patients are still under anesthesia rather than when they are in the recovery room. If the injury is identified in the operating room during the operation, the surgeon must first determine the degree or extent of injury. Minimal erythema and contusion (with an intact nerve)

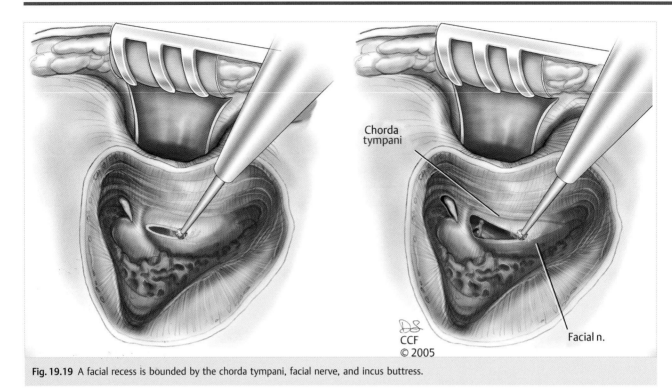

Fig. 19.19 A facial recess is bounded by the chorda tympani, facial nerve, and incus buttress.

does not require treatment other than possible oral high-dose steroids. Luckily the nerve is quite hardy and can be manipulated without much effect.[64,65] However, if the bruising/contusion is quite extensive, with significant swelling, then the nerve should be decompressed locally by removing bone (5 to 10 mm) on each side of the injury.[66] High-dose steroids should definitely be used in this instance, 60 to 80 mg each morning for 7 to 10 days. The patient may also need instruction in how to use ophthalmic drops and ointment and/or a moisture chamber at night. Opening the actual sheath tends to do more harm than good.[67,68]

Occasionally the nerve injury is more extensive, such that the nerve is fully or partially transected or a small divot (typically from a burr) is identified. This type of injury is emotionally troubling for both the patient and the surgeon. The surgeon always wants to believe the injury is not as bad as it is. Unfortunately, the injury is almost always more extensive than thought. This is true even when an objective observer is grading it. The classic algorithm is such that if less than one third of the nerve is cut, then the surgeon should decompress on either side of the injury.[69] If the injury is greater than one-third the diameter, then a repair is necessary. This gives the best chance of recovery to at least a House-Brackmann grade 3.[70,71]

Primary repair (end-to-end anastomosis) is preferred, as it requires only one anastomosis and should portend a better final House-Brackmann grade. However, if the defect is too big and cannot be made without tension, then a graft is necessary. Some extra length can be obtained by drilling out the stylomastoid foramen, but only a 1 or 2 mm at most; more than that disrupts the blood supply. Thus, the final outcome in this scenario is that there is not a clinically significant difference between one or two anastomosis.[67,72]

Prior to making the anastomosis, all bone spicules are cleaned from the nerve. The nerve repair is completed with 9–0 or 10–0 monofilament suture (▶ Fig. 19.20).

Laying the graft in the fallopian canal helps to keep it stable and immobile. If the nerve ends are stable, some surgeons will even use fibrin glue, Gelfoam, or Cargile to keep them together without suture.[67,68,73] In order to increase the surface area of the anastomosis, the ends should be cut at an oblique angle.[70,74] If a graft is required, either the great auricular or sural nerve should be used. Typically, for this type of repair, the great auricular should be able to provide more than enough length. In addition, it is typically accessible in the prepped-out field.[67] To obtain this nerve, a line is drawn from the mastoid tip to the angle of the jaw. A second line is drawn perpendicular to this first line starting at the mastoid tip. An incision is made onto the sternocleidomastoid muscle where the greater auricular nerve is found (▶ Fig. 19.21).[70]

Once the nerve is grafted, the patient and family need to be counseled on realistic expectations. Typically the first voluntary motion of the nerve might be detected at 6 to 9 months. Final recovery takes more than 1 year to occur, and the final outcome is usually a House-Brackmann grade of 3 or 4[72]; some synkinesis is common.[75]

If the facial nerve paralysis is detected in the recovery room, the surgeon has to critically ascertain whether the etiology is iatrogenic on his/her part or whether some other factor is responsible, such as injection of local anesthesia around the nerve or packing that is too tight. The packing should be loosened or removed, and then function will usually return in about 2 hours. If it does not return, then the surgeon must determine if it is full paralysis or very weak. Any voluntary movement indicates the nerve is not transected, and then the prognosis is excellent. The patient is treated with high-dose steroids and

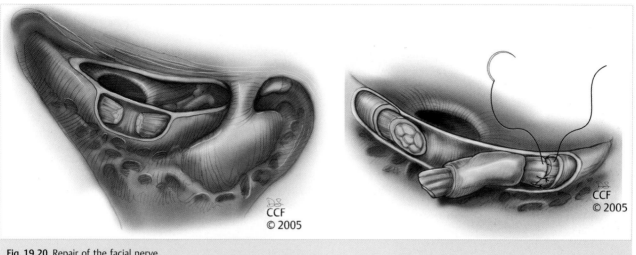

Fig. 19.20 Repair of the facial nerve.

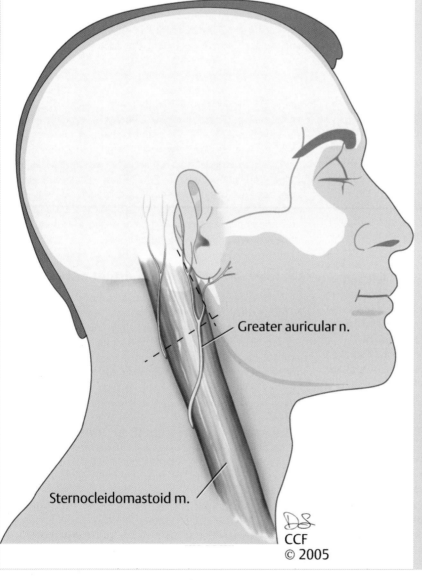

Greater auricular n.

Sternocleidomastoid m.

Fig. 19.21 Identifying the greater auricular nerve; dashed lines indicate the external landmarks (see text for details).

observed closely over the next few days. If the palsy should progress to complete paralysis, then the injury is more severe. After 72 hours from surgery, an electroneurography test (ENOG) can be performed. If the compound action potential is reduced by 95%, then the nerve can be explored in the next 1 to 3 days if all parties agree.[76,77] If the patient was determined to have complete paralysis in the recovery room, then the surgeon has to determine whether or not there is a chance that the nerve was compromised, and a reexploration should be performed. This reexploration can be done by the original surgeon, or, because of the emotional impact, the surgeon may elect to refer the patient to another otologist/neurotologist. The patient may be scanned and tested electrically (after 72 hours) if it is unlikely that the nerve was surgically injured, so the exploration can be delayed 1 to 3 days, but it should then proceed without undue delay.[77,78]

19.11.2 Vascular Injuries

The most common vascular injury involving tympanomastoidectomy surgery is sigmoid sinus injuries. Mild bleeding typically occurs from small, torn vessels on the sinus that are easily cauterized with bipolar cautery. A small laceration in the sigmoid sinus is easily treated with pressure because it is a low-pressure system. A piece of Gelfoam or Surgicel/Gelfoam is placed on the laceration and covered with a cottonoid. The area is left alone and the cottonoid is removed at the end of the procedure. A more substantial laceration requires more compression, usually extraluminally with Surgicel.[79] Intraluminal packing is another option, but to minimize the risk of embolization, a long tail of Surgicel is left posteriorly over the mastoid edge. Anesthesia is notified so that they can monitor and treat the patient quickly if signs of an air embolus are detected.

An injured jugular bulb can also bleed profusely. The bulb can be abnormally high (above the inferior annulus of the TM) in up to 7% of patients.[80] Occasionally, the high bulb may be dehiscent, making it more prone to injury. Again, pressure from Gelfoam or Surgicel is enough to control this bleeding. In the rare instance that this does not control the bleeding and the bleeding is profuse, then the internal jugular vein may be ligated in the neck and the sigmoid is packed extra- or intraluminally. Because the inferior petrosal vein may still cause bleeding via backflow, pressure on the bulb area must be maintained.

If bleeding occurs while raising the tympanomeatal flap, then Gelfoam or Surgicel is used to pack the middle ear onto the bulb. The flap is put back and the EAC is packed; the packing is kept in place for at least a week.[66,80] Injury during a myringotomy is typically controlled with EAC packing.

Carotid artery injury is exceedingly rare because a congenital dehiscent artery occurs less than 1% of the time.[81] The artery is normally covered by thick bone and lies medial to the eustachian tube, anteroinferior to the cochleariform process, and anteromedial to the cochlea. Preoperative scanning will detect any anomalies of the artery. When dissecting in this area, vigilance is necessary because the artery will not pulse normally in this area.[56]

Bleeding from the arterial wall is simply controlled with Surgicel because it arises from minor vessels along the wall. However, major bleeding must be controlled immediately by packing and pressure. Once hemorrhage is controlled, then definitive management can be decided: temporary balloon occlusion with secondary repair or grafting; permanent balloon occlusion or surgical ligation.[66,82] There is a risk of stroke with balloon occlusion, even in normal people.[83]

19.11.3 Dural Injury and Cerebrospinal Fluid Leak

During mastoid surgery it is common to expose the tegmen/dura because it is used as a landmark to perform safe mastoid surgery,[67] and exposure requires no further corrective action.[68] However, large defects may result in a meningoencephalocele over a long period of time, but even so, I would not recommend treatment immediately because the incidence of a meningoencephalocele occurring is so low. Dural violation, on the other hand, whether by drill, instruments, or cautery, does require some corrective action. The site of injury dictates the repair. Middle fossa tegmen dura is normally thick and associated with a significant amount of arachnoid tissue. This tissue actually helps form fibrous scar to seal a CSF leak. With small (1 cm) areas of injury, some bone is removed all around the site to allow placement of a fascia or muscle plug/graft.[66] A piece of Gelfoam can be used to help hold this graft in place after it is tucked under the bony edges. For large defects, a middle cranial fossa craniotomy with a fascia-bone-fascia graft sandwich is typically required to repair the dural defect.[56] Antibiotic coverage in all CSF leaks is recommended.

A CSF leak in the posterior fossa dura is more challenging because there is a paucity of arachnoid tissue in this area. Thus, even though fascia grafts are tucked in and around the bone circumferentially and Gelfoam is placed, the patient may require a lumbar drain and bed rest for 2 to 3 days.[68] Occasionally a posterior fossa leak requires sealing with connective tissue, bone wax, and abdominal fat graft. Consultation with neurosurgery is recommended if either a middle or posterior fossa leak cannot be resolved quickly with these efforts.

19.11.4 Semicircular Canal Fistula

It is more common to injure the membranous labyrinth when dissecting cholesteatoma off a dehiscent canal than it is to inadvertently drill into a semicircular canal. A drilling accident occurs less than 0.1% of the time.[84] Opening a bony canal itself does not necessarily lead to hearing loss. Significant damage more often occurs with suction into the vestibular system. If the bony labyrinth is entered, the surgeon should not perform suction but rather should seal the fistula with bone wax, fascia, or muscle.[85–87]

More commonly, the cholesteatoma erodes into the canal and causes a fistula.[88] Preoperative CT scanning usually identifies this pathology. If a labyrinthine fistula is suspected, the cholesteatoma sac contents should be removed and the matrix carefully inspected for deformity or blue coloration, indicating that the membranous labyrinth is exposed. If the fistula is small, then the sac may be removed by slow gentle movements and the fistula closed. If the fistula is larger, then leaving the matrix down over the fistula, to avoid inner ear trauma, should be considered. Either the canal wall is taken down and the matrix exteriorized, or the wall is left intact and the fistula is reassessed at a second-stage operation. Some fistulas can heal and some residual epithelium can simply disappear.[66] Definitive management is then decided at the second stage. Profound SNHL occurs in 3 to 22% of patients with disease-induced canal fistulas.[52] The surgeon should also keep in mind that if the lateral semicircular canal is involved, then the facial nerve is almost always exposed as well.

Oval window fistulization is more often iatrogenic from dissection of disease off the footplate and stapes, or the stapes can be dislocated when raising a tympanomeatal flap or manipulating the ossicular chain. During cholesteatoma surgery, it may be better to leave a little cholesteatoma and disease on the stapes and return in 6 to 9 months when it should be easier to remove (after it forms a small pearl) than to pursue total removal[66] or consider laser ablation. If the injury occurs and the footplate can be put back into position, it should be covered with connective tissue but one must make sure it does not sink into the vestibule. If the footplate is fistulized but the footplate is intact, then the fistula is sealed with fascia or muscle. Hearing loss and dizziness may occur in the short-term, but symptoms often improve with time.

Certainly, iatrogenic injuries occur. The key to avoidance is attention to detail. When injury does occur, the surgeon must know in advance how to handle it.

References

[1] Thorburn IA. Chronic disease of the middle ear. In: Scott-Brown WG, Balantyne JC, Groves J, eds. Diseases of the Ear, Nose and Throat, 2nd ed. London: Butterworth, 1965

[2] Procter B. Chronic otitis media and mastoiditis. In: Paparell M, Shumrick D, Gluckman J, Meyerhoff W, eds. Otolaryngology, vol 2, 3rd ed. Philadelphia: WB Saunders, 1991:1349–1376

[3] Weber PC, Roland PS, Hannley M et al. The development of antibiotic resistant organisms with the use of ototopical medications. Otolaryngol Head Neck Surg 2004; 130 Suppl: S89–S94

[4] Harker LA, Koontz FB. Bacteriology of cholesteatoma: clinical significance. Otolaryngol Head Neck Surg 1977; 84: 683–686

[5] Brook I. Aerobic and anaerobic bacteriology of cholesteatoma. Laryngoscope 1981; 91: 250–253

[6] Brook I. Bacteriology and treatment of chronic otitis media. Laryngoscope 1979; 89: 1129–1134

[7] Sheehy JL Chronic tympanomastoiditis. In: Gates G, ed. Current Therapy in Otolaryngology Head and Neck Surgery, 4th ed. Toronto: BC Decker 1990:19–22

[8] Cunningham M, Guardiani E, Kim HJ, Brook I. Otitis media. Future Microbiol 2012; 7: 733–753

[9] Saunders JE, Raju RP, Boone JL, Hales NW, Berryhill WE. Antibiotic resistance and otomycosis in the draining ear: culture results by diagnosis. Am J Otolaryngol 2011; 32: 470–476

[10] Fairbanks DN. Otic topical agents. Otolaryngol Head Neck Surg 1980; 88: 327–331

[11] Fairbanks DNF. Topical therapeutics for otitis media. Otolaryngol Head Neck Surg 1981; 89: 381–385

[12] Anderson CW, Stevens MH. Synchronous tuberculous involvement of both ears and the larynx in a patient with active pulmonary disease. Laryngoscope 1981; 91: 906–909

[13] Windle-Taylor PC, Bailey CM. Tuberculous otitis media: a series of 22 patients. Laryngoscope 1980; 90: 1039–1044

[14] Yu Z, Wang Z, Yang B, Han D, Zhang L. The value of preoperative CT scan of tympanic facial nerve canal in tympanomastoid surgery. Acta Otolaryngol 2011; 131: 774–778

[15] Tatlopinae A, Tuncel A, Ogredik EA et al. The role of CT scanning in chronic otitis media Eur Arch Otorhinolaryngol 2012; 269: 33–38

[16] Roland PS, Stewart MG, Hannley M et al. Consensus panel on role of potentially ototoxic antibiotics for topical middle ear use: introduction, methodology, and recommendations. Otolaryngol Head Neck Surg 2004; 130 Suppl: S51–S56

[17] Post JC. Genetics of otitis media. Adv Otorhinolaryngol 2011; 70: 135–140

[18] Loock JW. A randomised controlled trial of active chronic otitis media comparing courses of eardrops versus one-off topical treatments suitable for primary, secondary and tertiary healthcare settings. Clin Otolaryngol 2012; 37: 261–270

[19] Lee NH, Chang JW, Jung H, Im GT. Experience of Ras-related C3 botulineum toxin substrate (RAC-1) in human cholesteatoma. Eur Arch Otorhinolaryngol 2012

[20] Levenson MJ, Parisier SC, Chute P, Wenig S, Juarbe C. A review of twenty congenital cholesteatomas of the middle ear in children. Otolaryngol Head Neck Surg 1986; 94: 560–567

[21] Nelson M, Roger G, Koltai PJ et al. Congenital cholesteatoma: classification, management, and outcome. Arch Otolaryngol Head Neck Surg 2002; 128: 810–814

[22] Weber PC, Adkins WY, Jr. Congenital cholesteatomas in the tympanic membrane. Laryngoscope 1997; 107: 1181–1184

[23] Potsic WP, Samadi DS, Marsh RR, Wetmore RF. A staging system for congenital cholesteatoma. Arch Otolaryngol Head Neck Surg 2002; 128: 1009–1012

[24] Karmody CS, Byahatti SV, Blevins N, Valtonen H, Northrop C. The origin of congenital cholesteatoma. Am J Otol 1998; 19: 292–297

[25] Glasscock ME, Haynes DS, Storper I, et al. Surgery for chronic ear disease. In: Hughes GB, Pensak ML, eds. Clinical Otology, 2nd ed. New York: Thieme, 1997:215–232

[26] Nevoux J, Moya-Plana A, Chauvin P, Denoyelle F, Garabedian EN. Total ossiculoplasty in children: predictive factors and long-term follow-up. Arch Otolaryngol Head Neck Surg 2011; 137: 1240–1246

[27] Edfeldt L, Strömbäck K, Kinnefors A, Rask-Andersen H. Surgical treatment of adult cholesteatoma: long-term follow-up using total reconstruction procedure without staging. Acta Otolaryngol 2013; 133: 28–34

[28] Jackson CG. Cholesteatoma: the method of treatment. In: Gates GA, ed. Current Therapy in Otolaryngology Head and Neck Surgery, 4th ed. Toronto: BC Decker, 1990:23–28

[29] Jackson CG, Glasscock ME, III, Nissen AJ, Schwaber MK, Bojrab DI. Open mastoid procedures: contemporary indications and surgical technique. Laryngoscope 1985; 95: 1037–1043

[30] Glasscock ME, III, Jackson CG, Nissen AJ, Schwaber MK. Postauricular undersurface tympanic membrane grafting: a follow-up report. Laryngoscope 1982; 92: 718–727

[31] Storrs LA. Myringoplasty with the use of fascia grafts Arch Otolaryngol Head Neck Surg 1961; 74: 45–49

[32] Toynbee J. On the Use of an Artificial Membrane Tympanic in Cases of Deafness Dependent Upon Perforations in Destruction of the Natural Organ. London: J Churchill, 1853

[33] Berthold E. Ueber myringoplastick Wier Med Bull 1878; 1: 627

[34] Blake CJ. Transactions of the First Congress of the International Ontological Society. New York: D. Appelton, 1887

[35] Wullstein J. Funktionelle Operationen im mittelohr mit hilfe des freien spaltlappen-transplantates. Arch Ohren- Nasenkehlkopfheilkd 1952; 161: 422–435

[36] Zollner F. The principles of plastic surgery of the sound-conducting apparatus. J Laryngol Otol 1955; 69: 637–652

[37] Goodhill V. Tragal perichondrium and cartilage in tympanoplasty. Arch Otolaryngol 1967; 85: 480–491

[38] Glasscock ME, III. Tympanic membrane grafting with fascia: overlay vs. undersurface technique. Laryngoscope 1973; 83: 754–770

[39] Weber PC, Gantz BJ. Cartilage reconstruction of the scutum defects in canal wall up mastoidectomies. Am J Otolaryngol 1998; 19: 178–182

[40] Jansen C. Ulur Radikaoperationen Und Tympanoplastik Sitz Ber Fontbild, Arztekamm. Ob Vol 18, 1958

[41] Kessel J. Uber das Ausschneiden des Tromelfells, Hammers ad Ambosses bei Undurchgangigkeit det Tube. Arch Ohr Nas Kehlkophfheilk 1885; 22: 196

[42] Zaufal E. Technik der Trepanation des Prc. Mastoid Nach Kuster'schen Grundsatzen. Ohrenheilkd 1890; 30: 291

[43] Stacke L. Stacke's Operationsmethode. Arch Ohrenheilkd 1893; 35: 145

[44] Schwartze HH, Eysell CG. Uber die Kunstliche Eroffnung des Warzenfortsatzes. Arch Ohrenheilkd 1873; 7: 157

[45] Petit JL. Traite des Maladies Chirurgicales et des Opérations qui Leur Conviennent. Paris: Méquignon, 1790

[46] Hirsch BE, Kamerer DB, Doshi S. Single-stage management of cholesteatoma. Otolaryngol Head Neck Surg 1992; 106: 351–354

[47] Gantz BJ, Wilkinson EP, Hansen MR. Canal wall reconstruction tympanomastoidectomy with mastoid obliteration. Laryngoscope 2005; 115: 1734–1740

[48] Bondy G. Totalaufmeisselung mit Erhaltung von tromelfell und Gehorknockelchen. Monastsschr Ohrenheilk 1910; 44: 15

[49] Miller JJ, Weber PC, Patel S, Ramey J. Intracranial surgery: to shave or not to shave? Otol Neurotol 2001; 22: 908–911

[50] Sheehy JL. Surgery of chronic otitis media In: English G, ed. Otolaryngology, vol 1. Philadelphia: JB Lippincott, 1984

[51] Li PM, Linos E, Gurgel RK, Fischbein NJ, Blevins NH. Evaluating the utility of non-echo-planar diffusion-weighted imaging in the preoperative evaluation of cholesteatoma: a meta-analysis. Laryngoscope 2013; 123: 1247–1250

[52] Dawes PJ. Early complications of surgery for chronic otitis media. J Laryngol Otol 1999; 113: 803–810

[53] Kempf HG, Johann K, Lenarz T. Complications in pediatric cochlear implant surgery. Eur Arch Otorhinolaryngol 1999; 256: 128–132

[54] Greenberg JS, Manolidis S. High incidence of complications encountered in chronic otitis media surgery in a U.S. metropolitan public hospital. Otolaryngol Head Neck Surg 2001; 125: 623–627

[55] Miller JJ, Weber PC, Patel S, Ramey J. Intracranial surgery: to shave or not to shave? Otol Neurotol 2001; 22: 908–911

[56] Bellucci R. Iatrogenic surgical trauma in otology. J Laryngol Otol Suppl 1983; 8: 13–17

[57] May M, Wiet RJ. Iatrogenic injury–prevention and management In: May M, ed. The Facial Nerve. New York: Thieme, 1986:549–560

[58] Wiet RJ. Iatrogenic facial paralysis. Otolaryngol Clin North Am 1982; 15: 773–780

[59] Wiet RJ, Herzon GD. Surgery of the mastoid. In: Wiet RJ, Causse JB, eds. Complications in Otolaryngology Head and Neck Surgery. Philadelphia: BC Decker, 1986:25–31

[60] Roland PS, Meyerhoff WL. Intraoperative electrophysiological monitoring of the facial nerve: is it standard of practice? Am J Otolaryngol 1994; 15: 267–270

[61] Fenton JE, Fagan PA. Iatrogenic facial nerve injury. Laryngoscope 1995; 105: 444–445

[62] Baxter A. Dehiscence of the fallopian canal. An anatomical study. J Laryngol Otol 1971; 85: 587–594

[63] Schuknecht HF, Guyle AJ. Anatomy of the Temporal Bone with Surgical Implications. Philadelphia: Lea & Febiger, 1986

[64] Sheehy JL. The facial nerve in surgery of chronic otitis media. Otolaryngol Clin North Am 1974; 7: 493–503

[65] Neely JG. Surgery of acute infections and their complications In: Brackmann DE, Shelton C, Arriaga MA, eds. Otologic Surgery. Philadelphia: WB Saunders, 1994:201–210

[66] Wiet RJ, Harvet SA, Bauer GP. Management of complictions of chronic otitis media. In: Brackmann DE, Shelton C, Arriaga MA, eds. Otologic Surgery. Philadelphia: WB Saunders, 1994:257–276

[67] Smyth G, Gordon GDL, Toner JG. Mastoidectomy: canal wall down techniques In: Brackmann DE, Shelton C, Arriaga MA, eds. Otologic Surgery. Philadelphia: WB Saunders, 1994:225–239

[68] Paparella MM, Meyerhoff WL, Morris MS, Dacosta SS. Mastoidectomy and tympanoplasty. In: Paparell MM, Shumrick D, Gluckman JL, Meyerhoff WL, eds. Otolaryngology, vol 2, 3rd ed. Philadelphia: WB Saunders, 1991:1405–1439

[69] May M. Trauma to the facial nerve: external, surgical, iatrogenic. In: May M, Schaitkin BM, eds. The Facial Nerve, 2nd ed. New York: Thieme, 2000:367–382

[70] Adkins WY, Osguthorpe JD. Management of trauma of the facial nerve. Otolaryngol Clin North Am 1991; 24: 587–611

[71] Brackmann DE. Otoneurosurgical procedures. In: May M, ed. The Facial Nerve. New York: Thieme, 1986:589–618

[72] Fisch U, Rouleau M. Facial nerve reconstruction. J Otolaryngol 1980; 9: 487–492

[73] Fisch U,, Lanser mj. . Facial nerve grafting. Otolryngol Clin N Am 1991; 24: 691–708

[74] Yamamoto E, Fisch U. Experiments on facial nerve suturing. ORL J Otorhinolaryngol Relat Spec 1974; 36: 193–204

[75] Fisch U. Facial nerve grafting. Otolaryngol Clin North Am 1974; 7: 517–529

[76] Barrs DM. Facial nerve trauma: optimal timing for repair. Laryngoscope 1991; 101: 835–848

[77] May M. Facial reanimation after skull base trauma. In: May M, ed. The Facial Nerve. New York: Thieme, 1986:421–440

[78] McQuarrie IG, Grafstein B. Axon outgrowth enhanced by a previous nerve injury. Arch Neurol 1973; 29: 53–55

[79] Moloy PJ, Brackmann DE. Control of venous bleeding in otologic surgery. Laryngoscope 1986; 96: 580–582

[80] Graham MD. The jugular bulb: its anatomic and clinical considerations in contemporary otology. Laryngoscope 1977; 87: 105–125

[81] Goldman NC, Singleton GT, Holly EH. Aberrant internal carotid artery presenting as a mass in the middle ear. Arch Otolaryngol 1971; 94: 269–273

[82] Andrews JC, Valavanis A, Fisch U. Management of the internal carotid artery in surgery of the skull base. Laryngoscope 1989; 99: 1224–1229

[83] de Vries EJ, Sekhar LN, Janecka IP, Schramm VL, Jr, Horton JA, Eibling DE. Elective resection of the internal carotid artery without reconstruction. Laryngoscope 1988; 98: 960–966

[84] Palva T, Karja J, Palva A. Immediate and short-term complications of chronic ear surgery Arch Otolaryngol Head Neck Surg 1976; 102: 137–139

[85] Jahrsdoerfer RA, Johns ME, Cantrell RW. Labyrinthine trauma during ear surgery. Laryngoscope 1978; 88: 1589–1595

[86] Canalis RF, Gussen R, Abemayor E, Andrews J. Surgical trauma to the lateral semicircular canal with preservation of hearing. Laryngoscope 1987; 97: 575–581

[87] Cullen JR, Kerr AG. Iatrogenic fenestration of a semicircular canal: a method of closure. Laryngoscope 1986; 96: 1168–1169

[88] Moon IS, Kwon MO, Park CY et al. Surgical management of labyrinthine fistula in chronic otitis media with cholesteatoma. Auris Nasus Larynx 2012; 39: 261–264

20 Complications of Otitis Media

Kevin D. Brown, Samuel H. Selesnick, and Shan Tang

20.1 Introduction

Acute otitis media (AOM) is one of the most prevalent illnesses in children in the United States and a leading cause of health care visits and drug prescription. A 1989 prospective study demonstrated that 83% of children suffered at least one episode of AOM during their lifetime, whereas 46% of children had at least three episodes of AOM by age 3.[1] A recent review of the global burden of AOM reported the worldwide incidence rate of AOM to be 10.8% (i.e., 709 million cases per year), with 51% of these occurring in children under age 5. As with most infectious diseases, the incidence rate varies substantially between developed and developing areas, ranging from 3.6% in central Europe to 43% in sub-Saharan Africa.[2]

The use of antibiotic therapy in the management of AOM continues to be an active area of clinical investigation. The most recent clinical practice guidelines published in 2004 by the American Academy of Pediatrics and the American Academy of Family Physicians recommend that children younger than 6 months of age receive immediate antibiotic therapy, whereas children older than 6 months of age with nonsevere illness (mild otalgia and fever < 39°C) are initially observed without antibiotics.[3] The watchful-waiting policy is supported by studies that have shown marginal benefit from antibiotics for most children diagnosed with AOM.[4,5] However, recent studies that used more rigorous diagnostic criteria for AOM have demonstrated significantly lower rates of treatment failure in children 6 to 35 months of age who were given immediate antibiotic therapy compared to placebo.[6–8]

Acute otitis media that does not resolve may progress to a variety of complications, the most frequent of which is acute mastoiditis. Prior to the introduction of antibiotics, acute mastoiditis was the most common infectious condition requiring hospitalization among infants and children.[9] The incidence of acute mastoiditis has decreased substantially since the preantibiotic era, but some reviews published over the past two decades suggest that it may be rising once again.[10–12] The demographics of AOM and its sequelae continue to evolve, driven by factors such as antibiotic prescription patterns, development of antibiotic resistance, and use of pneumococcal vaccines.[13–16]

Complications from AOM can be organized into extracranial and intracranial areas of involvement, although one does not necessarily preclude the other. Extracranial complications can remain within the temporal bone or can extend beyond its confines.

Complications of Otitis Media

- Extracranial
  - Intratemporal
    - Mastoiditis
    - Ossicular erosion
    - Sensorineural hearing loss
    - Facial nerve paralysis
    - Labyrinthine fistula
    - Suppurative labyrinthitis
    - Petrous apicitis
  - Extratemporal
    - Subperiosteal abscess
    - Zygomatic abscess
    - Bezold abscess
    - Cervical/postauricular fistula
    - Extramastoid cholesteatoma
- Intracranial
  - Meningitis
  - Brain abscess
  - Subdural empyema
  - Epidural abscess
  - Sigmoid sinus septic thrombophlebitis
  - Otitic hydrocephalus
  - Meningoencephalocele

20.2 Extracranial Complications

20.2.1 Intratemporal Extension

Acute Mastoiditis

The discovery of antibiotics and their application to infectious diseases in the middle of the 20th century greatly reduced the frequency of progression of AOM to acute mastoiditis. Prior to the use of antibiotics, one quarter to one half of patients with AOM could be expected to develop acute mastoiditis.[17] In a review published in 2012, the incidence of acute mastoiditis was reported to be 1.62 to 1.88 per 100,000 person-years.[18]

Bacterial cultures obtained from myringotomy or mastoidectomy specimens in patients with acute mastoiditis most frequently grow *Streptococcus pneumoniae* or *Streptococcus pyogenes*. Other commonly reported causative organisms include *Staphylococcus aureus*, *Haemophilus influenzae*, coagulase-negative *Staphylococcus*, and *Pseudomonas aeruginosa*.[19–22] Of note, the widespread administration of the PCV7 pneumococcal conjugate vaccine over the past decade has led to an decrease in the disease burden of AOM and invasive pneumococcal disease caused by *S. pneumoniae* in general. At the same time, it is driving the increased prevalence of nonvaccine serotypes of *S. pneumoniae* including serotype 19A.[16,23] Recent evidence suggests that serotype 19A is more likely to demonstrate multidrug resistance and cause more severe disease compared to other serotypes.[24]

Acute mastoiditis is characterized by hyperemia of the mucosal lining of the mastoid air cells with development of fluid and pus within the air cells. Prolonged infection can lead to osteitis and subsequent destruction of the bony trabeculae that delineate the mastoid air cells. Loss of these bony trabeculae results in coalescence of the air cells, which become filled with pus. Once acute mastoiditis has progressed to the point of "coalescence," surgical management is required.[25] In the event that coalescent mastoiditis continues untreated, the process of bony erosion and abscess formation can extend to adjacent structures, resulting in a myriad of complications, many of which will be discussed in this chapter.

As mastoid air cells are contiguous with the middle ear space via the aditus ad antrum, so must mastoiditis be considered an extension of otitis media. Patients with mastoiditis typically present with the symptoms of AOM such as fever, ear pain, and conductive hearing loss. Purulent otorrhea arises in cases of tympanic membrane perforation. Physical examination reveals edema and erythema of the postauricular soft tissue with pain and tenderness over the mastoid process. Anterior and inferior displacement of the pinna often results in proptosis of the ear. Otoscopic examination may reveal fullness or "sagging" of the posterior superior external canal wall, secondary to periosteal thickening near the antrum. In addition, the tympanic membrane may show evidence of AOM; if the tympanic membrane is perforated, inflamed middle ear mucosa may be seen through the perforation.

Although acute mastoiditis is a clinical diagnosis, computed tomography (CT) can be helpful in identifying complications such as occult abscess, mastoid cortex dehiscence, or evidence of coalescence of mastoid cells.[22] Indications for CT include mental status changes or other signs of central nervous system involvement, meningitic symptoms, cranial nerve palsies, history of cholesteatoma, and lack of clinical improvement with appropriate management.[26,27] Opacification of the mastoid air cells and the middle ear space on CT can be observed due to mucosal edema as well as fluid or pus collection. Careful attention must be paid to the bony trabeculae defining the mastoid air cells. Haziness of these structures suggests demineralization and loss of integrity of the bony septa. This disease process may progress to complete destruction of the bone, resulting in coalescent mastoiditis and necessitating surgical intervention.

Cortical mastoidectomy (▶ Fig. 20.1) has been the traditional treatment of acute mastoiditis, but more recent reports have trended toward more conservative treatment. Reported rates of mastoidectomy utilized for the management of acute mastoiditis vary widely in the literature (9–88%), reflecting a lack of consensus in the management algorithm.[28] Some authors advocate initial treatment of uncomplicated acute mastoiditis with intravenous (IV) antibiotics alone.[29,30] Others endorse treating with a combination of IV antibiotics and myringotomy with or without a tube, reserving mastoidectomy for those patients with a poor response to initial conservative treatment.[28,31,32] Zanetti and Nassif[33] propose the following indications for initial treatment with mastoidectomy: exteriorized mastoid abscess in children aged > 30 months or weight > 15 kg, intracranial complications, cholesteatoma, and purulent otorrhea or granulation tissue.

Ossicular Erosion

Chronic otitis media (COM) commonly results in a conductive hearing loss. Conduction of sound through the middle ear is compromised by the presence of pus in the middle ear space;

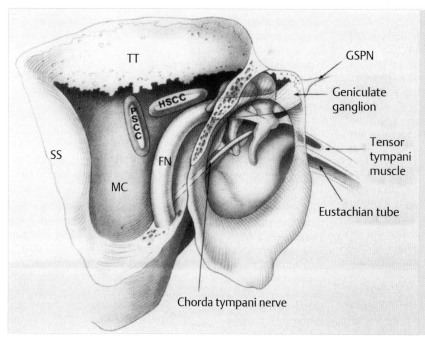

Fig. 20.1 Surgical anatomy of the middle ear and mastoid after a cortical mastoidectomy include the mastoid cavity (MC), the facial nerve (FN), the horizontal semicircular canal (HSCC), the posterior semicircular canal (PSCC), the sigmoid sinus (SS), the tegmen tympani (TT), and the greater superficial petrosal nerve (GSPN). (Used with permission from Selesnick SH, Jackler RK. Facial paralysis in suppurative ear disease. Oper Tech Otolaryngol–Head Neck Surg 1992;3:61–68.)

TT

GSPN

HSCC

Geniculate ganglion

P S C C

SS

FN

Tensor tympani muscle

MC

Eustachian tube

Chorda tympani nerve

however, damage to the ossicular chain may also contribute to the hearing loss. Typically, bony erosion occurs at the stapes suprastructure and the incus, whereas the malleus is less often involved. Treatment entails prosthetic reconstruction of the ossicular chain once the suppurative otitis media has been controlled. Other options for rehabilitation include direct round window placement of a vibrating mass transducer, a traditional hearing aid, or even a bone conduction hearing aid.

Sensorineural Hearing Loss

Sensorineural hearing loss has been positively correlated with the duration and severity of otitis media. This effect is most pronounced in high-frequency hearing.[34] The most commonly proposed theory is that pathological changes in the round window membrane can render it more permeable to bacterial toxins. Thus, the passage of chemical toxins and inflammatory mediators from the middle ear into the inner ear via the round window may damage the cochlear apparatus.[35,36] Fluorescence-labeled endotoxin introduced into the middle ear has been shown to accumulate in the basal turn of the cochlea, which is the area of the cochlea that contains the hair cells responsible for high-frequency hearing.[37] Studies detailing cochlear morphology in the setting of COM described loss of outer and inner hair cells and decrease in the area of the stria vascularis in the basal turn of the cochlea.[38,39]

Facial Nerve Paralysis

Facial nerve paralysis (FNP) is a rare complication of otitis media with a reported incidence of 0.16%.[40] The timing of the development of FNP after the onset of otitis media is important to consider, as it suggests the pathophysiology of the symptoms and more importantly, has implications for the treatment of the disease. The proposed mechanisms of AOM leading to FNP include direct involvement of the facial nerve by infection through bony dehiscences, fallopian canal osteitis with bone erosion and nerve involvement, inflammatory edema leading to compression and secondary ischemia, reactivation of a latent neurotropic virus (e.g., herpesvirus), reduced host immunologic response, and demyelination of the facial nerve by bacterial toxins.[41] FNP in the setting of AOM that is treated conservatively with antibiotics, corticosteroids, and myringotomy typically results in full recovery of facial function in 90 to 100% of patients, with recovery time varying from a few days up to 6 months.[41–43]

In contrast, the gradual onset of FNP that occurs in the setting of COM is more likely to be caused by progressive bony erosion that allows bacterial toxins direct access to the facial nerve (▶ Fig. 20.2). Bony erosion can also occur in the setting of cholesteatoma that has eroded through the fallopian canal and compresses the facial nerve directly. In these cases, mastoidectomy with facial nerve decompression is indicated.[43] The nerve should be identified, any granulation tissue should be exenterated, and the facial nerve should be decompressed several millimeters distal and proximal to the area of involvement. In cases of cholesteatoma invasion of the fallopian canal, all cholesteatoma must be removed to relieve pressure on the facial nerve. Intraoperative facial nerve monitoring may supply meaningful information.[44] Prognosis is generally poor, as most patients will

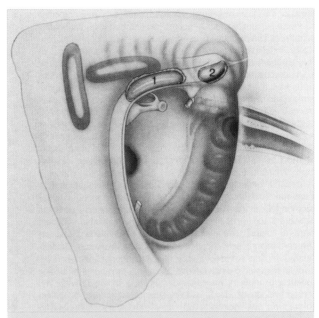

Fig. 20.2 Typical sites of facial nerve erosion by cholesteatoma and otitis media. The posterior portion of the tympanic segment and the second genu (1) and the anterior portion of the tympanic segment near the first genu (2) are most commonly affected.

still have residual paralysis in spite of surgical intervention.[43,45] One small case series of patients with FNP in the setting of COM without cholesteatoma showed that five of six patients had full recovery of facial nerve function after undergoing mastoidectomy with facial nerve decompression within 10 days of the onset of facial nerve dysfunction.[46] Outcomes are generally more favorable if the nerve is explored soon after the onset of FNP, but the window of opportunity for which facial nerve recovery can be maximized is unclear.[43]

Labyrinthine Fistula

The endosteal bone that forms the bony labyrinth is subject to damage from an inflammatory process that is engendered by infection or, more typically, by cholesteatoma. A fistula arises when the endosteal bone layer has been eroded, leaving only the endosteal membrane to separate the perilymphatic space from the infectious or cholesteatomatous process in the middle ear (▶ Fig. 20.3).[47] By virtue of cholesteatoma growth patterns most commonly involving the lateral semicircular canal, the lateral semicircular canal is more frequently involved than the superior or posterior semicircular canals, whereas the cochlea is rarely involved. A meta-analysis of 25 case series of mastoidectomies for chronic ear disease showed the incidence of labyrinthine fistula to be 7%, with 87% of these located in the lateral semicircular canal.[48]

Patients who develop labyrinthine fistulas typically present with dizziness and a chronically draining ear. Interestingly, the severity of symptoms depends on the rate of change in the size of the fistula rather than on the absolute size of the fistula.[49] A fistula test can be performed, although studies have suggested that this test is not highly sensitive or reliable. In a positive fistula test, positive pressure applied to the middle ear with a pneumatic otoscope results in nystagmus toward the ipsilateral

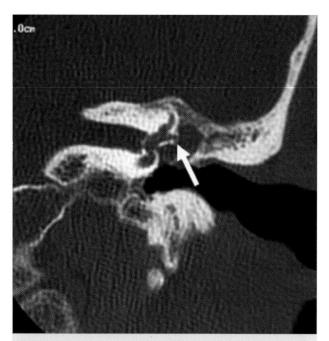

Fig. 20.3 Lateral semicircular canal fistula. In this coronal CT scan of the temporal bone, the endosteal bone covering the lateral-most aspect of the lateral semicircular canal (*white arrow*) has been eroded by an epitympanic cholesteatoma.

ear. When the pressure is reversed, the nystagmus is also reversed, and its fast component is directed toward the contralateral ear. Positive and negative pressures applied to the middle ear induce ampullopetal and ampullofugal movement of the endolymph, respectively (in the lateral semicircular canal), resulting in perception of rotation and resultant nystagmus. Labyrinthine fistulas involving the superior or posterior semicircular canals respond to fistula tests with pure vertical or complex nystagmus. The fistula test can be falsely positive with an abnormally mobile stapes. If the labyrinth is not functional, the fistula test can be falsely negative.

A patient in whom a labyrinthine fistula is suspected should undergo a CT scan of the temporal bone. The scan, in addition to suggesting the presence of cholesteatoma, is often useful in identifying a labyrinthine fistula. There are two general approaches to the surgical treatment of labyrinthine fistula in the literature. One school of thought advocates leaving a thin layer of cholesteatoma matrix over the fistula site and exteriorizing the cavity, theoretically incurring less risk of sensorineural hearing loss.[48] Gacek[47] recommends that the matrix of a small fistula (i.e., less than 2 mm in size) can be removed safely, whereas the matrix of a large fistula (greater than or equal to 2 mm) should be left over the fistula. The second school of thought advocates complete removal of cholesteatoma matrix over the fistula site with repair of the defect, thereby removing a potential nidus for infection and further bony erosion. Good hearing preservation has been reported after using materials such as bone wax, bone dust, and temporalis fascia to rapidly seal the open labyrinth.[50–54] A meta-analysis showed no significant difference in hearing results between patients in whom the matrix was removed (11% with decreased hearing and 5% with a dead ear postoperatively) and patients in

whom the matrix was left in situ (14% decreased hearing and 3% with a dead ear).[48]

Suppurative Labyrinthitis

Suppurative labyrinthitis is an uncommon complication of COM or mastoiditis that results from bacterial invasion of the inner ear via either the round or oval window or through a labyrinthine fistula created by cholesteatoma.[55] Initially, as bacterial toxins enter the inner ear, the labyrinth becomes irritated and hyperactive with ensuing nystagmus toward the infected ear. As bacteria enter the middle ear and frank purulence develops, the neuroepithelium of the inner ear becomes irreversibly damaged and inner ear function is lost. At this point, spontaneous nystagmus shifts away from the infected ear toward the opposite side. The onset of suppurative labyrinthitis is characterized by sudden profound sensorineural hearing loss and severe vertigo. Additionally, patients with suppurative labyrinthitis suffer from severe nausea and vomiting, dysequilibrium causing the body to fall in the direction opposite to the ear affected by labyrinthitis, and a tendency to reach past an intended target point during purposeful movements. Because perilymph is directly continuous with the cerebrospinal fluid, meningitis often ensues via the cochlear aqueduct.

Treatment consists of intravenous antibiotics and surgical drainage of purulence from the middle ear as well as debridement of granulomatous tissue or cholesteatoma. Restoration of labyrinthine and cochlear function is not a concern, as the inner ear damage is permanent. Rather, control and eradication of the infectious process is paramount in order to avert meningitis, which often presents with the classic signs of headache, fever, photophobia, and obtundation.

Petrous Apicitis

Petrous apex air cells exist in approximately 30% of normal temporal bones.[56] The petrous temporal bone can be divided into anterior and posterior regions by a plane passing through the axis of the modiolus (▶ Fig. 20.4). These two regions can be further subdivided into areas, each of which is pneumatized via different air cell tracts. The region anterior to the plane of the modiolus is subdivided into apical and peritubal areas, which lie posteromedial and anterolateral to the carotid canal, respectively. The region posterior to the plane of the modiolus is subdivided into supralabyrinthine and infralabyrinthine areas, which lie superior and inferior to the labyrinth, respectively (▶ Fig. 20.5).[57] In cases of COM or mastoiditis, the air cells of the petrous apex, like those of the mastoid, are subject to extension of inflammation and infection from the middle ear. As in mastoiditis, advancement of the disease process occurs by local extension through areas of bony erosion or by thrombophlebitic spread.

Petrositis presents with a triad of symptoms first described by Gradenigo[58] in 1904: retro-orbital pain, purulent otorrhea, and diplopia secondary to lateral rectus palsy. Irritation of the fifth cranial nerve within the Meckel cave can cause retro-orbital pain as well as a more generalized trigeminal neuralgia. Lateral rectus dysfunction is a result of inflammation of the sixth cranial nerve as it passes through the Dorello canal between the anteromedial petrous ridge and the posterior clinoid.[59] Other symptoms associated with petrositis include fever,

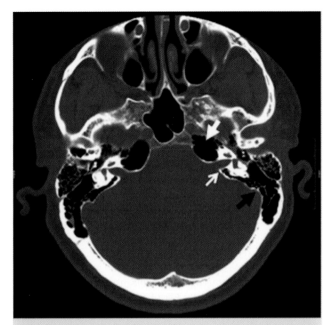

Fig. 20.4 Pneumatization of the petrous apex air cells. In this axial CT scan through the petrous apex of the temporal bones, anterior (*thick white arrow*) and posterior (*thin white arrow*) petrous apex air cells are well pneumatized and easily visualized. Perisinus mastoid air cells are also well pneumatized (*black arrow*).

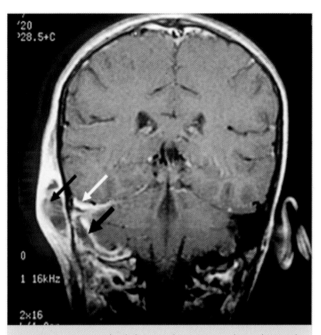

Fig. 20.5 Perisinus epidural abscess. This contrast-enhanced coronal T1-weighted magnetic resonance imaging demonstrates multiple intracranial complications of mastoiditis including focal meningitis (*thick white arrow*), sigmoid sinus thrombosis (*black arrow*), and perisinus epidural abscess (*thin white arrow*).

vertigo, hearing loss, and facial nerve dysfunction. Meningismus suggests intracranial extension of the infectious process.

Petrous apicitis is treated with intravenous antibiotics and surgical decompression and drainage of the petrous apex. A low threshold for surgical intervention must be maintained, as infection in the petrous apex has no natural route of drainage and thus has a greater likelihood of eroding through the confines of the petrous bone to involve the middle cranial fossa, the posterior cranial fossa, or the cavernous sinus. Surgical approaches to the petrous apex are as varied as the pneumatization tracts of the petrous apex air cells. Posterior approaches for the hearing ear include decompression through the (1) subarcuate tracts (through the superior semicircular canal),[60] (2) tracts along the sinodural angle (posterior to the superior semicircular canal and superior to the lateral semicircular canal), and (3) the infralabyrinthine tracts.[61] Anterior approaches can be made along (4) infracochlear tracts,[60] as well as (5) tracts anterior to the cochlea between the carotid artery and the middle fossa dura.[62] Surgical management of petrous apicitis includes a complete mastoidectomy, skeletonization of the semicircular canals, and exploration of all suspicious petrous air cell tracts. If the patient is deaf, a translabyrinthine approach offers the widest decompression.

20.2.2 Extratemporal Extension

The mucosal inflammation, fluid and pus collection, and bony destruction of mastoiditis can extend within and even out of the temporal bone via several routes. Most commonly, necrosis and demineralization of the mastoid bone allow for direct extension of the infectious process. Disease also can spread through healthy intact bone by thrombophlebitic or hematogenous dissemination. In cases of extratemporal extension, the surgeon also should be suspicious of concurrent intracranial complications.

Subperiosteal Abscess

First described by Bezold and Siebenmann[63] in 1908, the subperiosteal abscess represents lateral extension of acute mastoiditis through the thin bone of the lateral mastoid cortex typically superior to the insertion of the sternocleidomastoid muscle. The pinna is displaced anteriorly, inferiorly, and laterally, resulting in proptosis of the ear. Examination of the postauricular soft tissue reveals edema, erythema, and a deep fluctuance. Traditional surgical treatment consists of drainage via a postauricular incision and a simple mastoidectomy. Pus is encountered upon incising the periosteum superficial to the mastoid bone. A myringotomy also is performed, and the patient is treated with intravenous antibiotics. As with acute mastoiditis, there is a recent trend toward more conservative management. Several series published over the past decade have shown successful treatment of subperiosteal abscess using IV antibiotics, myringotomy tube insertion, and postauricular incision and drainage only, reserving mastoidectomy for the small minority of cases that do not respond to these conservative measures.[28,64–66]

Zygomatic Abscess

Rarely, extension of acute mastoiditis anteriorly via anterior air cells can lead to infectious involvement of the root of the zygoma. Perforation can occur anteriorly under the lower edge of the temporalis muscle, resulting in soft tissue edema and erythema of the cheek anterior to the ear. Management of a zygomatic abscess includes incision and drainage and antibiotics. Mastoidectomy is often necessary, though some patients may respond to conservative therapy alone.[67–69]

Bezold Abscess

Also described by Bezold and Siebenmann[63]at the beginning of the 20th century was extension of acute mastoiditis inferiorly to the mastoid tip. Perforation of the mastoid tip medial to the insertion of the sternocleidomastoid muscle results in the infectious process extending into the digastric groove and into deep neck spaces including the parapharyngeal space, the carotid sheath, and the retropharyngeal space. Unabated infection can extend into the mediastinum via the so-called danger space. Patients with a Bezold abscess usually present with diffuse edema of the lower mastoid area as well as a fluctuant neck mass. Surgical management includes drainage of the neck collection as well as cortical mastoidectomy with exenteration of air cells inferiorly to the mastoid tip. Careful identification and preservation of the facial nerve must be performed as the mastoid tip is approached. The neck must then be explored, and all involved deep neck spaces drained.

Cervical/Postauricular Fistula

Once the suppurative process of acute mastoiditis has eroded through its bony confines, it may extend through the soft tissue to the surface of the skin, forming a fistulous tract. A mastoid periosteal abscess may evolve into a postauricular fistula. Rarely, the deep neck space infection of a Bezold abscess can migrate to the skin surface and present as a cervical fistula. During surgical treatment of a postauricular or cervical fistula, the bony involvement is addressed with a simple mastoidectomy, any neck collection is drained, and the fistula is excised completely.

Extramastoid Cholesteatoma

Cholesteatoma represents cystic growth of keratinizing epithelium accompanied by an inflammatory process that is not necessarily infectious in nature but can demineralize and erode through the bony septa of the mastoid air cells as well as the lateral mastoid cortex. Therefore, extramastoid extension of a cholesteatoma should be considered an extramastoid complication of otitis media.[70] The cholesteatoma must be exenterated from all involved areas. As with the mastoidectomy for a Bezold abscess, the facial nerve must be identified and preserved as cholesteatoma is removed from areas near the mastoid tip.

20.3 Intracranial Complications

In the antibiotic era, intracranial complications of otitis media are quite rare. A 1995 review of 24,321 patients reported an intracranial complication rate of 0.36%.[71] Nevertheless, intracranial involvement, when it does occur, can be devastating; the same review reported a mortality rate of 18.4% in those patients who developed intracranial complications. Therefore, signs of meningismus or symptoms suggestive of intracranial pathology must be carefully noted particularly after antibiotic therapy has already begun.

20.3.1 Meningitis

Meningitis is one of the most common intracranial complications of otitis media.[71,72] Middle ear infections can progress to the brain by several routes: direct extension through bone eroded by inflammatory processes, through preformed pathways via the round window and the cochlear aqueduct, or by thrombophlebitic spread. Because these routes involve infection of intermediate areas between the inner ear and the meninges (i.e., mastoid air cells or inner ear), meningitis rarely occurs in the absence of another preexisting complication of otitis media.

Early meningitis presents as fever and persistent headache. As the disease progresses, patients may develop photophobia, lethargy, irritability, and neck stiffness. Patients with fully established disease become obtunded and develop seizure activity. Physical examination is often marked by a positive Kernig or Brudzinski sign. A Kernig sign is positive when the thigh is flexed at 90 degrees to the abdomen and the patient has subsequent difficulty extending at the knee secondary to pain. A Brudzinski sign is the involuntary flexion of the hips and knees when the neck is flexed.

Magnetic resonance imaging (MRI) of the brain with gadolinium contrast is the optimal imaging tool to confirm the diagnosis by meningeal enhancement. MRI scans also can identify the suppurative focus from which the meningitis arose as well as other intracranial complications of otitis media such as abscess formation or sigmoid sinus thrombosis. A lumbar puncture (LP) must be performed to establish the diagnosis as well as to determine the offending organism(s). An LP is performed only after cross-sectional imaging shows no abscess or hydrocephalus. Typically, an LP will show elevated opening pressure, elevated protein level, pleocytosis, and low glucose level.

Since the 1980s, the most common causes of bacterial meningitis in developed countries have been *S. pneumoniae*, *H. influenzae type b* (Hib), *Neisseria meningitidis*, group B *Streptococcus*, and *Listeria monocytogenes*.[73] The introduction of conjugate polysaccharide vaccines over the past few decades has dramatically altered the epidemiology of bacterial meningitis. Introduction of Hib vaccines reduced the percentage of childhood bacterial meningitis caused by *H. influenzae* from 73% in the early 1980s to only 16% in the early 1990s.[74] Between 1987 and 1999, the incidence of invasive Hib disease decreased by 99%.[75]

The heptavalent pneumococcal conjugate vaccine PCV7 was licensed in 2000 and is recommended by the Advisory Committee on Immunization Practices for all children in the United States 2 to 23 months of age who are at increased risk for pneumococcal disease.[76,77] A review of its effects on pneumococcal meningitis was published by Hsu et al[78] in 2009. These authors compared rates of pneumococcal meningitis between the 1998–1999 baseline period and 2004–2005. They found that the overall rate of pneumococcal meningitis decreased by 30% for all ages, with the largest decrease (64%) seen in the subgroup of patients under 2 years of age. The rate of meningitis caused by PCV7 serotypes decreased by 73%, whereas that caused by non-PCV7 serotypes increased by 60%. Again, these effects were most pronounced in children under 2 years of age.

They found a substantial decline in the incidence of pneumococcal meningitis due to serotypes that are resistant to antibiotics, likely because PCV7 has led to a reduction in the rates of nasopharyngeal carriage of, and disease caused by, penicillin-resistant isolates. Although penicillin resistance occurs mostly among PCV7-serotype isolates, the percentages of isolates of several non-PCV7 serotypes (including 19A) that are resistant to penicillin have increased.[78] The 10-valent and 13-valent pneumococcal conjugate vaccines (PCV10 and PCV13) are currently available, and the World Health Organization has endorsed their use in national immunization programs.[79]

Treatment of bacterial meningitis begins with stabilization of the patient and initiation of broad-spectrum intravenous antibiotics. Once the meningitic infection has been controlled, the suppurative focus must be surgically removed. Because otogenic meningitis rarely occurs in the absence of other complications of otitis media (e.g., mastoiditis, labyrinthitis, and petrous apicitis), concomitant complications need to be surgically addressed as well.

Brain Abscess

Brain abscesses are the leading cause of mortality among intracranial complications of otitis media.[71] Some series report that brain abscesses make up an even larger proportion of intracranial complications of otitis media than meningitis.[72,80] Cultures of otogenic brain abscesses typically yield mixed flora including anaerobes, Streptococcus species, Enterobacteriaceae (especially Proteus mirabilis), and Pseudomonas aeruginosa.[81] They can arise from hematogenous or thrombophlebitic extension of extradural infections. The development of a brain abscess usually occurs over the course of several days to several weeks. Initially, inflammation and edema of the white matter surrounding the infected vasculature manifests as encephalitis. The clinical presentation is very similar to that of meningitis, including persistent headache, moderate fever, chills, nausea, vomiting, neck stiffness, and altered mental status. An intermediate, quiescent phase ensues as the inflammatory process attempts to contain and encapsulate the focus of encephalitis by means of reactive gliosis. If successfully contained, the focus of infection may respond to antibiotics and be resorbed without need for surgical intervention. More frequently, infection progresses to an expanding granulomatous lesion with central necrosis and abscess formation. At this point, focal neurologic defects become apparent as the expanding abscess and its surrounding edema compress the brain. Although abscesses can occur anywhere in the brain, they are typically found in the ipsilateral temporal lobe or cerebellum.[71] Treatment of a brain abscess includes intravenous antibiotics and mastoidectomy in most cases, which may also be combined with neurologic surgical procedure. Neurosurgical drainage of the abscess is done concomitant with otologic decompression and debridement of the suppurative focus within the temporal bone.[72,80] Occasionally, in patients with severe symptoms, neurosurgical drainage and neurologic stabilization must be completed first, followed by the otologic procedure after the patient is stable.[71]

Subdural Empyema

Subdural empyema is a collection of pus between the dura mater and the arachnoid mater. Like brain abscesses, subdural empyemas can be seeded through thrombophlebitic spread; however, direct extension through bone also can occur. Subdural empyemas rarely result from otitis media, accounting for only 4% of intracranial complications of otitis media.[80] They occur more commonly as a complication of sinusitis.[82,83] Because a subdural empyema can track along a potential space, the infection progresses more rapidly than a brain abscess, and can extend throughout the subdural space until limited by specific boundaries such as the falx cerebri, tentorium cerebelli, and base of the brain. Initial symptoms can be mild and nonspecific such as fever, headache, and general malaise. As the infection progresses, however, signs of meningitis become apparent. Eventually, expansion of the empyema can compress the brain, leading to focal neurologic signs such as aphasia, hemianopsia, hemiplegia, or cranial nerve palsies.

Diagnosis of subdural empyema can be made by either CT scan or MRI scan. Treatment entails intravenous antibiotics, neurosurgical drainage of the empyema, and otologic surgical management of the middle ear and mastoid disease.

Epidural Abscess

Epidural abscess results from direct superior, posterior, or medial extension of coalescent mastoiditis through eroded bone into the middle or posterior fossa. In the middle fossa, purulence collects between the dura mater and the thin bony plate of the tegmen. Posterior fossa collections occur in the posterior petrous pyramid or just superior to the sigmoid sinus. Perisinus abscesses can lead to sigmoid sinus septic thrombophlebitis.[84] As with subdural empyema, epidural abscess is more often preceded by frontal sinusitis than by otitis media or mastoiditis.[83]

Epidural abscesses can initially be asymptomatic, or they can present insidiously with several days of fever, mental status changes, and neck pain. They typically do not involve the subjacent brain parenchyma.[85] Intracranial pressure is usually normal, and no focal neurologic deficits are observed until the abscess grows to a large size. An epidural abscess can readily be identified on CT or MRI (▶ Fig. 20.5). Once identified, the abscess can be drained and debrided via a cortical mastoidectomy approach. Management of the disease also includes intravenous antibiotics.

Sigmoid Sinus Septic Thrombophlebitis

A perisinus abscess can induce a mural thrombus within the sigmoid (a.k.a. lateral) sinus. The mural thrombus becomes infected and propagates to form an obliterating thrombus, occluding the lumen of the sinus. Fresh thrombus is formed and may cause propagation proximally to the internal jugular vein and distally to other dural sinuses including the cavernous sinus.[84] Infected thrombus can break off into the systemic circulation resulting in septic embolization. Obliterating thrombus also can predispose the affected vessels to perforation and subsequent hemorrhage. A mortality rate of up to 10% has been reported.[86]

The classic symptoms of sigmoid sinus septic thrombophlebitis (SSST) include "picket-fence" spiking fevers secondary to the dissemination of septic emboli into the systemic circulation, and the Griesinger sign, which is erythema and edema over the posterior mastoid secondary to thrombosis of a mastoid emissary vein.[87] With today's widespread use of antibiotics, the presentation of SSST is more attenuated and symptoms are less specific. Recent series report the most common signs and

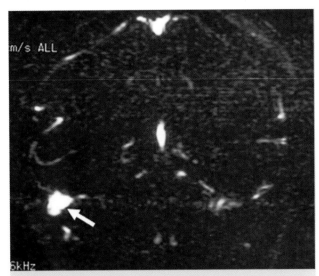

Fig. 20.6 Sigmoid sinus thrombosis. This magnetic resonance venogram demonstrates left-sided sigmoid sinus thrombosis. Note the enhancement consistent with flow in the right sigmoid sinus (*white arrow*) but absence of enhancement in the left sigmoid sinus.

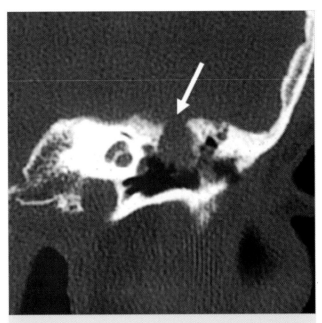

Fig. 20.7 This coronal CT scan of the temporal bone demonstrates erosion of the tegmen tympani by an epitympanic cholesteatoma (*white arrow*).

symptoms to be fever, headache, aural drainage, neck pain, otalgia, and mastoid tenderness.[84,88] Less common are meningeal signs, papilledema, ataxia, and cranial nerve palsies. MRI is the imaging method of choice for SSST.[89] A magnetic resonance venogram can be particularly helpful in identifying the degree of thrombus extension within the venous system (▶ Fig. 20.6).

Current treatment of SSST consists of intravenous antibiotics and surgical decompression with or without anticoagulation. Sitton and Chun[87] recently published a case series in combination with a literature review that encompassed data for a total of 26 patients with SSST. They report that most authors perform cortical mastoidectomy with or without myringotomy tube placement. Aspiration of the sigmoid sinus, thrombectomy, and internal jugular vein ligation are not frequently required. Nearly all patients (25/26) received anticoagulation with a combination of heparin, enoxaparin, and/or warfarin for a duration ranging from 3 weeks to 6 months. Five of the 25 patients that received anticoagulation had a bleeding complication, with severity ranging from self-limited epistaxis to postoperative hemorrhage/hematoma requiring transfusion. Although follow-up imaging performed 3 to 6 months after treatment showed clot resolution in only nine of the 26 patients, the majority of patients (23/26) experienced complete clinical recovery. The indications for anticoagulation remain unclear, largely because the small number of patients diagnosed with SSST precludes definitive outcome studies. One group suggests using anticoagulation in cases where there is evidence of thrombus progression, thrombus extension to other sites on initial examination (proximal jugular vein, transverse sinus, cavernous sinus), neurologic changes, persistent fevers, or embolic events.[90]

Otitic Hydrocephalus

Otitic hydrocephalus is a rare complication of otitis media that consists of elevated intracranial pressure without other focal neurologic abnormalities. The onset may be many weeks after

AOM or many years after the onset of chronic middle ear disease.[91] It is almost universally associated with sigmoid sinus thrombosis. The pathophysiology is poorly understood. One proposed mechanism is that nonobstructing mural thrombosis extending from the sigmoid sinus to the sagittal sinus directly interferes with the transfer of cerebrospinal fluid (CSF) to the venous sinus. An alternate hypothesis is that thrombus in the sigmoid sinus leads to impeded venous drainage into the neck, which then increases intracranial pressure either by direct transmission of the raised venous pressure to the CSF or by impeding CSF absorption by the arachnoid villi.[92]

Symptoms and signs include headache, drowsiness, blurred vision, nausea and vomiting, and occasionally diplopia. Examination may reveal papilledema and lateral rectus palsy due to cranial nerve VI stretch. Lumbar puncture reveals elevated CSF pressure with normal cytology and biochemistry. Treatment of otitic hydrocephalus includes management of the middle ear, mastoid, and sigmoid sinus disease as previously detailed in this chapter. Treatment is also directed toward relief of the elevated intracranial pressure with steroids, diuretics, and hyperosmolar agents.[91,93]

Meningoencephalocele

Herniation of the brain inferiorly into the mastoid cavity can occur when the integrity of the tegmen has been compromised. Tegmen compromise can occur by multiple mechanisms including congenital dehiscence, erosion by a chronically infected middle ear or cholesteatoma (▶ Fig. 20.7), or injury from a previous mastoidectomy. Meningoencephalic herniation (MEH) through the temporal bone commonly presents with CSF otorrhea or rhinorrhea or conductive hearing loss due either to impingement of the ossicular chain or to middle ear effusion. However, MEH secondary to COM is often masked by symptoms of the primary pathology and diagnosis of MEH may be diagnosed intraoperatively. CT scan of the temporal bone best defines the bony characteristics of the tegmen, whereas MRI is more ideal for distinguishing herniating brain tissue from cholesteatoma, granulation tissue, cholesterol granuloma, and other soft tissue masses.[94]

Treatment consists of surgical exploration of the mastoid cavity and repair of the tegmen. Common surgical approaches include transmastoid, middle cranial fossa, and combined transmastoid–middle cranial fossa. The transmastoid approach may be used for small defects limited to the tegmen mastoideum, whereas the middle cranial fossa and combined approaches are useful for larger defects and anteromedially located tegmental defects.[95,96] For cases with extensive middle ear destruction and limited possibility of reconstruction, Sanna et al[94] favor middle ear obliteration, which consists of blind sac closure of the external auditory canal, subtotal petrosectomy, and obliteration of the eustachian tube and surgical cavity.

20.4 Conclusion

The advent of antibiotic therapy has significantly decreased the incidence of complications of OM. Current trends toward decreasing the use of antibiotics for initial therapy of OM, the development of antibiotic resistance, and the introduction of new vaccine continue to change the face of AOM, COM, and their sequelae. Thus, the otolaryngologist must be increasingly vigilant and prepared for the diagnosis and management of these complications.

References

[1] Teele DW, Klein JO, Rosner BA. Epidemiology of otitis media during the first seven years of life in children in greater Boston: a prospective, cohort study. J Infect Dis 1989; 160: 83–94

[2] Monasta L, Ronfani L, Marchetti F et al. Burden of disease caused by otitis media: systematic review and global estimates. PLoS ONE 2012; 7: e36226

[3] American Academy of Pediatrics Subcommittee on Management of Acute Otitis Media. Diagnosis and management of acute otitis media. Pediatrics 2004; 113: 1451–1465

[4] Rovers MM, Glasziou P, Appelman CL et al. Antibiotics for acute otitis media: a meta-analysis with individual patient data. Lancet 2006; 368: 1429–1435

[5] Spiro DM, Arnold DH. The concept and practice of a wait-and-see approach to acute otitis media. Curr Opin Pediatr 2008; 20: 72–78

[6] Tähtinen PA, Laine MK, Huovinen P, Jalava J, Ruuskanen O, Ruohola A. A placebo-controlled trial of antimicrobial treatment for acute otitis media. N Engl J Med 2011; 364: 116–126

[7] Hoberman A, Paradise JL, Rockette HE et al. Treatment of acute otitis media in children under 2 years of age. N Engl J Med 2011; 364: 105–115

[8] Anwar AA, Lalwani AK. Should antibiotics be prescribed for acute otitis media? Laryngoscope 2012; 122: 4–5

[9] Thorne MC, Chewaproug L, Elden LM. Suppurative complications of acute otitis media: changes in frequency over time. Arch Otolaryngol Head Neck Surg 2009; 135: 638–641

[10] Hoppe JE, Köster S, Bootz F, Niethammer D. Acute mastoiditis—relevant once again. Infection 1994; 22: 178–182

[11] Katz A, Leibovitz E, Greenberg D et al. Acute mastoiditis in Southern Israel: a twelve year retrospective study (1990 through 2001). Pediatr Infect Dis J 2003; 22: 878–882

[12] Benito MB, Gorricho BP. Acute mastoiditis: increase in the incidence and complications. Int J Pediatr Otorhinolaryngol 2007; 71: 1007–1011

[13] Coco A, Vernacchio L, Horst M, Anderson A. Management of acute otitis media after publication of the 2004 AAP and AAFP clinical practice guideline. Pediatrics 2010; 125: 214–220

[14] Casey JR, Pichichero ME. Changes in frequency and pathogens causing acute otitis media in 1995–2003. Pediatr Infect Dis J 2004; 23: 824–828

[15] Fishman I, Sykes KJ, Horvat R, Selvarangan R, Newland J, Wei JL. Demographics and microbiology of otorrhea through patent tubes failing ototopical and/or oral antibiotic therapy. Otolaryngol Head Neck Surg 2011; 145: 1025–1029

[16] Stamboulidis K, Chatzaki D, Poulakou G et al. The impact of the heptavalent pneumococcal conjugate vaccine on the epidemiology of acute otitis media complicated by otorrhea. Pediatr Infect Dis J 2011; 30: 551–555

[17] Mygind H. Subperiosteal abscess of the mastoid region. Ann Otol Rhinol Laryngol 1910; 19: 259–265

[18] Pritchett CV, Thorne MC. Incidence of pediatric acute mastoiditis: 1997–2006. Arch Otolaryngol Head Neck Surg 2012; 138: 451–455

[19] Spratley J, Silveira H, Alvarez I, Pais-Clemente M. Acute mastoiditis in children: review of the current status. Int J Pediatr Otorhinolaryngol 2000; 56: 33–40

[20] Luntz M, Brodsky A, Nusem S et al. Acute mastoiditis—the antibiotic era: a multicenter study. Int J Pediatr Otorhinolaryngol 2001; 57: 1–9

[21] Ho D, Rotenberg BW, Berkowitz RG. The relationship between acute mastoiditis and antibiotic use for acute otitis media in children. Arch Otolaryngol Head Neck Surg 2008; 134: 45–48

[22] Lin HW, Shargorodsky J, Gopen Q. Clinical strategies for the management of acute mastoiditis in the pediatric population. Clin Pediatr (Phila) 2010; 49: 110–115

[23] Hsu KK, Shea KM, Stevenson AE, Pelton SI Massachusetts Department of Public Health. Changing serotypes causing childhood invasive pneumococcal disease: Massachusetts, 2001–2007. Pediatr Infect Dis J 2010; 29: 289–293

[24] Ongkasuwan J, Valdez TA, Hulten KG, Mason EO, Jr, Kaplan SL. Pneumococcal mastoiditis in children and the emergence of multidrug-resistant serotype 19A isolates. Pediatrics 2008; 122: 34–39

[25] Shambaugh GE, Glasscock ME. Surgery of the Ear. Philadelphia: WB Saunders, 1980:195–199

[26] Tamir S, Schwartz Y, Peleg U, Perez R, Sichel JY. Acute mastoiditis in children: is computed tomography always necessary? Ann Otol Rhinol Laryngol 2009; 118: 565–569

[27] Ida JB, Myer CM. Controversies in mastoiditis management. Clin Pediatr (Phila) 2010; 49: 611

[28] Taylor MF, Berkowitz RG. Indications for mastoidectomy in acute mastoiditis in children. Ann Otol Rhinol Laryngol 2004; 113: 69–72

[29] Geva A, Oestreicher-Kedem Y, Fishman G, Landsberg R, DeRowe A. Conservative management of acute mastoiditis in children. Int J Pediatr Otorhinolaryngol 2008; 72: 629–634

[30] Quesnel S, Nguyen M, Pierrot S, Contencin P, Manach Y, Couloigner V. Acute mastoiditis in children: a retrospective study of 188 patients. Int J Pediatr Otorhinolaryngol 2010; 74: 1388–1392

[31] Harley EH, Sdralis T, Berkowitz RG. Acute mastoiditis in children: a 12-year retrospective study. Otolaryngol Head Neck Surg 1997; 116: 26–30

[32] Psarommatis IM, Voudouris C, Douros K, Giannakopoulos P, Bairamis T, Carabinos C. Algorithmic management of pediatric acute mastoiditis. Int J Pediatr Otorhinolaryngol 2012; 76: 791–796

[33] Zanetti D, Nassif N. Indications for surgery in acute mastoiditis and their complications in children. Int J Pediatr Otorhinolaryngol 2006; 70: 1175–1182

[34] Papp Z, Rezes S, Jókay I, Sziklai I. Sensorineural hearing loss in chronic otitis media. Otol Neurotol 2003; 24: 141–144

[35] Juhn SK, Jung TTK, Lin J, Rhee CK. Effects of inflammatory mediators on middle ear pathology and on inner ear function. Ann N Y Acad Sci 1997; 830: 130–142

[36] Cureoglu S, Schachern PA, Rinaldo A, Tsuprun V, Ferlito A, Paparella MM. Round window membrane and labyrinthine pathological changes: an overview. Acta Otolaryngol 2005; 125: 9–15

[37] Takumida M, Anniko M. Localization of endotoxin in the inner ear following inoculation into the middle ear. Acta Otolaryngol 2004; 124: 772–777

[38] Cureoglu S, Schachern PA, Paparella MM, Lindgren BR. Cochlear changes in chronic otitis media. Laryngoscope 2004; 114: 622–626

[39] Joglekar S, Morita N, Cureoglu S et al. Cochlear pathology in human temporal bones with otitis media. Acta Otolaryngol 2010; 130: 472–476

[40] Pollock RA, Brown LA. Facial paralysis in otitis media. In: Graham MD, House WH, eds. Disorders of the Facial Nerve. New York: Raven Press, 1982:221–224

[41] Redaelli de Zinis LO, Gamba P, Balzanelli C. Acute otitis media and facial nerve paralysis in adults. Otol Neurotol 2003; 24: 113–117

[42] Popovtzer A, Raveh E, Bahar G, Oestreicher-Kedem Y, Feinmesser R, Nageris BI. Facial palsy associated with acute otitis media. Otolaryngol Head Neck Surg 2005; 132: 327–329

[43] Makeham TP, Croxson GR, Coulson S. Infective causes of facial nerve paralysis. Otol Neurotol 2007; 28: 100–103

[44] Selesnick SH, Jackler RK. Facial paralysis in suppurative ear disease. Oper Tech Otolaryngol – Head Neck Surg 1992; 3: 61–68

[45] Yetiser S, Tosun F, Kazkayasi M. Facial nerve paralysis due to chronic otitis media. Otol Neurotol 2002; 23: 580–588

[46] Harker LA, Pignatari SS. Facial nerve paralysis secondary to chronic otitis media without cholesteatoma. Am J Otol 1992; 13: 372–374

[47] Gacek RR. The surgical management of labyrinthine fistulae in chronic otitis media with cholesteatoma. Ann Otol Rhinol Laryngol 1974; 83: 10–, 1–19

[48] Copeland BJ, Buchman CA. Management of labyrinthine fistulae in chronic ear surgery. Am J Otolaryngol 2003; 24: 51–60

[49] Dawes JDK, Watson RT. Labyrinthine fistulae. J Laryngol Otol 1978; 92: 83–98

[50] Palva T, Ramsay H. Treatment of labyrinthine fistula. Arch Otolaryngol Head Neck Surg 1989; 115: 804–806

[51] Kobayashi T, Sato T, Toshima M, Ishidoya M, Suetake M, Takasaka T. Treatment of labyrinthine fistula with interruption of the semicircular canals. Arch Otolaryngol Head Neck Surg 1995; 121: 469–475

[52] Soda-Merhy A, Betancourt-Suárez MA. Surgical treatment of labyrinthine fistula caused by cholesteatoma. Otolaryngol Head Neck Surg 2000; 122: 739–742

[53] Magliulo G, Celebrini A, Cuiuli G, Parrotto D. Surgical management of the labyrinthine fistula complicating chronic otitis media with or without cholesteatoma. J Otolaryngol Head Neck Surg 2008; 37: 143–147

[54] Ueda Y, Kurita T, Matsuda Y, Ito S, Nakashima T. Surgical treatment of labyrinthine fistula in patients with cholesteatoma. J Laryngol Otol Suppl 2009; 31: 64–67

[55] Schuknecht HF. Pathology of the Ear. Philadelphia: Lea and Febiger, 1993

[56] Gulya AJ, Glasscock ME III, eds. Surgery of the ear. New York: BC Decker, 2002

[57] Allam AF, Schuknecht HF. Pathology of petrositis. Laryngoscope 1968; 78: 1813–1832

[58] Gradenigo G. Ueber circumscripte leptomeningitis mit spinalen symptomen . Arch Ohrenheilk. 1904; 51: 60–62

[59] Ezer H, Banerjee AD, Thakur JD, Nanda A. Dorello's canal for laymen: a Lego-like presentation. J Neurol Surg B Skull Base 2012; 73: 183–189

[60] Freckner P. Some remarks on the treatment of apicitis (petrositis) with or without Gradenigo's syndrome. Acta Otolaryngol (Stockh) 1932; 17: 97

[61] Farrior JB. Anterior hypotympanic approach for glomus tumor of the infratemporal fossa. Laryngoscope 1984; 94: 1016–1021

[62] Lempert J. Complete apicectomy (mastoidotympanoapicectomy). Arch Otolaryngol Head Neck Surg 1937; 25: 144–177

[63] Bezold F, Siebenmann F. Textbook of Otology (Holinger J, trans.). Chicago: E.H. Cosgrove, 1908:208

[64] Bauer PW, Brown KR, Jones DT. Mastoid subperiosteal abscess management in children. Int J Pediatr Otorhinolaryngol 2002; 63: 185–188

[65] Lahav J, Handzel O, Gertler R, Yehuda M, Halperin D. Postauricular needle aspiration of subperiosteal abscess in acute mastoiditis. Ann Otol Rhinol Laryngol 2005; 114: 323–327

[66] Bakhos D, Trijolet JP, Morinière S, Pondaven S, Al Zahrani M, Lescanne E. Conservative management of acute mastoiditis in children. Arch Otolaryngol Head Neck Surg 2011; 137: 346–350

[67] Tsai CJ, Guo YC, Tsai TL, Shiao AS. Zygomatic abscess complicating a huge mastoid cholesteatoma with intact eardrum. Otolaryngol Head Neck Surg 2003; 128: 436–438

[68] Weiss I, Marom T, Goldfarb A, Roth Y. Luc's abscess: the return of an old fellow. Otol Neurotol 2010; 31: 776–779

[69] Gurgel RK, Woodson EA, Lenkowski PW, Gubbels SP, Hansen MR. Zygomatic root abscess: a rare complication of otitis media. Otol Neurotol 2010; 31: 856–857

[70] Luetje CM. Extramastoid cholesteatoma in chronic ear disease: a report of two cases. Laryngoscope 1979; 89: 1755–1759

[71] Kangsanarak J, Navacharoen N, Fooanant S, Ruckphaopunt K. Intracranial complications of suppurative otitis media: 13 years' experience. Am J Otol 1995; 16: 104–109

[72] Isaacson B, Mirabal C, Kutz JW, Jr, Lee KH, Roland PS. Pediatric otogenic intracranial abscesses. Otolaryngol Head Neck Surg 2010; 142: 434–437

[73] Bottomley MJ, Serruto D, Sáfadi MA, Klugman KP. Future challenges in the elimination of bacterial meningitis. Vaccine 2012; 30 Suppl 2: B78–B86

[74] Dawson KG, Emerson JC, Burns JL. Fifteen years of experience with bacterial meningitis. Pediatr Infect Dis J 1999; 18: 816–822

[75] Watt JP, Levine OS, Santosham M. Global reduction of Hib disease: what are the next steps? Proceedings of the meeting Scottsdale, Arizona, September 22–25, 2002. J Pediatr 2003; 143 Suppl: S163–S187

[76] Advisory Committee on Immunization Practices. Preventing pneumococcal disease among infants and young children. Recommendations of the Advisory Committee on Immunization Practices (ACIP). MMWR Recomm Rep 2000; 49 RR-9: 1–35

[77] American Academy of Pediatrics, Committee on Infectious Diseases. American Academy of Pediatrics. Committee on Infectious Diseases. Policy statement: recommendations for the prevention of pneumococcal infections, including the use of pneumococcal conjugate vaccine (Prevnar), pneumococcal polysaccharide vaccine, and antibiotic prophylaxis. Pediatrics 2000; 106: 362–366

[78] Hsu HE, Shutt KA, Moore MR et al. Effect of pneumococcal conjugate vaccine on pneumococcal meningitis. N Engl J Med 2009; 360: 244–256

[79] WHO Publication. Pneumococcal vaccines WHO position paper - 2012 - recommendations. Vaccine 2012; 30: 4717–4718

[80] Penido NdeO, Borin A, Iha LC et al. Intracranial complications of otitis media: 15 years of experience in 33 patients. Otolaryngol Head Neck Surg 2005; 132: 37–42

[81] Arlotti M, Grossi P, Pea F et al. GISIG (Gruppo Italiano di Studio sulle Infezioni Gravi) Working Group on Brain Abscesses. Consensus document on controversial issues for the treatment of infections of the central nervous system: bacterial brain abscesses. Int J Infect Dis 2010; 14 Suppl 4: S79–S92

[82] Bernardini GL. Diagnosis and management of brain abscess and subdural empyema. Curr Neurol Neurosci Rep 2004; 4: 448–456

[83] DeMuri GP, Wald ER. Complications of acute bacterial sinusitis in children. Pediatr Infect Dis J 2011; 30: 701–702

[84] Kaplan DM, Kraus M, Puterman M, Niv A, Leiberman A, Fliss DM. Otogenic lateral sinus thrombosis in children. Int J Pediatr Otorhinolaryngol 1999; 49: 177–183

[85] Pradilla G, Ardila GP, Hsu W, Rigamonti D. Epidural abscesses of the CNS. Lancet Neurol 2009; 8: 292–300

[86] Ooi EH, Hilton M, Hunter G. Management of lateral sinus thrombosis: update and literature review. J Laryngol Otol 2003; 117: 932–939

[87] Sitton MS, Chun R. Pediatric otogenic lateral sinus thrombosis: role of anticoagulation and surgery. Int J Pediatr Otorhinolaryngol 2012; 76: 428–432

[88] Ropposch T, Nemetz U, Braun EM, Lackner A, Walch C. Low molecular weight heparin therapy in pediatric otogenic sigmoid sinus thrombosis: a safe treatment option? Int J Pediatr Otorhinolaryngol 2012; 76: 1023–1026

[89] Magliulo G, Terranova G, Cristofari P, Ronzoni R. Sigmoid sinus thrombosis and imaging techniques. Ann Otol Rhinol Laryngol 1996; 105: 991–993

[90] Bradley DT, Hashisaki GT, Mason JC. Otogenic sigmoid sinus thrombosis: what is the role of anticoagulation? Laryngoscope 2002; 112: 1726–1729

[91] Sadoghi M, Dabirmoghaddam P. Otitic hydrocephalus: case report and literature review. Am J Otolaryngol 2007; 28: 187–190

[92] Tomkinson A, Mills RG, Cantrell PJ. The pathophysiology of otitic hydrocephalus. J Laryngol Otol 1997; 111: 757–759

[93] Kuczkowski J, Dubaniewicz-Wybieralska M, Przewoźny T, Narozny W, Mikaszewski B. Otitic hydrocephalus associated with lateral sinus thrombosis and acute mastoiditis in children. Int J Pediatr Otorhinolaryngol 2006; 70: 1817–1823

[94] Sanna M, Fois P, Russo A, Falcioni M. Management of meningoencephalic herniation of the temporal bone: personal experience and literature review. Laryngoscope 2009; 119: 1579–1585

[95] Jackson CG, Pappas DG, Jr, Manolidis S et al. Brain herniation into the middle ear and mastoid: concepts in diagnosis and surgical management. Am J Otol 1997; 18: 198–205, discussion 205–206

[96] Mosnier I, Fiky LEL, Shahidi A, Sterkers O. Brain herniation and chronic otitis media: diagnosis and surgical management. Clin Otolaryngol Allied Sci 2000; 25: 385–391

21 Otosclerosis

Michael J. McKenna and Alicia M. Quesnel

21.1 Introduction

Otosclerosis is a bone disease that is unique to the human temporal bone.[1] One of the most common causes of acquired hearing loss, otosclerosis has a well-established hereditary predisposition, with approximately 50% of affected individuals having other known affected family members.[2] Otosclerosis occurs within the endochondral layer of the temporal bone, usually in certain sites of predilection that are associated with globuli interossei or so-called embryonic rests. The most common site of occurrence of otosclerosis is the fissula ante fenestram just anterior to the stapes footplate.[3,4] As the lesion enlarges and spreads, it encroaches on the stapes footplate and produces a conductive hearing loss (clinical otosclerosis). In some cases, the lesion may spread to involve the cochlea and result in an irreversible sensorineural hearing loss (SNHL).[5,6] However, the majority of lesions do not encroach on the footplate or cochlea; such lesions remain small and asymptomatic (histological otosclerosis).[7] The small histological foci are tenfold more common than the larger lesions that result in clinical manifestations.[8] Despite intensive investigation, the etiology of otosclerosis remains unknown.

21.2 Pathology

Histopathologically, the otosclerotic process is characterized by a wave of abnormal bone remodeling, resulting in the replacement of otic capsule bone with a hypercellular woven bone, which may undergo further remodeling, resulting in a mosaic sclerotic appearance. The initial remodeling process consists predominantly of mononuclear cells, including histiocytes and bone cells, many of which show degeneration with cellular lysis and release of cytoplastic contents.[9] There is a distinct absence of acute inflammatory cells.[10] Although the most common site of predilection is the fissula ante fenestram that lies in close proximity to the anterior portion of the stapes footplate, otosclerosis may also occur in other sites including the round window, sometimes resulting in round window obliteration. The degree of stapes footplate involvement from otosclerosis is highly variable. In the majority of cases, otosclerosis results in anterior stapes fixation without involvement of the footplate or the posterior annular ligament. In many cases, as the otosclerotic process begins to develop anterior to the footplate, the footplate becomes posteriorly displaced. This results in a jamming of the posterior footplate within the oval window and the development of a low-frequency conductive hearing loss (▶ Fig. 21.1).[11]

With bony fixation of the footplate, there is conductive hearing loss across all frequencies. This has long been recognized by stapes surgeons who, prior to the advent of the laser, were often reluctant to operate on patients without a negative Rinne test at 512 and 1024 Hz. These patients had a higher risk for footplate mobilization or a floating footplate upon down fracture of the stapes suprastructure. In some cases, the otosclerotic lesion may overgrow the footplate, resulting in obliterative otosclerosis.[12] It is not possible to differentiate between obliterative otosclerosis and bony ankylosis of the footplate without oval window obliteration on audiometric testing alone.

Large active otosclerotic lesions that involve the cochlear capsule and penetrate the cochlear endosteum can result in a progressive SNHL (▶ Fig. 21.2).[7,13] Until recently, there was no clear explanation for the cause of the SNHL in these patients. Temporal bone studies have failed to demonstrate a loss of sensory cells, both hair cells and spiral ganglion cells, in proportion to the degree of SNHL.[14,15] The only pathological correlation between SNHL and otosclerosis has been the penetration of the cochlear endosteum with hyalinization of the spiral ligament and atrophy of the stria vascularis.[16] Recent investigations have found that the spiral ligament, like the stria vascularis, is a dynamic organ that plays an important role in maintaining

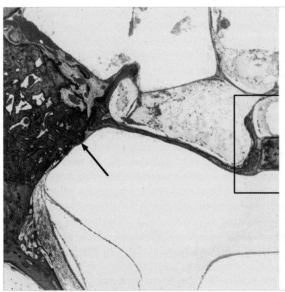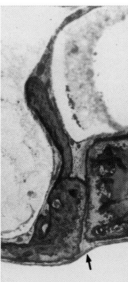

Fig. 21.1 Fixation of the footplate by an anterior focus of otosclerosis (*large arrow*). The otosclerotic process has also resulted in posterior displacement of the footplate. Inset: Higher magnification view of the posterior footplate, which has become jammed against the bony annulus (*small arrow*).

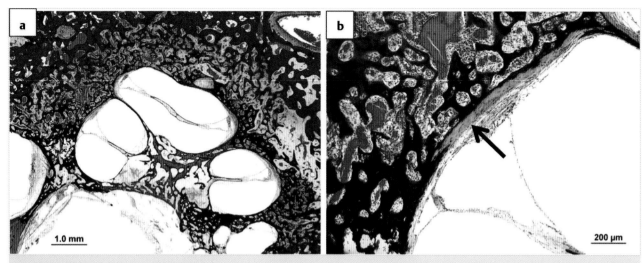

Fig. 21.2 Extensive foci of otosclerosis surrounding the cochlea in a temporal bone specimen from a patient with far advanced otosclerosis: (a) low power; (b) high power. There is hyalin deposition in the spiral ligament (*arrow*), where the otospongiosis has breached the cochlear endosteal layer.

normal cochlear physiology. It plays a critical role in the recirculation of potassium ions within the cochlea.[17] Disturbance of this function is one plausible explanation for the degree of SNHL that occurs in these patients.

21.3 Etiology

Although the precise etiology of otosclerosis has yet to be elucidated, significant progress has been made over the past 20 years. Fundamentally, otosclerosis is an active remodeling process of bone that occurs within the endochondral layer of the temporal bone, which under normal circumstances undergoes virtually no remodeling following development.[20–22] In this respect, the otic capsule is unique and different from all other bones in the body. To understand why this abnormal remodeling process occurs in the first place, it is important first to understand why the otic capsule is devoid of postdevelopmental remodeling. Zhender et al[23] have studied otic capsule remodeling in a number of species and have shown that remodeling in the otic capsule is markedly inhibited compared to other bones and that this inhibition is most prevalent in direct proximity to the inner ear.[24] These studies have led to the hypothesis that the inner ear itself may play a direct role in the inhibition of otic capsule remodeling by producing substances that diffuse into the surrounding bone and prevent remodeling. We have recently discovered that the spiral ligament produces a compound called osteoprotegerin (OPG) that is secreted into the perilymph and diffuses into the surrounding otic capsule bone.[25] OPG is a potent inhibitor of bone remodeling. It acts by inhibiting the recruitment, formation, and activity of osteoclasts that resorb bone. Knockout mice that lack OPG have active otic capsule remodeling that closely resembles otosclerosis.[26,27] We suspect that there are other factors involved in the inhibition of otic capsule remodeling other than OPG, although as of yet, they have not been clearly defined.

One hypothesis that has gained considerable support over the past 15 years is that otosclerosis may be related to a persistent measles virus infection within the otic capsule.[27] The evidence to support this hypothesis includes the demonstration of viral-like particles within osteoblasts and preosteoblasts in active otosclerotic lesions by electron microscopy, the demonstration of measles antigens within active lesions using immunohistochemical techniques, and the demonstration of measles virus gene products in active otosclerotic lesions using reverse transcription/polymerase chain reaction techniques.[28–35] This hypothesis would account for the fact that otosclerosis appears to involve only the human otic capsule, as measles virus affects only humans and closely related primates. It would also account for the significant decline in the incidence of new cases of otosclerosis, which is well correlated with the measles virus vaccination.[36,37]

Otosclerosis is most common among whites, uncommon among Asians, and extremely rare in blacks. Otosclerosis is estimated to occur histologically in 10% of the white population and results in hearing loss in approximately 0.5%.[6] The clinical prevalence of otosclerosis is estimated to be twice as common in females as in males.[38]

Familial aggregation of individuals affected by otosclerosis has been recognized for many years.[39,40] Most studies support a pattern of autosomal dominant transmission with incomplete penetrance in the range of 20 to 40%.[41] The most compelling evidence for an underlying genetic cause for otosclerosis comes from studies on monozygotic twins with clinical otosclerosis, in which concordance has been found in nearly all cases.[42] However, information does not exist on the genetic transmission of histological otosclerosis. It is not known whether the genetic basis of inheritance is related to the formation of an otosclerosis focus within the temporal bone or the tendency for a lesion to progress once it has begun, or both. Most studies on families with otosclerosis support a pattern of autosomal dominant transmission with incomplete penetrance. A study of 65 pedigrees with otosclerosis in Tunisia suggests that otosclerosis is primarily heterogenetic, and that in 13% of clinical cases studied the affected individuals carry a dominant gene with nearly complete penetrance.[43] Linkage analyses of large and unrelated families have revealed linkage to distinctly different loci, indicating that otosclerosis is heterogenetic.[44–49] The otosclerosis phenotype may result from several different gene defects. Each of the families that has been studied thus far is atypical in that the penetrance is nearly complete, with approximately half of all individuals in each family being affected. Although a strong familial component exists, several studies have reported that sporadic otosclerosis represents 40 to 50% of all clinical cases.

There is evidence to suggest that some cases of otosclerosis may be related to defects in expression of the COL1A1 gene. Association analysis using multiple polymorphic markers has revealed a significant association between both familial and sporadic cases of clinical otosclerosis and the COL1A1 gene.[49,50] The association has been found to increase from the 3' to the 5' region of the gene. Studies of the allelic expression of the CO-L1A1 gene in patients with clinical otosclerosis have revealed reduced expression of one COL1A1 allele in some cases, similar to that which has been described in many cases of type I osteogenesis imperfecta.[51,52] Type I osteogenesis imperfecta shares both clinical and histological similarities with otosclerosis. Approximately half of all patients with type I osteogenesis imperfecta develop hearing loss that is clinically indistinguishable from otosclerosis. It is also well known that some patients with clinical otosclerosis have blue sclera, a feature that is found in virtually all patients with type I osteogenesis imperfecta.[53] The histopathology of temporal bones from patients with type I osteogenesis imperfecta is identical to that observed in patients with otosclerosis.[54,55]

Although the etiology of otosclerosis is not clearly understood at present, the above studies have brought us much closer to understanding the basic nature of the disease. Otosclerosis is clearly a heterogenetic and possibly a multifactorial disease process. It is fundamentally a disturbance in the physiological pathways or factors that normally serve to inhibit otic capsule remodeling. As we develop a better understanding of the otic capsule physiology and the factors that account for its unique absence of remodeling, we will gain a better understanding of the processes that result in abnormal remodeling, including otosclerosis.

21.4 Diagnosis

21.4.1 History

Most often, otosclerosis results in a gradually progressive, conductive, or mixed hearing loss. In approximately 70% of cases, both ears are affected over time. Typically the age of onset is between 20 and 40. Juvenile onset is known to occur but is relatively uncommon and warrants further investigation of other possible causes. A progressive, purely SNHL may also occur as a result of otosclerosis, but this too is relatively rare and warrants investigation of other possible causes. In patients with a past history of infection, other possible causes of the conductive hearing loss need to be considered. A family history of hearing loss can be elicited in many cases. A family history of otosclerosis or another family member who has undergone a successful stapedectomy makes the diagnosis of otosclerosis far more likely.

When a careful history is taken, between 10 and 20% of patients will relate symptoms of dizziness or vertigo.[1,8] The symptoms are highly variable, ranging from benign paroxysmal positional vertigo, waxing and waning disequilibrium, and vertigo of the Ménière's type. In some cases, although uncommon,

otosclerosis may involve the endolymphatic duct, resulting in a hydrops and symptoms of Ménière's disease. This is important to recognize, as this is an absolute contraindication for stapedectomy, as hydrops may result in saccular dilatation predisposing the membranous labyrinth to injury upon fenestration of the footplate. For reasons that are unclear, some patients who have a history of giddiness or waxing and waning disequilibrium without true vertigo experience an improvement in their vestibular symptoms following stapedectomy.[18,19]

Some patients with superior canal dehiscence syndrome present with both conductive hearing loss and vestibular symptoms. The conductive hearing loss may closely mimic that seen in otosclerosis.[57] Often these patients complain of severe autophony. A diagnosis of superior canal dehiscence syndrome should be suspected in a patient with a low-frequency conductive hearing loss with bone conduction thresholds that rise above 0 dB. Acoustic reflex testing may also be helpful in differentiating otosclerosis from superior semicircular canal dehiscence (SSCD) syndrome as it should be present in SSCD and abnormal in otosclerosis.

21.4.2 Physical Examination

Otoscopic examination usually reveals normal-appearing tympanic membranes. Pneumo-otoscopy with magnification is helpful in both ruling out the presence of a middle ear effusion and assessing malleus mobility. The presence of tympanosclerosis or a retraction pocket should lead to the consideration of a conductive hearing loss of other causes. Occasionally, a vascular hue can be seen on the surface of the promontory, known as Schwartze's sign, which is the result of hyperemic middle ear mucosa over an area of active otosclerosis. Tuning fork tests, both Weber and Rinne, at 512 Hz and 1024 Hz should be performed. The results should be correlated with a complete audiogram.

21.5 Audiology

All patients undergo standard audiometry including pure-tone audiometry with air and bone testing and speech discrimination testing. It is important that true bone conduction thresholds be determined, as this information may be helpful in differentiating the conductive hearing loss in otosclerosis from that seen in SSCD. Patients with SSCD often demonstrate bone conduction thresholds above 0 dB, which will be missed if the audiologist stops testing at 0 dB. Until recently we had abandoned stapedial reflex testing as part of the standard audiometric evaluation in patients with conductive hearing loss. However, with the recognition that SSCD is a potential cause of conductive hearing loss and that patients with SSCD have normal acoustic reflex testing, we have begun testing the stapedial reflex in these patients.

Early in the development of conductive hearing loss from otosclerosis, patients typically demonstrate a low-frequency conductive loss that narrows in the high frequencies. This low-frequency conductive loss is related to the posterior displacement of the footplate as a result of an encroaching anterior otosclerotic lesion. The jammed footplate with impaired mobility maintains the capacity for transmission in the higher frequencies. With bony ankylosis of the footplate, the conductive hearing loss flattens across all frequencies.[56]

It is not unusual for patients with otosclerosis and conductive hearing loss to have a depression in the bone conduction thresholds that is most significant at 2,000 Hz, termed a Carhart notch, which is thought to represent an audiological artifact. It often resolves following a successful stapedectomy. For this reason, it is important that all patients who are tested postoperatively also have both air and bone thresholds tested.

Word recognition scores or speech discrimination is usually normal unless there is a significant sensorineural component to the hearing loss.

21.5.1 Imaging

Although imaging is not routinely necessary for the diagnosis of otosclerosis or prior to primary stapedectomy, it may be useful in certain situations. Imaging should be included in the evaluation of a patient with otosclerosis in any of the following circumstances: (1) the diagnosis is in question; (2) conductive hearing loss recurs after stapedectomy; (3) conductive hearing loss persists after stapedectomy; (4) vertigo is severe or persistent after stapedectomy; (5) the sensorineural component of the hearing loss requires evaluation; and (6) medical therapies are to be prescribed for otosclerosis-related SNHL.

Computed tomography (CT) is the most commonly employed imaging modality for the evaluation of otosclerosis. Modern CT, when used with a temporal bone imaging protocol and 0.5-mm slice thickness, provides excellent detail of the middle ear and otic capsule. Contemporary studies found that the sensitivity of CT for the diagnosis of clinical otosclerosis is greater than 90%, when compared to a diagnosis of otosclerosis based on otoscopic, audiological, or surgical findings.[57,58]

When the diagnosis of otosclerosis is in question, CT may be used to exclude other pathologies that cause conductive hearing loss, such as chronic otitis media and its sequelae, some traumatic ossicular discontinuities, middle ear masses, or third window lesions. Adhesions and lack of aeration in the middle ear, both of which suggest a diagnosis other than otosclerosis, can be easily seen by CT. Although the audiogram and vestibular evoked myogenic potential (VEMP) are important in the diagnosis of SSCD, CT usually definitively excludes this diagnosis.

Also, CT can help determine the cause of a recurrent conductive hearing loss and whether reexploration should be considered. A significantly lateralized piston, severe adhesions, and a middle ear effusion can be visualized on CT. More subtle marginalization or lateralization of the prosthesis may not be apparent. An air bubble in the vestibule (▶ Fig. 21.3) or a deep prosthesis causing post-stapedectomy vertigo may be demonstrated on CT. However, the ability to accurately determine prosthesis insertion depth on CT is limited. A recent study showed that CT tends to underestimate the vestibule insertion depth of stapes prostheses with fluoroplastic pistons, and overestimate the depth of those with stainless steel pistons.[59]

Otosclerosis may cause an SNHL when it involves the endosteal layer of the cochlea and causes hyalinization of the spiral ligament (▶ Fig. 21.2). Retrofenestral otosclerosis can be readily identified on CT, but it is more difficult to determine whether the retrofenestral focus has extended to the endosteal layer of the cochlea. Some studies have found that bone conduction

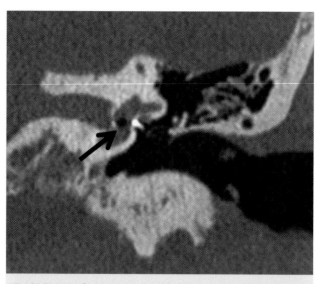

Fig. 21.3 Coronal noncontrast temporal bone computed tomography image from a patient who underwent stapedectomy for otosclerosis and developed a delayed perilymph fistula. The patient presented with severe vertigo and decrement in sensorineural hearing. There is an air bubble in the vestibule (*black arrow*).

thresholds correlate with CT findings of retrofenestral extension of otospongiosis,[60,61] whereas others have not.[62] The lack of uniformity in these results may be explained by comparison to the pathology, which indicates that CT can detect cochlear endosteal involvement by otosclerosis in 63% of affected temporal bones.[63]

21.6 Surgical Management by Stapedectomy

21.6.1 History of Otosclerosis Surgery

The history of otosclerosis surgery is among the most interesting and colorful chapters in all of otolaryngology. Any student of otology is strongly encouraged to read the biography of Howard House, *For the World to Hear*,[5,6] as it not only chronicles the history of otosclerosis surgery during the last century but also provides insight into the personalities of some of the great leaders in our field. Stapedectomy was first introduced as a treatment for otosclerosis in the late 1800s by Blake and Jack in Boston and shortly thereafter by DeRossi in Italy. Although the initial results were encouraging, there were cases of infection that resulted in meningitis and death and led to a condemnation of all stapes surgery by prominent leaders in the field. It was John Shea in 1956 who, with the benefit of improved instrumentation and employing the operating microscope, reintroduced stapedectomy using a polyethylene strut and vein graft. Although most otologists were skeptical at the time, within 10 years it became widely apparent that stapedectomy was the most reliable and safest technique for the restoration of hearing in patients with otosclerosis and stapes fixation. What followed was one of the most exciting periods in modern otology and occupied much of the agenda of the American Otological Society including papers and discussions.

There has been an evolution in the two fundamental steps of the operation including the fenestration of the oval window and the introduction of a prosthesis. The fenestration of the oval window evolved from a technique of total stapedectomy with removal of the stapes footplate with micro-picks, to partial stapedectomy, to the small fenestra technique, initially using micro-drills, and ultimately to the introduction of otologic lasers. Similarly, there has been an evolution in the development of prostheses from polyethylene tubes to fat and gel wires and ultimately to the piston prostheses of varying sizes and materials. Throughout this period, there have been significant improvements in the operating microscope including superior optics and brighter illumination. Although it is not clear what the future holds in terms of further technological innovations, with the advancements in robotic and computer technology, the evolution of stapes surgery will certainly continue.

21.6.2 Indications

In general there should be a conductive hearing loss of at least 25 dB in frequencies of 250 Hz to 1 kHz or higher as determined by both audiometry and the presence of a negative Rinne test at 512 Hz. The presence of a concomitant SNHL in the affected ear is not necessarily a contraindication for stapes surgery. It does, however, require some thoughtful consideration. If a hearing aid will still be required after successful stapedectomy, the procedure may be considered if it would result in improved performance with amplification. If both ears are involved, generally the poorer hearing ear is operated first. If the operation is a success, the patient may be a candidate for a contralateral stapedectomy a year later if the hearing in the operated ear has remained stable.

In some cases of advanced otosclerosis, it may be difficult on the basis of audiometry to determine whether or not a patient might benefit from a stapedectomy. Often the tuning-fork tests are more helpful than the audiogram under such circumstances. Often these patients have very poor speech discrimination scores preoperatively because of an inadequate presentation level, which is at the limit of the audiometer. These patients may demonstrate a dramatic improvement in their speech discrimination following stapedectomy.

21.6.3 Contraindications

Stapedectomy on an only hearing ear is almost always contraindicated. One exception may be a case of a profound mixed loss that is beyond the level of benefit of a conventional hearing aid. These patients would otherwise be considered cochlear implant candidates, and a stapedectomy may be considered as the first option prior to proceeding with implantation. Stapedectomy is contraindicated in cases of active infection of the middle ear or external auditory canal. It is also contraindicated in patients with tympanic membrane perforations. Patients in whom vestibular function is absolutely critical for their employment should be given special consideration. Stapedectomy is contraindicated in ears with Ménière disease and relatively contraindicated in patients with a contralateral otologic problem, which may threaten the hearing in their contralateral ear over time.

21.6.4 Informed Consent

All patients being considered for stapedectomy should be counseled regarding the potential benefits of amplification as a nonsurgical option to help improve their hearing. Patients should be made aware that there is no window of opportunity, and that a delay in deciding to proceed with surgery will not impact the eventual result. After describing the details of the surgical procedure in a manner that the patient can easily understand, all of the potential risks should be discussed, including failure of the surgery to improve hearing, by virtue of residual conductive hearing loss; creation of an SNHL, either partial or complete; vestibular dysfunction; perforation of the tympanic membrane; facial nerve dysfunction; disturbance in taste; development of a perilymph fistula; and late failure of the procedure. It is prudent to inform patients that some disturbance in taste related to manipulation of the chorda tympani nerve can be expected, as it occurs in most cases. Patients are reassured to know that this outcome was expected and is not a complication.

21.7 Primary Stapedectomy

21.7.1 Anesthesia

Primary stapedectomy can be performed with either local or general anesthesia. The primary advantage of local anesthesia is the time saved in putting patients to sleep and waking them up. There may be some advantage in monitoring vestibular symptoms, but this is certainly not borne out by differences in results with local and general anesthesia. General anesthesia provides assurance of absolute control of head motion and prevention of pain. In our recent experience, over half of our patients have selected general anesthesia.

21.8 Surgical Procedure

21.8.1 Positioning

The patient is placed in a supine head-hanging position with the head turned to the opposite shoulder. A downward tilt of the head of approximately 10 to 15 degrees helps bring the ear canal into a straight upright position and places the tympanic membrane in an approximate horizontal plane. A head rest that is separable from the remainder of the operating table is preferred to facilitate appropriate positioning. The headrest is fitted with a fastening mechanism for a self-retaining speculum holder with sufficient degrees of freedom to allow manipulation of the speculum during surgery. The external auditory meatus is injected in four quadrants with 1% Xylocaine with 1:100,000 epinephrine. The bony canal is then injected at the 12 o'clock and 6 o'clock positions with 2% Xylocaine with 1:50,000 epinephrine.

21.8.2 Exposure

A posterior tympanomeatal flap is developed such that there is some redundancy in the posterosuperior aspect to cover the area of bone that may be curetted to provide optimal

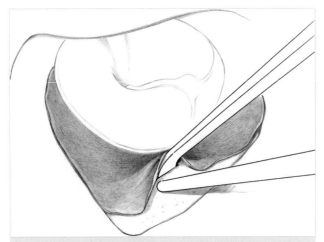

Fig. 21.4 Development of a posterior tympanomeatal flap. A triangular segment of meatal skin is incised with a roller knife and then elevated to the tympanic annulus. (Used with permission from Nadol JB Jr, McKenna MJ, eds. Surgery of the Ear and Temporal Bone, 2nd ed. Philadelphia: Lippincott Williams & Wilkins, 2005:276.)

visualization of the oval window (▶ Fig. 21.4). Bone is curetted from the posterosuperior portion of the tympanic annulus until both the pyramidal process and the tympanic segment of the facial nerve are easily visualized. Every effort should be made to preserve the chorda tympani nerve unless it severely obstructs access to the oval window niche. The round window is inspected and its patency should be noted in the operative report. The ossicular chain is palpated and the mobility of the malleus, incus, and stapes is established. The incudostapedial joint is separated with a joint knife (▶ Fig. 21.5).

The stapedial tendon is sectioned with the laser (▶ Fig. 21.6a). Any mucosal folds or adhesions are taken down with the laser until the crural arches and footplate are clearly visualized. Using a laser, a posterior crurotomy is accomplished at the junction of the posterior crus and the footplate (▶ Fig. 21.6b). If the anterior crus is visualized, this too is divided with the laser (▶ Fig. 21.6c). The suprastructure is then downfractured onto the promontory and removed from the middle ear. It is helpful to remove any remnant of the posterior crus extending above the level of the footplate because it will often obstruct introduction of the prosthesis later in the operation. A thick mucous membrane that obscures the footplate can also be coagulated with the laser (▶ Fig. 21.6d) to improve its exposure.

Prior to proceeding with fenestration of the footplate, it is important to control all mucosal bleeding that may occur as a result of removal of the suprastructure. Usually such bleeding will stop spontaneously over a period of a few minutes. If it does not, a small cotton ball soaked in epinephrine solution can be placed within the oval window niche until the bleeding ceases. Any bleeding during the process of fenestration will impair the surgeon's view and necessitate suctioning in proximity to an open vestibule, which can result in inner ear injury.

21.8.3 Fenestration

Fenestration is usually accomplished with the laser. Our experience has been with the argon and potassium titanyl phosphate

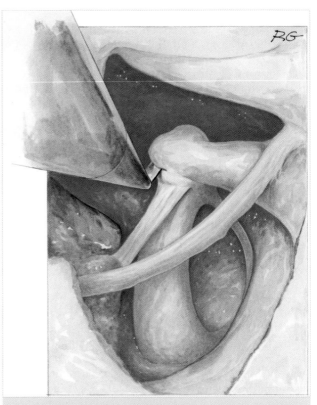

Fig. 21.5 Separation of the incudostapedial joint using a joint knife. (Used with permission from Nadol JB Jr, McKenna MJ, eds. Surgery of the Ear and Temporal Bone, 2nd ed. Philadelphia: Lippincott Williams & Wilkins, 2005:277.)

(KTP) lasers, both of which are in the visible range and can be passed through a fiberoptic cable and delivered with a handheld instrument. Others have had success with the carbon dioxide (CO_2) laser, which theoretically allows thermal energy dissipation in the liquid perilymph prior to reaching vestibular end organs with its wavelength of 10.6 μm. The CO_2 laser initially was mounted to the microscope and required a separate coaxial aiming beam, but is now available in the form of a handheld laser fiber. Advantages of the laser include (1) hemostatic properties; (2) precision that far exceeds that of other handheld instruments; (3) the ability to vaporize the posterior crus, therefore reducing the chance of a floating footplate; (4) the ability to create a precise fenestra in the footplate without excessive footplate or perilymph motion, thus minimizing the risk of acoustic trauma; and (5) the ability to fenestrate a floating footplate without the risk of depressing the footplate into the vestibule, which is an inherent risk of other fenestration techniques.

It has been our experience that neither the argon nor the KTP laser is effective in fenestrating thick footplates. If it is apparent that the footplate is thick and that the laser beam is not penetrating through the footplate as evidenced by a small amount of perilymph emanating through the central char, then fenestration is accomplished using the Skeeter drill and a 0.7-mm diamond bur. Because the argon and KTP lasers are delivered through a fiberoptic bundle, it becomes defocused at a very short distance beyond the tip of the probe. Therefore, to use the laser as a cutting tool, the tip of the probe needs to be in nearly direct contact with the bone. To use the laser as a coagulating

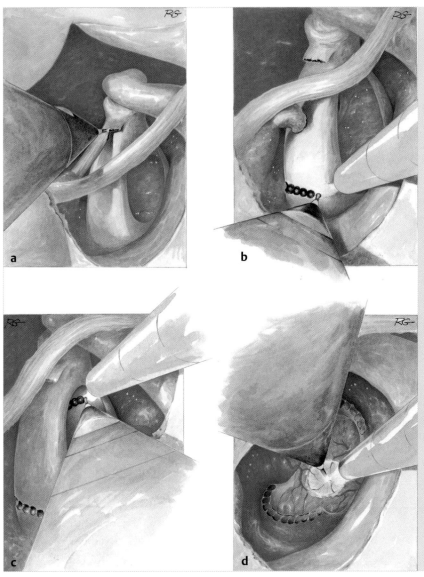

Fig. 21.6 Exposure of the stapes footplate using the handheld laser. (a) The stapedius tendon is separated. (b) A posterior crurotomy is performed. (c) If visible, the anterior crus is divided. (d) The laser beam is withdrawn approximately 2 mm from the footplate to coagulate thick mucosa overlying the lateral surface of the footplate. (Used with permission from Nadol JB Jr, McKenna MJ, eds. Surgery of the Ear and Temporal Bone, 2nd ed. Philadelphia: Lippincott Williams & Wilkins, 2005:277–279.)

instrument, the tip is withdrawn 2 to 3 mm, allowing the beam to defocus. The fiberoptic bundle delivers a spot size of approximately 200 μm. A rosette of laser spots is created in the thinnest portion of the footplate. The rosette should measure approximately 5 spot sizes in diameter in each dimension (▶ Fig. 21.7).

It is better to err on the side of a slightly large fenestra than to have one that is too small to admit a 0.6-mm piston and thus requires additional enlargement once the fenestra has been opened. To avoid thermal injury to the inner ear, 2 to 3 seconds is allowed between pulses to allow for the heat to dissipate. Once the rosette is created, the char is dispersed with a straight pick that is gently passed around the edges of the fenestra (▶ Fig. 21.8).

On occasion, a portion of the footplate may be relatively thicker and will remain intact, despite having been treated with the laser. Under such circumstances, the Skeeter drill with a 0.7-mm diamond bur is used gently to enlarge the fenestra. The diameter of the hole can be measured with either a measuring stick or a 0.6-mm footplate rasp, which should pass easily through the fenestra.

21.8.4 Measuring the Length of the Prosthesis

A measuring stick with a diameter of 0.6 mm and calibrated for length can be used to determine simultaneously the adequacy of the size of the fenestra and the required length of the piston prosthesis to be used. We utilize a 4-mm standard measuring stick and measure from the medial aspect of the long process of incus to the fenestra (▶ Fig. 21.9).

21.8.5 Placement and Attachment of the Prosthesis

The prostheses are available from several instrument suppliers in 3.25- to 4.75-mm lengths at increments of 0.25 mm. The combined length of the piston head and rod (exclusive of the loop) is used to identify the length of the prosthesis (▶ Fig. 21.10). The length of the prosthesis should be 0.25 mm longer than the measurement between the fenestra and the medial edge of the long process of the incus. In cases where it is

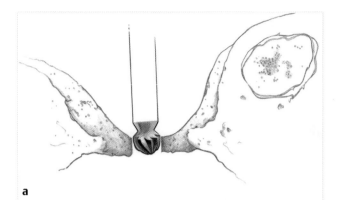

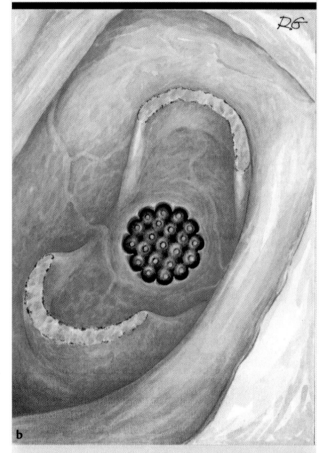

Fig. 21.7 Two methods of fenestration: (a) a microdrill with a 0.7-mm cutting bur and then a diamond bur is used fenestrate the footplate. (b) The laser is used to create a rosette of burn spots that should measure 5 spot sizes in diameter to create a 0.7-mm fenestra. Each burn spot has a black periphery representing charred bone, a more central halo of white representing vaporized bone, and a central pinhole representing complete fenestration, through which a small amount of perilymph can be seen to emanate. (Used with permission from Nadol JB Jr, McKenna MJ, eds. Surgery of the Ear and Temporal Bone. 2nd ed. Philadelphia: Lippincott Williams & Wilkins, 2005:280.)

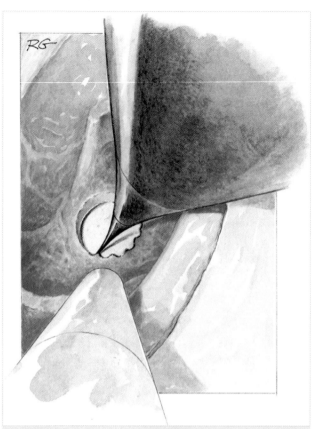

Fig. 21.8 The fenestra is completed using a straight pick to disperse the char. A 24-French gauge suction is held near but never over the fenestra. (Used with permission from Nadol JB Jr, McKenna MJ, eds. Surgery of the Ear and Temporal Bone. 2nd ed. Philadelphia: Lippincott Williams & Wilkins, 2005:281.)

anticipated that the prosthesis will require bending in order to accomplish a perpendicular entry into the fenestra, an additional 0.25 mm should be added.

Several stapes prostheses are commercially available and in current use. We are currently utilizing a Teflon piston with platinum wire and ribbon prosthesis. It is fashioned after the Schuknecht stainless steel wire Teflon piston and has the advantage of a platinum wire shaft and a platinum ribbon hook (▶ Fig. 21.11).

The wire allows easy alteration of the angulation once the prosthesis is in place and the platinum ribbon hook provides a wider purchase on the incus. In addition, the platinum is also somewhat easier to crimp because it does not have the metallic "memory" of stainless steel. The self-crimping nitinol prosthesis, with a loop made of nickel and titanium alloy attached to a fluoroplastic piston, was introduced in the past decade. The nitinol loop can be crimped by heat activation due to the shape memory properties of the alloy. It has the advantage of not requiring mechanical crimping and a very secure crimp can be accomplished by heating the wire with either a laser burst or a small bipolar forceps. Since 2005, multiple groups have reported hearing results equivalent to those with conventional prostheses.[58,64–67] Although there was initially a significant concern about potential allergic reactions to the nickel component of the alloy, this has not been a significant problem,[65] and the nitinol prostheses have been found to be highly biocompatible.[68]

The prosthesis is introduced by first grasping the open loop with a smooth alligator and adjusting the angle of the prosthesis with respect to the alligator in accordance with what the surgeon views when looking through the operating microscope.

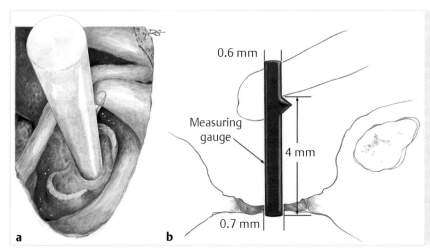

Fig. 21.9 Measuring the length of the prosthesis. (a) A measuring stick with a diameter of 0.6 mm and calibrated for length is placed just through the fenestra to determine its diameter and the required length of the piston prosthesis to be used. (b) We measure from the medial aspect of the long process of the incus to the fenestra. The 0.6-mm-diameter measuring stick should easily pass through a 0.7-mm-wide fenestra. A 4-mm standard measuring stick is shown. An additional 0.25 mm is added to allow for adequate penetration into the vestibule. Thus, in this example a 4.25 mm × 0.6 mm prosthesis would be needed. (Used with permission from Nadol JB Jr, McKenna MJ, eds. Surgery of the Ear and Temporal Bone, 2nd ed. Philadelphia: Lippincott Williams & Wilkins, 2005:281.)

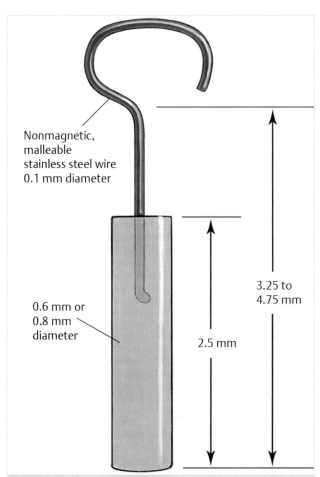

Fig. 21.10 The Teflon stainless steel wire prosthesis (designed in 1960 by H.F. Schuknecht and H. Terace) is commercially available in lengths from 3.25 to 4.75 mm and diameters of 0.6 or 0.8 mm. The nonmagnetic wire is MRI compatible. (Used with permission from Nadol JB Jr, McKenna MJ, eds. Surgery of the Ear and Temporal Bone, 2nd ed. Philadelphia: Lippincott Williams & Wilkins, 2005:282.)

prosthesis will be gently introduced into the fenestra and then around the long process of the incus. In some cases it is difficult to accomplish this with a single move and is best to gently place the prosthesis upright within the oval window niche. The loop can then be manipulated with either a straight pick or a small anterior hook such that it is properly positioned around the long process of the incus. The prosthesis should extend into the vestibule for approximately 0.25 mm. Some consider crimping the prosthesis the most difficult part of the stapedectomy procedure; hence, the rising popularity of the Nitinol or SMART prosthesis. A variety of crimping forceps are commercially available. Adjusting the microscope and the angle of introduction of the crimping forceps so that both blades of the forceps are easily visualized as it engages the loop facilitates crimping. The loop is gently engaged with both blades of the forceps and then crimped to the incus with sufficient firmness to create a stable linkage.

After the prosthesis is crimped, adjustments may be made in the angle of the prosthesis by bending the wire portion of the shaft with a right-angled hook to achieve optimal functional orientation within the fenestra. Usually this would entail a direct perpendicular drop into the fenestra. However, in cases of an overhanging facial nerve, the prosthesis can be bent inferiorly to avoid excessive contact with the nerve, which will impede its mobility. The prosthesis must move freely within the fenestra. This can be assessed by gently elevating the long process of the malleus while watching the motion of the prosthesis. If there is differential motion between the wire loop and incus, friction between the Teflon shaft and margins of the fenestra should be assumed and a modification of the angle made. Despite this, if the prosthesis does not have absolute freedom of movement at the level of the fenestra, the source of impedance must be identified or a good hearing result will not be achieved. Possibilities include a fenestra that is too small or a fleck of bone at the margin of the fenestra that is contacting the piston. The prosthesis should be removed, and the fenestra examined and enlarged if necessary with a small rasp. Once the prosthesis has been secured and the freedom of mobility confirmed, a small pledget of Gelfoam soaked in normal saline is placed around the base of the piston. In cases where the fenestra is significantly larger than the piston, a tissue graft is preferred. Subcutaneous fat from the postauricular area on the ear lobe can

Slightly loosening the grip on the prosthesis and gently tapping the prosthesis posteriorly against the annulus or anteriorly against the incus can further adjust this angle. Ideally, the

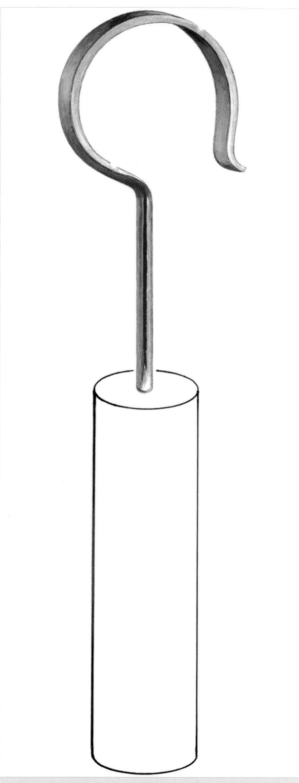

Fig. 21.11 The Massachusetts Eye and Ear Infirmary(MEEI) prosthesis is a modification of the Schuknecht piston prosthesis. The platinum ribbon hook affords a wider and more secure grasp onto the incus, while the cylindrical platinum wire shaft can be easily bent to any angle necessary for a perpendicular entry of the Teflon piston into the fenestra. Additionally, the platinum is relatively ease to crimp. (Used with permission from Nadol JB Jr, McKenna MJ, eds. Surgery of the Ear and Temporal Bone, 2nd ed. Philadelphia: Lippincott Williams & Wilkins, 2005:282.)

be harvested, cut into small pieces, and placed around the base of the piston with a straight pick. The tympanomeatal flap is then returned to its anatomic position and stabilized with either Gelfoam or silk packing. Antibiotic prophylaxis begun intraoperatively is generally continued for 1 week postoperatively while the packing is in place. Most patients are discharged from the hospital on the same day as their surgery. They are instructed to avoid any vigorous activity, keep water away from the ear, and refrain from blowing their nose.

21.8.6 Results

Expert results are usually defined as closure of the air–bone gap to 10 dB or less in 90% or more patients, with 1% or less incidence of profound SNHL (anacusis). Modifications of the technique, including the introduction of the small fenestra technique, application of the laser, and use of various materials for sealing the fenestra, and alterations in the stapes prostheses have not significantly improved hearing results.

21.9 Problems Encountered During and After Stapes Surgery

21.9.1 Intraoperative Problems and Complications

Exostoses of the External Auditory Canal

Small exostoses that do not impair the surgeon's ability to elevate a tympanomeatal flap and access the oval niche do not pose a problem and may be left intact. However, moderate or severe exostoses may severely limit exposure and should be managed as a separate procedure prior to performing a stapedectomy. In such cases, a stapedectomy can be performed at a later date once the healing of the external canal is complete.

21.9.2 Tears in the Tympanomeatal Flap

Tears in the tympanomeatal flap or tympanic membrane that occur during the elevation of the flap and drum should be repaired at the completion of the procedure. When this occurs, it has been our practice to harvest a piece of tragal perichondrium and use it as an underlay graft overlapping the defect by several millimeters. Although many of these tears may heal without grafting, the extra few minutes involved in harvesting the perichondrium and placing the graft will serve to prevent the need for another operation in most patients.

21.9.3 High Jugular Bulb

A superiorly located jugular bulb may come into juxtaposition with the tympanic annulus and is vulnerable to injury during elevation of the tympanomeatal flap. Thus, it is important that the flap be elevated with direct visualization especially when working inferiorly. Tears of the jugular bulb result in profuse bleeding and constitute an alarming, although not serious, complication. The bleeding can be controlled by elevating the head of the operating table and with the use of hemostatic packing such as Surgicel or Gelfoam. Modest pressure over the packing for a few minutes will generally result in cessation of the bleeding. If the bleeding is readily controlled, the operation may be continued. If, however, the tear is large and the bleeding is difficult to control, the procedure should be terminated.

21.9.4 Disarticulation of the Incus

Disarticulation or partial subluxation of the incus can occur during curetting or while separating the incudostapedial joint. If partial subluxation occurs, the operation may be completed, although the incus will be hypermobile and crimping will be more difficult. In most cases of partial subluxation, the incudomalleal joint will heal and the end result will be satisfactory. If, however, complete dislocation of the incus occurs as is evidenced by complete freedom of movement in both the medial to lateral and anterior to posterior dimensions, it is best to remove the incus and use a malleus attachment prosthesis.

21.9.5 Overhanging Facial Nerve

In rare cases, the facial nerve may be dehiscent and may completely fill the oval window niche. If the nerve is noted to be contacting the promontory inferior to the footplate with complete visual obstruction of the oval window, it is best to abort the procedure and replace the tympanomeatal flap. However, in the majority of cases of dehiscent overhanging facial nerves, the operation can be completed by using a microdrill and small diamond bur to create a fenestra that passes through the inferior aspect of the annular ligament. A small amount of bone can be removed over the promontory to facilitate exposure and free passage of the prosthesis. This technique of creating a marginal bur hole is similar to that used for removal of a floating footplate when the laser is not available. Unlike in the case of a marginal bur hole for a floating footplate, the fenestration may incorporate the inferior aspect of the fixed footplate. Often in cases of overhanging facial nerve, the wire of the prosthesis will need to be bent inferiorly to allow for perpendicular descent of the prosthesis into the bur hole and avoid contact with the facial nerve. Because of this requirement, a longer prosthesis is necessary.

21.9.6 Obliterative Otosclerosis of the Oval Window

Otosclerosis that obliterates the oval window niche cannot be easily managed or removed with the laser. However, the laser is helpful in cauterizing the surrounding mucosa to prevent any bleeding. Obliteration of the oval window niche with otosclerosis requires removal of the obliterating bone first by saucerization followed by fenestration (▶ Fig. 21.12). This is performed in incremental stages by first using a 1.0-mm diamond bur with gradual repeated drilling and saucerization until the bone has been thinned and the blue hue of the vestibule visualized. Final fenestration is then accomplished with the 0.7-mm diamond bur, which should be epicentered in the saucerized cavity. In these cases it is best to measure the distance between the incus and vestibule prior to fenestration, as it is often difficult to assess the depth of penetration of the measuring stick, once the fenestra has been created.

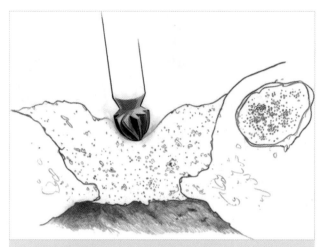

Fig. 21.12 Saucerization of obliterative otosclerosis of the oval window is incrementally performed starting with a 1-mm diamond bur to remove bone until the blue hue of the vestibule is seen. Final fenestration is then performed with either a 0.7-mm diamond bur or the laser. (Used with permission from Nadol JB Jr, McKenna MJ, eds. Surgery of the Ear and Temporal Bone, 2nd ed. Philadelphia: Lippincott Williams & Wilkins, 2005:292.)

21.9.7 Round Window Otosclerosis

Complete obliteration of the round window with otosclerosis can result in residual conductive hearing loss following stapedectomy. However, experience has shown that it is impossible to determine at surgery whether or not the round window niche is completely obliterated or partially obliterated. For this reason, it is advisable to complete the stapedectomy even in the presence of round window obliteration. Often, the hearing will be significantly improved despite the appearance of complete obliteration at surgery. However, if the hearing fails to improve postoperatively, revision surgery is not indicated. It is important that the surgeon examines the patency of the round window and notes this in the operative report. Past efforts to remove otosclerosis from the obliterated round window niche have universally resulted in SNHL and should never be attempted.

21.9.8 Persistent Stapedial Artery

During early development, the stapedial artery traverses the obturator foramen of the stapes and then regresses prior to birth. The remnant of this artery is often encountered at surgery as a small vessel that crosses the footplate and can be easily coagulated with the laser. This does not constitute a persistent stapedial artery. A true persistent stapedial artery may be found in 1 in 5,000 cases and in some cases may be of a caliber where it nearly fills the obturator foramen of the stapes. It cannot be safely coagulated with either a bipolar forceps or the laser. In most cases the persistent stapedial artery occupies the anterior half of the obturator foramen, leaving a potential space in the posterior half of the footplate where fenestration can be safely accomplished. If such is the case, stapedectomy may be performed using the technique described above. If there is a concern regarding the adequacy of the available footplate area to perform a stapedectomy, the procedure should be aborted.

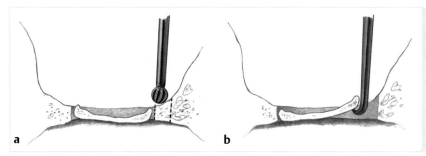

Fig. 21.13 Management of a floating or subluxed footplate with a marginal bur hole technique. (a) A marginal bur hole of 0.7-mm diameter, or less, is completed inferior to the annular ligament to allow for entry of a 0.3-mm angulated hook. (b) The hook is used to gently elevate and remove the footplate. (Used with permission from Nadol JB Jr, McKenna MJ, eds. Surgery of the Ear and Temporal Bone, 2nd ed. Philadelphia: Lippincott Williams & Wilkins, 2005:296.)

21.9.9 Malleus Ankylosis

Fixation of the malleus may be encountered at the time of primary stapedectomy, but in some cases it is clearly overlooked. When the malleus is rigidly fixed as a result of bony fixation in the epitympanum, the findings at surgery are not subtle and can be easily established by gentle palpation of the malleus. The incidence of malleus fixation is somewhat controversial. Studies of the temporal bone collection at the Massachusetts Eye and Ear Infirmary reveal an incidence of about 0.5%.[59] The condition does not appear to be related to otosclerosis.[60] Others have reported a higher incidence of malleus fixation and have attributed it to the underlying otosclerotic process, although the exact relationship is unclear.[61,62] When malleus fixation is encountered, the condition must be rectified if a satisfactory hearing result is to be obtained from stapedectomy. This is best accomplished by removal of the incus and the head of the malleus and reconstruction with a malleus attachment prosthesis.[69-72]

21.9.10 Gushers and Oozers

Occasionally, fenestration of the footplate results in the free flow of fluid from the vestibule into the middle ear. When the flow is torrential, it is often referred to as a perilymph gusher. A constant but persistent trickle of fluid that wells up through the fenestra is often called a perilymph oozer. Perilymph gushers occur as a result of a defect in the cribrose area of the internal auditory canal and are most often found in congenital anomalies of the inner ear. In many cases, the stapes fixation is likely of congenital origin as well. Perilymph oozers, on the other hand, are most often the result of a persistent cochlear aqueduct.[63] In most cases the occurrence of either a gusher or oozer is unanticipated. In the case of a perilymph gusher, it is nearly impossible to perform a stapedectomy until the flow of fluid has been curtailed. This very rapid flow of fluid through the vestibule is deleterious to the health of the inner ear and should be initially controlled by packing the fenestra with either a tissue graft, if immediately available, or a cotton pledget. The pressure head can then be lowered by placing a lumbar drain and removing spinal fluid. Stapedectomy should be accomplished using a tissue graft, either perichondrium or vein to prevent problems with persistent postoperative leakage. In the case of a perilymph oozer, lumbar drainage is usually not necessary. However, a tissue seal of perichondrium or vein should be utilized. If a perilymph gusher is anticipated, the lumbar drain should be placed prior to the fenestration to avoid the problems associated with turbulent flow through the vestibule.

21.9.11 Floating or Depressed Footplate

A floating footplate may occur in an ear with minimal stapes fixation and may result from down-fracture of the stapes suprastructure. It is a relatively rare occurrence with the use of the operating laser, which allows for the avoidance of mechanical force. If, during stapedectomy, the footplate is either mobilized or becomes free floating, the footplate may be fenestrated safely with the laser as long as the footplate is thin. If the laser is not available or the footplate is thick, the best option is to remove the footplate by first making a marginal bur hole inferior to the annular ligament. Once the bur hole has been completed, a small hook can be passed through it and under the inferior lip of the footplate. The footplate is then gently elevated and removed (▶ Fig. 21.13). The stapedectomy is then completed using a tissue seal consisting of perichondrium, vein, or small pieces of ear lobe fat packed around the base of the piston.

There is no good solution for the depressed footplate, one that has settled down into the vestibule. It is a near certainty that the patient will suffer immediate and protracted vertigo. A footplate that is depressed in a trapdoor or tilted configuration may sometimes be removed by engaging the nondepressed margin with a small hook at the crural remnant. If the footplate is totally depressed, no attempt should be made to remove it. A tissue graft and prosthesis should be introduced, although the results are highly variable.

21.10 Early Postoperative Complications

21.10.1 Facial Palsy

Facial paralysis following stapedectomy is alarming to both the patient and surgeon. There are two possible causes. The first is related to the use of local anesthesia at the time of surgery. If, after 3 hours, the facial paralysis persists, it is unlikely related to local anesthesia and almost certainly related to nerve trauma incurred at the time of surgery. If the operating surgeon is aware of the nerve having been manipulated or mildly traumatized at the time of surgery but is confident that the nerve is anatomically intact, then no intervention is necessary other than those necessary to prevent corneal exposure and perhaps a course of corticosteroids. If, however, the operating surgeon does not recall manipulating or traumatizing the nerve during the surgery, the patient should be returned to the operating room for facial nerve exploration and examination. In rare cases the facial nerve may pass inferior to the oval window and fan out over the promontory in a flattened configuration that is not easily recognized. If the continuity of the nerve is established, then observation is in order. If the nerve has been severely traumatized or transected, then repair with a short cable graft may be required. Fortunately, this is rarely necessary.

21.10.2 Otitis Media

Acute otitis media in the early postoperative period is a rare but worrisome complication. The patients are at high risk for developing suppurative labyrinthitis and meningitis. Patients should be admitted to the hospital and the packing removed. If there is suppuration in the ear canal, cultures should be taken and the patient started on broad-spectrum intravenous antibiotic coverage. Steroids may also be helpful in minimizing inner ear damage. Acute otitis media that occurs months following stapedectomy can be treated in the usual fashion with oral antibiotics.

21.10.3 Vertigo

The occurrence of vertigo either during surgery or immediately thereafter is indicative of a labyrinthine insult. This may be the result of air entering the vestibule during the procedure, blood within the vestibule, or mechanical trauma to the utricle that lies in close proximity to the oval window. These patients should remain within the hospital and should be managed with vestibular suppressants and steroids. Air within the vestibule usually resolves within 24 to 48 hours. Vertigo that is protracted beyond 48 hours is suggestive of a more serious insult and is often associated with SNHL. Even if these patients recover with a good hearing result, vestibular testing should be performed prior to considering a contralateral stapedectomy. Thoughtful consideration should be given to any patient in whom a stapedectomy is being considered when the contralateral ear has significantly reduced vestibular function.

21.10.4 Reparative Granuloma

Exuberant reactive granulation tissue in response to surgery or the placement of a foreign body (prosthesis) is a rare complication following stapedectomy.[74–76] The typical history is one of an uncomplicated procedure after which the patient does well for the first several days following surgery. Patients then develop symptoms of labyrinthitis with vertigo, spontaneous nystagmus toward the unoperated ear, and tinnitus. Usually the onset is between 5 days and 2 weeks. Examination of the ear upon removal of the packing often reveals an inflamed middle ear space without frank purulence. These patients are best served by returning them to the operating room for exploration of the ear under general anesthesia with the removal of the prosthesis and granulation tissue prior to sealing the fenestra with a tissue graft. In most cases there is a permanent SNHL. The vestibular symptoms usually resolve within a period of weeks. Steroids may also be helpful in reducing the degree of injury.

21.10.5 Delayed Facial Paralysis

Delayed facial paralysis following stapedectomy is an uncommon occurrence that may result from either minor trauma to the facial nerve during surgery with a delayed neurapraxia or possibly activation of a viral neuritis as is seen in Bell's palsy.

21.10.6 Sensorineural Hearing Loss

Sensorineural hearing loss following stapedectomy can occur immediately or in a delayed manner, anywhere from weeks to months following the procedure. Sensorineural hearing loss that occurs in the early postoperative period can be attributed to surgical trauma. The overall incidence in the hands of experienced surgeons is under 1%.[66] High-tone hearing loss above 4,000 Hz is likely related to acoustic trauma caused either by excessive manipulation of the footplate or the prosthesis.

21.10.7 Conductive Hearing Loss

Unexpected conductive hearing loss that occurs immediately following stapedectomy can be attributed to one or more of the following conditions: (1) malfunction of the prosthesis; (2) failure to recognize malleus fixation; (3) failure to recognize round window obliteration; (4) middle ear effusion or hemotympanum; or (5) the presence of an unrecognized superior canal dehiscence. In these cases, a high-resolution noncontrast CT scan may be helpful in ruling out superior canal dehiscence and round window obliteration. Ultimately, reexploration may be necessary to establish the cause.

21.11 Late Postoperative Complications

21.11.1 Perilymph Fistula

The development of a perilymph fistula can occur in either the early or late postoperative period. The classic symptoms are fluctuating SNHL and mild to moderate episodic unsteadiness. The diagnosis should be suspected in patients who have a positive fistula test or in whom Hallpike positional testing results in vertigo and nystagmus with the affected ear in a down position. Exploratory tympanotomy is indicated when a perilymph fistula is suspected.

21.11.2 Delayed-Onset Conductive Hearing Loss

The development of a delayed conductive hearing loss following a successful stapedectomy is relatively common. The exact incidence is unknown. We suspect that it is in the range of 5% of patients who have a successful stapedectomy. The most common cause is erosion of the long process of the incus at the prosthesis attachment site, which results in displacement of the prosthesis.[67] Other less common causes are new bone formation within the oval window niche, which restricts the movement of the prosthesis, and delayed round window obliteration.

21.11.3 Far Advanced Otosclerosis

It is well established that some patients with advanced otosclerosis develop a progressive irreversible SNHL. The diagnosis should be suspected in patients with known otosclerosis who develop a progressive SNHL and in patients who have a family history of otosclerosis. The loss is usually gradual and worse for the high frequencies. Many have used sodium fluoride in an effort to slow or stabilize the SNHL caused by otosclerosis, yet the efficacy of this treatment has not been well established. The only controlled prospective studies that have been done demonstrate a weak effect at best.[78] Some of the new biphosphate compounds that have been developed to treat other bone disorders including osteoporosis may prove to be of greater efficacy in preventing SNHL from otosclerosis.[79,80] Preliminary evaluation of a small cohort of patients treated with risedronate and zoledronate, third-generation bisphosphonates, suggests stabilization of progressive SNHL.[81] Treatment with systemic bisphosphonates must be weighed against the risks of the medication, which range from nausea and back pain to osteonecrosis of the mandible. Although difficult to conduct, studies on the medical treatment of otosclerosis-related SNHL are essential to further progress.

Patients with far advanced otosclerosis, who no longer receive benefit from conventional hearing aids, may be candidates for stapedectomy or cochlear implantation. Often, stapedectomy results in improvement of the hearing to levels that can benefit from conventional hearing aids, while avoiding the additional surgical risks, postoperative recovery, costs, and device maintenance associated with cochlear implantation.[82] The decision to proceed with stapedectomy or cochlear implantation in these patients should be based on the magnitude of the conductive component of hearing loss and the speech discrimination score. In these patients, however, reported speech discrimination scores may be very poor because of an inadequate presentation level, due to the limits of the audiometer. In this situation, an auscultation tube, which is placed with one end at the examiner's mouth and the other end in the patient's external auditory canal, can be a valuable tool. A patient's ability to

understand speech via an auscultation tube in the office suggests a higher likelihood of achieving serviceable hearing with stapedectomy. Additionally, the tuning fork examination is usually more helpful than the audiogram in determining whether to proceed with stapedectomy or cochlear implantation in these cases. Although stapedectomy should be considered first in patients with far advanced otosclerosis, these patients are also cochlear implant candidates and can be expected to achieve successful results with implantation.[83,84] There are several technical challenges specific to cochlear implantation in far advanced otosclerosis. Extensive otosclerosis may obliterate the round window or extend into the cochlear duct, necessitating a drill-out procedure for placement of the electrode. Cavitary otosclerotic foci around the cochlea increase the risk of transgression of the electrode through the cochlea into the internal auditory canal (▶ Fig. 21.14).

References

[1] Wang PC, Merchant SN, McKenna MJ, Glynn RJ, Nadol JB, Jr. Does otosclerosis occur only in the temporal bone? Am J Otol 1999; 20: 162–165

[2] Morrison AW. Genetic factors in otosclerosis. Ann R Coll Surg Engl 1967; 41: 202–237

[3] Nager GT. Histopathology of otosclerosis. Arch Otolaryngol 1969; 89: 341–363

[4] Lindsay JR. Histopathology of otosclerosis. Arch Otolaryngol 1973; 97: 24–29

[5] Ghorayeb BY, Linthicum FH, Jr. Otosclerotic inner ear syndrome. Ann Otol Rhinol Laryngol 1978; 87: 85–90

[6] Hueb MM, Goycoolea MV, Paparella MM, Oliveira JA. Otosclerosis: the University of Minnesota temporal bone collection. Otolaryngol Head Neck Surg 1991; 105: 396–405

[7] Schuknecht HF. Myths in neurotology. Am J Otol 1992; 13: 124–126

[8] Schuknecht HF, Kirchner JC. Cochlear otosclerosis: fact or fantasy. Laryngoscope 1974; 84: 766–782

[9] Guild SR. Histologic otosclerosis. Ann Otol Rhinol Laryngol 1944; 53: 246–267

[10] McKenna MJ, Gadre AK, Rask-Andersen H. Ultrastructural characterization of otospongiotic lesions in re-embedded celloidin sections. Acta Otolaryngol 1990; 109: 397–405

[11] Altermatt HJ, Gerber HA, Gaeng D, Müller C, Arnold W. [Immunohistochemical findings in otosclerotic lesions] HNO 1992; 40: 476–479

[12] Cherukupally SR, Merchant SN, Rosowski JJ. Correlations between pathologic changes in the stapes and conductive hearing loss in otosclerosis. Ann Otol Rhinol Laryngol 1998; 107: 319–326

[13] Schuknecht HF, Barber W. Histologic variants in otosclerosis. Laryngoscope 1985; 95: 1307–1317

[14] Kwok OT, Nadol JB, Jr. Correlation of otosclerotic foci and degenerative changes in the organ of Corti and spiral ganglion. Am J Otolaryngol 1989; 10: 1–12

[15] Nelson EG, Hinojosa R. Questioning the relationship between cochlear otosclerosis and sensorineural hearing loss: a quantitative evaluation of cochlear structures in cases of otosclerosis and review of the literature. Laryngoscope 2004; 114: 1214–1230

[16] Doherty JK, Linthicum FH, Jr. Spiral ligament and stria vascularis changes in cochlear otosclerosis: effect on hearing level. Otol Neurotol 2004; 25: 457–464

[17] Weber PC, Cunningham CD, III, Schulte BA. Potassium recycling pathways in the human cochlea. Laryngoscope 2001; 111: 1156–1165

[18] Cody DT, Baker HL, Jr. Otosclerosis: vestibular symptoms and sensorineural hearing loss. Ann Otol Rhinol Laryngol 1978; 87: 778–796

[19] Birch L, Elbrønd O. Stapedectomy and vertigo. Clin Otolaryngol Allied Sci 1985; 10: 217–223

[20] Frisch T, Sørensen MS, Overgaard S, Lind M, Bretlau P. Volume-referent bone turnover estimated from the interlabel area fraction after sequential labeling. Bone 1998; 22: 677–682

[21] Nadol JB, Jr. Pathoembryology of the middle ear. Birth Defects Orig Artic Ser 1980; 16: 181–209

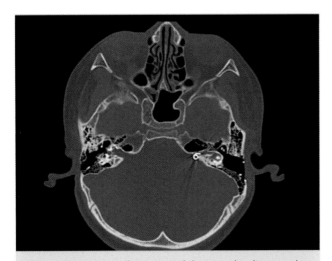

Fig. 21.14 Cavitary otosclerosis around the internal auditory canal (IAC) has replaced the normal bony partition between the IAC and cochlea in this patient with far advanced otosclerosis. This allowed the electrode of the cochlear implant to transgress the medial wall of the cochlea and pass into the internal auditory canal. (Courtesy of John W. House, MD.)

[22] Sørensen MS, Bretlau P, Jørgensen MB. Human perilabyrinthine bone dynamics. A functional approach to temporal bone histology. Acta Otolaryngol Suppl 1992; 496: 1–27

[23] Sørensen MS, Jørgensen MB, Bretlau P. Remodeling patterns in the bony otic capsule of the dog. Ann Otol Rhinol Laryngol 1991; 100: 751–758

[24] Zehnder AF, Kristiansen AG, Adams JC, Merchant SN, McKenna MJ. Osteoprotegerin in the inner ear may inhibit bone remodeling in the otic capsule. Laryngoscope 2005; 115: 172–177

[25] Zehnder AF, Kujawa SG, Kristiansen AG, Adams JC, McKenna MJ. Osteoprotegrin (OPG) knockout mice have abnormal otic capsule remodeling and progressive hearing loss. ARO Abstracts 2005; 28: 650

[26] McKenna MJ, Mills BG, Galey FR, Linthicum FH, Jr. Filamentous structures morphologically similar to viral nucleocapsids in otosclerotic lesions in two patients. Am J Otol 1986; 7: 25–28

[27] McKenna MJ, Mills BG. Immunohistochemical evidence of measles virus antigens in active otosclerosis. Otolaryngol Head Neck Surg 1989; 101: 415–421

[28] McKenna MJ, Mills BG. Ultrastructural and immunohistochemical evidence of measles virus in active otosclerosis. Acta Otolaryngol Suppl 1990; 470: 130–139, discussion 139–140

[29] McKenna MJ, Kristiansen AG, Haines J. Polymerase chain reaction amplification of a measles virus sequence from human temporal bone sections with active otosclerosis. Am J Otol 1996; 17: 827–830

[30] Niedermeyer HP, Arnold W, Neubert WJ, Höfler H. Evidence of measles virus RNA in otosclerotic tissue. ORL J Otorhinolaryngol Relat Spec 1994; 56: 130–132

[31] Niedermeyer HP, Arnold W. Otosclerosis: a measles virus associated inflammatory disease. Acta Otolaryngol 1995; 115: 300–303

[32] Arnold W, Niedermeyer HP, Lehn N, Neubert W, Höfler H. Measles virus in otosclerosis and the specific immune response of the inner ear. Acta Otolaryngol 1996; 116: 705–709

[33] Niedermeyer HP, Arnold W, Schuster M et al. Persistent measles virus infection and otosclerosis. Ann Otol Rhinol Laryngol 2001; 110: 897–903

[34] Karosi T, Kónya J, Szabó LZ, Sziklai I. Measles virus prevalence in otosclerotic stapes footplate samples. Otol Neurotol 2004; 25: 451–456

[35] Niedermeyer HP, Arnold W, Schwub D, Busch R, Wiest I, Sedlmeier R. Shift of the distribution of age in patients with otosclerosis. Acta Otolaryngol 2001; 121: 197–199

[36] Vrabec JT, Coker NJ. Stapes surgery in the United States. Otol Neurotol 2004; 25: 465–469

[37] Browning GG, Gatehouse S. The prevalence of middle ear disease in the adult British population. Clin Otolaryngol Allied Sci 1992; 17: 317–321

[38] Hammerschlag V. Zur frage der vererbbarkeit der otosklerose. Wien Klin Rdsch 1905; 19: 5–7

[39] Albrecht W. Über die vererbung der konstitutionell sporadischen taubstummheit der hereditären labyrithschwerhörigkeit und der otosklerose. Arch Ohren Nasen Kehlkopfheilkd 1923; 110: 15–48

[40] Sabitha R, Ramalingam R, Ramalingam KK, Sivakumaran TA, Ramesh A. Genetics of otosclerosis. J Laryngol Otol 1997; 111: 109–112

[41] Fowler EP. Otosclerosis in identical twins. A study of 40 pairs. Arch Otolaryngol 1966; 83: 324–328

[42] Ben Arab S, Bonaïti-Pellié C, Belkahia A. A genetic study of otosclerosis in a population living in the north of Tunisia. Ann Genet 1993; 36: 111–116

[43] Tomek MS, Brown MR, Mani SR et al. Localization of a gene for otosclerosis to chromosome 15q25-q26. Hum Mol Genet 1998; 7: 285–290

[44] Van Den Bogaert K, Govaerts PJ, Schatteman I et al. A second gene for otosclerosis, OTSC2, maps to chromosome 7q34-36. Am J Hum Genet 2001; 68: 495–500

[45] Chen W, Campbell CA, Green GE et al. Linkage of otosclerosis to a third locus (OTSC3) on human chromosome 6p21.3–22.3. J Med Genet 2002; 39: 473–477

[46] Van Den Bogaert K, Govaerts PJ, De Leenheer EM et al. Otosclerosis: a genetically heterogeneous disease involving at least three different genes. Bone 2002; 30: 624–630

[47] Van Den Bogaert K, De Leenheer EM, Chen W et al. A fifth locus for otosclerosis, OTSC5, maps to chromosome 3q22–24. J Med Genet 2004; 41: 450–453

[48] McKenna MJ, Kristiansen AG, Körkkö J. Sequence analysis of COC1A1 and COL1A2 genes in clinical otosclerosis: No evedence for mutations in the coding regions of the genes. Otorhinolaryngol Nova 2001; 11: 267–270

[49] McKenna MJ, Nguyen-Huynh AT, Kristiansen AG. Association of otosclerosis with Sp1 binding site polymorphism in COL1A1 gene: evidence for a shared genetic etiology with osteoporosis. Otol Neurotol 2004; 25: 447–450

[50] McKenna MJ, Kristiansen AG, Bartley ML, Rogus JJ, Haines JL. Association of COL1A1 and otosclerosis: evidence for a shared genetic etiology with mild osteogenesis imperfecta. Am J Otol 1998; 19: 604–610

[51] McKenna MJ, Kristiansen AG, Tropitzsch AS. Similar COL1A1 expression in fibroblasts from some patients with clinical otosclerosis and those with type I osteogenesis imperfecta. Ann Otol Rhinol Laryngol 2002; 111: 184–189

[52] Fowler EP. The incidence (and degrees) of blue scleras in otosclerosis and other ear disorders. Laryngoscope 1949; 59: 406–416

[53] Schuknecht HF. Pathology of the ear. Cambridge, MA: Harvard University Press, 1974

[54] Nager GT. Osteogenesis imperfecta of the temporal bone and its relation to otosclerosis. Ann Otol Rhinol Laryngol 1988; 97: 585–593

[55] Mikulec AA, McKenna MJ, Ramsey MJ et al. Superior semicircular canal dehiscence presenting as conductive hearing loss without vertigo. Otol Neurotol 2004; 25: 121–129

[56] Hyman S. For the World to Hear: A Biography of Howard P. House, M.D. Pasadena, CA: Hope Publishing House, 1990

[57] Lagleyre S, Sorrentino T, Calmels MN et al. Reliability of high-resolution CT scan in diagnosis of otosclerosis. Otol Neurotol 2009; 30: 1152–1159

[58] Shin YJ, Fraysse B, Deguine O, Cognard C, Charlet JP, Sévely A. Sensorineural hearing loss and otosclerosis: a clinical and radiologic survey of 437 cases. Acta Otolaryngol 2001; 121: 200–204

[59] Warren FM, Riggs S, Wiggins RH, III. Computed tomographic imaging of stapes implants. Otol Neurotol 2008; 29: 586–592

[60] Marx M, Lagleyre S, Escudé B et al. Correlations between CT scan findings and hearing thresholds in otosclerosis. Acta Otolaryngol 2011; 131: 351–357

[61] Wycherly BJ, Berkowitz F, Noone AM, Kim HJ. Computed tomography and otosclerosis: a practical method to correlate the sites affected to hearing loss. Ann Otol Rhinol Laryngol 2010; 119: 789–794

[62] Güneri EA, Ada E, Ceryan K, Güneri A. High-resolution computed tomographic evaluation of the cochlear capsule in otosclerosis: relationship between densitometry and sensorineural hearing loss. Ann Otol Rhinol Laryngol 1996; 105: 659–664

[63] Quesnel AM, Moonis G, Appel J et al. Correlation of computed tomography with histopathology in otosclerosis. Otol Neurotol 2013; 34: 22–28

[64] Rajan GP, Atlas MD, Subramaniam K, Eikelboom RH. Eliminating the limitations of manual crimping in stapes surgery? A preliminary trial with the shape memory Nitinol stapes piston. Laryngoscope 2005; 115: 366–369

[65] Fayad JN, Semaan MT, Meier JC, House JW. Hearing results using the SMart piston prosthesis. Otol Neurotol 2009; 30: 1122–1127

[66] Brown KD, Gantz BJ. Hearing results after stapedotomy with a nitinol piston prosthesis. Arch Otolaryngol Head Neck Surg 2007; 133: 758–762

[67] Sorom AJ, Driscoll CL, Beatty CW, Lundy L. Retrospective analysis of outcomes after stapedotomy with implantation of a self-crimping Nitinol stapes prosthesis. Otolaryngol Head Neck Surg 2007; 137: 65–69

[68] Roosli C, Schmid P, Huber AM. Biocompatibility of nitinol stapes prosthesis. Otol Neurotol 2011; 32: 265–270

[69] Nadol JB Jr, Schuknecht HF. Surgery for otosclerosis and fixation of the stapes. In: Nadol JB Jr, Mckenna MJ, eds. Surgery of the Ear and Temporal Bone, 2nd ed. Philadelphia: Lippincott Williams & Wilkins, 2005:273–303

[70] Harris JP, Mehta RP, Nadol JB. Malleus fixation: clinical and histopathologic findings. Ann Otol Rhinol Laryngol 2002; 111: 246–254

[71] Guilford FR, Anson BJ. Osseous fixation of the malleus. Trans Am Acad Ophthalmol Otolaryngol 1967; 71: 398–407

[72] Katzke D, Plester D. Idiopathic malleus head fixation as a cause of a combined conductive and sensorineural hearing loss. Clin Otolaryngol Allied Sci 1981; 6: 39–44

[73] Schuknecht HF, Reisser C. The morphologic basis for perilymphatic gushers and oozers. Adv Otorhinolaryngol 1988; 39: 1–12

[74] Kaufman RS, Schuknecht HF. Reparative granuloma following stapedectomy: a clinical entity. Ann Otol Rhinol Laryngol 1967; 76: 1008–1017

[75] Seicshnaydre MA, Sismanis A, Hughes GB. Update of reparative granuloma: survey of the American Otological Society and the American Neurotology Society. Am J Otol 1994; 15: 155–160

[76] Glasscock ME, III, Storper IS, Haynes DS, Bohrer PS. Twenty-five years of experience with stapedectomy. Laryngoscope 1995; 105: 899–904

[77] Han WW, Incesulu A, McKenna MJ, Rauch SD, Nadol JB, Jr, Glynn RJ. Revision stapedectomy: intraoperative findings, results, and review of the literature. Laryngoscope 1997; 107: 1185–1192

[78] Bretlau P, Salomon G, Johnsen NJ. Otospongiosis and sodium fluoride. A clinical double-blind, placebo-controlled study on sodium fluoride treatment in otospongiosis. Am J Otol 1989; 10: 20–22

[79] Kennedy DW, Hoffer ME, Holliday M. The effects of etidronate disodium on progressive hearing loss from otosclerosis. Otolaryngol Head Neck Surg 1993; 109: 461–467

[80] Brookler KH, Tanyeri H. Etidronate for the the neurotologic symptoms of otosclerosis: preliminary study. Ear Nose Throat J 1997; 76: 371–376, 379–381

[81] Quesnel AM, Seton M, Merchant SN, Halpin C, McKenna MJ. Third-generation bisphosphonates for treatment of sensorineural hearing loss in otosclerosis. Otol Neurotol 2012; 33: 1308–1314

[82] Lachance S, Bussières R, Côté M. Stapes surgery in profound hearing loss due to otosclerosis. Otol Neurotol 2012; 33: 721–723

[83] Semaan MT, Gehani NC, Tummala N et al. Cochlear implantation outcomes in patients with far advanced otosclerosis. Am J Otolaryngol 2012; 33: 608–614

[84] Muñoz-Fernández N, Morant-Ventura A, Achiques MT et al. Evolution of otosclerosis to cochlear implantation. Acta Otorrinolaringol Esp 2012; 63: 265–271

22 Temporal Bone Trauma

Brendan P. O'Connell, Paul R. Lambert, and May Y. Huang

22.1 Introduction

Temporal bone trauma occurs in 30 to 75% of head injuries.[1-7] Compared with the face and skull, the temporal bone is very dense and requires a tremendous amount of force to sustain fracture. The majority of temporal bone injuries are associated with multiple other traumas following motor vehicle accidents. Temporal bone trauma also may be associated with industrial accidents, recreational injuries, falls, assaults, or self-inflicted injuries. Types of temporal bone trauma include blunt trauma without fracture, blunt trauma with fracture, penetrating trauma, compressive injuries, and thermal injuries. Trauma may cause injury to specific parts of the external, middle, or inner ear in addition to other structures within the temporal bone. Frequently, the history of the type of temporal bone injury facilitates evaluation of the spectrum of potential sequelae.

22.2 Anatomic Considerations

The temporal bone is a wedge-shaped bone in the lateral skull base that is bordered by the middle fossa tegmen superiorly, the posterior fossa tegmen posteriorly, the temporomandibular joint anteriorly, the clivus and foramen magnum medially, and the infratemporal fossa inferiorly. The temporal bone is divided into four regions: squamous, petrous, mastoid, and tympanic. Its posterosuperior border is called the petrous ridge, which lies along the long axis of the temporal bone at about a 45-degree angle posterior to the midcoronal plane. The squamous portion articulates with the sphenoid bone anteriorly and the parietal bone posteriorly, thus forming the roof of the infratemporal fossa and the medial wall of the temporal fossa. At the base of the skull, the petrous and mastoid portions of the temporal bone lie lateral to the occipital bone at the foramen magnum. The petrous apex is separated from the clivus (the fusion of the occipital and sphenoid bones anterior to the foramen magnum) by the foramen lacerum. At the inferior aspect of the base of the skull medial to the styloid process lie the jugular and carotid foramina.

Vital structures that reside within the anatomic confines of the temporal bone include audiovestibular mechanoreceptors; cranial nerves V, VI, VII, and VIII; the sigmoid sinus; and the jugular bulb. Injury to these vital structures needs to be considered in evaluation of temporal bone trauma.

The seventh and eighth cranial nerves arise from the pons, enter the posterior aspect of the temporal bone at the porus acusticus, and then course laterally in the internal auditory canal toward the vestibule. The cochlea and semicircular canals lie anteroinferiorly and posterosuperiorly, respectively, in relation to the internal auditory canal.

The course of the facial or seventh nerve within the temporal bone can be described in segments: the meatal segment within the internal auditory canal, the labyrinthine segment within the internal auditory canal, the geniculate ganglion, the tympanic segment in the middle ear, and the mastoid segment. From the internal auditory canal the facial nerve passes through the facial hiatus into the labyrinthine segment of the fallopian canal. At the geniculate ganglion it gives off the greater superficial petrosal nerve (preganglionic parasympathetic innervation for lacrimation) and then turns posteroinferiorly (first genu) along the medial wall of the tympanic cavity. It passes superior to the cochleariform process and the oval window. Inferior to the horizontal semicircular canal it turns (second genu) into the mastoid segment. It gives off the stapedial branch and the chorda tympani branch (special visceral afferent innervation for taste and preganglionic parasympathetic innervation for submandibular and sublingual glands) before exiting the temporal bone through the stylomastoid foramen.

The trigeminal or fifth cranial nerve exits the pons and travels anterolaterally from the posterior fossa to the trigeminal ganglion by passing over the petrous apex just deep to the attachment of the tentorium cerebelli. Its branches exit the middle fossa via the superior orbital fissure, the foramen rotundum, and the foramen ovale.

The abducens or sixth cranial nerve travels forward from the pons through the dura over the clivus, passing through the Dorello canal at the petrous apex. The carotid artery enters the carotid canal at the inferior aspect of the petrous temporal bone (anterior to the jugular fossa), courses superiorly, and then turns anteromedially just medial to the cochlea and the eustachian tube. The internal carotid artery exits the petrous apex just above the foramen lacerum, ascends in the carotid siphon just lateral to the sella turcica, traverses the cavernous sinus, and enters the dura just medial to the anterior clinoid process.

The middle meningeal artery arises from the maxillary artery in the infratemporal fossa. It enters the temporal bone via the foramen spinosum, runs laterally in the dura over the middle fossa tegmen, and then branches into frontal and parietal branches. It gives rise to the superficial petrosal branch that enters the canal of the greater superficial petrosal nerve.

The sigmoid sinus extends from the transverse sinus to the jugular bulb, coursing from superior to inferior in the dura along the posterolateral aspect of the temporal bone. It receives the greater and lesser petrosal sinuses from the cavernous sinus, as well as the mastoid emissary vein. The jugular bulb lies medial to the vertical segment of the facial nerve and posterior to the ascending portion of the internal carotid artery.

22.3 Classifications of Types of Temporal Bone Trauma

22.3.1 Trauma with Fracture

Temporal bone fractures most commonly arise from blunt trauma. They have been traditionally classified as longitudinal or transverse, with respect to the long axis of the temporal bone as viewed from the middle fossa (▶ Fig. 22.1).

Longitudinal fractures are the most common fractures of the temporal bone, constituting approximately 70 to 90% of temporal bone fractures.[1-7] These fractures typically result from a direct blow to the temporal or parietal aspects of the head.

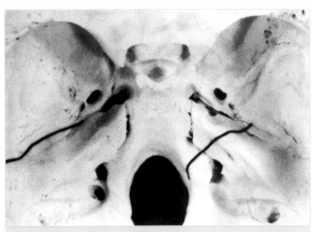

Fig. 22.1 Diagram of a longitudinal fracture (*left*) and a transverse temporal bone fracture (*right*) as viewed from the middle fossa.

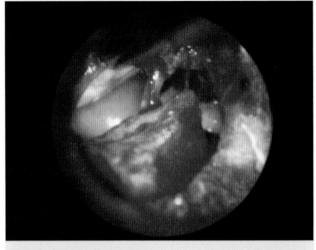

Fig. 22.2 Temporal bone fracture.

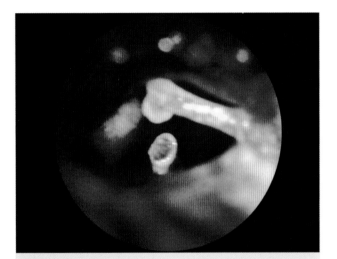

Fig. 22.3 Traumatic separation of the incus-stapes.

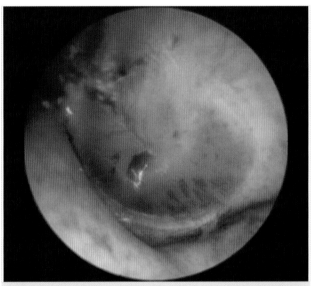

Fig. 22.4 Traumatic hemotympanum.

Symptoms at presentation include conductive hearing loss, bloody otorrhea, and loss of consciousness. Longitudinal fractures are bilateral in 8 to 29% of cases. The facial nerve is injured in approximately 15%. Due to the higher incidence of this type of fracture, however, facial nerve injury is most commonly caused by longitudinal fractures.

The longitudinal fracture line roughly parallels the long axis of the temporal bone in the coronal plane. Classically this fracture extends from the squamous portion of the temporal bone to the anterior portion of the petrous apex in the area of the foramen lacerum and foramen ovale. The fracture thus passes through the posterosuperior aspect of the external auditory canal, the tympanic membrane, and the roof of the middle ear (▶ Fig. 22.2; ▶ Fig. 22.3). These fractures commonly disrupt the ossicles or lacerate the skin of the ear canal, but usually spare the otic capsule. Fractures extending through the mastoid rather than the ear canal can result in hemotympanum without laceration of the tympanic membrane.

Transverse fractures are far less common, accounting for 20 to 30% of temporal bone fractures. Transverse fractures usually are associated with a blow to the occiput. Symptoms include profound sensorineural hearing loss (SNHL), vertigo, and severe head injury. In approximately 50% of these fractures, a facial paralysis occurs.[5,7–9]

The transverse fracture extends from the posterior fossa across the petrous pyramid to the foramen spinosum in a more sagittal plane. Transverse fractures extend through the internal auditory canal or the otic capsule. Fractures that arise near the porus acusticus can alternatively end at the oval or round window and produce hemotympanum without laceration of the tympanic membrane (▶ Fig. 22.4; ▶ Fig. 22.5).

Few temporal bone fractures are purely longitudinal or transverse. Between 50 and 75% of both pediatric and adult temporal bones could be classified as mixed in their axis of orientation.[4,7] In addition, there are not only two axes of orientation but also three planes of orientation by which to describe fractures. Fractures in the oblique plane of orientation are the most

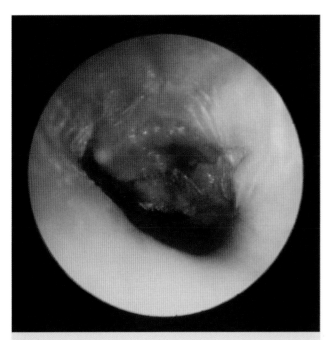

Fig. 22.5 Resolving traumatic hemotympanum.

common.[10-12] As seen from the middle fossa, oblique fractures extend roughly between the coronal and axial planes, across the mastoid cortex, external auditory canal, petrotympanic fissure, and glenoid fossa.

Although it is anatomically descriptive, the traditional radiographic classification of temporal bone fractures as longitudinal, transverse, oblique, or mixed has been criticized for its limited ability to predict potential complications of a fracture.[13-16]An alternative system of classification, intended to better predict clinical outcomes, has been proposed that categorizes fractures on the basis of otic capsule involvement. Otic capsule-violating fractures have a fracture line that disrupts either the cochlea or the labyrinth and generally result from a blow to the temporoparietal region. These fractures are rare, with reported rates of only 2.5 to 5.8%.[14,17] Conversely, otic capsule–sparing fractures do not involve the cochlea and the labyrinth; they typically result from a forceful blow to the occipital region.

In a retrospective review of 30 patients with temporal bone fractures, the otic capsule–based system demonstrated statistically significant predictive ability for adverse clinical outcomes, whereas the traditional radiographic classification system did not.[13] Patients with factures that violate the otic capsule are more likely to experience complications related to facial nerve injury, cerebrospinal fluid (CSF) leak, and SNHL than those with otic capsule sparing fractures.[13,14]Furthermore, patients with otic capsule–violating fractures demonstrate higher rates of associated intracranial complications, including epidural hematoma and subarachnoid hemorrhage.[14] The otic capsule–based system may have greater clinical utility than the traditional classification scheme given its ability to predict potential sequelae. Further investigation of larger patient populations is warranted.

As in adults, pediatric temporal bone fractures are commonly longitudinal or oblique.[18,19] The etiology of pediatric temporal bone fractures includes a higher incidence of falling from heights and automobile–pedestrian accidents. Facial nerve injury and CSF leak may be less common than in adults. The sites of temporal bone injury and their management are similar.

22.3.2 Penetrating Temporal Bone Trauma

The most common type of penetrating trauma affecting the temporal bone is a low-velocity gunshot wound.[20] Temporal bone injuries from the typical 0.22- to 0.38-mm caliber handgun are most commonly associated with a facial entrance wound rather than one on the side of the head. Mixed or comminuted fractures are most likely; there is no typical pattern of injury. Gunshot wounds of the temporal bone can create a wide variety of specific injuries including trauma to the major vessels, laceration of the dura, and destruction of the middle ear, inner ear, cranial nerves, and central nervous system. The facial nerve is injured in approximately 50% of cases. Usually the associated paralysis is immediate in onset and results from direct nerve injury.

22.4 Trauma Without Fracture

Injury to structures of the temporal bone can occur without temporal bone fracture. Such trauma is best enumerated by etiology. Barotrauma, thermal, foreign body, and compressive injuries frequently involve the external and middle ear. Concussive injuries or barotraumas more commonly involve the inner ear.

Blunt head trauma without fracture of the temporal bone may result in SNHL[2,21,22] from direct hair cell damage, disruption of inner ear membranes, or fracture of the oval window. A conductive hearing loss can result from ossicular damage or disruption of the tympanic membrane.

Foreign bodies used to remove cerumen, such as hair pins, cotton-tip applicators, pens, pencils, and toothpicks, can traumatize the external auditory canal or the tympanic membrane and result in localized laceration, hematoma, or infection. Injuries from foreign bodies can extend through the tympanic membrane to the middle and inner ear, causing hearing loss with or without vertigo.[23,24]

Compressive injuries to the ear can result from being slapped or struck on the side of the head or from falling on the water surface during water sports (e.g., waterskiing or diving). These incidents may result in laceration of the tympanic membrane. More significant compressive injuries result from blast injuries. Bomb explosions can cause disruption and implosion of the tympanic membrane as well as high-frequency SNHL due to disruption of the inner ear.[25,26]

Otitic barotrauma or aerotitis occurs when sudden and severe negative middle ear pressure results in trauma to the ear.[27-36] It can be precipitated by concurrent sinonasal inflammation. Symptoms typically include excruciating otalgia during descent while flying or ascent from underwater diving. Failure of the eustachian tube to open and adequately equilibrate middle ear pressure with atmospheric pressure causes hyperemia, edema, and ecchymosis of the middle ear mucosa with possible rupture of the tympanic membrane. Perilymph fistulas have also been reported after barotraumas, characterized by fluctuating SNHL and vertigo.[37-47]

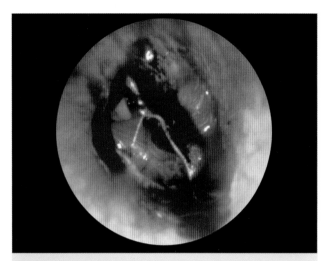

Fig. 22.6 Large traumatic perforation.

Thermal injuries involve the temporal bone as well. Hot slag injuries sustained during welding can cause a perforation of the tympanic membrane that is difficult to repair (▶ Fig. 22.6) as well as inner ear injury. Also, lightning bolt injuries to the temporal bone can occur from lightning conducted through a telephone to the ear. SNHL, vertigo, tinnitus, and facial paralysis potentially result from devitalized bone and soft tissue.[48-52]

22.5 Mechanisms of Injury

22.5.1 Auditory

Conductive hearing loss can arise from injury to the external auditory canal, tympanic membrane, or middle ear. Conductive hearing loss can become evident in the acute setting or on a delayed basis. Acutely, the ear canal often is filled with clotted blood, debris, or hematoma. The tympanic membrane may be lacerated, perforated, or completely disrupted. The middle ear may be filled with blood or CSF. The ossicular chain may be interrupted (▶ Fig. 22.7).

Incudostapedial joint separation is the most common ossicular injury, secondary to longitudinal temporal bone fracture.[4,53-60] Dislocation of the incus is the second most common finding, followed by fracture of the stapes superstructure. Fracture of the malleus is the least common. Delayed conductive hearing loss can be due to stenosis of the external auditory canal, or ossicular fixation. Ossicular fixation due to fibrous adhesion or bony ankylosis most commonly involves the head of the malleus and the body of the incus.

Severe head trauma of any type is associated with a high incidence of SNHL.[2,61,62] Approximately one third of patients with significant closed head injury experience hearing loss, and up to one half of them also have loss of consciousness. SNHL may result from injury to the inner ear, the eighth nerve, or the central auditory system. The inner ear and internal auditory canal may be directly involved, as in a transverse fracture. As many as one third of longitudinal fractures produce high-frequency SNHL, which is thought to arise from cochlear concussion.[63-70] Degeneration of the hair cells in the basal turn of the cochlea may be due either to production of a pressure wave being transmitted through bone to the cochlea or to sudden accelera-

tion–deceleration of the head with sudden movement of the stapes footplate. Disruption of the basilar membrane or tear of the oval window membrane with perilymph fistula may occur with excessive stapes footplate excursion. Traction on the eighth cranial nerve and brainstem contusion are more central etiologies for SNHL.

22.5.2 Vestibular

Benign paroxysmal positional vertigo is the most common form of disequilibrium after head injury.[21,22,68,69] It occurs in nearly half of patients with longitudinal temporal bone fractures and in one fifth of patients who suffer blunt head trauma without fracture. Typically the onset of symptoms immediately follows the injury. This clinical entity is thought to be due to disruption of the utricular macula. Detached otoconia enter the posterior semicircular canal and render the ampulla sensitive to gravity and thus changes in head position.[62,70-75]

Traumatic perilymph fistulas may result from fracture or subluxation of the stapes, penetrating trauma, and barotrauma.[27-47] Transverse fractures may directly involve the vestibule or semicircular canals and cause a leak of inner ear fluids.[76] A perilymph fistula (PLF) is a persistent, abnormal communication between the inner ear and middle ear or the mastoid. Trauma is the third most common cause of PLF, after iatrogenic injuries and idiopathic causes,[46] although the traumatic event can involve a relatively minor head injury. The defect is found in the oval window or the round window. Symptoms can include tinnitus, disequilibrium with or without vertigo, aural fullness, and SNHL that may be fluctuating. Patients often describe a popping sensation in the affected ear at the time the fistula occurs. Symptoms do not reliably predict the site of the fistula. The duration of symptoms is variable but can persist for months. Bilateral PLF is not uncommon.[43] The mechanisms of PLF formation are described as implosive or explosive. Implosive PLF, such as barotrauma, results in inward motion of the oval widow or round window. Explosive PLF results from increased intracranial pressure (e.g., the Valsalva maneuver) transmitted to the labyrinth, possibly by way of an abnormally patent cochlear aqueduct or internal auditory canal. Patients with congenital anomalies such as enlarged vestibular aqueduct are predisposed to PLF from minor head trauma.[44] Because the symptom complex caused by PLF is varied, the diagnosis of this entity can be difficult. A specific history of barotrauma or straining coincident with the onset of the symptoms provides some confidence in the diagnosis.

Injury to the labyrinth is more frequently caused by concussion of the labyrinth than by fracture. Concussive injury produces shock waves through the inner ear fluids that disrupt labyrinthine membranes.[63-67] Traction on the eighth nerve also may result in vestibular symptoms. Brainstem contusion or hemorrhage can involve vestibular nuclei, although trauma to the brainstem usually arises in conjunction with diffuse brain injury.[62,70-75,77] Isolated brainstem contusion is unusual. Typical presentation includes multiple cranial nerve palsies, elevated intracranial pressure, and focal neurologic signs.

22.5.3 Facial Nerve

In 80 to 90% of longitudinal fractures, the site of facial nerve trauma is located in the perigeniculate region or just distal to it in the tympanic segment (▶ Fig. 22.8).[5,8,9,78–80] Impingement from bone spicules is the most common mechanism of early-onset paralysis, followed by neural contusion. Transverse fractures usually injure the facial nerve in the labyrinthine portion, at or proximal to the geniculate ganglion. The geniculate region may be particularly sensitive to shearing forces in blunt head trauma; its bony covering is frequently dehiscent in this area compared with the surrounding labyrinthine and tympanic segments. In addition, the ganglion is tethered by the takeoff of the greater superficial petrosal nerve. Other mechanisms of injury to the intratemporal facial nerve include transection by fracture, hematoma within the nerve sheath, and edema with constriction in the fallopian canal.

Histopathologically, the extent of facial nerve injury can be classified as neurapraxia, axonotmesis, or neurotmesis.[81] Neurapraxia is defined as cessation of axoplasmic flow without degeneration of the axon. Axonotmesis describes degeneration of axons with maintenance of the endoneurial sheaths. In neurotmesis, the axons and their endoneurium degenerate. A more detailed classification of neural injuries has been presented by Sunderland,[82] who described five levels of injury based on the status of the endoneurium, perineurium, and epineurium. During the first 2 to 3 days of a complete paralysis, or before significant wallerian degeneration has occurred, electrical tests are not reliable in distinguishing between different levels of injury. Once axonal degeneration has occurred, electrical testing can differentiate neurapraxia from the other injury types. Electrical testing cannot distinguish between axonotmesis and neurotmesis, although the rapidity with which electrical excitability is lost can provide some indirect measure.[9,80,82–89] Any type of trauma to the facial nerve will cause a spectrum of neural injuries. If most of the nerve fibers are neurapraxic only, recovery will be excellent and occur rapidly. Recovery will also be excellent if the injury does not progress beyond the level of axonotmesis, although it will be delayed compared with the neurapraxic state, as regrowth of the axons to the motor end

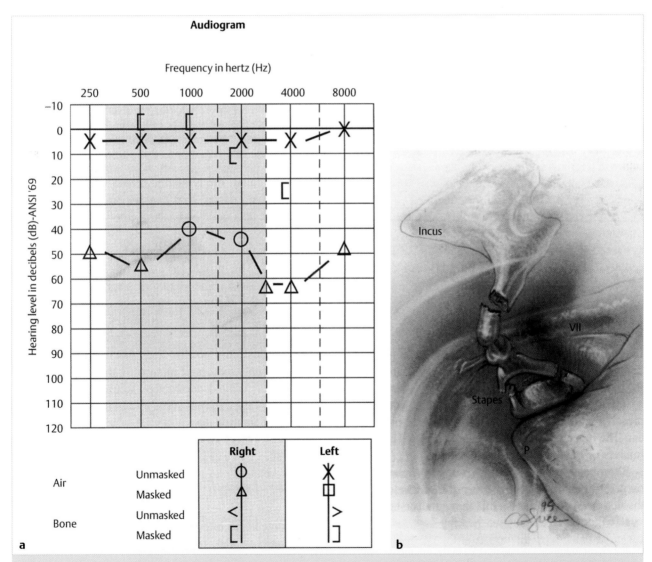

Fig. 22.7 (a) Audiogram showing persistent maximal conductive hearing loss many years after a fall. A computed tomography scan showed no temporal bone fracture. (b) Diagram of ossicular findings in same patient. Findings during middle ear exploration included fractures of the lenticular process of the incus and both crura of the stapes, as well as incudostapedial joint separation. A stapes prosthesis was successfully placed.

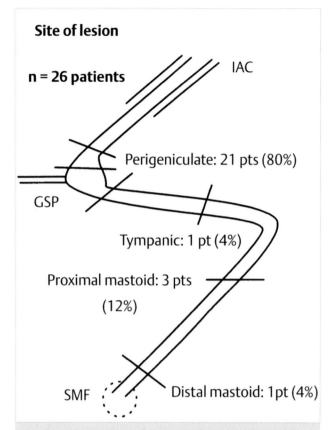

Fig. 22.8 Diagram of the middle fossa and mastoid exposure of the intratemporal facial nerve. The frequency of facial nerve injury is indicated at each site in 26 patients following longitudinal temporal bone fracture. IAC, internal auditory canal; GSP, greater superficial petrosal (nerve); SMF, stylomastoid foramen. (Adapted with permission from Lambert PR, Brackmann DE. Facial paralysis in longitudinal temporal bone fracture: a review of 26 cases. Laryngoscope 1984;94:1022–1026.)

plates occurs. Because the endoneurial tubules are lost in neurotmesis, regenerating axons will become misdirected, resulting in synkinesis, or encounter fibrosis, producing a residual weakness.

22.5.4 Intracranial

Intracranial injuries include trauma to the dura, brain parenchyma, and other neural or vascular structures. Fractures with dural tears or fractures through the otic capsule or internal auditory canal can result in leakage of CSF. Leaks can present as otorrhea, rhinorrhea (via the eustachian tube), or fluid behind an intact tympanic membrane. Multiple cranial nerves can be injured, including nerves V, VI, IX, X, XI, and XII. Introduction of air through the fracture into the cranial vault results in pneumocephalus. Mechanisms of brain injury include hemorrhage, contusion, infarct, and edema with increased intracerebral pressure. Herniation of brain through fractures results in encephalocele or meningoencephalocele. Bony fragments also can impinge directly on the brain and cause devitalization of the central nervous system.

22.5.5 Vascular

The location of hematomas can be extradural or subdural. In the region of the temporal bone, hematomas typically arise from injury to the middle meningeal artery. Direct vascular injury can be arterial or venous. Mechanisms of direct injury to the internal carotid arterial system include transection, laceration, thrombosis, aneurysm, and pseudoaneurysm formation. Fracture or penetrating injury in the mastoid area can lacerate or thrombose the sigmoid dural venous sinus. Associated venous injury includes avulsion of the superior or inferior petrosal sinuses, injury to the jugular bulb, or injury to the cavernous sinus.

22.6 Evaluation

Overall stabilization of the multiple-trauma patient precedes evaluation of specific temporal bone injuries. The history of the traumatic events and any loss of consciousness should be ascertained. Initial assessment is performed with emergency department personnel and includes level of consciousness, adequacy of the upper and lower airway, hemodynamic stability, and central neurologic deficits. The otolaryngologist may need to perform intubation, tracheotomy, or cricothyroidotomy emergently. Life-threatening injuries, such as shock, hemorrhage, expanding hematoma, tension pneumothorax, or cardiac arrhythmia, are the physician's first priority. In addition, the cervical spine must not be manipulated until instability has been ruled out by lateral neck plain films, preferably in flexion and extension. A pertinent medical history should be elicited from the patient or family members.

Examination of the head and neck can proceed once the patient has been stabilized. This examination must be performed deftly and thoroughly because many people may converge on the patient in the emergency room. Development of a methodical examination prevents the omission or repetition of part of the examination. It is suggested that one proceed from cranial to caudal, including the temporal bones. Examination of cranial nerves can be included with each region. Starting with the scalp and upper third of the face, rule out open skull or sinus fractures. Examine the reactivity and symmetry of the pupils and visual acuity. Check for restriction of extraocular motion, proptosis, enophthalmos, diplopia, and traumatic telecanthus. In the midface, rule out a nasal fracture, septal hematoma, CSF rhinorrhea, hypesthesia, asymmetry, malocclusion, and trismus. When evaluating the lower third and mandible, examine intraorally for fractures, edema, missing teeth, and hypesthesia. For each third of the face, take note of fractures (point tenderness, crepitus, and bony step-off), laceration, and facial motion. Examine lower cranial nerve function if possible, including the larynx and hypopharynx. Palpate the neck for trauma to the airway, hematoma, crepitus, and midline shift.

If there are no life-threatening emergencies, a focused history is taken and an examination of the temporal bone is performed. Pertinent history includes vertigo, hearing loss, otalgia, otorrhea, rhinorrhea, pulsatile tinnitus, and facial paralysis. Try to ascertain from other observers whether there was immediate or delayed onset of any facial paralysis. Vertigo may be episodic or intermittent, positional or spontaneous. On physical examination, look for postauricular ecchymosis or Battle's sign, which is consistent with temporal bone fracture. Periorbital ecchymosis or raccoon eyes are also indicative of a base of skull fracture. The auricle should be examined for external trauma, especially avulsion or denuded cartilage. The external auditory canal should be cleaned under an otomicroscope to facilitate examination. Signs of trauma in the external auditory canal include lacerations, ecchymoses, hematomas, and the presence of CSF. At the level of the tympanic membrane and the middle ear, document hemotympanum or other middle ear fluid (e.g., CSF), perforation, and any visible ossicular landmarks. If CSF otorrhea is seen, cleaning should stop and the ear should be packed to create a biological dressing.

Tuning forks can be useful for evaluation of hearing at the bedside. Lateralization of the tone to the afflicted ear is consistent with a conductive hearing loss and preservation of sensorineural function. Formal audiograms are usually obtained after the patient is otherwise stable and alert. Many conductive hearing losses will improve in the first few months, as middle ear fluid resolves or as loose ossicular connections restabilize. The conductive loss from persistent ossicular discontinuity will commonly exceed 30 to 45 dB. Ossicular discontinuity can result in a type AD (abnormally high peak admittance) tympanogram and the loss of stapedial reflexes in the affected ear.

The presence and directionality of any spontaneous nystagmus should be documented. Vertigo associated with spontaneous nystagmus or with decrease or absence of ipsilateral caloric response on electronystagmography (ENG) is indicative of injury to the peripheral vestibular system. The patient with positional or intermittent vertigo should be evaluated by positioning the head with the affected ear in the dependent position (Hallpike maneuver). Severe rotatory nystagmus lasting less than a minute with latency of onset and fatigability is consistent with benign paroxysmal positional vertigo. Symptoms of traumatic perilymph fistula include SNHL that may fluctuate, tinnitus, and vertigo. Delayed onset of symptoms can be difficult to distinguish from Ménière disease or delayed endolymphatic hydrops. A positive fistula test (using pneumatic otoscopy or ENG with an immittance device) can help confirm a suspected fistula, and the ENG may show ipsilateral caloric weakness.

The leak of clear watery fluid from the ear or from the nose, or clear fluid behind an intact tympanic membrane, indicates CSF leak. Flow will increase with the head hanging forward in the dependent position or with the Valsalva maneuver. Because otorrhea or rhinorrhea after trauma is typically mixed with bloody secretions, demonstration of the *ring sign* at the bedside adds support to the diagnosis. To demonstrate the ring sign, drop the fluid onto tissue paper and look for the CSF to spread and create a clear halo around the centrally located bloody secretion. Other methods of confirming a CSF leak include detection of leakage of fluorescein or radionuclides after placement of these substances into the subarachnoid space. The definitive test for identification of CSF is to analyze the fluid for the presence of β_2-transferrin.[90–104] Methods for the localization of persistent leaks have evolved over time. Iohexol high-resolution computed tomography (CT) scans have been successfully used to demonstrate site of leak. The CT or magnetic resonance imaging (MRI) may also show an encephalocele related to the fracture line, which may underlie the leak of CSF.

Most importantly, the function of all branches of the facial nerve should be evaluated for later comparison.[105] In cases of diminished or absent facial motion, symptoms of eye pain, diminished visual acuity, and epiphora should be noted. Corneal sensation and Bell's phenomenon should be documented. Central facial paralysis should not affect the forehead motion due to contralateral innervation. Extratemporal facial nerve injury should be suspected when there is sparing of some branches of the facial nerve or there is soft tissue injury medial to the lateral canthus of the eye.

If there is only facial paresis, no electrophysiological testing is warranted. Complete facial paralysis suggests an intratemporal injury and warrants electrophysiological testing. Commonly used tests include the maximal stimulation test (MST), electromyography (EMG), and electroneurography (ENoG). The Hilger stimulator can be used to deliver a suprathreshold nerve stimulus at the bedside; persistent normal facial motion after 48 to 72 hours postinjury helps to quantitate the degree and progression of wallerian degeneration. Following denervation, EMG will demonstrate fibrillation potentials. Recovery of facial movement will be preceded by the appearance of polyphasic reinnervation potentials on EMG.

Topognostic testing has been used to help determine the site of facial nerve injury, but it has not been consistently reliable. Topognostic testing and imaging may influence the surgical approach if exploration is indicated; however, most fractures require exploration of the perigeniculate area. An abnormal Schirmer lacrimation test may indicate facial nerve injury at or proximal to the greater superficial petrosal nerve (normal is 15 mm in 5 minutes). Stapedial reflexes should be obtained during the audiogram. An intact acoustic reflex with acute facial paralysis indicates a lesion in the mastoid or extratemporal segment of the facial nerve.

Temporal lobe injury may manifest as hemiplegia, expressive aphasia, seizures, or auditory, olfactory, or visual hallucinations. Central nervous system injuries include contusion of the brain parenchyma, edema, microvascular hemorrhage or infarct, and encephalopathy. These can be heralded by changes in level of consciousness, headache, seizures, loss of cognitive function, personality/behavioral changes, incoordination, spasticity/paralysis, or cranial nerve deficits. A funduscopic examination is important to rule out increased intracranial pressure manifested by papilledema.

High-resolution CT scan (1.5-mm-thick axial and coronal cuts) is the imaging technique of choice for radiographic evaluation of a temporal bone fracture (► Fig. 22.9).[12,106–108] This can usually be performed electively once the patient is stable, and it facilitates the diagnosis and prognosis of the structures injured in and around the temporal bone. The site of fracture, the site (s) of facial nerve injury, dislocation of ossicles, and the site of a CSF leak can often be determined. Penetrating trauma in this region may require an angiogram. The CT scan also is important in ruling out adjacent skull fractures, intracranial hematoma or hemorrhage, and parenchymal injury of the brain. Indications for immediate radiographic evaluation include open skull fractures, intracranial hemorrhage, blindness due to arterial occlusion, evidence of cavernous sinus injury, and any evidence of increased intracranial pressure.

A fracture of the carotid canal suggests possible vascular injury and should be investigated with CT angiography, magnetic

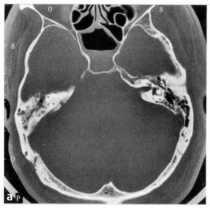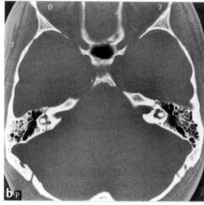

Fig. 22.9 (a) Axial CT scan image (bone window) of a left longitudinal temporal bone fracture due to a fall with loss of consciousness. (b) Axial scan image (bone window) of a right transverse temporal bone fracture sustained in a motor vehicle accident. The fracture traverses the labyrinth.

resoance angiography, or formal catheter angiography to rule out carotid artery injury.[109,110]

Surgical intervention specific to the temporal bone typically is based more on clinical findings and other diagnostic and prognostic tests (e.g., electrophysiological tests, audiometry) than on CT results.

22.7 Treatment

22.7.1 Auditory

Hemotympanum can result in up to a 30- to 45-dB conductive hearing loss initially. Usually, the hemotympanum is self-limited and clears by the fourth to sixth week. Myringotomy for drainage of the hemotympanum is not generally recommended due to the potential for infection.

Small traumatic perforations of the tympanic membrane often heal with conservative management over several weeks. Careful examination is needed to ensure that none of the perforation edges has become infolded, creating the risk for development of a cholesteatoma. A cigarette paper patch can be applied to a small perforation once the edges have been freshened. Unless there is gross contamination of the middle ear, antibiotic eardrops are not necessary. Keeping the ears free from water exposure is advised. For uncomplicated perforations that persist longer than several months, a variety of procedures can be offered to the patient. Similarly, fat myringoplasties have been employed with success. A type I tympanoplasty via a transcanal or postauricular approach traditionally has been recommended, especially if the perforation is large, difficult to visualize, or complicated by ossicular discontinuity or chronic infection.

Patients with persistent conductive hearing losses greater than 25 dB may be eligible for middle ear exploration with ossicular reconstruction. Hearing aids or conservative management are alternatives, depending on the patient's overall hearing status. Timing of the surgery is elective after hearing has stabilized; it is advisable to wait at least 3 months for any spontaneous healing to occur (suspected stapes fracture with PLF requires urgent surgery). Surgical options for a dislocated incus include incus interposition or transposition, or the use of an ossicular reconstruction prosthesis. Injuries involving the stapes footplate may necessitate repair by tissue graft or partial or total stapedectomy. Ossicular reconstruction can be accomplished by autograft (e.g., ossicle, bone, cartilage) or alloplastic material (e.g., stapes prosthesis, total or partial ossicular reconstruction prostheses). Fractured fragments dislocated into the vestibule are not removed due to the risk of SNHL.

Most patients with transverse fractures have a profound, irreversible SNHL. The majority of patients who have mild closed head injuries and have only low-frequency SNHL may recover hearing thresholds in the first couple of days; high-frequency losses are much less likely to recover. The vast majority of patients with temporal bone fractures and SNHL do not improve significantly with time. Moderate to severe losses may benefit from a hearing aid.

Patients with bilateral profound SNHL as a result of bilateral temporal bone fractures may be candidates for cochlear implantation. There are several reports of successful implantation with subsequent auditory rehabilitation in this subset of patients.[111–115] Pathological processes associated with temporal bone trauma and cognitive capacity of the patient as it relates to the ability to participate in postoperative aural rehabilitation should be considered prior to surgery.

Cochlear implantation in patients who have sustained temporal bone trauma can be challenging secondary to anatomic changes of the cochlea and the middle ear.[116] The presence of labyrinthitis ossificans, which most commonly occurs at the basal turn of the cochlea, can complicate round window electrode insertion and should be ruled out on preoperative high-resolution CT imaging. Other structural abnormalities such as middle ear granulation tissue and cochlear fibrosis are possible in the posttraumatic setting. Repeat imaging is obtained if there is a significant time delay between the initial CT scan after temporal bone trauma and the cochlear implantation. Intuitively, early implantation prevents the risk of cochlear ossification, which increases as time from injury increases; however, the optimal time after traumatic injury to perform cochlear implantation remains unclear.

In cases of deafness due to head trauma, it is critical to rule out auditory nerve disruption precluding successful cochlear implantation in that ear. MRI can provide valuable information in assessing the status of an intact vestibulocochlear nerve and a patent cochlear duct. Promontory stimulation testing to determine the functional integrity of the cochlear nerve should be considered in patients with no detectable pure tone thresholds in either ear on audiometric testing or radiographic evidence of fractures through the internal auditory canals. Otoacoustic emissions may also have utility in this setting as the presence of hair cell function suggests neural injury.[117]

Temporal bone fractures have been associated with a loss of spiral ganglion cells.[116] Animal models have demonstrated that implant stimulation of the afferent pathways begins at the level of the spiral ganglion cells.[118] Studies have failed to conclusively demonstrate that clinical performance with cochlear implants is directly related to the extent of survival of spiral ganglion cells, although this issue is controversial.[119,120] In fact, some groups have shown that there is an inverse relationship between survival of ganglion cells and performance.[121,122] The relationship between the absolute number of remaining spiral ganglion cells and successful cochlear implantation in the posttraumatic setting has not been studied.

Patients should be counseled preoperatively about the possibility of unintended facial nerve stimulation after implantation. Camilleri et al[123] reported two patients who experienced facial nerve stimulation after cochlear implantation; both were explanted and subsequently had the contralateral ear implanted. Camilleri's group postulated that current leaks from the electrode through low resistance fracture lines resulted in higher than expected rates of facial nerve stimulation. No difference in rates of other complications with cochlear implantation after temporal bone trauma and routine cochlear implantation has been reported.

Patients who have sustained trauma severe enough to cause bilateral profound SNHL often have other significant bodily injuries, in particular comorbid intracranial pathology. Impaired cognitive, behavioral, emotional, and physical function is not uncommon and can be a major impediment to cooperative participation in postoperative therapeutic rehabilitation. Although poor neurologic function does not preclude significant benefit that can be achieved by implantation, careful candidacy assessment is advised, as postimplant management can be challenging.[114,124]

Persistent nonpulsatile tinnitus after temporal bone trauma is usually associated with hearing loss and can be difficult to ameliorate. In patients who might otherwise benefit from a hearing aid, the aid may also mask tinnitus in the daytime. Background noise such as white noise or music from a radio can be used at night, or a more formal tinnitus masker can be fitted if there is sufficient residual inhibition.

22.7.2 Vestibular

The course of benign paroxysmal positional vertigo (BPPV) is usually self-limited with resolution of symptoms in 3 months.[62,70–75] Therapeutic maneuvers such as that of Epley may be efficacious and provide immediate resolution. Surgical interventions, such as singular neurectomy or vestibular nerve section, are rarely required.

Most of the symptoms of vestibular injury are self-limited and gradually resolve in 6 months. During that time the patient should be as active as possible and use the minimal amount of vestibular sedative needed, to facilitate central vestibular compensation. For severe continuous or prolonged episodes of vertigo, short courses of meclizine or diazepam may be helpful. Persistent vertigo or unsteadiness following head trauma suggests a possible central cause or failure of central compensation. In cases of failure of compensation, vestibular rehabilitation may be helpful. Surgical procedures for severe persistent symptoms of peripheral vestibular dysfunction would vestibular

nerve section (useful hearing) and a labyrinthectomy (no useful hearing).[125–130]

Urgent middle ear exploration is recommended to repair an obvious traumatic perilymph leak, to attempt hearing preservation, and to resolve disequilibrium.[37–47] Some otologists avoid urgent surgery for fear of doing more harm than good. There are no uniform criteria for selecting patients for middle ear exploration. A history of antecedent trauma, vertigo, and SNHL favor the diagnosis of PLF. Symptoms include tinnitus, vertigo with or without disequilibrium, aural fullness, and SNHL that may be fluctuating. The sensitivity of the fistula test may be as low as 60%,[43] so the diagnosis is based primarily on symptoms, a high index of clinical suspicion, and middle ear exploration. ENG may show abnormalities. The most common ENG finding is spontaneous nystagmus, which can be directed either away from or toward the affected ear. Positional nystagmus and ipsilateral vestibular hypofunction have been seen as well. Surgical repair of PLF will most likely improve vertigo; hearing and tinnitus can improve, according to some reports. The patient should be cautioned against the Valsalva maneuver, heavy lifting or straining, or flying for at least several weeks postrepair; scuba diving or other activities that can produce severe pressure changes within the ear may be contraindicated in the long term.

22.7.3 Facial Paralysis

Initial management of facial nerve dysfunction should include corneal protection. For significant lagophthalmos with incomplete eye closure, liberal use of eyedrops during the daytime is prescribed. Nightly application of ophthalmic ointment and eye protection (bubble protector, moisture chamber) are enforced to prevent exposure keratitis.

More definitive treatment is based on prognosis. Overall, facial nerve paresis (incomplete loss of facial nerve function) carries an excellent prognosis, and conservative management is recommended.[5,131–136] Electrical testing is not necessary in this setting. After paralysis, spontaneous nerve regeneration can be detectable by EMG as early as 3 weeks after injury. Reinnervation potentials usually precede the clinical return of motor function, which is usually apparent by 1 to 2 months. The role of steroids is unclear.

Clinical management of complete paralysis is based on electrophysiological testing.[9,80,82–89] Delay in the onset of the facial paralysis or the ability to stimulate the nerve more than 48 to 72 hours postinjury confirms that the nerve has not been transected. In either situation, however, the nerve still may be severely injured and require surgical intervention to maximize recovery potential. ENoG should be used to follow progression of neural degeneration for 2 to 3 weeks posttrauma (► Fig. 22.10). After 3 weeks, a false-negative response to ENoG may be due to asynchronous firing from regenerating axons. An EMG should be performed to rule out the presence of any voluntary potentials.

For complete facial nerve paralysis, early facial nerve exploration for decompression or repair is recommended if there is greater than 90% degeneration of the ENoG response within 2 weeks of onset of paralysis.[11,78,80,137–145] Studies have suggested that such rapid loss of electrical excitability indicates a severe injury in which a significant proportion of axons will progress

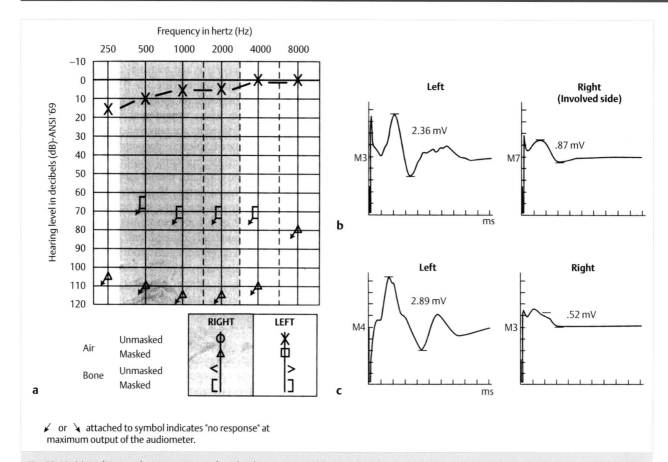

Fig. 22.10 (a) Audiogram demonstrating profound right sensorineural hearing loss due to a transverse temporal bone fracture. Associated findings included horizontal spontaneous nystagmus and complete facial paralysis. (b) Electroneurography of the right facial nerve in the same patient after a transverse temporal bone fracture. The amplitude of the compound action potential was 36% of the response from the contralateral facial nerve 8 days postinjury. (c) Serial electroneurography of the facial nerve showed a decrease in the amplitude of the compound muscle action potential to 18% within 3 weeks of injury. This patient did not undergo facial nerve exploration and began to show clinical return of function 1 month post-injury.

from axonotmesis to neurotmesis (▶ Fig. 22.11). EMG can be used to identify fibrillation potentials or polyphasic reinnervation potentials. Exploration for immediate-onset paralysis is indicated if there is obvious nerve transection, which is very likely in penetrating temporal bone trauma.

Although it is our bias to consider strongly surgical exploration for patients meeting the criteria noted above, we acknowledge that conclusive studies demonstrating the efficacy of facial nerve decompression are lacking. A recent systematic review on outcomes and management of facial paralysis secondary to temporal bone trauma was unable to definitely support either surgical or nonsurgical intervention. The authors highlighted the lack of high-quality evidence, heterogeneity of outcome measures, and incomplete data reporting in studies pertaining to this clinical entity.[146]

Brodie and Thompson[17] as well as other authors[147] have reported small series of patients who met the surgical criteria but were treated only with observation. Good recovery was reported in approximately 50 to 60% of these patients.

Patients with a complete paralysis who are initially seen several months after injury present a diagnostic dilemma, although decompression still may be indicated.[9,82,148,149] A history of sudden onset of facial paralysis suggests a more severe injury. An

EMG is obtained to detect evidence of reinnervation potentials or voluntary motor potentials. In this setting, failure to regenerate can be due to a transection injury or severe intraneural fibrosis. Exploration of the nerve at this time may optimize any chance for recovery. Nerve graft results seem better if performed within the first 12 months. In some instances, excision of a fibrotic segment with primary anastomosis or interposition graft as long as 12 to 18 months postinjury has resulted in recovery of facial tone and some mimetic movement. Viability of facial muscles should be confirmed by EMG fibrillation potentials. If more than 12 to 18 months have elapsed without clinical evidence of facial motion, substitution procedures (e.g., hypoglossal-to-facial anastomosis), muscle transpositions, or static sling procedures may be required.

The surgical approach to exploration and decompression of the facial nerve is based on the status of hearing and the anticipated sites of injury.[11,78,80,137–145] In most cases, exploration of the nerve needs to include the perigeniculate region. For most longitudinal temporal bone fractures, both middle cranial fossa and transmastoid explorations of the facial nerve are required (▶ Fig. 22.12). The nerve is exposed by a translabyrinthine approach in cases of a transverse fracture with severe to profound SNHL (▶ Fig. 22.13).

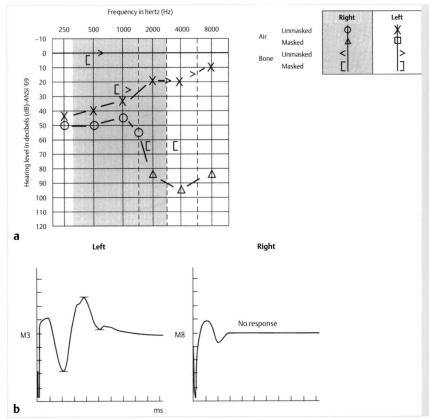

Fig. 22.11 (a) Audiogram after a mixed right temporal bone fracture showing right mixed hearing loss. (b) Electroneurography of the right facial nerve in the same patient showed no response 19 days postinjury, and there was no response to Hilger facial nerve stimulation. The patient underwent right facial nerve exploration and decompression via a middle fossa approach. The fracture had partially transected the labyrinthine segment of the facial nerve. Recovery of facial function 6 months later was poor, and this patient underwent a hypoglossal-to-facial nerve anastomosis.

Impinging bone fragments are removed and any intraneural hematoma evacuated. Nerve decompression usually extends from the meatal foramen to the vertical segment of the facial nerve. If greater than 50% of the cross-sectional area of the nerve has been lost, the injury should be treated as a complete transection. The traumatized region is completely excised and, if possible, rerouting of the nerve with primary anastomoses is accomplished. A greater auricular nerve graft is interposed if primary anastomosis without tension cannot be achieved.[150-154] Temporizing measures for eye protection include tarsorrhaphy or implantation of gold eyelid weight. These procedures are reversible if facial motion should return.

Exceptions to this management plan arise in the case of the neonate with complete facial paralysis. Neonatal facial paralysis is most commonly caused by birth trauma or by developmental neuromuscular anomalies. Facial paralysis following birth trauma has been associated with forceps delivery and with decompression of the head and face during prolonged or difficult spontaneous delivery. The temporal bone is softer in the neonate, and the facial nerve is more superficially located. Birth trauma results in compression or crushing of the facial nerve within the fallopian canal, but transection of the nerve has not been reported. Neonatal traumatic facial paralysis is usually unilateral and accompanied by facial ecchymosis, a Battle sign, or hemotympanum. In contrast, developmental anomalies presenting with facial paralysis are usually associated with maldevelopment of the face or ear and multiple or bilateral cranial nerve deficits, including abnormal eighth nerve findings.

Electrophysiological testing for neonatal facial paralysis should be done soon after birth. The primary clinical concern is documentation of the presence of neuromuscular integrity, to distinguish traumatic from developmental paralysis. Spontaneous and complete recovery occurs in greater than 90% of neonatal facial paralysis. Usually recovery is detectable within the first 4 weeks of life due to the excellent prognosis and the unlikelihood of nerve transection.[155-160] Observation and conservative management are recommended for 5 weeks before considering surgical exploration.

22.7.4 Intracranial

Treatment of parenchymal brain injury and intracranial complications depends on the site and the type of injury. Consultation with a neurologist or neurosurgeon should be obtained. Management of a confirmed CSF leak depends on duration, site, and presence of complications.[91-104] Conservative management is acceptable initially. Most leaks resolve spontaneously within the first 3 to 5 days after injury. Coverage with antibiotics is controversial and often not recommended, to prevent masking the early symptoms of meningitis or selecting for resistant organisms. Patients are initially treated with strict bed rest and head elevation; a lumbar drain may be necessary if this early conservative approach is unsuccessful. Leaks that persist beyond 10 to 14 days require surgical intervention due to the risk of meningitis. Surgical approaches to close a CSF leak depend on the site of leak and the hearing status. A transmastoid and middle fossa approach used alone or in combination allows both repair of the leak and reduction or resection of any encephalocele in cases of intact hearing. The transmastoid approach and repair with abdominal fat graft can be used if hearing has

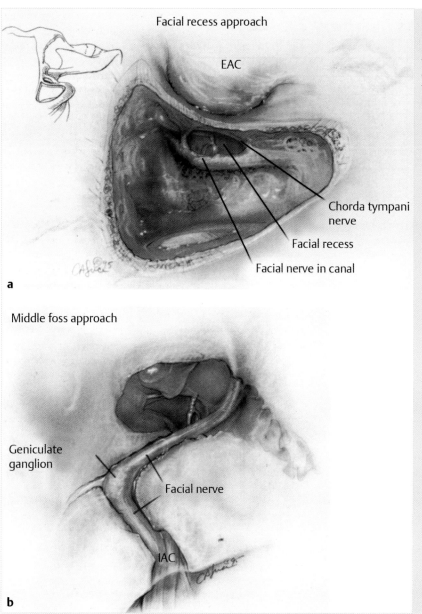

Facial recess approach

EAC

Chorda tympani nerve

Facial recess

Facial nerve in canal

a

Middle foss approach

Geniculate ganglion

Facial nerve

IAC

b

Fig. 22.12 (a) Diagram of the transmastoid facial recess approach to the facial nerve. This approach should be combined with the middle fossa approach (b) because of the high likelihood of coexisting injury to the mastoid segment of the nerve. EAC, external auditory canal; IAC, internal auditory canal.

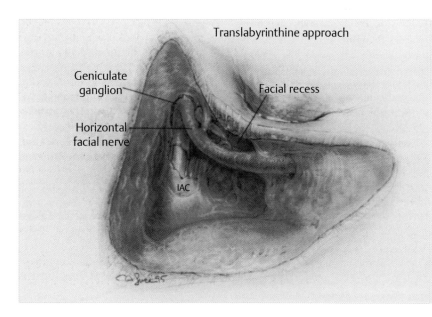

Translabyrinthine approach

Geniculate ganglion

Facial recess

Horizontal facial nerve

IAC

Fig. 22.13 Diagram of the translabyrinthine exposure of the facial nerve from the tympanic segment to the internal auditory canal (IAC), which can be used for transverse temporal bone fractures without residual hearing.

been lost, and obliteration of the eustachian tube and middle ear with soft tissue may be employed to isolate any dural dehiscence from the external environment.

22.7.5 Vascular

Intracranial vascular complications require neurosurgical consultation.[161-165] Hemorrhage from the sigmoid or petrosal sinuses can usually be managed by transmastoid exposure followed by extraluminal packing at the site of injury. Occasionally ligation of the internal jugular vein distally is also required. Arterial hemorrhage is most quickly managed by balloon occlusion or embolization.

22.8 Other Considerations

22.8.1 Recurrent Conductive Hearing Loss

Adhesions to the ossicles in the epitympanum and posterior mesotympanum as well as displacement of an ossicular prosthesis or repositioned incus may cause a conductive hearing loss during follow-up. Scarring in the external auditory canal leads to canal stenosis and secondary infection or cholesteatoma of the canal. Treatment of these conditions is primarily surgical, involving middle ear exploration and canaloplasty.

22.8.2 Cholesteatoma

Cholesteatoma may involve the pneumatized spaces of the temporal bone as a delayed complication of penetrating or blunt trauma, particularly after a longitudinal fracture.[166,167] The cholesteatoma primarily results from trapped or ingrown squamous epithelium of the external auditory canal. Treatment is surgical removal of the cholesteatoma from the canal, middle ear, or mastoid by transcanal or transmastoid approaches.

22.8.3 Delayed Endolymphatic Hydrops

Delayed endolymphatic hydrops with SNHL, episodic vertigo, aural fullness, and tinnitus can arise many years after transverse temporal bone and other fractures of the skull base.[76,168] Trauma or obstruction to the vestibular aqueduct is thought to be the mechanism responsible for hydrops.

22.8.4 Encephalocele

Temporal bone fractures heal primarily by fibrous union. The middle cranial fossa is usually sealed off from the ear within 3 to 4 weeks by a combination of mucosa, bone, and fibrous tissue from the endosteal and periosteal layers of the osseous labyrinth. An encephalocele or meningoencephalocele results from failure to adequately heal the fracture site and associated dural injury. If the dura is uninjured and the intracranial pressure remains within normal limits, then sizable middle fossa tegmen defects can be tolerated without formation of an encephalocele. In fact, spontaneous asymptomatic tegmen dehiscences frequently are found at surgery and at autopsy. Traumatic encephaloceles may be asymptomatic or may present in various

ways: a pulsatile soft mass in the external auditory canal that increases in size with Valsalva, recurrent meningitis, or herniation into the middle ear resulting in conductive hearing loss.[169-171]

Diagnosis of the tegmen defect is best accomplished by high-resolution axial and coronal CT scans, but the presence of central nervous system tissue and CSF in the herniated tissue is best identified on an MRI scan. Treatment is surgical reduction with excision of the herniated brain and repair of the tegmen defect. The surgical approach is transmastoid for small defects; this approach can be combined with a middle fossa approach for larger defects.

22.8.5 Otitic Meningitis

Meningitis can complicate a traumatic encephalocele or CSF leak.[91-94] Meningitis can also occur as a delayed consequence of a temporal bone fracture months or years later, even without a CSF leak. In such cases, incomplete healing of the fracture line provides a pathway for pathogens to access the CSF space. Recurrent meningitis is not unusual, and is usually associated with otitis media. One should look for a middle ear effusion that could represent an acute or resolving otitis media or CSF. Signs and symptoms of meningitis include fever, headache, meningismus, positive Kernig or Brudzinski sign, and changes in level of consciousness or mental status. Diagnosis is based on lumbar puncture with examination of the CSF for protein, glucose, Gram stain, cell count, and culture, after CT scan to rule out obstructive hydrocephalus. Intravenous antibiotics that provide central nervous system penetration and broad coverage of middle ear and upper respiratory organisms should be initiated immediately. Continued antibiotic treatment is based on culture results and sensitivities of the organisms, as well as the clinical response. Pneumococcus is the most frequent organism.

22.8.6 Pneumocephalus and Pneumolabyrinth

Pneumocephalus is a rare complication that denotes the entry of air into the cranial vault through a traumatic breach in the continuity of the dura and the bone.[172-175] Presenting symptoms can be vague. Headache, meningismus, aphasia, vomiting, visual alteration, decreased level of consciousness, hemiplegia, seizures, and other neurologic signs can occur. The diagnosis is readily made on CT scan. Uncomplicated pneumocephalus usually resolves spontaneously by resorption of the air. Persistent pneumocephalus or pneumocephalus associated with a persistent CSF leak is an indication for surgical repair of the defect. Tension pneumocephalus requires urgent surgical intervention. Entry of air into the labyrinth is also rare, but when seen on CT scan it indicates a fracture of the otic capsule or dislocation of the stapes.[176]

22.8.7 Temporomandibular Joint Trauma

The tympanic, petrous, and squamous portions of the temporal bone are situated about the posterior aspect of the glenoid fossa. Trauma to the mandible in cases of multiple trauma can result in posterior displacement of the mandibular condyle and thus results in a fracture of the external auditory canal. Uncommonly, there can be traumatic displacement of the condyle into the middle fossa with pneumocephalus, which must be emergently reduced and repaired. Fractures of the temporal bone can conversely extend into the glenoid fossa, resulting in air in the temporomandibular joint and joint dysfunction.[173-175,177-179]

22.8.8 Carotid-Cavernous Fistula

Carotid-cavernous fistula (CCF) may present immediately or years following a penetrating skull base trauma.[180] CCF can be classified as direct or indirect. Direct communication between the intracavernous internal carotid artery and the cavernous sinus is the most common type, and is most frequently caused by trauma. Indirect fistulas usually arise spontaneously and involve an abnormal connection between the cavernous sinus and the dural branches of either the internal or external carotid artery (middle meningeal artery, accessory meningeal artery, or the artery of the foramen rotundum). Symptoms usually result from shunting of blood into the superior ophthalmic vein, but can also present with a steal syndrome. Orbital findings include pulsatile proptosis or tinnitus, chemosis, lid edema, orbital bruit, ophthalmoplegia, glaucoma, decreased visual acuity, and severe epistaxis.

Diagnosis is based on angiography and imaging of the skull base. Direct CCF due to trauma requires intervention; progressive monocular blindness occurs in 50% of untreated cases. If facial nerve exploration is also needed, CCF repair should proceed first to avoid severe hemorrhage if fragments in the cavernous sinus are inadvertently manipulated. CCF can be surgically repaired by ligating the carotid proximally in the neck and distally at the supraclinoid carotid segment. Alternatively, the carotid artery can be preserved with selective embolization of the CCF.

References

[1] Murphy AG. The ear and cranial trauma. Arch Otolaryngol 1935; 21: 686–693

[2] Podoshin L, Fradis M. Hearing loss after head injury. Arch Otolaryngol 1975; 101: 15–18

[3] Singh SP, Adeloye A. Hearing loss in missile head injuries. J Laryngol Otol 1971; 85: 1183–1187

[4] Tos M. Prognosis of hearing loss in temporal bone fractures. J Laryngol Otol 1971; 85: 1147–1159

[5] Grove WE. Skull fractures involving the ear. A clinical study of 211 cases. Laryngoscope 1939; 49: 678–706

[6] Griffin JE, Altenau MM, Schaefer SD. Bilateral longitudinal temporal bone fractures: a retrospective review of seventeen cases. Laryngoscope 1979; 89: 1432–1435

[7] Proctor B, Gurdjian ES, Webster JE. The ear in head trauma. Laryngoscope 1956; 66: 16–59

[8] Fisch U. Facial paralysis in fractures of the petrous bone. Laryngoscope 1974; 84: 2141–2154

[9] Harker LA, McCabe BF. Temporal bone fractures and facial nerve injury. Otolaryngol Clin North Am 1974; 7: 425–431

[10] Ghorayeb BY, Yeakley JW. Temporal bone fractures: longitudinal or oblique? The case for oblique temporal bone fractures. Laryngoscope 1992; 102: 129–134

[11] McHugh HE. The surgical treatment of facial paralysis and traumatic conductive deafenss on fractures of the temporal bone. Ann Otol Rhinol Laryngol 1959; 68: 855–889

[12] Aguilar EA, III, Yeakley JW, Ghorayeb BY, Hauser M, Cabrera J, Jahrsdoerfer RA. High resolution CT scan of temporal bone fractures: association of facial nerve paralysis with temporal bone fractures. Head Neck Surg 1987; 9: 162–166

[13] Little SC, Kesser BW. Radiographic classification of temporal bone fractures: clinical predictability using a new system. Arch Otolaryngol Head Neck Surg 2006; 132: 1300–1304

[14] Dahiya R, Keller JD, Litofsky NS, Bankey PE, Bonassar LJ, Megerian CA. Temporal bone fractures: otic capsule sparing versus otic capsule violating clinical and radiographic considerations. J Trauma 1999; 47: 1079–1083

[15] Yanagihara N, Murakami S, Nishihara S. Temporal bone fractures inducing facial nerve paralysis: a new classification and its clinical significance. Ear Nose Throat J 1997; 76: 79–80, 83–86

[16] Ishman SL, Friedland DR. Temporal bone fractures: traditional classification and clinical relevance. Laryngoscope 2004; 114: 1734–1741

[17] Brodie HA, Thompson TC. Management of complications from 820 temporal bone fractures. Am J Otol 1997; 18: 188–197

[18] McGuirt WF, Jr, Stool SE. Temporal bone fractures in children: a review with emphasis on long-term sequelae. Clin Pediatr (Phila) 1992; 31: 12–18

[19] Williams WT, Ghorayeb BY, Yeakley JW. Pediatric temporal bone fractures. Laryngoscope 1992; 102: 600–603

[20] Duncan NO, III, Coker NJ, Jenkins HA, Canalis RF. Gunshot injuries of the temporal bone. Otolaryngol Head Neck Surg 1986; 94: 47–55

[21] Griffiths MV. The incidence of auditory and vestibular concussion following minor head injury. J Laryngol Otol 1979; 93: 253–265

[22] Barber HO. Head injury audiological and vestibular findings. Ann Otol Rhinol Laryngol 1969; 78: 239–252

[23] Silverstein H, Fabian RL, Stoll SE, Hong SW. Penetrating wounds of the tympanic membrane and ossicular chain. Trans Am Acad Ophthalmol Otolaryngol 1973; 77: ORL125–ORL135

[24] Arragg FG, Paparella MM. Traumatic fracture of the stapes. Laryngoscope 1964; 74: 1329–1332

[25] Kerr AG, Byrne JET. Concussive effects of bomb blast on the ear. J Laryngol Otol 1975; 89: 131–143

[26] Roberto M, Hamernik RP, Turrentine GA. Damage of the auditory system associated with acute blast trauma. Ann Otol Rhinol Laryngol Suppl 1989; 140: 23–34

[27] Armstrong HG, Heim JW. The effects of flight on the middle ear. JAMA 1937; 109: 417–421

[28] King PF. Otitic barotrauma. Proc R Soc Med 1966; 59: 543–554

[29] Bayliss GJ. Aural barotrauma in naval divers. Arch Otolaryngol 1968; 88: 141–147

[30] Soss SL. Sensorineural hearing loss with diving. Arch Otolaryngol 1971; 93: 501–504

[31] Freeman P, Edmonds C. Inner ear barotrauma. Arch Otolaryngol 1972; 95: 556–563

[32] Pullen FW, II, Rosenberg GJ, Cabeza CH. Sudden hearing loss in divers and fliers. Laryngoscope 1979; 89: 1373–1377

[33] Farmer JC, Thomas WG, Youngblood DG, Bennett PB. Inner ear decompression sickness. Laryngoscope 1976; 86: 1315–1327

[34] Gray RF, Barton RPE. Round window rupture. J Laryngol Otol 1981; 95: 165–177

[35] Fraser JG, Harborow PC. Labyrinthine window rupture. J Laryngol Otol 1975; 89: 1–7

[36] Althaus SR. Perilymph fistulas. Laryngoscope 1981; 91: 538–562

[37] Goodhill V. Ben H. Senturia lecture. Leaking labyrinth lesions, deafness, tinnitus and dizziness. Ann Otol Rhinol Laryngol 1981; 90: 99–106

[38] Feldmann H. Sudden hearing loss with delayed onset following head trauma. Acta Otolaryngol 1987; 103: 379–383

[39] Fee GA. Traumatic perilymphatic fistulas. Arch Otolaryngol 1968; 88: 477–480

[40] Tonkin JP, Fagan P. Rupture of the round window membrane. J Laryngol Otol 1975; 89: 733–756

[41] Kohut RI, Waldorf RA, Haenel JL, Thompson JN. Minute perilymph fistulas: vertigo and Hennebert's sign without hearing loss. Ann Otol Rhinol Laryngol 1979; 88: 153–159

[42] Thompson JN, Kohut KI. Perilymph fistulae: variability of symptoms and results of surgery. Otolaryngol Head Neck Surg 1979; 87: 898–903

[43] Goodhill V. Traumatic fistulae. J Laryngol Otol 1980; 94: 123–128

[44] Grimm RJ, Hemenway WG, Lebray PR, Black FO. The perilymph fistula syndrome defined in mild head trauma. Acta Otolaryngol Suppl 1989; 464: 1–40

[45] Paparella MM. Interactive inner-ear/middle-ear disease, including perilymphatic fistula. Acta Otolaryngol Suppl 1991; 485: 36–45

[46] Glasscock ME, III, Hart MJ, Rosdeutscher JD, Bhansali SA. Traumatic perilymphatic fistula: how long can symptoms persist? A follow-up report. Am J Otol 1992; 13: 333–338

[47] Seltzer S, McCabe BF. Perilymph fistula: the Iowa experience. Laryngoscope 1986; 96: 37–49

[48] Glasscock ME, III, McKennan KX, Levine SC. Persistent traumatic perilymph fistulas. Laryngoscope 1987; 97: 860–864

[49] Wright JW, Jr, Silk KL. Acoustic and vestibular defects in lightning survivors. Laryngoscope 1974; 84: 1378–1387

[50] Weiss KS. Otologic lightning bolts. Am J Otolaryngol 1980; 1: 334–337

[51] Jones DT, Ogren FP, Roh LH, Moore GF. Lightning and its effects on the auditory system. Laryngoscope 1991; 101: 830–834

[52] Bergstrom L, Neblett LW, Sando I, Hemenway WG, Harrison GD. The lightning-damaged ear. Arch Otolaryngol 1974; 100: 117–121

[53] Youngs R, Deck J, Kwok P, Hawke M. Severe sensorineural hearing loss caused by lightning. A temporal bone case report. Arch Otolaryngol Head Neck Surg 1988; 114: 1184–1187

[54] Hough JV. Restoration of hearing loss after head trauma. Ann Otol Rhinol Laryngol 1969; 78: 210–226

[55] Does IE, Bottema T. Posttraumatic conductive hearing loss. Arch Otolaryngol 1965; 82: 331–339

[56] Wright JW, Jr, Taylor CE, Bizal JA. Tomography and the vulnerable incus. Ann Otol Rhinol Laryngol 1969; 78: 263–279

[57] Cannon CR, Jahrsdoerfer RA. Temporal bone fractures. Review of 90 cases. Arch Otolaryngol 1983; 109: 285–288

[58] Spector GJ, Pratt LL, Randall G. A clinical study of delayed reconstruction in ossicular fractures. Laryngoscope 1973; 83: 837–851

[59] Hough JV, Stuart WD. Middle ear injuries in skull trauma. Laryngoscope 1968; 78: 899–937

[60] Bellucci RJ. Traumatic injuries of the middle ear. Otolaryngol Clin North Am 1983; 16: 633–650

[61] Strohm M. Trauma of the middle ear. Clinical findings, postmortem observations and results of experimental studies. Adv Otorhinolaryngol 1986; 35: 1–254

[62] Schuknecht HF, Davison RC. Deafness and vertigo from head injury. AMA Arch Otolaryngol 1956; 63: 513–528

[63] Schuknecht HF. A clinical study of auditory damage following blows to the head. Ann Otol Rhinol Laryngol 1950; 59: 331–358

[64] Makishima K, Snow JB. Pathogenesis of hearing loss in head injury. Studies in man and experimental animals. Arch Otolaryngol 1975; 101: 426–432

[65] Makishima K, Sobel SF, Snow JB, Jr. Histopathologic correlates of otoneurologic manifestations following head trauma. Laryngoscope 1976; 86: 1303–1314

[66] Lindsay JR, Zajtchuk J. Concussion of the inner ear. Ann Otol Rhinol Laryngol 1970; 79: 699–709

[67] Schuknecht HF. Mechanism of inner ear injury from blows to the head. Ann Otol Rhinol Laryngol 1969; 78: 253–262

[68] Kirikae I, Eguchi K, Okamoto M, Nakamura K. Histopathological changes in the auditory pathway in cases of fatal head injury. Acta Otolaryngol 1969; 67: 341–349

[69] Rantanen T, Aantaa E, Salmivalli A et al. Audiometric and electronystagmographic studies of patients with traumatic skull injuries. Acta Otolaryngol 1966; 224 suppl: 256–259

[70] Pearson BW, Barber HO. Head injury. Some otoneurologic sequelae. Arch Otolaryngol 1973; 97: 81–84

[71] Dix MR, Hallpike CS. The pathology, symptomatology and diagnosis of certain common disorders of the vestibular system. Ann Otol Rhinol Laryngol 1952; 61: 987–1016

[72] Schuknecht HF. Cupulolithiasis. Arch Otolaryngol 1969; 90: 765–778

[73] Parker DE, Covell WP, von Gierke HE. Exploration of vestibular damage in guinea pigs following mechanical stimulation. Acta Otolaryngol 1968; 239: 239–, 7

[74] Cawthorne T. Positional nystagmus. Ann Otol Rhinol Laryngol 1954; 63: 481–490

[75] Cawthorne TE, Hallpike CS. A study of the clinical features and pathological changes within the temporal bones, brain stem and cerebellum of an early case of positional nystagmus of the so-called benign paroxysmal type. Acta Otolaryngol 1957; 48: 89–103, discussion, 103–105

[76] Gordon N. Post-traumatic vertigo, with special reference to positional nystagmus. Lancet 1954; 266: 1216–1218

[77] Rizvi SS, Gibbin KP. Effect of transverse temporal bone fracture on the fluid compartment of the inner ear. Ann Otol Rhinol Laryngol 1979; 88: 741–748

[78] Windle WF, Groat RA, Fox CA. Experimental structural alterations in the brain during and after concussion. Surg Gynecol Obstet 1944; 79: 561–572

[79] Lambert PR, Brackmann DE. Facial paralysis in longitudinal temporal bone fractures: a review of 26 cases. Laryngoscope 1984; 94: 1022–1026

[80] Travis LW, Stalnaker RL, Melvin JW. Impact trauma of the human temporal bone. J Trauma 1977; 17: 761–766

[81] Coker NJ, Kendall KA, Jenkins HA, Alford BR. Traumatic intratemporal facial nerve injury: management rationale for preservation of function. Otolaryngol Head Neck Surg 1987; 97: 262–269

[82] Sunderland S. Nerve and Nerve Injuries, 2nd ed. New York: Churchill-Livingstone, 1978

[83] Esslen E. Electrodiagnosis of facial palsy. In: Miehlke A, ed. Surgery of the Facial Nerve, 2nd ed. Philadelphia: WB Saunders, 1973:45–51

[84] May M, Harvey JE, Marovitz WF, Stroud M. The prognostic accuracy of the maximal stimulation test compared with that of the nerve excitability test in Bell's palsy. Laryngoscope 1971; 81: 931–938

[85] Fisch U. Prognostic value of electrical tests in acute facial paralysis. Am J Otol 1984; 5: 494–498

[86] Hughes GB. Electroneurography: objective prognostic assessment of facial paralysis. Am J Otol 1982; 4: 73–76

[87] Kamerer DB. Intratemporal facial nerve injuries. Otolaryngol Head Neck Surg 1982; 90: 612–615

[88] Coker NJ, Fordice JO, Moore S. Correlation of the nerve excitability test and electroneurography in acute facial paralysis. Am J Otol 1992; 13: 127–133

[89] Coker NJ. Facial electroneurography: analysis of techniques and correlation with degenerating motoneurons. Laryngoscope 1992; 102: 747–759

[90] Lewis BI, Adour KK, Kahn JM, Lewis AJ. Hilger facial nerve stimulator: a 25-year update. Laryngoscope 1991; 101: 71–74

[91] McGuirt WF, Jr, Stool SE. Cerebrospinal fluid fistula: the identification and management in pediatric temporal bone fractures. Laryngoscope 1995; 105: 359–364

[92] Dula DJ, Fales W. The "ring sign": is it a reliable indicator for cerebral spinal fluid? Ann Emerg Med 1993; 22: 718–720

[93] Ryall RG, Peacock MK, Simpson DA. Usefulness of beta 2-transferrin assay in the detection of cerebrospinal fluid leaks following head injury. J Neurosurg 1992; 77: 737–739

[94] Fransen P, Sindic CJ, Thauvoy C, Laterre C, Stroobandt G. Highly sensitive detection of beta-2 transferrin in rhinorrhea and otorrhea as a marker for cerebrospinal fluid (C.S.F.) leakage. Acta Neurochir (Wien) 1991; 109: 98–101

[95] Irjala K, Suonpää J, Laurent B. Identification of CSF leakage by immunofixation. Arch Otolaryngol 1979; 105: 447–448

[96] Miller RH. Cerebrospinal fluid rhinorrhea and otorrhea. Clin Neurosurg 1972; 19: 263–270

[97] Hicks GW, Wright JW, Jr, Wright JW, III. Cerebrospinal fluid otorrhea. Laryngoscope 1980; 90 Suppl 25: 1–25

[98] Dandy WE. Treatment of rhinorrhea and otorrhea. Arch Surg 1944; 49: 75–85

[99] Calcaterra TC, Rand RW. Tympanic cavity obliteration for cerebrospinal otorhinorrhea. Arch Otolaryngol 1973; 97: 388–390

[100] MacGee EE, Cauthen JC, Brackett CE. Meningitis following acute traumatic cerebrospinal fluid fistula. J Neurosurg 1970; 33: 312–316

[101] Klastersky J, Sadeghi M, Brihaye J. Antimicrobial prophylaxis in patients with rhinorrhea or otorrhea: a double-blind study. Surg Neurol 1976; 6: 111–114

[102] Pollak AM, Pauw BK, Marion MS. Temporal bone histopathology: residents' quiz. Otogenic pneumococci meningitis after transverse temporal bone fracture during childhood. Am J Otolaryngol 1991; 12: 56–58

[103] Oberascher G. Cerebrospinal fluid otorrhea—new trends in diagnosis. Am J Otol 1988; 9: 102–108

[104] Westmore GA, Whittam DE. Cerebrospinal fluid rhinorrhoea and its management. Br J Surg 1982; 69: 489–492

[105] Leech PJ, Paterson A. Conservative and operative management for cerebrospinal-fluid leakage after closed head injury. Lancet 1973; 1: 1013–1016

[106] House JW. Facial nerve grading systems. Laryngoscope 1983; 93: 1056–1069

[107] Schubiger O, Valavanis A, Stuckmann G, Antonucci F. Temporal bone fractures and their complications. Examination with high resolution CT. Neuroradiology 1986; 28: 93–99

[108] Kahn JB, Stewart MG, Diaz-Marchan PJ. Acute temporal bone trauma: utility of high-resolution computed tomography. Am J Otol 2000; 21: 743–752

[109] McKinney A, Ott F, Short J, McKinney Z, Truwit C. Angiographic frequency of blunt cerebrovascular injury in patients with carotid canal or vertebral foramen fractures on multidetector CT. Eur J Radiol 2007; 62: 385–393

[110] York G, Barboriak D, Petrella J, DeLong D, Provenzale JM. Association of internal carotid artery injury with carotid canal fractures in patients with head trauma. AJR Am J Roentgenol 2005; 184: 1672–1678

[111] Zanetti D, Campovecchi CB, Pasini S. Binaural cochlear implantation after bilateral temporal bone fractures. Int J Audiol 2010; 49: 788–793

[112] Simons JP, Whitaker ME, Hirsch BE. Cochlear implantation in a patient with bilateral temporal bone fractures. Otolaryngol Head Neck Surg 2005; 132: 809–811

[113] Serin GM, Derinsu U, Sari M et al. Cochlear implantation in patients with bilateral cochlear trauma. Am J Otolaryngol 2010; 31: 350–355

[114] Greenberg SL, Shipp D, Lin VY, Chen JM, Nedzelski JM. Cochlear implantation in patients with bilateral severe sensorineural hearing loss after major blunt head trauma. Otol Neurotol 2011; 32: 48–54

[115] Chung JH, Shin MC, Min HJ, Park CW, Lee SH. Bilateral cochlear implantation in a patient with bilateral temporal bone fractures. Am J Otolaryngol 2011; 32: 256–258

[116] Morgan WE, Coker NJ, Jenkins HA. Histopathology of temporal bone fractures: implications for cochlear implantation. Laryngoscope 1994; 104: 426–432

[117] Fujimoto C, Ito K, Takano S, Karino S, Iwasaki S. Successful cochlear implantation in a patient with bilateral progressive sensorineural hearing loss after traumatic subarachnoid hemorrhage and brain contusion. Ann Otol Rhinol Laryngol 2007; 116: 897–901

[118] Clopton BM, Spelman FA, Miller JM. Estimates of essential neural elements for stimulation through a cochlear prosthesis. Ann Otol Rhinol Laryngol Suppl 1980; 89: 5–7

[119] Blamey P. Are spiral ganglion cell numbers important for speech perception with a cochlear implant? Am J Otol 1997; 18 Suppl: S11–S12

[120] Khan AM, Handzel O, Burgess BJ, Damian D, Eddington DK, Nadol JB, Jr. Is word recognition correlated with the number of surviving spiral ganglion cells and electrode insertion depth in human subjects with cochlear implants? Laryngoscope 2005; 115: 672–677

[121] Fayad JN, Linthicum FH, Jr. Multichannel cochlear implants: relation of histopathology to performance. Laryngoscope 2006; 116: 1310–1320

[122] Nadol JB, Jr, Shiao JY, Burgess BJ et al. Histopathology of cochlear implants in humans. Ann Otol Rhinol Laryngol 2001; 110: 883–891

[123] Camilleri AE, Toner JG, Howarth KL, Hampton S, Ramsden RT. Cochlear implantation following temporal bone fracture. J Laryngol Otol 1999; 113: 454–457

[124] Coligado EJ, Wiet RJ, O'Connor CA, Ito V, Sahgal V. Multichannel cochlear implantation in the rehabilitation of post-traumatic sensorineural hearing loss. Arch Phys Med Rehabil 1993; 74: 653–657

[125] Haberkamp TJ, Harvey SA, Daniels DL. The use of gadolinium-enhanced magnetic resonance imaging to determine lesion site in traumatic facial paralysis. Laryngoscope 1990; 100: 1294–1300

[126] Gotten N. Survey of one hundred cases of whiplash injury after settlement of litigation. J Am Med Assoc 1956; 162: 865–867

[127] Toglia JU, Rosenberg PE, Ronis ML. Posttraumatic dizziness; vestibular, audiologic, and medicolegal aspects. Arch Otolaryngol 1970; 92: 485–492

[128] Tuohimaa P. Vestibular disturbances after acute mild head injury. Acta Otolaryngol Suppl 1978; 359: 3–67

[129] Ylikoski J, Palva T, Sanna M. Dizziness after head trauma: clinical and morphologic findings. Am J Otol 1982; 3: 343–352

[130] Gacek RR. Transection of the posterior ampullary nerve for the relief of benign paroxysmal positional vertigo. Ann Otol Rhinol Laryngol 1974; 83: 596–605

[131] Garcia-Ibanez E, Garcia-Ibanez JL. Middle fossa vestibular neurectomy: a report of 373 cases. Otolaryngol Head Neck Surg 1980; 88: 486–490

[132] Turner JWA. Facial palsy in closed head injuries. Lancet 1944; 246: 756–757

[133] Potter JM. Facial palsy following head injury. J Laryngol Otol 1964; 78: 654–657

[134] Curtin JM. Fracture of the skull and intratemporal lesions affecting the facial nerve. Adv Otorhinolaryngol 1977; 22: 202–206

[135] Kettel K. Peripheral facial paralysis in fractures of the temporal bone; indications for surgical repair of the nerve; report of cases in which the Balance and Duel operation was used. Arch Otolaryngol 1950; 51: 25–41, illust

[136] McKennan KX, Chole RA. Facial paralysis in temporal bone trauma. Am J Otol 1992; 13: 167–172

[137] Adegbite AB, Khan MI, Tan L. Predicting recovery of facial nerve function following injury from a basilar skull fracture. J Neurosurg 1991; 75: 759–762

[138] Adour KK, Boyajian JA, Kahn ZM, Schneider GS. Surgical and nonsurgical management of facial paralysis following closed head injury. Laryngoscope 1977; 87: 380–390

[139] Alford BR, Sessions RB, Weber SC. Indications for surgical decompression of the facial nerve. Laryngoscope 1971; 81: 620–635

[140] Fisch U. Total facial nerve decompression and electroneurography. In: Silverstein H, Norrell H, eds. Neurologic Surgery of the Ear. Birmingham, AL: Aesculapis, 1977:chapter 4

[141] Sillman JS, Niparko JK, Lee SS, Kileny PR. Prognostic value of evoked and standard electromyography in acute facial paralysis. Otolaryngol Head Neck Surg 1992; 107: 377–381

[142] Yanagihara N. Transmastoid decompression of the facial nerve in temporal bone fracture. Otolaryngol Head Neck Surg 1982; 90: 616–621

[143] May M, Klein SR. Facial nerve decompression complications. Laryngoscope 1983; 93: 299–305

[144] Fisch U, Esslen E. Total intratemporal exposure of the facial nerve. Pathologic findings in Bell's palsy. Arch Otolaryngol 1972; 95: 335–341

[145] House WF, Crabtree JA. Surgical exposure of petrous portion of seventh nerve. Arch Otolaryngol 1965; 81: 506–507

[146] Nash JJ, Friedland DR, Boorsma KJ, Rhee JS. Management and outcomes of facial paralysis from intratemporal blunt trauma: a systematic review. Laryngoscope 2010; 120 Suppl 4: S214

[147] Chang CY, Cass SP. Management of facial nerve injury due to temporal bone trauma. Am J Otol 1999; 20: 96–114

[148] May M. Total facial nerve exploration: transmastoid, extralabyrinthine, and subtemporal indications and results. Laryngoscope 1979; 89: 906–917

[149] Brodsky L, Eviatar A, Daniller A. Post-traumatic facial nerve paralysis: three cases of delayed temporal bone exploration with recovery. Laryngoscope 1983; 93: 1560–1565

[150] Felix H, Eby TL, Fisch U. New aspects of facial nerve pathology in temporal bone fractures. Acta Otolaryngol 1991; 111: 332–336

[151] Coker NJ. Management of traumatic injuries to the facial nerve. Otolaryngol Clin North Am 1991; 24: 215–227

[152] Fisch U. Facial nerve grafting. Otolaryngol Clin North Am 1974; 7: 517–529

[153] Fisch U, Lanser MJ. Facial nerve grafting. Otolaryngol Clin North Am 1991; 24: 691–708

[154] Barrs DM. Facial nerve trauma: optimal timing for repair. Laryngoscope 1991; 101: 835–848

[155] Fisch U, Dobie RA, Gmür A, Felix H. Intracranial facial nerve anastomosis. Am J Otol 1987; 8: 23–29

[156] McHugh HE. Facial paralysis in birth injury and skull fractures. Arch Otolaryngol 1963; 78: 443–455

[157] Grundfast KM, Guarisco JL, Thomsen JR, Koch B. Diverse etiologies of facial paralysis in children. Int J Pediatr Otorhinolaryngol 1990; 19: 223–239

[158] Orobello P. Congenital and acquired facial nerve paralysis in children. Otolaryngol Clin North Am 1991; 24: 647–652

[159] Bergman I, May M, Stool S, Wessel HB. Neonatal traumatic facial palsy. Laryngoscope 1986; 96: 381–384

[160] Kumari S, Bhargava SK, Choudhury P, Ghosh S. Facial palsy in newborn: clinical profile and long-term follow-up. Indian Pediatr 1980; 17: 917–922

[161] Smith JD, Crumley RL, Harker LA. Facial paralysis in the newborn. Otolaryngol Head Neck Surg 1981; 89: 1021–1024

[162] du Trevou M, Bullock R, Teasdale E, Quin RO. False aneurysms of the carotid tree due to unsuspected penetrating injury of the head and neck. Injury 1991; 22: 237–239

[163] Meder JF, Gaston A, Merienne L, Godon-Hardy S, Fredy D. Traumatic aneurysms of the internal and external carotid arteries. One case and a review of the literature. J Neuroradiol 1992; 19: 248–255

[164] Chandrasekaran S, Zainal J. Delayed traumatic extradural haematomas. Aust N Z J Surg 1993; 63: 780–783

[165] Goodwin JR, Johnson MH. Carotid injury secondary to blunt head trauma: case report. J Trauma 1994; 37: 119–122

[166] Pollanen MS, Deck JH, Blenkinsop B, Farkas EM. Fracture of temporal bone with exsanguination: pathology and mechanism. Can J Neurol Sci 1992; 19: 196–200

[167] Freeman J. Temporal bone fractures and cholesteatoma. Ann Otol Rhinol Laryngol 1983; 92: 558–560

[168] Bottrill ID. Post-traumatic cholesteatoma. J Laryngol Otol 1991; 105: 367–369

[169] Clark SK, Rees TS. Posttraumatic endolymphatic hydrops. Arch Otolaryngol 1977; 103: 725–726

[170] Golding-Wood DG, Williams HO, Brookes GB. Tegmental dehiscence and brain herniation into the middle ear cleft. J Laryngol Otol 1991; 105: 477–480

[171] Ramsden RT, Latif A, Lye RH, Dutton JEM. Endaural cerebral hernia. J Laryngol Otol 1985; 99: 643–651

[172] Kamerer DB, Caparosa RJ. Temporal bone encephalocele—diagnosis and treatment. Laryngoscope 1982; 92: 878–882

[173] Andrews JC, Canalis RF. Otogenic pneumocephalus. Laryngoscope 1986; 96: 521–528

[174] Tarlov IM, Mule J. Traumatic pneumocephalus associated with cerebrospinal otorrhea. Am J Roentgenol Radium Ther 1946; 56: 179–184

[175] Lunsford LD, Maroon JC, Sheptak PE, Albin MS. Subdural tension pneumocephalus. Report of two cases. J Neurosurg 1979; 50: 525–527

[176] Weissman JL, Curtin HD. Pneumolabyrinth: a computed tomographic sign of temporal bone fracture. Am J Otolaryngol 1992; 13: 113–114

[177] Betz BW, Wiener MD. Air in the temporomandibular joint fossa: CT sign of temporal bone fracture. Radiology 1991; 180: 463–466

[178] Engevall S, Fischer K. Dislocation of the mandibular condyle into the middle cranial fossa: review of the literature and report of a case. J Oral Maxillofac Surg 1992; 50: 524–527

[179] Avrahami E. CT of intact but nonfunctioning temporomandibular joints following temporal bone fracture. Neuroradiology 1994; 36: 142–143

[180] Roland JT, Jr, Hammerschlag PE, Lewis WS, Choi I, Berenstein A. Management of traumatic facial nerve paralysis with carotid artery cavernous sinus fistula. Eur Arch Otorhinolaryngol 1994; 251: 57–60

23 Hereditary Hearing Impairment

Matthew J. Provenzano and John H. Greinwald Jr.

23.1 Introduction

Few areas of medicine have been as dramatically affected by advances in molecular genetics as clinical otology and the diagnosis and management of patients with hereditary hearing impairment (HHI). Research has elucidated genes responsible for some of the most common forms of HHI; widely available laboratory assays can identify mutations in these genes. Traditional diagnostic testing, often uninformative, has been replaced with improved testing that can reveal the genetic basis of the hearing loss. This improved diagnostic ability has tremendous clinical relevance for the approximately 28 million Americans, nearly 1 to 6 per 1,000 live births, suffering from hearing impairment.[1] Furthermore, nearly 5% of children will have a demonstrable hearing loss by 18 years of age, with that incidence reaching 60% by age 70.[2] America's aging population and increasing prevalence of hearing loss requires more accurate, efficient, and cost-effective diagnosis and management of patients with hearing loss. This chapter illustrates how molecular medicine translates into the field of clinical otology, particularly the care of patients with HHI.

23.2 Basic Principles in Genetics

A meaningful discussion about the genetic mechanisms of HHI requires a review of some basic terminology. Genes, housed on 23 pairs of chromosomes, can be separated into three distinct regions: (1) the actual coding sequence(s) (called *exons*) that contain the information for synthesizing proteins; (2) interspersed (noncoding) DNA between these exons (called *introns*); and (3) regulatory regions of DNA before (*upstream*) and after (*downstream*) the exons. The upstream areas contain specific regions called *promoters* that bind regulatory proteins and serve as molecular switches that turn on *transcription* (messenger RNA [mRNA] production). The cellular mechanism then *translates* the mRNA into specific proteins that carry out the actual function of that gene.

Mutations of the DNA sequence can significantly alter *transcription* and *translation*. *Nonsense* mutations result in premature termination of DNA *transcription*; no mRNA or protein is synthesized. In contrast, *missense* mutations results in synthesis of a protein with an abnormal structure. In this case, the abnormal protein may not function properly, thereby contributing to a disease process.

Other relevant terminology can best be explained by discussing a specific example of genetic hearing impairment: Gap junction beta 2 (*GJB2*)-related HHI. (*GJB2*-related hearing loss is discussed in greater detail later in this chapter). *GJB2* refers to the specific gene located on chromosome 13 at a *locus* (position on the chromosome) designated 13q11; "13" refers to the 13th chromosome, with "q11" further specifying a position along the long arm of that chromosome. Every person carries two copies of the *GJB2* gene in every cell of the body. One copy (or *allele*) of the *GJB2* gene is inherited from the biological mother and the second from the biological father. Several variants of the *GJB2*

gene exist. If both alleles of the *GJB2* gene are identical, then the individual is *homozygous* at the *GJB2* locus. If the alleles are different, then the individual is *heterozygous* for *GJB2*. A person's *genotype* describes the genetic composition of an individual, whereas *phenotype* describes the person's physical characteristics. In the case of HHI, the patient's genotype (i.e., which alleles of the *GJB2* gene a person carries) largely determines the onset and degree of hearing impairment (i.e., the phenotype).

Each copy of our DNA (aka alleles) can function in a *dominant* or *recessive* manner depending on whether the presence of a single allele can determine the phenotype (dominant) or whether two copies are required to produce a phenotype (recessive). In most cases of *GJB2*-related hearing impairment, both copies of a person's *GJB2* gene need to be abnormal in order to cause a hearing impairment; this is a case of autosomal recessive inheritance. In other autosomal dominant processes, one abnormal copy of the gene, even in the presence of one normal allele, is sufficient to produce a phenotype. Dominant traits typically present in each generation, whereas recessive traits usually do not. A parent heterozygous for a dominant allele will pass it to an offspring 50% of the time regardless of the genotype of the other parent. In contrast, recessive traits require that both parents be either homozygous or heterozygous for that allele. There is a 25% chance that the offspring will receive a recessive allele from each heterozygous parent.

The phenomenon of *penetrance* complicates this simple, mendelian inheritance pattern. *Penetrance* describes the phenomenon whereby the same gene may manifest a variety of different phenotypes. In some autosomal dominant disorders, a patient may carry an abnormal gene but not display any physical abnormalities (incomplete penetrance). Furthermore, dominant disorders also can show *variable expressivity* whereby different family members who carry the same abnormal gene can present with different phenotypic manifestations. In the case of HHI, this might present as varying degrees of hearing impairment in family members all carrying the same genetic abnormality.

Sex-linked or X-linked traits demonstrate a different inheritance pattern due to males carrying only one X chromosome whereas females have two. For example, an X-linked recessive trait can lack phenotypic expression if carried in a heterozygous female. However, male offspring of this female would have a 50% chance of inheriting the gene. Expression of the gene would occur in the male child, given the lack of a second X chromosome. The female offspring of an X-linked female carrier has a 50% risk of also being a carrier. An affected male could not pass along the gene to his son as only the Y chromosome is transferred from male to male. This affected father, by passing along the affected X chromosome, would make his daughter a carrier.

Abnormalities that involve portions of or an entire nonsex chromosome, as opposed to individual genes, can also lead to phenotypic changes. Most chromosomal abnormalities result in clinical conditions with developmental delays and a spectrum of congenital anomalies. For instance, Trisomy 21 (Down syndrome) is caused by the presence of a complete third copy of chromosome 21. Sex chromosome duplication tends to be associated with milder phenotypes such as Klinefelter syndrome (47, XXY or XYY) or Turner syndrome (45 XO).

Perturbations in DNA packaging within the chromosomes can also lead to phenotypic abnormalities. DNA winds around protein bundles called histones. Chemical modifications to these histones determine the orientation of the DNA relative to the proteins. Tight DNA packaging prevents the transcription mechanisms from accessing the DNA, thereby preventing gene expression. A more relaxed orientation allows for transcription and eventual translation into a functioning protein. Additional modifications to the DNA itself, particularly placement of a methyl group on cytosine, can also prevent transcription. These changes in packaging and DNA orientation create a situation whereby phenotypic changes can occur in the context of a preserved DNA sequence; gene expression changes based on DNA availability and not DNA mutations. These changes to DNA packaging and gene expression, in the absence of genetic mutations, is called epigenetics. Evidence now demonstrates that these epigenetic modifications play important roles in various disease processes and may contribute to HHI.[3]

An exhaustive review of molecular genetics and its contribution to hearing impairment vastly exceeds the space limitations of this chapter. For further reading in these areas, the reader is referred to resources such as the Hereditary Hearing Loss Homepage (www.hereditaryhearingloss.org).

23.3 Autosomal Recessive Disorders

An autosomal recessive mode of inheritance pattern accounts for most genetic hearing disorders. Furthermore, for those hearing impairments presenting in childhood, roughly 80% will be inherited recessively. Approximately 80 to 90% of HHI is not associated with a specific syndrome. From a clinical perspective, this poses significant challenges in the evaluation and management of an otherwise healthy-appearing child presenting with sensorineural hearing impairment (SNHI). Although most children will not have any other anomalies, a thorough evaluation is necessary to identify syndromic patients that could require alternative evaluation and management pathways.

A common scenario is to identify an isolated child with SNHI in a family with no known history of HHI. The medical evaluation of such a patient requires methodical history taking, complete physical examination, ancillary testing, and genetic evaluation in order to differentiate nongenetic versus genetic causes of hearing impairment. The sections below describe different categories of autosomal recessive, autosomal dominant, sex-linked, mitochondrial mutations, and chromosomal abnormality-related and epigenetic perturbations leading to HHI. To further structure the discussion, each category is then subdivided into syndromic and nonsyndromic forms of HHI where appropriate.

23.3.1 Autosomal Recessive Nonsyndromic Hearing Impairment

Autosomal recessive nonsyndromic hearing impairment (ARN-SHI) is a genetically heterogeneous disorder. As an illustration,

41 loci for ARNSHI have already been reported. The nomenclature for these genetic loci uses the prefix DFNB; DFN indicates deafness, and B indicates an autosomal recessive mode of inheritance. In contrast, the prefix DFNA would indicate deafness transmitted in an autosomal dominant (A) fashion. To date, a large number of genes involved with ARNSHI have been identified (▶ Table 23.1); DFNB1 (the first autosomal recessive disorder) is responsible for 30 to 40% of all cases of ARNSHI.

DFNB1

Gap junction beta 2 (GJB2), located at the DFNB1 locus, encodes for a protein called Connexin 26.[4-7] Connexin 26 represents one of a family of gap junction proteins that form intercellular channels that allow low molecular weight molecules to travel from cell to cell. In the inner ear, Connexin 26 is one of several gap junction proteins expressed in the epithelia lining of the cochlea. It is likely involved in potassium recycling critical to hair cell function.

Although GJB2-related HHI has been identified in most regions of the world, certain ethnic backgrounds and populations display different rates of specific GJB2 mutations. For example, deletion of a guanine residue at nucleotide position 35 (35delG) is one of the most common mutations found in patients with ARNSHI and is particularly common in those of European descent. In contrast, a deletion of a thymine at position 167 (167delT) is much more common in Ashkenazi Jewish populations, whereas a 235delC mutation is more frequently identified in Asian patients.

Overall, DFNB1 is believed to cause 20% of all childhood HHI. The severity of hearing loss is directly proportional to the likelihood that DFNB1 mutations are responsible for the impairment. Among children with hearing thresholds greater than 70 dB, almost 40% will have DFNB1 mutations. The rate of DFNB1 mutations drops to 10 to 15% for those patients with less severe hearing loss. The high frequency of heterozygous carriers of deafness-causing GJB2 mutations in the Caucasian United States population, estimated at 1 in 40, further illustrates the clinical relevance of DFNB1. This high carrier rate, taken together with the relatively small gene size, makes genetic screening and molecular diagnosis of GJB2-related hearing loss extremely feasible and attractive.

Multiple mutations can also occur simultaneously on different chromosomes, a state known as double heterozygosity. Concomitant mutations in gap junction beta 6 (GJB6) and GJB2 demonstrate this phenomenon. A large deletion of the GJB6 upstream region has been found by itself to produce a severe hearing impairment phenotype.[8] However, the greater significance of GJB6 mutations may lie in the fact that as many as 10% of patients with ARNSHI and GJB2 mutation also carry a large deletion of GJB6. The co-localization of GJB2 and GJB6 to the same region of chromosome 13 may indicate that these genes share a common regulatory region. These various mutations demonstrate the importance of gap junction genes in HHI despite their function remaining somewhat nebulous.

Interestingly, work has demonstrated that specific GJB2 mutations correlate with the degree of hearing impairment.[9] As an example, patients with two nonsense mutations (biallelic nonsense mutations, e.g., 35delG/35delG) have an extremely high likelihood of ultimately demonstrating a bilateral severe to

Table 23.1 Genetic Defects Associated with Hearing Impairment

Gene (Protein)	Locus	Mode of Inheritance/Syndrome	Phenotype
CDH23 (cadherin 23)	DFNB12	ARNSHL	Sensorineural hearing loss (SNHL)
	Usher 1C	AR syndromic	Congenital hearing loss, retinitis pigmentosa, and variable vestibular areflexia
COCH (cochlin)	DFNA9	ADNSHL	Onset of hearing loss occurs between ages 20 to 30; profound at high frequencies, and displays variable progression to anacusis by ages 40 to 50; vestibular dysfunction is variable
COL2A1 (collagen 2A1) *COL11A2* (collagen11A2) *COL11A1* (collagen 11A1)	Stickler	AR syndromic	Ocular, Pierre Robin sequence, SNHL
COL4A3 (collagen4A3) *COL4A4* (collagen 4A3) *COL4A5* (collagen 4A5)	Alport	X-linked AR syndromic AD syndromic	Progressive, high-frequency, sensorineural deafness, nephritis
DDP (deafness/dystonia peptide)	DDP (previously called DFN1)	XL syndromic	Early-onset deafness with mental retardation in adulthood
DIAPH1 (diaphanous)	DFNA1	ASNSHL	Fully penetrant, nonsyndromic sensorineural progressive low-frequency hearing loss
EDNRB (endothelin receptor)	Waardenburg type 4	AD syndromic	Combined with Hirschsprung disease
EYA1 (eyes absent 1)	Branchio-otorenal (BOR)	AD syndromic	Hearing loss is usually stable; may be conductive, sensorineural, or mixed; 2% of children with profound deafness have BOR syndrome
GJB2 (connexin 26)	DFNA3	ADNSHL	Severe to profound SNHL
	DFNB1	ARNSHL	Stable mild to profound SNHL
GJB6 (connexin 30)	DFNA4	ARNSHL	Severe to profound SNHL
ICERE-1 (inversely correlated with estrogen receptor expression)	DFNA5	ADNSHL	Progressive hearing loss starting in the high frequencies
KVLQT1 (potassium-gated voltage channels) *KCNE1* (potassium channel, voltage-gated, risk-related subfamily, member 1	Jervell and Lange-Nielsen	AR syndromic	Severe to profound hearing loss, prolonged QT interval, syncope
MITF (microphthalmia associated transcription factor)	Waardenburg type 2	AD syndromic	Same as type I but without dystopia canthorum
MYO1A (myosin 1A)	DFNA48	ADNSHL	Bilateral moderate to severe hearing loss
MYO7A (myosin 7A)	DFNB2 DFNA11 Usher 1B	ARNSHL ADNSHL AR syndromic	Profound congenital deafness, vestibular areflexia, and progressive retinitis pigmentosa; flat audiogram at young ages and some progression at the high frequencies
MYO15 (Myosin 15)	DFNB3	ARNSHL	Profound deafness
NDP (Norrin)	Norrie	X-linked syndromic	Ocular symptoms (pseudotumor of the retina, retinal hyperplasia, hypoplasia, and necrosis of the inner layer of the retina, cataracts, phthisis bulbi, progressive SNHL, and mental retardation
OTOF (Otoferlin)	DFNB9	ARNSHL	Severe to profound SNHL
PAX3 (paired box gene 3)	Waardenburg type 1	AD syndromic	Pigmentary abnormalities of hair, iris, and skin (often white forelock and heterochromia iridis); sensorineural deafness, dystopia canthorum (lateral displacement of the inner canthus of each eye)
	Waardenburg type 3		Type 1 and upper limb abnormalities
POU3F4 (POU domain 3, transcription factor 4)	DFN 3	X-linked	Fixed stapes

Table 23.1 continued

Gene (Protein)	Locus	Mode of Inheritance/Syndrome	Phenotype
POU4F3 (POU domain 4, transcription factor 3)	DFNA15	ADNSHL	Progressive hearing loss
SLC26A4 (Pendrin)	DFNB4	ARNSHL	EVAS, Mondini, Goiter, SNHL
	Pendred	AR syndromic	
TCOF1 (Treacle)	Treacher Collins	AD syndromic	Coloboma of the lower eyelid, micrognathia, microtia, hypoplasia of the zygomatic arches, macrostomia, hearing loss
TECTA (α-Tectorin)	DFNA8/12 DFNB21	ADNSHL ARNSHL	Prelingual severe to profound sensorineural deafness
USH1C (USH1C)	DFNB21 Usher 1C	ARNSHL AR syndromic	Profound congenital deafness, vestibular areflexia, and progressive retinitis pigmentosa
USH2A (USH2A)	Usher 2A	AR syndromic	
tRNA$^{ser(UCN)}$	tRNA$^{ser(UCN)}$	Mitochondrial	Mild to severe, can be progressive
12rRNA	12rRNA	Mitochondrial	Mild to severe, usually associated with aminoglycoside exposure

ARSNHL, autosomal recessive sensorineural hearing loss; ADSNHL, autosomal dominant sensorineural hearing loss; AR syndromic, autosomal recessive syndromic; AD syndromic, autosomal dominant syndromic; EVAS, enlarged vestibular aqueduct syndrome.

Source: Data from Van Camp G, Smith RJH. Hereditary hearing loss homepage. For a more comprehensive and current list of genes related to nonsyndromic and common syndromic hearing impairment, refer to this website. Additional information about these genes can be obtained from the online mendelian inheritance in man website (http://www.ncbi.nlm.nih.gov/entrez/query.fcgi?db=omim).

profound hearing impairment. In contrast, patients with two missense mutations (e.g., M34T/M34T) are much more likely to demonstrate mild to moderate hearing impairment. These prognostic factors carry tremendous relevance for those patients identified through universal newborn hearing screening programs. Management for these hearing-impaired newborns will be dictated in part by their hearing prognosis. Strategies seek to maximize the infant's hearing and language skill development and to take advantage of early windows of opportunity; this may include cochlear implantation at 12 months of age for severely impaired children. By obtaining *GJB2* genotyping shortly after confirming a hearing impairment, clinicians can identify those infants likely to demonstrate severe-to-profound hearing impairments. These children may require earlier and more intense interventions to reach their full communicational potential.

Detection of specific genetic mutations responsible for HHI presents a clinically useful and necessary first step in translating molecular genetics to patient care. Published data demonstrate how molecular information can be incorporated into clinical practice in order to improve diagnosis and cost-effectiveness.[10] For pediatric patients with ARNSHI and hearing thresholds greater than 60 dB, *GJB2* testing is recommended as the first line of evaluation. Hearing thresholds less than 60 dB should initially be evaluated by temporal bone computed tomography (CT), with *GJB2* reserved for those patients with nondiagnostic imaging. Newer high-throughput sequencing platforms are revolutionizing the evaluation of children with SNHI. For the example, the Otoseq™ platform can detect nearly 90% of the genetic causes of SNHI in a single test and will likely become the first line testing platform for all patients.

Otoferlin

Mutations to the gene *Otoferlin (OTOF)* also contribute to ARN-SHI.[11,12] *OTOF* mutations have been associated with a specific form of hearing impairment known as auditory neuropathy or auditory dyssynchrony (AD). AD is audiometrically characterized by an abnormal auditory brainstem response (ABR) with decreased waveforms but retained cochlear microphone. Preservation of otoacoustic emissions (OAEs) in these patients suggests intact outer hair cell function. These patients can have mild to profound hearing loss. It is estimated that 5 to 10% of patients with SNHI have AD. The optimal management of these patients remains challenging, as some do not benefit from traditional amplification or other assistive listening devices. Through an improved understanding of the molecular genetics and biology of AD, improved therapies may become apparent.

23.3.2 Autosomal Recessive Syndromic Hearing Impairment

Jervell and Lange-Nielsen Syndrome

Jervell and Lange-Nielsen (JLN) syndrome represents a rare but very significant form of syndromic HHI. Infants with JLN are typically identified with a severe-to-profound congenital hearing impairment. The patients also carry a significant risk for QT-interval prolongation that can cause episodes of syncope or sudden cardiac death. If properly identified, these infants' cardiac condition can be managed with beta-blockers. Accordingly, a clinician can detect a potentially life-threatening cardiac condition by obtaining an electrocardiogram on infants with severe-to-profound SNHI. Other patients with SNHI and unexplained seizures or a family history of syncope or sudden death should similarly be sent for an electrocardiogram and possible cardiologic evaluation. Genetically, some cases of JLN can be attributed to mutations of a potassium channel gene, *KVLQT1*.[13] Mutations of *KCNE1* have also been identified in some families with JLN,[14] indicating again that the causes of ARNSHI can be heterogeneous.

Pendred Syndrome and Enlarged Vestibular Aqueduct Syndrome

Although the association of goiter and SNHI have been known since the late 1800s, the molecular basis for Pendred syndrome (euthyroid goiter and SNHI)[15,16] was not elucidated until the 1990s.[17–19] The Pendred syndrome gene (*PDS*), also referred to as *SLC26A4* (solute carrier family 26, member 4), encodes for the anion transporter Pendrin protein. *PDS* mutations in patients with enlarged vestibular aqueduct syndrome (EVAS) have been reported to be identified in as many as 50% of some Asian EVAS populations.[20] In the United States, *PDS* mutations are found in approximately 5 to 10% of patients with EVAS. The hearing impairment in Pendred syndrome varies in both severity and age of onset. Some patients display a profound loss from birth, whereas others show later-onset SNHI of lesser severity. Diagnostic imaging studies routinely show cochlear hypoplasias (Mondini-type deformities) in concert with enlarged vestibular aqueducts. However, mutations of the *PDS* gene have been identified in some patients with isolated unilateral or bilateral enlarged vestibular aqueducts on CT imaging.[21]

Previously, the diagnostic test for Pendred syndrome was an abnormal perchlorate discharge test that identified iodine organification defects common in these patients. However, neither the sensitivity nor specificity for this assay has been definitively determined. Thyroid function testing for patients with suspected Pendred syndrome is still routinely recommended. Typically, goiter does not manifest until 8 years of age or later; exogenous thyroid hormone therapy is often the most appropriate therapy. Genetic testing for *PDS* mutations provides another manner for identifying these patients. Roughly 1 to 2% of patients with severe-to-profound hearing impairment can be attributed to *PDS* mutations. For families with the full Pendred phenotype (i.e., hearing impairment and euthyroid goiter), there is little evidence of genetic heterogeneity.

In comparison to classic Pendred syndrome, EVAS can also present with varying degrees of SNHI but without goiter. These patients typically present with a flat or down-sloping audiometric hearing loss pattern and either SNHI or mixed hearing impairment. The cause of a common low-frequency conductive hearing loss component is not known. Progressive hearing impairment, seen in roughly 25% of patients with EVAS, has been commonly associated with head trauma. Because of this phenomenon, patients should be counseled regarding the avoidance of specific activities or sports in which head trauma could be routinely anticipated. Approximately 5 to 10% of patients report vestibular symptoms. CT findings show either isolated enlargement of the vestibular aqueducts or incomplete partitioning of the cochlea. Genetically, these patients will have no mutations or one mutation in PDS. The latter likely represents an example of

digenic inheritance, as the phenotype is intermediary between patients with two mutations in PDS and those with none.[22]

Usher Syndrome

Usher syndrome, characterized by retinitis pigmentosa and hearing impairment, accounts for roughly half of the deaf and blind persons in the United States. Although Usher syndrome has been clinically recognized for over a century, only recently have the molecular genetic underpinnings for this disorder been identified. Linkage studies have shown this disorder to be genetically heterogeneous, with different genetic loci responsible for at least three clinically discrete subtypes of Usher syndrome. The severity and progression of the hearing impairment, in conjunction with the extent of vestibular system dysfunction, determine the different Usher subtypes.[23–26] Type 1 Usher's patients (USH1) display congenital profound SNHI and absent vestibular function. Usher type 2 (USH2) patients show moderate SNHI and normal vestibular function. Usher type 3 patients (USH3) have progressive hearing loss and variable degrees of vestibular dysfunction. Notably, USH3 has primarily been reported in Norwegian cohorts.

As reflected in ▶ Table 23.1, several different causative genes have been identified for USH1, and at least three have been confirmed for USH2. USH1 is most commonly the result of mutations in the Myosin VII gene (*MYO7A*), an unconventional myosin necessary for normal stereocilia formation and function in hair cells. Quite differently, USH2 is frequently caused by mutations of USH2A that encode for an extracellular matrix protein (usherin).[27] The exact function of USHA remains to be elucidated.

Patients with Usher syndrome require a multidisciplinary evaluation. An ophthalmologic consultation is requisite. Electroretinographic studies can reveal abnormalities in patients as early as the second or third year of life, earlier than funduscopic exams can reveal any lesions. Early diagnosis can impact the medical management of, and educational interventions for, an affected child.[28]

23.4 Autosomal Dominant Disorders

At least 20 genes have already been identified that can produce an autosomal dominant HHI. In addition, another 18 loci associated with autosomal dominant HHI have been mapped to specific chromosomal locations. As such, advances in molecular genetics have greatly enhanced our understanding of the causes and mechanisms of HHI. Autosomal dominant, nonsyndromic hearing impairment loci are designated DFNA followed by a number indicating the order of discovery of the genetic locus (e.g., DFNA1). Diagnosing an autosomal dominant HHI in patients with a classic dominant inheritance pattern and a distinct phenotype is fairly straightforward. However, variable expressivity (as described above) may lead to different affected members of the same family displaying different types of hearing impairment, making determination of the inheritance pattern difficult. Newer high-throughput platforms containing all the autosomal dominant genes will likely be able to diagnose most families with this pattern of inheritance.

23.4.1 Autosomal Dominant Nonsyndromic Hearing Impairment

The vast majority of patients with autosomal dominant nonsyndromic hearing impairments (ADNSHI) show progressive hearing impairment at around 20 to 30 years of age. Some forms of ADNSHI, such as DFNA10 and DFNA13, may not manifest until significantly older ages.[29,30] The degree of hearing loss progression and the audiometric pattern can be variable in ADNSHI. For example, almost all DFNA-associated hearing impairments are typically progressive but incomplete, with patients usually performing well with hearing aids/amplification. However, both DFNA3 and DFNA8/12 can be congenital in onset and stable. Rarely, ADNSHI progresses to profound deafness (i.e., DFNA1) and can requiring cochlear implantation.

▶ Table 23.1 presents summary data on genes and loci associated with ADNSHI. As noted with their autosomal recessive counterparts, the autosomal dominant genes are significantly heterogeneous. Some encode for voltage-gated potassium channels (KCNQ4, DNFA2), various Connexins (including Connexin 26, 30, and 31, which map to the DFNA2, DFNA11, and DFNB1 loci), Tecta (a tectorial membrane component), COL11A2 (a collagen gene responsible for DFNA13), transcription factors (for example, POU4F3, DFNA15), developmentally important genes (HDIA1, causing DFNA1), unconventional myosins (MYO7A, causing DFNA11, in addition to DFNB2 and USH1B) and structural binding proteins (e.g., COCH, DFNA9). Several DFNA loci represent novel genes with unknown functions (e.g., DFNA5).[31–36]

Some genes such as GJB2 or MYO7A can be either dominant or negative depending on the mutation. MYO7A mutations have been reported in Usher syndrome, DFNA11, and DFNB2. The molecular biology and mechanisms responsible for these genotype-phenotype correlations remain unclear.

Work on DFNA9 and the COCH also provide one of the first genes linked to vestibular disorders.[37] By examining the functions of COCH, investigators may be able to gain insight into the molecular processes causing this disorder.

23.4.2 Autosomal Dominant Syndromic Hearing Impairment

Melnick-Fraser or Branchio-Otorenal Syndrome

Characterized by anomalies of the branchial-derived structures, renal anomalies and hearing impairment, branchio-otorenal (BOR) syndrome has been reported to affect as many as 2% of children in schools for the deaf.[38] Phenotypically, the hearing impairment in BOR syndrome can be conductive due to abnormalities of the auricle, external auditory canal, or middle ear ossicles. However, SNHI or mixed hearing impairment is also seen and can be due to a spectrum of cochlear hypoplasias or dysplasias. Up to 40% of patients with BOR demonstrate cochlear abnormalities on high-resolution CT scanning. External ear defects can include ear pits, microtia, periauricular skin tags,

and appendages. Cervical cysts and sinuses due to branchial cleft anomalies similarly present in a highly variable fashion. The renal anomalies can be mild and asymptomatic or severe with agenesis and renal failure. The potential for significant renal comorbidities mandates that children with hearing impairment, ear anomalies, and branchial cleft lesions receive a complete renal evaluation.

Genotypically, BOR syndrome has been linked to mutations of the EYA1 gene on chromosome 8q13.[39] EYA1 is an evolutionarily conserved gene first identified in Drosophila as the eyeless gene. This gene appears to be specifically involved in morphogenesis of the ear, branchial structures, and kidney.[40,41] The criteria for BOR syndrome can be broken down into major and minor criteria; the diagnosis is based on the patient exhibiting three major criteria, two major and two minor criteria, or one major criteria and an affected first-degree relative.[42] Some genetic heterogeneity of BOR syndrome is suggested by the fact that only 15% of affected individuals show EYA1 mutations. However, this low rate of association could be a function of misdiagnosis of the BOR syndrome; more precise and rigorous criteria for clinically diagnosing BOR syndrome would greatly improve the accuracy of diagnosis. Using more stringent criteria for BOR syndrome, up to 40% of patients can be found to carry mutations of the EYA1 gene.

Neurofibromatosis

Two distinct forms of neurofibromatosis have been clinically and genetically defined: neurofibromatosis 1 (NF1, or classic neurofibromatosis), and neurofibromatosis 2 (NF2, or central neurofibromatosis). Although both forms of neurofibromatosis are associated with skin lesions (café-au-lait spots) and multiple neurofibromas, NF2 is distinguished by bilateral vestibular schwannomas. The molecular genetics of NF1 and NF2 highlight how seemingly similar clinical diseases sharing multiple features derive from very distinct genetic defects. The gene responsible for NF1 is caused by a neural growth factor, neurofibromin, that maps to chromosome 17q11.[43] In contrast, NF2 is caused by mutations of schwannomin, a classic tumor suppressor gene, located on chromosome 22q12.[44] Genetic data also highlight the critical importance of precise clinical diagnosis; clinical findings may make it difficult to distinguish between two diseases that appear clinically similar but are genetically diverse.

Neurofibromatosis 1, also referred to as von Recklinghausen disease, is a relatively common disease affecting roughly 1 in 3,000 persons per year. Diagnostic criteria for NF1 include multiple café-au-lait spots, cutaneous and plexiform neurofibromas, pseudarthrosis, Lisch nodules, and optic gliomas. Although not as common as skin lesions, central and peripheral nervous system neurofibromas do occur in NF1; these lesions can cause blindness, hearing impairment, and mental retardation. Hearing needs to be routinely monitored, as approximately 5% will develop vestibular schwannomas. Any changes in hearing would warrant diagnostic imaging such as gadolinium-enhanced magnetic resonance imaging (MRI) to rule out retrocochlear pathology.

Bilateral vestibular schwannomas are the hallmark feature of NF2. Although typically slow-growing lesions, these tumors can be detected as early as the second decade of life. Although tinnitus and vestibular symptoms can be identified in many young adults, these lesions may remain asymptomatic for years. The optimal method and timing of treatment remains controversial, as facial nerve function, hearing, and vestibular symptoms must be weighed against one another.[45,46] In addition to vestibular schwannomas, other central nervous system lesions need to be ruled out in patients with any neurologic symptoms or deficits.

For both NF1 and NF2, early diagnosis and counseling can greatly improve the overall management. Genetic testing for neurofibromin and schwannomin now provide objective data for prenatal counseling and asymptomatic family members at risk for NF1 or NF2.[47]

Otosclerosis

Typically presenting as a gradually progressive conductive hearing loss, otosclerosis appears to be inherited in an autosomal dominant manner with penetrance estimated between 25 and 40%. Mean age of onset for hearing impairment is in the third decade of life, with women being more frequently affected than men. Some authors have reported an exacerbation of hearing loss during pregnancy, prompting speculation that hormonal regulation or additional factors may modify the phenotypic manifestation of this disease.[48] Additional research has also identified measles virus particles in affected otosclerotic bone, suggesting a potential role for the viral genome in the pathogenesis of otosclerosis.[49] However, others have disputed this finding.[48] Pathological examination of otosclerotic temporal bones reveals replacement of normal bone in the middle and inner ear by otosclerotic bone. This bony remodeling leads to stapes footplate fixation and subsequent progressive conductive hearing loss. If the otosclerotic process involves the cochlea, SNHI can develop.

As with many of the other HHI disorders discussed in this chapter, otosclerosis is a genetically heterogeneous disease with at least four different associated loci from mapping studies: OTSC1 (chromosome 15q26), OTSC2 (7q34–36), OTSC3 (6p21–22), and OTSC4 (3q22–24).[49–53]

Stickler Syndrome

In addition to SNHI or a mixed sensorineural and conductive hearing impairment, individuals affected by Stickler syndrome may demonstrate a number of non-otolaryngological ailments. These include hypermobility and enlargement of joints associated with early-onset arthritis, severe near-sightedness possibly leading to retinal detachment, cataracts, Robin sequence–like facial dysmorphology, and spondyloepiphyseal dysplasia. Approximately 80% of individuals have impaired hearing, with 15% overall showing a progressive pattern.

Likely due to genetic heterogeneity with variable expressivity, three different types of Stickler syndrome have been identified. Stickler syndrome type 1 (STL1) is the classically described syndrome associated with mutations of the collagen 2A1 (CO-L2A1) gene. The STL1 phenotype includes cleft palate, midface hypoplasia, progressive myopia, vitreoretinal degeneration, variable degrees of hearing loss, joint degeneration, abnormal epiphyseal development, and irregularities of the vertebral bodies.

Different mutations of COL2A1 can result in more severe disease associated with progressive SNHI (e.g., Kniest syndrome and spondyloepiphyseal dysplasia congenita).[54] Stickler syndrome type 2 (STL2) is caused by mutations of a different collagen gene (COL11A1) but manifests with the same craniofacial and hearing abnormalities as those seen in STL1. Stickler syndrome type 3 (STL3) is caused by mutations in the COL11A2 gene and results in a slightly milder form of the syndrome largely lacking the ophthalmologic abnormalities. Patients with STL3 typically demonstrate palatal and joint abnormalities but rarely have near-sightedness or vitreoretinal degeneration. Gene expression patterns help explain the differences between STL3 and STL1/2 phenotypes. All of the organs affected in STL1 and STL2 express the two collagen genes (COL2A1 and COL11A1). In contrast, STL3 is caused by mutations of COL11A2, which is not expressed in the vitreous,[54] explaining the lack of ophthalmologic symptoms.

Treacher Collins Syndrome (Mandibulofacial Dysostosis)

Treacher Collins syndrome involves abnormalities of the jaw, face, and ears. There is significant variability in the phenotype. Bilateral microtia and aural atresia are common. Approximately 30% of children with Treacher Collins demonstrate ossicular abnormalities that contribute to the conductive hearing loss. Individuals may demonstrate either pure conductive hearing loss or mixed hearing loss due to inner ear malformations. The degree of SNHI, ranging from mild to severe, largely depends on the degree of inner ear dysplasia. Although defects of vestibular apparatus can also be noted on CT scanning, clinically significant vestibular disorders are rare. Hypoplastic zygomas result in the downward slanting palpebral fissures characteristic of Treacher Collins syndrome. Bilateral colobomas and a symmetric hypoplastic mandible are also commonly observed.

Many individuals affected by Treacher Collins syndrome demonstrate mutations of TCOF1. This gene is normally expressed during early craniofacial development. Although typically inherited in an autosomal dominant fashion, new mutations of TCOF1 are identified in as many as 60% of affected individuals.[55]

Waardenburg Syndrome

Waardenburg syndrome is classically described as hearing impairment, a white forelock, heterochromic iridis, dystopia canthorum, and synophrys. However, Waardenburg syndrome highlights the phenomenon of variable expressivity in hereditary disorders. For example, pigmentary abnormalities traditionally associated with Waardenburg syndrome include the white forelock, heterochromic iridis, premature graying, and vitiligo. Yet only 20 to 30% of individuals affected by Waardenburg syndrome demonstrate a white forelock, with variable age of initial onset. Similar variability also occurs for the craniofacial features.

Although variability makes clinical phenotyping challenging, studies have established a number of different types of Waardenburg syndrome.[56] Waardenburg syndrome 1 (WS1) is distinguished from WS2 by the presence of dystopia canthorum (absent in WS2). Hearing loss also differentiates WS1 and WS2. Although more than half of WS2 patients demonstrate SNHI, only about 20% of WS1 patients do so. Interestingly, enlarged vestibular aqueducts have been reported in as many as 50% of Waardenburg patients.[57] WS3 and WS4 occur far less frequently than WS1 and WS2. WS3, also referred to as Klein-Waardenburg syndrome, is characterized by bony malformations of the hands and forearms in addition to the abnormalities seen in WS1. WS4, also referred to as Waardenburg-Shah syndrome, can be distinguished by its association with Hirschsprung disease; it has either an autosomal recessive or autosomal dominant transmission pattern.

The phenotypic variability of Waardenburg syndrome speaks to the diversity of associated genetic mutations. Pax3, MITF, EDNRB, and EDN3 mutations have all been reported in Waardenburg syndrome. However, the vast majority of cases of WS1 are associated with mutations of the *PAX3* gene located on 2q37. A critical regulator of face and inner ear morphogenesis, *PAX3* has been extensively studied. Mouse models carrying a targeted mutation of *PAX3* result in a phenotype with pigmentary and eye abnormalities similar to the WS phenotype.[58,59] Interestingly, hearing loss is not observed in these mice unless they are homozygous for *PAX3* mutations. In contrast, WS2 has been associated with mutation of the microphthalmia associated transcription factor (MITF) in up to 20% of individuals.[60] A novel mutation of SNAI2[57] has also been identified as causative. Studies have demonstrated that MITF can potentially activate the promoter of SNAI2, thereby providing a mechanism by which both genes produce a similar phenotype. WS3 has also been associated with *PAX3* mutations whereas endothelin-B receptor (EDNRB) and endothelin-3 (EDN3) mutations are associated with WS4.[58,61,62]

23.5 Sex-Linked Disorders

Sex-linked HHI accounts for 1 to 2% of all cases. However, due to the nature of X-linked disorders, up to 5% of nonsyndromic profound SNHI in males can be attributed to sex-linked disorders. To date, no genes on the Y chromosome have been implicated in hearing loss. Accordingly, the following discussion focuses solely on X-linked conditions.

23.5.1 Sex-Linked Nonsyndromic Hearing Impairment

Of the four loci identified on the X chromosome, the best studied is the DFN3 locus that encodes for the transcription factor POU3F4. The HHI observed in this syndrome is typically mixed and progressive in nature. Mutations of POU3F4 result in stapes fixation and are associated with an increased risk of perilymphatic gusher during stapes surgery.[63] Preoperative CT scanning demonstrating abnormal enlargement of the internal auditory canal or deficient bone at the base of the cochlea warrants conservative nonsurgical management of the conductive hearing loss in order to avoid a stapes "gusher" and profound hearing loss postoperatively.

23.5.2 Sex-Linked Syndromic Hearing Impairment

Norrie Syndrome

Norrie syndrome is a fairly rare neurodevelopmental disorder characterized by a rapidly progressive vision loss with exudative vitreoretinopathy and ocular degeneration that result in microphthalmia. Progressive SNHL begins between the ages of 20 and 30 years and affects almost one third of patients. In some families, progressive mental deterioration is also observed. Linkage studies have identified *NDP* as the gene responsible for Norrie syndrome. The gene product, norrin, is very similar to developmentally important transforming growth factor-β. Mutations of *NDP* alone can cause progressive mental retardation.[64,65] The variable neurocognitive deterioration seen in these patients may be explained by large deletions of the *NDP* region that include contiguous monoamine oxidase genes.

Otopalatodigital Syndrome

Hypertelorism, craniofacial defects of the supraorbital region, a flattened midface, small nose, and cleft palate are the typical head and neck manifestations of otopalatodigital syndrome. In addition, affected persons are short in stature. Additional features include very broad fingers and toes, digits of variable length, and extremely wide-spaced first and second toes. Associated ossicular abnormalities lead to a conductive hearing loss typically amenable to surgical reconstruction or amplification. Linkage studies have mapped the genetic locus to Xq28.[66]

Wildervanck Syndrome

Wildervanck syndrome has been described as fused cervical vertebrae, SNHI or a mixed hearing impairment, and abducens nerve palsy. Lack of lateral rectus function results in retraction of the eye on lateral gaze. This finding is commonly known as Duane retraction syndrome and is caused by abnormalities between the cranial nerves controlling extraocular movement and the brainstem. Hearing loss in Wildervanck syndrome is almost always seen in women, and suggests that the trait is possibly X-linked dominant or perhaps lethal in males. Isolated Duane retraction syndrome also carries a small risk of SNHI (approximately 10%).[67]

Alport Syndrome

Alport syndrome, the classic ear and kidney disorder, consists of progressive glomerulonephritis and progressive SNHI. Renal disease typically progresses to renal failure and can present with microhematuria as early as infancy. Males are affected much more severely than females. If not managed early and effectively, death can occur by the third decade due to uremia. Loss of hearing may not begin until the mid-20 s with a somewhat variable rate of progression. Up to 85% of cases are associated with mutations of the *COL4A5* gene.[68] However, mutation of an autosomal type 4 collagen gene can also produce a recessive form of Alport syndrome that also is more severe in males.

Deafness Dystonia Syndrome

This extremely rare disorder is a neurodegenerative syndrome originally described as a nonsyndromic disorder (DFN1). However, refined clinical evaluation of these individuals reveals a more accurate clinical syndrome composed of myopia, cortical blindness, dystonia, fractures, and cognitive deterioration along with progressive SNHI. Mutations of the *DDP* gene, hypothesized to be important in the process of mitochondrial protein transport, have been identified in individuals affected by deafness dystonia syndrome.[69,70]

23.6 Mitochondrial DNA Disorders

In discussing mitochondrial genetic disorders, it is important to highlight the significant differences between nuclear chromosomes and mitochondrial DNA. Mitochondria are intracellular organelles largely responsible for generating energy in the form of adenosine triphosphate (ATP). Uniquely, mitochondria contain their own relatively small circular loops of DNA approximately 16 kilobases (kb) in length. This small mitochondrial genome contains the genes for mitochondrial proteins required for oxidative phosphorylation and ATP generation. Each mitochondrion contains anywhere from two to 10 copies of this small genome. Spontaneous mutations are more common in mitochondrial genomes than the nuclear genome, possibly due to a less efficient DNA repair mechanism in mitochondria.

Mitochondrial genetics are also significantly different from nuclear genetics in that mitochondria are transmitted via the ovum and not the sperm. As a result, the entire mitochondrial genome transfers from mother to offspring. Furthermore, it is relevant to note that each cell may contain as many as several hundred mitochondria. If the mother is *homoplasmic* for a mitochondrial mutation, all of the offspring are affected and it is likely that all or most of the mitochondria carry DNA with a specific mutation. In contrast, if only a small percentage of the mitochondria carry abnormal genomes (*heteroplasmy*), the phenotype may be modified and different tissues within the same person can carry differing fractions of mutated mitochondria.

23.6.1 Mitochondrial Nonsyndromic Hearing Impairment

Several mitochondrial genetic mutations have recently been identified that result in nonsyndromic SNHI. Many of these mutations occur in genes encoding for a ribosomal RNA 12S component or for transfer RNA genes. Persons carrying these mutations typically show mild and occasionally progressive hearing impairment. Perhaps of greater significance, however, is work demonstrating that patients carrying certain mitochondrial DNA mutations are predisposed to aminoglycoside antibiotic–induced SNHI.[71] This finding carries important clinical relevance given that about 2% of the hearing-impaired population and 0.5% of the general population in the United States harbor mitochondrial mutations. Mutations at mitochondrial loci A1555G, 961, and 1494 have all been linked to aminoglycoside-induced hearing loss; A1555G is the most common.

To further highlight the clinical significance of mitochondrial genetic predisposition to aminoglycoside-induced hearing loss, it is worthwhile to examine the use of gentamicin in the neonatal populations. Approximately half the low birth weight infants are exposed to gentamicin at least once during their neonatal period. Almost all extremely low birth weight infants receive one or more courses of gentamicin. In these populations, the prevalence of predisposing mitochondrial DNA mutations may be 1 or 2%. Accordingly, screening high-risk infants for 12S rRNA mutations could potentially identify those likely to develop an irreversible SNHI.

The mechanism by which aminoglycosides and mitochondrial DNA mutations produce hearing loss has recently been elucidated to a greater extent. Aminoglycoside binds to the 16S rRNA of bacteria. Mutations of the human 12S rRNA result in a ribosomal RNA remarkably similar to the bacterial 16S rRNA, thereby making it amenable to binding with aminoglycoside antibiotics and subsequently causing ototoxicity.[72,73]

23.6.2 Mitochondrial Syndromic Hearing Impairment

Mitochondrial disorders are often marked by progressive neuromuscular degeneration with ataxia, likely resulting from deficient mitochondrial energy production in the affected muscles and neural tissues. Ophthalmoplegia and SNHI are also routinely seen in these syndromic mitochondrial disorders.

MELAS

The abbreviation MELAS refers to mitochondrial encephalopathy, lactic acidosis, and stroke. Clinical variability in this syndrome is common. SNHI occurs in roughly one third of patients, with other symptoms including intermittent vomiting, limb weakness, partial visual loss, seizures, headaches, diabetes, short stature, heart problems, and renal insufficiency. Mutations of a transfer RNA (tRNA) have been associated with this syndrome.[74]

MIDD

The abbreviation MIDD refers to maternally inherited diabetes and deafness. As in MELAS, mutations of the tRNA[lys] have been identified in patients with MIDD. Other large genetic deletions, insertions, and point mutations in a tRNA[glu] have been reported.[69,75]

Kearns-Sayre Syndrome

Kearns-Sayre syndrome (KSS) is characterized by ataxia, short stature, ophthalmoplegia, retinopathy, delayed puberty, and SNHI. Myopathy, encephalopathy, and cardiomyopathy are also frequently present. The syndrome has mitochondrial causes; point mutations and large gene rearrangements are often causative.[76]

MERRF

Myoclonic epilepsy with ragged red fibers (MERFF) is typified by epilepsy, ataxia, and SNHI. Some individuals develop optic atrophy as well. As with KSS, a number of genetic abnormalities are responsible for this disease. Various mutations affecting the gene *MTTK* tRNA[lys] have been associated with MERRF.[76]

23.7 Epigenetic Causes of Hearing Loss

Epigenetics encompasses a variety of chromatin modifications leading to changes in gene expression. Work has demonstrated that epigenetic modifications play important roles in a variety of biological processes. Embryology and development employ a number of epigenetic mechanisms. Malignancy formation and epigenetics have also been extensively studied. Given the importance of this molecular process, it seems logical that it would be involved with possible causes of hearing loss. However, epigenetic hearing loss has been studied much less than other causes. Despite the relative prematurity of this field, evidence demonstrates that epigenetics likely plays a direct or indirect role in the development of some forms of hearing loss.[3]

Many of the diseases discussed in this chapter may have epigenetic connections. Histone modifications and DNA methylation may be important in vestibular Schwannoma formation.[77] Stickler syndrome also has epigenetic connections. The collagen genes *COL2A1* and *COL11A1*, aside from harboring genetic mutations, also undergo certain histone modifications that change their expression patterns.[78] It is not currently known whether these modifications are as important in hearing loss development as their mutation counterparts. There is also evidence that some of the causes of hearing loss not discussed in this chapter may have an epigenetic connection. Beckwith-Wiedemann syndrome, a disease marked by multiple abnormalities including hearing loss, has been associated with an epigenetic imprinting error on the gene *KCNQ1OT1*.[79] Changes to DNA methylation have also been connected to facioscapulohumeral muscular dystrophy, another disorder associated with hearing loss.[80]

References

[1] Yoshinaga-Itano C, Sedey AL, Coulter DK, Mehl AL. Language of early- and later-identified children with hearing loss. Pediatrics 1998; 102: 1161–1171

[2] Lin FR, Thorpe R, Gordon-Salant S, Ferrucci L. Hearing loss prevalence and risk factors among older adults in the United States. J Gerontol A Biol Sci Med Sci 2011; 66: 582–590

[3] Provenzano MJ, Domann FE. A role for epigenetics in hearing: establishment and maintenance of auditory specific gene expression patterns. Hear Res 2007; 233: 1–13

[4] Rabionet R, Gasparini P, Estivill X. Molecular genetics of hearing impairment due to mutations in gap junction genes encoding beta connexins. Hum Mutat 2000; 16: 190–202

[5] Wilcox SA, Saunders K, Osborn AH et al. High frequency hearing loss correlated with mutations in the GJB2 gene. Hum Genet 2000; 106: 399–405

[6] Kelsell DP, Dunlop J, Stevens HP et al. Connexin 26 mutations in hereditary non-syndromic sensorineural deafness. Nature 1997; 387: 80–83

[7] Kelley PM, Harris DJ, Comer BC et al. Novel mutations in the connexin 26 gene (GJB2) that cause autosomal recessive (DFNB1) hearing loss. Am J Hum Genet 1998; 62: 792–799

[8] Del Castillo IM-PM, Moreno-Pelayo MA, Del Castillo FJ et al. Prevalence and evolutionary origins of the del(GJB6-D13S1830) mutation in the DFNB1 locus in hearing-impaired subjects: a multicenter study. Am J Hum Genet 2003; 73: 1452–1458

[9] Lim LH, Bradshaw JK, Guo Y et al. Genotypic and phenotypic correlations of DFNB1-related hearing impairment in the Midwestern United States. Arch Otolaryngol Head Neck Surg 2003; 129: 836–840

[10] Preciado DA, Lim LH, Cohen AP et al. A diagnostic paradigm for childhood idiopathic sensorineural hearing loss. Otolaryngol Head Neck Surg 2004; 131: 804–809

[11] Yasunaga S, Grati M, Cohen-Salmon M et al. A mutation in OTOF, encoding otoferlin, a FER-1-like protein, causes DFNB9, a nonsyndromic form of deafness. Nat Genet 1999; 21: 363–369

[12] Varga R, Kelley PM, Keats BJ et al. Non-syndromic recessive auditory neuropathy is the result of mutations in the otoferlin (OTOF) gene. J Med Genet 2003; 40: 45–50

[13] Neyroud N, Tesson F, Denjoy I et al. A novel mutation in the potassium channel gene KVLQT1 causes the Jervell and Lange-Nielsen cardioauditory syndrome. Nat Genet 1997; 15: 186–189

[14] Schulze-Bahr E, Wang Q, Wedekind H et al. KCNE1 mutations cause jervell and Lange-Nielsen syndrome. Nat Genet 1997; 17: 267–268

[15] Reardon W, OMahoney CF, Trembath R, Jan H, Phelps PD. Enlarged vestibular aqueduct: a radiological marker of pendred syndrome, and mutation of the PDS gene. QJM 2000; 93: 99–104

[16] Reardon W, Coffey R, Phelps PD et al. Pendred syndrome—100 years of underascertainment? QJM 1997; 90: 443–447

[17] Everett LA, Glaser B, Beck JC et al. Pendred syndrome is caused by mutations in a putative sulphate transporter gene (PDS). Nat Genet 1997; 17: 411–422

[18] Sheffield VC, Kraiem Z, Beck JC et al. Pendred syndrome maps to chromosome 7q21–34 and is caused by an intrinsic defect in thyroid iodine organification. Nat Genet 1996; 12: 424–426

[19] Usami S, Abe S, Weston MD, Shinkawa H, Van Camp G, Kimberling WJ. Non-syndromic hearing loss associated with enlarged vestibular aqueduct is caused by PDS mutations. Hum Genet 1999; 104: 188–192

[20] Wu CC, Chen PJ, Hsu CJ. Specificity of SLC26A4 mutations in the pathogenesis of inner ear malformations. Audiol Neurootol 2005; 10: 234–242

[21] Greinwald J, DeAlarcon A, Cohen A et al. Significance of unilateral enlarged vestibular aqueduct. Laryngoscope 2013; 123: 1537–1546

[22] Madden C, Halsted M, Meinzen-Derr J et al. The influence of mutations in the SLC26A4 gene on the temporal bone in a population with enlarged vestibular aqueduct. Arch Otolaryngol Head Neck Surg 2007; 133: 162–168

[23] Weil D, Blanchard S, Kaplan J et al. Defective myosin VIIA gene responsible for Usher syndrome type 1B. Nature 1995; 374: 60–61

[24] Smith RJ, Lee EC, Kimberling WJ et al. Localization of two genes for Usher syndrome type I to chromosome 11. Genomics 1992; 14: 995–1002

[25] Kimberling WJ, Weston MD, Möller C et al. Localization of Usher syndrome type II to chromosome 1q. Genomics 1990; 7: 245–249

[26] Chaïb H, Kaplan J, Gerber S et al. A newly identified locus for Usher syndrome type I, USH1E, maps to chromosome 21q21. Hum Mol Genet 1997; 6: 27–31

[27] Eudy JD, Weston MD, Yao S et al. Mutation of a gene encoding a protein with extracellular matrix motifs in Usher syndrome type IIa. Science 1998; 280: 1753–1757

[28] Russ SA, Dougherty D, Jagadish P. Accelerating evidence into practice for the benefit of children with early hearing loss. Pediatrics 2010; 126 Suppl 1: S7–S18

[29] McGuirt WT, Prasad SD, Griffith AJ et al. Mutations in COL11A2 cause nonsyndromic hearing loss (DFNA13). Nat Genet 1999; 23: 413–419

[30] O'Neill ME, Marietta J, Nishimura D et al. A gene for autosomal dominant late-onset progressive non-syndromic hearing loss, DFNA10, maps to chromosome 6. Hum Mol Genet 1996; 5: 853–856

[31] Kubisch C, Schroeder BC, Friedrich T et al. KCNQ4, a novel potassium channel expressed in sensory outer hair cells, is mutated in dominant deafness. Cell 1999; 96: 437–446

[32] Lynch ED, Lee MK, Morrow JE, Welcsh PL, León PE, King MC. Nonsyndromic deafness DFNA1 associated with mutation of a human homolog of the Drosophila gene diaphanous. Science 1997; 278: 1315–1318

[33] Govaerts PJ, De Ceulaer G, Daemers K et al. Clinical presentation of DFNA8-DFNA12. Adv Otorhinolaryngol 2002; 61: 60–65

[34] Verhoeven K, Van Camp G, Govaerts PJ et al. A gene for autosomal dominant nonsyndromic hearing loss (DFNA12) maps to chromosome 11q22–24. Am J Hum Genet 1997; 60: 1168–1173

[35] Vahava O, Morell R, Lynch ED et al. Mutation in transcription factor POU4F3 associated with inherited progressive hearing loss in humans. Science 1998; 279: 1950–1954

[36] Brown MR, Tomek MS, Van Laer L et al. A novel locus for autosomal dominant nonsyndromic hearing loss, DFNA13, maps to chromosome 6p. Am J Hum Genet 1997; 61: 924–927

[37] Usami S, Takahashi K, Yuge I et al. Mutations in the COCH gene are a frequent cause of autosomal dominant progressive cochleo-vestibular dysfunction, but not of Meniere's disease. Eur J Hum Genet 2003; 11: 744–748

[38] Chen A, Francis M, Ni L et al. Phenotypic manifestations of branchio-oto-renal syndrome. Am J Med Genet 1995; 58: 365–370

[39] Abdelhak S, Kalatzis V, Heilig R et al. A human homologue of the Drosophila eyes absent gene underlies branchio-oto-renal (BOR) syndrome and identifies a novel gene family. Nat Genet 1997; 15: 157–164

[40] Zou D, Silvius D, Fritzsch B, Xu PX. Eya1 and Six1 are essential for early steps of sensory neurogenesis in mammalian cranial placodes. Development 2004; 131: 5561–5572

[41] Kalatzis V, Sahly I, El-Amraoui A, Petit C. Eya1 expression in the developing ear and kidney: towards the understanding of the pathogenesis of Branchio-Oto-Renal (BOR) syndrome. Dev Dyn 1998; 213: 486–499

[42] Chang EH, Menezes M, Meyer NC et al. Branchio-oto-renal syndrome: the mutation spectrum in EYA1 and its phenotypic consequences. Hum Mutat 2004; 23: 582–589

[43] Skuse GR, Kosciolek BA, Rowley PT. Molecular genetic analysis of tumors in von Recklinghausen neurofibromatosis: loss of heterozygosity for chromosome 17. Genes Chromosomes Cancer 1989; 1: 36–41

[44] Wolff RK, Frazer KA, Jackler RK, Lanser MJ, Pitts LH, Cox DR. Analysis of chromosome 22 deletions in neurofibromatosis type 2-related tumors. Am J Hum Genet 1992; 51: 478–485

[45] Woodson EA, Dempewolf RD, Gubbels SP et al. Long-term hearing preservation after microsurgical excision of vestibular schwannoma. Otol Neurotol 2010; 31: 1144–1152

[46] Meyer TA, Canty PA, Wilkinson EP, Hansen MR, Rubinstein JT, Gantz BJ. Small acoustic neuromas: surgical outcomes versus observation or radiation. Otol Neurotol 2006; 27: 380–392

[47] Terzi YK, Oguzkan-Balci S, Anlar B, Aysun S, Guran S, Ayter S. Reproductive decisions after prenatal diagnosis in neurofibromatosis type 1: importance of genetic counseling. Genet Couns 2009; 20: 195–202

[48] Schrauwen I, Van Camp G. The etiology of otosclerosis: a combination of genes and environment. Laryngoscope 2010; 120: 1195–1202

[49] Niedermeyer HP, Arnold W. Otosclerosis: a measles virus associated inflammatory disease. Acta Otolaryngol 1995; 115: 300–303

[50] Van Den Bogaert K, De Leenheer EM, Chen W et al. A fifth locus for otosclerosis, OTSC5, maps to chromosome 3q22–24. J Med Genet 2004; 41: 450–453

[51] Van Den Bogaert K, Govaerts PJ, De Leenheer EM et al. Otosclerosis: a genetically heterogeneous disease involving at least three different genes. Bone 2002; 30: 624–630

[52] Van Den Bogaert K, Govaerts PJ, Schatteman I et al. A second gene for otosclerosis, OTSC2, maps to chromosome 7q34-36. Am J Hum Genet 2001; 68: 495–500

[53] Di Leva F, D'Adamo AP, Strollo L et al. Otosclerosis: exclusion of linkage to the OTSC1 and OTSC2 loci in four Italian families. Int J Audiol 2003; 42: 475–480

[54] Snead MP, Yates JR. Clinical and Molecular genetics of Stickler syndrome. J Med Genet 1999; 36: 353–359

[55] Conte C, D'Apice MR, Rinaldi F, Gambardella S, Sangiuolo F, Novelli G. Novel mutations of TCOF1 gene in European patients with Treacher Collins syndrome. BMC Med Genet 2011; 12: 125

[56] Pingault V, Ente D, Dastot-Le Moal F, Goossens M, Marlin S, Bondurand N. Review and update of mutations causing Waardenburg syndrome. Hum Mutat 2010; 31: 391–406

[57] Sánchez-Martín M, Rodríguez-García A, Pérez-Losada J, Sagrera A, Read AP, Sánchez-García I. SLUG (SNAI2) deletions in patients with Waardenburg disease. Hum Mol Genet 2002; 11: 3231–3236

[58] Hoth CF, Milunsky A, Lipsky N, Sheffer R, Clarren SK, Baldwin CT. Mutations in the paired domain of the human PAX3 gene cause Klein-Waardenburg syndrome (WS-III) as well as Waardenburg syndrome type I (WS-I). Am J Hum Genet 1993; 52: 455–462

[59] Tassabehji M, Read AP, Newton VE et al. Waardenburg's syndrome patients have mutations in the human homologue of the Pax-3 paired box gene. Nature 1992; 355: 635–636

[60] Hughes AE, Newton VE, Liu XZ, Read AP. A gene for Waardenburg syndrome type 2 maps close to the human homologue of the microphthalmia gene at chromosome 3p12-p14.1. Nat Genet 1994; 7: 509–512

[61] Edery P, Attié T, Amiel J et al. Mutation of the endothelin-3 gene in the Waardenburg-Hirschsprung disease (Shah-Waardenburg syndrome). Nat Genet 1996; 12: 442–444

[62] Attié T, Till M, Pelet A et al. Mutation of the endothelin-receptor B gene in Waardenburg-Hirschsprung disease. Hum Mol Genet 1995; 4: 2407–2409

[63] Schild C, Prera E, Lüblinghoff N, Arndt S, Aschendorff A, Birkenhäger R. Novel mutation in the homeobox domain of transcription factor POU3F4 associated with profound sensorineural hearing loss. Otol Neurotol 2011; 32: 690–694

[64] Berger W, Meindl A, van de Pol TJ et al. Isolation of a candidate gene for Norrie disease by positional cloning. Nat Genet 1992; 1: 199–203

[65] Chen ZY, Hendriks RW, Jobling MA et al. Isolation and characterization of a candidate gene for Norrie disease. Nat Genet 1992; 1: 204–208

[66] Robertson SP, Walsh S, Oldridge M, Gunn T, Becroft D, Wilkie AO. Linkage of otopalatodigital syndrome type 2 (OPD2) to distal Xq28: evidence for allelism with OPD1. Am J Hum Genet 2001; 69: 223–227

[67] Eisemann ML, Sharma GK. The Wildervanck syndrome: cervico-oculo-acoustic dysplasia. Otolaryngol Head Neck Surg (1979) 1979; 87: 892–897

[68] Barker DF, Hostikka SL, Zhou J et al. Identification of mutations in the COL4A5 collagen gene in Alport syndrome. Science 1990; 248: 1224–1227

[69] Jin H, May M, Tranebjaerg L et al. A novel X-linked gene, DDP, shows mutations in families with deafness (DFN-1), dystonia, mental deficiency and blindness. Nat Genet 1996; 14: 177–180

[70] Tranebjaerg L, Hamel BC, Gabreels FJ, Renier WO, Van Ghelue M. A de novo missense mutation in a critical domain of the X-linked DDP gene causes the typical deafness-dystonia-optic atrophy syndrome. Eur J Hum Genet 2000; 8: 464–467

[71] Bai YH, Ren CC, Gong XR, Meng LP. A maternal hereditary deafness pedigree of the A1555G mitochondrial mutation, causing aminoglycoside ototoxicity predisposition. J Laryngol Otol 2008; 122: 1037–1041

[72] Prezant TR, Agapian JV, Bohlman MC et al. Mitochondrial ribosomal RNA mutation associated with both antibiotic-induced and non-syndromic deafness. Nat Genet 1993; 4: 289–294

[73] Zhao H, Li R, Wang Q et al. Maternally inherited aminoglycoside-induced and nonsyndromic deafness is associated with the novel C1494T mutation in the mitochondrial 12S rRNA gene in a large Chinese family. Am J Hum Genet 2004; 74: 139–152

[74] Kaufmann P, Koga Y, Shanske S et al. Mitochondrial DNA and RNA processing in MELAS. Ann Neurol 1996; 40: 172–180

[75] van den Ouweland JM, Lemkes HH, Ruitenbeek W et al. Mutation in mitochondrial tRNA(Leu)(UUR) gene in a large pedigree with maternally transmitted type II diabetes mellitus and deafness. Nat Genet 1992; 1: 368–371

[76] Kokotas H, Petersen MB, Willems PJ. Mitochondrial deafness. Clin Genet 2007; 71: 379–391

[77] Lassaletta L, Bello MJ, Del Río L et al. DNA methylation of multiple genes in vestibular schwannoma: Relationship with clinical and radiological findings. Otol Neurotol 2006; 27: 1180–1185

[78] Wilkin DJ, Liberfarb R, Davis J et al. Rapid determination of COL2A1 mutations in individuals with Stickler syndrome: analysis of potential premature termination codons. Am J Med Genet 2000; 94: 141–148

[79] Chiesa N, De Crescenzo A, Mishra K et al. The KCNQ1OT1 imprinting control region and non-coding RNA: new properties derived from the study of Beckwith-Wiedemann syndrome and Silver-Russell syndrome cases. Hum Mol Genet 2012; 21: 10–25

[80] van Overveld PG, Lemmers RJ, Sandkuijl LA et al. Hypomethylation of D4Z4 in 4q-linked and non-4q-linked facioscapulohumeral muscular dystrophy. Nat Genet 2003; 35: 315–317

24 Nonhereditary Hearing Loss

Edwin M. Monsell and Eric L. Slattery

24.1 Introduction

Approximately 36 million adults in the United States have some degree of sensorineural hearing loss (SNHL).[1] The two most common causes of hearing loss are advanced age and exposure to toxic noise.

24.2 Presbycusis

Presbycusis refers to hearing impairment associated with aging. It commonly presents in the elderly patient with progressive, bilateral SNHL. Presbycusis results from a progressive loss of sensory hair cells and other changes in the auditory system. Because the human auditory system lacks the ability to regenerate these highly specialized structures, function declines. Differentiating the factors leading to presbycusis is difficult. Noise exposure, metabolic effects, toxic exposures, and genetics all likely contribute. Despite a varied etiology, presbycusis generally follows clinical patterns that are helpful in diagnosis and management. Hearing loss has been linked to depression and cognitive decline in the elderly as an independent risk factor[2,3]; however, it is less clear that amplification would prevent or reduce cognitive decline.[4]

24.2.1 Epidemiology

The prevalence of hearing loss increases with age. In the Framingham study, approximately 50% of male respondents aged 65 to 69 years reported some hearing loss. The report of hearing loss increased to 80% between the ages of 85 and 90 years.[5] This study also reported higher audiometric thresholds with increasing age, especially in high frequencies. It has been estimated that 10% of the general population has hearing loss severe enough to impair communication, increasing to 40% at age 65 years and above.[6] The 1999–2004 National Health and Nutritional Examination Survey (NHANES) data showed that 49% of Americans between the ages of 60 and 69 years had either a unilateral or bilateral pure-tone hearing threshold average (0.5, 1, 2, and 4 kHz) of 25 dB or greater.[7] In this same study, 77% of adults age 60 to 69 years had either a unilateral or bilateral pure-tone high-frequency threshold average (2, 3, and 6 kHz) of 25 dB or greater. Furthermore, the 2005–2006 cycle of the NHANES, which also incorporated audiometric data for individuals older than 70 years ($N = 717$), showed a 63% prevalence of SNHL of 25 dB or greater (mean of thresholds at 0.5, 1, 2, and 4 kHz) in the better ear.[8] The prevalence of SNHL is expected to increase as the United States population ages. About 20% of the U.S. population is expected to be older than 65 years of age by 2030.[9]

Hearing loss associated with aging is not expressed uniformly in the geriatric population. Men generally have greater prevalence and severity of hearing loss than women, especially in speech frequencies and in high frequencies.[5] Presbycusis usually reflects a gradual decline in hearing sensitivity, but is highly variable in its age of onset and rate of progression.

Among the 1,662 subjects in the Framingham cohort, word recognition declined more rapidly in men than in women and was poorer in men than in women at all ages.[5] Jerger et al[10] suggested that a "gender reversal" phenomenon may exist in that women exhibit poorer hearing below 1 kHz, whereas men seem to hear worse above 1 kHz as they age. The prevalence of presbycusis has been shown to vary with socioeconomic and ethnic background. African Americans have consistently been shown to have a lower incidence of hearing loss in the elderly population.[11,12] No mechanism for this effect has been confirmed.[13]

24.2.2 Etiology and Pathophysiology

Many factors have been implicated in the pathogenesis of presbycusis, including genetic predispositions, occupational exposures, diet, cardiovascular disease, smoking, alcohol abuse, and head trauma.[14–16] Although noise-induced hearing loss is often considered a separate entity from presbycusis, these classifications likely overlap in clinical practice, with noise exposure being another component in age-related hearing loss. Rosenhall et al[16] studied hearing levels at ages 70 to 85 years in a longitudinal study and found a weak correlation between hearing loss and smoking, alcohol abuse, and head trauma in men, and between hearing loss and intake of pharmaceutical agents (especially salicylates) in women. Gates et al[14] found a small but statistically significant association between SNHL and cardiovascular disease in the elderly that is greater for women than for men and more prevalent in low than in the high frequencies.

By examining histopathological specimens from patients with audiometric data, Schuknecht[17] identified four variants of presbycusis: sensory, neural, metabolic or strial, and conductive. In this original study, 11.9% of patients had sensory presbycusis, 30.7% had neural presbycusis, 34.6% had strial presbycusis, and 22.8% had conductive presbycusis. Schuknecht[18] later reported that 25% of all cases of presbycusis showed no specific histopathological correlates of hearing loss. He classified these as cases of indeterminate presbycusis. It has been postulated that the malfunction in these cases is caused by impairment of cochlear mechanics, altered biochemistry, or tissue changes that cannot be demonstrated by light microscopy.[19,20] A subclassification of seven types of presbycusis has been suggested, based in part on studies that attempted to relate histopathological findings and audiometric shapes. The seven types are sensory, neural, strial, cochlear conductive, indeterminate, central presbycusis, and middle ear aging. Probably each case includes a mixture of pathophysiological mechanisms. Pearlman[21] proposed a working clinical definition of "classic presbycusis" defined by the following: (1) bilaterally symmetric SNHL; (2) absent or partial recruitment; (3) a negative history for noise exposure; and (4) phonemic regression.[22] Not all cases of presbycusis will show these classic features.

Sensory Presbycusis

Sensory presbycusis is associated with a steeply down-sloping audiometric configuration beginning just above the speech frequencies, with slow deterioration of hearing sensitivity beginning in middle age.[23,24] This audiometric configuration is associated with degeneration of the organ of Corti. The lesion is often restricted to the mid-basal turn of the cochlea, has sharply defined boundaries, and may involve only the outer hair cells or both the outer and inner hair cells. A sensory lesion restricted to the outer hair cells causes up to a 50-dB threshold elevation for those frequencies having their tonotopic locus within the area of the lesion.[19] Advanced lesions show loss of supporting cells, further degeneration of hair cells, and replacement by epithelioid cells.[18,25,26] Sometimes mild sensory lesions occur at frequencies higher than the speech frequencies, and discrimination scores are well preserved.

Neural Presbycusis

In neural presbycusis, first-order neurons (spiral ganglion cells) are lost, often with preservation of sensory cells.[18,25,26] Although a severe sensory lesion that involves the sustentacular elements of the organ of Corti may be associated with retrograde degeneration of cochlear neurons,[19] neuronal degeneration does not necessarily further aggravate a sensory hearing loss, because the neural loss is obscured by the preexisting hair cell loss.[19] The typical audiometric pure-tone pattern in neural presbycusis is a down-sloping high-frequency configuration, relatively more flat than that seen in sensory presbycusis. Speech frequencies are affected, and there exists a decline in speech discrimination scores that is disproportionate to the degree of pure-tone hearing loss. Thus, neural presbycusis may be a cause of phonemic regression, that is, a decrease in speech understanding out of proportion to the pure-tone level of hearing loss. Histopathological studies showed that neurons are lost throughout the cochlea but more are lost in the basal turn.[18,27] In primary neuronal degeneration, word recognition scores are affected when the number of primary auditory neurons exceeds 50% of the neonatal normal level.[28]

Strial Presbycusis

Because the stria vascularis has no tonotopic organization, its atrophy affects thresholds at all frequencies equally, resulting in a flat audiometric shape. It has been suggested that strial atrophy results in degradation of endolymph.[19] Experimental animal data suggest a reduction of the endolymphatic potential in the presence of strial atrophy.[29,30] Speech discrimination scores are well preserved, often not declining until the pure-tone average exceeds 50 dB.[18] A flat audiometric configuration with good word recognition suggests the presence of strial atrophy as an isolated lesion.[31] The pattern of atrophy may be patchy or uniform, or may occur predominantly in the apical half of the cochlea. Large intracellular vacuoles, cystic structures, and/or basophilic deposits may be seen.[18,32] The volumetric loss of stria vascularis must exceed 30% before pure-tone thresholds are affected.[33]

Cochlear Conductive and Indeterminate Presbycusis

Cochlear conductive presbycusis refers to an age-related decrease in pure-tone sensitivity and word discrimination score

with no histopathological findings.[31] Hearing loss usually starts in midlife and progresses slowly. It has been proposed that this hearing loss results from excessive stiffness of the basilar membrane with impaired mechanical-electrical transduction of sound energy.[31] The greatest effect on hearing sensitivity would be expected to be at the basal end, where the basilar membrane is shortest. The resulting audiometric configuration would be a down-sloping linear pattern.

Frequency selectivity, which is important in the understanding of human speech, refers to the ability of the ear to discriminate between two simultaneously occurring sounds of different spectral composition. Using psychoacoustic tuning curves, Matschke[34] found that frequency selectivity mainly concerns frequencies above 2 kHz and is significantly impaired by progressive loss of outer hair cells in the basal parts of the cochlea in aging. Although pure-tone audiograms showed high-frequency hearing loss in midlife, frequency selectivity was not significantly disturbed before age 60.[34] Another study did not demonstrate a statistically significant correlation between speech discrimination and frequency selectivity.[35] These studies suggest that explanations of indeterminate presbycusis based on light microscopy may not be taking into account the contribution of central auditory factors to auditory disability. Contemporary immunohistological techniques may show abnormalities not detectable by ordinary light microscopy, for example, loss of ion channels within the stria vascularis, and might lower the percentage of cases classified as cochlear conductive or indeterminate presbycusis.[36]

Middle Ear Aging

Degenerative changes in the middle ear can also influence hearing in the elderly. Nixon et al[37] showed that a mean air–bone gap of 12 dB occurred in a group of elderly patients, typically at 2,000 to 4,000 Hz. They proposed that hearing loss resulted from loosening of the ligaments and articulations of the ossicles. Belal and Stewart[38] also demonstrated arthritis and ankylosis of the ossicles with aging in histopathological preparations. Aging ear canals lose some of their rigidity. The resulting collapse under the audiologist's headphones may result in a false air–bone gap. This phenomenon may be avoided by placing a short length of rigid plastic tubing in the external ear canal or by using insert earphones.

Central Presbycusis

Central presbycusis is the loss of auditory performance that reflects a progressive deterioration in the integrative and synthesizing functions of the central auditory nervous system.[39] Studies of central auditory deficits in aging populations have been confounded by the effects of aging on the auditory periphery.[40] Nonetheless, several studies suggested a strong relationship between hearing ability and central auditory function.[40–42] Clinical presentation of central effects include poor speech recognition when matched for peripheral sensitivity.[43,44] Temporal gap detection, often tested as the threshold of detecting the onset of two voices separated by a defined gap, often increases with age.[45] Data suggest that brainstem changes in glycinergic neurotransmission in the dorsal nuclei of the cochlear nucleus, along with alterations in γ-aminobutyric acid (GABA)-related neural function in the inferior colliculus, may play a role in decreased temporal processing of auditory information.[46,47]

24.2.3 Clinical Presentation and Diagnosis

Patients can be screened for hearing loss by the history, screening audiometry, or a validated questionnaire. Patients are more likely to report difficulty understanding speech than an inability to hear. Unilateral auditory complaints or the presence of other inner ear symptoms such as vertigo or aural fullness should be pursued with prompt investigation. Medical examination by a qualified physician and comprehensive audiometry are necessary to identify the type and cause of hearing loss. Common causes of hearing loss in the elderly include Ménière's disease, vestibular schwannomas and other tumors, chronic infection, noise exposure, otosclerosis, autoimmune inner ear disease, sudden hearing loss, and ototoxicity.

Paget disease of bone is an important treatable cause of hearing loss that occurs in the middle-aged and elderly.[48] A high-frequency sensory loss and a low-frequency air–bone gap are characteristic when the temporal bone is involved.[49,50] Treatment, which is associated with little or no morbidity, may stabilize the process,[51] although it is uncertain whether established pagetic hearing loss can be reversed. Patients may be screened for Paget disease with a test for serum alkaline phosphatase, and the diagnosis may be confirmed by high-resolution computed tomography (CT) imaging of the temporal bones.[52]

24.2.4 Management

The human inner ear lacks the ability to replace cells following loss, and currently no regenerative treatment exists.[53] There is no known medical or surgical treatment that is successful for true presbycusis. Due to this constraint, management of presbycusis focuses on prevention of further hearing loss along with rehabilitation. Prevention includes maintaining good cardiovascular health, given that hypertension, hyperlipidemia, and diabetes may be associated with more prevalent or severe age-related hearing loss.[36] Prevention also includes protection from noise exposure, which is discussed below.

Rehabilitation includes educating and counseling the patient. Education of family members and friends about strategies to maximize communication with the hearing-impaired individual can be of tremendous value. Simple measures such as maintaining face-to-face clear speaking is helpful. Being able to see a speaker's face helps with interpretation by facial expression and lip reading. Manipulating the environment to decrease competing sounds also increases speech recognition.

Amplification with hearing aids often is indicated once hearing thresholds show a moderate loss. Hearing aid technology has improved significantly in the last several decades. Multichannel digital technology has permitted the development of enhanced capabilities for noise reduction, compression, speech clarity, and localization. Modern hearing aids offer the option of improved connectivity with telephones, MP3 players, and specially equipped public venues. When optimal amplification is inadequate for speech comprehension in everyday life, cochlear implantation may be indicated.

24.3 Noise-Induced Hearing Loss

Exposure to noise is a common and well-characterized etiology for SNHL in industrialized societies. Despite higher awareness and better compliance with protection from noise, millions of people continue to suffer from this avoidable source of hearing loss, and many more are at risk. Acoustic trauma is distinguished from noise-induced hearing loss (NIHL) as hearing loss caused by abrupt damage to the ear from intense sound, such as from close proximity to munitions or explosives.

24.3.1 Epidemiology

During and after the Second World War, many cases of NIHL came to light due to exposure to exploding munitions and the increased availability of audiometric testing. Epidemiological studies in the decades that followed helped define the extent of hearing loss, and led to the establishment of safety guidelines. In the United States in 1998 the National Institute of Occupational Safety and Health (NIOSH), which acts as an advisory board for the Occupational Safety and Health Administration (OSHA), estimated that toxic noise exposure is at least partly responsible for hearing loss in half of Americans with hearing loss.[54] Data cited in the 2006 NHANES survey found that 13% of 5,418 participants aged 20 to 69 displayed threshold shifts consistent with NIHL. Using these data, the NIDCD estimated as many as 26 million Americans have some hearing loss attributable to noise exposure, and approximately 10 million Americans have significant impairment due to NIHL.[55]

24.3.2 Etiology and Pathophysiology

Humans are particularly susceptible to NIHL from sound at frequencies in the audible spectrum. Since the 1960s, sound level meters have incorporated a weighting standard, called the A-network, which has a relationship of frequency to sound pressure level similar to an inversion of the human audibility curve; that is, the frequencies between 500 and 8,000 Hz receive the heaviest weighting. Such measurements reflect the relative risk that measured sounds could damage human hearing, and are expressed in dBA. Damage to human hearing may occur when one is subjected to 8-hour daily exposures of continuous sound at 85 dBA.[56]

It is accepted that higher sound intensities may be safe if the duration of exposure is shorter. Three-dBA and 5-dBA trading rules have been established by various professional and regulatory bodies. For example, with a 5-dBA trading rule, if 80 dBA is established as the acceptable level of sound exposure for an 8-hour work shift, 85 dBA would be acceptable for 4 hours, 90 dB for 2 hours, and 95 dBA for 1 hour.[54] OSHA has adopted a 5-dB trading rule.[57] Other groups support a more conservative trading rule.[58,59]

A noise-induced temporary threshold shift (TTS) is defined as the reversible increase in the threshold of audibility for an ear at a given frequency following exposure to noise. A true TTS must be distinguished from physiological phenomena of sensory adaptation, such as residual masking.[60] In experimental studies, a TTS is often measured 2 minutes after cessation of the noise, with most TTS resolved by 15 minutes after exposure.[61] OSHA requires hearing conservation programs to test hearing sensitivity at least 14 hours after exposure to noise to establish a worker's baseline hearing levels.[57] Loss of hearing following this reversible period of the TTS is termed a permanent threshold shift (PTS).

Permanent threshold shift was studied in detail by Passchier-Vermeer, who followed patients after 10 years of noise exposure.[62] Data were corrected for presbycusis. No PTS was seen for noise exposure of 80 dB or less in an 8-hour day. Noise of 85 dB produced 10 dB PTS at 4,000 Hz; 90-dB noise produced a 20-dB shift at 4,000 Hz, but none in the speech range (500, 1,000, and 2,000 Hz). Noise intensity greater than 90 dB produced shifts greater than 20 dB, including the speech range.[62] Laboratory and field studies have resulted in the development of tables that predict levels of noise-induced PTS.[62]

Numerous histopathological studies examining acoustic effects on the inner ear have shown that various cells are damaged from noise exposure. Early studies, reviewed by Saunders et al,[63] showed that hair cells (outer hair cells being more susceptible than inner hair cells) and spiral ganglion cells were lost with PTS, and that ultrastructural damage (e.g., damage to the stereocilia of outer hair cells) without cell loss occurred even when only a TTS occurred from sound exposure. When a TTS occurs, this damage is repaired. With PTS, loss of hair cells appears both in the expected tonotopic area of the basilar membrane correlating to the frequency of noise exposure, but also at the most basal (high frequency) area or "hook" region of the cochlea.[64,65] Behavioral and audiometric data correlate with this upward frequency shift of hair cell loss from noise. Cells not directly related to mechanotransduction (supporting cell, fibrocytes of the spiral ligament, and cells in the stria vascularis) are also damaged by noise exposure.[66]

Damage from noise exposure appears to occur at least in part by oxidative metabolic stress.[67–69] Increased metabolic demand is thought to increase the oxidative environment by ischemia followed by reperfusion and production of mitochondrial free radicals.[70,71] A variety of oxidative species have been described after noise exposure.[72,73]

Synaptic uncoupling between inner hair cells and afferent neurons has also been demonstrated with noise exposure.[74,75] Excitotoxicity of afferent from glutamate excess release from inner hair cells with noise exposure has been hypothesized as the mechanism for synaptic damage, with glutaminergic analogues causing synaptic loss in guinea pigs.[76,77] From these pharmacologically induced toxicity studies it appeared that synapses reformed after the glutaminergic excitotoxicity. Studies of synaptic loss following noise exposure in mice and guinea pigs showed that synapses were reduced considerably without much new synapse formation, even with TTS.[78]

Heat stress, mild noise, and hypoxia ("preconditioning") have been shown to reduce inner ear damage caused by noise exposure.[79–81] Administration to mice of low doses of kanamycin, an ototoxic aminoglycoside, prior to noise exposure also appears to decrease inner ear damage.[82] The mechanisms of protection are unknown, although an increase of blood flow, heat shock proteins, antioxidants, and glucocorticoids have all been hypothesized to be responsible. The understanding of this mechanism may lead to protective strategies in the future.

24.3.3 Clinical Presentation and Diagnosis

The diagnosis of NIHL follows from the clinical history and supportive audiometric data. The physical examination helps in excluding other causes of hearing loss. NIHL is usually bilaterally symmetrical, but asymmetries of up to 15 dB are not uncommon.[83] If asymmetric loss is present without a clear reason (e.g., left hearing loss with right-handed shooting of recreational, non-military weapons), other causes of asymmetric hearing loss should be considered. In pure NIHL, profound hearing loss is rare. Low-frequency thresholds are rarely higher than 40 dB, and high-frequency thresholds are rarely higher than 75 dB. NIHL does not progress after cessation of noise exposure.[83] After 15 years of continuous exposure, NIHL may continue to progress, but at a much slower rate.[56,84]

There may be several reasons why the 3- to 6-kHz region of the cochlea is most affected when the ear is exposed to high levels of broadband noise. The acoustic resonances of the ear canal and middle ear enhance the sensitivity to sounds from 1 to 4 kHz.[85] The acoustic reflex attenuates sound at frequencies below 2 kHz.[86] It is possible that mechanical forces may be stronger in the 3- to 6-kHz region due to the geometry of the cochlea, or that its blood supply may be more tenuous there.[25,87] The theory of special vulnerability of this region is supported by the fact that hearing loss in head trauma also affects this region preferentially.[56]

In evaluating claims for compensation for occupational hearing loss, it is necessary to confirm the presence of hearing loss, its magnitude, and possible etiologies, including functional hearing loss. It is essential to determine whether occupational noise exposure likely exceeded a time-weighted average of 80 to 85 dB. One must also allocate the proportion of hearing loss that may be attributed to presbycusis versus NIHL.[56,88]

24.3.4 Management

Because there is no effective treatment for established NIHL, the most effective management currently is avoidance. Environmental controls to minimize noise include reduction of noise at the source, reduction of noise transmitted through the building structure, and revision of work procedures to minimize duration of noise exposure.[89] If noise exposure is unavoidable, ear protectors may at least reduce the level of exposure.[89–91] If properly used, the most effective muffs and plugs may attenuate ambient sound by as much as 30 to 32 dB. Ear plugs designed to provide equal attenuation of sounds across the frequency spectrum ("musician's ear plugs") may allow workers to hear coworkers' speech while providing up to 20 to 25 dB of attenuation in noisy environments.

The Committee on Hearing and Equilibrium of the American Academy of Otolaryngology–Head and Neck Surgery (AAO-HNS) established guidelines for initiating a hearing conservation program.[89] These recommendations included difficulty communicating by speech in the presence of noise, the presence of tinnitus after working in noise for several hours, or a temporary loss of hearing that lasts for several hours after exposure to noise. NIHL has prompted the development of otologic referral criteria for workers exposed to industrial noise.[92–97] If hearing loss continues to progress despite appropriate measures, it may be necessary for the physician to recommend job reassignment.[59]

Audiological and medical referral criteria for occupational hearing conservation programs were established by the Medical Aspects of Noise Committee of the American Council of Otolaryngology.[98] Workers should be referred according to these criteria: if the average hearing level at 500, 1,000, 2,000, and 3,000 Hz is greater than 30 dB; if there is more than 15-dB difference in average hearing between the ears at 500, 1,000, and 2,000 Hz or more than 30 dB at 3,000, 4,000, and 6,000 Hz; if there is a change from previous audiograms of more than 15 dB in the speech range, 20 dB at 3,000 Hz, or 30 dB at 4,000 to 6,000 Hz; or if variable or inconsistent responses are measured.[99]

Medical criteria for referral include significant, persistent, or recurrent otologic symptoms.[98] The percentage hearing handicap is a binaural assessment that may be calculated using guidelines of the Committee on Hearing and Equilibrium of the AAO-HNS. The average of the hearing thresholds at 500, 1,000, 2,000, and 3,000 Hz should be calculated for each ear, and the percent impairment for each ear may be then calculated by multiplying by 1.5 the amount by which the above-average hearing threshold level exceeds 25 dB (up to a maximum of 92 dB). The hearing handicap may then be calculated by multiplying smaller percentage (better ear) by 5, adding this figure to the larger percentage, and dividing the total by 6.[99] This percentage hearing handicap can then be applied to statutes and rules pertaining to occupational hearing loss.[99–101]

Noise exposure may occur from motor vehicles, power tools, or firearms, during work or recreation. It is quite easy for portable headphone audio devices to exceed current OSHA recommendations for industrial noise exposure. Similarly, sound levels measured at popular music concerts often exceed 95 dB. TTSs have been measured frequently in conjunction with music players and concerts.[102–105] Nonetheless, guidelines for recreational sound exposure have not been established. Much needs to be done to communicate the risks of recreational noise exposure.

Clinicians have long been concerned about the risk of over-amplification by hearing aids. To ensure that NIHL does not occur from a hearing aid, the output levels from the aid must be such that they would not cause injury to a person with normal hearing.[106] This constraint may be difficult to satisfy for users with severe to profound SNHL. In these patients, some risk of hearing damage must be accepted in exchange for the advantage gained from the use of a hearing aid.[84,106]

24.3.5 Acoustic Trauma

Acoustic trauma is distinct from other forms of NIHL in that it refers to sudden mechanical disruption of auditory structures from bursts of intense acoustic energy (i.e., impulse noise). Because impulse pressure waves have a much faster rise time than the neural response in the auditory system, impulse sounds are seldom accurately perceived, and middle ear protective reflexes are ineffective. Sound intensity levels above 180 dB can rupture or produce hemorrhages within the human tympanic membrane or disrupt or fracture the ossicular chain.[107] Impact noise

greater than a 140-dB peak sound pressure level may result in a PTS from a single exposure. Some early models of cordless telephones incorporated the ringer into the receiver, resulting in cases of acoustic trauma. Because the noise source was in the low-frequency region, a low-frequency NIHL was produced. These devices have been redesigned to eliminate this risk.[108-110]

Antioxidants have long been thought to have promising chemoprotective properties by neutralizing reactive oxygen species produced by damaging the inner ear.[111] The most studied of these compounds is N-acetylcysteine, which has been shown to have protective effects both in animal models and in humans.[55] More studies elucidating dose, timing, and durability of the effect need to be performed.

24.4 Sudden Sensorineural Hearing Loss

Sudden sensorineural hearing loss (SSNHL) has been defined in one study as 30 dB or more SNHL occurring in at least three contiguous audiometric frequencies within 3 days or less.[112] Slower loss over more than 3 days usually is described as "rapidly progressive," slowly progressive, or stable.[113] SSNHL was first described by De Kleyn[114] in 1944. The etiology is often idiopathic, although other etiologies may be present in up to 15 to 30% of cases and should be investigated.[115] The weight of evidence is that early treatment may be beneficial. Thus, it is important that physicians in primary care and emergency facilities be aware of this diagnosis.

24.4.1 Epidemiology

It has been estimated that the incidence of sudden hearing loss occurs in approximately 5 to 20 of 100,000 persons per year.[116] SSNHL accounts for approximately 1% of all cases of SNHL.[117] The highest incidence of SSNHL occurs between the ages of 40 and 55 years, and has no gender predilection.[118–120] Bilateral loss occurs in about 5% of cases.[121]

24.4.2 Etiology and Clinical Presentation

A recent meta-analysis examining the etiology of SSNHL reviewing 23 studies reported that 71% of SSNHL was idiopathic.[115] Among the attributed causes 12.8% were infectious (usually defined by demonstrating seroconversion), 4.7% other otologic disease, 4.2% trauma, 2.8% vascular or hematologic, 2.3% neoplastic, and 2.2% other sources.

Although an infectious etiology, particularly viral, has long been thought to play a major role in SSNHL, objective evidence of acute damage of the inner ear from viral infection is lacking.[122] There is a 5 to 65% prevalence of previous viral illness in patients with sudden hearing loss.[123–126] Most studies examining etiology have focused on seroconversion rates in patients with SSNHL; there are no studies proving causality as defined by Koch postulates. In 1983 Wilson et al[126] found seroconversion to mumps, rubeola, varicella zoster, cytomegalovirus, and influenza B viruses in 63% of 122 patients with SSNHL and in 40% of controls. Perhaps the strongest evidence for viral etiology comes from identification of viruses in the inner ear using indirect immunofluorescence. Cytomegalovirus, mumps, and rubeola have been identified in inner ears of patients suffering from SSNHL.[127] The proposed mechanism of viral-induced damage is from either direct invasion of cells in the inner ear, with subsequent reactivation or by systemic inflammatory events.[128]

Other potential causes of SSNHL include neoplasm. Up to 1 to 10% of SSNHL has been described due to vestibular schwannoma, other cerebellopontine angle tumors, and leukemia with intracochlear hemorrhage.[129,130] Vascular phenomena such as embolic events have been hypothesized, although they are likely to be uncommon contributors given the high rate (up to 65%) of full or partial recovery.[119] Experimental data suggested irreversible damage to the inner ear following quite brief interruption or impairment of cochlear blood flow.[131] Furthermore, SSNHL is not more prevalent in the elderly or those with cardiovascular risk factors.[119] Connective tissue, which was observed in the cochlea after vascular occlusion in experimental models, is rarely seen in temporal bones examined histopathologically following SSNHL.[132–134] Although sudden breaks in the membranous labyrinth have been suggested to contribute to SSNHL, both clinical and histopathological studies do not support this as a common cause.[132,135] More recently, a stress response theory has been postulated, suggesting that an inflammatory cascade within the inner ear from cytokines and transcription factors leads to damage.[132]

Histopathological studies of temporal bones from individuals with SSNHL have demonstrated atrophy of the organ of Corti, stria vascularis, and tectorial membrane.[136,137] Changes were most often seen in the basal turn of the cochlea; however, in some specimens, all turns of the cochlea were involved. The degeneration of neural structures appeared significantly less than that in structures of the cochlea, with vascular channels appearing to be open in all specimens.

24.4.3 Clinical Presentation and Diagnosis

Sudden SNHL should be considered an otologic urgency. Usually the otoscopic examination is normal. Mild low-frequency losses have the best prognosis.[138] Spontaneous improvement is often followed by further recovery. The presence of vertigo is a poor prognostic finding, often corroborated by abnormal vestibular function testing.

Laboratory blood tests, including the fluorescent treponemal antibody-absorption (FTA-Abs) test, and tests seeking confirmation of autoimmunity, such as sedimentation rate, C-reactive protein, rheumatoid factor, and antinuclear antibody, are nearly always noncontributory. Serum heat shock protein 70 antibody has been shown to be higher in patients with SSNHL and may suggest an autoimmune etiology.[139] Magnetic resonance imaging studies of the head are important if trauma, tumor, or other central nervous system (CNS) causes are suspected, and to rule out vestibular schwannoma, even if hearing improves.

The natural history of SSNHL is highly variable. It has been estimated that 65% of patients with SSNHL spontaneously improve.[138] Because most spontaneous improvement occurs in the first 2 weeks after onset, the prognosis is worse the longer the symptoms last. Studies are prone to selection bias in that patients might not all be seen in the same stage of disease. In 15% of patients, the hearing loss progresses.[140]

24.4.4 Management

Sudden SNHL is usually treated with oral corticosteroids. This practice became established in 1980 following the report by Wilson et al,[141] who followed 33 patients treated with steroids in a randomized placebo-controlled study. Some received dexamethasone, 4.5 mg twice daily for 4 days, followed by a short tapering dose; others received methylprednisolone, 16 mg for 3 days, which was tapered for the next 8 days. Although the study design contained several flaws, preliminary results suggested that steroids had statistically significant benefits in the recovery of hearing in patients with moderate hearing losses. Moskowitz et al[142] confirmed the findings of Wilson et al in 36 patients treated with dexamethasone, 0.75 mg four times daily for 3 days, followed by a tapering dose during a total of 12 days. Conversely, Byl[116] found no treatment benefit in an 8-year prospective study of 225 patients with SNHL. A retrospective study examining 266 patients treated with steroids showed a significant improvement in patients with pure-tone averages greater than 60 dB, but no significant difference in the group with less than 60 dB pure-tone average.[143] The treatment that has been the most widely accepted is corticosteroids, such as prednisone, 1 mg/kg of lean body mass per day for 7 to 14 days.[144,145] If hearing levels improve and the medication is well tolerated, the course of treatment may be extended.

Intratympanic steroids have also been used. In a recent large randomized, controlled study, intratympanic methylprednisolone was given in four 40-mg doses over 2 weeks compared to oral prednisone 60 mg per day for 14 days with a 5-day tapering dose. In this study, intratympanic methylprednisone was not inferior to oral prednisone.[146] Thus, in patients with contraindications to systemic steroids, such as poorly controlled diabetes, intratympanic steroid treatment may be considered.

Four randomized controlled trials and numerous retrospective series were recently reviewed.[147] Most of the series had small numbers of subjects. They also had varying operational definitions of treatment success. Most studies reported some improvement in hearing levels, leading the authors to support the use of intratympanic steroids as salvage treatment.

A meta-analysis of six randomized controlled trials showed that hyperbaric oxygen treatment resulted in significantly increased hearing levels.[148] Good prognostic factors included early initiation of therapy and worse hearing levels at the time of treatment. A recent small randomized controlled trial comparing the combination of steroid and hyperbaric oxygen ($N = 36$) versus steroid therapy alone ($N = 21$) found no evidence favoring the combined therapy.[149] It should be noted that hyperbaric oxygen does not currently have a Food and Drug Administration (FDA)-approved indication in the United States, and is costly and time consuming. Up to 46% of patients treated will experience eustachian tube dysfunction, and 7% of patients treated will have clinically significant barotrauma.[147,150,151] Other studies have found no evidence for the use of antiviral therapy, vasoactive substances, or antioxidants, and, thus, these treatments are not supported by current clinical practice guidelines.[147,152]

Rehabilitation includes amplification, CROS (contralateral routing of signal), BiCROS (bilateral routing of signal), and bone conduction hearing devices, some of which are semi-implantable.

24.5 Ototoxicity

Ototoxicity is "the tendency of certain therapeutic agents and other chemical substances to cause functional impairment and cellular degeneration of the tissues of the inner ear, and especially of the end organs and neurons of the cochlear and vestibular divisions of the eighth cranial nerve."[153] Ototoxicity is distinguished from neurotoxicity, the process by which drugs and other substances may alter hearing or equilibrium by acting at the level of the brainstem or central connections of the cochlear and vestibular nuclei. Ototoxicity has been recognized since the late 1800s, when it was observed that quinine and acetylsalicylic acid (ASA) produced dizziness, tinnitus, and hearing loss. Since this time a number of drugs have been shown or suspected to have ototoxic potential (see box below). The auditory toxicity of aminoglycosides, cisplatin, loop diuretics, and salicylates will be discussed.

Ototoxic Medications

- Definite ototoxicity:
  - Aminoglycosides
  - Cisplatin/carboplatin
  - Loop diuretics (furosemide/ethacrynic acid)
  - Aspirin
  - Quinine
- Possible ototoxicity:
  - Vancomycin
  - Erythromycin
  - Vincristine

24.5.1 Aminoglycosides

The aminoglycosides are highly polar, polycationic compounds, predominantly 4,6-diglycosylated 2-deostreptamines. The first aminoglycoside, streptomycin, was isolated from the soil bacterium *Streptomyces*.[154] Later, another derivative, dihydrostreptomycin, was developed.[155] Other *Streptomyces*-derived aminoglycosides include kanamycin and tobramycin.[156] Gentamicin, the first aminoglycoside derived from *Micromonospora*, was isolated. The suffix "-micin"—spelled with the letter "i" instead of "y"—was used to denote this different origin.[157] Since then, numerous other aminoglycosides have been isolated, including the semisynthetic amikacin.[158]

The antibacterial activity of aminoglycosides results from binding to the 30S ribosomal subunit, resulting in inhibition of protein synthesis by the microbe. Activity is strongest against gram-negative and enterococcal species. As early as 1945, it was observed that 2 to 3 g/day of streptomycin would damage or destroy vestibular function in 2 to 4 weeks.[159,160] Dihydrostreptomycin was quickly abandoned in most parts of the world due to its cochleotoxicity.[155] Hearing loss has been reported as long as 5 months after discontinuation of dihydrostreptomycin,

and after a patient has received as little as 4 g total dose.[160] In industrialized nations aminoglycosides are seldom used except for treatment of resistant forms of tuberculosis (streptomycin) or severe gram-negative infections (gentamicin). Aminoglycosides are inexpensive to manufacture and have long shelf lives, so they are still widely used in third-world countries.

Pathophysiology

The highly polar nature of the aminoglycosides accounts for their water solubility, renal excretion, and difficulty with traversing plasma membranes passively. They must be transported actively or engulfed by pinocytosis to reach the interior of cells. Only 1 to 3% of the oral dose is absorbed. Aminoglycosides have very strong tissue-binding properties, and may be found in the urine of patients with normal renal function as long as 20 days after the cessation of therapy.[161] Animal experiments indicated that the serum half-life of aminoglycosides is approximately 80 minutes.[161] The concentration of aminoglycoside in the perilymph rose slowly, reaching its peak 2 to 5 hours after injection, at a level 3 to 5% of peak serum level.[162] The half-life of aminoglycoside in the perilymph occurred between 3 and 15 hours after parenteral administration.[161,162] Ototoxicity did not correlate with drug concentration in inner ear tissue or fluids, and inner ear fluid concentrations at no time exceeded serum levels.[163–166] Gentamicin was localized in hair cells for weeks to months after administration, even without electrophysiological signs of ototoxicity.[167] Ototoxicity did not correlate with nephrotoxicity; furthermore, damage to the auditory and vestibular systems occurred somewhat independently. In animals exposed to aminoglycosides the loss of hair cells of the organ of Corti was most severe in the basal turn of the cochlea and was progressively less severe toward the apex. The inner row of the outer hair cells was affected first, followed by the outer two rows with increased exposure to the drug. The inner hair cells and the rest of the organ of Corti were damaged only in cases of severe toxicity. Evidence of damage to other cochlear structures has also been noted, including the stria vascularis, spiral ligament, spiral prominence, outer sulcus, and Reissner's membrane.[160] Damage to auditory nerve fibers can occur secondary to the changes in the hair cells; however, ganglion cell bodies do not seem to be affected directly.[168,169] Histological and clinical cases of asymmetric and unilateral cochleotoxicity have been reported.[170]

Electrochemical studies of animal models of cochlear toxicity demonstrated that aminoglycosides produced a reduction in the endolymphatic potential and cationic content of endolymph.[171] Reductions of the levels of adenosine triphosphatase and succinic acid dehydrogenase were found in the stria vascularis and may affect the composition of endolymph.[172,173]

Animal studies of aminoglycoside toxicity suggested that type I hair cells of the crista ampullaris were damaged earlier than the type II cells. The summit of the crista appeared to be the area damaged first, followed by the sloping regions. The hair cells of the saccule appeared to be less sensitive to aminoglycoside toxicity than those of the utricle.[161] Loss of vestibular hair cells, type I more than type II, and vacuolization of the remaining hair cells, have been described in the cristae.[170,174] Hair cell loss and vacuolization have also been observed in the maculae of the utricle and saccule.[174]

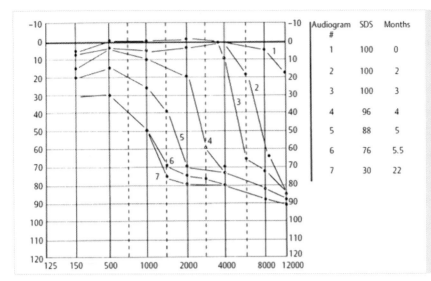

Fig. 24.1 A family of audiometric curves showing progressive hearing loss in a 41-year-old woman treated with amikacin for a life-threatening, disseminated atypical mycobacterial infection that was sensitive only to that drug. Treatment was stopped after 4 months, but the hearing loss continued to progress, with an eventual loss of speech discrimination score (SDS) to 30% at 22 months after the beginning of treatment. (Courtesy of Edwin M. Monsell, MD, PhD.)

Following delivery of aminoglycosides into the perilymph, evidence suggested that aminoglycosides entered hair cells through the mechanoelectrical transduction channels on stereocilia bundles.[175–177] Evidence implicated oxygen and nitrogen free radical species as the primary mechanism of permanent cellular injury in aminoglycoside ototoxicity.[178,179] Binding of aminoglycosides to ribosomal RNA in mitochondria of hair cells was hypothesized to cause uncoupling of the electron transport chain and free radical production.[180] Support for this hypothesis comes from observation of decreased function in gram-positive bacteria not normally susceptible to aminoglycosides with expression of the human A1555G ribosome mutation, known to cause increased ototoxicity.[181] Cell signaling, including mitogen-activated protein (MAP) kinases, has been shown to be involved in aminoglycoside damage. JNK, a MAP kinase, was activated. Inhibition of this pathway increased hair cell survival.[182] Interestingly, another MAP kinase, ERK1/2, was shown to be increased in supporting cells, and inhibition of this molecule showed increased hair cell survival.[183] Cell death occurred primarily by apoptosis and appeared to use the mitochondrially driven intrinsic apoptotic pathway.[184,185]

Clinical Presentation and Diagnosis

It has been estimated that ototoxicity due to aminoglycoside use ranges in prevalence from 2 to 15% of patients treated with systemic courses, with values of 2.4% for netilmicin, 6.1% for tobramycin, 8.6% for gentamicin, and 13.9% for amikacin in a survey of prospective studies.[186] The ototoxicity of gentamicin and amikacin were compared in a prospective study.[162] Drug dosages were modified to keep plasma levels within the recommended range. Cochlear toxicity was defined as a 15-dB or greater loss of pure-tone sensitivity at two or more frequencies in one or both ears. Vestibular toxicity was defined as a decrease of at least 50% in the peak slow-phase velocity after caloric stimulation. In the gentamicin-treated group, 7% of patients developed cochlear toxicity and 4% developed vestibular toxicity. Only half the patients in these categories were symptomatic at the time of testing. Unilateral toxicity, reversible losses, and onset of toxicity after discontinuation of the drug were all observed. In the amikacin-treated group, 9% of patients developed

cochlear toxicity and 6% developed vestibular toxicity. Less than half of the patients in either category were symptomatic when losses were determined.

Gentamicin and tobramycin were compared in a prospective study.[161] Toxicity was defined as SNHL of 20 dB or greater or reduction by 33% or more of slow-phase nystagmus velocity 90 seconds after irrigation. Cochlear toxicity developed in 16.4% of patients receiving gentamicin and in 15.3% of patients receiving tobramycin. High-frequency SNHL was demonstrated in this study similar to that observed by the authors (▶ Fig. 24.1).

Vestibular toxicity developed in 15.1% of patients receiving gentamicin and in 4.6% of patients receiving tobramycin. Decreased pure-tone sensitivity was unilateral in 91% of patients. Toxicity was first noted 3 to 35 days after the onset of therapy. Fifty-five percent of the patients recovered their loss of pure-tone sensitivity within 6 months. Nonrecovery was associated with hearing losses greater than 25 dB, delayed onset, immediate onset that progressed despite discontinuation of the drug, and continuation of the drug after the onset of toxicity. In cases of vestibular toxicity, the mean depression of slow-phase velocity was 45%. The mean time of appearance of vestibular toxicity was 11.5 days after the onset of treatment. Fifty-three percent of patients recovered within 9 months.[161] Most patients who developed cochlear or vestibular ototoxicity were asymptomatic. Less than 5% of patients reported any symptoms; these included decreased hearing, tinnitus, otalgia, and imbalance. Development of symptoms did not correlate well with measurable ototoxicity.[161]

Black et al[187] conducted a prospective study of amikacin ototoxicity in a group of 44 patients. Significant hearing loss was defined as a 15-dB or more loss of pure-tone sensitivity. Significant hearing loss was detected in 24% of the patients, half of whom had unilateral hearing loss. Audiometric recovery was documented in 23% of this group. Hearing loss occurred mostly in frequencies of 8 kHz or higher; however, in 25% of the patients frequencies as low as 2 kHz were involved. No patient complained of vertigo. Eighty-four percent of the patients who developed hearing loss were asymptomatic.

Although these three studies reported different rates of ototoxicity, they agreed on several points: (1) Aminoglycoside ototoxicity could be unilateral and reversible. (2) Aminoglycoside cochlear toxicity was not confined to frequencies above 8 kHz. (3) Most patients who developed measurable ototoxicity were asymptomatic at the time of discovery. (4) Gentamicin, previously thought to be primarily vestibulotoxic, also caused cochlear toxicity. (5) Gentamicin, tobramycin, and amikacin could cause ototoxicity after they were withdrawn (▶ Fig. 24.1).

Proposed risk factors for aminoglycoside-induced ototoxicity have included the type of aminoglycoside, concomitant exposure to other ototoxic drugs (loop diuretics, chemotherapeutic agents), noise exposure, duration of therapy, total dose, plasma level, perilymph level, age, sex, hepatic dysfunction, renal dysfunction, bacteremia, dehydration, and hyperthermia.[155] Fee's[161] series demonstrated three factors that were associated with increased risk of ototoxicity from gentamicin and tobramycin: duration of therapy greater than 10 days, decreased pure-tone sensitivity on the initial audiogram, and "severe illness." Risk factors included duration of therapy longer than 10 days, administration of greater than 15 g of amikacin, previous exposure to aminoglycosides, peak serum levels greater than 32 μg/mL, and trough levels greater than 10 μg/mL. Two large retrospective studies, which together included more than 5,000 patients, demonstrated the influence of previous aminoglycoside exposure and high daily doses.[188,189]

A familial tendency for increased aminoglycoside susceptibility to ototoxicity has been reported.[190] A mitochondrial mutation A1555G in the 12S rRNA gene was shown to be associated with this form of increased susceptibility.[191,192]

24.5.2 Cisplatin

Cisplatin (cis-diamminedichloroplatinum II) is a potent cell cycle agent used to treat a wide variety of solid tumors. Recognized side effects include ototoxicity, neurotoxicity, nephrotoxicity, gastrointestinal toxicity, and myelosuppression.[193] Most patients treated with cisplatin experience tinnitus, and many have symptomatic SNHL.[193–196] Carboplatin is less ototoxic than cisplatin.[197]

Pathophysiology

Animal studies demonstrated a loss of pure-tone auditory sensitivity initially in the high frequencies.[198] In both guinea pigs and rhesus monkeys, this loss was reversible in its early stages.[198–200] Histopathological examination of animal temporal bones after induction of cisplatin ototoxicity showed primarily a loss of outer hair cells in the cochlea. These changes were most pronounced in the region of the basal turn. Ultrastructural changes in the stria vascularis, affecting mostly the marginal cells, were reported.[201] In addition, collapse of the Reissner membrane in the basal turn was noted.[198] Clinical vestibular ototoxicity by cisplatin has not been confirmed to date, although cisplatin is clearly ototoxic to vestibular organs in culture.[202,203] Oxygen free radical species have been implicated in toxicity. Cisplatin has been shown to increase activation of NOX3 with subsequent production of reactive oxygen species.[204,205]

Cytokine release has been reported with auditory cell lines following exposure to cisplatin with inhibition leading to increased survival.[206] Platinated adducts, thought to induce

cisplatin's toxicity in tumor cells, were reported within cells of the inner ear, including hair cells and marginal cells.[207,208] Cell death occurred through apoptosis.[209]

Clinical Presentation

Tinnitus and high-frequency hearing loss are common symptoms associated with cisplatin ototoxicity. Early clinical studies suggested that cisplatin produced an irreversible, dose-related SNHL in the 4- to 8-kHz range in approximately 11% of patients.[194,195,210] In a prospective study of 32 patients receiving cisplatin, Reddel et al[196] found that 47% developed an SNHL of 15 dB or greater after receiving a mean cumulative dose of 203 mg/m². The incidence and degree of hearing loss increased with increasing cumulative doses of cisplatin. Although loss of pure-tone sensitivity initially was worse in the 6- to 8-kHz range, losses in the 3- to 4-kHz range became evident as cumulative doses increased. In other studies, patients followed 12 to 18 months after discovery of hearing loss did not show evidence of reversibility.[193] It was shown that up to 75 to 100% of patients treated with cisplatin have audiometric changes, but that these losses are not necessarily symptomatic.[211] Although children were observed to be less susceptible than adults to ototoxicity from aminoglycosides, they were found to be at higher risk for ototoxicity from cisplatin.[212] Bolus administration of cisplatin has been associated with significantly greater incidence of hearing loss than slow infusion over 2 hours.[195]

Instances of presumed vestibular toxicity, as evidenced by vertigo and disequilibrium, also have been reported in patients receiving cisplatin, though confirmation through vestibular testing has been inconclusive.[193,213] Symptoms of vestibular toxicity may be overlooked or minimized in debilitated cancer patients.

24.5.3 Loop Diuretics

Furosemide and ethacrynic acid are members of a family of drugs called "loop diuretics" because they produce diuresis by blocking reabsorption of sodium and chloride in the proximal renal tubule. Other members of this group include bumetanide, piretanide, azosemide, triflocin, and indapamide. These drugs are excreted almost entirely by the kidney. Furosemide is the most commonly used loop diuretic in the United States and is often used to treat congestive heart failure.

Pathophysiology

Animal experiments demonstrated that furosemide and ethacrynic acid produced a dose-related, reversible reduction in the endocochlear potential.[214,215] Intravenous furosemide increased the endolymphatic sodium concentration and decreased the potassium concentration.[215] Behavioral studies in guinea pigs confirmed that these changes correlated with temporary alterations in auditory sensitivity.[216] The renal target of furosemide is the Na-K-2Cl transporter, which has been shown to exist in the inner ear. Inactivation of the transporter caused hearing loss and a decrease in endolymph production.[217]

Histological changes observed in animal temporal bones were mostly in the stria vascularis, and included intercellular edema, capillary narrowing, and degeneration of the intermediate cell layer.[214,216,218] Degenerative changes of the outer hair cells, primarily in the basal turn, were also observed, but less consistently.[160,215] Degeneration of both type I and type II hair cells in the ampullae and maculae of the vestibular labyrinth were reported.[219]

Clinical Presentation

Ethacrynic acid and furosemide produced transient or permanent hearing loss following either oral or intravenous administration.[215,220] Reversible hearing loss appeared to be more common.[221] When reversible, hearing loss generally recovered within 30 minutes to 54 hours.[221] Reversible tinnitus and vertigo also were reported after administration of loop diuretics.[215] Clinical studies also suggested that rapid intravenous infusion of furosemide increased the incidence of ototoxicity.[218]

Patients at greatest risk for loop diuretic ototoxicity were those with renal compromise, possibly those receiving aminoglycoside antibiotics, and premature infants.[218,221] Because loop diuretics are eliminated by glomerular filtration, renal impairment prolongs the serum half-life. This increase in serum half-life may permit elevation of perilymph concentration of these drugs, thereby increasing their ototoxicity.[221]

24.5.4 Salicylates and Quinine

The ototoxic potential of acetylsalicylic acid (ASA) has been recognized at least since 1899, when it was first used to treat rheumatic fever.[220] Before it was possible to measure serum drug levels, hearing loss, tinnitus, and vertigo were used to establish the dosage of ASA used in the treatment of gout and rheumatic fever.[222]

Pathophysiology

Acetylsalicylic Acid

Usually no unequivocal histopathological abnormalities are found in ASA ototoxicity; biochemical abnormalities are suspected.[222–226] Recent studies have pointed to the importance of subcisternal organelles in outer hair cells in the active cochlear amplifier and in outer hair cell motility. They demonstrated the reversible disruption of this mechanism by ASA. A recent study provided evidence that high-dose salicylates may cause tinnitus through activation of postsynaptic N-methyl-D-aspartate (NMDA) receptors.[227]

Quinine

Quinine is an alkaloid compound derived from the bark of the cinchona tree, native to certain parts of South America.[221] Its traditional use was to treat malaria. It has largely been replaced by less toxic synthetic drugs. Quinine also is employed in the treatment of nocturnal leg cramping. Quinidine, its stereoisomer, sometimes is used in the treatment of cardiac arrhythmias.[220] The cinchona alkaloids are eliminated primarily by hepatic degradation and eliminated by glomerular filtration. Plasma levels fall rapidly upon termination of therapy, and only negligible concentrations can be detected after 24 hours.

Animal Experiments

Animal experiments have demonstrated capillary constriction in the stria vascularis, suprastrial ligament, tympanic lip, and basilar membrane of the guinea pigs' temporal bones following the induction of cochlear toxicity with quinine.[153] Atrophy of the stria vascularis with decreased cellularity and vacuolization were observed as well as degenerative changes of the organ of Corti.[228]

Clinical Presentation

Hearing loss and tinnitus are two symptoms most commonly associated with salicylate ototoxicity. Both appear reversible; recovery usually occurs after 24 to 72 hours.[226] Doses above 4 g per day of aspirin are associated with either a flat or high-frequency SNHL of up to 40 dB.[222,229] Patients receiving high doses of quinine (approximately 2 g/day), or a single dose in cases of hypersensitivity, may develop a toxicity syndrome known as cinchonism: tinnitus, decreased hearing, vertigo, headache, nausea, and disturbed vision.[220] These symptoms generally resolve rapidly upon withdrawal of the drug; however, cases of irreversible hearing loss and tinnitus have been reported.[153]

24.5.5 Management of Ototoxicity

Because a uniform method of monitoring for all drugs is not reasonable or practical, we suggest that monitoring for ototoxicity be individualized to the patient and the drug. During monitoring of cochlear function, particular attention should be paid to pure-tone thresholds at 4 kHz and above, because a decrease in sensitivity to high-frequency sounds is the most sensitive auditory change for most ototoxic agents. Otoacoustic emissions show promise as another method for monitoring.[230] If clinical circumstances permit, vestibular tests may be considered even after a patient has received aminoglycosides for several days, as the earliest reported incidence of ototoxicity was 5 days after beginning therapy.[162]

When a patient is referred for evaluation of possible ototoxicity, the otolaryngologist-audiologist team should identify possible ototoxicity and make appropriate recommendations based on clinical findings and test results. In many cases, there are no alternatives to the ototoxic medication. It may be appropriate for the physician prescribing the ototoxic medication to renew the discussion of informed consent if the medication is to be continued.

The rapid administration of bolus doses of ototoxic drugs and their concomitant administration (especially loop diuretics combined with aminoglycosides) should be avoided. A positive family history of hearing loss from aminoglycosides may help prevent deafness in other family members due to the A1555G mitochondrial mutation.[231]

Much work has been done concerning aminoglycoside dosing, challenging some prior assumptions. It is now accepted that efficacy, safety, and ototoxicity are not significantly different for once-daily versus thrice-daily dosing and may be improved with the former.[232–236] Furthermore, ototoxicity seems to be predicted best by the total (cumulative) dose rather than by serum peak and trough levels or any other factor.[237] Adjusting the dose of aminoglycosides according to creatinine clearance rather than serum level is suggested.[237] Even when these precautions are taken, there may still be an important role for monitoring cochlear and vestibular function, because, as detailed above for aminoglycosides and cisplatin, only a small number of patients develop symptoms at the time they have measurable ototoxicity.

The use of topical otic drops containing neomycin continues to be widespread. Despite appropriate concern, hearing loss from the use of topical neomycin is remarkably rare, especially when it is used in the treatment of chronic suppurative otitis media. Reasonable caution in the use of ototopical neomycin is advisable, although difficult to define.

Compounds that hold promise for otoprotection for aminoglycoside and cisplatin ototoxicity have been reviewed recently.[238,239] Thiol-containing compounds, sulfhydryl compounds, D-methionine, N-acetylcysteine, caspase inhibitors, and intratympanic steroids, many of which act to decrease reactive oxygen species, may have preventive value. Clinical trials are needed to determine the clinical effectiveness and safety of chemoprotective strategies. The phosphonic acid derivative fosfomycin has been shown to be protective of ototoxicity and does not inhibit tumoricidal activity in vitro.[240,241] However, nausea from fosfomycin may limit its use in some patient populations. As described above with aminoglycosides, preconditioning of nonlethal stress to the inner ear (such other ototoxins, heat, etc.) may have a protective role.

24.5.6 Central Auditory Toxicity

The concept of central auditory toxicity arose with the recognition that hyperbilirubinemia, such as occurs in kernicterus, can be toxic to the brainstem central auditory system. Abnormal auditory brainstem responses (ABRs) are often recorded in this disorder, indicating delay in the normal process of postnatal maturation of the ABR. Central auditory toxicity from the artemisinins, a relatively new class of antimalarial compounds, was suspected, but ruled out in a recent clinical trial.[242]

Auditory neuropathy spectrum is a collection of disorders of mostly unknown etiology. These children are often graduates of neonatal intensive care units.[243,244] They are functionally deaf or severely hearing impaired, but have normal otoacoustic emissions, indicating normal hair cell function.

24.6 Miscellaneous Other Causes of Sensorineural Hearing Loss

24.6.1 Hypoxemia

Many experimental studies have documented inner ear pathology following vascular occlusion. Kimura and Perlman[245] found rapid, progressive loss of hair cells after arterial occlusion of the labyrinthine artery. First inner hair cells, then outer, supporting, and strial cells degenerated. Eventually, the labyrinth ossified. Inner hair cells appeared to be more sensitive than outer hair cells to mild hypoxia over an extended period time.[246] Venous occlusion also produced strial damage, hair cell loss, and hemorrhagic lesions.[247,248] Anoxia appeared to potentiate noise-induced hearing loss.[249,250]

Many medical conditions can predispose to vascular occlusion, in which isolated hearing loss has been reported, including leukemia,[250–252] Buerger's disease,[253] macroglobulinemia,[253] fat embolism,[254] cardiac bypass,[255–258] sickle cell disease,[259,260] cryoglobulinemia,[261,262] nonotologic surgery,[263] Hand-Schüller-Christian disease,[264] and vasculitis.[265] Hypoxemia without vascular occlusion has been associated with a high risk of SNHL in infants.[266]

24.6.2 Diabetes Mellitus

Whether diabetes mellitus results in hearing loss through vascular impairment, metabolic pathways, or both, or not at all is a continuing and unresolved controversy. In the 1999–2004 NHANES, patients with diabetes were noted to have a higher association with hearing loss.[267] Hearing loss has been reported in diabetes mellitus,[268–273] though in some reports there was also significant generalized vascular disease.[274] There is evidence suggesting that hypertensive end-organ disease of the cochlea may be amplified by coexisting diabetes, with increased hearing loss in the 4- to 8-Hz range.[275] It has been suggested that SNHL may result from diabetic neuropathy.[276] Other investigators were unable to establish an association between diabetes and SNHL.[275,277–284] Although the duration of diabetes has not been correlated with the degree of hearing loss,[269,285] the severity of diabetes may be.[269] No relationship was found between insulin dose or a family history of diabetes versus SNHL.[285]

Wackym and Linthicum[284] examined temporal bones of eight diabetics who had significantly more hearing loss than age- and sex-matched controls. Microangiopathy was found in the endolymphatic sac, stria vascularis, and basilar membrane in patients with diabetes. SNHL was strongly correlated with involvement of endolymphatic sac and basilar membrane vessels. Earlier histological studies showed vascular changes consistent with atherosclerosis in the stria vascularis and basement membrane, but no degeneration of the organ of Corti.[275,284]

24.7 Infection and Sensorineural Hearing Loss

24.7.1 Viral Infection

Viruses have been implicated in many hearing disorders, but establishing causation has been difficult. The presumed role of viruses in SSNHL was discussed above. Serum viral titers can establish the presence of viral infection. Cytomegalovirus (CMV), mumps, and rubeola were identified in inner ears of patients suffering from SHL.[127,138] CMV[286–288] and mumps[289,290] were cultured from inner ear fluids. Rubeola inclusion bodies were identified in the inner ear.[291]

Rubella has been closely related epidemiologically with SNHL.[292,293] Other viruses implicated in SNHL include herpes simplex, varicella zoster, Epstein-Barr virus, hepatitis virus, variola, adenovirus, influenza and parainfluenza, polio virus, encephalitis virus, and infectious mononucleosis.[286,294] Severe SNHL with encephalitis following vaccination with live measles virus was reported.[295] There have been nine reports of SNHL after measles, mumps, and rubella (MMR) immunization.[296] Careful review revealed that in three cases the deafness was unrelated to MMR immunization and in six cases the cause was unknown. It is still unproven that MMR can be an etiology.[296] Hall and Richards[297] considered the possibility of mumps in 33 children with profound acquired unilateral SNHL. Fifteen gave a history of mumps, 12 of whom contracted the infection between the last normal and first abnormal hearing tests.

Cytomegalovirus infection is currently reported as the most common cause of congenital viral-induced deafness.[298] The incidence of congenital CMV has been estimated at about 0.7%, although this likely is an underestimate.[299] Approximately 10 to 15% of those born with congenital CMV had SNHL.[300] An association has been shown between congenital CMV infection (CMV viremia detected by polymerase chain reaction [PCR] in early infancy) and increased likelihood for SNHL.[301] In a randomized controlled trial, none of 25 neonates with congenital CMV treated with ganciclovir had abnormal hearing levels estimated by ABR, versus seven of 17 untreated controls, who did show worse hearing levels.[302]

Temporal bone pathology in viral-induced hearing loss generally consisted of strial atrophy with hair cell loss. Labyrinthitis and auditory nerve inflammation also were reported.[286,290,291,294,303,304] A large review of 52 pairs of infant and children temporal bones demonstrated no evidence of CMV endolabyrinthitis, even in a single case with extensive congenital CMV infection.[298,310] SNHL has been associated with Reye syndrome.[305]

Human Immunodeficiency Virus

Human immunodeficiency virus (HIV), the causative agent of acquired immunodeficiency syndrome (AIDS), was associated with multiple otologic findings.[306,307] In one study 57% of AIDS patients and 45% of non-AIDS HIV-infected individuals had abnormal results in various audiological, vestibular, and electrophysiological tests, whereas only 12% of the seronegative control group showed abnormalities.[307] SNHL was reported in 21 to 49% of infected individuals.[308–310]

Sensorineural hearing loss has been attributed to direct infection by HIV, opportunistic infection (bacterial, viral, parasitic, and fungal), CNS disease, malignancies (i.e., lymphoma and Kaposi's sarcoma), and ototoxic therapy.[308,311] Reactivation of varicella, CMV, and latent syphilis, along with cryptococcus, may affect the eighth cranial nerve.[308] Audiological evaluation of individuals separated according to Centers for Disease Control and Prevention (CDC) guidelines of HIV progression, showed a worsening of hearing at all ranges tested in later stages of the disease, especially at 500, 2,000, and 8,000 Hz.[306] Soucek and Michaels[312] reported hearing impairment > 20 dB in 69% of HIV subjects. Almost all impaired patients displayed diminished otoacoustic emissions, suggesting impairment of outer hair cell function. Delayed and desynchronized latencies between intervals I and V of brainstem auditory-evoked responses have been reported in HIV, suggesting CNS dysfunction.[307,311,313,314] CNS findings usually appear early in the progression of the disease, often during HIV's subclinical phase.[315–318]

Temporal bone histopathological studies have shown multiple abnormalities in patients with HIV. Findings included severe petrositis with marrow replacement, mastoiditis, ossicular destruction, precipitations in the perilymphatic and endolymphatic spaces of the vestibule and of the semicircular canals, and subepithelial elevation of the sensory epithelium of the saccule and utricle.[319] Large aggregations of HIV-like particles were found around the tectorial membrane and in endolymphatic structures, suggesting these extracellular areas may be able to support HIV or opportunistic infection.[320] Ultrastructural investigation showed shortened and fused cilia of the hair cells. Pathological changes consistent with viral infection occurred in hair cells and supporting cells of the cochlea.[320] Similar HIV-like particles, inclusion bodies, and other viral ultrastructural changes were observed in vestibular structures such as the labyrinthine wall, supporting cells, maculae, and cristae.[320] The inner ear has been shown to have changes suggestive of CMV infection, Kaposi sarcoma in the eighth cranial nerve, and fungal infection by disseminated *Cryptococcus*.[321]

Otitis media, usually with effusion, chronic otitis media, acute otitis media, otitis externa, and progression of latent otosyphilis have all been described at higher frequencies in HIV patients.[309,312,322,323] Histological studies have also shown otitis media, which may have been a pre-terminal event in some cases.[323]

Ototoxicity due to antiretroviral therapy, including azidothymidine (AZT), dideoxyinosine (DDI), and dideoxycytidine (DDC), has been described. Hearing loss and tinnitus due to these agents can present with sudden or gradual onset.[308,324] Auditory dysfunction from these drugs may be caused by a reduction in mitochondrial DNA.[325–327] It has been suggested that drug effects may compound synergistically with age-related and possibly HIV-related mitochondrial DNA reduction to cause hearing loss.[324,328–330]

24.7.2 Otitic Syphilis

Syphilitic inner ear disease results from vasculitis and obliterative endarteritis.[331,332] Pathology of syphilitic labyrinthitis consists of diffuse osteitis, severe endolymphatic hydrops, and degeneration of the membranous labyrinth.[332] Electrocochleographic features of hydropic syphilitic lesions resembled those in Ménière disease.[333]

The diagnosis of otitic syphilis may be straightforward when the patient presents with primary or secondary disease and acute ear symptoms; however, the majority of patients presented with late disease, delayed otologic symptoms, and otherwise normal physical examinations.[334–336] Despite a sensitivity of 100% and a specificity of 98%, the predictive value of a positive FTA-Abs (or microhemagglutination-*Treponema pallidum* [MHA-TP]) is still only 22% in an otologic population because the prevalence of disease is so low.[337] The FTA-Abs assay reliably indicates an immunologic history of exposure to *Treponemal pallium* or to a cross-reacting antigen. It does not distinguish between active and treated disease. A Western blot assay can eliminate the possibility of a false-positive result and can confirm whether the infection is active.[338] This assay can be used to refute the diagnosis by demonstrating that the FTA-Abs result was falsely positive for syphilis or that the infection is inactive.[338] Because the predictive value of a positive test is so low and the sensitivity of the FTA-Abs is twice as great as the sensitivity of the rapid plasma reagin (RPR), the RPR is considered an inadequate screening test for suspect patients in otology.[337]

Treatment of otologic syphilis combines penicillin and steroids.[336,339,340] Because most patients have latent disease in which the spirochete replicates more slowly (up to 90 days), prolonged penicillin treatment is necessary.[341] Otosyphilis can and does present at any stage of HIV infection and should be considered in seropositive patients presenting with otologic complaints.[342] Physicians should consult reliable sources for current recommendations for antibiotics, dosage, and duration of therapy.

24.7.3 Bacterial Infection and Sensorineural Hearing Loss

There is an association between otitis media and SNHL.[343-345] Bacterial meningitis frequently results in SNHL and deafness. The prevalence of SNHL was reported to be 11% of 47 patients followed prospectively.[346] Late-onset hearing loss was not observed in this study; however, one patient developed progressive hearing loss. Both bilateral and unilateral hearing losses were noted. The degree of hearing loss varied from mild to profound, with no consistent audiometric pattern. Statistical analysis revealed that patients in the hearing-impaired group and normal-hearing group did not differ significantly in the types of therapy they received. Since the advent of the septivalent anti-pneumococcus vaccine, the incidence of bacterial meningitis has dropped dramatically to a point where meningitis is no longer a common cause of profound SNHL in children.[347,348]

References

[1] National Institutes of Health. Quick Statistics, 2010. http://www.nidcd.nih.gov/health/statistics/Pages/quick.aspx

[2] Herbst KG, Humphrey C. Hearing impairment and mental state in the elderly living at home. BMJ 1980; 281: 903–905

[3] Uhlmann RF, Larson EB, Rees TS, Koepsell TD, Duckert LG. Relationship of hearing impairment to dementia and cognitive dysfunction in older adults. JAMA 1989; 261: 1916–1919

[4] Thomas PD, Hunt WC, Garry PJ, Hood RB, Goodwin JM, Goodwin JS. Hearing acuity in a healthy elderly population: effects on emotional, cognitive, and social status. J Gerontol 1983; 38: 321–325

[5] Gates GA, Cooper JC, Jr, Kannel WB, Miller NJ. Hearing in the elderly: the Framingham cohort, 1983–1985. Part I. Basic audiometric test results. Ear Hear 1990; 11: 247–256

[6] Ries PW. Prevalence and characteristics of persons with hearing trouble: United States, 1990–91. Vital Health Stat 10 1994: 1–75

[7] Agrawal Y, Platz EA, Niparko JK. Prevalence of hearing loss and differences by demographic characteristics among US adults: data from the National Health and Nutrition Examination Survey, 1999–2004. Arch Intern Med 2008; 168: 1522–1530

[8] Lin FR. Hearing loss and cognition among older adults in the United States. J Gerontol A Biol Sci Med Sci 2011; 66: 1131–1136

[9] Department of Health and Human Services. 2011. http://www.aoa.gov/aoaroot/aging_statistics/index.aspx.

[10] Jerger J, Chmiel R, Stach B, Spretnjak M. Gender affects audiometric shape in presbyacusis. J Am Acad Audiol 1993; 4: 42–49

[11] Cooper JC, Jr. Health and Nutrition Examination Survey of 1971–75: Part I. Ear and race effects in hearing. J Am Acad Audiol 1994; 5: 30–36

[12] Helzner EP, Cauley JA, Pratt SR et al. Race and sex differences in age-related hearing loss: the Health, Aging and Body Composition Study. J Am Geriatr Soc 2005; 53: 2119–2127

[13] Lin FR, Maas P, Chien W, Carey JP, Ferrucci L, Thorpe R. Association of skin color, race/ethnicity, and hearing loss among adults in the USA. J Assoc Res Otolaryngol 2012; 13: 109–117

[14] Gates GA, Cobb JL, D'Agostino RB, Wolf PA. The relation of hearing in the elderly to the presence of cardiovascular disease and cardiovascular risk factors. Arch Otolaryngol Head Neck Surg 1993; 119: 156–161

[15] Rosen S, Bergman M, Plester D, El-Mofty A, Satti MH. Presbycusis study of a relatively noise-free population in the Sudan. Ann Otol Rhinol Laryngol 1962; 71: 727–743

[16] Rosenhall U, Sixt E, Sundh V, Svanborg A. Correlations between presbyacusis and extrinsic noxious factors. Audiology 1993; 32: 234–243

[17] Schuknecht HF. Presbycusis. Laryngoscope 1955; 65: 402–419

[18] Schuknecht HF. Pathology of the Ear, 2nd ed. Philadelphia: Lea & Febiger, 1993

[19] Schuknecht HF. Auditory and cytocochlear correlates of inner ear disorders. Otolaryngol Head Neck Surg 1994; 110: 530–538

[20] Nadol JB, Jr. Electron microscopic findings in presbycusic degeneration of the basal turn of the human cochlea. Otolaryngol Head Neck Surg 1979; 87: 818–836

[21] Pearlman RC. Presbycusis: the need for a clinical definition. Am J Otol 1982; 3: 183–186

[22] Gaeth J. A Study of Phonemic Regression Associated with Hearing Loss. Evanston, IL: Northwestern University, 1948

[23] Schuknecht HF. Pathology of the Ear, 2nd ed. Philadelphia: Lea & Febiger, 1992

[24] Zunehmendern A. Ein nues gestez. Arch Ohr Waskehlkheilk 1899; 32: 53

[25] Crowe S, Guild S, Polvogt L. Observations on Pathology of High Tone Deafness. Baltimore: Johns Hopkins Hospital, 1934:315–379

[26] Saxen A. Pathologie und klinik der aterschinerhorigkcit nacht unter suchungen von fund aiero Saxen. Acta Otolaryngol Suppl (Stockh) 1937; 23: 19

[27] Bredberg G. Cellular pattern and nerve supply of the human organ of Corti. Acta Otolaryngol 1968 Suppl 236–1

[28] Pauler M, Schuknecht HF, Thornton AR. Correlative studies of cochlear neuronal loss with speech discrimination and pure-tone thresholds. Arch Otorhinolaryngol 1986; 243: 200–206

[29] Gratton MA, Schmiedt RA, Schulte BA. Age-related decreases in endocochlear potential are associated with vascular abnormalities in the stria vascularis. Hear Res 1996; 94: 116–124

[30] Gratton MA, Schulte BA. Alterations in microvasculature are associated with atrophy of the stria vascularis in quiet-aged gerbils. Hear Res 1995; 82: 44–52

[31] Schuknecht HF. Further observations on the pathology of presbycusis. Arch Otolaryngol 1964; 80: 369–382

[32] Schuknecht HF, Watanuki K, Takahashi T et al. Atrophy of the stria vascularis, a common cause for hearing loss. Laryngoscope 1974; 84: 1777–1821

[33] Pauler M, Schuknecht HF, White JA. Atrophy of the stria vascularis as a cause of sensorineural hearing loss. Laryngoscope 1988; 98: 754–759

[34] Matschke RG. Frequency selectivity and psychoacoustic tuning curves in old age. Acta Otolaryngol Suppl 1990; 476: 114–119

[35] Bonding P. Frequency selectivity and speech discrimination in sensorineural hearing loss. Scand Audiol 1979; 8: 205–215

[36] Gates GA, Mills JH. Presbycusis. Lancet 2005; 366: 1111–1120

[37] Nixon JC, Glorig A, High WS. Changes in air and bone conduction thresholds as a function of age. J Laryngol Otol 1962; 76: 288–298

[38] Belal A, Stewart TJ. Pathologocal changes in the middle ear joints. Ann Otol Rhinol Laryngol 1974; 83: 159–167

[39] Welsh LW, Welsh JJ, Healy MP. Central presbycusis. Laryngoscope 1985; 95: 128–136

[40] Gatehouse S. The contribution of central auditory factors to auditory disability. Acta Otolaryngol Suppl 1990; 476: 182–188

[41] van Rooij JC, Plomp R. Auditive and cognitive factors in speech perception by elderly listeners. Acta Otolaryngol Suppl 1990; 476: 177–181

[42] Rizzo SR, Jr, Gutnick HN. Cochlear versus retrocochlear presbyacusis: clinical correlates. Ear Hear 1991; 12: 61–63

[43] Dubno JR, Horwitz AR, Ahlstrom JB. Recovery from prior stimulation: masking of speech by interrupted noise for younger and older adults with normal hearing. J Acoust Soc Am 2003; 113: 2084–2094

[44] Frisina RD. Subcortical neural coding mechanisms for auditory temporal processing. Hear Res 2001; 158: 1–27

[45] Walton JP. Timing is everything: temporal processing deficits in the aged auditory brainstem. Hear Res 2010; 264: 63–69

[46] Caspary DM, Milbrandt JC, Helfert RH. Central auditory aging: GABA changes in the inferior colliculus. Exp Gerontol 1995; 30: 349–360

[47] Milbrandt JC, Albin RL, Turgeon SM, Caspary DM. GABAA receptor binding in the aging rat inferior colliculus. Neuroscience 1996; 73: 449–458

[48] Lutman ME. Hearing disability in the elderly. Acta Otolaryngol Suppl 1990; 476: 239–248

[49] Harner SG, Rose DE, Facer GW. Paget's disease and hearing loss. Otolaryngology 1978; 86: ORL-869–ORL-874

[50] Monsell EM, Cody DD, Bone HG et al. Hearing loss in Paget's disease of bone: the relationship between pure-tone thresholds and mineral density of the cochlear capsule. Hear Res 1995; 83: 114–120

[51] el Sammaa M, Linthicum FH, Jr, House HP, House JW. Calcitonin as treatment for hearing loss in Paget's disease. Am J Otol 1986; 7: 241–243

[52] Baraka ME. Rate of progression of hearing loss in Paget's disease. J Laryngol Otol 1984; 98: 573–575

[53] Alvarado DM, Hawkins RD, Bashiardes S et al. An RNA interference-based screen of transcription factor genes identifies pathways necessary for sensory regeneration in the avian inner ear. J Neurosci 2011; 31: 4535–4543

[54] National Institute of Occupational Safety and Health. Criteria for a Recommended Standard: Occupational Noise Exposure. Washington, DC: NIOSH, 1998

[55] Kopke RD, Jackson RL, Coleman JK, Liu J, Bielefeld EC, Balough BJ. NAC for noise: from the bench top to the clinic. Hear Res 2007; 226: 114–125

[56] Dobie RA. Medical-Legal Evaluation of Hearing Loss. New York: Van Nostrand Reinhold, 1993

[57] Occupational Safety and Health Administration, Department of Labor. Occupational Noise Exposure. Hearing Conservation Amendment Final Rule, 1983

[58] National Institutes of Health. Noise and Hearing Loss. Bethesda, MD: NIH, 1990

[59] Standardization, I.I.O.f.S., Standard 1999.2. 1989

[60] Meister F. Der einfluss ein winkdauer bei der beschallung des ohers. Larmbekamfung 1973; 10: 89–91

[61] Ward WD. Temporary threshold shift and damage-risk criteria for intermittent noise exposures. J Acoust Soc Am 1970; 48: 561–574

[62] Passchier-Vermeer , W . Hearing Loss due to continuous exposure to steady-state broad-band noise. J Acoust Soc Am. 19 74; 56: 1585–15–93

[63] Saunders JC, Dear SP, Schneider ME. The anatomical consequences of acoustic injury: A review and tutorial. J Acoust Soc Am 1985; 78: 833–860

[64] Fried MP, Dudek SE, Bohne BA. Basal turn cochlear lesions following exposure to low-frequency noise. Trans Sect Otolaryngol Am Acad Ophthalmol Otolaryngol 1976; 82: 285–298

[65] Liberman MC, Beil DG. Hair cell condition and auditory nerve response in normal and noise-damaged cochleas. Acta Otolaryngol 1979; 88: 161–176

[66] Wang Y, Hirose K, Liberman MC. Dynamics of noise-induced cellular injury and repair in the mouse cochlea. J Assoc Res Otolaryngol 2002; 3: 248–268

[67] Lim DJ, Melnick W. Acoustic damage of the cochlea. A scanning and transmission electron microscopic observation. Arch Otolaryngol 1971; 94: 294–305

[68] Henderson D, Hamernik RP. Biologic bases of noise-induced hearing loss. Occup Med 1995; 10: 513–534

[69] Slepecky N. Overview of mechanical damage to the inner ear: noise as a tool to probe cochlear function. Hear Res 1986; 22: 307–321

[70] Lamm K, Arnold W. The effect of blood flow promoting drugs on cochlear blood flow, perilymphatic pO and auditory function in the normal and noise-damaged hypoxic and ischemic guinea pig inner ear. Hear Res 2000; 141: 199–219

[71] Poderoso JJ, Boveris A, Cadenas E. Mitochondrial oxidative stress: a self-propagating process with implications for signaling cascades. Biofactors 2000; 11: 43–45

[72] Ohlemiller KK, Wright JS, Dugan LL. Early elevation of cochlear reactive oxygen species following noise exposure. Audiol Neurootol 1999; 4: 229–236

[73] Yamane H, Nakai Y, Takayama M et al. The emergence of free radicals after acoustic trauma and strial blood flow. Acta Otolaryngol Suppl 1995; 519: 87–92

[74] Spoendlin H. Primary structural changes in the organ of Corti after acoustic overstimulation. Acta Otolaryngol 1971; 71: 166–176

[75] Robertson D. Functional significance of dendritic swelling after loud sounds in the guinea pig cochlea. Hear Res 1983; 9: 263–278

[76] Pujol R, Puel JL. Excitotoxicity, synaptic repair, and functional recovery in the mammalian cochlea: a review of recent findings. Ann N Y Acad Sci 1999; 884: 249–254

[77] Puel JL, Ruel J, Gervais d'Aldin C, Pujol R. Excitotoxicity and repair of cochlear synapses after noise-trauma induced hearing loss. Neuroreport 1998; 9: 2109–2114

[78] Kujawa SG, Liberman MC. Adding insult to injury: cochlear nerve degeneration after "temporary" noise-induced hearing loss. J Neurosci 2009; 29: 14077–14085

[79] Yoshida N, Kristiansen A, Liberman MC. Heat stress and protection from permanent acoustic injury in mice. J Neurosci 1999; 19: 10116–10124

[80] Yoshida N, Liberman MC. Sound conditioning reduces noise-induced permanent threshold shift in mice. Hear Res 2000; 148: 213–219

[81] Niu X, Canlon B. Protective mechanisms of sound conditioning. Adv Otorhinolaryngol 2002; 59: 96–105

[82] Fernandez EA, Ohlemiller KK, Gagnon PM, Clark WW. Protection against noise-induced hearing loss in young CBA/J mice by low-dose kanamycin. J Assoc Res Otolaryngol 2010; 11: 235–244

[83] ACOM Noise and Hearing Conservation Committee. Occupational noise-induced hearing loss. J Occup Med 1989; 31: 996

[84] Standardization., I.I.O.f.S., Acoustics-Determination of Occupational Noise Exposure and Estimation of Noise-Induced Hearing Impairment. 1999

[85] Pierson LL, Gerhardt KJ, Rodriguez GP, Yanke RB. Relationship between outer ear resonance and permanent noise-induced hearing loss. Am J Otolaryngol 1994; 15: 37–40

[86] Borg E, Nilsson R. Acoustic reflex in industrial noise. In: Silman S, ed. The Acoustic Reflex: Basic Principles and Clinical Applications. Orlando, FL: Academic Press, 1984:413–440

[87] Schuknecht HF, Tonndorf J. Acoustic trauma of the coch ea from ear surgery. Laryngoscope 1960; 70: 479–505

[88] Osguthorpe J, Klein J, eds. Hearing Compensation Evaluation, vol I. Alexandria, VA: American Academy of Otolaryngology-Head and Neck Surgery Foundation, 1989

[89] Catlin Doerfler L, Linthicum FH, Jr. Guide for conservation of hearing and noise. Trans Am Acad Ophthalmol Otolaryngol Suppl: 197

[90] Berger EH. The performance of hearing protectors in industrial noise environments. Sound Vibrat 1980: 14–17

[91] Dancer A, Grateau P, Cabanis A et al. Effectiveness of earplugs in high-intensity impulse noise. J Acoust Soc Am 1992; 91: 1677–1689

[92] Dobie RA. Time for action in hearing conservation. Otolaryngol Head Neck Surg 1983; 91: 347–349

[93] Alberti PW, Blair RL. Occupational hearing loss: an Ontario perspective. Laryngoscope 1982; 92: 535–539

[94] Dobie RA, Archer RJ. Results of otologic referrals in an industrial hearing conservation program. Otolaryngol Head Neck Surg 1981; 89: 294–301

[95] Dobie RA. Otologic referral criteria. Otolaryngol Head Neck Surg 1982; 90: 598–601

[96] Fox MS. Workmen's compensation hearing loss claims. Laryngoscope 1980; 90: 1077–1081

[97] Dobie RA. Industrial audiometry and the otologist. Laryngoscope 1985; 95: 382–385

[98] Otolaryngology AC American Council of Otolaryngology. The otologic referral criteria for occupational hearing conservation programs. Medical Aspects of noise Committee. Otolaryngol Clin North Am 1979; 12: 635–636

[99] Catlin FI American Academy of Otolaryngology Committee on Hearing and Equilibrium. Guide for the evaluation of hearing handicap. Otolaryngol Clin North Am 1979; 12: 655–663

[100] Department of Defense. Instruction Bulletin 6055, 1978

[101] Fox M. Hearing loss statutes in the United States and Canada. Natl Saf News 1972; 105: 55–56

[102] Yassi A, Pollock N, Tran N, Cheang M. Risks to hearing from a rock concert. Can Fam Physician 1993; 39: 1045–1050

[103] Drake-Lee AB. Beyond music: auditory temporary threshold shift in rock musicians after a heavy metal concert. J R Soc Med 1992; 85: 617–619

[104] Turunen-Rise I, Flottorp G, Tvete O. A study of the possibility of acquiring noise-induced hearing loss by the use of personal cassette players (walkman). Scand Audiol Suppl 1991; 34: 133–144

[105] Lee PC, Senders CW, Gantz BJ, Otto SR. Transient sensorineural hearing loss after overuse of portable headphone cassette radios. Otolaryngol Head Neck Surg 1985; 93: 622–625

[106] Macrae JH. Prediction of deterioration in hearing due to hearing aid use. J Speech Hear Res 1991; 34: 661–670

[107] Von Gierke HE. Effects of sonic boom on people: review and outlook. J Acoust Soc Am 1966; 39: S43–S50

[108] Singleton GT, Whitaker DL, Keim RJ, Kemker FJ. Cordless telephones: a threat to hearing. Ann Otol Rhinol Laryngol 1984; 93: 565–568

[109] Orchik DJ, Schumaier DR, Shea JJ, Moretz WH, Jr. Intensity and frequency of sound levels from cordless telephones. A pediatric alert. Clin Pediatr (Phila) 1985; 24: 688–690

[110] Gerling IJ, Jerger JF. Cordless telephones and acoustic trauma: a case study. Ear Hear 1985; 6: 203–205

[111] Le Prell CG, Yamashita D, Minami SB, Yamasoba T, Miller JM. Mechanisms of noise-induced hearing loss indicate multiple methods of prevention. Hear Res 2007; 226: 22–43

[112] Schreiber BE, Agrup C, Haskard DO, Luxon LM. Sudden sensorineural hearing loss. Lancet 2010; 375: 1203–1211

[113] Terayama Y, Ishibe Y, Matsushima J. Rapidly progressive sensorineural hearing loss (rapid deafness). Acta Otolaryngol Suppl 1988; 456: 43–48

[114] De Kleyn A. Sudden complete or partila loss of function of the octavus system in apparently normal persons. Acta Otolaryngol 1944; 32: 407–429

[115] Chau JK, Lin JR, Atashband S, Irvine RA, Westerberg BD. Systematic review of the evidence for the etiology of adult sudden sensorineural hearing loss. Laryngoscope 2010; 120: 1011–1021

[116] Byl FM, Jr. Sudden hearing loss: eight years' experience and suggested prognostic table. Laryngoscope 1984; 94: 647–661

[117] Ben-David Y, Danino J, Podoshin L. Idiopathic sudden deafness. Ear Nose Throat J 1982; 61: 54–60

[118] Shaia FT, Sheehy JL. Sudden sensori-neural hearing impairment: a report of 1,220 cases. Laryngoscope 1976; 86: 389–398

[119] Mattox DE, Simmons FB. Natural history of sudden sensorineural hearing loss. Ann Otol Rhinol Laryngol 1977; 86: 463–480

[120] Fetterman BL, Luxford WM, Saunders JE. Sudden bilateral sensorineural hearing loss. Laryngoscope 1996; 106: 1347–1350

[121] Oh JH, Park K, Lee SJ, Shin YR, Choung YH. Bilateral versus unilateral sudden sensorineural hearing loss. Otolaryngol Head Neck Surg 2007; 136: 87–91

[122] Stokroos RJ, Albers FW. The etiology of idiopathic sudden sensorineural hearing loss. A review of the literature. Acta Otorhinolaryngol Belg 1996; 50: 69–76

[123] Jaffe BF. Clinical studies in sudden deafness. Adv Otorhinolaryngol 1973; 20: 221–228

[124] Rowson KE, Hinchcliffe R. A virological and epidemiological study of patients with acute hearing loss. Lancet 1975; 1: 471–473

[125] Veltri RW, Wilson WR, Sprinkle PM, Rodman SM, Kavesh DA. The implication of viruses in idiopathic sudden hearing loss: primary infection or reactivation of latent viruses? Otolaryngol Head Neck Surg 1981; 89: 137–141

[126] Wilson WR, Veltri RW, Laird N, Sprinkle PM. Viral and epidemiologic studies of idiopathic sudden hearing loss. Otolaryngol Head Neck Surg 1983; 91: 653–658

[127] Cole RR, Jahrsdoerfer RA. Sudden hearing loss: an update. Am J Otol 1988; 9: 211–215

[128] Merchant SN, Durand ML, Adams JC. Sudden deafness: is it viral? ORL J Otorhinolaryngol Relat Spec 2008; 70: 52–60, discussion 60–62

[129] Ramos HV, Barros FA, Yamashita H, Penido NdeO, Souza AC, Yamaoka WY. Magnetic resonance imaging in sudden deafness. Braz J Otorhinolaryngol 2005; 71: 422–426

[130] Suzuki H, Mori T, Hashida K et al. Prediction model for hearing outcome in patients with idiopathic sudden sensorineural hearing loss. Eur Arch Otorhinolaryngol 2011; 268: 497–500

[131] Perlman HB, Kimura R, Fernandez C. Experiments on temporary obstruction of the internal auditory artery. Laryngoscope 1959; 69: 591–613

[132] Merchant SN, Adams JC, Nadol JB, Jr. Pathology and pathophysiology of idiopathic sudden sensorineural hearing loss. Otol Neurotol 2005; 26: 151–160

[133] Perlman HB, Kimura R. Experimental obstruction of venous drainage and arterial supply of the inner ear. Ann Otol Rhinol Laryngol 1957; 66: 537–546

[134] Belal A, Jr. The effects of vascular occlusion on the human inner ear. J Laryngol Otol 1979; 93: 955–968

[135] Schuknecht HF, Donovan ED. The pathology of idiopathic sudden sensorineural hearing loss. Arch Otorhinolaryng 1986; 243: 1–15

[136] Schuknecht HF, Kimura RS, Naufal PM. The pathology of sudden deafness. Acta Otolaryngol 1973; 76: 75–97

[137] Beal DD, Hemenway WG, Lindsay JR. Inner ear pathology of sudden deafness. Histopathology of acquired deafness in the adult coincident with viral infection. Arch Otolaryngol 1967; 85: 591–598

[138] Mattox DE. Medical management of sudden hearing loss. Otolaryngol Head Neck Surg (1979) 1980; 88: 111–113

[139] Park SN, Yeo SW, Park KH. Serum heat shock protein 70 and its correlation with clinical characteristics in patients with sudden sensorineural hearing loss. Laryngoscope 2006; 116: 121–125

[140] Simmons B. Sudden sensorineural hearing loss, In: English G, ed. Otolaryngology. Hagerstown, MD: Harper and Row, 1976

[141] Wilson WR, Byl FM, Laird N. The efficacy of steroids in the treatment of idiopathic sudden hearing loss. A double-blind clinical study. Arch Otolaryngol 1980; 106: 772–776

[142] Moskowitz D, Lee KJ, Smith HW. Steroid use in idiopathic sudden sensorineural hearing loss. Laryngoscope 1984; 94: 664–666

[143] Chen CY, Halpin C, Rauch SD. Oral steroid treatment of sudden sensorineural hearing loss: a ten year retrospective analysis. Otol Neurotol 2003; 24: 728–733

[144] Veldman JE, Hanada T, Meeuwsen F. Diagnostic and therapeutic dilemmas in rapidly progressive sensorineural hearing loss and sudden deafness. A reappraisal of immune reactivity in inner ear disorders. Acta Otolaryngol 1993; 113: 303–306

[145] Moscicki RA, San Martin JE, Quintero CH, Rauch SD, Nadol JB, Jr, Bloch KJ. Serum antibody to inner ear proteins in patients with progressive hearing loss. Correlation with disease activity and response to corticosteroid treatment. JAMA 1994; 272: 611–616

[146] Rauch SD, Halpin CF, Antonelli PJ et al. Oral vs intratympanic corticosteroid therapy for idiopathic sudden sensorineural hearing loss: a randomized trial. JAMA 2011; 305: 2071–2079

[147] Stachler RJ, Chandrasekhar SS, Archer SM et al. American Academy of Otolaryngology-Head and Neck Surgery. Clinical practice guideline: sudden hearing loss. Otolaryngol Head Neck Surg 2012; 146 Suppl: S1–S35

[148] Bennett M, Kertesz T, Yeung P. Hyperbaric oxygen therapy for idiopathic sudden sensorineural hearing loss and tinnitus: a systematic review of randomized controlled trials. J Laryngol Otol 2005; 119: 791–798

[149] Cekin E, Cincik H, Ulubil SA, Gungor A. Effectiveness of hyperbaric oxygen therapy in management of sudden hearing loss. J Laryngol Otol 2009; 123: 609–612

[150] Fernau JL, Hirsch BE, Derkay C, Ramasastry S, Schaefer SE. Hyperbaric oxygen therapy: effect on middle ear and eustachian tube function. Laryngoscope 1992; 102: 48–52

[151] Körpinar S, Alkan Z, Yiğit O et al. Factors influencing the outcome of idiopathic sudden sensorineural hearing loss treated with hyperbaric oxygen therapy. Eur Arch Otorhinolaryngol 2011; 268: 41–47

[152] Rauch SD. Clinical practice. Idiopathic sudden sensorineural hearing loss. N Engl J Med 2008; 359: 833–840

[153] Hawkins J. Drug ototoxicity. In: Keidel W, Neff SW, eds. Handbook of Sensory Physiology. New York: Springer, 1976:704–748

[154] Jones D, Metzger HJ, Schatz A, Waksman SA. Control of gram-negative bacteria in experimental animals by streptomycin. Science 1944; 100: 103–105

[155] Black FO, Pesznecker SC. Vestibular ototoxicity. Clinical considerations. Otolaryngol Clin North Am 1993; 26: 713–736

[156] Higgins CE, Kastner RE. Nebramycin, a new broad-spectrum antibiotic complex. II. Description of Streptomyces tenebrarius. Antimicrob Agents Chemother (Bethesda) 1967; 7: 324–331

[157] Weinstein MJ, Wagman GH, Oden EM, Marquez JA. Biological activity of the antibiotic components of the gentamicin complex. J Bacteriol 1967; 94: 789–790

[158] Kawaguchi H, Naito T, Nakagawa S, Fujisawa KI. BB-K 8, a new semisynthetic aminoglycoside antibiotic. J Antibiot (Tokyo) 1972; 25: 695–708

[159] Rizzi MD, Hirose K. Aminoglycoside ototoxicity. Curr Opin Otolaryngol Head Neck Surg 2007; 15: 352–357

[160] Schuknecht HF. Pathology of the Ear. Cambridge, MA: Harvard University Press, 1974

[161] Fee WE, Jr. Aminoglycoside ototoxicity in the human. Laryngoscope 1980; 90 Suppl 24: 1–19

[162] Lerner SA, Matz GJ. Aminoglycoside ototoxicity. Am J Otolaryngol 1980; 1: 169–179

[163] Ohtani I, Ohtsuki K, Aikawa T, Sato Y, Anzai T, Ouchi J. Mechanism of protective effect of fosfomycin against aminoglycoside ototoxicity. Auris Nasus Larynx 1984; 11: 119–124

[164] Ohtsuki K, Ohtani I, Aikawa T et al. The ototoxicity and the accumulation in the inner ear fluids of the various aminoglycoside antibiotics. Ear Res Jpn 1982; 13: 85–87

[165] Tran Ba Huy P, Bernard P, Schacht J. Kinetics of gentamicin uptake and release in the rat. Comparison of inner ear tissues and fluids with other organs. J Clin Invest 1986; 77: 1492–1500

[166] Dulon D, Aran JM, Zajic G, Schacht J. Comparative uptake of gentamicin, netilmicin, and amikacin in the guinea pig cochlea and vestibule. Antimicrob Agents Chemother 1986; 30: 96–100

[167] Hiel H, Bennani H, Erre JP, Aurousseau C, Aran JM. Kinetics of gentamicin in cochlear hair cells after chronic treatment. Acta Otolaryngol 1992; 112: 272–277

[168] Huizing EH, de Groot JC. Human cochlear pathology in aminoglycoside ototoxicity—a review. Acta Otolaryngol Suppl 1987; 436: 117–125

[169] Hinojosa R, Lerner SA. Cochlear neural degeneration without hair cell loss in two patients with aminoglycoside ototoxicity. J Infect Dis 1987; 156: 449–455

[170] Johnsson LG, Hawkins JE, Jr, Kingsley TC, Black FO, Matz GJ. Aminoglycoside-induced cochlear pathology in man. Acta Otolaryngol Suppl 1981; 383: 1–19

[171] Mendelsohn M, Katzenberg I. The effect of kanamycin on the cation content of the endolymph. Laryngoscope 1972; 82: 397–403

[172] Iinuma T, Mizukoshi O, Daly JF. Possible effects of various ototoxic drugs upon the ATP-hydrolyzing system in the stria vascularis and spiral ligament of the guinea pig. Laryngoscope 1967; 77: 159–170

[173] Musabeck K, Schatzle W. Experimentelle studien zur ototoxicitate des dihydrostreptomycins. Hr Nos u Kehlk Heilik 1962; 181: 41–48

[174] Keene M, Hawke M, Barber HO, Farkashidy J. Histopathological findings in clinical gentamicin ototoxicity. Arch Otolaryngol 1982; 108: 65–70

[175] Richardson GP, Forge A, Kros CJ, Fleming J, Brown SD, Steel KP. Myosin VIIA is required for aminoglycoside accumulation in cochlear hair cells. J Neurosci 1997; 17: 9506–9519

[176] Gale JE, Marcotti W, Kennedy HJ, Kros CJ, Richardson GP. FM1–43 dye behaves as a permeant blocker of the hair-cell mechanotransducer channel. J Neurosci 2001; 21: 7013–7025

[177] Alharazneh A, Luk L, Huth M et al. Functional hair cell mechanotransducer channels are required for aminoglycoside ototoxicity. PLoS ONE 2011; 6: e22347

[178] Schacht J. Mechanism for aminiglycoside ototoxicity: basic science research. In: Roland P, Rutka J, eds. Ototoxicity. Hamilton, Ontario: BC Decker, 2004:93–100

[179] Forge A, Schacht J. Aminoglycoside antibiotics. Audiol Neurootol 2000; 5: 3–22

[180] Warchol ME. Cellular mechanisms of aminoglycoside ototoxicity. Curr Opin Otolaryngol Head Neck Surg 2010; 18: 454–458

[181] Hobbie SN, Akshay S, Kalapala SK, Bruell CM, Shcherbakov D, Böttger EC. Genetic analysis of interactions with eukaryotic rRNA identify the mitoribosome as target in aminoglycoside ototoxicity. Proc Natl Acad Sci U S A 2008; 105: 20888–20893

[182] Matsui JI, Gale JE, Warchol ME. Critical signaling events during the aminoglycoside-induced death of sensory hair cells in vitro. J Neurobiol 2004; 61: 250–266

[183] Lahne M, Gale JE. Damage-induced activation of ERK1/2 in cochlear supporting cells is a hair cell death-promoting signal that depends on extracellular ATP and calcium. J Neurosci 2008; 28: 4918–4928

[184] Cunningham LL, Matsui JI, Warchol ME, Rubel EW. Overexpression of Bcl-2 prevents neomycin-induced hair cell death and caspase-9 activation in the adult mouse utricle in vitro. J Neurobiol 2004; 60: 89–100

[185] Matsui JI, Haque A, Huss D et al. Caspase inhibitors promote vestibular hair cell survival and function after aminoglycoside treatment in vivo. J Neurosci 2003; 23: 6111–6122

[186] Kahlmeter G, Dahlager JI. Aminoglycoside toxicity - a review of clinical studies published between 1975 and 1982. J Antimicrob Chemother 1984; 13 Suppl A: 9–22

[187] Black RE, Lau WK, Weinstein RJ, Young LS, Hewitt WL. Ototoxicity of amikacin. Antimicrob Agents Chemother 1976; 9: 956–961

[188] Neu HC, Bendush CL. Ototoxicity of tobramycin: a clinical overview. J Infect Dis 1976; 134 Suppl: S206–S218

[189] Jackson GG, Arcieri G. Ototoxicity of gentamicin in man: a survey and controlled analysis of clinical experience in the United States. J Infect Dis 1971; 124 Suppl: S130–S137

[190] Prazic M, Salaj B, Subotic R. Familial Sensitivity to Streptomycin. J Laryngol Otol 1964; 78: 1037–1043

[191] Higashi K. Unique inheritance of streptomycin-induced deafness. Clin Genet 1989; 35: 433–436

[192] Prezant TR, Agapian JV, Bohlman MC et al. Mitochondrial ribosomal RNA mutation associated with both antibiotic-induced and non-syndromic deafness. Nat Genet 1993; 4: 289–294

[193] Chapman P. Rapid onset hearing loss after Cisplatinum therapy: case reports and literature review. J Laryngol Otol 1982; 96: 159–162

[194] Kovach JS, Moertel CG, Schutt AJ, Reitemeier RG, Hahn RG. Phase II study of cis-diamminedichloroplatinum (NSC-119875) in advanced carcinoma of the large bowel. Cancer Chemother Rep 1973; 57: 357–359

[195] Lippman AJ, Helson C, Helson L, Krakoff IH. Clinical trials of cis-diamminedichloroplatinum (NSC-119875). Cancer Chemother Rep 1973; 57: 191–200

[196] Reddel RR, Kefford RF, Grant JM, Coates AS, Fox RM, Tattersall MH. Ototoxicity in patients receiving cisplatin: importance of dose and method of drug administration. Cancer Treat Rep 1982; 66: 19–23

[197] Gratton MA, Smyth B. Ototoxicity of platinum compounds. In: Roland P, Rutka J, eds. Ototoxicity. Hamilton, Ontario: BC Decker, 2004:60–75

[198] Komune S, Asakuma S, Snow JB, Jr. Pathophysiology of the ototoxicity of cis-diamminedichloroplatinum. Otolaryngol Head Neck Surg 1981; 89: 275–282

[199] Fleischman RW, Stadnicki SW, Ethier MF, Schaeppi U. Ototoxicity of cis-dichlorodiammine platinum (II) in the guinea pig. Toxicol Appl Pharmacol 1975; 33: 320–332

[200] Stadnicki SW, Fleischman RW, Schaeppi U, Merriam P. Cis-dichlorodiammineplatinum (II) (NSC-119875): hearing loss and other toxic effects in rhesus monkeys. Cancer Chemother Rep 1975; 59: 467–480

[201] Kohn S, Fradis M, Pratt H et al. Cisplatin ototoxicity in guinea pigs with special reference to toxic effects in the stria vascularis. Laryngoscope 1988; 98: 865–871

[202] Schmitt NC, Rubel EW, Nathanson NM. Cisplatin-induced hair cell death requires STAT1 and is attenuated by epigallocatechin gallate. J Neurosci 2009; 29: 3843–3851

[203] Slattery EL, Warchol ME. Cisplatin ototoxicity blocks sensory regeneration in the avian inner ear. J Neurosci 2010; 30: 3473–3481

[204] Bánfi B, Malgrange B, Knisz J, Steger K, Dubois-Dauphin M, Krause KH. NOX3, a superoxide-generating NADPH oxidase of the inner ear. J Biol Chem 2004; 279: 46065–46072

[205] Rybak LP, Whitworth CA, Mukherjea D, Ramkumar V. Mechanisms of cisplatin-induced ototoxicity and prevention. Hear Res 2007; 226: 157–167

[206] So H, Kim H, Lee JH et al. Cisplatin cytotoxicity of auditory cells requires secretions of proinflammatory cytokines via activation of ERK and NF-kappaB. J Assoc Res Otolaryngol 2007; 8: 338–355

[207] Thomas JP, Lautermann J, Liedert B, Seiler F, Thomale J. High accumulation of platinum-DNA adducts in strial marginal cells of the cochlea is an early event in cisplatin but not carboplatin ototoxicity. Mol Pharmacol 2006; 70: 23–29

[208] van Ruijven MW, de Groot JC, Hendriksen F, Smoorenburg GF. Immunohistochemical detection of platinated DNA in the cochlea of cisplatin-treated guinea pigs. Hear Res 2005; 203: 112–121

[209] Watanabe K, Inai S, Jinnouchi K, Baba S, Yagi T. Expression of caspase-activated deoxyribonuclease (CAD) and caspase 3 (CPP32) in the cochlea of cisplatin (CDDP)-treated guinea pigs. Auris Nasus Larynx 2003; 30: 219–225

[210] Piel IJ, Meyer D, Perlia CP, Wolfe VI. Effects of cis-diamminedichloroplatinum (NSC-119875) on hearing function in man. Cancer Chemother Rep 1974; 58: 871–875

[211] McKeage MJ. Comparative adverse effect profiles of platinum drugs. Drug Saf 1995; 13: 228–244

[212] Rybak LP. Mechanisms of cisplatin ototoxicity and progress in otoprotection. Curr Opin Otolaryngol Head Neck Surg 2007; 15: 364–369

[213] Schaefer SD, Wright CG, Post JD, Frenkel EP. Cis-platinum vestibular toxicity. Cancer 1981; 47: 857–859

[214] Rybak LP. Pathophysiology of furosemide ototoxicity. J Otolaryngol 1982; 11: 127–133

[215] Arnold W, Nadol JB, Jr, Weidauer H. Ultrastructural histopathology in a case of human ototoxicity due to loop diuretics. Acta Otolaryngol 1981; 91: 399–414

[216] Quick CA, Hoppe W. Permanent deafness associated with furosemide administration. Ann Otol Rhinol Laryngol 1975; 84: 94–101

[217] Delpire E, Lu J, England R, Dull C, Thorne T. Deafness and imbalance associated with inactivation of the secretory Na-K-2Cl co-transporter. Nat Genet 1999; 22: 192–195

[218] Bosher SK. Ethacrynic acid ototoxicity as a general model in cochlear pathology. Adv Otorhinolaryngol 1977; 22: 81–89

[219] Matz GJ, Hinojosa R. Histopathology following use of ethacrynic acid. Surg Forum 1973; 24: 488–489

[220] Goodman L, Gilman A. The Pharmacological Basis of Therapeutics. New York: Macmillan, 1975

[221] Gallagher KL, Jones JK. Furosemide-induced ototoxicity. Ann Intern Med 1979; 91: 744–745

[222] Myers EN, Bernstein JM. Salicylate ototoxicity; a clinical and experimental study. Arch Otolaryngol 1965; 82: 483–493

[223] Hawkins J. Iatrogenic toxic deafness in children. In: McConnell F, Ward P, eds. Symposium on Deafness in Childhood. Nashville: Vanderbilt University Press, 1967

[224] Bernstein JM, Weiss AD. Further observations on salicylate ototoxicity. J Laryngol Otol 1967; 81: 915–925

[225] Perez de Moura LF, Hayden RC, Jr. Salicylate ototoxicity. A human temporal bone report. Arch Otolaryngol 1968; 87: 368–372

[226] Jung TT, Rhee CK, Lee CS, Park YS, Choi DC. Ototoxicity of salicylate, nonsteroidal antiinflammatory drugs, and quinine. Otolaryngol Clin North Am 1993; 26: 791–810

[227] Ruel J, Chabbert C, Nouvian R et al. Salicylate enables cochlear arachidonic-acid-sensitive NMDA receptor responses. J Neurosci 2008; 28: 7313–7323

[228] Ruedi L, Furrer W, Luthy F, Nager G, Tschirren B. Further observations concerning the toxic effects of streptomycin and quinine on the auditory organ of guinea pigs. Laryngoscope 1952; 62: 333–351

[229] McCabe PA, Dey FL. The effect of aspirin upon auditory sensitivity. Ann Otol Rhinol Laryngol 1965; 74: 312–325

[230] Campbell KC, Durrant J. Audiologic monitoring for ototoxicity. Otolaryngol Clin North Am 1993; 26: 903–914

[231] Fischel-Ghodsian N. Genetic factors in aminoglycoside ototoxicity. In: Roland P, Rutka J, eds. Ototoxicity. Hamilton, Ontario: BC Decker, 2004: 144–152

[232] Barclay ML, Begg EJ, Hickling KG. What is the evidence for once-daily aminoglycoside therapy? Clin Pharmacokinet 1994; 27: 32–48

[233] Gølloe AM, Graudal N, Christensen HR, Kampmann JP. Aminoglycosides: single or multiple daily dosing? A meta-analysis on efficacy and safety. Eur J Clin Pharmacol 1995; 48: 39–43

[234] Tulkens PM. Pharmacokinetic and toxicological evaluation of a once-daily regimen versus conventional schedules of netilmicin and amikacin. J Antimicrob Chemother 1991; 27 Suppl C: 49–61

[235] Smyth AR, Bhatt J. Once-daily versus multiple-daily dosing with intravenous aminoglycosides for cystic fibrosis. Cochrane Database Syst Rev 2012; 2: CD002009

[236] Nordström L, Lerner SA. Single daily dose therapy with aminoglycosides. J Hosp Infect 1991; 18 Suppl A: 117–129

[237] Beaubien AR, Ormsby E, Bayne A et al. Evidence that amikacin ototoxicity is related to total perilymph area under the concentration-time curve regardless of concentration. Antimicrob Agents Chemother 1991; 35: 1070–1074

[238] Xie J, Talaska AE, Schacht J. New developments in aminoglycoside therapy and ototoxicity. Hear Res 2011; 281: 28–37

[239] Rybak LP, Mukherjea D, Jajoo S, Ramkumar V. Cisplatin ototoxicity and protection: clinical and experimental studies. Tohoku J Exp Med 2009; 219: 177–186

[240] Schweitzer VG, Dolan DF, Abrams GE, Davidson T, Snyder R. Amelioration of cisplatin-induced ototoxicity by fosfomycin. Laryngoscope 1986; 96: 948–958

[241] Olson JJ, Truelson JM, Street N. In vitro interaction of cisplatin and fosfomycin on squamous cell carcinoma cultures. Arch Otolaryngol Head Neck Surg 1994; 120: 1253–1257

[242] Carrasquilla G, Barón C, Monsell EM et al. Randomized, prospective, three-arm study to confirm the auditory safety and efficacy of artemether-lumefantrine in Colombian patients with uncomplicated Plasmodium falciparum malaria. Am J Trop Med Hyg 2012; 86: 75–83

[243] Saluja S, Agarwal A, Kler N, Amin S. Auditory neuropathy spectrum disorder in late preterm and term infants with severe jaundice. Int J Pediatr Otorhinolaryngol 2010; 74: 1292–1297

[244] Smith RJ, Zimmerman B, Connolly PK, Jerger SW, Yelich A. Screening audiometry using the high-risk register in a level III nursery. Arch Otolaryngol Head Neck Surg 1992; 118: 1306–1311

[245] Kimura R, Perlman HB. Arterial obstruction of the labyrinth. I. Cochlear changes. Ann Otol Rhinol Laryngol 1958; 67: 5–24

[246] Sawada S, Mori N, Mount RJ, Harrison RV. Differential vulnerability of inner and outer hair cell systems to chronic mild hypoxia and glutamate ototoxicity: insights into the cause of auditory neuropathy. J Otolaryngol 2001; 30: 106–114

[247] Belal A, Jr. Pathology of vascular sensorineural hearing impairment. Laryngoscope 1980; 90: 1831–1839

[248] Kimura R, Perlman HB. Extensive venous obstruction of the labyrinth. A. Cochlear changes. Ann Otol Rhinol Laryngol 1956; 65: 332–350

[249] Chen GD. Effect of hypoxia on noise-induced auditory impairment. Hear Res 2002; 172: 186–195

[250] Chen GD, Liu Y. Mechanisms of noise-induced hearing loss potentiation by hypoxia. Hear Res 2005; 200: 1–9

[251] Druss JG. Aural manifestations of leukemia. Arch Otolaryngol 1945; 42: 267–274

[252] Schuknecht HF, Igarashi M, Chasin WD. Inner ear hemorrhage in leukemia. A case report. Laryngoscope 1965; 75: 662–668

[253] Kirikae I, Nomura Y, Shitara T, Kobayashi T. Sudden deafness due to Buerger's disease. Arch Otolaryngol 1962; 75: 502–505

[254] Jaffe BF. Sudden deafness—a local manifestation of systemic disorders: fat emboli, hypercoagulation and infections. Laryngoscope 1970; 80: 788–801

[255] Shapiro MJ, Purn JM, Raskin C. A study of the effects of cardiopulmonary bypass surgery on auditory function. Laryngoscope 1981; 91: 2046–2052

[256] Plasse HM, Mittleman M, Frost JO. Unilateral sudden hearing loss after open heart surgery: a detailed study of seven cases. Laryngoscope 1981; 91: 101–109

[257] Young IM, Mehta GK, Lowry LD. Unilateral sudden hearing loss with complete recovery following cardiopulmonary bypass surgery. Yonsei Med J 1987; 28: 152–156

[258] Ness JA, Stankiewicz JA, Kaniff T, Pifarre R, Allegretti J. Sensorineural hearing loss associated with aortocoronary bypass surgery: a prospective analysis. Laryngoscope 1993; 103: 589–593

[259] Orchik DJ, Dunn JW. Sickle cell anemia and sudden deafness. Arch Otolaryngol 1977; 103: 369–370

[260] Friedman EM, Herer GR, Luban NL, Williams I. Sickle cell anemia and hearing. Ann Otol Rhinol Laryngol 1980; 89: 342–347

[261] Nomura Y, Tsuchida M, Mori S, Sakurai T. Deafness in cryoglobulinemia. Ann Otol Rhinol Laryngol 1982; 91: 250–255

[262] Barr DP, Reader GG, Wheeler CH. Cryoglobulinemia; report of two cases with discussion of clinical manifestations, incidence and significance. Ann Intern Med 1950; 32: 6–29, illust

[263] Millen SJ, Toohill RJ, Lehman RH. Sudden sensorineural hearing loss: operative complication in non-otologic surgery. Laryngoscope 1982; 92: 613–617

[264] Tos M. A survey of Hand-Schüller-Christian's disease in otolaryngology. Acta Otolaryngol 1966; 62: 217–228

[265] Hughes GB, Kinney SE, Barna BP, Calabrese LH. Practical versus theoretical management of autoimmune inner ear disease. Laryngoscope 1984; 94: 758–767

[266] Salamy A, Eldredge L, Tooley WH. Neonatal status and hearing loss in high-risk infants. J Pediatr 1989; 114: 847–852

[267] Bainbridge KE, Hoffman HJ, Cowie CC. Diabetes and hearing impairment in the United States: audiometric evidence from the National Health and Nutrition Examination Survey, 1999 to 2004. Ann Intern Med 2008; 149: 1–10

[268] Ma F, Gómez-Marín O, Lee DJ, Balkany T. Diabetes and hearing impairment in Mexican American adults: a population-based study. J Laryngol Otol 1998; 112: 835–839

[269] Kurien M, Thomas K, Bhanu TS. Hearing threshold in patients with diabetes mellitus. J Laryngol Otol 1989; 103: 164–168

[270] Celik O, Yalçin S, Celebi H, Oztürk A. Hearing loss in insulin-dependent diabetes mellitus. Auris Nasus Larynx 1996; 23: 127–132

[271] Dalton DS, Cruickshanks KJ, Klein R, Klein BE, Wiley TL. Association of NIDDM and hearing loss. Diabetes Care 1998; 21: 1540–1544

[272] de España R, Biurrun O, Lorente J, Traserra J. Hearing and diabetes. ORL J Otorhinolaryngol Relat Spec 1995; 57: 325–327

[273] Kakarlapudi V, Sawyer R, Staecker H. The effect of diabetes on sensorineural hearing loss. Otol Neurotol 2003; 24: 382–386

[274] Jorgensen MB, Buch NH. Studies on inner-ear function and cranial nerves in diabetics. Acta Otolaryngol 1961; 53: 350–364

[275] Costa OA. Inner ear pathology in experimental diabetes. Laryngoscope 1967; 77: 68–75

[276] Friedman SA, Schulman RH, Weiss S. Hearing and diabetic neuropathy. Arch Intern Med 1975; 135: 573–576

[277] Wilson WR, Laird N, Moo-Young G, Soeldner JS, Kavesh DA, MacMeel JW. The relationship of idiopathic sudden hearing loss to diabetes mellitus. Laryngoscope 1982; 92: 155–160

[278] Sieger A, White NH, Skinner MW, Spector GJ. Auditory function in children with diabetes mellitus. Ann Otol Rhinol Laryngol 1983; 92: 237–241

[279] Miller JJ, Beck L, Davis A, Jones DE, Thomas AB. Hearing loss in patients with diabetic retinopathy. Am J Otolaryngol 1983; 4: 342–346

[280] Harner SG. Hearing in adult-onset diabetes mellitus. Otolaryngol Head Neck Surg 1981; 89: 322–327

[281] Parving A, Elberling C, Balle V, Parbo J, Dejgaard A, Parving HH. Hearing disorders in patients with insulin-dependent diabetes mellitus. Audiology 1990; 29: 113–121

[282] Duck SW, Prazma J, Bennett PS, Pillsbury HC. Interaction between hypertension and diabetes mellitus in the pathogenesis of sensorineural hearing loss. Laryngoscope 1997; 107: 1596–1605

[283] Jorgensen MB. The inner ear in diabetes mellitus. Histological studies. Arch Otolaryngol 1961; 74: 373–381

[284] Wackym PA, Linthicum FH, Jr. Diabetes mellitus and hearing loss: clinical and histopathologic relationships. Am J Otol 1986; 7: 176–182

[285] Cullen JR, Cinnamond MJ. Hearing loss in diabetics. J Laryngol Otol 1993; 107: 179–182

[286] Davis LE, Johnsson LG. Viral infections of the inner ear: clinical, virologic, and pathologic studies in humans and animals. Am J Otolaryngol 1983; 4: 347–362

[287] Strauss M, Davis GL. Viral disease of the labyrinth. I. Review of the literature and discussion of the role of cytomegalovirus in congenital deafness. Ann Otol Rhinol Laryngol 1973; 82: 577–583

[288] Pappas DG. Hearing impairments and vestibular abnormalities among children with subclinical cytomegalovirus. Ann Otol Rhinol Laryngol 1983; 92: 552–557

[289] Westmore GA, Pickard BH, Stern H. Isolation of mumps virus from the inner ear after sudden deafness. BMJ 1979; 1: 14–15

[290] Smith GA, Gussen R. Inner ear pathologic features following mumps infection. Report of a case in an adult. Arch Otolaryngol 1976; 102: 108–111

[291] Bordley JE, Kapur YP. Histopathologic changes in the temporal bone resulting from measles infection. Arch Otolaryngol 1977; 103: 162–168

[292] Lindsay JR, Caruthers DG, Hemenway WG, Harrison S. Inner ear pathology following maternal rubella. Ann Otol Rhinol Laryngol 1953; 62: 1201–1218

[293] Wild NJ, Sheppard S, Smithells RW, Holzel H, Jones G. Onset and severity of hearing loss due to congenital rubella infection. Arch Dis Child 1989; 64: 1280–1283

[294] Beg JA. Bilateral sensorineural hearing loss as a complication of infectious mononucleosis. Arch Otolaryngol 1981; 107: 620–622

[295] Brodsky L, Stanievich J. Sensorineural hearing loss following live measles virus vaccination. Int J Pediatr Otorhinolaryngol 1985; 10: 159–163

[296] Stewart BJ, Prabhu PU. Reports of sensorineural deafness after measles, mumps, and rubella immunisation. Arch Dis Child 1993; 69: 153–154

[297] Hall R, Richards H. Hearing loss due to mumps. Arch Dis Child 1987; 62: 189–191

[298] Strauss M. A clinical pathologic study of hearing loss in congenital cytomegalovirus infection. Laryngoscope 1985; 95: 951–962

[299] Dollard SC, Grosse SD, Ross DS. New estimates of the prevalence of neurological and sensory sequelae and mortality associated with congenital cytomegalovirus infection. Rev Med Virol 2007; 17: 355–363

[300] Grosse SD, Ross DS, Dollard SC. Congenital cytomegalovirus (CMV) infection as a cause of permanent bilateral hearing loss: a quantitative assessment. J Clin Virol 2008; 41: 57–62

[301] Bradford RD, Cloud G, Lakeman AD et al. National Institute of Allergy and Infectious Diseases Collaborative Antiviral Study Group. Detection of cytomegalovirus (CMV) DNA by polymerase chain reaction is associated with hearing loss in newborns with symptomatic congenital CMV infection involving the central nervous system. J Infect Dis 2005; 191: 227–233

[302] Kimberlin DW, Lin CY, Sánchez PJ et al. National Institute of Allergy and Infectious Diseases Collaborative Antiviral Study Group. Effect of ganciclovir therapy on hearing in symptomatic congenital cytomegalovirus disease involving the central nervous system: a randomized, controlled trial. J Pediatr 2003; 143: 16–25

[303] Zajtchuk JT, Matz GJ, Lindsay JR. Temporal bone pathology in herpes oticus. Ann Otol Rhinol Laryngol 1972; 81: 331–338

[304] Suboti R. Histopathological findings in the inner ear caused by measles. J Laryngol Otol 1976; 90: 173–181

[305] Hinojosa R, Lindsay JR. Inner ear degeneration in Reye's syndrome. Arch Otolaryngol 1977; 103: 634–640

[306] Chandrasekhar SS, Connelly PE, Brahmbhatt SS, Shah CS, Kloser PC, Baredes S. Otologic and audiologic evaluation of human immunodeficiency virus-infected patients. Am J Otolaryngol 2000; 21: 1–9

[307] Hausler R, Vibert D, Koralnik IJ, Hirschel B. Neuro-otological manifestations in different stages of HIV infection. Acta Otolaryngol Suppl 1991; 481: 515–521

[308] Gurney TA, Murr AH. Otolaryngologic manifestations of human immunodeficiency virus infection. Otolaryngol Clin North Am 2003; 36: 607–624

[309] Kohan D, Rothstein SG, Cohen NL. Otologic disease in patients with acquired immunodeficiency syndrome. Ann Otol Rhinol Laryngol 1988; 97: 636–640

[310] Rarey KE. Otologic pathophysiology in patients with human immunodeficiency virus. Am J Otolaryngol 1990; 11: 366–369

[311] Lalwani AK, Sooy CD. Otologic and neurotologic manifestations of acquired immunodeficiency syndrome. Otolaryngol Clin North Am 1992; 25: 1183–1197

[312] Soucek S, Michaels L. The ear in the acquired immunodeficiency syndrome: II. Clinical and audiologic investigation. Am J Otol 1996; 17: 35–39

[313] Welkoborsky HJ, Lowitzsch K. Auditory brain stem responses in patients with human immunotropic virus infection of different stages. Ear Hear 1992; 13: 55–57

[314] Hart CW, Cokely CG, Schupbach J, Dal Canto MC, Coppleson LW. Neurotologic findings of a patient with acquired immune deficiency syndrome. Ear Hear 1989; 10: 68–76

[315] Bankaitis AE. The effects of click rate on the auditory brain stem response (ABR) in patients with varying degrees of HIV-infection: a pilot study. Ear Hear 1995; 16: 321–324

[316] Castello E, Baroni N, Pallestrini E. Neurotological auditory brain stem response findings in human immunodeficiency virus-positive patients without neurologic manifestations. Ann Otol Rhinol Laryngol 1998; 107: 1054–1060

[317] Pagano MA, Cahn PE, Garau ML et al. Brain-stem auditory evoked potentials in human immunodeficiency virus-seropositive patients with and without acquired immunodeficiency syndrome. Arch Neurol 1992; 49: 166–169

[318] Reyes-Contreras L, Silva-Rojas A, Ysunza-Rivera A, Jiménez-Ruíz G, Berruecos-Villalobos P, Romo-Gutiérrez G. Brainstem auditory evoked response in HIV-infected patients with and without AIDS. Arch Med Res 2002; 33: 25–28

[319] Chandrasekhar SS, Siverls V, Sekhar HK. Histopathologic and ultrastructural changes in the temporal bones of HIV-infected human adults. Am J Otol 1992; 13: 207–214

[320] Pappas DG, Jr et al. Ultrastructural findings in the cochlea of AIDS cases. Am J Otol 1994; 15: 456–465

[321] Michaels L, Soucek S, Liang J. The ear in the acquired immunodeficiency syndrome: I. Temporal bone histopathologic study. Am J Otol 1994; 15: 515–522

[322] Linstrom CJ, Pincus RL, Leavitt EB, Urbina MC. Otologic neurotologic manifestations of HIV-related disease. Otolaryngol Head Neck Surg 1993; 108: 680–687

[323] Morris MS, Prasad S. Otologic disease in the acquired immunodeficiency syndrome. Ear Nose Throat J 1990; 69: 451–453

[324] Simdon J, Watters D, Bartlett S, Connick E. Ototoxicity associated with use of nucleoside analog reverse transcriptase inhibitors: a report of 3 possible cases and review of the literature. Clin Infect Dis 2001; 32: 1623–1627

[325] Brinkman K, ter Hofstede HJ, Burger DM, Smeitink JA, Koopmans PP. Adverse effects of reverse transcriptase inhibitors: mitochondrial toxicity as common pathway. AIDS 1998; 12: 1735–1744

[326] Lewis W, Dalakas MC. Mitochondrial toxicity of antiviral drugs. Nat Med 1995; 1: 417–422

[327] Brinkman K, Kakuda TN. Mitochondrial toxicity of nucleoside analogue reverse transcriptase inhibitors: a looming obstacle for long-term antiretroviral therapy? Curr Opin Infect Dis 2000; 13: 5–11

[328] Johns DR. Seminars in medicine of the Beth Israel Hospital, Boston. Mitochondrial DNA and disease. N Engl J Med 1995; 333: 638–644

[329] Shigenaga MK, Hagen TM, Ames BN. Oxidative damage and mitochondrial decay in aging. Proc Natl Acad Sci U S A 1994; 91: 10771–10778

[330] Simonetti S, Chen X, DiMauro S, Schon EA. Accumulation of deletions in human mitochondrial DNA during normal aging: analysis by quantitative PCR. Biochim Biophys Acta 1992; 1180: 113–122

[331] McNulty JS, Fassett RL. Syphilis: an otolaryngologic perspective. Laryngoscope 1981; 91: 889–905

[332] Belal A, Jr, Linthicum FH, Jr. Pathology of congenital syphilitic labyrinthitis. Am J Otolaryngol 1980; 1: 109–118

[333] Nagasaki T, Watanabe Y, Aso S, Mizukoshi K. Electrocochleography in syphilitic hearing loss. Acta Otolaryngol Suppl 1993; 504: 68–73

[334] Zoller M, Wilson WR, Nadol JB, Jr, Girard KF. Detection of syphilitic hearing loss. Arch Otolaryngol 1978; 104: 63–65

[335] Balkany TJ, Dans PE. Reversible sudden deafness in early acquired syphilis. Arch Otolaryngol 1978; 104: 66–68

[336] Hendershot EL. Luetic deafness. Otolaryngol Clin North Am 1978; 11: 43–47

[337] Hughes GB, Rutherford I. Predictive value of serologic tests for syphilis in otology. Ann Otol Rhinol Laryngol 1986; 95: 250–259

[338] Birdsall HH, Baughn RE, Jenkins HA. The diagnostic dilemma of otosyphilis. A new western blot assay. Arch Otolaryngol Head Neck Surg 1990; 116: 617–621

[339] Pillsbury HC, Shea JJ. Luetic hydrops—diagnosis and therapy. Laryngoscope 1979; 89: 1135–1144

[340] Patterson ME. Congenital luetic hearing impairment. Treatment with prednisone. Arch Otolaryngol 1968; 87: 378–382

[341] Hughes GB, Haberkamp TJ. Other auditory disorders. In: Textbook of Clinical Otology. New York: Thieme, 1985

[342] Smith ME, Canalis RF. Otologic manifestations of AIDS: the otosyphilis connection. Laryngoscope 1989; 99: 365–372

[343] Aviel A, Ostfeld E. Acquired irreversible sensorineural hearing loss associated with otitis media with effusion. Am J Otolaryngol 1982; 3: 217–222

[344] Paparella MM, Goycoolea MV, Meyerhoff WL. Inner ear pathology and otitis media. A review. Ann Otol Rhinol Laryngol Suppl 1980; 89: 249–253

[345] Paparella MM, Morizono T, Le CT et al. Sensorineural hearing loss in otitis media. Ann Otol Rhinol Laryngol 1984; 93: 623–629

[346] Berlow SJ, Caldarelli DD, Matz GJ, Meyer DH, Harsch GG. Bacterial meningitis and sensorineural hearing loss: a prospective investigation. Laryngoscope 1980; 90: 1445–1452

[347] HHS-CDC news. HHS-CDC news: Direct and indirect effects of routine vaccination of children with 7-valent pneumococcal conjugate vaccine on incidence of invasive pneumococcal disease—US, 1998–2003. Ann Pharmacother 2005; 39: 1967–1968

[348] Young NM, Tan TQ. Current techniques in management of postmeningitic deafness in children. Arch Otolaryngol Head Neck Surg 2010; 136: 993–998

25 Benign Neoplasms of the Temporal Bone

Peter L. Santa Maria, Lawrence R. Lustig, and Robert K. Jackler

25.1 Introduction

The benign tumors of the temporal bone comprise a diverse spectrum of lesions that have largely been responsible for defining the specialty of neurotology and skull base surgery. In spite of their benign histopathological characteristics, however, these lesions may be locally destructive. Prompt diagnosis and treatment is therefore necessary to prevent further worsening of audiological, vestibular, facial, or lower cranial nerve dysfunction that is so common upon presentation (▶ Table 25.1).

25.2 Schwannoma

The most common tumor of the temporal bone and cerebellopontine angle is the schwannoma, accounting for 6% of all intracranial tumors, and 91% of all tumors in and around the temporal bone.[1,2] Schwannomas are benign tumors of the nerve sheath, which historically have also been referred to as neuromas, neurofibromas, neurinomas, and neurilemmomas.[3] Within the temporal bone, schwannomas arise in three anatomic loci: the internal auditory canal (IAC) from the eighth cranial nerve, the fallopian canal from the seventh cranial nerve, and the jugular foramen from cranial nerves IX to XI.

25.2.1 Vestibular Schwannoma/ Acoustic Neuroma

Vestibular schwannomas, more commonly known as acoustic neuromas (ANs), are the most commonly occurring schwannoma of the temporal bone, and by inference, the most commonly encountered tumor in otology. An overwhelming majority of ANs arise de novo as a solitary lesion. Diagnosis typically occurs after the sixth decade, with a slightly higher incidence in females.[4] Neurofibromatosis type 2 (NF2), accounting for only 5% of tumors, is associated with bilateral ANs and tends to present earlier in life (▶ Fig. 25.1).

Recent studies suggest that undiagnosed ANs may be present in as many as 2 in 10,000 of the population.[5] Schwannomas, as their name implies, are derived from Schwann cells. Their point of origin is repeatedly described in the literature as arising at the transition zone between central and peripheral myelin, known as the Obersteiner-Redlich zone, though one small series indicates that most vestibular nerve schwannomas may in fact originate lateral to the glial–schwannian junction of the nerve.[6,7] The tumors arise with an equal frequency from the superior and inferior divisions of the vestibular nerve, and usually originate within the medial portion of the IAC, though a fraction arise extrameatally or in the lateral IAC.[8]

Table 25.1 Primary Temporal Bone Neoplasms

Site	Benign	Malignant
Pinna	Hemangioma	Basal cell carcinoma
		Squamous cell carcinoma
		Melanoma
EAC	Osteoma	Squamous cell carcinoma
	Neurofibroma	Adenoid-cystic carcinoma
Middle ear	Adenoma	Squamous cell carcinoma (rare)
	Glomus tympanicum	Rhabdomyosarcoma
	Schwannoma (CN VII)	
Mastoid	Adenoma	Squamous cell carcinoma (rare)
	Schwannoma (CN VII)	Papillary adenocarcinoma
IAC	Schwannoma (CN VIII >> VII)	
	Meningioma-ossifying hemangioma	
Jugular foramen	Glomus jugulare meningioma	
	Schwannoma (CN IX–XII)	
Petrous apex	Chondroma	Chondrosarcoma
		Chordoma
		Metastases

CN, cranial nerve; EAC, external auditory canal; IAC, internal auditory canal.

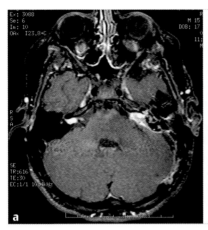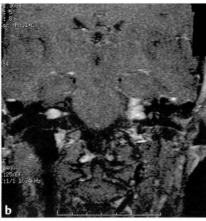

Fig. 25.1 A patient with neurofibromatosis type 2 (NF2) and bilateral vestibular schwannomas. (a) The T1-weighted magnetic resonance imaging (MRI) scan with gadolinium enhancement in the axial plane shows a characteristic tumor of the right internal auditory canal with a small cerebellopontine angle component. The tumor on the left, which has the appearance of a meningioma with dural tail enhancement, was found to be a vestibular schwannoma at surgery. (b) The coronal view shows the tumors in this same patient.

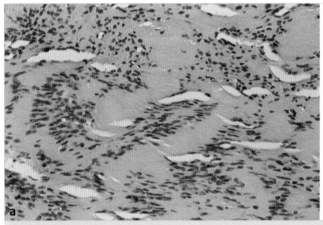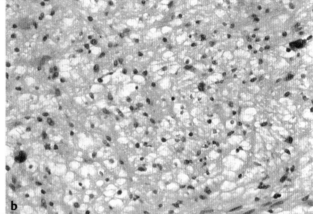

Fig. 25.2 Histopathology of vestibular schwannomas. These hematoxylin and eosin (H&E) stains demonstrate the two common types of histopathology seen in vestibular schwannomas. (a) The Antoni A pattern consists of densely packed spindle-shaped cells with darkly staining nuclei. When they appear in a whorled configuration it is referred to as a Verocay body. (b) The Antoni B pattern consists of a more diffusely arranged cell pattern with increased pleomorphism. This pattern tends to predominate in larger tumors, though any tumor may contain one or both patterns. The clinical significance of these two patterns is unclear.

The elucidation of the underlying genetics of ANs is derived from the study of NF2 patients. The specific defect for NF2 leading to bilateral ANs has been genetically mapped to chromosome 22.[9] The gene product, termed *merlin*, is believed to be a tumor-suppressor gene, requiring both copies of the gene to be dysfunctional for tumorigenesis to occur. NF2 patients are therefore born with one defective gene, leading to a lifelong propensity toward AN development. Patients with sporadically arising ANs, by contrast, have acquired defects of both gene copies, leading to the formation of tumor.[10,11] The precise role of the *merlin* gene product remains unclear, but has been shown to exert its activity by inhibiting phosphatidylinositol 3-kinase.[12,13]

There has been considerable interest in the media over the possible role of mobile phones in acoustic neuromas and other brain tumors. Despite there being dominance in handedness and ear side of phone use, the tumor itself does not show laterality. The Danish cohort study of almost 3 million and the Interphone study have shown no correlation.[14,15] A large Japanese epidemiological study suggested there was an increased risk if the average call duration was more than 20 minutes; however, there was a large recall bias.[16]

Macroscopically, ANs are smooth-walled gray or yellowish masses. Though they have been traditionally described as being well encapsulated, studies indicate that they do not possess a true capsule.[17] Microscopically, two morphological patterns can be discerned. The Antoni A pattern consists of densely packed spindle-shaped cells with darkly staining nuclei. When they appear in a whorled configuration, it is referred to as a Verocay body. The Antoni B pattern consists of a more diffusely arranged cell pattern with increased pleomorphism (▶ Fig. 25.2). Any tumor may contain one or both patterns. The clinical significance of these two patterns is unclear, though the Antoni B type tends to predominate in larger tumors. The immunoperoxidase stain S-100 is positive and is used to confirm the diagnosis of schwannoma.[18–20]

The majority of ANs are benign and slow-growing tumors. Though the average growth rate for tumors has been estimated to be between 0.1 and 0.2 cm in diameter per year, the range is variable, and 10 to 15% have a growth rate greater than 1 cm per year.[21,22] The growth rate has been shown to be related to the concentration of vascular endothelial growth factor.[23] The growth of acoustic neuromas can be classified into four stages: intracanalicular, cisternal, brainstem compressive, and hydrocephalic (▶ Fig. 25.3).[4]

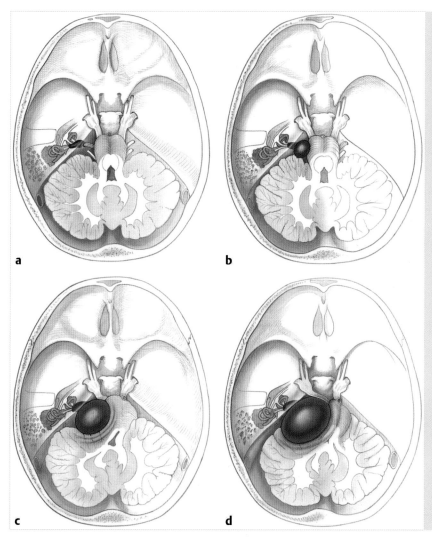

a

b

c

d

The clinical presentation of patients with AN reflects the tumor growth patterns. Asymmetrical sensorineural hearing loss, occurring in 95% of patients, is believed to be secondary to direct compression of the tumor on cranial nerve VIII within the IAC, or due to compression of the nerve's vascular supply. The hearing loss is sudden in onset in about one fourth of cases.[4] Additional symptoms include high-pitched, continuous, asymmetrical tinnitus; vertigo; disequilibrium and ataxia (up to 70% incidence in larger tumors); facial sensory disturbances (50%); facial twitching (10%); headaches (40%); nystagmus; and decreased corneal reflexes.[4] Unilateral tonal tinnitus is often used as screening criteria. Magnetic resonance imaging (MRI) scans performed in this group will only detect an acoustic neuroma in around 1 in 200 patients.[24] Audiometric testing typically reveals asymmetrical sensorineural hearing loss predominating in the high frequencies, though this configuration is not strictly found. If a threshold to define asymmetrical hearing loss is used at ≥ 15 dB between 2 and 8 kHz, 91% of acoustic neuromas would be detected.[25] Word recognition scores often are out of proportion to the degree of pure-tone hearing thresholds.

A number of other tests are often used but are not specific. Worsening word recognition with louder volume (PB [phonetically balanced] rollover) is a sign of retrocochlear pathology. There is usually either an absent stapedial reflex or a reflex

decay, but this is not sufficiently reliable to be of much diagnostic value.[26] Auditory brainstem response (ABR) testing is also used to assist in identifying retrocochlear pathology. The presence of a wave I and absence of waves II to V is the most specific finding for AN, though one must be wary of both false-positive (> 80%) and false-negative (12–18%) ABRs.[27,28] Abnormalities in vestibular testing are sometimes claimed to localize which vestibular nerve is affected with videonystagmography (VNG), with caloric irrigation being a test for the superior vestibular nerve, and cervical vestibular evoked myogenic potentials (cVEMPs) being a test for the inferior vestibular nerve. In practice they do not correlate with tumor location, as a growing tumor may cause more dysfunction on a neighboring nerve than the nerve of origin.

Contrast-enhanced MRI provides the gold standard for the diagnosis of the AN, which is able to detect tumors as small as 1 mm. The MRI features of AN are summarized in ▶ Table 25.2. The well-demarcated lesions are isointense on T1-weighted images and demonstrate some signal increase on T2-weighted images with areas of heterogeneity (▶ Fig. 25.4).[29]

After gadolinium administration, enhancement is striking, more so than most other benign extraaxial tumors.[30] High-resolution computed tomography (CT), though not as sensitive as MRI for small tumors, reliably demonstrates a smoothly

Table 25.2 MRI Features of Acoustic Neuroma vs. Meningioma

	Acoustic Neuroma	Meningioma
T1	Isointense or hypointense, gadolinium enhancement	Isointense or hypointense, gadolinium enhancement
T2	Hypointense	Hypointense
Appearance	More homogeneous	More heterogeneous
Angle at the petrous bone	Acute	Obtuse
Dural tail	No	Yes
Relationship to IAC	Centered, expands it	Eccentric
Hyperostosis	No	Maybe

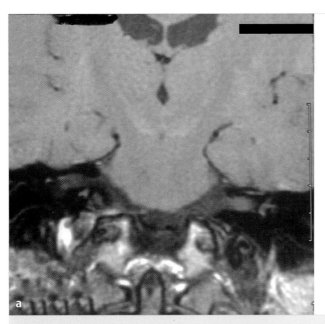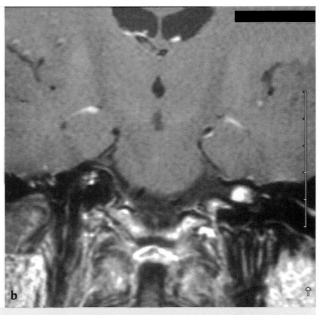

Fig. 25.4 A coronal MRI of a small left intracanalicular vestibular schwannoma measuring about 8 mm. The tumor is barely visible on the T1-weighted images without gadolinium enhancement (a), whereas with gadolinium (b) the tumor is markedly enhanced.

marginated, contrast-enhancing mass within the cerebellopontine angle (CPA) in tumors over 1.5 cm in diameter (▶ Fig. 25.5).[30]

Although the tumors are slow growing and benign, in most cases treatment is recommended because growth may lead to multiple cranial neuropathies, brainstem compression, hydrocephalus, and death. In selected cases, a conservative "watch and wait" approach may be appropriate, such as in the elderly or medically infirm, or if it is the choice of a compliant patient.[31,32] The natural history shows that up to 75% of tumors will show no growth,[33] and therefore a period of observation is reasonable at initial presentation. Significant growth, defined as growth by 2 mm or more in any dimension, is an indication for treatment. During observation the patient may still develop a hearing loss even without tumor growth.[34] Future treatment of a larger tumor if growth occurs increases the risk of potential complications.

The first priority of surgery or radiation therapy is to alleviate the risk of progressive intracranial tumor growth, and it is secondarily concerned with preservation of facial nerve function

and sparing of useful hearing. A variety of techniques have been employed to achieve these ends, including the translabyrinthine, retrosigmoid, and middle fossa approaches. The decision of which to use depends on the tumor size, its depth of penetration within the IAC, the degree of hearing loss, and the experience of the surgical team (▶ Table 25.3).[35,36]

A recent surgical trend also includes near-total tumor resection (remnant ≤ 2.5 mm in length and ≤ 2 mm thick) followed by expectant observation in an effort to improve facial nerve outcomes.[37] In such a scenario, recurrences have been shown to be about 3%. Intraoperative cranial nerve monitoring is routinely employed to assist with neural preservation during tumor resection. The results after surgery are dependent on the experience of the surgical team.[38] The expected mortality is less than 2% in most major centers, with tumor-related mortality limited to those with large tumors. Complications occur in about 20% of cases, and most commonly include cerebrospinal fluid (CSF) leakage, meningitis, and chronic headache.[39–41] Less common are traumatic parenchymal injury from intraoperative retraction, arterial or venous cerebral infarct, postoperative hemorrhage into the CPA, and air embolism.[42,43] Anatomically the facial nerve is preserved in 82 to 97% of cases, with an overwhelming majority having grade 1 or 2 facial nerve function 1 year after surgery. Whether anatomic preservation correlates with postoperative nerve function, however, is subject to debate.[44,45] Stimulating the facial nerve at the end of the case with a threshold of ≤ 0.05 mA has been shown to predict facial nerve

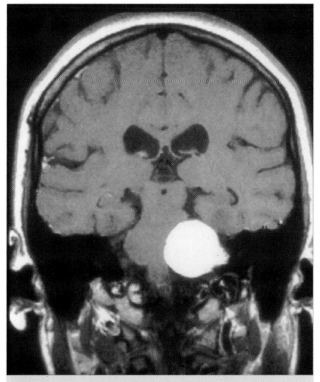

Fig. 25.5 A 4-cm vestibular schwannoma with brainstem compression is shown in this coronal T1-weighted MRI scan with gadolinium enhancement.

function of 93 to 100% of grade 1 to 2 at 12 months.[46] Hearing preservation surgery may be attempted for tumors with less than a 1.5 cm intracranial component and that meet the "50/ 50" rule, with a speech reception threshold less than 50 dB and a word recognition score of greater than 50%, though these rules are not strict and are even now being redefined and broadened.[47–50] Though results vary widely from center to center, useful hearing is commonly preserved in about one fourth of cases attempted, though in the most favorable tumors hearing preservation may be as high as 70% in experienced centers.[51,52]

Stereotactic radiosurgery (gamma knife) is being increasingly employed in a growing number of centers as an alternative to surgery for tumors < 3 cm in size, resulting in acceptable morbidity and a similar spectrum of functional deficits, though the long-term control rates have not yet been conclusively established. For those patients unable to tolerate the risk of surgery, stereotactic radiation may represent a viable alternative.[53–57] This technique relies on conformal radiation dose plans with steep radiation falloff to minimize injury to vital surrounding structures.[58] There is also growing acceptance that for large tumors, a subtotal resection of tumor, leaving the tumor capsule behind to preserve existing cranial nerve function, followed by radiation or gamma knife treatment, represents an alternative treatment option.[59] Several larger series with adequate (10 years or greater) follow-up have shown that following single-dose radiotherapy, 20 to 25% of tumors remain stable, 50 to 75% of tumors shrink in size, and 2 to 13% show further growth.[60–63] However, these rates need to be tempered by the observation that in untreated tumors followed over a 3-year period, 50% of tumors remain stable, 14% shrink, and 37% enlarge.[64] There may be transient growth in the year following treatment in 15 to 30% or stabilization at a higher volume after initial growth in 5 to 10%.[65]

Tumor control is less likely in patients with NF2 or with predominantly cystic tumors.[58] Though older dosing regimens were associated with a 37% incidence of facial palsy, newer dosing algorithms are rarely associated with facial nerve weakness

Table 25.3 Surgical Approaches for the Management of Acoustic Neuroma

Approach	Indications	Advantages	Disadvantages
Retrosigmoid	Good hearing and minimal IAC component (not involving lateral third of IAC)	Excellent exposure	Increased incidence of postoperative headaches (15% moderate to severe)
		Hearing preservation possible	Higher incidence of CSF leak (15%)
		Familiar to neurosurgeon	Need for more vigorous cerebellar retraction (+ hydrocephalus) Difficult fundus exposure
Translabyrinthine/anterosigmoid	Any size + no hearing	Lower surgical morbidity Most direct route More facial nerve reconstructive options Limited cerebellar retraction	Inability to preserve hearing
Middle fossa	Good hearing + minimal CPA component	Superior hearing preservation results	Increased risk of transient facial neurapraxia
			Unsuitable for tumors with large CPA component Temporal lobe retraction (not tolerated well in patients > 65 years)

CPA, cerebellopontine angle; CSF, cerebrospinal fluid.

following stereotactic radiotherapy (0.5–8% permanent).[62,66] Loss of serviceable hearing (> 50% speech reception threshold and < 50% word recognition scores) has been shown to occur in 30 to 50% of cases in the 2 years following treatment.[62,63,66–69] However, should a patient undergo stereotactic radiotherapy for a vestibular schwannoma and subsequently need surgical resection for a continually growing tumor, the facial nerve function preservation rates are not as good as compared with when there was no prior radiotherapy.[70,71] There is always a risk of a radiation-induced malignancy, with a small number of reported cases in the literature.[72–74] Radiotherapy for these lesions should be used cautiously in younger individuals.

The major dilemma in vestibular schwannoma management are young healthy patients with good hearing: to treat or wait and re-scan in 6 to 12 months. The patients are likely to need treatment at some point in their lifetime. First, patients must understand that the least risk to immediate hearing is to do nothing; however, even small tumors can suddenly cause hearing to drop. Only 38% of patients can expect good hearing at 10 years if there is a reduction in word recognition at presentation; 69% of those with 100% word recognition at presentation can expect good hearing at 10 years.[75] Also, in theory, facial nerve injury during surgery is greater if the tumor grows in the 6- to 12-month follow-up interval. Even the risk of partial but significant hearing loss with gamma knife (about 25% chance) outweighs most other considerations. Wait and re-scan has become the standard for initial management of intracanalicular schwannomas for many neurotologists. One major exception is significant dizziness attacks, which are best managed by tumor surgery that sections the vestibular nerve. Tumors that are larger at presentation or that present with tinnitus are more likely to show growth over time.[76]

Anti–vascular endothelial growth factor (VEGF) therapies, such as bevacizumab, are currently under clinical trials in NF2 patients, with promising results of tumor stabilization, possible tumor shrinkage, and hearing recovery in a subset of patients. In a recent review of 31 patients, 90% had stable or improved hearing after 1 year of treatment and 61% at 3 years; 87% of patients had stable or decreased tumor size after 1 year of treatment and 54% at 3 years.[77] VEGF is expressed in 100% of acoustic neuromas[78] and plays a role in tumor angiogenesis and vessel permeability, and anti-VEGF therapies normalize the schwannoma vasculature.[79] Adverse effects of anti-VEGF therapies include hypertension, proteinuria, thromboembolism, impaired wound healing, and bleeding.[80] Because of this increase in bleeding, any surgery must be postponed for at least 6 weeks after cessation of the drug. A decision to cease treatment comes with the potential for rapid rebound growth.[81,82] Other emerging therapies include epidermal growth factor receptor (EGFR) inhibitors, which may stabilize growth or reduce the growth rate of rapidly growing tumors.[83]

25.2.2 Jugular Foramen Schwannoma

Though schwannomas are the second most common lesion of the jugular foramen, after glomus tumors, overall they are relatively rare, representing about 3% of all intracranial schwannomas.[84,85] Schwannomas presenting in this region arise from cranial nerves IX to XII. As with vestibular schwannomas, these tumors probably occur at the transition zone between the central

and peripheral myelin. Histologically, the tumors resemble vestibular schwannomas.[86]

Three tumor growth patterns have been recognized for jugular foramen schwannomas.[87] Tumors arising in the distal portion of the foramen may expand inferiorly out of the skull base. More proximally arising tumors can expand into the posterior fossa. Others arise in the middle of the foramen and either expand primarily into bone or become bilobed, with an expansion both out of the skull base and into the posterior fossa.

The most common presenting symptoms are hoarseness, swallowing difficulties, and vertigo.[84–87] Other symptoms may include shoulder weakness, headache, nausea, vomiting, facial numbness or spasm, dysphagia, and visual disturbances. On exam, cranial nerve X is dysfunctional in 63% of cases presenting, and may be accompanied by deficits of cranial nerves IX (55%), XI (41%), and XII (36%).[88] Cranial nerve V and VII dysfunction is less common on examination, as are hemifacial spasm, nystagmus, ataxia, and papilledema.[84]

High-resolution CT typically demonstrates a well-demarcated, smoothly marginated expansion of the foramen walls (▶ Fig. 25.6). MRI is superior for diagnosis, and demonstrates a lesion isointense to brain parenchyma on contrast-enhanced T1-weighted images, whereas T2-weighted images usually reveal a high signal intensity. The addition of gadolinium causes a marked signal increase. Differentiation from paragangliomas is made possible by noting the morphologically smooth manner of bony erosion as compared with a more irregular pattern with glomus tumors and meningiomas. In contrast to glomus tumors, flow voids are notably absent.[85] Angiography is often

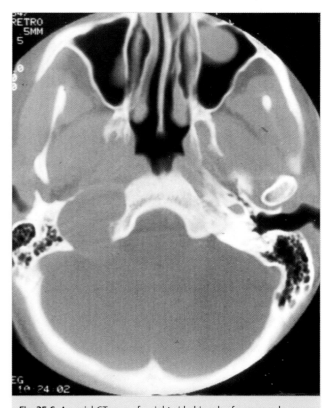

Fig. 25.6 An axial CT scan of a right-sided jugular foramen schwannoma. Note the smooth enlargement of the jugular foramen. The patient presented with headaches, hoarseness, and dysphagia.

undertaken under the presumption that the tumor is a paraganglioma; it is of little use diagnostically for schwannomas unless one anticipates a possible surgical need to evaluate the carotid or jugulosigmoid venous systems.[85]

As with vestibular schwannomas, the treatment is primarily surgical.[89] Because of the variability of tumor presentation, the surgical approach must be individualized. Techniques for exposure of the jugular foramen have become increasingly routine in recent years.[89–92] Jugular foramen schwannomas, because they often have an intracranial component, frequently require a transjugular posterior fossa craniotomy. Surgery may lead to worsening of existing dysfunction or new paralysis of cranial nerves IX to XI, leading to postoperative hoarseness, dysphagia, and shoulder weakness in many cases.[88,93–95] Vocal cord medialization procedures can help compensate for paralytic laryngeal dysfunction. Preservation of periosteum covering cranial nerves reduces lower cranial nerve dysfunction postoperatively.[96] Stereotactic radiotherapy has also been used in this patient group either as primary therapy or to treat the tumor remnant, with early reports of good tumor control.[97–100]

25.2.3 Facial Nerve Schwannoma

Schwannomas of the facial nerve are uncommon lesions, accounting for only 1.2% of all temporal bone tumors.[1] Though its true incidence is not known, one study was able to identify only one case out of 1,400 temporal bones analyzed.[101] Schwannomas have been identified along the entire course of the facial nerve, although intratemporal tumors appear to be much more common than the intracranial variety.[102,103] Within the temporal bone, the most common sites of involvement, in decreasing frequency, are the geniculate ganglion, horizontal and vertical segments, IAC, and labyrinthine segment. Involvement of multiple segments of the facial nerve are almost twice as common as a single segment (64% compared to 36%).[104] A small percentage display an unusual multicentricity evidenced by multiple discrete intraneural connections, sometimes described as a string of pearls.[105] The tendency for growth longitudinally along the lumen of the fallopian canal may lead to tumor prolapse into the middle ear, IAC, and CPA, and out of the stylomastoid foramen.

In contrast to ANs, facial nerve schwannomas tend to be slower growing and are often present for years before detection.[106] However, because of the facial nerve's intimate relationship with the sensory organs, otic capsule erosion is more common, occurring in up to 30% of cases.[103]

Facial nerve dysfunction (palsy or twitch) is the hallmark of the clinical presentation. It occurs due to compression of the nerve within the fallopian canal. The most common pattern is slowly progressive palsy, often accompanied by hyperfunction manifested as a limited twitch or a full hemifacial spasm. Recurrent acute paralytic episodes with partial or even complete recovery may also occur. Patients are commonly misdiagnosed with Bell's palsy with the first episode of paralysis. Successive bouts of palsy then ensue, with increasingly poorer facial nerve function. This presentation of recurrent, progressively more severe episodes of facial palsy is a classic characteristic of facial nerve schwannoma. The facial nerve is surprisingly resistant to compression. It has been estimated that 50% of facial nerve fibers must degenerate before clinical signs of a palsy are detected.[106,107] In one study of 48 patients with facial nerve neuromas, 26 presented with normal facial function.[103] Thus, patients without functional recovery from an idiopathic facial paralysis after 3 months or with a history of recurrent Bell palsy should have an enhanced MRI scan to search for tumor or facial nerve pathology.[106]

Patients may also present with normal facial nerve function and a conductive hearing loss.[103] Additional presenting symptoms include vertigo from a labyrinthine fistula and sensorineural hearing loss from cochlear invasion.[67,108–110] Prolonged pain should also raise one's suspicion for a diagnosis other than idiopathic facial palsy.[103,105,106] Examination of the ear may demonstrate a mass behind the drum in up to 29% of cases.[106] Because biopsy of a facial nerve schwannoma in the middle ear usually results in a facial paralysis, appropriate imaging studies are recommended prior to biopsy of any middle ear tumor. Site-of-lesion tests, such as the Schirmer test of lacrimation and stapedial reflex testing, although theoretically attractive, are not completely reliable and have been made largely obsolete by CT and MRI.

Radiographically, facial nerve schwannomas are similar to those arising in other portions of the temporal bone. They are hypointense on T1 images, hyperintense on T2 images, and show marked enhancement with gadolinium. An enhancing enlargement of varying thickness along a large segment of facial nerve is considered highly suggestive of schwannoma. Although high-resolution CT can identify these tumors due to their osseous erosion, MRI is a more sensitive diagnostic tool.[111]

Surgical resection and grafting has been the traditional management; however, this has changed to include observation, bony decompression, or stereotactic radiation with the goal of maintaining facial nerve function for as long as possible.[60,108–110] Resection and grafting lead to at best a House-Brackmann grade of 3 (facial weakness at rest with good eye closure), and therefore patients are often managed in other ways until their facial function deteriorates to this level.[112–115] To approach these lesions surgically, lesions limited to the transverse or descending portions of the nerve, a tympanomastoid approach may be used.[116] Lesions that involve the labyrinthine segment, IAC, or geniculate ganglion require the addition of an extradural middle cranial fossa approach. If cochlear function has been destroyed, a translabyrinthine approach may be utilized.[106] Surgical options include complete resection, debulking, or decompression.[112] At surgery, it is occasionally possible to remove a facial nerve schwannoma with preservation of its nerve of origin. More commonly, however, nerve repair with an interposition graft is needed. This may be accomplished with either a greater auricular or sural nerve graft. In general, those patients with long-standing facial nerve paralysis (> 12 months) tend to have poorer postoperative facial nerve function. Because a common presentation for facial nerve schwannomas is a conductive hearing loss, it is not uncommon to first identify these tumors intraoperatively during an exploratory tympanotomy with the intent of performing a stapedectomy. In such a scenario, if a soft tissue mass is identified leaning on or eroding the stapes superstructure at tympanotomy, the surgeon should halt the procedure and perform imaging studies, and not biopsy the lesion. The use of stereotactic radiotherapy is a recent development in treating facial nerve schwannomas. Studies so far are limited by very small sample size, but they report good tumor control and facial nerve function.[117–119] Radiation injury to the cochlea is always a concern in these patients.

Facial nerve schwannomas in the IAC usually present with sensorineural rather than conductive hearing loss. They may mimic acoustic neuromas in clinical presentation but tend to produce facial nerve symptoms earlier than would be expected of acoustic neuromas of similar size. Facial nerve schwannomas in the IAC are managed in the same way with observation, radiation, or surgery, with the ultimate goal of preserving function for as long as possible. Surgery for IAC facial nerve schwannomas can provides an opportunity for tumor removal and excellent facial nerve outcomes (House-Brackmann grade 1 or 2 in 90%).[120–122]

25.3 Paraganglioma (Glomus Tumor)

The most common tumor of the middle ear and second most common tumor found in the temporal bone is the paraganglioma, more commonly known as a glomus tumor but occasionally referred to as a chemodectoma.[123] Paraganglia, the origin of these tumors, exist throughout the temporal bone, including on the jugular dome, the promontory of the middle ear, and along Jacobson's and Arnold's nerves, and account for the predilection of glomus tumors toward these anatomic sites.[124] The term *glomus* was mistakenly attached to these tumors when it was believed that their origin was similar to true glomus (arteriovenous) complexes, and though now recognized as inaccurate, the nomenclature has persisted.[125]

Although most glomus tumors appear to arise sporadically, there are reports of families with several members affected by glomus tumors, with an unusual *genomic imprinting* mode of inheritance.[126,127] In this manner of transmission, tumors occur only in the offspring of an affected female when there is transmittance of the gene through a carrier male, accounting for the observed tumor occurrence in "skipped" generations.[128] So far there have been 10 genes associated with paragangliomas with or without pheochromocytoma. These include *VHL* (von Hippel–Lindau), *NF1* (neurofibromatosis type 1), *RET* (multiple endocrine neoplasia type 2), mutations in any of the succinate dehydrogenase complex subunit genes (*SDHA, SDHB, SDHC, SDHD*) or the subunit cofactor (*SDHAF2*), and two newly identified genes (*TMEM127* and *MAX*).[129–131] This is helpful to remember as the "disease of 10's," with 10% familial cases and 10 genes implicated. There is a clear predilection for these tumors to arise in females, and patients usually present after the fifth decade of life.[123–126,128,132]

Glomus tumors are typically reddish-purple, vascular, and lobulated masses. Histologically they resemble normal paraganglia with clusters of chief cells, characteristically termed *zellballen* (literally translated as "cell balls") in a highly vascular stroma. This pattern is enhanced on silver staining, which is useful diagnostically. Sustentacular cells and nerve axons, seen in the normal paraganglion, are rarely seen in the tumor, however.[133,134]

Glomus tumors contain the neural crest cell-derived chief cells, which are included in the diffuse neuroendocrine system (DNES). They almost always contain catecholamines, but this is clinically significant in only 1 to 3% of glomus tumors.[125,134,135]

Nevertheless it is reasonable to perform preoperative evaluation in all patients, searching for the presence of catecholamine-producing tumors, because life-threatening intraoperative hypertension is possible if preoperative alpha- and beta-blockade are not administered. Elevation of urine catecholamine levels (three to five times normal) requires differentiation from pheochromocytomas, and occasionally may require selective renal vein sampling for adequate diagnosis.[136]

Glomus tumors involving the temporal bone are divided into two categories based on their anatomic location. Other classification schemes further subdivide these tumors according to size and extent of invasion (▶ Table 25.4).[136] Those arising along the course of the Jacobson nerve and involving primarily the tympanic cavity are termed *glomus tympanicum*. Paragangliomas arising from the dome of the jugular bulb and involving the jugular foramen and related structures are termed *glomus jugulare*. Both types are marked by slow, progressive growth, spreading via the pathways of least resistance, such as the temporal bone air-cell tracts, neural foramina, vascular channels, bony haversian systems, and the eustachian tube.[136–139] Advanced lesions of either type have the ability to invade cranial nerves.[140] However, the clinical presentation and operative management of each may be markedly different, and thus each is discussed individually. *Glomus vagale* tumors arise beneath the cranial base in proximity to cranial nerve X. A small minority of vagale tumors involve the temporal bone via retrograde spread through the jugular foramen.

The appearance of a paraganglioma on MRI reflects its highly vascular nature. Glomus tumors are isointense on T1-weighted images and brightly enhance with gadolinium. They typically show numerous signal voids due to the numerous vascular channels within, giving them a "salt and pepper" appearance.[141,142] On T2-weighted images, they demonstrate increased signal intensity in the solid portions of the tumor, with persistent flow void in the vascular portions.[29] Because paragangliomas can be multiple, some advocate that the imaging study should be carried down to the level of the carotid bifurcation to determine if multiple tumors exist.[143] Angiography is an additional important aspect of the evaluation of glomus tumors, but should be deferred until the preoperative period when both diagnostic and therapeutic (embolization) measures can be accomplished in a single study. The study allows the determination of the arterial supply, degree of vascularity, degree of arteriovenous shunting, evidence of major venous sinus occlusion, and confirmation of the diagnosis. Another advantage of angiography is that it can single-handedly evaluate both the internal and external carotid systems for evidence of multiple early lesions. Embolization is usually performed at the time of angiography as a preoperative maneuver to limit surgical blood loss.[144,145] Magnetic resonance angiography and venography are newer modalities that can also aid in the diagnosis of vascular lesions of the temporal bone including glomus tumors. The role of these newer radiographic modalities in the evaluation of glomus tumors is currently being defined.[146]

25.3.1 Glomus Tympanicum

Glomus tympanicum is a paraganglioma that arises from the promontory of the middle ear. Because of the vascularity of these tumors, pulsatile tinnitus is often the first presenting

Table 25.4 Classification Schemes for Glomus Tumors

Tumor	Description
Glasscock/Jackson Classification of Glomus Tumors *Glomus tympanicum*	
Type I	Small mass limited to the promontory
Type II	Tumor completely filling the middle ear space
Type III	Tumor filling the middle ear and extending into the mastoid
Type IV	Tumor filling the middle ear, extending into the mastoid or through the tympanic membrane to fill the external auditory canal; +/− internal carotid artery involvement
Glomus jugulare	
Type I	Small tumors involving the jugular bulb, middle ear, and mastoid
Type II	Tumor extending under the internal auditory canal; might have intracranial extension
Type III	Tumor extending into petrous apex; might have intracranial extension
Type IV	Tumor extending beyond petrous apex into clivus or infratemporal fossa; might have intracranial extension
Fisch Classification of Glomus Tumors	
Type A	Tumors limited to the middle ear cleft (glomus tympanicum)
Type B	Tumors limited to the tympanomastoid area with no bone destruction in the infralabyrinthine compartment of the temporal bone
Type C	Tumors involving the infralabyrinthine compartment with extension into the petrous apex
Type D1	Tumors with intracranial extension ≤ 2 cm in diameter
Type D2	Tumors with intracranial extension > 2 cm in diameter

Data from Jackson CG. Skull base surgery. Am J Otol 1981;3:161–171; and Oldring D, Fisch U. Glomus tumors of the temporal region: surgical therapy. Am J Otol 1979;1:7–18.

symptom.[137] Further growth causes conductive hearing loss as ossicular mobility is inhibited, which occurs in approximately half of all patients.[136] Continued expansion may cause the glomus tympanicum to erode laterally through the drum, mimicking a friable, bleeding polyp, or it may expand medially causing facial nerve dysfunction, sensorineural hearing loss, or vertigo.[123–126,128,133–138] Rarely, it may present as a eustachian tube mass or epistaxis.[147–149] In one large series of 71 patients, the presenting symptoms, in order of decreasing frequency, were pulsatile tinnitus (76%), hearing loss (conductive 52%, mixed 17%, sensorineural 5%), aural pressure/fullness (18%), vertigo/dizziness (9%), external canal bleeding (7%), and headache (4%).[138] Brown's sign, which consists of a pulsatile, purple-red middle ear mass that blanches with positive pneumatic otoscopy, is a frequently mentioned distinguishing sign but is of little clinical value.[150]

The differentiation between tympanicum and jugulare tumors is not always possible by physical examination alone because both lesions typically involve the middle ear.[136] Furthermore, other vascular lesions of the middle ear, such as an aberrant carotid artery or a high-riding jugular bulb, may mimic a glomus tumor, and thus radiographic evaluation prior to biopsy or surgical intervention is important. Temporal bone CT can identify an intact plate of bone at the lateral aspect of the jugular fossa, indicating that a tumor is limited to the middle ear and aiding its identification as a glomus tympanicum. CT is also useful for evaluating the degree of bony erosion and

the tumor's relationship to surrounding temporal bone structures.[136–138,140,143] MRI, although not as good as CT at evaluating bony changes within the temporal bone, is superior in identifying the extent of the tumor and defining the relationship of tumor to surrounding structures once it has extended beyond the confines of the middle ear.[151] Both MRI and CT are therefore recommended when differentiating glomus tumors from mimicking vascular lesions.[152] MRI is particularly useful in determining hypotympanic extension and planning the surgical approach.[153] Angiography, although useful for larger lesions, is not required for small glomus tympanicum tumors limited to the middle ear. The blood supply is usually from the inferior tympanic branch of the ascending pharyngeal artery.

Surgery is the principal mode of therapy for glomus tympanicum tumors. Patients with small lesions limited to the promontory that can be completely visualized by otoscopy and are confined to the mesotympanum on CT scan can be approached via a transcanal incision and a tympanomeatal flap to expose the middle ear. Larger lesions are best exposed postauricularly via an extended facial recess approach.[154] Occasionally very large tumors (large Fisch class B) require subtotal petrosectomy and blind sac closure.[155] Using these methods, complete tumor removal can be achieved in greater than 90% of cases.[138] Lasers are often used to assist with resection of these vascular tumors.[156] Closure of the air–bone gap can be expected in a majority of patients, whereas about 10% suffer some sensorineural worsening.

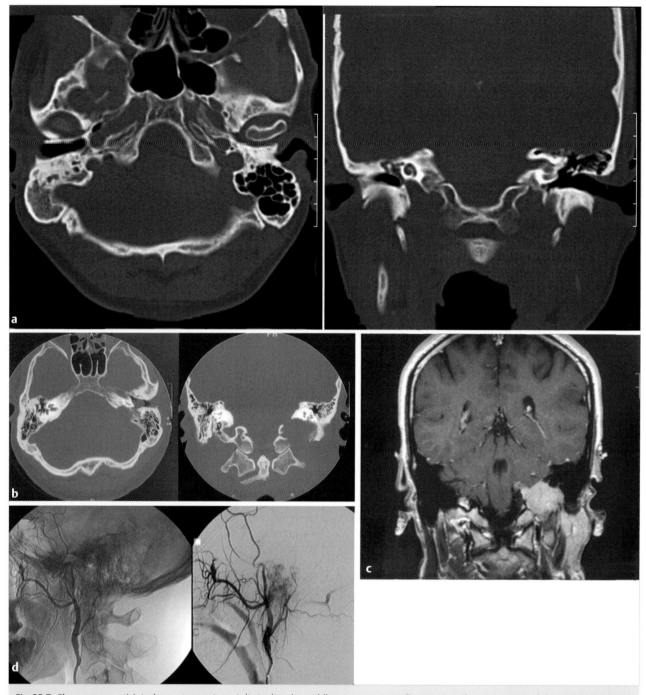

Fig. 25.7 Glomus tumors. (a) A glomus tympanicum is limited to the middle ear space, typically arising on the promontory of the cochlea. Both the axial (*left*) and coronal (*right*) views demonstrate opacification within the right middle ear space. A clear bony demarcation between the hypotympanum and jugular foramen/dome of the jugular bulb can be seen, which allows this tumor to be distinguished from a glomus jugulare. (b) In contrast, a glomus jugulare can erode through the hypotympanum, presenting in the middle ear in a similar fashion. However, in this case, the middle ear presentation is the "tip of the iceberg," as shown in axial (*left*) and coronal (*right*) CT images of this left glomus jugulare. (c) A T1-weighted MRI scan from the patient shown in b, demonstrating the tumor's intracranial extent. (d) Preoperative angiography, employed just prior to embolization to minimize blood loss in these highly vascular tumors, demonstrates the feeding vessels, which are often branches of the ascending pharyngeal artery.

25.3.2 Glomus Jugulare

Glomus jugulare tumors arise from paragangliomas situated near the dome of the jugular bulb or the proximal portions of the Arnold or Jacobson nerves. In contrast to the small confines of the middle ear where growth of a glomus tympanicum causes early symptoms, growth of a tumor in the jugular foramen region may remain clinically silent for years. Patients may not seek medical attention until the tumor has caused dysfunction of the lower cranial nerves or grown into the middle ear causing symptoms similar to a glomus tympanicum (pulsatile tinnitus, hearing loss). Growth of the glomus jugulare may carry the tumor into the neck intraluminally within the jugular vein, into the lower reaches of the posterior cranial fossa, or proximally into the sigmoid or even transverse sinus (▶ Fig. 25.7).[123,139] Middle fossa extension is, however, rare.

Due to these tumors' proximity to the hearing apparatus, pulsatile tinnitus, hearing loss, otalgia, and aural fullness are the most frequent presenting symptoms.[138] Because cranial nerves IX to XI lie adjacent to the jugular bulb, they are frequently involved, as discovered upon the patient's clinical presentation, and lead to symptoms such as hoarseness and dysphagia.[132,135,136,138,157,158] Vertigo, facial weakness, and headache are additional presenting symptoms. The thin plate of bone separating the dome of the jugular bulb from the middle ear is frequently eroded by tumor, enabling access into the middle ear. This accounts for the finding of a middle ear mass or external auditory canal mass on exam in about 70% of patients, despite its origin within the jugular foramen.[138] Though a cranial nerve X deficit is the most commonly encountered cranial nerve deficit upon presentation (24% of cases), cranial nerves VII through XII are susceptible to injury depending on the size and location of the lesion.[88,132,135,136,138,157,158] Because cranial nerve XII is least likely to be involved with tumor, its dysfunction is usually indicative of more extensive disease.[88]

The radiographic appearance of a glomus jugulare is similar to that of the glomus tympanicum, yet there are a few important distinctions. As mentioned above, an intact plate of bone at the lateral aspect of the jugular fossa indicates that the tumor is limited to the middle ear and probably not a glomus jugulare. Further, the carotid crest, a vertically oriented triangular wedge of bone between the jugular bulb and the *carotid artery,* is often eroded with a glomus jugulare, a sign considered to be pathognomonic by many. Both of these findings can be demonstrated by high-resolution CT (▶ Fig. 25.7). MRI is important in defining the extent of tumor, particularly intracranially (posterior fossa) and extracranially (upper neck), and assists with surgical planning. The tumor appearance is similar to that of a glomus tympanicum, though generally much more extensive.

Angiography is also very important during the evaluation of glomus jugulare and its vascular supply (▶ Fig. 25.7). Because an angiogram is needed immediately prior to surgical resection with embolization of the feeding vessels, the angiogram should be held off until just prior to surgery to avoid the need for a second angiogram. Although the inferior tympanic branch of the ascending pharyngeal artery or the stylomastoid artery (from occipital or postauricular arteries) is often the main blood supply, there is almost any variation possible. When there is significant supply from the internal carotid system (caroticotympanic) or the vertebral-basilar system, embolization carries significant risk.[159,160] These large vascular lesions also commonly involve the sigmoid sinus and inferior petrosal sinus. Some surgeons arrange preoperative embolization of the inferior petrosal sinus to control bleeding when opening the jugular bulb.[161] The intrapetrous carotid genu is usually eroded in larger lesions, although it rarely becomes occluded. Blood loss during tumor resection can be significant; thus preoperative embolization can help with intraoperative hemostasis. Most surgeons would not recommend carotid resection for these benign tumors; rather, a small remnant is left and potentially treated if it regrows with stereotactic radiation.

Treatment of the glomus jugulare can be complicated due to its origin in a surgically difficult location and its ability to involve a variety of critical neurovascular structures. Further, some argue that equal results can be obtained treating these lesions with either surgery or radiation therapy. Reports suggest, however, that with contemporary techniques there is an acceptably low disability rate following surgical resection, with a low probability of tumor recurrence and a good quality of life.[138,139,158,162,163] Depending on the size and location of the tumor, it may be approached by a canal-wall-up or canal-wall-down mastoidectomy, an infratemporal fossa approach, a translabyrinthine approach, a transcochlear approach, or a combination of any of the above.[164] The transjugular approach, consisting of a lateral craniotomy conducted through a partial petrosectomy traversing the jugular fossa combined with resection of the sigmoid sinus and jugular bulb, which often have been occluded by disease, is another popular approach.[165] Because larger tumors tend to infiltrate cranial nerves, larger tumors are associated with a higher incidence of postoperative neural deficits.[157] One of the key surgical principles involves exposing the jugular fossa and gaining control of the vessels above and below the lesion. Facial nerve rerouting may be required for larger tumors with evidence of carotid erosion, though a majority of tumors can be resected with the facial nerve left in situ using the fallopian bridge technique.[90] Surgical complications most commonly include CSF leak (12%) and aspiration (in up to one third).[138,166] New postoperative lower cranial deficits as a result of surgery can occur in up to one half of cases.[90] There are also rare reports of death associated with surgery due to complications of lower cranial nerve palsy, such as aspiration.[167] In many of these cases, rehabilitation with speech therapy, vocal cord medialization procedures, and facial nerve reanimation techniques can offer adequate functional outcomes.

Radiation therapy is advocated in some centers as a first-line therapy for advanced glomus jugulare tumors or advanced patient age.[168–174] A recent meta-analysis of 19 studies was conducted with a total of 335 patients treated with radiotherapy reporting up to 95% tumor control in the medium term.[175] These data do not distinguish between those tumors that would have grown and those that would have remained stable. The lack of long-term follow-up means that radiation should be advised with caution in young patients. Growth despite radiation leads to an increased risk to surrounding cranial nerves.[176] There are no adequately controlled clinical trials comparing the two modalities, although there are limited studies comparing both modalities.[170] The possibility of a rare but lethal radiation-induced tumor of the temporal bone must also be factored into the clinical decision to use this modality.[177] Thus, although most agree that radiation is indicated for incompletely resected tumors or those with positive surgical margins, the superiority of either modality still remains in question, and treatment must be individualized.[178–180]

Having presented the advantages and disadvantages of surgery versus gamma knife/fractionated stereotactic radiotherapy for glomus jugulare, the issue can be more clearly stated: If you were 60 + years old with a 5-cm tumor eroding the base of your skull, filling the middle ear, extending anteriorly toward the carotid artery and eustachian tube, but not (yet) affecting cranial nerves VII, IX, or X, what would you do? A traditional surgical approach would be translabyrinthine-transcochlear with anterior rerouting of the facial nerve, intra/extraluminal packing of the lateral sinus, ligation of the internal jugular vein, and systematic removal of all tumor following primarily the course of the internal carotid artery. When the tumor in the jugular bulb is removed, packing the petrosal sinuses must be tight to ensure hemostasis, which in turn can traumatize nerves IX to XI. For the sake of discussion, we will ignore issues of reconstructing the wound. In most cases, the patient is deaf (and temporarily dizzy), with a temporary facial paralysis that will never return completely to normal, often with vocal palsy/paralysis and dysphagia with the risk of possible aspiration pneumonia, and with reduced mobility of the shoulder. Moreover, despite perioperative embolization, hemorrhage and multiple transfusions can be dramatic, and not infrequently some tumor is left behind.

Some institutions support surgery in those patients who preoperatively already have lower cranial nerve deficits.[1,55,1,59,164] Another approach to management is to debulk those portions of tumor that do not incur cranial nerve deficits to attain a size more easily treated by gamma knife. Finally, a reasonable option is to treat the entire tumor with gamma knife or fractionated stereotactic radiosurgery in hopes of preventing tumor growth and postpone deficits. In this latter option, the main issue is timing of radiation therapy, which remains controversial.

This management dilemma is hotly debated by many experienced neuro-otologists. Quality-of-life issues have swayed *many* former surgeons toward radiation therapy.

25.4 Meningioma

Meningiomas, the second most common brain tumors in adults, accounting for up to one fifth of all intracranial neoplasms, are the second most common tumor of the central nervous system (CNS) after gliomas.[181,182] In spite of this prevalence, they account for only 10% of the tumors involving the CPA.[183] These slow-growing, benign tumors are growths of dural fibroblasts, pial cells, and arachnoid villi. They preferentially arise along the major venous sinuses and their contributing veins, at neural foramina, and from arachnoid cells anywhere along the arachnoid membrane (▶ Fig. 25.8).[184]

The etiology of meningiomas remains uncertain, though an association with progesterone levels and breast cancer has been demonstrated.[185] Genetically, cytogenetic losses on chromosomes 1, 7, 10, and 14 and telomerase activation have been observed in clinically aggressive meningiomas, whereas monosomy 22 has been shown to be a common early molecular event in tumor formation.[182] Several candidate growth regulatory genes have been identified, including the NF2 gene *merlin*, tumor suppressor in lung cancer-1 (*TSLC1*), protein 4.1B, and *p53/MDM2* and S6-*kinase* genes.[182] Meningiomas have a clear association with NF2, and it has been estimated that one fifth of adolescents with a meningioma have NF2. There is also a four times higher incidence of meningiomas in patients who have received radiation therapy to the head.[186,187]

Meningiomas almost always involve the temporal bone secondarily due to spread from an adjacent region.[183,188–190] Most reports of primary middle ear meningiomas date from before the era of modern imaging when it was difficult to distinguish

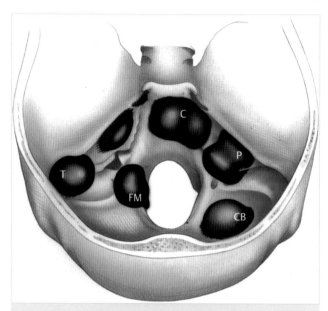

Fig. 25.8 Meningioma of the skull base. Common areas of meningioma occurrence within the skull base that may impinge on the temporal bone are shown. These include the posterior petrous pyramid (P), tentorium (T), clivus (C), cerebellum (CB), and foramen magnum (FM).

the point of origin.[181,184–186,188–190] It is thus likely that many of these older reports actually described intracranial meningiomas that secondarily invaded the structures of the temporal bone.[191] Today, the vast majority demonstrably have a dural origin, with several potential pathways to the middle ear. Those meningiomas that have been described as arising primarily from within the temporal bone were believed to arise from the internal auditory meatus and canal, the jugular foramen, the geniculate ganglion, and the sulcus of the greater and lesser superficial petrosal nerves.[181,184–186,188–190] Extratemporal meningiomas are far more common, and usually originate at the CPA attached to the posterior surface of the petrous pyramid. Tumors arising in this location account for up to 7 to 12% of all meningiomas.[183,192] In decreasing frequency, the other sites of origin of extratemporal meningiomas are the tentorium, clivus, cerebellar convexity, and foramen magnum. A majority of these extratemporal meningiomas of the posterior fossa arise from the porus acusticus or adjacent to the superior petrosal sinus.[184] Once an extratemporal meningioma has invaded the temporal bone, additional spread is common; about 40% will have spread extratemporally into the nasopharynx, retromaxillary space, retromandibular space, cervical space, parapharyngeal space, sphenoid sinus, pterygopalatine fossa, or the orbit.[184] Rarely, a meningioma will reside entirely within the IAC, mimicking an AN in both its clinical and radiographic presentation, with diagnosis only being made on histopathology.[190,193,194] Meningiomas in the jugular foramen mimic glomus jugulare tumors.[195]

The presence of a dural tail and the absence of flow voids are important features in differentiating a meningioma from other jugular foramen tumors.[196] Meningiomas tend to be lobulated, tough, white-gray masses that are well circumscribed and that indent the adjacent nervous tissue, often growing "en-plaque" to cover a wide surface of the cranial base. Hyperostosis of the

Table 25.5 World Health Organization Classification of Meningiomas

Grade 1	Grade 2	Grade 3
Meningothelial meningioma	Chordoid meningioma	Papillary meningioma
Fibrous (fibroblastic) meningioma	Clear cell meningioma	Rhabdoid meningioma
Transitional (mixed) meningioma	Atypical meningioma	Anaplastic meningioma
Psammomatous meningioma		
Angiomatous meningioma		
Microcystic meningioma		
Secretory meningioma		
Lymphoplasmacyte-rich meningioma		
Metaplastic meningioma		

adjacent skull or penetration into adjacent bone is sometimes found. Histologically, four subcategories can be identified. *Syncytial* or *meningotheliomatous* lesions (55%) consist of an irregular arrangement of epithelial-like cells with abundant cytoplasm. *Fibroblastic* lesions (15%) demonstrate palisading spindle cells with interwoven reticulin collagen fibers and occasional psammoma bodies. *Transitional* tumors (30%) have features of both with prominent psammoma bodies, whereas *angioblastic* tumors (5%) are highly cellular with poorly defined cell cytoplasm.[192,193,197] The World Health Organization grading scale for meningioma is shown in ▶ Table 25.5.

Meningiomas involving the temporal bone, in keeping with other meningiomas, affect women by a ratio of 2:1 and commonly are diagnosed in the middle and later decades of life.[184] The symptoms at presentation, in order of decreasing frequency, are progressive hearing loss, headaches, vertigo, tinnitus, otorrhea, otalgia, facial weakness or loss of taste, diplopia or visual disturbances, dysphagia, dysarthria, dysphonia, nausea and vomiting, facial pain or paresthesias, exophthalmos, lower limb hemiparesis or paraparesis, and periauricular swelling or neck mass.[184,190] Meningiomas may also gain access to the middle ear, mimicking an otitis media,[198] with a hyperemic tympanic membrane, granulation tissue, facial nerve involvement, and conductive hearing loss. In contrast to patients with an AN, who uniformly present with hearing loss, only 60% of patients with meningiomas involving the temporal bone present with hearing loss.[199] For meningiomas primarily involving the jugular foramen, the chief presenting symptoms and signs are pulsatile tinnitus, a middle ear mass, and dysfunction of the lower cranial nerves manifesting as hoarseness, dysphagia, and dysarthria.[200]

Magnetic resonance imaging with gadolinium is currently the most effective radiological study for diagnosis, as it differentiates meningiomas from the more common ANs (▶ Fig. 25.9). On T1-weighted images, meningiomas are isointense to slightly hypointense in relation to surrounding brain tissue. Their appearance on T2-weighted images is highly variable, though they tend to be less intense than ANs. There is moderate enhancement with gadolinium.[201] Whereas ANs tend to involve the entire IAC, forming an acute angle with the posterior surface of the petrous bone, meningiomas tend to be broad based, project asymmetrically into the IAC, and occasionally have

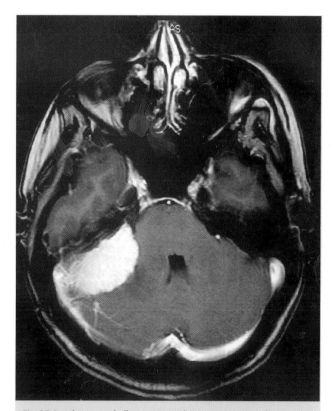

Fig. 25.9 A large cerebellopontine angle meningioma, as demonstrated by this axial, T1-weighted MRI scan with gadolinium enhancement. The tumor shows characteristic features of a meningioma, including dural "tails."

calcifications or cystic changes and a dural "tail" sign.[202,203] If the MRI appearance is suspicious for a highly vascular tumor, then angiography with embolization is indicated, and also helps to differentiate a meningioma from a glomus tumor.[200] High-resolution CT may be of value in determining bony involvement.[194,204,205]

Although meningiomas are benign tumors, they are locally destructive and have the ability to invade cranial nerves. Surgical excision, therefore, is the treatment of choice. Conservative management may be selected in smaller lesions, in the elderly, or in those unable to tolerate surgical excision. The surgical approach is determined by several factors, including the size, the location relative to other critical neurovascular structures, and the status of hearing. The propensity of meningiomas to spread within the osseous haversian canals necessitates a surgical resection of adjacent bone to ensure tumor eradication. Surgical routes employed vary according to the anatomic peculiarities of each tumor, and include the middle fossa, suboccipital, translabyrinthine, transcochlear, combined translabyrinthine-suboccipital, and transtentorial approaches.[192,206,207] Hearing preservation is much more likely in CPA meningiomas as compared with ANs. Therefore, a labyrinth-sparing procedure is chosen for CPA meningiomas when the hearing is good, regardless of the tumor size. Hearing preservation is successful in about one third or more of cases.[208,209] Most surgeons prefer a subtotal resection in attempt to preserve cranial nerve function.[2,9,2,10] Surgery for meningiomas in the jugular foramen has a high incidence (61%) of new lower cranial nerve palsy.[211] This includes a rate of up to 50% new vocal cord palsy.[195]

The role of radiotherapy is controversial.[212–214] Although there is an increasing trend to use radiotherapy as a primary treatment modality, it is more commonly used following a subtotal tumor resection.[214,215] Stereotactic radiosurgery, or gamma knife, is also being increasingly used as a viable treatment option for skull base meningiomas.[212,216–218]

Because meningiomas tend to invade cranial nerves and encircle other critical neurovascular structures, complete excision is often difficult. Even with gross total resection, recurrence rates approach 30% in some series.[219] Long-term follow-up is thus warranted after tumor extirpation with periodic radiological evaluation.

25.5 Adenomatous Tumors

Adenomatous tumors involving the temporal bone are rare lesions.[220] In the medical literature prior to the 1990s, all adenomatous tumors of the middle ear and temporal bone were grouped together, making historical comparisons difficult. Two distinct clinical and histopathological subtypes have since been identified: a *mixed pleomorphic cell* pattern and a *papillary* pattern.[221] *Carcinoid* tumors are also recognized by some as a distinct clinical subtype of adenomatous tumors, though others group these tumors with the mixed pleomorphic cell type. Adenomatous tumors also include some lesions that have previously been reported as "ceruminomas," an ambiguous and misleading term used to describe a diverse group of glandular tumors of the middle ear and mastoid.[222]

25.5.1 Mixed Pleomorphic Cell Pattern (Mucosal Adenoma)

Mixed tumors are the more common and benign of the two major subtypes of adenomas and are always confined to the middle ear and mastoid. This pattern demonstrates acinar, solid, trabecular, and carcinoid-like histopathological features. Some bone involvement is always seen, and cholesteatoma or inflammation is nearly always present. Rarely, the otic capsule or facial nerve may be involved. These tumors are believed to arise from the poorly differentiated basement membrane cells within the normal mucosa of the middle ear, promontory, and eustachian tube.[221–223]

The majority of patients with mixed pleomorphic tumors of the middle ear are male, and typically present between the ages of 20 and 60. These tumors are commonly diagnosed preoperatively as chronic otitis media.[224] Rarely, they have been reported to involve the adjacent posterior fossa.[225] Conductive hearing loss is often present as a result of tumor growth occluding the sound-transducing mechanism, whereas otorrhea, facial nerve weakness, and tinnitus are variably present. Examination typically demonstrates a soft tissue middle ear mass. High-resolution CT scans conform to the clinical exam, and usually demonstrate a soft tissue middle ear and mastoid mass without associated bone destruction.

Because these lesions are commonly confused with chronic otitis media, the diagnosis is often made intraoperatively during a mastoidectomy and tympanoplasty. Despite the benign implication of their diagnosis, however, the mixed pleomorphic pattern tumors have a high likelihood of recurrence, with the ability to invade bone and soft tissue. Thus, complete surgical resection is necessary for cure, and long-term follow-up is mandatory to evaluate for recurrence.[223]

25.5.2 Papillary Pattern (Endolymphatic Sac Adenoma)

Adenomatous tumors with a papillary pattern are rarer and more aggressive lesions.[220] Historically, these lesions have also been called endolymphatic sac tumors, Heffner's tumors, low-grade papillary adenocarcinoma, and aggressive papillary middle ear tumors. In contrast to their more benign counterpart, these papillary neoplasms typically demonstrate adjacent bone invasion and extension into the petrous apex. Involvement of the facial nerve and middle or posterior cranial fossa dura is also commonly seen.[221,223,226–228] The tumors are neuroectodermal in origin,[229] and have been traditionally believed to arise in the endolymphatic sac, with subsequent extension into the posterior fossa and endolymphatic duct, providing access to the vestibule, mastoid process, and retrofacial air cells and facial nerve.[230,231] There are a few reported cases without apical petrous temporal bone invasion, suggesting they do not always arise from the endolymphatic sac.[232] Other possible sites of origin include epithelia of the middle ear, mastoid, or ectopic choroid plexus.[227] Histologically, these tumors are composed of a single- to double-layered epithelial lining with a variable cytoplasm and hyalinization. They show neuroectodermal staining (cytokeratin, S100, glial fibrillary acidic protein [GFAP], vimentin).[229] All papillary tumors invade adjacent bone and demonstrate glandular features that suggest the origin is from endolymphatic sac.[221,223,229,230,233]

Clinically, these tumors may behave aggressively locally and have a lethal potential. In one study, these tumors had an incidence of 11% in patients von Hippel–Lindau disease, leading some authors to suggest patients with this tumor should have screening for von Hippel–Lindau.[227,234] There is a female preponderance, and patients usually present at between 20 and 60 years of age. Symptoms at presentation include hearing loss and facial nerve paralysis, vertigo, and tinnitus.[134] Sometimes it may present with Ménière syndrome.[230] On high-resolution CT

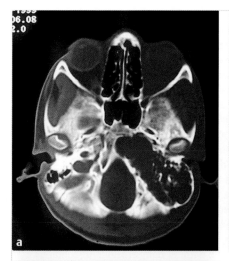
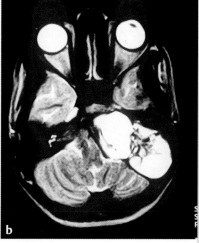
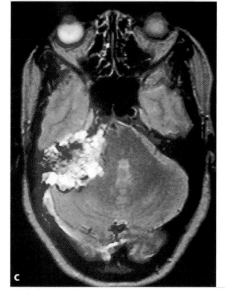

Fig. 25.10 An endolymphatic sac adenoma, which has also been classified as a low-grade adenocarcinoma, can be locally destructive. CT (a) and MRI (b) demonstrate a large endolymphatic sac tumor in the same patient that was locally destructive but not invasive. (c) An MRI scan demonstrates a right-sided endolymphatic sac tumor from another patient.

scanning, the lesions are typically located near the vestibular aqueduct, centered between the sigmoid sinus and the IAC. Involvement of the IAC, jugular bulb, and mastoid is common, as is erosion of the bone toward the vestibule of the labyrinth (▶ Fig. 25.10).[221,223,230] Despite their benign histology, there are two reports of metastasis to the spine.[235,236]

Treatment is primarily surgical, with complete excision and adequate margins the surgical goal. This is usually accomplished via a translabyrinthine approach, which removes the dura, jugular bulb, and any involved cranial nerves.[237] Being highly vascular, often preoperative embolization is used.[227] Postoperative radiation is controversial because there is still debate about whether the tumor is malignant or benign and whether it displays clinical or pathological features or both. With gross total surgical removal, a 90% cure rate has been reported. When radiation therapy is used after incomplete tumor extirpation, only 50% respond, though the numbers reported are very small and not statistically valid.[221,223,230,237,238]

25.5.3 Carcinoid Tumor

Although some believe that all carcinoid tumors of the middle ear should be classified as mixed pleomorphic adenomatous tumors, others consider them to be a unique histopathological subtype of adenomatous tumors.[239–241] The first case was reported in 1980 by Murphy et al,[242] and less than 20 additional cases have been reported since then.[239,240,243–247] Carcinoid tumors are slow-growing but locally invasive lesions found in the middle ear. These rare lesions are believed to arise from the enterochromaffin cells of the endocrine system, and thus have the ability to secrete a variety of peptide hormones. Unlike similar lesions in other parts of the body, however, middle ear carcinoid tumors do not secrete large amounts of these hormones and thus are not associated with the systemic manifestations of carcinoid syndrome, such as flushing, wheezing, abdominal cramps, and diarrhea.[241]

Histologically, the tumors demonstrate ribbons and cords of trabecular, cuboidal cells. Argyrophil staining is positive in 80% of cases. Immunohistochemical stains are positive for cytokeratin AE-1, AE-3, serotonin, and neuron-specific enolase. Electron microscopy shows neurosecretory granules.[241]

Tumors present in both sexes between the second and sixth decades. Patients typically present with conductive hearing loss and the feeling of ear blockage. Tinnitus and transient facial paresis have also been described. Examination often demonstrates an intact but bulging drum. However, in less than half of all cases will a middle ear mass actually be seen. CT scan is useful for identifying the extent of middle ear involvement, as well as the status of the ossicles and facial nerve. Bony erosion or destruction is never seen.[239–241,243–247]

Definitive therapy involves complete tumor excision. Because the ossicles are frequently enveloped by tumor, which may extend into the mastoid, the surgeon should be prepared to perform a tympanomastoidectomy and ossicular reconstruction concurrently. With adequate excision, recurrence is unlikely. There is one documented case of metastasis to the neck.[248] The role of radiotherapy is controversial, and currently is only considered after incomplete tumor excision or when the tumor has spread beyond the middle ear and mastoid.[241]

25.5.4 Glandular Tumors of the External Auditory Canal

The general term *ceruminoma* has been applied to a diverse spectrum of tumors originating from the glandular structures of the external auditory canal. The rarity of these lesions has contributed to this use of one term for different tumors. The most extensive review of the topic comprises only 32 cases over a 32-year period.[222] In fact, these tumors represent a variety of glandular tumors ranging from benign to malignant. The benign tumors include *ceruminomous adenomas*, similar to the mixed-pleomorphic pattern of the middle ear; *pleomorphic adenomas*, which are salivary gland choristomas (see below); and *cylindromas*, which are exceedingly rare tumors arising from the pilosebaceous units of the external canal.[222] One study evaluating the ultrastructure of these tumors demonstrated apocrine caps, microvilli, cell junctions, secretory granules, vacuoles, lipid droplets, and siderosomes, which are the characteristic features of apocrine glands.[249] Presentation of the benign ceruminomous adenoma typically includes external auditory canal obstruction with hearing loss. Treatment for benign tumors includes conservative local excision with a skin graft to the operative site. Radiotherapy is not necessary.[222]

25.5.5 Choristomas

Choristoma is the pathological term given to a benign cohesive mass of aberrant tissue or scattered cells in an inappropriate anatomic location. It is an extremely rare lesion in the temporal bone.[250] Although most reports are of salivary gland choristomas, neural, sebaceous, and cartilaginous choristomas have also been described.[251–258] It has been postulated that salivary gland tissue becomes trapped during fusion of the tympanic, mastoid, and squamous portions of the temporal bone, leading to the formation of salivary choristomas.[252,254] Neural rests of tissue are believed to gain access to the middle ear via Hyrtl (tympanomeningeal) fissures during development, giving rise to the less common neural choristoma.[251–253] A commonly accepted theory of brain heterotopia is that it is a variant of an encephalocele in which a pedicle, directly connecting the neuroglial tissue with the subarachnoid or ventricular spaces, has detached and has eventually been absorbed or become vestigial.[256]

Microscopically, choristomas of the middle ear are characterized by well-formed serous and mucous acini arranged randomly or in a lobular formation. Mucinous microcysts and fibroadipose tissue components have also been described.[250] Macroscopically, the tumors are lobulated and firm. Occasionally the tumor is attached to the middle ear by a fine stalk.

Choristomas have been reported in patients ranging in age from 5 to 52 years and there is no sex predilection. The most common location of a middle ear choristoma is in association with the facial nerve and is often associated with developmental anomalies of the facial nerve, facial canal,[259] and ossicular chain, particularly an absent or malformed incus or stapes.[260] Because of this frequent association, a second branchial arch embryological etiology has been proposed.[261]

Although tumors have been described in all ages, they typically present in the first two decades.[254] These benign tumors grow slowly and tend to produce few symptoms other than a conductive hearing loss in the affected ear, correlating with the degree of ossicular involvement. CT typically demonstrates a middle ear mass lesion without bony erosion. Angiography fails to demonstrate a tumor blush typically seen with vascular tumors of this region, further aiding in their differentiation.

Treatment is determined by the size and location of the tumor. Small tumors or those attached solely by a thin stalk may be readily excised. Larger or broad-based tumors, however, must be approached with a degree of caution. Because of its frequent association with the facial nerve, temporary or permanent palsy has been reported postoperatively in 25% of cases after tumor resection.[260] Attempts at ossiculoplasty to correct the conductive hearing loss have yielded success in approximately two thirds of cases. Because there is often little to no tumor growth over time and there is no reported evidence of malignant degeneration, conservative management with serial examinations is acceptable in those wishing to forgo surgery.[262]

25.6 Hemangiomas and Vascular Malformations

Historically, the literature on benign vascular tumors has lacked a rational or consistent nomenclature, and has contributed to widespread misunderstanding of these lesions.[263] The term *hemangioma* has historically been used to describe any vascular lesion, and is commonly preceded by descriptive but confusing and unhelpful terms such as *strawberry, cavernous*, and *capillary*. In 1982 a new system of classification of vascular tumors was developed based on the clinical behavior and growth characteristics of these lesions. The classification groups vascular tumors under two categories: *hemangiomas* and *vascular malformations*.[264] Hemangiomas usually present during the first month of life, and are characterized by a rapid growth period (proliferative phase) followed by a slow period of involution. Hemangiomas are further categorized on the basis of depth within the dermis, as cutaneous (entirely within papillary dermis), subcutaneous (into the reticular dermis or subcutaneous fat), or compound (containing elements of both).[264,265] In contrast, vascular malformations are always present at birth, and grow in proportion to body growth without regression. They can be arterial, capillary, venous, lymphatic, or any combination of these. Some authors have further divided these vascular malformations into low-flow lesions (venous malformations) and high-flow lesions (arteriovenous malformations).[263]

Unfortunately, the otologic literature does not differentiate between these two types of lesions, making clinical comparisons difficult.[266] To add a further element of confusion, some authors have reported that vascular lesions of the temporal bone frequently contain elements of both hemangiomas and vascular malformations.[267] However, a majority of the vascular lesions of the temporal bones are probably not hemangiomas but rather subcategories of vascular malformations. Histologically, hemangiomas are characterized by endothelial hyperplasia and an increase in the number of mast cells during the proliferative phase, followed by fibrosis, fatty infiltration, decreased cellularity, and normalization of the mast cell count during involution of the lesion. In contrast, vascular malformations are collections of abnormal vessels with normal endothelium and mast cell counts.[263] Using these histological criteria, the term *cavernous hemangioma*, frequently used to describe lesions in the otologic literature, is more appropriately classified as a vascular malformation. Alternatively, the term *capillary hemangioma* probably describes a true hemangioma, but this has not been reported in the temporal bone.[266,268,269]

Vascular malformations of the temporal bone are rare entities, composing less than 1% of all temporal bone tumors.[1,270] The overwhelming majority of these lesions present within the IAC or at the geniculate ganglion.[270–274] Rarely, they may arise within the middle ear, external auditory canal, or tympanic membrane.[267–270,275–280] Tumor predilection for this region is believed to be due to the extensive blood supply surrounding the Scarpa ganglion and the geniculate ganglion. A majority of tumors are smaller than 1 cm at the time of presentation.[267–270,281]

Patients typically present after the third decade of life. When the geniculate ganglion is the site of origin, a seventh cranial nerve dysfunction (weakness or twitch) is nearly always present. Overall, facial nerve dysfunction is present in about 80% of temporal bone vascular malformations, and is usually the reason patients seek medical attention.[270]Other symptoms noted on clinical presentation include hemifacial spasm, tinnitus, conductive hearing loss (more commonly with geniculate ganglion malformations), progressive sensorineural hearing loss (more commonly with IAC tumors), and vertigo.[270,271,282]

Radiographically, high-resolution CT and MRI define the lesion and provide complementary information. MRI demonstrates all tumors within the IAC and some tumors near the geniculate.[271] The lesions appear hyperintense on T2-weighted images, and tend to be more hyperintense than are acoustic schwannomas.[270,282,283] Some geniculate ganglion lesions are difficult to visualize on MRI, but intratumoral calcium can be detected on high-resolution CT.[283] Venous malformations of the geniculate region may be differentiated from other temporal bone tumors based on radiographic appearances. A focal, enhancing lesion of the geniculate ganglion that is sessile on the middle fossa floor, erodes bone diffusely, has irregular margins, and contains flecks of calcification is most likely a meningioma. Facial nerve schwannomas typically cause smoothly marginated expansion and tend to be less focal, extending along the fallopian canal longitudinally. Hemangiomas produce facial nerve symptoms at a smaller size than facial nerve neuromas. The pathophysiology behind this appears to be a vascular steal mechanism where blood is taken away from the nerve trunk to the tumor.[284]

The treatment of choice is surgical excision, with removal by drill of normal bony margins. The choice of surgical approach depends on the tumor location and size, but a middle fossa, transmastoid, or translabyrinthine approach is commonly employed. Because of the destructive nature of these benign tumors, intratemporal facial nerve grafting is frequently required. Facial nerve repairs are more often required for geniculate vascular malformations than for those originating within the IAC.[267,270,271,282,283] When facial paralysis is of recent origin, or partial function remains, the native facial nerve can often be preserved. In long-standing complete palsies, however, a graft is almost always required.

Surgery is generally successful at eradicating lesions, with a low likelihood of recurrence after complete excision. Results of facial nerve function following repair are good (House-Brackmann grade 3–4/6) except when nerve repair is delayed more than one year from the onset of the palsy.[267,270,282,283] If integrity of the facial nerve is preserved, patients can recover to a House-Brackmann grade 1 or 2 in 72%.[285] For patients undergoing middle fossa or transmastoid procedures, approximately two thirds can expect postoperative hearing preservation to within 10 dB of preoperative speech thresholds.[267]

25.7 Langerhans Cell Histiocytosis (Eosinophilic Granuloma)

Langerhans cell histiocytosis, previously referred to as histiocytosis X and reticuloendotheliosis, is a group of diseases with widely disparate clinical manifestations but all characterized by an accumulation of proliferating cells similar to Langerhans cells.[286] Historically the disease has been categorized into a spectrum of three diseases. *Eosinophilic granuloma* is the most mild form, and consists of multifocal bony erosions limited to the skull, long bones, ribs, vertebrae, pelvis, maxilla, and mandible.[287,288] The temporal bone is the most common site of the cranial base.[289] *Hand-Schüller-Christian syndrome* and *Letterer-Siwe disease* are the more chronic and severe forms of Langerhans cell histiocytosis, respectively, and are both marked by multiorgan involvement.[290] The underlying pathology in all three diseases is proliferating Langerhans cells, a histiocyte involved in cell-mediated immunity, osteoclastic activity, and eosinophilic infiltration.[287] It is unknown what causes the abnormal proliferation or even whether the Langerhans cells are normal or pathological. Proposed theories for the genesis of the disease cite metabolic, genetic, infectious, neoplastic, and immunologic causes.[287,288,290]

The eosinophilic granuloma consists of a soft friable red mass containing histiocytes, eosinophils, lymphocytes, plasma cells, and multinucleated giant cells. The presence of histiocytes, with characteristic Birbeck granules (trilaminar rod-shapes organelles within the nuclear cytoplasm) seen under electron microscopy is considered diagnostic.[291]

Solitary eosinophilic granuloma most commonly appears in children over 5 years of age and in young adults, in contrast to the more severe systemic forms of Langerhans cell histiocytosis, which tend to occur in infants and young children.[287] Temporal bone lesions have been described within the lateral mastoid and the petrous apex, and may also involve the entire temporal bone. Otologic involvement in Langerhans cell histiocytosis has been estimated from 15 to 61% of patients, and may be the sole presenting symptom in 5 to 25% of children.[292,293] The lesions typically present as a painful postauricular soft tissue swelling. Otorrhea, granulation tissue within the external auditory canal, and otitis externa are also common at presentation, making differentiation from routine chronic otitis media difficult.[288,294] Conductive hearing loss by either soft tissue obstruction or, less commonly, ossicular erosion may also be present. Sensorineural hearing loss from destruction of the bony labyrinth has also been described.[292] Facial palsy may be associated with the more severe forms of Langerhans cell histiocytosis in about 3% of cases.[295]

Skull and plain radiographs demonstrate destructive, osteolytic lesions of the temporal bone, which is commonly mistaken for suppurative mastoiditis, cholesteatoma, or a metastatic osteolytic lesion.[292] A CT scan revealing a destructive lesion with well-defined soft tissue margins is typical and is helpful in demarcating the areas of temporal bone involvement.[289] On MRI, the lesion is usually hypointense on T1- and T2-weighted images, but highlights with gadolinium.[288]

Once the diagnosis is made, treatment consists of conservative curettage.[288,292] The use of radiotherapy has fallen out of favor and is generally reserved for postsurgical residual disease or recurrence.[293] Intralesional steroid injections have also been successful in some reported cases.[296] When there is multisystem involvement, chemotherapy and intravenous steroids are advocated.[288]

When the disease is limited to the temporal bone, the eosinophilic granuloma typically resolves after local excision or radiation without recurrence.[293] Surgery usually consists of curetting the bony cavity created by the tumor. However, the disease may progress to a more disseminated form, and thus close follow-up observation is warranted.[288] With multisystem, nonosseous involvement, the prognosis is much poorer, with mortality reported at about 40%.[292]

References

[1] Brackmann DE, Bartels LJ. Rare tumors of the cerebellopontine angle. Otolaryngol Head Neck Surg 1980; 88: 555–559

[2] Mahaley MS, Jr, Mettlin C, Natarajan N, Laws ER, Jr, Peace BB. Analysis of patterns of care of brain tumor patients in the United States: a study of the Brain Tumor Section of the AANS and the CNS and the Commission on Cancer of the ACS. Clin Neurosurg 1990; 36: 347–352

[3] Ahn MS, Jackler RK, Lustig LR. The early history of the neurofibromatosis. Evolution of the concept of neurofibromatosis type 2. Arch Otolaryngol Head Neck Surg 1996; 122: 1240–1249

[4] Selesnick SH, Jackler RK, Pitts LW. The changing clinical presentation of acoustic tumors in the MRI era. Laryngoscope 1993; 103: 431–436

[5] Lin D, Hegarty JL, Fischbein NJ, Jackler RK. The prevalence of "incidental" acoustic neuroma. Arch Otolaryngol Head Neck Surg 2005; 131: 241–244

[6] Sterkers JM, Perre J, Viala P, Foncin JF. The origin of acoustic neuromas. Acta Otolaryngol 1987; 103: 427–431

[7] Xenellis JE, Linthicum FH, Jr. On the myth of the glial/schwann junction (Obersteiner-Redlich zone): origin of vestibular nerve schwannomas. Otol Neurotol 2003; 24: 1

[8] Jackler RK. Acoustic neuroma (vestibular schwannoma). In: Jackler RK, ed. Neurotology. St. Louis: Mosby, 1994

[9] Seizinger BR, Martuza RL, Gusella JF. Loss of genes on chromosome 22 in tumorigenesis of human acoustic neuroma. Nature 1986; 322: 644–647

[10] Wolff RK, Frazer KA, Jackler RK, Lanser MJ, Pitts LH, Cox DR. Analysis of chromosome 22 deletions in neurofibromatosis type 2-related tumors. Am J Hum Genet 1992; 51: 478–485

[11] Lanser MJ, Sussman SA, Frazer K. Epidemiology, pathogenesis, and genetics of acoustic tumors. Otolaryngol Clin North Am 1992; 25: 499–520

[12] Grönholm M, Teesalu T, Tyynelä J et al. Characterization of the NF2 protein merlin and the ERM protein ezrin in human, rat, and mouse central nervous system. Mol Cell Neurosci 2005; 28: 683–693

[13] Rong R, Tang X, Gutmann DH, Ye K. Neurofibromatosis 2 (NF2) tumor suppressor merlin inhibits phosphatidylinositol 3-kinase through binding to PIKE-L. Proc Natl Acad Sci U S A 2004; 101: 18200–18205

[14] Schüz J, Steding-Jessen M, Hansen S et al. Long-term mobile phone use and the risk of vestibular schwannoma: a Danish nationwide cohort study. Am J Epidemiol 2011; 174: 416–422

[15] INTERPHONE Study Group. Acoustic neuroma risk in relation to mobile telephone use: results of the INTERPHONE international case-control study. Cancer Epidemiol 2011; 35: 453–464

[16] Sato Y, Akiba S, Kubo O, Yamaguchi N. A case-case study of mobile phone use and acoustic neuroma risk in Japan. Bioelectromagnetics 2011; 32: 85–93

[17] Kuo TC, Jackler RK, Wong K, Blevins NH, Pitts LH. Are acoustic neuromas encapsulated tumors? Otolaryngol Head Neck Surg 1997; 117: 606–609

[18] Rutka J. Controversies in the histopathology of acoustic neuromas and their biological behavior. In: Tos M, Thomsen J, eds. Proceedings of the First International Conference on Acoustic Neuroma. Amsterdam: Kugler, 1992:199–202

[19] Hebbar GK, McKenna MJ, Linthicum FH, Jr. Immunohistochemical localization of vimentin and S-100 antigen in small acoustic tumors and adjacent cochlear nerves. Am J Otol 1990; 11: 310–313

[20] Nager GT. Acoustic neurinomas. Pathology and differential diagnosis. Arch Otolaryngol 1969; 89: 252–279

[21] Nedzelski JM, Schessel DA, Pfleiderer A, Kassel EE, Rowed DW. Conservative management of acoustic neuromas. Otolaryngol Clin North Am 1992; 25: 691–705

[22] Bederson JB, von Ammon K, Wichmann WW, Yasargil MG. Conservative treatment of patients with acoustic tumors. Neurosurgery 1991; 28: 646–650, discussion 650–651

[23] Cayé-Thomasen P, Werther K, Nalla A et al. VEGF and VEGF receptor-1 concentration in vestibular schwannoma homogenates correlates to tumor growth rate. Otol Neurotol 2005; 26: 98–101

[24] Dawes PJ, Basiouny HE. Outcome of using magnetic resonance imaging as an initial screen to exclude vestibular schwannoma in patients presenting with unilateral tinnitus. J Laryngol Otol 1999; 113: 818–822

[25] Gimsing S. Vestibular schwannoma: when to look for it? J Laryngol Otol 2010; 124: 258–264

[26] Kanzaki J, Ogawa K, Ogawa S, Yamamoto M, Ikeda S, O-Uchi T. Audiological findings in acoustic neuroma. Acta Otolaryngol Suppl 1991; 487: 125–132

[27] Wilson DF, Hodgson RS, Gustafson MF, Hogue S, Mills L. The sensitivity of auditory brainstem response testing in small acoustic neuromas. Laryngoscope 1992; 102: 961–964

[28] Weiss MH, Kisiel DL, Bhatia P. Predictive value of brainstem evoked response in the diagnosis of acoustic neuroma. Otolaryngol Head Neck Surg 1990; 103: 583–585

[29] Hasso AN, Ledington JA. Imaging modalities for the study of the temporal bone. Otolaryngol Clin North Am 1988; 21: 219–244

[30] Breger RK, Papke RA, Pojunas KW, Haughton VM, Williams AL, Daniels DL. Benign extraaxial tumors: contrast enhancement with Gd-DTPA. Radiology 1987; 163: 427–429

[31] Shin YJ, Fraysse B, Cognard C et al. Effectiveness of conservative management of acoustic neuromas. Am J Otol 2000; 21: 857–862

[32] Raut VV, Walsh RM, Bath AP et al. Conservative management of vestibular schwannomas—second review of a prospective longitudinal study. Clin Otolaryngol Allied Sci 2004; 29: 505–514

[33] Nikolopoulos TP, Fortnum H, O'Donoghue G, Baguley D. Acoustic neuroma growth: a systematic review of the evidence. Otol Neurotol 2010; 31: 478–485

[34] Stangerup SE, Tos M, Thomsen J, Caye-Thomasen P. Hearing outcomes of vestibular schwannoma patients managed with "wait and scan": predictive value of hearing level at diagnosis. J Laryngol Otol 2010; 124: 490–494

[35] Jackler RK, Pitts LH. Selection of surgical approach to acoustic neuroma. Otolaryngol Clin North Am 1992; 25: 361–387

[36] Colletti V, Fiorino F. Middle fossa versus retrosigmoid-transmeatal approach in vestibular schwannoma surgery: a prospective study. Otol Neurotol 2003; 24: 927–934

[37] Bloch DC, Oghalai JS, Jackler RK, Osofsky M, Pitts LH. The fate of the tumor remnant after less-than-complete acoustic neuroma resection. Otolaryngol Head Neck Surg 2004; 130: 104–112

[38] Thomsen J, Tos M, Harmsen A. Acoustic neuroma surgery: results of translabyrinthine tumour removal in 300 patients. Discussion of choice of approach in relation to overall results and possibility of hearing preservation. Br J Neurosurg 1989; 3: 349–360

[39] Mosek AC, Dodick DW, Ebersold MJ, Swanson JW. Headache after resection of acoustic neuroma. Headache 1999; 39: 89–94

[40] Sanna M, Falcioni M, Rohit . Cerebro-spinal fluid leak after acoustic neuroma surgery. Otol Neurotol 2003; 24: 524

[41] Schaller B, Baumann A. Headache after removal of vestibular schwannoma via the retrosigmoid approach: a long-term follow-up-study. Otolaryngol Head Neck Surg 2003; 128: 387–395

[42] Wiet RJ, Teixido M, Liang JG. Complications in acoustic neuroma surgery. Otolaryngol Clin North Am 1992; 25: 389–412

[43] Sanna M, Khrais T, Russo A, Piccirillo E, Augurio A. Hearing preservation surgery in vestibular schwannoma: the hidden truth. Ann Otol Rhinol Laryngol 2004; 113: 156–163

[44] Lalwani AK, Butt FY, Jackler RK, Pitts LH, Yingling CD. Facial nerve outcome after acoustic neuroma surgery: a study from the era of cranial nerve monitoring. Otolaryngol Head Neck Surg 1994; 111: 561–570

[45] Kartush JM, Lundy LB. Facial nerve outcome in acoustic neuroma surgery. Otolaryngol Clin North Am 1992; 25: 623–647

[46] Marin P, Pouliot D, Fradet G. Facial nerve outcome with a peroperative stimulation threshold under 0.05 mA. Laryngoscope 2011; 121: 2295–2298

[47] Shelton C. Hearing preservation in acoustic tumor surgery. Otolaryngol Clin North Am 1992; 25: 609–621

[48] Chee GH, Nedzelski JM, Rowed D. Acoustic neuroma surgery: the results of long-term hearing preservation. Otol Neurotol 2003; 24: 672–676

[49] Friedman RA, Kesser B, Brackmann DE, Fisher LM, Slattery WH, Hitselberger WE. Long-term hearing preservation after middle fossa removal of vestibular schwannoma. Otolaryngol Head Neck Surg 2003; 129: 660–665

[50] Yates PD, Jackler RK, Satar B, Pitts LH, Oghalai JS. Is it worthwhile to attempt hearing preservation in larger acoustic neuromas? Otol Neurotol 2003; 24: 460–464

[51] Sanna M. Hearing preservation: a critical review of the literature. In: Tos M, Thomsen J, eds. Proceedings of the First International Conference on Acoustic Neuroma. Amsterdam: Kluger, 1992:631–638

[52] Friedman WA, Foote KD. Linear accelerator-based radiosurgery for vestibular schwannoma. Neurosurg Focus 2003; 14: e2

[53] Wiet RJ, Zappia JJ, Hecht CS, O'Connor CA. Conservative management of patients with small acoustic tumors. Laryngoscope 1995; 105: 795–800

[54] Rowe JG, Radatz M, Walton L, Kemeny AA. Stereotactic radiosurgery for type 2 neurofibromatosis acoustic neuromas: patient selection and tumour size. Stereotact Funct Neurosurg 2002; 79: 107–116

[55] Bolsi A, Fogliata A, Cozzi L. Radiotherapy of small intracranial tumours with different advanced techniques using photon and proton beams: a treatment planning study. Radiother Oncol 2003; 68: 1–14

[56] Chakrabarti I, Apuzzo ML, Giannotta SL. Acoustic tumors: operation versus radiation—making sense of opposing viewpoints. Part I. Acoustic neuroma: decision making with all the tools. Clin Neurosurg 2003; 50: 293–312

[57] De Salles AA, Frighetto L, Selch M. Stereotactic and microsurgery for acoustic neuroma: the controversy continues. Int J Radiat Oncol Biol Phys 2003; 56: 1215–1217

[58] Link MJ, Driscoll CL, Foote RL, Pollock BE. Radiation therapy and radiosurgery for vestibular schwannomas: indications, techniques, and results. Otolaryngol Clin North Am 2012; 45: 353–366, viii–ixviii–ix.

[59] Iwai Y, Yamanaka K, Ishiguro T. Surgery combined with radiosurgery of large acoustic neuromas. Surg Neurol 2003; 59: 283–289, discussion 289–291

[60] Chung JW, Ahn JH, Kim JH, Nam SY, Kim CJ, Lee KS. Facial nerve schwannomas: different manifestations and outcomes. Surg Neurol 2004; 62: 245–252, discussion 452

[61] Hasegawa T, Kida Y, Kobayashi T, Yoshimoto M, Mori Y, Yoshida J. Long-term outcomes in patients with vestibular schwannomas treated using gamma knife surgery: 10-year follow up. J Neurosurg 2005; 102: 10–16

[62] Lunsford LD, Niranjan A, Flickinger JC, Maitz A, Kondziolka D. Radiosurgery of vestibular schwannomas: summary of experience in 829 cases. J Neurosurg 2005; 102 Suppl: 195–199

[63] Wowra B, Muacevic A, Jess-Hempen A, Hempel JM, Müller-Schunk S, Tonn JC. Outpatient gamma knife surgery for vestibular schwannoma: definition of the therapeutic profile based on a 10-year experience. J Neurosurg 2005; 102 Suppl: 114–118

[64] Walsh RM, Bath AP, Bance ML, Keller A, Tator CH, Rutka JA. The natural history of untreated vestibular schwannomas. Is there a role for conservative management? Rev Laryngol Otol Rhinol (Bord) 2000; 121: 21–26

[65] Pollock BE. Management of vestibular schwannomas that enlarge after stereotactic radiosurgery: treatment recommendations based on a 15 year experience. Neurosurgery 2006; 58: 241–248, discussion 241–248

[66] Roche PH, Noudel R, Régis J. Management of radiation/radiosurgical complications and failures. Otolaryngol Clin North Am 2012; 45: 367–374, ix

[67] Chung HT, Ma R, Toyota B, Clark B, Robar J, McKenzie M. Audiologic and treatment outcomes after linear accelerator-based stereotactic irradiation for acoustic neuroma. Int J Radiat Oncol Biol Phys 2004; 59: 1116–1121

[68] Flickinger JC, Kondziolka D, Niranjan A, Lunsford LD. Results of acoustic neuroma radiosurgery: an analysis of 5 years' experience using current methods. J Neurosurg 2001; 94: 1–6

[69] Régis J, Pellet W, Delsanti C et al. Functional outcome after gamma knife surgery or microsurgery for vestibular schwannomas. J Neurosurg 2002; 97: 1091–1100

[70] Limb CJ, Long DM, Niparko JK. Acoustic neuromas after failed radiation therapy: challenges of surgical salvage. Laryngoscope 2005; 115: 93–98

[71] Slattery WH, III, Brackmann DE. Results of surgery following stereotactic irradiation for acoustic neuromas. Am J Otol 1995; 16: 315–319, discussion 319–321

[72] Karampelas I, Alberico RA, Plunkett RJ, Fenstermaker RA. Intratumoral hemorrhage after remote subtotal microsurgical resection and gamma knife radiosurgery for vestibular schwannoma. Acta Neurochir (Wien) 2007; 149: 313–316, discussion 316–317

[73] Lustig LR. Radiation-induced tumors of the temporal bone. In: Jackler RK, Driscoll CL, eds. Tumors of the Ear and Temporal Bone. Philadelphia: Lippincott Williams & Wilkins, 2000

[74] Tanbouzi Husseini S, Piccirillo E, Taibah A, Paties CT, Rizzoli R, Sanna M. Malignancy in vestibular schwannoma after stereotactic radiotherapy: a case report and review of the literature. Laryngoscope 2011; 121: 923–928

[75] Stangerup SE, Thomsen J, Tos M, Cayé-Thomasen P. Long-term hearing preservation in vestibular schwannoma. Otol Neurotol 2010; 31: 271–275

[76] Agrawal Y, Clark JH, Limb CJ, Niparko JK, Francis HW. Predictors of vestibular schwannoma growth and clinical implications. Otol Neurotol 2010; 31: 807–812

[77] Plotkin SR, Merker VL, Halpin C et al. Bevacizumab for progressive vestibular schwannoma in neurofibromatosis type 2: a retrospective review of 31 patients. Otol Neurotol 2012; 33: 1046–1052

[78] Komotar RJ, Starke RM, Sisti MB, Connolly ES. The role of bevacizumab in hearing preservation and tumor volume control in patients with vestibular schwannomas. Neurosurgery 2009; 65: N12

[79] Wong HK, Lahdenranta J, Kamoun WS et al. Anti-vascular endothelial growth factor therapies as a novel therapeutic approach to treating neurofibromatosis-related tumors. Cancer Res 2010; 70: 3483–3493

[80] Shord SS, Bressler LR, Tierney LA, Cuellar S, George A. Understanding and managing the possible adverse effects associated with bevacizumab. Am J Health Syst Pharm 2009; 66: 999–1013

[81] Batchelor TT, Sorensen AG, di Tomaso E et al. AZD2171, a pan-VEGF receptor tyrosine kinase inhibitor, normalizes tumor vasculature and alleviates edema in glioblastoma patients. Cancer Cell 2007; 11: 83–95

[82] Mautner VF, Nguyen R, Knecht R, Bokemeyer C. Radiographic regression of vestibular schwannomas induced by bevacizumab treatment: sustain under continuous drug application and rebound after drug discontinuation. Ann Oncol 2010; 21: 2294–2295

[83] Plotkin SR, Halpin C, McKenna MJ, Loeffler JS, Batchelor TT, Barker FG, II. Erlotinib for progressive vestibular schwannoma in neurofibromatosis 2 patients. Otol Neurotol 2010; 31: 1135–1143

[84] Tan LC, Bordi L, Symon L, Cheesman AD. Jugular foramen neuromas: a review of 14 cases. Surg Neurol 1990; 34: 205–211

[85] Horn K, Hankinson H. Tumors of the jugular foramen. In: Jackler RK, Brackman D, eds. Neurotology. St. Louis: Mosby, 1994:1059–1068

[86] Gacek RR. Pathology of jugular foramen neurofibroma. Ann Otol Rhinol Laryngol 1983; 92: 128–133

[87] Kaye AH, Hahn JF, Kinney SE, Hardy RW, Jr, Bay JW. Jugular foramen schwannomas. J Neurosurg 1984; 60: 1045–1053

[88] Lustig LR, Jackler RK. The variable relationship between the lower cranial nerves and jugular foramen tumors: implications for neural preservation. Am J Otol 1996; 17: 658–668

[89] Ramina R, Maniglia JJ, Fernandes YB et al. Jugular foramen tumors: diagnosis and treatment. Neurosurg Focus 2004; 17: E5

[90] Pensak ML, Jackler RK. Removal of jugular foramen tumors: the fallopian bridge technique. Otolaryngol Head Neck Surg 1997; 117: 586–591

[91] Van Calenbergh F, Noens B, Delaere P et al. Jugular foramen schwannoma: surgical experience in six cases. Acta Chir Belg 2004; 104: 435–439

[92] Wilson MA, Hillman TA, Wiggins RH, Shelton C. Jugular foramen schwannomas: diagnosis, management, and outcomes. Laryngoscope 2005; 115: 1486–1492

[93] Bulsara KR, Sameshima T, Friedman AH, Fukushima T. Microsurgical management of 53 jugular foramen schwannomas: lessons learned incorporated into a modified grading system. J Neurosurg 2008; 109: 794–803

[94] Chibbaro S, Mirone G, Makiese O, Bresson D, George B. Dumbbell-shaped jugular foramen schwannomas: surgical management, outcome and complications on a series of 16 patients. Neurosurg Rev 2009; 32: 151–159, discussion 159

[95] Fukuda M, Oishi M, Saito A, Fujii Y. Long-term outcomes after surgical treatment of jugular foramen schwannoma. Skull Base 2009; 19: 401–408

[96] Sutiono AB, Kawase T, Tabuse M et al. Importance of preserved periosteum around jugular foramen neurinomas for functional outcome of lower cranial nerves: anatomic and clinical studies. Neurosurgery 2011; 69 Suppl Operative: ons230–ons240, discussion ons240

[97] Peker S, Sengöz M, Kılıç T, Pamir MN. Gamma knife radiosurgery for jugular foramen schwannomas. Neurosurg Rev 2012; 35: 549–553, discussion 553

[98] Choi CY, Soltys SG, Gibbs IC et al. Stereotactic radiosurgery of cranial nonvestibular schwannomas: results of single- and multisession radiosurgery. Neurosurgery 2011; 68: 1200–1208, discussion 1208

[99] Martin JJ, Kondziolka D, Flickinger JC, Mathieu D, Niranjan A, Lunsford LD. Cranial nerve preservation and outcomes after stereotactic radiosurgery for jugular foramen schwannomas. Neurosurgery 2007; 61: 76–81, discussion 81

[100] Fayad JN, Keles B, Brackmann DE. Jugular foramen tumors: clinical characteristics and treatment outcomes. Otol Neurotol 2010; 31: 299–305

[101] Jung TT, Jun BH, Shea D, Paparella MM. Primary and secondary tumors of the facial nerve. A temporal bone study. Arch Otolaryngol Head Neck Surg 1986; 112: 1269–1273

[102] Dort JC, Fisch U. Facial nerve schwannomas. Skull Base Surg 1991; 1: 51–56

[103] O'Donoghue GM, Brackmann DE, House JW, Jackler RK. Neuromas of the facial nerve. Am J Otol 1989; 10: 49–54

[104] Kertesz TR, Shelton C, Wiggins RH, Salzman KL, Glastonbury CM, Harnsberger R. Intratemporal facial nerve neuroma: anatomical location and radiological features. Laryngoscope 2001; 111: 1250–1256

[105] Janecka IP, Conley J. Primary neoplasms of the facial nerve. Plast Reconstr Surg 1987; 79: 177–185

[106] O'Donoghue G. Tumors of the facial nerve. In: Jackler RK, ed. Neurotology. St. Louis: Mosby, 1994

[107] Saito H, Saito S, Sano T, Kagawa N, Hizawa K, Tatara K. Immunoreactive somatostatin in catecholamine-producing extra-adrenal paraganglioma. Cancer 1982; 50: 560–565

[108] Peco MT, Palacios E. Intracranial and intratemporal facial nerve schwannoma. Ear Nose Throat J 2002; 81: 312

[109] Sarma S, Sekhar LN, Schessel DA. Nonvestibular schwannomas of the brain: a 7-year experience. Neurosurgery 2002; 50: 437–448, discussion 438–439

[110] Ulku CH, Uyar Y, Acar O, Yaman H, Avunduk MC. Facial nerve schwannomas: a report of four cases and a review of the literature. Am J Otolaryngol 2004; 25: 426–431

[111] Parnes LS, Lee DH, Peerless SJ. Magnetic resonance imaging of facial nerve neuromas. Laryngoscope 1991; 101: 31–35

[112] Wilkinson EP, Hoa M, Slattery WH, III et al. Evolution in the management of facial nerve schwannoma. Laryngoscope 2011; 121: 2065–2074

[113] Presutti L, Grammatica A, Alicandri-Ciufelli M, Marchioni D, Cunsolo EM. Facial nerve schwannoma. Otol Neurotol 2009; 30: 683–685

[114] Kim CS, Chang SO, Oh SH, Ahn SH, Hwang CH, Lee HJ. Management of intratemporal facial nerve schwannoma. Otol Neurotol 2003; 24: 312–316

[115] Marzo SJ, Zender CA, Leonetti JP. Facial nerve schwannoma. Curr Opin Otolaryngol Head Neck Surg 2009; 17: 346–350

[116] Liu R, Fagan P. Facial nerve schwannoma: surgical excision versus conservative management. Ann Otol Rhinol Laryngol 2001; 110: 1025–1029

[117] Nishioka K, Abo D, Aoyama H et al. Stereotactic radiotherapy for intracranial nonacoustic schwannomas including facial nerve schwannoma. Int J Radiat Oncol Biol Phys 2009; 75: 1415–1419

[118] Kida Y, Yoshimoto M, Hasegawa T. Radiosurgery for facial schwannoma. J Neurosurg 2007; 106: 24–29

[119] Litre CF, Gourg GP, Tamura M et al. Gamma knife surgery for facial nerve schwannomas. Neurosurgery 2007; 60: 853–859, discussion 853–859

[120] Mowry S, Hansen M, Gantz B. Surgical management of internal auditory canal and cerebellopontine angle facial nerve schwannoma. Otol Neurotol 2012; 33: 1071–1076

[121] Perez R, Chen JM, Nedzelski JM. Intratemporal facial nerve schwannoma: a management dilemma. Otol Neurotol 2005; 26: 121–126

[122] Lee JD, Kim SH, Song MH, Lee HK, Lee WS. Management of facial nerve schwannoma in patients with favorable facial function. Laryngoscope 2007; 117: 1063–1068

[123] Spector GJ, Maisel RH, Ogura JH. Glomus tumors in the middle ear. I. An analysis of 46 patients. Laryngoscope 1973; 83: 1652–1672

[124] Guild SR. The glomus jugulare, a nonchromaffin paraganglion, in man. Ann Otol Rhinol Laryngol 1953; 62: 1045–1071concld.

[125] Gulya AJ. The glomus tumor and its biology. Laryngoscope 1993; 103 Suppl 60: 7–15

[126] Heutink P, van der Mey AG, Sandkuijl LA et al. A gene subject to genomic imprinting and responsible for hereditary paragangliomas maps to chromosome 11q23 qter. Hum Mol Genet 1992; 1: 7–10

[127] Heth J. The basic science of glomus jugulare tumors. Neurosurg Focus 2004; 17: E2

[128] van der Mey AG, Maaswinkel-Mooy PD, Cornelisse CJ, Schmidt PH, van de Kamp JJ. Genomic imprinting in hereditary glomus tumours: evidence for new genetic theory. Lancet 1989; 2: 1291–1294

[129] Fishbein L, Nathanson KL. Pheochromocytoma and paraganglioma: understanding the complexities of the genetic background. Cancer Genet 2012; 205: 1–11

[130] Gimenez-Roqueplo AP, Dahia PL, Robledo M. An update on the genetics of paraganglioma, pheochromocytoma, and associated hereditary syndromes. Horm Metab Res 2012; 44: 328–333

[131] Semaan MT, Megerian CA. Current assessment and management of glomus tumors. Curr Opin Otolaryngol Head Neck Surg 2008; 16: 420–426

[132] Alford BR, Guilford FR. A comprehensive study of tumors of the glomus jugulare. Laryngoscope 1962; 72: 765–805

[133] Batsakis J. Tumors of the Head and Neck: Clinical and Pathological Considerations 2nd ed. Baltimore: Williams & Wilkins, 1979

[134] Glenner G, Grimley P. Tumors of the extra-adrenal paraganglion system (including chemoreceptors). In: Atlas of Tumor Pathology. Washington DC: Armed Forces Institute of Pathology, 1974:1–90

[135] Gulya AJ. Paraneoplastic disorders. In: Jackler RK, Brackman D, eds. Neurotology. St. Louis: Mosby, 1994:535–542

[136] Jackson CG. Neurotologic skull base surgery for glomus tumors. Diagnosis for treatment planning and treatment options. Laryngoscope 1993; 103 Suppl 60: 17–22

[137] House WF, Glasscock ME, III. Glomus tympanicum tumors. Arch Otolaryngol 1968; 87: 550–554

[138] Woods CI, Strasnick B, Jackson CG. Surgery for glomus tumors: the Otology Group experience. Laryngoscope 1993; 103 Suppl 60: 65–70

[139] Jackson CG, Kaylie DM, Coppit G, Gardner EK. Glomus jugulare tumors with intracranial extension. Neurosurg Focus 2004; 17: E7

[140] Makek M, Franklin DJ, Zhao JC, Fisch U. Neural infiltration of glomus temporale tumors. Am J Otol 1990; 11: 1–5

[141] Olsen WL, Dillon WP, Kelly WM, Norman D, Brant-Zawadzki M, Newton TH. MR imaging of paragangliomas. AJR Am J Roentgenol 1987; 148: 201–204

[142] Motamedi K, Seeger LL. Benign bone tumors. Radiol Clin North Am 2011; 49: 1115–1134, vv.

[143] Arriaga MA, Lo WW, Brackmann DE. Magnetic resonance angiography of synchronous bilateral carotid body paragangliomas and bilateral vagal paragangliomas. Ann Otol Rhinol Laryngol 1992; 101: 955–957

[144] Dowd C, Halback V, Higashida R, Heishima G. Diagnostic and therapeutic angiography. In: Jackler RK, Brackman D, eds. Neurotology. St. Louis: Mosby, 1994:399–436

[145] Moret J, Picard L. Vascular architecture of tympanojugular glomus tumors. Semin Intervent Radiol 1987; 4: 291–308

[146] Sismanis A, Smoker WR. Pulsatile tinnitus: recent advances in diagnosis. Laryngoscope 1994; 104: 681–688

[147] Lum C, Keller AM, Kassel E, Blend R, Waldron J, Rutka J. Unusual eustachian tube mass: glomus tympanicum. AJNR Am J Neuroradiol 2001; 22: 508–509

[148] Tatla T, Savy LE, Wareing MJ. Epistaxis as a rare presenting feature of glomus tympanicum. J Laryngol Otol 2003; 117: 577–579

[149] Ibrahimov M, Yilmaz M, Mamanov M, Korkut N. Glomus tympanicum: an unusual cause of epistaxis. J Craniofac Surg 2012; 23: 1224–1225

[150] Brown LA. Glomus jugulare tumor of the middle ear; clinical aspects. Laryngoscope 1953; 63: 281–292

[151] Lo WW, Solti-Bohman LG, Lambert PR. High-resolution CT in the evaluation of glomus tumors of the temporal bone. Radiology 1984; 150: 737–742

[152] Amin MF, Ameen NF. Diagnostic efficiency of multidetector computed tomography versus magnetic resonance imaging in differentiation of head and neck paragangliomas from other mimicking vascular lesions: comparison with histopathologic examination. Eur Arch Otorhinolaryngol 2012; 27: 27

[153] Alaani A, Chavda SV, Irving RM. The crucial role of imaging in determining the approach to glomus tympanicum tumours. Eur Arch Otorhinolaryngol 2009; 266: 827–831

[154] Jackson CG. Basic surgical principles of neurotologic skull base surgery. Laryngoscope 1993; 103 Suppl 60: 29–44

[155] Sanna M, Fois P, Pasanisi E, Russo A, Bacciu A. Middle ear and mastoid glomus tumors (glomus tympanicum): an algorithm for the surgical management. Auris Nasus Larynx 2010; 37: 661–668

[156] Durvasula VS, De R, Baguley DM, Moffat DA. Laser excision of glomus tympanicum tumours: long-term results. Eur Arch Otorhinolaryngol 2005; 262: 325–327

[157] Jackson CG, Cueva RA, Thedinger BA, Glasscock ME, III. Cranial nerve preservation in lesions of the jugular fossa. Otolaryngol Head Neck Surg 1991; 105: 687–693

[158] Jackson CG. Glomus tympanicum and glomus jugulare tumors. Otolaryngol Clin North Am 2001; 34: 941–970, vii

[159] Sanna M, Shin SH, De Donato G et al. Management of complex tympanojugular paragangliomas including endovascular intervention. Laryngoscope 2011; 121: 1372–1382

[160] Sawlani V, Browing S, Sawhney IM, Redfern R. Posterior circulation stroke following embolization of glomus tympanicum?relevance of anatomy and anastomoses of ascending pharyngeal artery. A case report. Interv Neuroradiol 2009; 15: 229–236

[161] Warren FM, III, McCool RR, Hunt JO et al. Preoperative embolization of the inferior petrosal sinus in surgery for glomus jugulare tumors. Otol Neurotol 2011; 32: 1538–1541

[162] Miman MC, Aktas D, Oncel S, Ozturan O, Kalcioglu MT. Glomus jugulare. Otolaryngol Head Neck Surg 2002; 127: 585–586

[163] House JW, Fayad JN. Glomus jugulare. Ear Nose Throat J 2004; 83: 800

[164] Sanna M, Flanagan S. The combined transmastoid retro- and infralabyrinthine transjugular transcondylar transtubercular high cervical approach for resection of glomus jugulare tumors. Neurosurgery 2007; 61: E1340–, author reply E1340

[165] Oghalai JS, Leung MK, Jackler RK, McDermott MW. Transjugular craniotomy for the management of jugular foramen tumors with intracranial extension. Otol Neurotol 2004; 25: 570–579, discussion 579

[166] Cheesman AD, Kelly AM. Rehabilitation after treatment for jugular foramen lesions. Skull Base 2009; 19: 99–108

[167] Makiese O, Chibbaro S, Marsella M, Tran Ba Huy P, George B. Jugular foramen paragangliomas: management, outcome and avoidance of complications in a series of 75 cases. Neurosurg Rev 2012; 35: 185–194, discussion 194

[168] Bari ME, Kemeny AA, Forster DM, Radatz MW. Radiosurgery for the control of glomus jugulare tumours. J Pak Med Assoc 2003; 53: 147–151

[169] Foote RL, Pollock BE, Gorman DA et al. Glomus jugulare tumor: tumor control and complications after stereotactic radiosurgery. Head Neck 2002; 24: 332–338, discussion 338–339

[170] Gottfried ON, Liu JK, Couldwell WT. Comparison of radiosurgery and conventional surgery for the treatment of glomus jugulare tumors. Neurosurg Focus 2004; 17: E4

[171] Pollock BE. Stereotactic radiosurgery in patients with glomus jugulare tumors. Neurosurg Focus 2004; 17: E10

[172] Saringer W, Khayal H, Ertl A, Schoeggl A, Kitz K. Efficiency of gamma knife radiosurgery in the treatment of glomus jugulare tumors. Minim Invasive Neurosurg 2001; 44: 141–146

[173] Sheehan J, Kondziolka D, Flickinger J, Lunsford LD. Gamma knife surgery for glomus jugulare tumors: an intermediate report on efficacy and safety. J Neurosurg 2005; 102 Suppl: 241–246

[174] Hurmuz P, Cengiz M, Ozyigit G et al. Robotic stereotactic radiosurgery in patients with unresectable glomus jugulare tumors. Technol Cancer Res Treat 2012; 10: 10

[175] Guss ZD, Batra S, Limb CJ et al. Radiosurgery of glomus jugulare tumors: a meta-analysis. Int J Radiat Oncol Biol Phys 2011; 81: e497–e502

[176] Chen PG, Nguyen JH, Payne SC, Sheehan JP, Hashisaki GT. Treatment of glomus jugulare tumors with gamma knife radiosurgery. Laryngoscope 2010; 120: 1856–1862

[177] Lustig LR, Jackler RK, Lanser MJ. Radiation-induced tumors of the temporal bone. Am J Otol 1997; 18: 230–235

[178] Miller JP, Semaan M, Einstein D, Megerian CA, Maciunas RJ. Staged gamma knife radiosurgery after tailored surgical resection: a novel treatment paradigm for glomus jugulare tumors. Stereotact Funct Neurosurg 2009; 87: 31–36

[179] Fayad JN, Schwartz MS, Brackmann DE. Treatment of recurrent and residual glomus jugulare tumors. Skull Base 2009; 19: 92–98

[180] Miller JP, Semaan MT, Maciunas RJ, Einstein DB, Megerian CA. Radiosurgery for glomus jugulare tumors. Otolaryngol Clin North Am 2009; 42: 689–706

[181] Nager GT, Masica DN. Meningiomas of the cerebello-pontine angle and their relation to the temporal bone. Laryngoscope 1970; 80: 863–895

[182] Lusis E, Gutmann DH. Meningioma: an update. Curr Opin Neurol 2004; 17: 687–692

[183] Ferlito A, Devaney KO, Rinaldo A. Primary extracranial meningioma in the vicinity of the temporal bone: a benign lesion which is rarely recognized clinically. Acta Otolaryngol 2004; 124: 5–7

[184] Nager GT, Heroy J, Hoeplinger M. Meningiomas invading the temporal bone with extension to the neck. Am J Otolaryngol 1983; 4: 297–324

[185] Lesch KP, Gross S. Estrogen receptor immunoreactivity in meningiomas. Comparison with the binding activity of estrogen, progesterone, and androgen receptors. J Neurosurg 1987; 67: 237–243

[186] Modan B, Baidatz D, Mart H, Steinitz R, Levin SG. Radiation-induced head and neck tumours. Lancet 1974; 1: 277–279

[187] Frisch CD, Carlson ML, Link MJ. Synchronous head and neck tumors after low-dose radiation to the temporal bone. Otol Neurotol 2012; 33: e3–e4

[188] Roberti F, Sekhar LN, Kalavakonda C, Wright DC. Posterior fossa meningiomas: surgical experience in 161 cases. Surg Neurol 2001; 56: 8–20, discussion 20–21

[189] Selesnick SH, Nguyen TD, Gutin PH, Lavyne MH. Posterior petrous face meningiomas. Otolaryngol Head Neck Surg 2001; 124: 408–413

[190] Thompson LD, Bouffard JP, Sandberg GD, Mena H. Primary ear and temporal bone meningiomas: a clinicopathologic study of 36 cases with a review of the literature. Mod Pathol 2003; 16: 236–245

[191] Chang CY, Cheung SW, Jackler RK. Meningiomas presenting in the temporal bone: the pathways of spread from an intracranial site of origin. Otolaryngol Head Neck Surg 1998; 119: 658–664

[192] Singh A, Selesnick S. Meningiomas of the posterior fossa and skull base. In: Jackler RK, Brackman D, eds. Neurotology, 2nd ed. St. Louis: Mosby, 2005:792–840

[193] Langman AW, Jackler RK, Althaus SR. Meningioma of the internal auditory canal. Am J Otol 1990; 11: 201–204

[194] Laudadio P, Canani FB, Cunsolo E. Meningioma of the internal auditory canal. Acta Otolaryngol 2004; 124: 1231–1234

[195] Gilbert ME, Shelton C, McDonald A et al. Meningioma of the jugular foramen: glomus jugulare mimic and surgical challenge. Laryngoscope 2004; 114: 25–32

[196] Macdonald AJ, Salzman KL, Harnsberger HR, Gilbert E, Shelton C. Primary jugular foramen meningioma: imaging appearance and differentiating features. AJR Am J Roentgenol 2004; 182: 373–377

[197] Morris J, Schoen W. The nervous system. In: Robbins SL, Cotran RS, Kumar V, eds. Pathologic Basis of Disease, 5th ed. Philadelphia: WB Saunders, 1984

[198] Shihada R, Lurie M, Luntz M. Skull base meningiomas mimicking otitis media. J Laryngol Otol 2012; 126: 619–624

[199] Laird FJ, Harner SG, Laws ER, Jr, Reese DF. Meningiomas of the cerebellopontine angle. Otolaryngol Head Neck Surg 1985; 93: 163–167

[200] Molony TB, Brackmann DE, Lo WW. Meningiomas of the jugular foramen. Otolaryngol Head Neck Surg 1992; 106: 128–136

[201] Curati WL, Graif M, Kingsley DP, King T, Scholtz CL, Steiner RE. MRI in acoustic neuroma: a review of 35 patients. Neuroradiology 1986; 28: 208–214

[202] Lalwani AK, Jackler RK. Preoperative differentiation between meningioma of the cerebellopontine angle and acoustic neuroma using MRI. Otolaryngol Head Neck Surg 1993; 109: 88–95

[203] Wilms G, Plets C, Goossens L, Goffin J, Vanwambeke K. The radiological differentiation of acoustic neurinoma and meningioma occurring together in the cerebellopontine angle. Neurosurgery 1992; 30: 443–445, discussion 445–446

[204] Itoh T, Harada M, Ichikawa T, Shimoyamada K, Katayama N, Tsukune Y. A case of jugular foramen chordoma with extension to the neck: CT and MR findings. Radiat Med 2000; 18: 63–65

[205] Rinaldi A, Gazzeri G, Callovini GM, Masci P, Natali G. Acoustic intrameatal meningiomas. J Neurosurg Sci 2000; 44: 25–32

[206] Zhu W, Mao Y. Combined supratentorial and infratentorial approaches for removal of petroclival meningiomas. World Neurosurg 2011; 75: 422–423

[207] Leonetti JP, Anderson DE, Marzo SJ, Origitano TC, Schuman R. Combined transtemporal access for large (> 3 cm) meningiomas of the cerebellopontine angle. Otolaryngol Head Neck Surg 2006; 134: 949–952

[208] Glasscock M, Minor L, McMenomey S. Meningiomas of the cerebellopontine angle. In: Jackler RK, Brackman D, eds. Neurotology. St. Louis: Mosby, 1994:795–821

[209] Baugh A, Hillman TA, Shelton C. Combined petrosal approaches in the management of temporal bone meningiomas. Otol Neurotol 2007; 28: 236–239

[210] Nanda A, Javalkar V, Banerjee AD. Petroclival meningiomas: study on outcomes, complications and recurrence rates. J Neurosurg 2011; 114: 1268–1277

[211] Sanna M, Bacciu A, Falcioni M, Taibah A, Piazza P. Surgical management of jugular foramen meningiomas: a series of 13 cases and review of the literature. Laryngoscope 2007; 117: 1710–1719

[212] Chamberlain MC, Blumenthal DT. Intracranial meningiomas: diagnosis and treatment. Expert Rev Neurother 2004; 4: 641–648

[213] Milker-Zabel S, Zabel A, Schulz-Ertner D, Schlegel W, Wannenmacher M, Debus J. Fractionated stereotactic radiotherapy in patients with benign or atypical intracranial meningioma: long-term experience and prognostic factors. Int J Radiat Oncol Biol Phys 2005; 61: 809–816

[214] Tonn JC. Microneurosurgery and radiosurgery–an attractive combination. Acta Neurochir Suppl (Wien) 2004; 91: 103–108

[215] Barbaro NM, Gutin PH, Wilson CB, Sheline GE, Boldrey EB, Wara WM. Radiation therapy in the treatment of partially resected meningiomas. Neurosurgery 1987; 20: 525–528

[216] Kondziolka D, Lunsford LD, Flickinger JC. The role of radiosurgery in the management of chordoma and chondrosarcoma of the cranial base. Neurosurgery 1991; 29: 38–45, discussion 45–46

[217] Liscák R, Kollová A, Vladyka V, Simonová G, Novotný J, Jr. Gamma knife radiosurgery of skull base meningiomas. Acta Neurochir Suppl (Wien) 2004; 91: 65–74

[218] Flannery TJ, Kano H, Lunsford LD et al. Long-term control of petroclival meningiomas through radiosurgery. J Neurosurg 2010; 112: 957–964

[219] Mirimanoff RO, Dosoretz DE, Linggood RM, Ojemann RG, Martuza RL. Meningioma: analysis of recurrence and progression following neurosurgical resection. J Neurosurg 1985; 62: 18–24

[220] Polinsky MN, Brunberg JA, McKeever PE, Sandler HM, Telian S, Ross D. Aggressive papillary middle ear tumors: a report of two cases with review of the literature. Neurosurgery 1994; 35: 493–497, discussion 497

[221] Benecke JE, Jr, Noel FL, Carberry JN, House JW, Patterson M. Adenomatous tumors of the middle ear and mastoid. Am J Otol 1990; 11: 20–26

[222] Mills RG, Douglas-Jones T, Williams RG. 'Ceruminoma'–a defunct diagnosis. J Laryngol Otol 1995; 109: 180–188

[223] Batsakis JG. Adenomatous tumors of the middle ear. Ann Otol Rhinol Laryngol 1989; 98: 749–752

[224] Xenellis J, Mountricha A, Maragoudakis P et al. A histological examination in the cases of initial diagnosis as chronic otitis media with a polypoid mass in the external ear canal. Auris Nasus Larynx 2011; 38: 325–328

[225] Peters BR, Maddox HE, III, Batsakia JG. Pleomorphic adenoma of the middle ear and mastoid with posterior fossa extension. Arch Otolaryngol Head Neck Surg 1988; 114: 676–678

[226] Batsakis JG, el-Naggar AK. Papillary neoplasms (Heffner's tumors) of the endolymphatic sac. Ann Otol Rhinol Laryngol 1993; 102: 648–651

[227] Richards PS, Clifton AG. Endolymphatic sac tumours. J Laryngol Otol 2003; 117: 666–669

[228] Stendel R, Suess O, Prosenc N, Funk T, Brock M. Neoplasm of endolymphatic sac origin: clinical, radiological and pathological features. Acta Neurochir (Wien) 1998; 140: 1083–1087

[229] Luff DA, Simmons M, Malik T, Ramsden RT, Reid H. Endolymphatic sac tumours. J Laryngol Otol 2002; 116: 398–401

[230] Heffner DK. Low-grade adenocarcinoma of probable endolymphatic sac origin A clinicopathologic study of 20 cases. Cancer 1989; 64: 2292–2302

[231] Poe DS, Tarlov EC, Thomas CB, Kveton JF. Aggressive papillary tumors of temporal bone. Otolaryngol Head Neck Surg 1993; 108: 80–86

[232] Tysome JR, Harcourt J, Patel MC, Sandison A, Michaels L. Aggressive papillary tumor of the middle ear: a true entity or an endolymphatic sac neoplasm? Ear Nose Throat J 2008; 87: 378–393

[233] Noel FL, Benecke JE, Jr, Carberry JN, House JW, Patterson M. Adenomas of the mastoid and middle ear. Otolaryngol Head Neck Surg 1991; 104: 133–134

[234] Panchwagh J, Goel A, Shenoy A. Bilateral endolymphatic sac papillary carcinoma. Br J Neurosurg 1999; 13: 79–81

[235] Tay KY, Yu E, Kassel E. Spinal metastasis from endolymphatic sac tumor. AJNR Am J Neuroradiol 2007; 28: 613–614

[236] Bambakidis NC, Rodrigue T, Megerian CA, Ratcheson RA. Endolymphatic sac tumor metastatic to the spine. Case report. J Neurosurg Spine 2005; 3: 68–70

[237] Li JC, Brackmann DE, Lo WW, Carberry JN, House JW. Reclassification of aggressive adenomatous mastoid neoplasms as endolymphatic sac tumors. Laryngoscope 1993; 103: 1342–1348

[238] Timmer FC, Neeskens LJ, van den Hoogen FJ et al. Endolymphatic sac tumors: clinical outcome and management in a series of 9 cases. Otol Neurotol 2011; 32: 680–685

[239] Devaney KO, Ferlito A, Rinaldo A. Epithelial tumors of the middle ear–are middle ear carcinoids really distinct from middle ear adenomas? Acta Otolaryngol 2003; 123: 678–682

[240] Torske KR, Thompson LD. Adenoma versus carcinoid tumor of the middle ear: a study of 48 cases and review of the literature. Mod Pathol 2002; 15: 543–555

[241] Krouse JH, Nadol JB, Jr, Goodman ML. Carcinoid tumors of the middle ear. Ann Otol Rhinol Laryngol 1990; 99: 547–552

[242] Murphy GF, Pilch BZ, Dickersin GR, Goodman ML, Nadol JB, Jr. Carcinoid tumor of the middle ear. Am J Clin Pathol 1980; 73: 816–823

[243] Bläker H, Dyckhoff G, Weidauer H, Otto HF. Carcinoid tumor of the middle ear in a 28-year-old patient. Pathol Oncol Res 1998; 4: 40–43

[244] Mooney EE, Dodd LG, Oury TD, Burchette JL, Layfield LJ, Scher RL. Middle ear carcinoid: an indolent tumor with metastatic potential. Head Neck 1999; 21: 72–77

[245] Nikanne E, Kantola O, Parviainen T. Carcinoid tumor of the middle ear. Acta Otolaryngol 2004; 124: 754–757

[246] Shibosawa E, Tsutsumi K, Ihara Y, Kinoshita H, Koizuka I. A case of carcinoid tumor of the middle ear. Auris Nasus Larynx 2003; 30 Suppl: S99–S102

[247] Chan KC, Wu CM, Huang SF. Carcinoid tumor of the middle ear: a case report. Am J Otolaryngol 2005; 26: 57–59

[248] Pellini R, Ruggieri M, Pichi B, Covello R, Danesi G, Spriano G. A case of cervical metastases from temporal bone carcinoid. Head Neck 2005; 27: 644–647

[249] Schenk P, Handisurya A, Steurer M. Ultrastructural morphology of a middle ear ceruminoma. ORL J Otorhinolaryngol Relat Spec 2002; 64: 358–363

[250] el-Naggar AK, Pflatz M, Ordóñez NG, Batsakis JG. Tumors of the middle ear and endolymphatic sac. Pathol Annu 1994; 29: 199–231

[251] Gulya AJ, Glasscock ME, III, Pensak ML. Neural choristoma of the middle ear. Otolaryngol Head Neck Surg 1987; 97: 52–56

[252] Nelson EG, Kratz RC. Sebaceous choristoma of the middle ear. Otolaryngol Head Neck Surg 1993; 108: 372–373

[253] Gyure KA, Thompson LD, Morrison AL. A clinicopathological study of 15 patients with neuroglial heterotopias and encephaloceles of the middle ear and mastoid region. Laryngoscope 2000; 110: 1731–1735

[254] Rinaldo A, Ferlito A, Devaney KO. Salivary gland choristoma of the middle ear. A review. ORL J Otorhinolaryngol Relat Spec 2004; 66: 141–147

[255] Martinez-Peñuela A, Quer S, Beloqui R, Bulnes MD, Martinez-Peñuela JM. Glial choristoma of the middle ear: report of 2 cases. Otol Neurotol 2011; 32: e26–e27

[256] Uğuz MZ, Arslanoğlu S, Terzi S, Etit D. Glial heterotopia of the middle ear. J Laryngol Otol 2007; 121: e4

[257] Enoz M, Suoglu Y. Salivary gland choristoma of the middle ear. Laryngoscope 2006; 116: 1033–1034

[258] Lee FP. Cartilaginous choristoma of the bony external auditory canal: a study of 36 cases. Otolaryngol Head Neck Surg 2005; 133: 786–790

[259] Anderhuber W, Beham A, Walch C, Stammberger H. Choristoma of the middle ear. Eur Arch Otorhinolaryngol 1996; 253: 182–184

[260] Kartush JM, Graham MD. Salivary gland choristoma of the middle ear: a case report and review of the literature. Laryngoscope 1984; 94: 228–230

[261] Abadir WF, Pease WS. Salivary gland choristoma of the middle ear. J Laryngol Otol 1978; 92: 247–252

[262] Vasama JP, Ramsay H, Markkola A. Choristoma of the middle ear. Otol Neurotol 2001; 22: 421–422

[263] Jackson IT, Carreño R, Potparic Z, Hussain K. Hemangiomas, vascular malformations, and lymphovenous malformations: classification and methods of treatment. Plast Reconstr Surg 1993; 91: 1216–1230

[264] Mulliken JB, Glowacki J. Hemangiomas and vascular malformations in infants and children: a classification based on endothelial characteristics. Plast Reconstr Surg 1982; 69: 412–422

[265] Waner M, Suen JY, Dinehart S. Treatment of hemangiomas of the head and neck. Laryngoscope 1992; 102: 1123–1132

[266] Buchanan DS, Fagan PA, Turner J. Cavernous haemangioma of the temporal bone. J Laryngol Otol 1992; 106: 1086–1088

[267] Shelton C, Brackmann DE, Lo WW, Carberry JN. Intratemporal facial nerve hemangiomas. Otolaryngol Head Neck Surg 1991; 104: 116–121

[268] Glasscock ME, III, Smith PG, Schwaber MK, Nissen AJ. Clinical aspects of osseous hemangiomas of the skull base. Laryngoscope 1984; 94: 869–873

[269] Mazzoni A, Pareschi R, Calabrese V. Intratemporal vascular tumours. J Laryngol Otol 1988; 102: 353–356

[270] Dufour JJ, Michaud LA, Mohr G, Pouliot D, Picard C. Intratemporal vascular malformations (angiomas): particular clinical features. J Otolaryngol 1994; 23: 250–253

[271] Barrera JE, Jenkins H, Said S. Cavernous hemangioma of the internal auditory canal: a case report and review of the literature. Am J Otolaryngol 2004; 25: 199–203

[272] Aquilina K, Nanra JS, Brett F, Walsh RM, Rawluk D. Cavernous angioma of the internal auditory canal. J Laryngol Otol 2004; 118: 368–371

[273] Gjuric M, Koester M, Paulus W. Cavernous hemangioma of the internal auditory canal arising from the inferior vestibular nerve: case report and review of the literature. Am J Otol 2000; 21: 110–114

[274] Lenarz M, Durisin M, Kamenetzki P, Becker H, Kreipe HH, Lenarz T. Cavernous hemangioma of the internal auditory canal. Eur Arch Otorhinolaryngol 2007; 264: 569–571

[275] Tokyol C, Yilmaz MD. Middle ear hemangioma: a case report. Am J Otolaryngol 2003; 24: 405–407

[276] Reeck JB, Yen TL, Szmit A, Cheung SW. Cavernous hemangioma of the external ear canal. Laryngoscope 2002; 112: 1750–1752

[277] Limb CJ, Mabrie DC, Carey JP, Minor LB. Hemangioma of the external auditory canal. Otolaryngol Head Neck Surg 2002; 126: 74–75

[278] Hecht DA, Jackson CG, Grundfast KM. Management of middle ear hemangiomas. Am J Otolaryngol 2001; 22: 362–366

[279] Jang CH, Choi HS, Hong YS, Cho YB. Cavernous hemangioma of the tympanic membrane. Clin Exp Otorhinolaryngol 2011; 4: 109–111

[280] Bijelic L, Wei JL, McDonald TJ. Hemangioma of the tympanic membrane. Otolaryngol Head Neck Surg 2001; 125: 272–273

[281] Fisch U, Ruttner J. Pathology of intratemporal tumors involving the facial nerve. In: Fisch U, ed. Facial Nerve Surgery. Birmingham: Aesculapius, 1977:448–456

[282] Eby TL, Fisch U, Makek MS. Facial nerve management in temporal bone hemangiomas. Am J Otol 1992; 13: 223–232

[283] Lo WW, Shelton C, Waluch V et al. Intratemporal vascular tumors: detection with CT and MR imaging. Radiology 1989; 171: 445–448

[284] Piccirillo E, Agarwal M, Rohit , Khrais T, Sanna M. Management of temporal bone hemangiomas. Ann Otol Rhinol Laryngol 2004; 113: 431–437

[285] Semaan MT, Slattery WH, Brackmann DE. Geniculate ganglion hemangiomas: clinical results and long-term follow-up. Otol Neurotol 2010; 31: 665–670

[286] Badalian-Very G, Vergilio JA, Fleming M, Rollins BJ. Pathogenesis of Langerhans cell histiocytosis. Annu Rev Pathol 2012; 6: 6

[287] Goldsmith AJ, Myssiorek D, Valderrama E, Patel M. Unifocal Langerhans' cell histiocytosis (eosinophilic granuloma) of the petrous apex. Arch Otolaryngol Head Neck Surg 1993; 119: 113–116

[288] Cunningham MJ, Curtin HD, Jaffe R, Stool SE. Otologic manifestations of Langerhans' cell histiocytosis. Arch Otolaryngol Head Neck Surg 1989; 115: 807–813

[289] Neilan RE, Kutz JW, Jr. Langerhans cell histiocytosis of the temporal bone. Otol Neurotol 2012; 33: e31–e32

[290] Nolph MB, Luikin GA, Histiocytosis X. Otolaryngol Clin North Am 1982; 15: 635–648

[291] Aricò M, Danesino C. Langerhans' cell histiocytosis: is there a role for genetics? Haematologica 2001; 86: 1009–1014

[292] McCaffrey TV, McDonald TJ. Histiocytosis X of the ear and temporal bone: review of 22 cases. Laryngoscope 1979; 89: 1735–1742

[293] Bayazit Y, Sirikci A, Bayaram M, Kanlikama M, Demir A, Bakir K. Eosinophilic granuloma of the temporal bone. Auris Nasus Larynx 2001; 28: 99–102

[294] DeRowe A, Bernheim J, Ophir D. Eosinophilic granuloma presenting as chronic otitis media: pitfalls in the diagnosis of aural polyps in children. J Otolaryngol 1995; 24: 258–260

[295] Tos M. Facial palsy in Hand-Schüller-Christian's disease. Arch Otolaryngol 1969; 90: 563–567

[296] Fradis M, Podoshin L, Ben-David J, Grishkan A. Eosinophilic granuloma of the temporal bone. J Laryngol Otol 1985; 99: 475–479

26 Cystic Lesions of the Petrous Apex

Laura Brainard, Todd A. Hillman, and Douglas A. Chen

26.1 Introduction

Cystic lesions of the petrous apex are uncommon temporal bone pathologies that include cholesterol granuloma, cholesteatoma, mucocele, and other, rarer lesions. This chapter reviews petrous apex anatomy, differential diagnosis of cystic lesions, and surgical approaches to the petrous apex.

26.2 History

It is useful to examine the history of petrous apicitis, because it is through the diagnosis and treatment of petrous apicitis that otologic surgeons gained an understanding of the anatomy and surgical approaches to the petrous apex, many of which are still used today in treating cystic lesions of the petrous apex.

Historically, there was a progression of surgical management of petrous apicitis, with earlier surgeons favoring more conservative, less invasive approaches, and later surgeons, with the benefit of advanced surgical skills, anatomic understanding, and extensive study, undertaking more invasive approaches to the skull base. Initial surgical approaches included various approaches to the floor of the middle cranial fossa, allowing inspection of the superior surface of the petrous pyramid and treatment of suppurative disease that had erupted through the petrous bone, but did not allow inspection within the petrous apex. Spurred on by the continued high rate of progression to meningitis and almost certain death associated with that complication, surgeons became more aggressive, developing petrous apicotomy procedures that enabled limited exploration of the petrous apex. Other surgeons, still not satisfied, developed approaches that skeletonized the petrous carotid, and, most aggressively, involved removal of a significant portion of the carotid canal.

In the preantibiotic era, suppurative petrous apicitis was a common and often fatal outcome of chronic otitis media. In the early 1900s, shortly after Gradenigo published a report in 1904 describing the triad of signs that have come to bear his name, many case reports of patients presenting with Gradenigo syndrome followed, both confirming Gradenigo's theory and describing treatment approaches and clinical outcomes.[1] It was generally understood that Gradenigo syndrome was a circumscribed serous meningitis, originating from petrous apex osteomyelitis that had begun as an acute otitis media. In certain instances, this localized meningitis resolved spontaneously, but in others, it progressed to brain abscess, with signs of increased intracranial pressure (headache, vomiting, drowsiness, spontaneous nystagmus). The challenge in distinguishing an otitic meningitis from the circumscribed meningitis of Gradenigo syndrome was no small task, which one surgeon likened to "solv[ing] the same kind of riddle as 'what has web feet, feathers, and barks like a dog'."[2] Although some patients received surgical treatments and had rapid clinical improvement with resolution of the characteristic diplopia, facial pain, and otorrhea, others were successfully treated with observation after limited mastoidectomy, although with a more protracted clinical course. Many patients died, with the nature of disease elucidated only on postmortem evaluation, or in spite of correct diagnosis, but with inadequate treatment, or treatment performed after the onset of meningitis. Other cases presented in a delayed fashion after relatively minor ear symptoms, or an indolent, nonspecific course. Without the benefit of modern day radiology (computed tomography [CT]/magnetic resonance imaging [MRI]/nuclear medicine scans), the surgeons at that time had to rely heavily on clinical history, presentation, simple X-rays and suspicion of underlying petrous apex disease, in spite of sometimes minor mastoid and ear findings. Their understanding of the relationship of cranial nerves (CNs) V and VI to the petrous apex and to the mastoid air-cell tracts allowed them to operate on the ear for what sometimes presented as "eye" symptoms, or for meningitis presenting remotely from onset of ear symptoms.[3]

In attempts to better understand the spread of disease from the mastoid and middle ear to the petrous apex, both macroscopic and microscopic postmortem temporal bone evaluations were performed. Macroscopic evaluations favored peritubal cells and the carotid canal as routes of infectious spread, whereas microscopic evaluation favored the perilabyrinthine route.[4] In 1906, Lombard poured mercury into the petrous tip of a patient who had died from meningitis following an acute otitis media. The mercury, when poured into the healthy side, followed a sublabyrinthine route into the middle ear. Autopsy evaluation of the diseased side showed that the infection had also spread via the sublabyrinthine route. In 1938, Lindsay presented the pathological findings of 28 meningitis deaths from the preceding 7 years, in which temporal bones were available for review. Of the 28 cases, eight originated from suppuration of the petrous apex. Five of the eight had been treated with simple or radical mastoidectomy before succumbing to meningitis. His microscopic evaluation of the postmortem bones led him to an understanding of which air-cell tracts were involved in spread of infection to the petrous apex. It also became apparent that access to the involved anterior petrous apex was not possible through the standard transmastoid route.[5]

The initial surgical treatments of petrous apicitis included middle fossa craniotomy, radical mastoidectomy, labyrinthectomy, and paracentesis. Following fistulous tracts of pus toward the petrous apex helped otologic surgeons deepen their understanding of the complicated anatomy and navigate safely to the seat of infection. Many surgical approaches were developed in this way, including the infralabyrinthine, subarcuate, pericarotid, and infracochlear approaches. In 1931, Eagleton presented a paper describing his approach to suppurative petrous apicitis, which he called "unlocking the petrous pyramid." The exact surgical procedure varied depending on the fistulous tracts he identified intraoperatively, but all involved developing drainage pathways to the petrous apex, as well as ipsilateral common carotid artery ligation. Unlike Lempert, who maintained that petrous apicitis was not an osteomyelitis, Eagleton maintained that it was; the bone marrow spaces in the petrous apex were similar to those in long bones, and, as with treatment of osteomyelitis in long bones, drainage was all that was necessary. The blood supply of these regions and the marrow were thought to have reparative properties, in contrast to mastoiditis, which was thought not to be an osteomyelitis and required complete removal of all involved bony spaces.[6]

In 1932, Ramadier presented to the Anatomical Society of Paris a novel approach to the petrous apex, which, at the time of presentation, he had performed successfully on a dozen patients; he called it exploration of the petrous apex by the carotid canal route. This approach involved a radical mastoidectomy, removal of the anterior bony external canal wall, and anterior displacement of the temporomandibular joint. He argued that because the carotid artery presented the greatest danger in the petrous apex, the best way to protect it was to expose it, putting it under the control of direct visualization. Additionally, he found that the carotid artery could serve as a guide, leading him to the most medial aspect of the anterior petrous apex. Well aware that it was often impossible to definitively verify the presence of a petrous apex osteomyelitis, he continued to put great hope in radiology, which at that time was only able to give very limited information.[7]

Four years later, in 1936, Lempert presented the "complete apicectomy." Similar to, but more extensive than, Ramadier's approach, he emphasized removal of bone of the carotid canal, and separation of the base of the petrous pyramid from the laterally positioned tympanic and mastoid segments of the temporal bone, to enable complete inspection of all three sides of the petrous pyramid and the entire petrous carotid from the vertical segment at the skull base to the vertical segment at the foramen lacerum. He criticized Ramadier's technique as being a mere apicotomy, insufficient for eradicating disease in the petrous apex, and insufficient for drainage, once the skeletonized petrous carotid fell back into place, obscuring the drainage tract that had been created. Lempert was concerned with the 20% of patients with petrous apicitis who, failing simple mastoidectomy, died from meningitis. His feeling was that those who were successfully treated with limited surgery or with observation, did not truly have suppurative apicitis. For this reason, he was adamant that all patients with radiographic and clinical evidence of suppurative apicitis be treated with aggressive surgery; he was opposed to what he called a laissez-faire attitude, couched as "conservative otology." Even so, many of his patients presented with advanced disease, with signs of meningitis, and died even after "successful" surgery, some from meningitis, some from surgical complications, including cerebral embolus, after alternating postoperative injections of Pregl's iodine solution and acriflavine base (an antiseptic, used as a modern-day antifungal in fish tanks) into the exposed petrous carotid artery. Lempert's paper illustrates quite vividly the struggle of early otologists, not only to diagnose and learn how best to treat petrous apicitis, but also to develop at a common language for the anatomy and classification of the disease:

I find in reviewing my experience with the treatment of petrositis, that I passed through a transitional period, beginning with complete inactivity, a laissez faire attitude, masquerading as conservative otology. This was due to lack of knowledge of what to do in these cases other than a mastoidectomy. Then followed a second stage, with a sort of rationalizing self-defense conservatism, when I began to comprehend the pathologic picture of petrositis but did not know how to approach the lesion surgically. A third stage ensued when I became cognizant of the work of Eagleton, Kopetzky

and Almour, Frenckner and Ramadier, who described surgical procedures for drainage of suppurative apicitis. At this point I decided to employ the Kopetzky and Almour technic, because it appeared to me to be the simplest and safest of all those described, and it surgically drains any lesion of suppurative apicitis encountered in pneumatized bone.[8]

In trying to save patients from the all too often fatal complications of otitis media, the early surgeons developed surgical approaches to the petrous apex, which, although used rarely for this reason today, are used in the treatment of cystic lesions of the petrous apex, whose presentation is often more subtle and less life-threatening than its infectious counterpart.

26.3 Anatomy

The French term for petrous apex, *la pointe du rocher*, literally, "point of the rock," is an apt descriptor. As anyone who has ever harvested a temporal bone can attest, the petrous bone is the most compact and medial part of the temporal bone. Its location, as well as the vital structures, both neural and vascular, that pass through and adjacent to the petrous apex, are what makes accessing this region so challenging (▶ Fig. 26.1).

The petrous apex is defined as that part of the temporal bone that is anteromedial to the inner ear and lateral to the petro-occipital fissure.[9] It is described as a three-sided, truncated pyramid, with the base facing laterally and the point of the pyramid

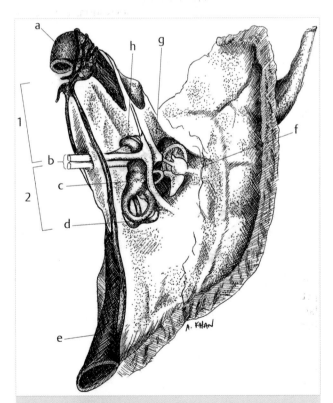

Fig. 26.1 Anterior (1) and posterior (2) petrous apex. (a) Carotid artery; (b) internal auditory canal; (c) vestibule; (d) semicircular canals; (e) internal jugular vein; (f) middle ear structures; (g) Eustachian tube; (h) cochlea.

angling anteriorly, medially, and slightly upward. It is situated between the greater wing of the sphenoid anterolaterally and the occipital bone/clivus posteromedially. It is divided by a line in the coronal plane through the internal auditory canal (IAC) into the anterior and posterior petrous apex. The petrous apex is an integral part of the skull base, providing support for the cranial contents and housing the sensory organs of the temporal bone, as well as the facial and carotid canals.[10]

The base of the pyramid is the bony labyrinth, and includes the semicircular canals and the cochlea. Anteriorly, the base includes the semicanal of the tensor tympani muscle and the internal carotid artery (ICA).

The three-sided pyramid has anterior, inferior, and posterior surfaces. The anterior surface, sometimes referred to as the superior surface, serves as the posterior and medial floor of the middle cranial fossa. The arcuate eminence, located on the anterior surface, indicates the location of the superior semicircular canal, albeit inconsistently. The lesser petrosal nerve exits the tympanic canaliculus and runs anteriorly toward the foramen ovale where it exits the cranium to synapse at the otic ganglion. Medial to this, and not quite parallel, the greater superficial petrosal nerve arises from the anterior aspect of the geniculate ganglion and courses anteriorly, exiting the facial hiatus to emerge on the floor of the middle cranial fossa. It courses anteriorly toward the foramen lacerum, where it joins with the deep petrosal nerve and ultimately synapses at the pterygopalatine ganglion. Medially lies a depression for the trigeminal ganglion (Meckel's cave) and just anterior to this, the foramen lacerum and the carotid canal from which the ICA emerges on its way toward the cavernous sinus anteriorly.

The posterior surface of the petrous apex forms the anterior border of the posterior cranial fossa. The medial opening of the IAC, the porus acusticus, is located here, as is a small depression for the endolymphatic sac. Anteriorly, near the apex, the midportion of the abducens nerve travels with the inferior petrosal sinus through Dorello's canal, a tight fold of dura, the superior border of which is known as the petroclival, petrosphenoidal, or Gruber's ligament.[11] This ligament courses medially from the tip of the petrous apex to the ipsilateral posterior clinoid process.[12] The proximity of the abducens nerve to the petrous apex is clinically significant because it accounts for the CN VI palsy that accompanies some petrous apex lesions and forms part of the classic Gradenigo triad of signs: abducens palsy, ipsilateral facial pain, and otorrhea. The posterior surface of the temporal bone is "framed" by venous sinuses. The superior petrosal sinus, which drains the cavernous sinus into the lateral venous sinus, runs in the superior petrosal sulcus at the junction of the posterior and middle fossa dural plates, at the border between the anterior and posterior surfaces of the petrous bone. The inferior petrosal sinus, which drains the cavernous sinus into the jugular bulb, runs in the petro-occipital suture line, at the inferior border of the posterior surface.

The inferior surface of the petrous bone is located between the occipital bone and the greater wing of the sphenoid, forming a significant part of the skull base. The ICA enters the petrous apex anteriorly, coursing vertically through the carotid canal toward the genu, where it curves anteromedially to form the horizontal segment heading toward the cavernous sinus. Just lateral to it lie the eustachian tube and the tensor tympani muscle. Posterior and medial to the carotid canal, the jugular fossa forms a depression on the inferior surface of the petrous bone where the jugular bulb sits. They are separated from one another by the jugulocarotid canal. The jugular foramen, located on the inferior and medial surface of the petrous bone, is formed by the occipital and petrous bones; it is where CNs IX, X, and XI exit the skull base.[13]

The petrous apex is variably pneumatized. Reports vary from 10 to 15% of cadaveric specimens,[14] to 35% of CT scans studied.[15] There is usually symmetric pneumatization of temporal bones, and the asymmetry, when present, can be a source of clinical confusion. The bony portion of the petrous apex may be diploic (marrow-filled) or sclerotic. Poorly aerated petrous apices contain more bone marrow than those that are well aerated, although most do contain some bone marrow.

The blood supply to the petrous apex is from periosteal loops supplied by branches of the carotid plexus.

26.3.1 Internal Carotid Artery

The internal carotid artery is arguably the most important structure in the petrous apex. Because many of the surgical approaches used to access this region involve dissection along the ICA, or, in some cases, skeletonization and lateralization of the ICA, it is critical that the operating surgeon appreciate the anatomic relationships and characteristics of the ICA. The wall of the intracranial ICA is much thinner, and correspondingly more susceptible to injury than its cervical counterpart. As the ICA enters the temporal bone at the skull base, it loses its thick, muscular, medial layer and resembles the intracranial and intracavernous ICA. The wall thickness of the ICA decreases from a minimum of 1 mm in the neck to 0.030–0.062 mm in the cranium. For this reason, when performing pericarotid dissection, it is advisable, if at all possible, to leave a thin shell of bone to protect the carotid from injury. Likewise, the surgeon should be mindful of the high rate (~80%) of dorsal (endocranial) and (~35%) ventral (exocranial) dehiscences of the petrous carotid.[16] The ICA is closely associated with the cochlea, lying just anterior to it. The distance between the membranous cochlea and the ICA ranges from 0.33 to 3.7 mm; thus, the decision to dissect between these two structures carries with it the potential for sensorineural hearing loss.[17] The actual incidence of ICA injury is low and the transcanal infracochlear approach has not been associated with significant carotid injury or hearing loss.

26.4 Clinical Presentation

As the pioneers of the petrous apex discovered through their experience with petrous apicitis, the clinical presentation of petrous apex lesions reflects the involved, adjacent anatomy. The signs and symptoms of petrous apex lesions are widely variable, ranging from asymptomatic to highly symptomatic with multiple cranial neuropathies. The presentation depends on the size, location, and nature of the lesion. Asymptomatic lesions are found incidentally on imaging obtained for evaluation of unrelated symptoms.[18] Symptomatic cystic petrous apex lesions can cause hearing loss, facial twitching, otalgia, nausea, lightheadedness, vertigo, tinnitus, facial hypesthesia, and, less frequently, CN VI and VII palsies with associated diplopia and facial weakness.[19,20] Lower cranial neuropathies involving CNs IX, X, XI, and XII have also been described. Patients can also present with headache or aural pressure. Conductive hearing loss can be due to eustachian tube compression, whereas sensorineural hearing loss is seen with involvement of the IAC or inner ear. Otorrhea and ophthalmoplegia can occur with extension into cavernous sinus, but this is rare. In petrous apex cholesterol granulomas, hearing loss and vertigo are the most common presenting symptoms, occurring in up to 50% of symptomatic patients, followed by tinnitus and headache.[21]

The clinical examination may or may not be normal, with the specific patient presentation depending on the location, extent and nature of the lesion. Tympanic membrane retraction, middle ear effusion, otorrhea, hypesthesia in the distribution of the mandibular branch of the trigeminal nerve, imbalance, and, rarely, palsy of CNs VI or VII have been described.

26.5 Imaging

Prior to modern imaging techniques, petrous apex lesions could not be diagnosed until they were large enough to be symptomatic. CT and MRI, used together, are key in the diagnosis and surgical planning of cystic lesions of the petrous apex. Accurate preoperative diagnosis is important because different cystic lesions require different surgical approaches. Incorrect preoperative diagnosis has led to unnecessarily extensive surgery. Although cholesterol granuloma is amenable to drainage and permanent fistulization, cholesteatoma is not, requiring, instead, complete excision or marsupialization.[22] In addition to noting the MRI and contrast enhancement characteristics of a given lesion, it is useful to note whether the lesion is expansile, if the bony architecture is intact, if the edges of the lesion are smooth or scalloped, if the surrounding bone is expanded and remodeled or eroded, if the lesion enhances, and to identify the relationship of the lesion to the petrous ICA and otic capsule.[23]

Petrous apex lesions can be divided into solid and cystic lesions. Included in the differential diagnosis of cystic lesions of the petrous apex are cholesterol granuloma, cholesteatoma, mucocele, anatomic variants (asymmetric pneumatization, giant air cells, petrous carotid artery dehiscence), arachnoid cyst, and trapped fluid. Solid tumors include mesenchymal tumors (chondroma, chondrosarcoma, osteoclastoma, fibrous dysplasia), eosinophilic granuloma (Langerhans histiocytosis), schwannoma, paraganglioma, meningioma, lymphoma, sarcoma, hemangioma, and metastatic lesions. One retrospective case review reported on 66 petrous apex lesions over 20 years, 61% of which were cholesterol granuloma, 9% cholesteatoma, and 6% chondrosarcoma, the most common solid tumor of the petrous apex.[21]

Cholesterol granuloma, the most common petrous apex cystic lesion, appears on CT as a smooth, sharply marginated, expansile ovoid lesion with erosion of adjacent bony structures (▶ Fig. 26.2).

Medial expansion beyond the petro-occipital fissure is common, and can involve the lateral clivus and jugular tubercle. Inferior extension erodes into the hypoglossal canal and the foramen magnum. Anterior expansion causes bowing, thinning, and erosion of the horizontal carotid canal, the sphenoid sinus, and the cavernous sinus. Posterior expansion leads to bulging into the posterior fossa, but without dural involvement. Superior expansion, although less common, is characterized

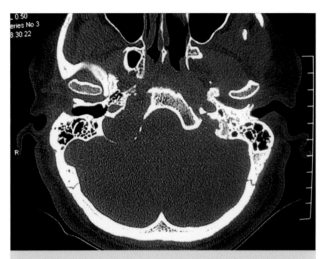

Fig. 26.2 Computed tomography scan of a cholesterol granuloma, showing smoothly expansile cystic lesion with bony erosion.

by minimal bulging into the middle fossa.[19] Cortical bone remodeling, such as that seen with bowing of the horizontal carotid canal or sphenoid walls, is suggestive of slow growth. Eustachian tube dysfunction can occur when compressed by an expanding lesion and may result in mastoid air-cell opacification. In one study, extension beyond the petrous apex was most likely to occur (in order of decreasing frequency) into the carotid canal, clivus, or middle fossa floor (▶ Table 26.1).[21]

Although confusion may arise based on similar CT appearance of cholesterol granuloma, mucocele, and cholesteatoma, the MRI appearance of cholesterol granuloma is unique because it is hyperintense to brain on both T1- and T2-weighted imaging (▶ Fig. 26.3), whereas the other two are hyperintense on T2 only. CT imaging is necessary for surgical planning and to distinguish cholesteatoma and mucocele from retained secretions and asymmetric pneumatization in which the retained bony architecture is characteristic, as distinct from cholesteatoma and mucocele in which the bony architecture is eroded. Diffusion-weighted imaging (DWI) is necessary to distinguish arachnoid cyst from cholesteatoma, because CT, T1-, and T2-weighted imaging characteristics are identical. Arachnoid cyst is hypointense on DWI, whereas cholesteatoma is hyperintense on DWI.

An effusion is bright on T2-weighted MRI, with variable signal on T1-weighted (brighter with higher protein concentration), and appears as a nonexpansile, fluid-attenuated opacification of the air cells, with preservation of bony septa on CT. For retained fluid that is bright on both T1- and T2-weighted MRI, CT shows intact bony architecture of the petrous apex, but interval imaging helps to rule out an incipient cholesterol granuloma if suspicion exists.

26.6 Pathology

26.6.1 Cholesterol Granuloma

Cholesterol granuloma of the petrous apex, the most common cystic lesion of the petrous apex, was first reported in the

Table 26.1 Imaging Features of Cystic Lesions of the Petrous Apex[5,22,27,36,38,41]

Lesion	CT	MRI
Cholesterol granuloma	Smooth, expansile, rim enhancing (occasionally)	↑ T1 ↑ T2 nonenhancing ↑ DWI
Cholesteatoma	Smooth or scalloped, punched-out borders; bony destruction; nonenhancing	↓ T1 ↑ T2 nonenhancing ↑ DWI ↑ FLAIR
Mucocele	Smooth, expansile, nonenhancing	↓ T1, ↑ T2 rim enhancing only
Petrous apex effusion	Nonexpansile, preserved bony trabeculae; nonenhancing	↓ → ↑ T1, ↑ T2 ↓ DWI
Arachnoid cyst	Smooth, expansile, nonenhancing	↓ → ↑ T1, ↑ T2 ± rim enhancement; homogeneous ↓ DWI ↓ FLAIR
Asymmetric pneumatization/bone marrow asymmetry	Smooth or scalloped; preserved bony trabeculae; no bony destruction	↑ T1, ↓ T2 nonenhancing
Petrous apicitis	Irregular borders; bony destruction; rim enhancement	↓ T1, ↑ T2 rim enhancement
Internal carotid aneurysm	Smooth, expansile, enhancement contiguous with petrous carotid	↓ T1, ↓ → ↑ T2 rim enhancement with flow-void artifacts

DWI, diffusion-weighted imaging; FLAIR, fluid-attenuated inversion recovery imaging.

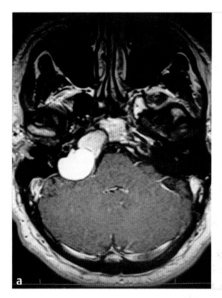 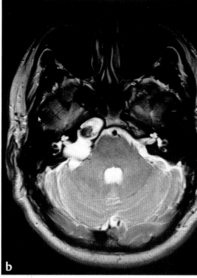

Fig. 26.3 Magnetic resonance imaging (MRI) of cholesterol granuloma of the petrous apex. (a) Hyperintense on T1-weighted MRI. (b) Hyperintense on T2-weighted MRI.

English-language literature in 1943, and cited again in several subsequent case reports, but was not recognized as a distinct clinical entity of the petrous apex until the mid-1980s.[24] Before that it had been called congenital epidermoid, epidermoid cyst, and giant cholesterol cyst.[25,26] It is an expansile, round or ovoid cyst with a fibrous capsule filled with yellowish or brownish fluid. Histologically, it contains breakdown products of blood and chronic inflammation: multinucleated giant cells with cholesterol clefts, hemosiderin-laden macrophages, fibrous tissue, chronic inflammatory cells, and blood vessels in varying proportions.[19] There is an equal distribution between males and females and bilaterality has been reported in 16 to 19% of cholesterol granuloma patients.[27] The average age at presentation is around 40 years.[21,28]

Cholesterol granuloma is an uncommon lesion that forms in exceptionally well-aerated petrous apices. Hemorrhage into the air-cell system occurs, and anaerobic breakdown of blood incites a foreign body reaction to cholesterol crystals, characterized giant cell reaction, fibrosis, and vessel proliferation. When the vessels rupture, additional cholesterol crystals are released and the process continues. Progressive granuloma formation and bony resorption ensues. What leads to the initial hemorrhage is not certain, but two theories have been elaborated to explain the formation of cholesterol granuloma: the obstruction-vacuum theory and the exposed marrow theory.[27] According to the former, mucosal swelling leads to chronic obstruction of the petrous apex air-cell spaces. Resorption of trapped gas leads to the development of negative pressure within the air-cell spaces, which in turn causes blood vessels to rupture. The lack of a drainage pathway results in pooling of blood with ultimate breakdown of blood cells and accumulation of cholesterol crystals. Thus begins the formation of cholesterol granuloma.[19]

However, several problems with the obstruction-vacuum theory have been cited: (1) the observation that although impaired ventilation is very common, cholesterol granuloma formation is rare and is found more commonly in well-aerated, not poorly aerated petrous apices; (2) a lack of correlation with underlying eustachian tube dysfunction and chronic effusion; (3) the observation that once the cholesterol granuloma forms, the negative pressure impetus for hemorrhage, and therefore the source of hemorrhage (inflamed mucosa), no longer exists; and (4) the tendency for recurrence after surgical drainage and stenting.[27]

The more recently proposed exposed marrow theory suggests that, in young adults, as the budding mucosa invades and replaces hematopoietic marrow, the bony interface becomes deficient and the mucosal air-cell lining and the vascular marrow are in direct contact. When hemorrhage from the marrow occurs (due to an as yet undetermined inciting event), it coagulates in the mucosal cells and occludes outflow pathways. Continued hemorrhage from the exposed marrow causes cyst expansion over time. This theory helps to explain the occurrence of cholesterol granuloma formation in the well-pneumatized petrous apex. In addition, it differentiates between cholesterol granuloma of the mastoid and middle ear, which is associated with poor pneumatization, and cholesterol granuloma of the petrous apex, which is not. Histopathological evidence now exists to support the exposed marrow theory of petrous apex cholesterol granuloma formation.[29]

26.6.2 Cholesteatoma

Cholesteatoma of the petrous apex is the second most common lesion of the petrous apex, accounting for 4 to 9% of petrous apex lesions. It consists of stratified squamous epithelial lining surrounding desquamated keratin. Primary or congenital cholesteatoma is thought to arise from epithelial rests in the temporal bone or cerebellopontine angle during development. Secondary cholesteatoma of the petrous apex is an extension of middle ear or mastoid disease into the petrous apex. The secondary cholesteatoma is typically accompanied by examination findings and a history consistent with chronic otitis media, and is therefore less likely to present a diagnostic dilemma. Because the imaging characteristics are similar to arachnoid cyst, it is important to distinguish them preoperatively. This can be done with MRI fluid-attenuated inversion recovery (FLAIR) imaging sequencing or DWI.

Although cholesterol granuloma and cholesteatoma are often found together in the middle ear and mastoid, this has not been observed in the petrous apex.[19] However, there is a case report of coexisting middle ear cholesteatoma and a giant petrous apex cholesterol granuloma.[30]

26.6.3 Mucocele and Petrous Apex Effusion

Mucocele and petrous apex effusion, or retained mucus, are thought to occur in the petrous apex air cells when the air cells become obstructed. In the case of mucocele, the reported symptoms include vertigo, sensorineural hearing loss, and tinnitus. Petrous apex mucocele requires treatment only when symptomatic, ideally with drainage to the mastoid or sphenoid sinus.[31] Although retained fluid of the petrous apex has generally been thought of as a "leave it alone" lesion of the petrous apex,[32] more recently it has been associated with a variety of symptoms, including previous meningitis, retro-orbital pain and pressure, progressive sensorineural hearing loss, aural pressure, hemifacial spasm, and atypical positional vertigo. Symptom resolution has occurred with treatment, ranging from medical management with antibiotics and steroids to surgical intervention for drainage of the trapped fluid.[33]

26.6.4 Arachnoid Cyst

Arachnoid cyst, also referred to as invasive cerebrospinal fluid (CSF) cyst and petrous apex cephalocele,[34] is a benign cyst composed of arachnoid membranes filled with CSF. Congenital arachnoid cysts are thought to derive from splitting or duplication of the arachnoid membrane, whereas acquired cysts may be due to surgery, trauma, complicated otitis media, or cranial irradiation. Noncommunicating cysts are theorized to expand from fluid produced by the arachnoid membrane, and communicating cysts by a communication with normal CSF spaces via a unidirectional valve mechanism.[35] They are expansile lesions that may show bony erosion of the petrous apex. Comprising only 1% of intracranial masses, they are uncommonly located within or adjacent to the temporal bone; 11% are in the cerebellopontine angle. Sixty to 70% of symptomatic arachnoid cysts are diagnosed in childhood. Most commonly, they are asymptomatic lesions found on imaging obtained for other purposes. Headache, the most common "presenting" symptom, is often not caused by the arachnoid cyst. On the other hand, headache may be a symptom of intracranial hypertension caused by the cyst; it is important to try to identify if the cyst is causing the headache. As with other lesions of the petrous apex, the symptoms depend on the location of the lesion. Middle fossa arachnoid cysts are mostly within the Meckel cave and may present with facial dysesthesias, whereas those located in the cerebellopontine angle may present with imbalance, progressive sensorineural hearing loss, tinnitus, seizures, and other cranial neuropathies. Symptoms often do not correlate with the size of the lesion.

Because of the risks associated with treatment, asymptomatic lesions can be followed with serial imaging, although some surgeons advocate removal of even asymptomatic lesions for fear of infection and formation of subdural collections. Not all symptoms resolve or improve with surgical treatment; 50 to 70% of symptomatic patients improve after treatment.[36] Peripetrosal arachnoid cysts have also been reported in association with vestibular schwannoma. It is important to distinguish these lesions from cholesteatoma and mucocele because, although the CT and T1- and T2-weighted MRI characteristics are similar, the surgical approaches are very different. Diffusion-weighted imaging is useful for this purpose, as cholesteatoma is hyperintense and arachnoid cyst is hypointense.

Heavily weighted T2 imaging, FLAIR, is also useful in differentiating cholesteatoma, which is hyperintense, from arachnoid cyst, which is hypointense, because the FLAIR sequence is able to suppress signal arising from CSF such that it remains black.[37–39] Although far less common than either cholesterol granuloma or cholesteatoma of the petrous apex, peripetrosal arachnoid cysts have been described and are important to keep in the differential diagnosis of cystic lesions of the petrous apex.[40] There has been more than one report of preoperative misdiagnosis of arachnoid cyst as cholesteatoma, leading to unnecessarily extensive surgery.[41]

26.6.5 Asymmetric Pneumatization

Asymmetric pneumatization is an anatomic variant that is often confused with pathology on imaging. The bone marrow appears hyperintense on nonenhanced T1-weighted MRI, but does not have any associated bony destruction or expansion on CT. In addition, the bony septa are intact. Approximately 30% of temporal bones have a pneumatized petrous apex, and 6.8% of patients have some degree of asymmetry.[22,42]

26.6.6 Aneurysms

Aneurysms of the petrous carotid are extremely rare, but have been reported and are worth mentioning in the context of cystic lesions of the petrous apex because improper preoperative diagnosis could lead to catastrophic management decisions. On CT they show contrast enhancement in continuity with the petrous carotid. Arteriography is definitive. Aneurysms show mixed signal intensity on T2-weighted MRI with rim enhancement and flow voids on gadolinium-enhanced MRI. Presenting symptoms are variable and have been reported to include pain, dysfunction of CNs V to X and XII, Horner syndrome, otorrhagia, epistaxis, purulent otorrhea, and bruit. In one series of seven patients with petrous carotid aneurysm, one had a saccular aneurysm and the remaining six had fusiform aneurysms with intraluminal thrombus. All seven patients had resolution of the presenting symptoms after treatment: carotid artery occlusion in six, and aneurysm obliteration in the one patient with a saccular aneurysm. There was only one minor complication, a self-limited ipsilateral visual loss in a hypercoagulable patient. There have been several reports of death due to open surgical biopsy of carotid aneurysm mistaken for a glomus tumor.[43]

26.7 Management

26.7.1 Conservative

Observation of cholesterol granuloma is a reasonable option for asymptomatic patients, older patients, and those who are in poor health and unable to undergo general anesthesia. In one retrospective review of 27 patients with petrous apex cholesterol granuloma, 12 patients had incidentally found asymptomatic cholesterol granulomas, found on imaging obtained for other reasons, primarily chronic rhinosinusitis. They were managed with a wait-and-see approach. Of this group, over a mean

follow-up of 56 months, only one patient showed an increase in size of the lesion and all patients remained asymptomatic.[28] These patients are followed with serial CT/MRI.

26.7.2 Surgery

Surgery is the treatment of choice for patients with cholesterol granuloma who are symptomatic at presentation, become symptomatic after a period of observation, or whose lesions show growth after a period of observation.

The choice of surgical approach is informed by the location of the lesion, relationship to neurovascular structures including anatomic variations (e.g., high jugular bulb), hearing status, as well as the surgeon's skill and experience. This is not a new concept. When surgeons were developing approaches to the petrous apex for petrous apicitis, they found, for example, that although the posterior petrous apex was best approached via fistulous tracts of the sinodural angle, through the subarcuate fossa, or through the infralabyrinthine approach, the anterior petrous apex was more readily accessed via approaches such as radical mastoidectomy, infracochlear approach, and middle fossa craniotomy.[17]

Cystic lesions of the petrous apex are unique in that, although they are deep within the skull base, they are amenable to drainage with permanent fistulization through the mastoid and middle ear (▶ Fig. 26.4).

Unlike solid tumors, which may require complete resection, cystic lesions, with the exception of cholesteatoma, do not. In contrast to cholesteatoma, cholesterol granuloma has an "inactive" fibrous capsule and lacks an epithelial lining that acts as the source of continued disease. Although complete removal of cholesteatoma is a widely agreed upon goal, there is some disagreement as to whether total cyst wall removal is necessary for cholesterol granuloma. Both sides have their proponents, with those favoring simple drainage and stenting citing decreased surgical risk and low recurrence rates,[25,44,45] and those favoring total removal citing risk of recurrence and the inability to control injury to the petrous carotid through less invasive techniques. Nevertheless, most would probably agree that the creation of a permanent fistula tract is the less morbid procedure with acceptable success rates. For this reason, and in spite of the risk of recurrence, it is reasonable to approach cystic lesions in a more conservative fashion. In addition, cases of cholesterol granuloma of the petrous apex have been described in which the cyst has skeletonized surrounding structures, including the petrous carotid, the jugular bulb, and the IAC. Attempting to completely remove the fibrous capsule in these instances could result in further neurologic deficit, CSF leak, or vascular injury.[24] Stenting of the surgically created fistula tract has become standard because of the tendency for stenosis of the surgical site when left unstented. Silastic has been successfully used for this purpose. In one study, four of five patients who required revision surgery had not been previously stented. The fifth had a stent that became occluded by fibrous tissue.[44]

Surgical approaches to petrous apex cholesterol granuloma reported in the literature are numerous: transcanal infracochlear; transmastoid infralabyrinthine; middle fossa craniotomy; and translabyrinthine, suboccipital, transsphenoidal endoscopic and infratemporal fossa types A and B with or without a transotic approach. The first three are the most common.[27]

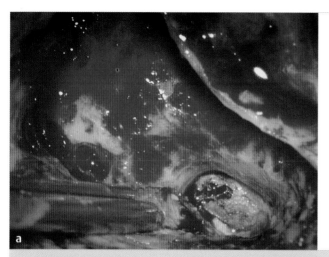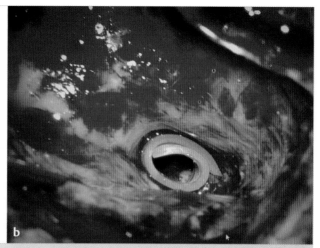

Fig. 26.4 Intraoperative images of cholesterol granuloma of the petrous apex. (a) Cyst capsule as seen via infralabyrinthine approach. (b) Cholesterol granuloma after drainage and stenting with Silastic sheeting.

In the case of serviceable preoperative hearing, hearing preservation is the goal, and many of the described approaches enable this goal. The transmastoid infralabyrinthine (IL) approach involves a postauricular approach, complete mastoidectomy, and skeletonization of the sigmoid sinus and posterior fossa dura. The limits of dissection are the sigmoid sinus and posterior fossa dura posteriorly, the posterior semicircular canal superiorly, the vertical segment of the facial nerve anteriorly and laterally, and the jugular bulb inferiorly. If the position of the cholesterol granuloma and the anatomy are favorable for the IL approach, hearing can be preserved and the ICA and ossicular chain are not at risk. This approach enables direct drainage of the cyst into the mastoid cavity. On the other hand, a high jugular bulb may not allow for safe access via this route; it is also not amenable to more anteriorly placed cysts.[46] In one series of six patients who underwent the IL approach for drainage of cholesterol granuloma, one patient lost serviceable hearing postoperatively.[44]

The transcanal infracochlear (IC) approach involves a standard postauricular approach, transection of the membranous external auditory canal, and elevation of a superiorly based tympanomeatal flap. The external auditory canal is enlarged inferiorly and anteriorly to provide access to the hypotympanum. Dissection is carried out in an anteromedial direction, inferior to the cochlea and posterior to the ICA. Once the cyst is identified and drained, a silicone catheter is placed from the cyst cavity into the middle ear.[47] The external auditory canal defects are filled with bone *pâté*. The risks include vascular injury and hearing loss (both conductive and sensorineural), although these complications have not been widely reported. Of 18 patients who underwent this approach for drainage of a cholesterol granuloma, one had a resultant tympanic membrane perforation.[44] As long as the plane of dissection remains inferior to the round window, the otic capsule is not violated, and there is no hearing or vestibular injury. The anterior limit of dissection is the petrous carotid artery. The IC approach enables dependent drainage into a well-aerated area of the middle ear near the eustachian tube, preservation of the conductive mechanism of the external and middle ear, and reexploration via an inferior myringotomy, if necessary.[44]

This approach is useful in cases where a high jugular bulb precludes the use of the infralabyrinthine approach. In another series of 12 patients, there were no major operative complications.[21] It also provided the highest rate of postsurgical aeration of the cyst cavity as demonstrated on postsurgical imaging, with the average time interval between surgery and the most recent imaging study being 60.4 months.[44] Nevertheless, it may be intimidating to drill in the space bordered by three structures you want to preserve (internal jugular vein (IJ), ICA, and cochlea). With this in mind, recent work has been done investigating the feasibility of computer-assisted surgery (CAS) in cholesterol granuloma surgery. In one study CAS decreased operative time and provided intraoperative localization of the ICA, facial nerve, and the cyst.[48] In another study, aimed at "mating" a robotic system with CT- or MRI-guided imaging, the mean circular fenestration in pneumatized temporal bones was 5.7 ± 0.6 mm, adequate for performing infracochlear fenestration and perhaps explaining why no major complications have been reported with this approach.[45]

Another of the hearing preservation approaches, the middle fossa craniotomy, is useful for those lesions that involve the anterior surface of the petrous pyramid, because this approach enables dissection along the floor of the middle fossa floor. Once the lesions are identified, a stent can be placed from the cyst cavity to the epitympanic or mastoid cavity, although concerns have been raised about the long-term patency of such a stent. This approach has also been described as enabling complete cyst wall removal with fat-packing of the cyst cavity; some maintain that filling the cyst space with fat prevents recurrence. Although rare, this approach has the associated risks that come with temporal lobe retraction: bleeding, stroke, and death. There have been reports of postoperative CSF leak, bleeding, and meningitis for middle fossa craniotomy performed for drainage of cholesterol granuloma.[49]

The preauricular subtemporal approach is a hearing-preservation approach that allows for wide access to the petrous apex. It is used mostly for petrous apex tumors and has a high rate of total tumor removal (85%) and hearing preservation, but has associated new-onset cranial neuropathies (CNs III to VII).[50] This approach could also be used for access to an anteriorly situated cystic lesion of the petrous apex, but would be more suited to a lesion requiring total excision, such as petrous apex cholesteatoma.

Although less invasive approaches are favored by most surgeons, and the debate over the necessity of total cyst wall is mostly historical, the infratemporal fossa types A and B approaches provide access to the petrous apex when the jugular bulb precludes the use of the infralabyrinthine or infracochlear approach. It has associated morbidity of temporary facial paralysis, maximal conductive hearing loss, and some difficulty with mastication because it involves anterior transposition of the facial nerve, blind sac closure of the ear canal, exposure and inferior retraction of the mandibular condyle, and sectioning of the mandibular division of the trigeminal nerve. On the other hand, it provides adequate space for operation, control of the ICA, and the possibility of complete cyst wall removal from the clivus and sphenoid sinus. Packing of the cavity with fat after complete cyst removal has also been described (for both cholesterol granuloma and cholesteatoma) and has a very low recurrence rate.[28]

The endoscopic endonasal approaches (EEAs) to the petrous apex offer a minimally invasive alternative to the middle fossa and transtemporal approaches that enable preservation of hearing and vestibular function, and drainage and stenting of cystic lesions.[51] The facial nerve is not at risk, and the location of the surgical fenestration enables an in-office endoscopic follow-up examination. The transsphenoid approach to the petrous apex was first described in 1977 by Montgomery,[52] and Fucci et al[53] were the first to describe the endoscopic transsphenoidal approach. It has since evolved to incorporate the use of image guidance, and many case reports have been published attesting to the viability of the endoscopic transsphenoidal approach.[54] This approach now includes the transsphenoidal transclival approach, the transsphenoidal transclival approach with paraclival ICA lateralization, and the transpterygoid infrapetrous or sublacerum approach.[46] The approach involves a four-handed, two-surgeon procedure, with posterior septectomy, removal of the anterior face of the sphenoid sinus, and identification of the ICA, optic nerve prominences, pituitary fossa, and clivus. The lesion is accessed by drilling medial to the ICA and lateral to the clival dura. The cyst is opened, drained, and stented.[55] Not all endoscopic surgeons use a stent; some prefer to create a permanent fistula tract with the use of a pedicled nasoseptal flap; yet others simply rely on a large osteotomy. The more lateral the lesion, the more expanded the approach must be, involving bony dissection inferior to the petrous carotid in cases where the lesion is lateral and extends inferior to the intrapetrous carotid. Image guidance helps to guide surgical dissection and avoid injuring the important surrounding neurovascular structures. Of 16 patients who underwent an EEA to the petrous apex, all had improvement of one or more of their presenting symptoms, and two (12.5%), who had not had initial stent placement, experienced recurrence requiring reoperation and stent placement (mean follow-up 20 months). Complications included eustachian tube dysfunction with chronic serous otitis media, dry eye from vidian nerve transection, transient ipsilateral CN VI palsy, and severe epistaxis. Optic nerve injury, chronic sphenoid sinusitis, and, as with many of the petrous apex approaches, ICA injury are potential complications of this approach.[56,57]

One study compared an expanded EEA to the IC approach using cadaveric specimens and radiographic imaging. The authors divided the petrous apex into three areas—superior, anteroinferior, and posteroinferior—with each segment correlating with a different section of the petrous ICA. Performing surgery on cadaveric specimens and comparing high-resolution CT scans, the authors determined that the EEA provided access to the superior and anteroinferior petrous apex in all specimens and to the posteroinferior petrous apex in 90% of cases. The IC approach, on the other hand, provided access to the anteroinferior petrous apex in 80% of cases, to the posteroinferior petrous apex in 60%, and to the superior petrous apex in none, because access was blocked by the cochlea. Additionally, the radiographically calculated drainage window that is possible via EEA was three times larger than that made possible by the IC approach.[58]

The translabyrinthine and transotic approaches are reserved for patients with large, symptomatic lesions and no serviceable hearing. They provide wide exposure of the petrous apex. They are also useful in cases of recurrence or where complete excision is more important, such as with cholesteatoma.

Postsurgically, many preoperative symptoms resolve, whereas others stabilize. Less frequently, there is additional deficit. Resolution of CN VI palsy, facial twitching, facial hypesthesia, and facial weakness have been reported.[19,24] In one report, 82% of patients showed improvement of symptoms after surgery, and 89% of those who had preoperative CN deficits recovered normal function.[44] In another, 83% of preoperative CN deficits resolved postoperatively. The persistent deficits included CN V and a grade 2/6 CN VII.[49]

Recurrence of cholesterol granuloma after surgical drainage is considered when symptoms recur. Cyst cavity aeration and decreased size are indicators of long-term efficacy of treatment; however, lack of aeration of the cyst cavity alone does not imply failure of treatment, because this has been practically difficult to achieve.[44] Additionally, cyst size tends to remain stable after surgery, so a cyst that remains the same size is also not indicative of failure. Recurrence rates of 14 to 16% have been reported.[27] Another study, with mean follow-up of 90.7 months, showed recurrence rates of 18% for those patients who had stents placed and 83% for those without stent placement. Overall, revision surgery rate was 41%, higher than previously reported, possibly due to longer follow-up.[29] Recurrence has been associated with a failed drainage pathway, either plugging of stents or stenosis of surgical fenestrations, and not with failure to remove the cyst wall.[44] Stent placement is more likely to maintain drainage pathway patency, but is not guaranteed to do so. Reoperation should be considered for patients with recurrence who are symptomatic or whose lesions are growing.

When symptomatic, arachnoid cysts, radiographically similar to cholesteatoma on both MRI and CT, are amenable to a variety of surgical interventions, including shunting, open excision, open or neuroendoscopic fenestration, or marsupialization. Surgical drainage via a middle cranial fossa-transpetrous approach with partial or complete removal of the arachnoid wall has been advocated as a less invasive, highly successful strategy for arachnoid cysts of the anterior petrous apex,[36] whereas marsupialization via a posterior fossa approach has been recommended for symptomatic arachnoid cysts of the posterior petrous apex.[34]

As previously mentioned, petrous apex cholesteatoma is distinct from other cystic lesions of the petrous apex because it requires more extensive surgery to achieve complete excision.[59] Cholesteatoma expands into the areas of least resistance, but also invades surrounding structures, such as the clivus, sphenoid sinus, and rhinopharynx.[60] Slow-growing petrous apex cholesteatomas often remain symptomatic until they involve the facial nerve or the labyrinth. These patients frequently present with hearing loss and facial weakness. Otorrhea and vertigo are also common.[61] Sanna et al[62] developed a classification system for petrous apex cholesteatomas (supralabyrinthine, infralabyrinthine, massive, infralabyrinthine-apical, and apical) that reflects both the location and extent of disease and is used to guide surgical management. Although hearing preservation and facial nerve preservation are desirable, disease eradication takes precedence, and both hearing and facial nerve continuity are sacrificed as necessary. In one study of 13 petrous apex cholesteatomas, 69% of which were classified as congenital, all patients presented with hearing loss, both conductive and sensorineural, and 46% of patients presented with a facial nerve weakness (House-Brackmann grades 4 to 6). Intraoperative findings in this study revealed invasion of the cochlea (54%), semicircular canals (39%), and encasement of the facial nerve (46%). All but three patients underwent destructive procedures (translabyrinthine, subtotal petrosectomy with labyrinthectomy, and transotic approach). Four patients required surgical management of the facial nerve, including greater auricular nerve interposition graft and hypoglossal-facial nerve anastomosis.[63] During the 18 to 110 months of follow-up, there were no recurrences. In another series of 10 patients with petrous apex cholesteatoma, 40% were classified as congenital, 80% presented with moderate to profound sensorineural hearing loss, 50% with facial nerve dysfunction, and 20% with preceding bacterial meningitis. This highlights the more aggressive nature of the disease and the corresponding more aggressive surgical approaches called for in cases of petrous apex cholesteatoma.

Although complete extirpation is the goal, it is not always possible. Failing this, marsupialization with close follow-up provides an acceptable alternative.[64,65] One author favored complete removal and cavity obliteration following subtotal petrosectomy with exteriorization via a modified transcochlear approach reserved for those cases where complete matrix removal from intact neurovascular structures was not possible or where maintenance of good preoperative hearing or facial nerve function precluded complete matrix removal. The benefit of cavity obliteration with autologous fat is protection of exposed neurovascular structures (dura, ICA, facial nerve) from infection and prevention of large draining cavities. In either case, long-term follow-up is necessary, to monitor for occult recurrence in cases of cavity obliteration and for cavity maintenance in cases of exteriorization.[66]

26.8 Conclusion

Cystic lesions of the petrous apex require a high index of suspicion to diagnose. MRI and CT are necessary for diagnosis and surgical planning. In those patients who are asymptomatic, it is reasonable to follow them with serial imaging. In those with symptomatic or expanding lesions, careful surgical planning,

carried out in an interdisciplinary team fashion when called for, is required. Determination of the surgical approach is based on the nature of the lesion, hearing and facial nerve status, the anatomic relations between the lesion and the surrounding neurovascular structures, and the ability to achieve permanent drainage. Because of the risk of recurrence, regardless of surgical approach, long-term follow-up is required with serial imaging.

References

[1] Frenckner P. Some remarks on the treatment of apicitis (petrositis) with or without Gradenigo's Syndrome. Acta Otolaryngol (Stockh) 1932; 17: 97–120

[2] Adelstein LJ. Gradenigo's syndrome and brain abscess secondary to otitis media—differential diagnosis report of cases. Cal West Med 1931; 34: 23–26

[3] Estcourt HG. Gradenigo's syndrome. Proc R Soc Med 1926; 19: 29–31

[4] Kopetzky SJ, Almour R. The suppuration of the petrous pyramid: pathology, symptomatology and surgical treatment. Ann Otol Rhinol Laryngol 1930; 39: 996–1016

[5] Lindsay JR. Suppuration in the petrous pyramid—some views on its surgical management. Ann Otol Rhinol Laryngol 1938; 47: 3–36

[6] Eagleton WP. Unlocking the petrous apex for localized bulbar (pontile) meningitis secondary to suppuration of the petrous apex. Arch Otolaryngol Head Neck Surg 1931; 13: 386–422

[7] Ramadier J. Exploration de la pointe du roches par la voie du canal carotidien. Ann d'Oto-laryngol 1933; 4: 422–444

[8] Lempert J. Complete apicectomy (mastoidotympanoapicectomy), new technique for complete apical exenteration of apical carotid portion of pertous pyramid. Arch Otolaryngol 1937; 25: 144–177

[9] Connor SE, Leung R, Natas S. Imaging of the petrous apex: a pictorial review. Br J Radiol 2008; 81: 427–435

[10] Rhoton AJ. 3D anatomy and surgical approaches of the temporal bone and adjacent areas. Neurosurgery 2007; 61: 1–250

[11] Tubbs RS, Radcliff V, Shoja MM et al. Dorello canal revisited: an observation that potentially explains the frequency of abducens nerve injury after head injury. World Neurosurg 2012; 77: 119–121

[12] Chapman PR, Shah R, Curé JK, Bag AK. Petrous apex lesions: pictorial review. AJR Am J Roentgenol 2011; 196 Suppl: WS26–WS37, Quiz S40–S43

[13] Caldemeyer KS, Mathews VP, Azzarelli B, Smith RR. The jugular foramen: a review of anatomy, masses, and imaging characteristics. Radiographics 1997; 17: 1123–1139

[14] Gulya AJ. Glasscock-Shambaugh Surgery of the Ear, 6th ed. Shelton, CT: People's Medical Publishing House–USA, 2010

[15] Virapongse C, Sarwar M, Bhimani S, Sasaki C, Shapiro R. Computed tomography of temporal bone pneumatization: 1. Normal pattern and morphology. AJR Am J Roentgenol 1985; 145: 473–481

[16] Hearst MJ, Kadar A, Keller JT, Choo DI, Pensak ML, Samy RN. Petrous carotid canal dehiscence: an anatomic and radiographic study. Otol Neurotol 2008; 29: 1001–1004

[17] Chole RA. Petrous apicitis: surgical anatomy. Ann Otol Rhinol Laryngol 1985; 94: 251–257

[18] Leonetti JP, Shownkeen H, Marzo SJ. Incidental petrous apex findings on magnetic resonance imaging. Ear Nose Throat J 2001; 80: 200–202, 205–206

[19] Lo WW, Solti-Bohman LG, Brackmann DE, Gruskin P. Cholesterol granuloma of the petrous apex: CT diagnosis. Radiology 1984; 153: 705–711

[20] Brodkey JA, Robertson JH, Shea JJ, III, Gardner G. Cholesterol granulomas of the petrous apex: combined neurosurgical and otological management. J Neurosurg 1996; 85: 625–633

[21] Muckle RP, De la Cruz A, Lo WM. Petrous apex lesions. Am J Otol 1998; 19: 219–225

[22] Arriaga MA, Brackmann DE. Differential diagnosis of primary petrous apex lesions [review]. Am J Otol 1991; 12: 470–474. Erratum in Am J Otol 1992;13:297

[23] Curtin HD, Som PM. The petrous apex. Otolaryngol Clin North Am 1995; 28: 473–496

[24] Graham MD, Kemink JL, Latack JT, Kartush JM. The giant cholesterol cyst of the petrous apex: a distinct clinical entity. Laryngoscope 1985; 95: 1401–1406

[25] Thedinger BA, Nadol JB Jr, Montgomery WW, Thedinger BS, Greenberg JJ. Radiographic diagnosis, surgical treatment, and long-term follow-up of cholesterol granulomas of the petrous apex. Laryngoscope 1989; 99: 896–907

[26] Latack JT, Graham MD, Kemink JL, Knake JE. Giant cholesterol cysts of the petrous apex: radiologic features. AJNR Am J Neuroradiol 1985; 6: 409–413

[27] Jackler RK, Cho M. A new theory to explain the genesis of petrous apex cholesterol granuloma. Otol Neurotol 2003; 24: 96–106, discussion 106

[28] Sanna M, Dispenza F, Mathur N, De Stefano A, De Donato G. Otoneurological management of petrous apex cholesterol granuloma. Am J Otolaryngol 2009; 30: 407–414

[29] Hoa M, House JW, Linthicum FH, Jr. Petrous apex cholesterol granuloma: maintenance of drainage pathway, the histopathology of surgical management and histopathologic evidence for the exposed marrow theory. Otol Neurotol 2012; 33: 1059–1065

[30] Brand R, Shihada R, Segev Y, Doweck I, Brackmann D, Luntz M. Coexisting middle ear cholesteatoma and giant petrous apex cholesterol granuloma. Otol Neurotol 2012; 33: e25–e26

[31] DeLozier HL, Parkins CW, Gacek RR. Mucocele of the petrous apex. J Laryngol Otol 1979; 93: 177–180

[32] Moore KR, Harnsberger HR, Shelton C, Davidson HC. Leave me alone" lesions of the petrous apex. AJNR Am J Neuroradiol 1998; 19: 733–738

[33] Arriaga MA. Petrous apex effusion: a clinical disorder. Laryngoscope 2006; 116: 1349–1356

[34] Isaacson B, Coker NJ, Vrabec JT, Yoshor D, Oghalai JS. Invasive cerebrospinal fluid cysts and cephaloceles of the petrous apex. Otol Neurotol 2006; 27: 1131–1141

[35] Cheung SW, Broberg TG, Jackler RK. Petrous apex arachnoid cyst: radiographic confusion with primary cholesteatoma. Am J Otol 1995; 16: 690–694

[36] Cristobal R, Oghalai JS. Peripetrosal arachnoid cysts. Curr Opin Otolaryngol Head Neck Surg 2007; 15: 323–329

[37] Kuzma BB, Goodman JM. Epidermoid or arachnoid cyst? Surg Neurol 1997; 47: 395–396

[38] Alkilic-Genauzeau I, Boukobza M, Lot G, George B, Merland JJCT. [CT and MRI features of arachnoid cyst of the petrous apex: report of 3 cases] J Radiol 2007; 88: 1179–1183

[39] Chang P, Fagan PA, Atlas MD, Roche J. Imaging destructive lesions of the petrous apex. Laryngoscope 1998; 108: 599–604

[40] Batra A, Tripathi RP, Singh AK, Tatke M. Petrous apex arachnoid cyst extending into Meckel's cave. Australas Radiol 2002; 46: 295–298

[41] Achilli V, Danesi G, Caverni L, Richichi M. Petrous apex arachnoid cyst: a case report and review of the literature. Acta Otorhinolaryngol Ital 2005; 25: 296–300

[42] Roland PS, Meyerhoff WL, Judge LO, Mickey BE. Asymmetric pneumatization of the petrous apex. Otolaryngol Head Neck Surg 1990; 103: 80–88

[43] Halbach VV, Higashida RT, Hieshima GB et al. Aneurysms of the petrous portion of the internal carotid artery: results of treatment with endovascular or surgical occlusion. AJNR Am J Neuroradiol 1990; 11: 253–257

[44] Brackmann DE, Toh EH. Surgical management of petrous apex cholesterol granulomas. Otol Neurotol 2002; 23: 529–533

[45] Leung R, Samy RN, Leach JL, Murugappan S, Stredney D, Wiet G. Radiographic anatomy of the infracochlear approach to the petrous apex for computer-assisted surgery. Otol Neurotol 2010; 31: 419–423

[46] Zanation AM, Snyderman CH, Carrau RL, Gardner PA, Prevedello DM, Kassam AB. Endoscopic endonasal surgery for petrous apex lesions. Laryngoscope 2009; 119: 19–25

[47] Giddings NA, Brackmann DE, Kwartler JA. Transcanal infracochlear approach to the petrous apex. Otolaryngol Head Neck Surg 1991; 104: 29–36

[48] Caversaccio M, Panosetti E, Ziglinas P, Lukes A, Häusler R. Cholesterol granuloma of the petrous apex: benefit of computer-aided surgery. Eur Arch Otorhinolaryngol 2009; 266: 47–50

[49] Fong BP, Brackmann DE, Telischi FF. The long-term follow-up of drainage procedures for petrous apex cholesterol granulomas. Arch Otolaryngol Head Neck Surg 1995; 121: 426–430

[50] Leonetti JP, Anderson DE, Marzo SJ, Origitano TC, Schuman R. The preauricular subtemporal approach for transcranial petrous apex tumors. Otol Neurotol 2008; 29: 380–383

[51] Jaberoo MC, Hassan A, Pulido MA, Saleh HA. Endoscopic endonasal approaches to management of cholesterol granuloma of the petrous apex. Skull Base 2010; 20: 375–379

[52] Montgomery WW. Cystic lesions of the petrous apex: transsphenoid approach. Ann Otol Rhinol Laryngol 1977; 86: 429–435

[53] Fucci MJ, Alford EL, Lowry LD, Keane WM, Sataloff RT. Endoscopic management of a giant cholesterol cyst of the petrous apex. Skull Base Surg 1994; 4: 52–58

[54] Dhanasekar G, Jones NS. Endoscopic trans-sphenoidal removal of cholesterol granuloma of the petrous apex: case report and literature review. J Laryngol Otol 2011; 125: 169–172

[55] Edkins O, Lubbe D, Taylor A. Endoscopic trans-sphenoidal drainage of petrous apex cholesterol granulomas. S Afr J Surg 2010; 48: 94–96

[56] Paluzzi A, Gardner P, Fernandez-Miranda JC et al. Endoscopic endonasal approach to cholesterol granulomas of the petrous apex: a series of 17 patients: clinical article. J Neurosurg 2012; 116: 792–798

[57] Sade B, Batra PS, Scharpf J, Citardi MJ, Lee JH. Minimally invasive endoscopic endonasal management of skull base cholesterol granulomas. World Neurosurg 2012; 78: 683–688

[58] Scopel TF, Fernandez-Miranda JC, Pinheiro-Neto CD et al. Petrous apex cholesterol granulomas: endonasal versus infracochlear approach. Laryngoscope 2012; 122: 751–761

[59] Angeli SI, De la Cruz A, Hitselberger W. The transcochlear approach revisited. Otol Neurotol 2001; 22: 690–695

[60] Pandya Y, Piccirillo E, Mancini F, Sanna M. Management of complex cases of petrous bone cholesteatoma. Ann Otol Rhinol Laryngol 2010; 119: 514–525

[61] Omran A, De Denato G, Piccirillo E, Leone O, Sanna M. Petrous bone cholesteatoma: management and outcomes. Laryngoscope 2006; 116: 619–626

[62] Sanna M, Pandya Y, Mancini F, Sequino G, Piccirillo E. Petrous bone cholesteatoma: classification, management and review of the literature. Audiol Neurootol 2011; 16: 124–136

[63] Song JJ, An YH, Ahn SH et al. Surgical management options and postoperative functional outcomes of petrous apex cholesteatoma. Acta Otolaryngol 2011; 131: 1142–1149

[64] Glasscock ME III, Woods CI III, Poe DS, Patterson AK, Welling DB. Petrous apex cholesteatoma. Otolaryngol Clin North Am 1989; 22: 981–1002

[65] Horn KL, Shea JJ III, Brackmann DE. Congenital cholesteatoma of the petrous pyramid. Arch Otolaryngol 1985; 111: 621–622

[66] Pyle GM, Wiet RJ. Petrous apex cholesteatoma: exteriorization vs. subtotal petrosectomy with obliteration. Skull Base Surg 1991; 1: 97–105

27 Malignant Tumors of the Temporal Bone

Christine H. Heubi and Myles L. Pensak

27.1 Introduction

Malignant tumors of the temporal bone are often diagnosed at late stages of disease and portend a dismal prognosis. Symptoms are often analogous with those of chronic suppurative ear disease, and, thus, in the absence of a high suspicion for malignancy, are treated as such. Electrophysiological and neuroradiological investigations may assist in the suggestion of malignant characteristics, and this heightened suspicion, combined with contemporary skull base surgical techniques, adjuvant radiotherapy, and chemotherapy, may improve survival rates over time. This chapter summarizes the pathobiology of temporal bone malignancies, the current literature on management options available at this time, and pain management options for palliative treatment for patients with these tumors.

27.2 Relevant Anatomy of the Temporal Bone

The temporal bone is positioned between the middle and posterior cranial fossa and is constituted of four distinct segments: petrous, squamous, mastoid, and tympanic.[1] The petrous portion of the temporal bone contributes to the skull base of both the middle and posterior fossa, and is directed anteriorly and medially, juxtaposing the clivus and sphenoid. The squamous portion contributes to the lateral skull enclosing the temporal lobe of the brain. The mastoid portion contributes to the inferolateral skull base, and both enlarges and pneumatizes over the first few years of life to eventually overlie the stylomastoid foramen. The tympanic segment, although poorly developed at birth, forms the majority of the bony external auditory canal (EAC) and grows to maturity by age 3. The foramen of Huschke delineates the inadequate closure of the tympanic ring anteriorly.

Pneumatization of the petrous and mastoid portions of the temporal bone varies widely. The mesotympanum defines the largest pneumatized space and communicates directly with the eustachian tube anteriorly. This space communicates with the mastoid central air-cell tract via the aditus ad antrum, which then in turn may lead to perilabyrinthine, retrofacial, perisinus, apical, epitympanic, and sinodural air-cell tracts.[2]

Although there are many natural barriers to tumor spread within the temporal bone, some specific anatomic relationships within this region may assist in the extension of malignancy. The natural cleavage planes within the fibroelastic cartilage of the EAC, the fissures of Santorini, may allow delivery of tumor anteriorly to the parotid gland and posteriorly to the soft tissue lateral to the mastoid process. Incomplete closure of the foramen of Huschke also permits anterior spread into the parotid and glenoid fossa. If tumor invades the middle ear space, and thus the mesotympanum, there is the potential for spread anteriorly through the eustachian tube to the infratemporal fossa and parapharyngeal space. This area also provides unimpeded access to all areas of the petrous bone through the central air-cell tract. Although the bony partitions of the temporal bone may act as a barrier to direct tumor spread, as bony erosion

occurs over time, access is allowed anteriorly toward the infratemporal fossa, inferiorly toward the jugular fossa, superiorly into the middle cranial vault, or posteriorly toward the posterior fossa.

Although there are recognized pathways of lymphatic drainage from the area around the temporal bone, metastatic spread from the area is not common.[3–6] When lymphadenopathy occurs, it is often associated with a secondary inflammatory process rather than with direct tumor involvement, but metastases have been reported in 10 to 15% of cases.[7,8]

Lymph nodes within the parotid and preauricular region receive drainage from the conchal cowl, cartilaginous canal, tragus, and fossa triangularis. Infraauricular lymph nodes receive drainage from the lobule and antitragus. Postauricular or deep jugulodigastric lymphatics, along with spinal accessory lymphatics, receive drainage from the helix and antihelix. The EAC lymphatics drain anteriorly into the preauricular and parotid lymph nodes, inferiorly into the upper cervical and deep internal jugular nodes, and posteriorly into the postauricular nodes. The middle ear has a reticular lymphatic network surrounding the eustachian tube and draining into the upper jugular and retropharyngeal lymph nodes. The inner ear has no known lymphatic drainage.

27.3 Clinical Presentation and Assessment

Often indistinguishable from chronic suppurative otitis, patients with temporal bone malignancies commonly present with aural discharge, fullness, and hearing loss. Although bloody drainage may occur, it is more concerning in conjunction with pain. Symptoms more alarming for malignancy are cranial neuropathies, including facial paralysis and cochleovestibular deficits. Signs of meningeal involvement, including severe headache, may be late findings. ▶ Fig. 27.1 lists the signs and symptoms found in the University of Cincinnati tumor registry recorded for patients with malignant temporal bone tumors from 1984 to 2005.

A complete history and neurotologic examination is essential in the evaluation of a temporal bone tumor. Audiometric, electrophysiological, and neuroradiological studies may also assist in defining the extent of tumor growth and the involvement of surrounding structures. Baseline studies can elaborate the etiology of hearing loss; audiometrics, including discrimination scores and acoustic reflexes, along with auditory brainstem response (ABR), may be used to assess retrocochlear pathology. Impedance assessments and tympanometry may help define middle ear involvement. Electronystagmography, rotation chair analysis, and platform posturography are of limited value, but will be abnormal if the integrity of the vestibular apparatus has been compromised.

High-resolution computed tomography (CT) and magnetic resonance imaging (MRI) are used in combination to give a radiological assessment of the temporal bone, as each adds a unique perspective. In the setting of malignancy, CT is utilized to evaluate the location of the mass in relation to the osseous temporal bone, to describe patterns of bony destruction, and to determine involvement of specific structures (▶ Fig. 27.1).

Integrity of the otic capsule, facial nerve canal, tegmen, jugular bulb, carotid canal, and the ossicular chain are important structures that are best evaluated with CT. High-resolution CT is currently performed utilizing multidetector CT scanners, which acquire the raw CT data in a helical fashion. This results in a data set that can be reconstructed at sub-centimeter slice thickness in multiple planes without loss of image quality. More precise imaging of the aforementioned structures is therefore allowed, as each structure may be better visualized on a certain imaging plane.[9–13]

Magnetic resonance imaging is utilized to evaluate the location of a mass, with particular focus on intracranial extension, dural or parenchymal involvement, perineural or foraminal spread, and extratemporal extension (▶ Fig. 27.2). Furthermore, signal intensities on different pulse sequences can better characterize the mass and help narrow the differential diagnosis.[9,11,14,15] Specific attention should be paid to both the involvement

and patency of the carotid artery and dural venous sinuses. On contrast-enhanced CT, the normally opacified vasculature can be identified and any encasement, stenosis, or occlusion should be documented. On conventional MRI, vasculature is identified by the loss of signal intensity due to flowing blood, specifically on T2-weighted images, also known as flow voids. Magnetic resonance angiography and venography techniques can be employed to address the presence of flow signal with the arterial or venous system respectively.

Catheter-directed angiography is infrequently used in the workup of temporal bone malignancies, except in cases where the carotid needs to be sacrificed for en-bloc surgical resection. In these cases, preoperative catheter directed angiography with the balloon occlusion test is performed in conjunction with single photon emission computed tomography (SPECT) perfusion imaging in order to determine cerebral artery collateral flow and tolerance for carotid artery sacrifice.[16]

Staging criteria for temporal bone malignancy has been published, but there is no universally accepted system. Although the American Joint Committee on Cancer uses the same staging system that has been applied to cutaneous malignancies at other sites, the unique anatomy of the temporal bone makes these criteria inadequate. Proposed staging systems have focused on tumor size and clinical appearance, as well as CT appearance of tumors.[14,17,18] ▶ Table 27.2 and ▶ Table 27.3 list the proposed staging systems from Arriaga et al and Pensak et al, respectively. Nakagawa et al modified the Pittsburgh staging system to include tumors with infratemporal fossa involvement in the T3 category.[19]

27.4 Pathology of Temporal Bone Malignancies

Squamous cell carcinoma (SCC) accounts for approximately 85% of malignancies of the EAC and petrous bone, although basal cell carcinoma (BCC) accounts for the majority of lesions on the pinna.[20–23] Other primary tumors of the temporal bone include glandular tumors, rhabdomyosarcomas, regionally invasive cancers, and metastatic disease, altogether accounting for the other 15% of tumors found in this region.[24–26] ▶ Table 27.4 lists

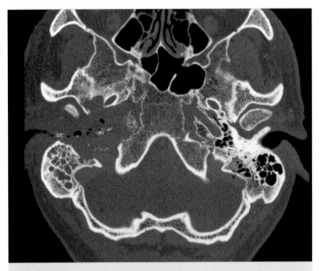

Fig. 27.1 Extensive bone erosion is noted in this high-resolution axial computed tomography (CT) of the temporal bone.

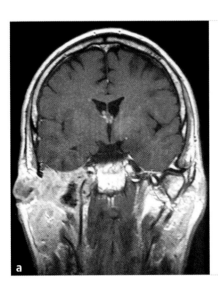
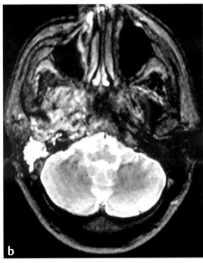

Fig. 27.2 Significant infratemporal fossa invasion is reflected by loss of soft tissue planes on magnetic resonance imaging (MRI) scan in both coronal (a) and axial (b) planes.

benign, aggressive benign, and malignant tumors of the temporal bone.

The box below lists malignant tumors of metastatic origin found to invade the temporal bone.

Metastatic Temporal Bone Tumors

- Breast carcinoma
- Lung carcinoma
- Renal carcinoma
- Thyroid carcinoma
- Gastrointestinal/hepatocellular adenocarcinoma
- Osteoblastoma
- Non-Hodgkin lymphoma
- Leukemia
- Melanoma

27.4.1 Squamous Cell Carcinoma

Squamous cell carcinoma most frequently appears within the cartilaginous portion of the EAC.[27–33] SCC presents in the fifth to sixth decade of life, and patients often have a history of chronic aural drainage, pain, and hearing loss. Misdiagnosis as suppurative otitis media or otitis externa accounts for these patients' initially being treated with multiple courses of topical and systemic antibiotics without symptom resolution prior to a biopsy being performed. As tumor extension occurs, chronic otalgia and cranial nerve damage (sensorineural hearing loss, facial weakness) become evident. Chewing and swallowing may become involved with tumor extension into the glenoid fossa and infratemporal fossa. Although significant local growth of these tumors may be evident at diagnosis, regional lymphatic metastases are infrequent.

Although no etiologic factors have been found to explain SCC of the EAC, the most commonly cited risk factor is chronic otitis media. In addition, the other conditions examined include radiotherapy to the area, chronic otitis externa, cholesteatoma, and lymphoproliferative disorders. Human papillomavirus (HPV) has also been linked to SCC of the temporal bone as part of the multistep process in the development of malignancy.[34] In the past, a select group of these patients had the common history of being radium-dial painters in watch factories, or of having received radium water or salts for therapeutic reasons.[35] In regard to auricular tumors, SCC is the second most common tumor found; risk factors include sun exposure and local trauma.

On inspection, these tumors frequently appear granular and are quite friable with ill-defined borders. Manipulation may provoke bleeding, thus heightening suspicion and leading to biopsy.

27.4.2 Basal Cell Carcinoma

Basal cell carcinoma often presents on the helical rim, and can be found anywhere in the periauricular area.[17,33,36–40] These

Table 27.1 Signs and Symptoms of Malignant Temporal Bone Tumors and the Percentage of Patients in Whom They Are Found

Signs		Symptoms	
Canal mass or lesion	92%	Pain	72%
Aural drainage	84%	Hearing loss	66%
Periauricular swelling	29%	Pruritis	42%
Facial paralysis	20%	Bleeding	24%
Neck nodes	8%	Headache	20%
Temporal mass	6%	Tinnitus	20%
		Facial numbness	10%
		Vertigo	8%
		Hoarseness	4%

Table 27.3 University of Cincinnati Grading System for Temporal Bone Tumors

Grade	
Grade I	Tumor in a single site, ≤ 1 cm
Grade II	Tumor in a single site, > 1 cm
Grade III	Transannular tumor extension
Grade IV	Mastoid or petrous air-cell invasion
Grade V	Periauricular or contiguous extension (extratemporal/dural invasion)
Grade VI	Neck adenopathy, distant anatomic site, or infratemporal fossa extension

Table 27.2 Pittsburgh Staging System for Malignant External Auditory Canal Tumors

T1	Tumor limited to external auditory canal without bony erosion or evidence of soft tissue extension
T2	Tumor with limited external auditory canal bony erosion (not full thickness) or radiographic finding consistent with limited (< 0.5 cm) soft tissue involvement
T3	Tumor eroding the osseous external auditory canal (full thickness) with limited (< 0.5 cm) soft tissue involvement or tumor involving the middle ear or mastoid or patients presenting with facial paralysis
T4	Tumor eroding cochlea, petrous apex, medial wall of the middle ear, carotid canal, jugular foramen, or dura, or with extensive (> 0.5 cm) soft tissue involvement.
N status	Involvement of lymph nodes is a poor prognostic finding and automatically places patient in an advanced stage (either stage III [T1N1] or stage IV [T2-T4N1])
M status	Distant metastasis indicates a poor prognosis and immediately places patient in stage IV

Table 27.4 Benign, Aggressive Benign, and Malignant Temporal Bone Tumors

Benign	Aggressive Benign	Malignant
Meningioma, low grade	Chondroblastoma	Squamous cell
Schwannoma	Plasmacytoma	Basal cell
Paraganglioma	Hemangiopericytoma	Melanoma
Osteoma	Hemangioendothelioma	Ceruminous gland tumor
Adenoma	Meningioma, high grade	Adenoid cystic
Chordoma		Endolymphatic sac tumor
Lipoma		Rhabdomyosarcoma
		Ewing's sarcoma
		Chondrosarcoma
		Adenocarcinoma
		Chondrosarcoma
		Glioma
		Astrocytoma
		Medulloblastoma
		Neuroblastoma

tumors are associated with excessive sun exposure and are found with high prevalence in older Caucasian men. These tumors erode perichondrium and periosteum as they enlarge, and often set up conditions conducive to secondary infection at the site. These lesions spread to the temporal bone by extension to the EAC, a path commonly seen in lesions originating in preauricular skin or the conchal bowl.

Basal cell tumors often grow more slowly than SCCs, but are still able to deeply infiltrate surrounding tissues if left to progress. As these lesions do not illicit pain until deeply infiltrating, they are often neglected, and late diagnosis ensues. However, they carry a better prognosis than that of SCCs, and are more likely to be resectable.

The most common variant of BCC is the nodular type; this variant as well as the superficial and ulcerative variants is less aggressive than the morpheaform and basaloid variants. Because of their common location on the auricle, these tumors are often removed with the assistance of Mohs micrographic surgery in an effort to minimize the removal of noninvolved tissues. This method has been shown to be effective as long as there is no involvement of the EAC.

27.4.3 Melanoma

Melanoma is very rarely found in the temporal bone.[41] It carries a poor prognosis and often presents at advanced stages. Surgical resection, if possible, followed by radiotherapy, is the treatment of choice.

27.4.4 Glandular Tumors

Despite the fact that the skin of the EAC contains ceruminous, modified apocrine, and sebaceous glands, glandular tumors of the EAC are very uncommon.[18,25,41–46] More frequently, regionally invasive salivary gland tumors extending from the parotid gland are encountered. Of glandular tumors, adenoid cystic carcinoma is the most frequently encountered. Despite its propensity for neural invasion, surgery with preservation of the facial nerve has become the mainstay of treatment. However, wide margins at the time of resection are advised, and some authors argue that the treatment of choice for these patients is lateral temporal bone resection along with superficial parotidectomy. Neck dissection in any patient with radiographic evidence of lymphadenopathy is also advocated. In addition, postoperative radiotherapy is suggested, particularly given the high rate of local recurrence. As is common in adenoid cystic carcinoma in any location of the head and neck, many patients succumb to metastatic disease, often in the lung, years after primary resection. Tumors such as high-grade adenocarcinoma, high-grade mucoepidermoid, and acinic cell carcinoma continue to be dealt with in an aggressive fashion with nerve sacrifice when involved.

Primary low-grade adenocarcinoma of the endolymphatic sac and aggressive papillary cystadenoma are found to invade the temporal bone. These are very rare tumors, but have been diagnosed in clinical connection with von Hippel–Lindau (VHL) disease. Certain mutations within the *VHL* gene locus have been shown to correlate with loss of a tumor suppressor gene, both in familial and sporadic VHL. It is thought that further genetic research may be able to predict solely with genetic testing which VHL patients will develop endolymphatic sac tumors.

27.4.5 Rhabdomyosarcoma

Rhabdomyosarcoma is the most common malignant tumor of soft tissue in the pediatric population.[47–50] The embryonal variant is the most common variant to be found in the head and neck, and 4 to 7% of these lesions involve the temporal bone. The most common presenting signs and symptoms are a mass in the auricular region, a polyp in the EAC, otorrhea, otalgia, and facial nerve weakness. Many patients present in a delayed manner given the similarity of symptoms to that of chronic suppurative otitis media. More specifically, 20% of children diagnosed with this lesion have metastatic spread at the time of presentation. As a result, a high degree of suspicion is necessary in children who present with these signs and symptoms, particularly aural polyp and nerve palsy. The lungs are the most common site of metastatic spread, and a chest X-ray, as well as a bone scan, should be included in the workup. Lesions that demonstrate invasion of the bone or cranial involvement have significantly lower 5-year survival rates.

Multimodal treatment for rhabdomyosarcoma has improved outcomes significantly. Multidrug chemotherapy with radiation is the mainstay of treatment. In light of improved 5-year survival with multimodal treatment, complete surgical excision has become unnecessary. Surgery is reserved for biopsy, removal of small lesions, or debulking of disease.

27.4.6 Ewing Sarcoma

Ewing sarcoma is a very uncommon tumor of the temporal bone.[51] To date, six case reports have been published that describe the clinical course of the disease. In each of these publications, children and young adults aged 5 months to 17 years were affected. Patients presented with a variety of symptoms including headache, syncope, facial paralysis, and emesis, as well as signs of increased intracranial pressure. These patients were treated with a combination of surgical resection, chemotherapy, and radiotherapy. With improved chemotherapeutic agents used in multimodal therapy, overall survival for patients with Ewing's sarcoma has increased significantly.

27.4.7 Metastatic Tumors

Metastatic spread to the temporal bone is rare; however, a variety of tumors have been diagnosed within the temporal bone.[52–68] Breast cancer, followed by lung and kidney, are the most common. Prognosis varies based on the histopathology, but it is typically poor. In addition, hematopoietic lesions including lymphoma and leukemia may invade the temporal bone. Plasmacytoma may also be found in this region, and manifests as a granular, friable mass in the middle ear or mastoid.

Malignant or highly aggressive benign intracranial tumors may occasionally invade the temporal bone, including seeding from meningeal carcinomatosis in rare cases. Primary brain tumors with invasion into the temporal bone may include medulloblastoma, neuroblastoma, malignant meningioma, and choroids plexus tumors.

27.5 Clinical Management

Once a malignancy involving the temporal bone has been recognized, it is important to determine the resectability of the tumor, along with the functional status of the patient. Limitations of both CT and MRI may prevent distinguishing between tumor and inflammatory process or cholesterol granuloma within the air-cell system and petrous apex, making it difficult to fully evaluate the extent of the tumor. Overall, management of temporal bone malignancies requires a multidisciplinary approach. The treatment plan for these tumors depends both on the extent of the lesion and the pathology. In general, surgery is the mainstay of treatment, regardless of the pathology. In addition, postoperative radiation therapy is advocated depending on the stage of the disease and extent of resection.[69]

Historically, findings of gross intraparenchymal brain invasion, extensive infratemporal fossa involvement, or extension along the internal carotid artery to the cavernous sinus exclude surgical intervention in patients.[70–73] However, due to the lack of other efficacious primary treatment modalities, many surgeons consider the only contraindications to resection to be significant medical comorbidities, advanced local disease, and metastatic spread.[41]

Advances in microvascular reconstruction now allow patients who undergo extensive resections to have improved cosmetic and functional outcomes. Patients with severe intercurrent systemic disease, especially cardiopulmonary in origin, may not tolerate the extended surgical intervention necessary for tumor resection. Palliative radiation may be offered as a treatment option in these cases.[74–77]

Total en-bloc resection of the temporal bone has been advocated for the treatment of temporal bone malignancies, but a piecemeal approach has also been developed due to studies displaying the improbability of not violating tumor margins during surgical excision.[78,79] Although debate continues as to which approach shows the best clinical outcomes, some standard surgical options have been traditionally outlined for resection of disease.

27.5.1 Wedge Resection

If tumor is exclusively located on the auricle without extension into the temporal bone noted, a wedge resection is often adequate treatment.[80] Mohs microsurgical techniques also offer an alternative that spares noninvolved tissue in these smaller tumors.[40] Briefly, the skin surrounding the lesion and the underlying auricular cartilage is removed. The defect may be closed primarily or with the application of a split-thickness skin graft.

27.5.2 Sleeve Resection

Lesions in the ear canal lateral to the bony–cartilaginous junction may be amenable to a composite sleeve resection (▶ Fig. 27.3).[81,82] With this technique, a medial incision is completed initially to ensure that the bony–cartilaginous region is not involved. Then, a lateral cut is made to encompass the lesion, surrounding skin, and underlying cartilage. This is removed and reconstruction may utilize split-thickness skin grafting.

27.5.3 Lateral Temporal Bone Resection

Lesions of the ear canal that lie juxtaposed to the bony cartilaginous junction or extend medially without gross violation of the tympanic annulus may be treated with a lateral temporal bone resection (▶ Fig. 27.3).[83–87] This may be performed in

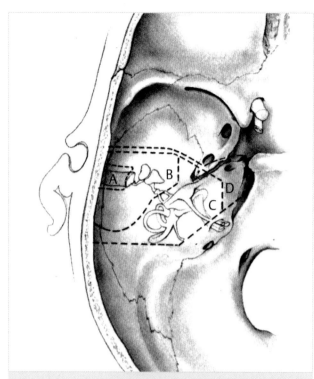

Fig. 27.3 Lesions lateral to the cartilaginous bony external auditory canal junction (A) are amenable to sleeve resection. Extension to the bony external auditory canal (B) that does not violate the middle ear or mastoid is often managed with a lateral temporal bone resection. The margins of a subtotal temporal bone resection (C) are shown extending to the internal auditory canal medially. In a total temporal bone resection, the petrous apex (D) is taken. Some authors have advocated sacrifice of the internal carotid artery.

conjunction with a parotidectomy for completeness. A superiorly or postauricularly based flap is created to isolate the non-involved auricle centered around an "apple core" circumscribing the lesion. A cortical mastoidectomy and extended facial recess are drilled. The incudostapedial joint is separated and the roof of the middle ear is dissected from the tegmen plate. The zygomatic root is sectioned and the floor is separated just lateral to the facial nerve, jugular bulb, and internal carotid artery. The skin and cartilage of the auricle as well as the EAC, tympanic ring and membrane, and malleus–incus complex are removed. A split-thickness skin graft with bolster packing is used for closure.

27.5.4 Subtotal Temporal Bone Resection

This resection removes the temporal bone lateral to the internal carotid artery, medially to the internal auditory canal (IAC), and inferiorly to the jugular foramen, leaving only the petrous apex.[88–90] A temporal craniotomy is performed to allow access to the IAC and demonstrate the absence of tumor along the floor of the middle fossa. Tumor may be resected if it involves dura only, but if extension into the temporal lobe parenchyma is found, the tumor is considered inoperable. The temporal lobe is identified superiorly, and the posterior fossa is uncovered posteriorly. The carotid artery and jugular veins are identified

within the neck and followed superiorly to the skull base. The jugular bulb and sigmoid sinus are also completely unroofed with a mastoidectomy. Anteriorly, the facial nerve is identified within the parotid gland. The mandibular condyle is sectioned and the bone is severed cleanly from the middle fossa dura superiorly, internal carotid artery anteroinferiorly, and the IAC medially. Often, piecemeal removal of residual areas of tumor is necessary after this resection.

In the past, closure of defects was accomplished by cervicofacial rotational flaps, split-thickness skin grafts, and regional pedicled flaps. More recently, free flaps have been shown to be superior, particularly in regard to efficacy, availability, and match of the defect size.[91] The radial forearm free flap and the anterolateral thigh flap are ideal choices for reconstruction. Based on the experience with 73 free tissue transfers in lateral temporal bone defects, Rosenthal et al[91] proposed a classification system based on depth and width of the defect to aid in reconstruction. In their series, when a lateral temporal bone resection was performed, with or without an auriculectomy, the radial forearm free flap or anterolateral thigh flap was found to offer excellent cosmetic and functional results. Cervicofacial rotation flaps and regional flaps were reserved for superficial defects.

27.5.5 Total Temporal Bone Resection

This resection includes the petrous apex with the removed specimen.[92–96] The petrous apex is isolated from the cavernous sinus at the anterior medial aspect of the bony carotid artery. The carotid is then mobilized anterior and medially during resection, or may be resected with the specimen. Resection of the carotid artery requires specific preoperative planning. Radiographic evaluation to determine options for sacrifice of the artery is essential.

27.6 Radiation Therapy

Radiation therapy is used in conjunction with surgical excision to treat temporal bone malignancies.[41,74–77] The radiation protocol is individualized to each patient, with specific regard to tumor pathology, extent of resection, and structures to be included in the radiation field. The dosage at the surgical site is typically 60 Gy, and can be increased if the surgical margins are positive. If used as primary treatment for a patient deemed to be a poor surgical candidate, the dosage is increased to 70 Gy. Preauricular, postauricular, and subdigastric nodes are usually encompassed within the radiation field setup. Given the rarity of temporal bone malignancies, there are few centers with adequate numbers to evaluate treatment protocols. In a series of 33 patients published by Zhang et al,[97] radiation alone yielded a 5-year survival of 28.7%, whereas combined surgery and radiation yielded 59.6%.

Intensity-modulated radiation therapy (IMRT), as an adjunct to external beam radiation, has been trialed on selected tumors of the head and neck, including temporal bone carcinoma. Proper dosimetry and accurate target volume delineation has led to excellent reported local freedom from progression rates.[98]

More recently, IMRT has been trialed as the primary modality for postoperative radiotherapy. It offers the advantage of targeted dose administration while sparing surrounding structures, a concept that is ideal for radiotherapy administered near the brain. To date, only one study has been published with outcomes using this treatment modality, and further investigation is needed.[69]

Primary radiotherapy is indicated in palliation and eradication of pain from bony metastasis in head and neck cancer. Pain relief has been reported in 70 to 90% of patients treated for bony metastasis in this manner.[99] Others question the use of radiotherapy for pain and feel that the same results may be achieved with proper analgesics.[36]

Complications of radiotherapy are well recognized and can range from minor to severe. Radiation of the auricle may cause desquamation, irritation, dryness, and necrosis of the remaining cartilage. Within the EAC, thickening of the canal epithelium and tympanic membrane have been documented, along with loss of cerumen glands leading to severe dryness. Within the middle ear, eustachian tube dysfunction may lead to effusion. Osteoradionecrosis may occur at the bony EAC, mastoid, or skull base due to devascularization of the bone. Radiation-induced tumors, parenchymal brain necrosis, and carotid artery pseudoaneurysm, although extremely rare, may occur following radiation to the temporal bone.[100–102]

27.7 Chemotherapy

Chemotherapeutic regimens are the mainstay of treatment for pediatric rhabdomyosarcoma with adjuvant radiation and surgery when indicated.[48] Single- and multidrug regimens of chemotherapy are being used in SCC of the head and neck, particularly in patients with advanced disease or metastatic disease. Treatment protocols are tailored to the tumor type.[103] Unfortunately, the use of chemotherapeutic agents has not yet been shown to significantly impact survival rates.

More recent studies have looked at the use of concurrent superselective intraarterial chemotherapy combined with radiotherapy for advanced-stage SCC of the temporal bone, with encouraging results. Further studies are needed, but this may represent an effective treatment option in late-stage disease.[104]

For locally advanced or metastatic BCC, vismodegib, a small-molecule inhibitor of the hedgehog pathway, represents a new treatment option. The effectiveness of this drug, as demonstrated by randomized controlled trials, is based on the finding that dysregulation of the hedgehog signaling pathway has been identified in the majority of BCCs.[105]

27.8 Pain Management and Quality of Life

Patients diagnosed with temporal bone malignancies may present with pain. Pain may be attributed to the primary tumor mass, bony erosion, or compromise of vascular and nervous structures as the tumor infiltrates areas around the temporal bone, such as the cerebellopontine angle, infratemporal fossa, temporomandibular joint, or upper cervical region. Unfortunately, cancer pain is often underestimated and undertreated.[106] The treatment options available, usually consisting of combination surgery and radiation therapy, have been found to cause significant increases in pain when evaluated using quality-of-life survey techniques.[107] Myofascial spasm may also contribute to discomfort after surgical disruption of normal functional muscle groups.

Pharmacological management of pain in the head and neck region includes identification and control of both somatic and neuropathic pain. Somatic pain control guidelines have been adopted by the World Health Organization and outline treatment plans beginning with mild analgesics plus nonsteroidal antiinflammatory drugs, progressing to mild opiates, and finally to opioid analgesics.[108] Effective treatment for neuropathic pain may begin with amitriptyline and carbamazepine. Nerve blocks, especially for malignancies involving the cranial nerves and sympathetic/parasympathetic chains, may be indicated for effective pain management.[109]

27.9 Conclusion

Diagnosis and management of temporal bone malignancy continues to be a formidable challenge, despite advances in microsurgical techniques, imaging, and radiotherapy. Although tumors limited to the auricle or confined to the EAC portend relatively favorable prognosis, it is often not possible preoperatively to fully appreciate tumor extent. Temporal bone resection is difficult, and may not allow for en-bloc excision of malignancy. Establishment of clean margins is further encumbered by inadequate tumor volume in frozen section specimens, sampling error, and significant quantities of bone in the sample specimen. There is significant variability in survival data for temporal bone malignancies. Studies are limited in sample size and variability of tumor pathology. In general, the literature offers support for 5-year survival rates ranging from 28 to 66%.[41,110,111] However, a study of 35 patients reported a 5-year survival rate of 77%.[112]

In cases where complete resection is questioned, or for advanced lesions, adjunctive radiation therapy may be employed. Although there has been agreement that radiation therapy alone has proven ineffective for complete treatment of temporal bone malignancy, its use in the postoperative period has been shown in some studies to increase survivorship in patients once gross tumor has been removed. Chemotherapy has been indicated in only a limited set of tumor types.

Surgical and adjuvant intervention for temporal bone malignancy represents a possibility for life-sustaining treatment in light of a rare and dire tumor, especially after frequent delay in diagnosis. Advances in imaging, the implementation of free flap reconstruction, and improved radiotherapy regiments provide improved management strategies for patients. High suspicion for these tumors, along with adequate assessment and treatment, can potentially provide favorable outcomes despite the often poor prognosis accompanying diagnosis.

References

[1] Anson BJ, Donaldson JA, Eds. Surgical Anatomy of the Temporal Bone. Philadelphia: WB Saunders, 1981
[2] Schuknecht H. Pathology of the Ear, 2nd ed. Philadelphia: Lea & Febiger, 1993
[3] Lewis JS. Surgical management of tumors of the middle ear and mastoid. J Laryngol Otol 1983; 97: 299–311

[4] Goodwin WJ, Jesse RH. Malignant neoplasms of the external auditory canal and temporal bone. Arch Otolaryngol 1980; 106: 675–679

[5] Kinney SE, Wood BG. Malignancies of the external ear canal and temporal bone: surgical techniques and results. Laryngoscope 1987; 97: 158–164

[6] Chung SJ, Pensak ML. Tumors of the temporal bone. In: Jackler R, Brackmann D, eds. Neurotology, 2nd ed. Philadelphia: Elsevier Mosby, 2005

[7] Pensak ML. Skull base surgery. In: Glasscock ME, Shambaugh GE, eds. Surgery of the Ear. Philadelphia: WB Saunders, 1990:503–533

[8] Arena S, Keen M. Carcinoma of the middle ear and temporal bone. Am J Otol 1988; 9: 351–356

[9] Chapman PR, Shah R, Curé JK, Bag AK. Petrous apex lesions: pictorial review. AJR Am J Roentgenol 2011; 196 Suppl: WS26–WS37, Quiz S40–S43

[10] Phillips GS, LoGerfo SE, Richardson ML, Anzai Y. Interactive Web-based learning module on CT of the temporal bone: anatomy and pathology. Radiographics 2012; 32: E85–E105

[11] Friedman DP, Rao VMMR. MR and CT of squamous cell carcinoma of the middle ear and mastoid complex. AJNR Am J Neuroradiol 1991; 12: 872–874

[12] Jäger L, Bonell H, Liebl M et al. CT of the normal temporal bone: comparison of multi- and single-detector row CT. Radiology 2005; 235: 133–141

[13] Swartz JD, Russell KB, Wolfson RJ, Marlowe FI. High resolution computed tomography in evaluation of the temporal bone. Head Neck Surg 1984; 6: 921–931

[14] Ball JB, Jr, Pensak ML. Fundamentals of magnetic resonance imaging. Am J Otol 1987; 8: 81–85

[15] Ozgen B, Oguz KK, Cila A. Diffusion MR imaging features of skull base osteomyelitis compared with skull base malignancy. AJNR Am J Neuroradiol 2011; 32: 179–184

[16] American Society of Interventional and Therapeutic Neuroradiology. Carotid artery balloon test occlusion.[Suppl] AJNR Am J Neuroradiol 2001; 22 Suppl: S8–S9

[17] Pensak ML, Gleich LL, Gluckman JL, Shumrick KA. Temporal bone carcinoma: contemporary perspectives in the skull base surgical era. Laryngoscope 1996; 106: 1234–1237

[18] Stell PM, McCormick MS. Carcinoma of the external auditory meatus and middle ear. Prognostic factors and a suggested staging system. J Laryngol Otol 1985; 99: 847–850

[19] Nakagawa T, Natori Y, Kumamoto Y, et al. Squamous cell carcinoma of the external auditory canal and middle ear: Proposal of modification of Pittsburgh TNM staging system. American Otological Society 138th Annual Meeting 2005, Boca Raton, Florida

[20] Batsakis JG, ed. Tumors of the Head and Neck, 2nd ed. Baltimore: Williams & Wilkins, 1979

[21] Gacek RR, Goodman M. Management of malignancy of the temporal bone. Laryngoscope 1977; 87: 1622–1634

[22] Clairmont AA, Conley JJ. Primary carcinoma of the mastoid bone. Ann Otol Rhinol Laryngol 1977; 86: 306–309

[23] Bloom BJ, Smith RN. Case records of the Massachusetts General Hospital. Weekly clinicopathological exercises. Case 29-2002. A 17-year-old boy with acute mitral regurgitation and pulmonary edema. N Engl J Med 2002; 347: 921–928

[24] Wiatrak BJ, Pensak ML. Rhabdomyosarcoma of the ear and temporal bone. Laryngoscope 1989; 99: 1188–1192

[25] Pulec JL. Glandular tumors of the external auditory canal. Laryngoscope 1977; 87: 1601–1612

[26] Perzin KH, Gullane P, Conley J. Adenoid cystic carcinoma involving the external auditory canal. A clinicopathologic study of 16 cases. Cancer 1982; 50: 2873–2883

[27] Lewis JS. Squamous carcinoma of the ear. Arch Otolaryngol 1973; 97: 41–42

[28] Tucker WN. Cancer of the middle ear. Cancer 1965; 18: 642–650

[29] Lewis JS. A guide to cancer of the ear. CA Cancer J Clin 1977; 27: 42–46

[30] Arena S, Keen M. Carcinoma of the middle ear and temporal bone. Am J Otol 1988; 9: 351–356

[31] Conley J, Schuller DE. Malignancies of the ear. Laryngoscope 1976; 86: 1147–1163

[32] Crabtree JA, Britton BH, Pierce MK. Carcinoma of the external auditory canal. Laryngoscope 1976; 86: 405–415

[33] Ahmad I, Das Gupta AR. Epidemiology of basal cell carcinoma and squamous cell carcinoma of the pinna. J Laryngol Otol 2001; 115: 85–86

[34] Jin YT, Tsai ST, Li C et al. Prevalence of human papillomavirus in middle ear carcinoma associated with chronic otitis media. Am J Pathol 1997; 150: 1327–1333

[35] Beal DD, Lindsay JR, Ward PH. Radiation induced carcinoma of the mastoid. Arch Otolaryngol 1965; 81: 9–16

[36] Adams GL, Paparella MM, el-Fiky FM. Primary and metastatic tumors of the temporal bone. Laryngoscope 1971; 81: 1273–1285

[37] Parkin JL, Stevens MH. Basal cell carcinoma of the temporal bone. Otolaryngol Head Neck Surg 1979; 87: 645–647

[38] Harwood AR, Keane TJ. Malignant tumors of the temporal bone and external ear: medical and radiation therapy. In: Alberti PW, Reuben RJ, eds. Otologic Medicine and Surgery, vol 2. London: Churchill Livingstone, 1988

[39] Spector JG. Management of temporal bone carcinomas: a therapeutic analysis of two groups of patients and long-term followup. Otolaryngol Head Neck Surg 1991; 104: 58–66

[40] Glied M, Berg D, Witterick I. Basal cell carcinoma of the conchal bowl: interdisciplinary approach to treatment. J Otolaryngol 1998; 27: 322–326

[41] Casper KA, Pensak M. Surgery for malignant lesions. In: Gulya AJ, Minor LB, Poe DS, eds. Glasscock-Shambaugh Surgery of the Ear. Shelton, CT: People's Medical Publishing House, 2010:751–764

[42] Cannon CR, McLean WC. Adenoid cystic carcinoma of the middle ear and temporal bone. Otolaryngol Head Neck Surg 1983; 91: 96–99

[43] Choo D, Shotland L, Mastroianni M et al. Endolymphatic sac tumors in von Hippel-Lindau disease. J Neurosurg 2004; 100: 480–487

[44] Irving RM. The molecular pathology of tumours of the ear and temporal bone. J Laryngol Otol 1998; 112: 1011–1018

[45] Kawahara N, Kume H, Ueki K, Mishima K, Sasaki T, Kirino T. VHL gene inactivation in an endolymphatic sac tumor associated with von Hippel-Lindau disease. Neurology 1999; 53: 208–210

[46] Dong F, Gidley PW, Ho T, Luna MA, Ginsberg LE, Sturgis EM. Adenoid cystic carcinoma of the external auditory canal. Laryngoscope 2008; 118: 1591–1596

[47] Feldman BA. Rhabdomyosarcoma of the head and neck. Laryngoscope 1982; 92: 424–440

[48] Raney RB, Jr, Lawrence W, Jr, Maurer HM et al. Rhabdomyosarcoma of the ear in childhood. A report from the Intergroup Rhabdomyosarcoma Study-I. Cancer 1983; 51: 2356–2361

[49] Durve DV, Kanegaonkar RG, Albert D, Levitt G. Paediatric rhabdomyosarcoma of the ear and temporal bone. Clin Otolaryngol Allied Sci 2004; 29: 32–37

[50] Sbeity S, Abella A, Arcand P, Quintal MC, Saliba I. Temporal bone rhabdomyosarcoma in children. Int J Pediatr Otorhinolaryngol 2007; 71: 807–814

[51] Kadar AA, Hearst MJ, Collins MH, Mangano FT, Samy RN. Ewing's sarcoma of the petrous temporal bone: case report and literature review. Skull Base 2010; 20: 213–217

[52] Zechner G, Altmann F. The temporal bone in leukemia. Histological studies. Ann Otol Rhinol Laryngol 1969; 78: 375–387

[53] Harbert F, Liu JC, Berry RG. Metastatic malignant melanoma to both VIIIth nerves. J Laryngol Otol 1969; 83: 889–898

[54] Hoshino T, Hiraide F, Nomura Y. Metastatic tumour of the inner ear: a histopathological report. J Laryngol Otol 1972; 86: 697–707

[55] Maddox HE, III. Metastatic tumors of the temporal bone. Ann Otol Rhinol Laryngol 1967; 76: 149–165

[56] Stucker FJ, Holmes WF. Metastatic disease of the temporal bone. Laryngoscope 1976; 86: 1136–1140

[57] Paparella MM, el-Fiky FM. Ear involvement in malignant lymphoma. Ann Otol Rhinol Laryngol 1972; 81: 352–363

[58] Takahara T, Sando I, Bluestone CD, Myers EN. Lymphoma invading the anterior eustachian tube. Temporal bone histopathology of functional tubal obstruction. Ann Otol Rhinol Laryngol 1986; 95: 101–105

[59] Thomas JR, Davis WE. Breast carcinoma metastatic to the temporal bone. Mo Med 1975; 72: 77–78

[60] Brown NE, O'Brien DA, Megerian CA. Metastatic hepatocellular carcinoma to the temporal bone in a post-liver transplant patient. Otolaryngol Head Neck Surg 2004; 130: 370–371

[61] Ruenes R, Palacios E. Plasmacytoma of the petrous temporal bone. Ear Nose Throat J 2003; 82: 672

[62] Koral K, Curran JG, Thompson A. Primary non-Hodgkin's lymphoma of the temporal bone. CT findings. Clin Imaging 2003; 27: 386–388

[63] Chang CY, O'Halloran EK, Fisher SR. Primary non-Hodgkin's lymphoma of the petrous bone: case report. Otolaryngol Head Neck Surg 2004; 130: 360–362

[64] Musacchio M, Mont'Alverne F, Belzile F, Lenz V, Riquelme C, Tournade A. Posterior cervical haemangiopericytoma with intracranial and skull base extension. Diagnostic and therapeutic challenge of a rare hypervascular neoplasm. J Neuroradiol 2003; 30: 180–187

[65] Ohba S, Kurokawa R, Yoshida K, Kawase T. Metastatic adenocarcinoma of the dura mimicking petroclival meningioma—case report. Neurol Med Chir (Tokyo) 2004; 44: 317–320

[66] Kim HL, Im SA, Lim GY et al. High grade hemangioendothelioma of the temporal bone in a child: a case report. Korean J Radiol 2004; 5: 214–217

[67] Gaudet EL, Jr, Nuss DW, Johnson DH, Jr, Miranne LS, Jr. Chondroblastoma of the temporal bone involving the temporomandibular joint, mandibular condyle, and middle cranial fossa: case report and review of the literature. Cranio 2004; 22: 160–168

[68] Streitmann MJ, Sismanis A. Metastatic carcinoma of the temporal bone. Am J Otol 1996; 17: 780–783

[69] Chen WY, Kuo SH, Chen YH et al. Postoperative intensity-modulated radiotherapy for squamous cell carcinoma of the external auditory canal and middle ear: treatment outcomes, marginal misses, and perspective on target delineation. Int J Radiat Oncol Biol Phys 2012; 82: 1485–1493

[70] Arena S. Treatment of carcinoma of the temporal bone. Am J Otol 1983; 5: 56–61

[71] Conley JJ, Schuller DE. Malignancies of the ear. Laryngoscope 1976; 86: 1147–1163

[72] Ariyan S, Sasaki CT, Spencer D. Radical en bloc resection of the temporal bone. Am J Surg 1981; 142: 443–447

[73] Graham MD, Sataloff RT, Kemink JL, Wolf GT, McGillicuddy JE. Total en bloc resection of the temporal bone and carotid artery for malignant tumors of the ear and temporal bone. Laryngoscope 1984; 94: 528–533

[74] Million RR, Cassisi NJ. Temporal bone. In: Million RR, Cassisi NJ, eds. Management of Head and Neck Cancer: a Multidisciplinary Approach. Philadelphia: JB Lippincott, 1984

[75] Wang CC. Radiation therapy in the management of carcinoma of the external auditory canal, middle ear, or mastoid. Radiology 1975; 116: 713–715

[76] Gabriele P, Magnano M, Albera R et al. Carcinoma of the external auditory meatus and middle ear. Results of the treatment of 28 cases. Tumori 1994; 80: 40–43

[77] Korzeniowski S, Pszon J. The results of radiotherapy of cancer of the middle ear. Int J Radiat Oncol Biol Phys 1990; 18: 631–633

[78] Lewis JS. Surgical management of tumors of the middle ear and mastoid. J Laryngol Otol 1983; 97: 299–311

[79] Neely JG, Forrester M. Anatomic considerations of the medial cuts in the subtotal temporal bone resection. Otolaryngol Head Neck Surg 1982; 90: 641–645

[80] Bailin PL, Levine HL, Wood BG, Tucker HM. Cutaneous carcinoma of the auricular and periauricular region. Arch Otolaryngol 1980; 106: 692–696

[81] Kinney SE, Wood BG. Malignancies of the external ear canal and temporal bone: surgical techniques and results. Laryngoscope 1987; 97: 158–164

[82] Krepsi YP, Levine TM. Management and therapy of tumors of the temporal bone. In: Alberti PW, Reuben RJ, eds. Otologic Medicine and Surgery. New York: Churchill-Livingstone, 1988

[83] Schramm VL. Temporal bone resection. In: Sekhar LN, Schramm VL, eds. Tumors of the Cranial Base: Diagnosis and Treatment. Mount Kisco, NY: Futura, 1987

[84] Arena S. Tumor surgery of the temporal bone. Laryngoscope 1974; 84: 645–670

[85] Conley JJ. Cancer of the middle ear. Trans Am Otol Soc 1965; 53: 189–207

[86] Goodwin WJ, Jesse RH. Malignant neoplasms of the external auditory canal and temporal bone. Arch Otolaryngol 1980; 106: 675–679

[87] Kinney SE, Wood BG. Surgical treatment of skull-base malignancy. Otolaryngol Head Neck Surg 1984; 92: 94–99

[88] Hilding DA, Selker R. Total resection of the temporal bone for carcinoma. Arch Otolaryngol 1969; 89: 636–645

[89] Kinney SE. Clinical evaluation and treatment of ear tumors. In: Thawley E, Panje WR, eds. Comprehensive Management of Head and Neck Tumors. Philadelphia: WB Sauders, 1987

[90] Lewis JS. Temporal bone resection. Review of 100 cases. Arch Otolaryngol 1975; 101: 23–25

[91] Rosenthal EL, King T, McGrew BM, Carroll W, Magnuson JS, Wax MK. Evolution of a paradigm for free tissue transfer reconstruction of lateral temporal bone defects. Head Neck 2008; 30: 589–594

[92] Wu BT, Wang FT. Long-term observation of total temporal bone resection in carcinoma of the middle ear and temporal bone. Chin Med J (Engl) 1984; 97: 205–210[Engl]

[93] Sekhar LN, Schramm VL Jr, et al. Operative management of large neoplasms of the lateral and posterior cranial base. In: Sekhar LN, Schramm VL, eds. Tumors of the Cranial Base: Diagnosis and Treatment. Mount Kisco, NY: Futura, 1987

[94] Lesser RW, Spector GJ, Devineni VR. Malignant tumors of the middle ear and external auditory canal: a 20-year review. Otolaryngol Head Neck Surg 1987; 96: 43–47

[95] Stucker FJ, Holmes WF. Metastatic disease of the temporal bone. Laryngoscope 1976; 86: 1136–1140

[96] Tabb HG, Komet H, McLaurin JW. Cancer of the external auditory canal: treatment with radical mastoidectomy and irradiation. Laryngoscope 1964; 74: 634–643

[97] Zhang B, Tu G, Xu G, Tang P, Hu Y. Squamous cell carcinoma of temporal bone: reported on 33 patients. Head Neck 1999; 21: 461–466

[98] Lee N, Xia P, Fischbein NJ, Akazawa P, Akazawa C, Quivey JM. Intensity-modulated radiation therapy for head-and-neck cancer: the UCSF experience focusing on target volume delineation. Int J Radiat Oncol Biol Phys 2003; 57: 49–60

[99] Buckley JG, Ferlito A, Shaha AR, Rinaldo A. The treatment of distant metastases in head and neck cancer—present and future. ORL J Otorhinolaryngol Relat Spec 2001; 63: 259–264

[100] Hsieh ST, Guo YC, Tsai TL, Li WY, Lin CZ. Parosteal osteosarcoma of the mastoid bone following radiotherapy for nasopharyngeal carcinoma. J Chin Med Assoc 2004; 67: 314–316

[101] Wang PC, Tu TY, Liu KD. Cystic brain necrosis and temporal bone osteoradionecrosis after radiotherapy and surgery in a patient of ear carcinoma. J Chin Med Assoc 2004; 67: 487–491

[102] Auyeung KM, Lui WM, Chow LCK, Chan FL. Massive epistaxis related to petrous carotid artery pseudoaneurysm after radiation therapy: emergency treatment with covered stent in two cases. AJNR Am J Neuroradiol 2003; 24: 1449–1452

[103] de Mulder PH. The chemotherapy of head and neck cancer. Anticancer Drugs 1999; 10 Suppl 1: S33–S37

[104] Sugimoto H, Ito M, Yoshida S, Hatano M, Yoshizaki T. Concurrent superselective intra-arterial chemotherapy and radiotherapy for late-stage squamous cell carcinoma of the temporal bone. Ann Otol Rhinol Laryngol 2011; 120: 372–376

[105] Sekulic A, Migden MR, Oro AE et al. Efficacy and safety of vismodegib in advanced basal-cell carcinoma. N Engl J Med 2012; 366: 2171–2179

[106] Greipp ME. Undermedication for pain: an ethical model. ANS Adv Nurs Sci 1992; 15: 44–53

[107] Whale Z, Lyne PA, Papanikolaou P. Pain experience following radical treatment for head and neck cancer. Eur J Oncol Nurs 2001; 5: 112–120

[108] World Health Organization. Cancer pain relief and palliative care: report of a WHO expert committee. Geneva: WHO, 1990

[109] Vecht CJ, Hoff AM, Kansen PJ, de Boer MF, Bosch DA. Types and causes of pain in cancer of the head and neck. Cancer 1992; 70: 178–184

[110] Dean NR, White HN, Carter DS et al. Outcomes following temporal bone resection. Laryngoscope 2010; 120: 1516–1522

[111] Gidley PW, Roberts DB, Sturgis EM. Squamous cell carcinoma of the temporal bone. Laryngoscope 2010; 120: 1144–1151

[112] Moore MG, Deschler DG, McKenna MJ, Varvares MA, Lin DT. Management outcomes following lateral temporal bone resection for ear and temporal bone malignancies. Otolaryngol Head Neck Surg 2007; 137: 893–898

28 Vestibular Disorders

Mitchell K. Schwaber

28.1 Introduction

Dizziness is a term used to describe a myriad of patient perceptions, including light-headedness, syncope, disequilibrium, panic attacks, motion intolerance, visual disturbances, and true vertigo. It is the clinician's responsibility to determine which of these perceptions the patient is experiencing by obtaining a careful history, often using descriptions in layman's terms. True vertigo is characterized by the perception that the external world is spinning, whirling, or swaying, and it is usually indicative of a vestibular disorder. Furthermore, true vertigo is usually accompanied by nystagmus. On the other hand, patients with nonvestibular dizziness more often perceive a sensation of movement or disorientation within their head, rather than the perception of the external world spinning. Also, nonvestibular dizziness is rarely accompanied by nystagmus. Chapter 14 discusses other features that can be helpful in differentiating vestibular and nonvestibular dizziness.

Once the clinician has established that the patient is indeed experiencing vertigo, the next step is to further characterize the nature, severity, and triggers for the episodes, in an effort to diagnose the likely cause.

28.2 Episodic Vertigo

Most experienced clinicians can determine the likely etiology of the vestibular complaint with a brief history and exam. The major diagnostic entities include (1) Ménière disease; (2) recurrent vestibular neuritis; (3) benign positional vertigo; (4) migraine associated vertigo; (5) posttraumatic vertigo, including labyrinthine fracture and perilymph fistula; (6) superior semicircular canal dehiscence; and (7) vertigo associated with otitis media. Each of these conditions has unique features that should lead to easy recognition by most clinicians. These features as well as additional information concerning diagnosis and contemporary treatment options are reviewed in greater detail in this chapter. Furthermore, a number of miscellaneous entities including disembarking syndrome, vascular loop syndrome, multiple sclerosis and various cerebellar stroke syndromes, labyrinthine artery occlusion, vestibular ototoxicity, and inferior vestibular neuritis are briefly discussed also.

28.3 Ménière Syndrome and Ménière Disease

Ménière syndrome is defined as the clinical disorder associated with the histopathological finding of endolymphatic hydrops. Clinically, Ménière syndrome includes the following features: recurrent, spontaneous episodic vertigo; hearing loss; aural fullness; and tinnitus. Under the most recent guidelines of the American Academy of Otolaryngology–Head and Neck Surgery (AAO-HNS),[1] either tinnitus or fullness or both must be present on the affected side to establish the diagnosis. Recognized causes of Ménière syndrome include (1) idiopathic, also known as Ménière disease; (2) posttraumatic, following head injury or ear surgery; (3) postinfectious or delayed-onset Ménière syndrome following a viral infection, usually mumps or measles; (4) late-stage syphilis; and (5) classic Cogan syndrome with episodic vertigo, hearing loss, and interstitial keratitis, without syphilis. To these five entities, many clinicians add labyrinthine artery occlusion, which can often appear to be the onset of Ménière syndrome.

Although Ménière disease is by far the most common cause of Ménière syndrome and the terms are often used interchangeably, it should be remembered that a patient has an idiopathic etiology only when the known causes have been excluded.

28.3.1 Clinical Presentation

Ménière disease is characterized by a history of increasing ear fullness with roaring tinnitus, followed by a sensation of blocked hearing. If the symptoms further worsen, a definitive vertigo spell may occur within a few minutes. Alternatively, patients may note the sudden onset of vertigo with little or no warning. Friberg et al[2] found that the disorder begins with hearing loss alone in 42%, vertigo alone in 11%, vertigo with hearing loss in 44%, and tinnitus alone in 3%. In addition, there are now several reports of Ménière disease beginning as positional vertigo.[3]

The definitive vertigo spell is spontaneous rotational vertigo lasting 20 minutes or longer, with accompanying nausea, vomiting, and other autonomic symptoms. Most vertigo episodes last from 2 to 4 hours, although some can last for more than 6 hours. During the episode of vertigo, horizontal or horizontal-rotary nystagmus is *always* present. Following the vertigo episode, the patient may note that the hearing in the involved ear is markedly diminished. Disequilibrium may follow the definitive episode and may last for several days. Although the clinician might strongly suspect that the patient has Ménière disease, definitive diagnosis depends on the occurrence of two or more definitive episodes lasting 20 minutes or longer.

The hearing loss that occurs with Ménière disease typically begins with acoustic distortion that can be best described as a tinny quality to the signal. Another description is that only the higher-intensity peaks of certain frequencies are heard, whereas the rest of the frequencies are somewhat clipped or muffled. Loudness recruitment or loudness intolerance is also noted early in the illness, and is usually described by the patient as ordinary sounds being painfully loud in the affected ear. Early in the illness, many patients experience fluctuating hearing, with recovery beginning within a few hours of the episode. Hearing recovery may occur several days or months after a severe episode of vertigo. Either a shift of 15 dB or more in the average threshold of 0.5, 1, 2, or 3 kHz or a shift in speech discrimination of 15% is considered a significant change.

The hearing loss that accompanies Ménière disease typically follows one of three forms[1]: (1) a low-frequency sensorineural

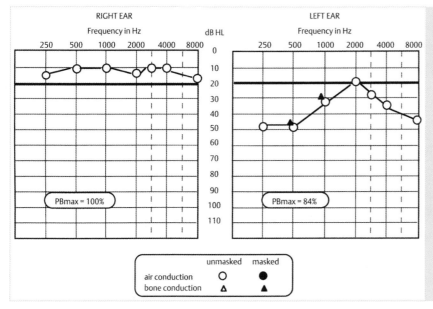

Fig. 28.1 Audiogram of patient with Ménière disease. The left ear shows the typical audiometric pattern of early Ménière disease. PBmax, maximum-phonetic balance, or word-recognition, score.

loss that is greatest at 250 Hz, 500 Hz, and at 1 kHz, with normal threshold at 2 kHz, and a sensorineural loss above 2 kHz (▶ Fig. 28.1); (2) a flat, moderately severe sensorineural loss at 500 Hz, 1 kHz, 2 kHz, and 3 kHz; or (3) in patients with bilateral hearing loss, an asymmetry of greater than 25 dB in one ear. Most patients with Ménière disease, however, do experience a loss of hearing in the affected ear that slowly worsens over time, although it is extremely rare for a patient to lose all of the hearing in the ear. For most patients with Ménière disease, the hearing threshold usually stabilizes at 50 to 60 dB levels, with a flat configuration ("burned out ear").

Aural pressure, positional vertigo, and roaring tinnitus are extremely common between definitive episodes of severe vertigo, as is instability with fast movements as well as a constant rocking sensation. Following the onset, there may be a period of remission that can confuse the clinical picture. Over time, however, Ménière disease progresses from an early stage, through a middle stage, to a late or burn-out stage.

Ménière disease also presents in several atypical clinical forms, including the Lermoyez variant, the otolithic crisis of Tumarkin or "drop attacks," cochlear Ménière disease, vestibular Ménière disease, and delayed-onset Ménière syndrome. The Lermoyez variant is associated with hearing improvement before, during, or after the vertigo episode. The otolithic crisis or drop attack is characterized by a sudden falling that is often accompanied by sudden firing of the extensor muscles of the extremities. The otolithic crisis is thought to represent firing of primitive muscle reflexes in response to sudden decompression of the saccule or utricle.

Cochlear and vestibular Ménière disease may represent early or possible Ménière disease, although the Committee on Hearing and Equilibrium[1] has recommended that the use of these terms be discontinued. Cochlear Ménière disease is characterized by the auditory symptoms of Ménière disease, but none of the vestibular symptoms. Cochlear Ménière disease is thought to represent endolymphatic hydrops (ELH) confined to the cochlear duct. Vestibular Ménière disease is characterized by the vestibular symptoms of Ménière disease without the auditory symptoms. Although many of these patients progress to

the classic form, other clinical entities include migraine and recurrent vestibular neuritis.[4–6]

Delayed-onset Ménière syndrome or postinfectious Ménière syndrome represents a distinct clinical entity, in which a patient with a long-standing unilateral sensorineural hearing loss begins to experience episodic vertigo indistinguishable from classic Ménière disease. There are two forms of the illness, ipsilateral and contralateral, indicating which ear is thought to be causing the problem. In the ipsilateral form, the deafened ear is usually found to have a caloric weakness on electronystagmography (ENG) testing. In the contralateral form, the better hearing ear begins to show fluctuating sensorineural levels, and on caloric testing shows a significant weakness. Schuknecht et al[7] identified features in the temporal bones of these patients that suggested that these findings are due to a subclinical viral infection in childhood, but many clinicians feel delayed contralateral endolymphatic hydrops is immune or autoimmune related.

The incidence of Ménière disease varies considerably in the various populations in which it has been studied.[8] In the United States the incidence has been reported as between 15 and 40 per 100,000 per year, whereas in the United Kingdom the incidence is reported as 157 per 100,000. The incidence in Sweden is reported as 50 per 100,000. The symptoms of Ménière disease typically start at age 35 to 45, although later onset certainly occurs. There does seem to be a slight female-to-male preponderance, although the true incidence in males is probably underreported.

One third of all patients have bilateral Ménière disease, and the vast majority becomes symptomatic in the other ear within the first 3 years of onset. Several reports suggest that Ménière disease, in particular bilateral Ménière disease, might be an immunologically related disorder.[9,10] Hereditary, viral, noise, and allergic factors have also been identified, although their exact significance remains to be determined.[11–13]

28.3.2 Histopathology

Hallpike and Cairns[14] and Yamakawa[15] first reported the histopathological finding of ELH in the temporal bones of patients

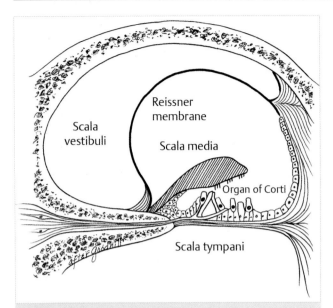

Fig. 28.2 Histopathology of Ménière disease, demonstrating displacement of the Reissner membrane and disruption of the organ of Corti by endolymphatic hydrops.

with symptoms suggestive of Ménière syndrome. Most of the distention is seen in the cochlear and saccular ducts (▶ Fig. 28.2), although occasionally the walls of the utricle and the ampullae are distorted. In some cases, the Reissner membrane is so distended that the space of the scala vestibulae is completely taken up by the scala media. Ruptures of the membranous labyrinth, fistulas between the endolymph and perilymph, collapse of the membranous labyrinth, and vestibular fibrosis further characterize the histopathological picture of ELH.[16]

Recently, Shimizu et al[17] reported the temporal bone findings in subjects with Ménière disease compared to normals. This study demonstrated that in Ménière disease, blockage of the endolymphatic duct and saccular duct were significant findings. The utriculo-endolymphatic valve and the ductus reuniens were not found to be indicative of Ménière disease.

Altmann and Kornfield[18] noted that only minimal histopathological changes are seen in the sensory epithelia of these cases. However, other investigators have identified a variety of ultrastructural abnormalities including loss of inner and outer hair cells, and spiral ligament fibrocytes,[19] as well as decreased strial vascularity.[20]

Endolymphatic hydrops has been documented at autopsy in a wide variety of disorders,[21] including acoustic trauma, autoimmune inner ear disease, chronic otitis media, Cogan syndrome, congenital deafness, fenestration of the otic capsule, leukemia, Mondini dysplasia, otosclerosis, serious labyrinthitis, syphilis, temporal bone trauma, and viral labyrinthitis.

28.3.3 Pathophysiology

The exact mechanism by which idiopathic ELH occurs remains unproven, although it has become a central theory that ELH causes the symptoms of Ménière syndrome. Specifically, this theory states that it is the increased pressure that causes the ear fullness, the hyperacusis and distorted hearing, and the

unsteadiness and disequilibrium. Furthermore, the theory holds that, if the membranous labyrinth breaks, the patient then suffers a severe episode of vertigo, with a decline in hearing and resultant tinnitus.

In contrast, Rauch et al,[22] in reviewing the temporal bone collection of the Massachusetts Eye and Ear Infirmary, have suggested that ELH does not cause the symptoms of Ménière syndrome, but rather is an epiphenomenon. These investigators theorize that ELH is perhaps an indicator of inner ear membrane dysfunction or failure, and that some other factors usually affect fluid management within the inner ear. Altered fluid management then produces both symptoms of ELH. Similar conclusions were reached by Swart and Schuknecht,[23] who reported the results of long-term destruction of the endolymphatic sac in monkeys.

Although the central role of ELH in Ménière syndrome remains controversial, several pathophysiological mechanisms have been proposed to explain its development. The most prevalent theory of pathophysiology of ELH is that the distention of the endolymphatic system occurs because of excessive accumulation of endolymph, primarily due to altered resorption by the endolymphatic duct and sac.[24] Altered resorption could be due to perisaccular and vestibular epithelial fibrosis,[25-28] altered glycoprotein metabolism,[29,30] viral infection of the inner ear,[7,31, 32] or immune-mediated injury.[33,34] In addition, anatomic abnormalities in the bony structures surrounding the endolymphatic duct might also influence the development of ELH.[28,35] A bony abnormality might cause only a marginal obstruction of the duct, but when added to these other factors would result in a much more severe obstruction to endolymph flow.

Gartner et al[36] used polymerase chain reaction to study the Scarpa ganglion of patients undergoing vestibular neurectomy for Ménière disease. Although herpes simplex and varicella zoster virus were found in the geniculate ganglion of most subjects, they were not found in the Scarpa ganglion of Ménière disease patients. In addition, when Ménière disease patients are treated with antiviral therapy, there has been no demonstrable effect. However, it should be noted that the lack of response to therapy is not evidence of pathophysiology.

As a corollary to the theory of excessive accumulation of endolymph, increased endolymphatic pressure is thought by many to cause the symptoms in these cases.[37,38] Furthermore, Zenner et al[39] have demonstrated experimentally that the hearing loss and tinnitus of ELH could be caused by ruptures of the membranes lining the endolymphatic space, so that potassium-rich endolymph intoxicates the sensory and neural structures. As a result of this potassium influx into the perilymph, the outer hair cells are depolarized, with shortening and loss of motility. Both fluctuating and chronic hearing loss in Ménière syndrome can be explained by this model.

Gibson[40] has proposed a new mechanism for vertigo: the endolymph drains too rapidly from the cochlear duct, which results in overfilling of the utricle and the semicircular canals. Stretching of the cristae then results in attacks of vertigo.

Other data tend to contradict the pressure hypothesis in ELH. For one thing, although various hearing abnormalities are commonly demonstrated[38] in experimental hydrops, vestibular dysfunction is rarely observed in these models. Also, Long and Morizono[41] measured the pressure gradients in experimental hydrops using microelectrode recording techniques, and found differences between endolymph and perilymph pressure that approximated 0.5 mm Hg. These investigators suggested that as pressure gradients increased, various corrective mechanisms such as an ion balance, endolymph secretion, and absorption are modulated to return the gradient to 0 mm Hg.

Kitahara et al,[42] in a series of elegant pressure studies using artificial endolymph, demonstrated that the auditory and vestibular abnormalities found in ELH most likely arise from biochemical rather than pressure alterations. Juhn et al[43] essentially concluded the same in their review of the subject. Following obliteration of the endolymphatic duct of guinea pigs, experimental findings, in addition to ELH, include a decrease in the endocochlear potential,[44] an increase in intracochlear calcium,[45] alterations in potassium permeability and in the inhibition of the electrogenic transport processes,[46] and increased endolymphatic fluid protein content.[47]

In summary, evidence exists that the symptoms of Ménière disease may be due to membranous ruptures or to some alteration in the biochemical gradients within the endolymphatic space. Undoubtedly, our theories of the pathophysiology of Ménière disease will seem rather naive in the future. At this writing, however, most investigators believe that idiopathic ELH or Ménière disease is a multifactorial illness, and that individuals might have more than one factor simultaneously contributing to the development of this problem.

28.3.4 Evaluation

The single most important step in the evaluation of the patient with recurrent vertigo and hearing loss is the medical history. An experienced clinician can often formulate the most likely diagnosis through history alone, and if Ménière syndrome is suspected, the history should then focus on the exclusion of other conditions that can mimic this disorder. Specifically, the diagnoses of perilymph fistula, chronic labyrinthitis, syphilis, acoustic tumor, and labyrinthine/cerebellar artery occlusion should be excluded.

Perilymph fistula is usually associated with sudden, severe sensorineural loss with disequilibrium, and only occasional vertigo episodes. However, fluctuating hearing loss and ear fullness can also be seen with this disorder. Most cases of perilymph fistula are associated with straining, barometric pressure changes, or trauma, although definitive exclusion can only be accomplished through surgical exploration in some cases.

Chronic labyrinthitis should be suspected if the patient gives a history of ear drainage, ear pain, or prior ear surgery. Late-stage syphilitic labyrinthitis should be suspected in any patient with prior treatment for syphilis and with slowly progressive sensorineural hearing loss and progressive disequilibrium. Late-stage syphilitic labyrinthitis can also be clinically indistinguishable from Ménière disease, with the only differentiating point being positive serology tests. Autoimmune inner ear syndrome should be suspected in patients with rapidly progressive or bilateral sensorineural hearing loss with episodic vertigo. These patients may have other autoimmune disorders such as systemic lupus erythematosa, rheumatoid arthritis, or vasculitis. Acoustic tumor cases are characterized by progressive unilateral sensorineural hearing loss, decreased speech discrimination, tinnitus, and disequilibrium rather than episodic vertigo.

On completing the initial history, the details of the illness including onset, associated symptoms, and duration and frequency of vertigo episodes, and the provoking factors should be determined. The presence of roaring tinnitus, ear fullness, and fluctuating hearing loss, and their relationship to the episodic vertigo should also be noted. The past medical history, the response to any prior treatments, and the family history of illness should then be recorded. Any related medical illnesses, such as adult-onset diabetes mellitus, migraine, or vascular insufficiency, in addition to their treatments, are then noted.

The next step in the evaluation of the patient with suspected Ménière syndrome is to perform the otolaryngological and head and neck examination. Any external or middle ear disease is noted, as are any related findings. Attention is then turned to the neurotologic examination. Spontaneous nystagmus, usually with the fast component beating away from the affected ear, is often visible with Frenzel glasses. Head-shake nystagmus is then elicited by having the patient rapidly shake the head back and forth 15 to 20 times, and then observing spontaneous nystagmus beating away from the affected ear. The Romberg, Quix, and rapid turning tests often show a drift toward the affected side, particularly if the patient has recently experienced vertigo. The Hennebert sign should be sought or a fistula test should be performed with either a pneumatic otoscope or by compressing the tragus into the ear canal. A deviation of the eyes away from the ear being tested is considered to be an objective positive test and is noted in some Ménière disease patients. A sensation of sway may be reported by the patient and is considered to be a subjectively positive symptom of dysfunction.

The audiometric evaluation of these patients includes a pure-tone audiogram with speech discrimination testing, tympanometry and immittance testing, and acoustic reflex decay testing. The pattern of results seen with Ménière disease was described earlier (see Clinical Presentation). If the initial evaluation suggests the possibility of Ménière disease, additional studies to confirm the diagnosis may be obtained, including dehydration testing, electrocochleography (ECochG), and vestibular evoked myogenic potentials (VEMPs).

Dehydration tests are performed using furosemide 20 to 40 mg p.o. This agent causes rapid diuresis, and as a result improved hearing thresholds can be noted in patients with early Ménière disease.[48] Although this information proves useful in some circumstances, most clinicians do not routinely use this study because of the unpleasant side effects of the test as well as the availability of other diagnostic studies.

Electrocochleography[49] uses computerized signal-averaging techniques to record the electrical signals from the cochlea and the auditory nerve in response to an auditory signal. Electrodes used for this study include transtympanic needles placed on the promontory of the cochlea, tympanic membrane electrodes, and ear canal electrodes. The major advantage of all three is an improved signal-to-noise ratio, so that the action potential or $N - 1$ is accentuated. With a variety of stimuli, including clicks and tone bursts with alternating polarity, the summating potential (SP) and action potential (AP) are further accentuated. Ménière disease is characterized by an enhanced SP, and, relative to the amplitude of the AP, an increased SP/AP ratio (▶ Fig. 28.3).

An SP/AP ratio above 0.40 is thought by many clinicians to indicate ELH,[49] although the test-retest reliability and specificity of this value remains in question.[50] This information is helpful

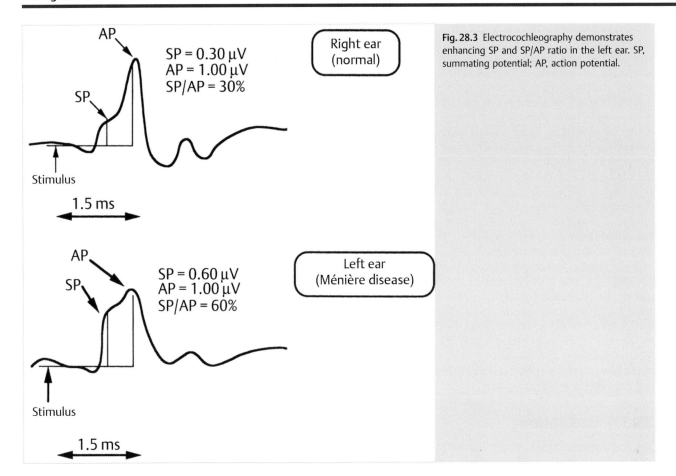

Fig. 28.3 Electrocochleography demonstrates enhancing SP and SP/AP ratio in the left ear. SP, summating potential; AP, action potential.

in cases where the diagnosis is not certain, such as differentiating nonhydropic sensorineural loss from early Ménière disease, and in the evaluation of the opposite ear in suspected bilateral Ménière disease.[51]

Vestibular testing provides limited though useful information in the evaluation of Ménière disease patients. Vestibular studies commonly employed include ENG, rotational testing, and computerized dynamic platform posturography (CDP). Vestibular function in Ménière disease patients fluctuates and is extremely variable, and as a result test data may be completely normal even in cases with active episodic vertigo. ENG enables separate evaluation of each labyrinth, and abnormalities including decreased caloric response and positional nystagmus are noted in 50% of Ménière disease patients.[52] ENG can be helpful to confirm the presence of a vestibular disorder, either by documentation of a deficit or by reproducing the symptoms for the patient.

Standard rotary chair testing has limited usefulness in the evaluation of patients with unilateral Ménière disease, because it evaluates both labyrinths simultaneously. During an acute vertigo episode, rotational testing can show an altered vestibular-ocular reflex (VOR), specifically phase shift, decreased gain, and an asymmetric response. However, between episodes, rotary chair testing is usually normal. However, O'Leary and Davis[53] have reported that with active head rotation or so-called vestibular autorotation in the vertical plane, Ménière disease patients typically demonstrate markedly increased gain. Rotational testing can be extremely helpful in the evaluation of compensation following vestibular surgery, bilateral vestibular disorders, and gentamicin treatment. When compensation has

occurred, the VOR symmetry and gain are usually within the normal range.

The VEMP can be used to evaluate the status of the saccule and the inferior vestibular nerve. The VEMP actually measures the contractions of the sternocleidomastoid muscle in response to acoustic stimulation of the saccule, that is, the sacculocolic reflex. VEMPs are records using a 750-Hz tone burst, at 95 dB HL. The stimulus rate is 4.3/second, with masking in the contralateral ear. The response is recorded using electrodes placed on the sternocleidomastoid muscle, which is placed under stretch tension. Usually 200 responses are averaged, and the threshold response is sought by lowering the signal intensity in 10 dB steps.

The VEMP response is a biphasic wave recorded between 13 and 23 ms after the stimulus, and its peaks are labeled P_{13} and P_{23}, respectively. Alternatively, these two waves are labeled P1 and N1, as noted in ▸ Fig. 28.4. The amplitude varies between 10 and 300 μV. The asymmetric ratio between sides utilizes a formula similar to that used for ENG. The peak-to-peak amplitude (A) is measured for both the left and right ears, A_L and A_R, respectively:

See the formula below.

$$\text{Asymmetric ratio (AR)} = \frac{A_L - A_R}{A_L + A_R} \times 100$$

A percent difference greater than 40% is considered significant.

In approximately half of patients with active Ménière disease,[54] the VEMP is asymmetric on the side of the affected ear; this is thought to indicate saccular hydrops,[55] but no definitive data have yet proved this point. However, an asymmetric VEMP

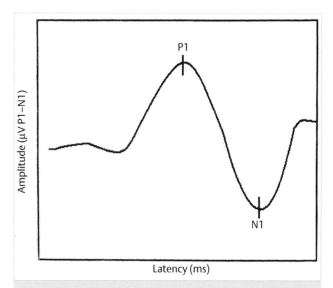

Fig. 28.4 Vestibular evoked myogenic potential. P1 and N1 denote the peaks of biphasic waveforms.

does indicate abnormal vestibular function, and therefore may confirm a history of Ménière syndrome or early ELH. Lin et al[56] have reported the value of VEMP in detecting early and asymptomatic saccular hydrops, and as a predictor of bilateral Ménière disease. Approximately 25% of asymptomatic ears have a hydropic pattern, when the opposite ear has definite Ménière disease.

The CDP is useful in determining if a patient in fact has vestibular dysfunction,[52] in measuring compensation after vestibular surgery, and in providing objective data to confirm the presence of a vestibular handicap. It is also useful in determining the proper physical therapy regimen for patients with stabilized vestibular deficits. However, it does not lateralize the side in Ménière disease nor does it provide pathognomonic findings to confirm Ménière disease.

Laboratory evaluation of patients with Ménière syndrome is aimed at excluding several readily identifiable disorders that can affect the patient with Ménière syndrome. These laboratory studies include fluorescent treponemal antibody absorption (FTA-Abs) or microhemagglutination–*Treponema pallidum* (MHA-TP) to exclude syphilis, fasting blood glucose to exclude adult-onset diabetes mellitus, cholesterol and triglyceride studies, and thyroid function tests. In addition, a large number of clinicians routinely obtain laboratory studies to exclude immune-related illnesses, particularly in bilateral Ménière syndrome. These studies include the sedimentation rate, antinuclear antibody, rheumatoid factor, antineutrphil cytoplasmic antibody (ANCA) tests, and, in some cases of atopy, the radioallergosorbent test (RAST).[21] If there is a strong suspicion of autoimmune inner ear syndrome, specific testing with humoral heat shock protein-70 (HSP-70) or cellular cochilin-tomoprotein (COCH) testing protein testing may be obtained. Many clinicians use a positive response to corticosteroid trial to denote a positive test for these disorders.

On rare occasions acoustic tumors can present with episodic vertigo. If, during the course of evaluating patients with suspected Ménière syndrome, the clinical features or audiometric or vestibular findings suggest the possibility of an acoustic tumor or another mass lesion, additional imaging studies should be performed. These studies should also be performed prior to any definitive surgical procedure. Diagnostic imaging usually includes magnetic resonance imaging (MRI) scans—either a focused internal auditory canal study (fast spin echo) or a contrasted study with gadolinium agents. In some cases, auditory brainstem responses or high-resolution computed tomography (CT) scans of the temporal bone might provide additional information.

Nakashima et al[57] have described the use of a 3-tesla MRI scan with intratympanic diluted gadolinium contrast to image Ménière disease patients. After perfusing the middle ear with an eightfold dilution of gadolinium, the contrast agent passed through the round window membrane into the scala tympani. Using a three-dimensional (3D) fluid-attenuated inversion recovery (FLAIR) technique, the scala media and scala tympani compartments could be readily seen. In patients with Ménière disease, there was only a small thin amount of gadolinium noted in scala tympani, as the scala media had expanded and taken up much of the space. Undoubtedly, further advances in imaging as well as clinical correlation of this finding will determine if intratympanic contrasted MRI scans have a role in these patients. For example, Gürkov et al[58] recently prospectively compared the results of ECochG studies, the duration of Ménière disease, and the degree of hearing loss with the degree of ELH as detected on MRI following intratympanic gadolinium administration. In this study, the degree of hydrops significantly correlated with positive ECochG findings, hearing loss, duration of illness, and saccular abnormalities as measured on VEMPs.

28.3.5 Classification and Staging

The Committee on Hearing and Equilibrium[1] of the AAO-HNS updated the diagnosis and classification of Ménière disease, as noted in the box below.

Diagnosis of Ménière Disease

- Certain Ménière disease
  - Definite Ménière disease, plus histopathological confirmation
- Definite Ménière disease
  - Two or more definitive spontaneous episodes of vertigo 20 minutes or longer
  - Audiometrically documented hearing loss on at least one occasion
  - Tinnitus or aural fullness in the treated ear
  - Other causes excluded
- Probable Ménière disease
  - One definitive episode of vertigo
  - Audiometrically documented hearing loss on at least one occasion
  - Tinnitus or aural fullness in the treated ear
  - Other causes excluded
- Possible Ménière disease
  - Episodic vertigo of the Ménière type without documented hearing loss, or
  - Sensorineural hearing loss, fluctuating or fixed, with disequilibrium but without definitive episodes

Other causes excluded

The diagnosis takes into account the certainty of the clinical diagnosis and includes possible, probably, definite, and certain Ménière disease. A single definitive episode of vertigo with documented hearing loss is considered probably Ménière disease, whereas multiple episodes with hearing loss are definite Ménière disease. In staging Ménière disease, the committee recommends that the stage be related to the hearing level only, as noted in ▶ Table 28.1. This staging system is in contrast to prior staging systems that were based on the frequency of vertigo episodes. The hearing level is based on a four-tone average of 0.5, 1, 2, and 3 kHz, obtained from the worst audiogram in the prior 6 months.

As a practical matter, it is most helpful to break down the course of Ménière disease in a way that the patient can understand. This means describing three clinical phases of the disease including early, middle, and late, as noted in ▶ Table 28.2.

In early Ménière disease, the hearing actively fluctuates, as does the fullness and tinnitus. The vertigo in these patients is infrequent and there may be long periods of remission associated with this phase. The middle phase is characterized by a fixed, flat sensorineural loss with reasonably good discrimination. These patients often have severe episodic vertigo that is accompanied by nausea, vomiting, ear blockage or fullness, and increased tinnitus. There may also be some positional vertigo and unsteadiness in this phase. The late phase is also known as the "burned-out" phase, and in this phase the hearing loss is fixed, and the discrimination is poor. In this phase, however, the patient complains of unsteady episodes and occasionally drop attacks or transient vertigo episodes; that is, there is no longer any severe vertigo episodes. Furthermore, it is helpful to discuss with the patient the finding that the usual course of this illness is to go to the late phase over the course of 10 to 15 years; that is, if the symptoms can be controlled, the patient will eventually stop having vertigo episodes. Describing this course is also helpful in sorting out the treatment options that the patient should consider.

28.3.6 Management of Early Phase Ménière Disease

The management of early-phase Ménière disease is directed at decreasing the fluid volume of the endolymph, increasing the circulation of the inner ear, or altering the immune reactivity or blockage of the endolymphatic duct.[21] None of these proposed regimens has ever been shown in the double-blind controlled study to be effective.[59] Despite that fact, most clinicians utilize one or more of these management strategies in an effort to alter the natural history of the disorder (▶ Table 28.3).

The most common management strategy is the use of a low-sodium diet and diuretic to decrease endolymph volume.[21] It is possible that this treatment strategy actually affects the inner

Table 28.1 Staging of Definite and Certain Ménière Disease*

Stage	Four-Tone Average (dB)
1	≤ 25
2	26–40
3	41–70
4	> 70

*Staging is based on the four-tone average (arithmetic mean rounded to the nearest whole number) of the pure-tone thresholds at 0.5, 1, 2, and 3 kHz of the worst audiogram during the interval 6 months before treatment. This is the same audiogram that is used as the baseline valuation to determine hearing outcome from treatment. Staging should be applied only to cases of definite or certain Ménière disease.

Table 28.2 Clinical Phases of Ménière Disease

	Early	Middle	Late
Hearing	Fluctuates	Fixed flat	Fixed flat
Discrimination	Good	Decreased	Poor
Tinnitus/fullness	Fluctuates	Constant	Constant
Vertigo	Infrequent	Severe	None
Unsteadiness/positional vertigo	None	Occasional	Frequent

Table 28.3 Management of Ménière Disease

Early Phase	Middle Phase	Late Phase
Diet	Vestibular suppressants	Vestibular suppression
Diuretic	Intratympanic gentamicin perfusion	Intratympanic gentamicin perfusion
Vasodilator therapy	Gentamicin deafferentation	Transmastoid labyrinthectomy
Vestibular suppressants	Vestibular nerve section	Vestibular rehab therapy
Short course of steroids	Vestibular rehab therapy	
Intratympanic steroid perfusion		
Endolymphatic sac surgery		
Pressure pulse treatment		

ear through an unrecognized indirect mechanism, such as altering the ionic balance in some way. For most clinicians, a low-sodium diet is targeted at 1,500 to 2,000 mg of sodium per day. This can be achieved by avoiding table salt and using a salt substitute, and avoiding obviously salty foods such as pickles, salty snacks, salty meats, and pizza. To this diet is added a diuretic, usually a combination of hydrochlorothiazide 25 mg and triamterene 37.5 mg, taken daily, with potassium supplements as needed. Occasionally, furosemide 20 to 40 mg per day is recommended, although daily potassium supplementation is required with this drug. The vast majority of patients tolerate this regimen quite well, although muscle cramps, itching, and weakness do occur. In cases where significant side effects occur, the dose can be decreased to one half. Alternatively, a carbonic anhydrase diuretic can be prescribed. Vertigo control varies between 50 and 70% with this regimen.[59]

Vasodilator therapy is based on the belief by many clinicians that Ménière disease is related to decreased inner ear blood flow. In this treatment strategy, the patient is instructed to avoid caffeine and nicotine completely. A vasodilating drug such as niacin, papaverine, or β-histamine is prescribed to improve the blood flow.[21] Lastly, the patient is told to avoid stressful situations and to begin a walking program for aerobic conditioning and for stress control. Although the effectiveness of this regimen in controlling Ménière disease can be questioned, it is extremely beneficial to the patient both physically and psychologically and has few side effects.

A third treatment strategy is to alter the immune response, using either corticosteroids or allergic desensitization. These agents act by decreasing inflammation, and theoretically they alter the fluid mechanics of the inner ear. Whether the endolymphatic sac function or the autoimmune response to inner ear membranes is actually changed is a matter of conjecture.

A course of corticosteroids is often recommended[21] for patients with (1) active unilateral Ménière disease with episodic vertigo unresponsive to vestibular suppressives and low-salt diet with diuretics, (2) Ménière disease with a sudden decrease in hearing threshold, or (3) bilateral Ménière disease. This treatment strategy typically takes one of two forms. The first is to use a dose pack of methylprednisolone, dexamethasone, or another corticosteroid. Although the regimen is convenient, questions have arisen as to whether the duration and dose are sufficient to suppress the immune response. The second regimen is to use prednisone 60 to 80 mg per day for 7 days, with a tapered dose over the next 7 days. Response to either regimen would indicate steroid responsiveness, in which case further prolonged use can be discussed with the patient. The side effects of short-term steroid use include appetite stimulation, irritability, heartburn and digestive disorder, and insomnia. The indigestion can be readily controlled using an antacid or an H2 blocker.

28.3.7 Intratympanic Dexamethasone Perfusion

If the patient has demonstrated oral steroid responsiveness or if the patient has a history of diabetes mellitus type 2, the clinician should consider intratympanic dexamethasone perfusion (ITDP) as the next step in management. Barrs et al[60] found that 52% of patients have relief of vertigo for 3 months with intratympanic dexamethasone given weekly for 4 weeks. Barrs et al noted the lower cost, ease of administration in the office, and low complication rate in recommending ITDP for persistent vertigo. Doyle et al[61] found that 76% of patients had at least temporary vertigo control with intratympanic dexamethasone (16 mg/mL). Neither group of authors found any improvement in hearing loss or tinnitus with this treatment.

Most clinicians perform ITDP in the office under local anesthesia. The drum is anesthetized using phenol on a small applicator in a location on the superior aspect of the drum. Dexamethasone (4–10 mg/mL) is slowly injected into the middle ear via a 25-gauge spinal needle passed through the spot treated with phenol. The steroid is slowly injected and approximately 0.5 mL is usually perfused to fill the middle ear. The patient reclines for 15 to 20 minutes to enable absorption. There is usually some transient mild vertigo triggered by the steroid that rapidly stops. The number of perfusions traditionally varied from one to three a week, but the current physician preference seems to be to perform the procedure daily for 3 days. Some clinicians fill the middle ear with a cellulose or hyaluronic acid matrix soaked with dexamethasone. Recently, Piu et al[62] reported a micronized drug delivery polymer that may allow a sustained release to the inner ear.

Vestibular suppressives and antiemetics also play a significant role in the management of patients with early Ménière syndrome. Vestibular suppressives are drugs with variable anticholinergic, sedative, and antiemetic effects that can be used to lessen the severity of the vertigo as well as the associated autonomic effects.[21] Some of the most useful are meclizine 12.5 to 25 mg p.o. t.i.d., dimenhydrinate 25 mg p.o. or p.r. every 6 to 8 hours, and oral diazepam 2.5 to 5 mg p.o. b.i.d. or t.i.d. The major side effect of these drugs is drowsiness, and the patient should avoid the use of alcohol or other nervous system depressants when taking them. Patients should also avoid driving while taking vestibular suppressives. Glycopyrrolate (Robinul) 1 or 2 mg p.o. b.i.d. or metoclopramide (Reglan) 10 mg p.o. b.i.d. is an effective antinauseant with few side effects (Baxter Pharmaceutical, Deerfield, IL). Antinauseants can be used on a continuous basis, whereas most vestibular suppressives should be used only as indicated.

Gates et al[63] have described a new medical treatment for early Ménière disease using a device to deliver transtympanic micropressure to the inner ear (Meniett, Medtronic Corp., Minneapolis, MN). The treatment theoretically lowers fluid pressure in the inner ear, and is self-administered by the patient two or three times per day. The physician places a tympanostomy tube, and instructs the patient as to how to place the ear plug that delivers the micropressure pulses. The Meniett device reportedly does have short-term efficacy, and appears to be safe. It is primarily used for patients who wish to avoid surgery, such as deafferentation procedures, and is helpful in the management of patients with bilateral Ménière disease. Some control of tinnitus and vertigo occurs in 50 to 60% of cases, and in the author's experience usually lasts for up to 18 months.

Some Ménière disease patients continue to have severe debilitating vertigo despite oral or suppository medication. In these cases, hospitalization is often indicated for rehydration and for intravenous therapy to lessen the symptoms. Ondansetron 4 to 8 mg can be given intravenously, very slowly over 60 minutes. Although the drug is effective in stopping acute nausea, it does cause drowsiness. Alternatively, diazepam 5 to 10 mg intravenously is also effective in controlling the episode of vertigo in these cases.

28.3.8 Endolymphatic Sac Surgery

Few procedures in otologic surgery have been as controversial as endolymphatic sac surgery. Opinions regarding the efficacy of this procedure vary from those who conclude that the procedure is effective in over 80% of cases to those who believe that the procedure is no better than a placebo or sham procedure.[64-69] Despite this controversy, most clinicians recommend endolymphatic surgery because it is a nondestructive procedure that can be performed on an outpatient basis. Endolymphatic sac surgery offers the possibility of vertigo control with little risk of morbidity. Theoretically, endolymphatic sac surgery improves the function of a scarified endolymphatic sac or opens a blocked endolymphatic duct. As a consequence, the pressure in the endolymphatic space is thought to decrease. Alternatively, endolymphatic sac surgery might cause a temporary subclinical labyrinthitis that perhaps alters the pattern of Ménière disease.

Most clinicians recommend endolymphatic sac surgery for Ménière disease cases in which the hearing continues to fluctuate and for early-phase Ménière disease. Endolymphatic sac surgery is recommended when the patient has life-altering vertigo, occurring once a month or more often. Some clinicians recommend endolymphatic sac surgery only in cases where an enlarged summating potential or an increased SP/AP ratio is observed on ECochG. In most cases, intratympanic steroid perfusion is performed at the same time as endolymphatic sac surgery. This technique is described above. In some cases, gentamicin is diluted to 10 mg/mL concentration, and this solution is used to fill the middle ear. Diluted gentamicin perfusion is chosen when the exact phase of the Ménière disease is not entirely clear.

The endolymphatic sac is exposed after performing a simple mastoidectomy through a postauricular incision. The endolymphatic sac is found embedded in the dura posteroinferior to the posterior semicircular canal (▶ Fig. 28.5a). It extends down inferiorly, under the vertical segment of the facial nerve and toward the top of the jugular bulb. The superior margin of the endolymphatic sac is defined by a line that extends the plane of the lateral semicircular canal and runs perpendicular to the posterior semicircular canal, the so-called Donaldson line. In most Ménière disease cases, the endolymphatic sac is placed a little more inferior than in normals. Once identified, the sac can be decompressed by removing the overlying bone, or it can be opened (▶ Fig. 28.5b) and its lumen probed. Currently the author prefers to decompress the sac and the posterior fossa dura plate, without opening the sac. Alternatively, the sac can be shunted into the mastoid, using a variety of tubing or sheeting materials. The incision is closed with buried absorbable sutures and the wound dressed.

The patient is followed at increasing intervals over the next 6 months. In cases where the procedure is effective, vertigo episodes are absent or occur significantly less often. Ear fullness and tinnitus are usually improved in the majority of patients also. In some patients, the hearing threshold markedly improves or stabilizes, although this occurs less often than vertigo improvement.

28.3.9 Management of the Middle Phase of Ménière Disease

The middle phase of Ménière disease is characterized by a flat sensorineural hearing loss, good discrimination scores, and, in some cases, severe episodic vertigo. There may also be positional vertigo. In most cases, these patients have been on early-phase therapy, including medical management, vestibular and nausea suppressants, and, in some cases, intratympanic steroid perfusion (ITSP). If the history suggests that there has been a recent decline in hearing, it is reasonable to consider endolymphatic sac surgery with ITSP for middle-phase patients.

However, middle-phase patients are often very frustrated by the lack of control of their episodic vertigo. Patients who have had two or three episodes of vertigo in the prior 3 months have life-altering vertigo and are ready to proceed with more aggressive management, such as deafferentation. The author prefers a step-wise approach to these patients, including (1) office-based diluted intratympanic gentamicin perfusion (ITGP); (2) middle ear exploration (MEE) with full-strength gentamicin perfusion, with simultaneous endolymphatic sac decompression; and (3) vestibular nerve section. The rationale and approach are discussed above (▶ Table 28.2).

28.3.10 Intratympanic Gentamicin Perfusion

Intratympanic gentamicin perfusion is performed on an outpatient basis, in the clinic setting, with local anesthesia. The gentamicin (40 mg/mL) is diluted with 1 part gentamicin and 3 parts normal saline for a final concentration of gentamicin 10 mg/mL. In this procedure, gentamicin penetrates the round window, mixes in the perilymph of the scala tympani, and travels through the cochlea, ultimately reaching the sensory neuroepithelia of the vestibule and the semicircular canals. Because gentamicin is relatively more vestibulotoxic than it is cochleotoxic, this results in a mild vestibular deficit without hearing loss. With diluted gentamicin, a vestibular deficit occurs in approximately 50% of patients, with a very low incidence of sensorineural hearing loss. In addition, there may be additional effects of the gentamicin on the labyrinth, including decreased endolymph production, although this remains unproven.

When the gentamicin causes vestibular deficit, the episodic vertigo is significantly modified, and the episodes are described as mostly a sense of unsteadiness. The need for vestibular suppressives is markedly diminished in these cases, an effect that usually lasts for months to years.

Intratympanic gentamicin perfusion is performed through the tympanic membrane under microscopic vision. After anesthetizing the tympanic membrane (▶ Fig. 28.6) using a 25-gauge spinal needle, the solution is slowly infused into the middle ear. After the middle ear is filled, the patient remains in the supine position with the head partly turned to allow the drug to make contact with the round window membrane. Patients may feel a slight vertigo sensation during the perfusion because of the caloric effect of the solution, and may also feel a slight burning sensation.

Intratympanic gentamicin perfusion is performed once a week until an effect is noted. The gentamicin effect can be seen

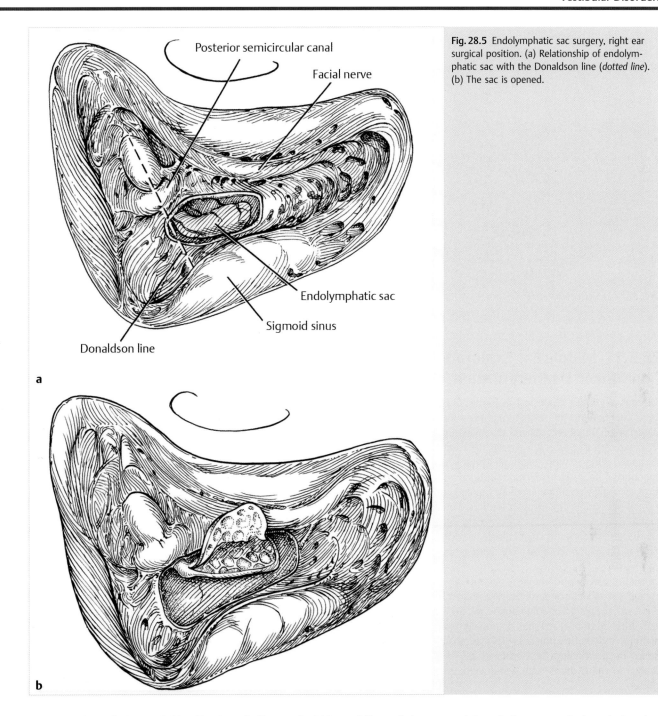

Posterior semicircular canal

Facial nerve

Endolymphatic sac

Sigmoid sinus

Donaldson line

a

b

Fig. 28.5 Endolymphatic sac surgery, right ear surgical position. (a) Relationship of endolymphatic sac with the Donaldson line (*dotted line*). (b) The sac is opened.

with a single perfusion, and this effect is typically noted within 5 days. When the gentamicin effect occurs, patients typically note a pulling or swaying sensation or a sense of disequilibrium. Spontaneous nystagmus away from the treated ear can also be seen with Frenzel glasses at this point. If the gentamicin effect is noted or if a hearing loss occurs, ITGP is discontinued. Most patients demonstrate the gentamicin effect with one to three perfusions. Some clinicians give a single perfusion and wait a full month to gauge the effect.

Despite the best efforts of the clinician, approximately 15% of patients have no improvement following two ITGPs. This is thought to be due to a variety of factors, including blockage of the round window niche by tissue or inflammatory scarring,

failure of the gentamicin solution to reach the window because of a narrow niche, or a lack of viscosity with the solution. Several approaches to this problem have been reported including the placement of a micro-wick device to transmit the drug to the window, the use of hyaluronic acid with the gentamicin solution, and the placement of oxycellulose gelatin through the drum into the middle ear to act as a reservoir. Plontke[70] reported the visualization of the round window using a small, 1.2-mm endo-otoscope introduced through the tympanic membrane. He suggests that this procedure be performed at the time of the initial ITGP, and if a secondary blockage is found, the patient should then have a formal MEE.

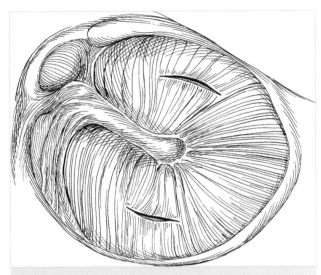

Fig. 28.6 Transtympanic gentamicin perfusion, right ear, surgical position.

28.3.11 Middle Ear Exploration with Gentamicin Deafferentation

Alternatively, most clinicians, including Crane et al,[71] recommend that patients not responding have either MEE or vestibular nerve section. I recommend that patients who fail in-office ITGP undergo MEE with full-strength gentamicin application to the round window with gelatin pledgets. At this setting, a tympanomeatal flap is elevated and the round window is inspected for a secondary membrane, which can be gently removed with a small right-angled instrument without damaging the primary round window membrane. A secondary membrane accounts for the vast majority of ITGP failures, according to Crane et al. Packing the round window niche with gelatin and then instilling full-strength (40 mg/mL) gentamicin usually creates a significant deafferentation in these patients, and there is a slightly greater risk of sensorineural hearing loss. At the same setting, I prefer to include an endolymphatic sac decompression, which adds little additional risk but potentially reverses some of the hydrops and the hearing loss. This approach is further reinforced by the findings of Fiorino et al,[72,73] who reported no change in the hydrops with gentamicin, on the basis of MRI studies.

28.3.12 Retrosigmoid Vestibular Nerve Section

Retrosigmoid vestibular nerve section (RVNS) is an effective procedure for the control of episodic vertigo with preservation of hearing (▶ Fig. 28.7). It is indicated for patients with hearing better than 70 dB HL and discrimination better than 30%. Following Silverstein's and Norrell's introduction of the retrolabyrinthine approach to vestibular nerve section, the procedure has undergone a slow evolution to the current approach.[74] RVNS offers superior, readily obtained exposure of the cochleovestibular nerve with a low incidence of complications. The ease and rapidity of the exposure makes RVNS the preferred approach over the middle fossa vestibular nerve section for the vast majority of clinicians. The vestibular nerve can be selectively sectioned through the retrosigmoid approach, and, if necessary, the internal auditory canal can be drilled for additional exposure of the branches. However, a complete or near-complete vestibular nerve section can be performed in virtually every case with this exposure. RVNS requires hospitalization for several days after surgery, in addition to an overnight stay in the intensive care unit for monitoring. As a consequence, RVNS is also a more costly procedure for the control of episodic vertigo.

An RVNS is indicated in patients with unilateral Ménière disease and with a fixed or stable sensorineural loss in the serviceable range. It is much more effective for the episodic vertigo of Ménière disease than other vestibular disorders, perhaps as a result of better patient selection.[74] RVNS can also be employed if other procedures such as ITGP or endolymphatic sac surgery have failed. Successful elimination of episodic vertigo occurs in nearly 90% of cases. Neither the hearing nor the ELH appears to be altered by the procedure.

The procedure is performed with the patient in the supine position with the head turned away and secured in Mayfield pins. At the inception of the procedure, the patient is given mannitol 100 g, furosemide 40 mg, and Solu-Cortef 125 mg intravenously. These drugs, coupled with hyperventilation of the patient, result in decreased cerebrospinal fluid (CSF) volume and pressure. A C-shaped incision (or standard suboccipital incision) is made behind the ear and the skin and musculoperiosteum are elevated to the level of the mastoid. Several mastoid emissary veins must be controlled during this process. The posterior portion of the mastoid is opened with the drill to identify the location of the sigmoid sinus. The bony plate immediately behind the sigmoid sinus is outlined with the drill, removed, and set aside for replacement at closure. This exposes dura for about 5 cm in length and width, behind the sigmoid sinus and below the transverse sinus. The dura is opened in a cruciate fashion, and the dural leaves are retracted with sutures. The blade of the self-retaining retractor is used to gently retract the cerebellum from inferior. After draining the CSF from the basal cistern, the cerebellum can usually be retracted to provide adequate exposure of the cochleovestibular nerve. The arachnoid surrounding the nerve is gently dissected to further expose the cochleovestibular and facial nerves.

The cleavage plane between the vestibular and cochlear portions of the nerve is then identified, and usually a small blood vessel runs in the plane. The superior half of the nerve or the vestibular portion is sectioned using a 90-degree back-cutting knife and microscissors. In most cases, the bundles within the nerve clearly differentiate the vestibular portion. Care is taken to avoid injuring the facial nerve. On completing the nerve section, the subarachnoid space is inspected for bleeding, and if none is seen, the dura is closed. Either the bone plate is replaced or cranioplasty is performed. Then the incision is closed in multiple layers.

28.3.13 Middle Fossa Vestibular Nerve Section

This procedure has advantages over the RVNS. The middle fossa approach is primarily extradural and offers the opportunity to visualize the separate nerve bundles discretely (▶ Fig. 28.8). As a result, some clinicians are of the opinion that the middle fossa

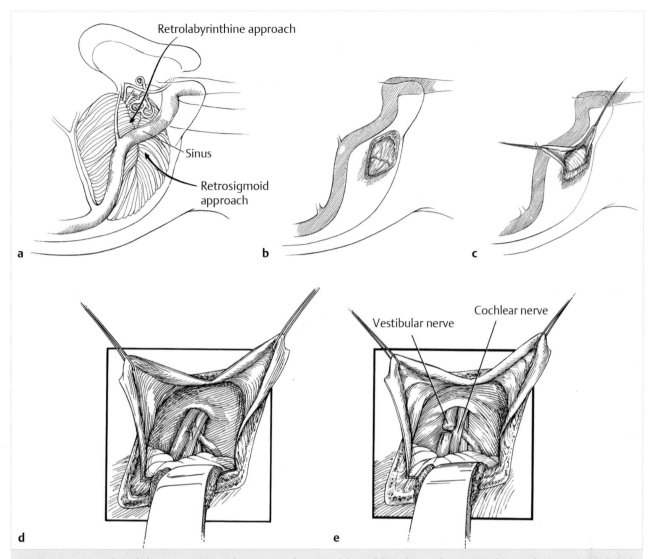

Fig. 28.7 Retrosigmoid vestibular nerve section, right ear, surgical position. (a) Retrolabyrinthine and retrosigmoid approaches are compared. (b) Bone removal. (c) Dural opening. (d) Cochleovestibular nerve demonstrating cleavage plane between divisions. (e) Vestibular nerve (superior portion of eighth nerve complex) is sectioned.

approach enables a more complete and thorough nerve section. However, the middle fossa exposure is somewhat more difficult as compared with RVNS, including the orientation of the procedure as well as the greater difficulty sectioning the inferior vestibular nerve, and probably slightly higher risk of hearing loss and facial palsy.

28.3.14 Management of Late-Phase Ménière Disease

The late phase of Ménière disease is sometimes referred to as the "burned out" phase. It is characterized by severe hearing loss, poor speech understanding, and episodes of unsteadiness as opposed to vertigo. Some patients, however, have occasional vertigo episodes, positional vertigo, and "drop attacks" or the crisis of Tumarkin. In general vestibular suppressants, supportive therapy, and vestibular rehabilitation control most of the symptoms. In some cases, the vestibular symptoms become incapacitating and the clinician should consider deafferentation.

Late-phase Ménière patients tend to be older, so that preoperative assessment of vestibular function and the ability of the patient to compensate for the procedure are indicated. ENG testing usually gives valuable information as to the degree of vestibular weakness in the involved ear as well as the normal one. An assessment of gait, coordination, and agility by the clinician or by a physical therapist is also useful. Furthermore, the physical therapist can prepare the patient for gait training, walking aids, and the planned postoperative therapy at the visit. If the opposite ear is abnormal or if the potential for compensation is poor, recovery is much less predictable and the clinician should not proceed with deafferentation. Deafferentation in late-phase Ménière patients can be performed in two ways: ITGP or transmastoid labyrinthectomy. ITGP, which was discussed earlier, offers some advantages, including that it is performed on an outpatient basis with local anesthesia, and it entails a low risk of complications, a slower onset, and a gradual deafferentation. The slower deafferentation is better tolerated in some patients,

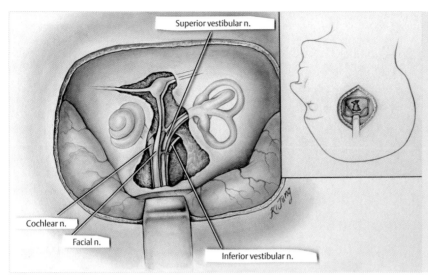

Fig. 28.8 Middle fossa vestibular nerve section. Right ear, surgical position. The superior and inferior vestibular nerves are cut.

Superior vestibular n.

Cochlear n.

Facial n.

Inferior vestibular n.

and preservation of residual hearing may be helpful in sound localization.

28.3.15 Transmastoid Labyrinthectomy

A traditional procedure for Ménière disease, transmastoid labyrinthectomy (TML), cures a high percentage of patients with episodic vertigo without entailing an intracranial procedure. By removing the vestibular neuroepithelium, the vestibular function in the operated ear is completely ablated. This results in control of vertigo in more than 90% of cases. Unfortunately, the hearing is also lost with this procedure. Patient selection may play a significant role in the outcome of TML, as the clinician is much more likely to recommend this procedure to those patients with unequivocal unilateral vestibular dysfunction. Generally, a preoperative ENG must show normal caloric function in the opposite ear. TML usually requires postoperative hospitalization until the patient can tolerate oral intake and can ambulate with assistance. Transcanal labyrinthectomy is an alternative procedure to TML, and although it can be performed with less exposure, it is difficult to be certain that all of the sensory neuroepithelium has been removed with this procedure. Translabyrinthine vestibular nerve section is an alternative to TML, which adds the section of the vestibular nerve to the removal of the sensory neuroepithelium. Translabyrinthine vestibular nerve section, as compared with TML, is associated with greater complications, including headache and CSF leak, without any noticeable improvement in results.

Transmastoid labyrinthectomy is indicated in patients with unilateral Ménière disease and severe sensorineural hearing loss. Most clinicians use a hearing criteria of a pure-tone average greater than 70 dB and speech discrimination worse than 30%. These criteria are flexible, however, and under certain circumstances a clinician might use a pure-tone average of 50 dB and speech discrimination of 50%. Factors that might influence these criteria are hearing loss in the contralateral ear, older age, and prior otologic procedures. Additionally, the certainty that TML stops the vertigo episodes and the rapidity with which it does so are distinct advantages for many patients.

Transmastoid labyrinthectomy is performed through a postauricular incision (▶ Fig. 28.9). After completing a simple mastoidectomy, the semicircular canals are carefully identified by removing the surrounding air cells. The location of the vertical segment of the facial nerve is also verified. The lateral, superior, and upper half of the posterior semicircular canals are opened, with care taken to avoid injury to the tympanic segment and second genu of the facial nerve. On opening the ampullated ends of the lateral and superior canals, the sensory neuroepithelium is removed. The bridge of bone between the crura of the lateral canal is then opened, allowing removal of the utricle and the saccule. The inferior portion of the posterior semicircular canal, under the vertical segment of the facial nerve, is carefully opened and the posterior canal ampulla is removed. After careful inspection to be certain of the complete removal, the postauricular incision is closed with buried absorbable sutures.

Other procedures are no longer performed by most clinicians, including streptomycin perfusion of the lateral semicircular canal or of the middle ear.[75] Cochleosacculotomy is performed infrequently in elderly patients with Ménière disease who would otherwise be candidates for TML. In each of these procedures, the incidence of sensorineural hearing loss is extremely high. In addition, a critical review of the data regarding the use of microvascular decompression of the cochleovestibular nerve has led to the conclusion by most clinicians that this procedure is not effective for episodic vertigo of Ménière disease.[76,77]

If vestibular surgery results in stable vestibular function, the patient may benefit from vestibular rehabilitation. Vestibular exercises can help in the early stages of vestibular compensation after a deafferentation procedure. Specific vestibular rehabilitation therapy can also aid in vestibular compensation, and particularly in cases with persistent disequilibrium. After 4 to 6 weeks, most patients are able to return to all of the activities of daily living including work, driving, and exercise.

28.4 Perilymph Fistula

A patient with a perilymph fistula (PLF) can present with symptoms virtually indistinguishable from those of Ménière syndrome. There are four recognized patterns of this disorder: (1) vertigo episodes without hearing loss; (2) hearing loss without vertigo; (3) a Ménière syndrome pattern; and (4) a

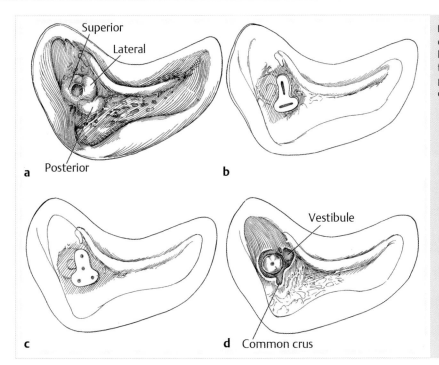

a — Superior, Lateral, Posterior
b
c
d — Vestibule, Common crus

Fig. 28.9 Transmastoid labyrinthectomy. Right ear, surgical position. (a) The labyrinth is skeletonized. (b) The lateral and posterior canals are fenestrated. (c) Deeper bone removal reveals two pairs of "snake eyes." (d) The superior canal is opened and followed to the vestibule.

miscellaneous pattern with disequilibrium but not episodic vertigo.[78] Unlike Ménière syndrome, PLF is usually associated with either an implosive or an explosive event, such as straining or causing the ear to pop. PLF also occurs after stapedectomy. It should be noted, however, that spontaneous PLFs have been discovered at the time of endolymphatic sac surgery for classic Ménière disease.

Middle ear exploration is recommended to repair an obvious traumatic perilymph leak, to attempt hearing preservation, and to resolve the disequilibrium. There are no uniform criteria for selecting patients for middle ear exploration, but a history of antecedent trauma, vertigo, and sensorineural hearing loss favors the diagnosis of PLF. The diagnosis is based primarily on the presentation of the symptom complex and a high index of clinical suspicion.

Most patients demonstrate a positive fistula test; that is, pneumatic pressure on the tympanic membrane triggers a brief sense of movement and perhaps eye deviation. Recently, in an effort to find a diagnostic marker, a variety of proteins associated with perilymph fluid have been studied, including β_2-transferrin, B-trace protein, and cochlin-tomoprotein. Of these, cochlin-tomoprotein appears to be the most promising with regard to sensitivity and specificity.[79] Cochlin-tomoprotein is a perilymph-specific protein, although assays are not readily available at this time. In the future, a positive cochlin-tomoprotein assay will likely be a strong indication for surgical exploration.

Middle ear exploration is performed through a transcanal approach. Either perichondrium or temporalis fascia is used to seal the round (or oval) window. Surgical repair of PLF will most likely improve vertigo; hearing and tinnitus can improve according to some reports. After surgery the patient should be cautioned against heavy lifting or straining for several weeks.

28.4.1 Superior Semicircular Canal Dehiscence

Superior semicircular canal dehiscence (SSCD) is a syndrome characterized by vertigo and oscillopsia induced by loud sounds or by stimuli that change middle ear or intracranial pressure (► Fig. 28.10; ► Fig. 28.11).[80] Specifically, the Tullio phenomenon (visual distortion caused by loud sounds), the Hennebert sign, and Valsalva maneuvers all elicit vestibular symptoms. These findings are thought to be caused by the excessive movement of perilymph, as a result of a defect in the bony semicircular canal.

Approximately 70% of patients have an air–bone gap on the affected side, and the tuning fork tests typically confirm this finding. Some of these patients have undergone exploration of the middle ear for possible stapedectomy, at which time a mobile stapes footplate was found. The explanation for the air–bone gap is an increased sensitivity to bone conduction, again caused by increased perilymph movement with skull vibration. Stapes reflexes are present.

The VEMP is very useful in the evaluation of patients suspected to have SSCD. As described earlier, the VEMP records the sacculocolic reflex, specifically recording the contractions of the sternocleidomastoid muscle. The response is typically recorded at 95-dB levels, but in cases of SSCD the response can be recorded at 65- to 75-dB HL levels in the affected ear. In addition, patients with an air–bone gap would not be expected to have a response at such lower thresholds. Theoretically, acoustic stimulation of the saccule is increased by excessive perilymph movement, resulting in increased response of the sternocleidomastoid muscle.

High-resolution temporal bone CT scans are used to document the presence of SSCD. Using coronal views in the plane of the superior canal, the bony labyrinth is specifically visualized

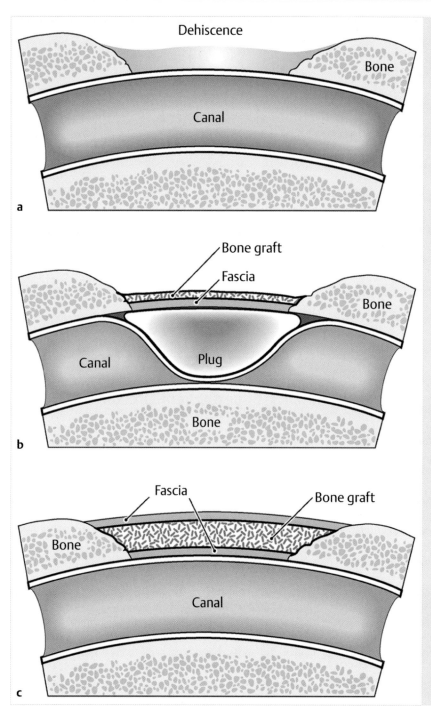

Fig. 28.10 (a) The bony dehiscence of the superior semicircular canal. (b) Plugging of the canal with soft tissue and covering the defect with fascia and bone graft. (c) Resurfacing of the canal.

and inspected for thinning or dehiscence. The affected ear is also compared with the contralateral side, using 0.5-mm cuts. Minor[80] has reported that CT scans of the temporal bone have 100% sensitivity, 99% specificity, and a positive predictive rate of 93%. However, Vrabek (personal communication) has presented findings that suggest 9% of all normals have thin bone over the superior semicircular canal.

Most patients with SSCD have mild to moderate symptoms, which can be managed with an ear plug or avoidance of loud sounds. However, some patients are debilitated by their symptoms, and in these cases surgical repair should be considered. Two approaches have been reported: (1) resurfacing of the de-

hiscence with bone or bone cement, and (2) soft tissue plugging of the canal to diminish the excessive perilymph movement. Minor[80] recommends superior canal occlusion or plugging through either a middle fossa or transmastoid approach.

Today, most clinicians prefer the transmastoid approach to occlude the superior canal.[81] The procedure is technically similar to that described for the posterior canal later in this chapter. Although this approach does carry a small risk of hearing loss, nearly 90% of patients report relief of their vestibular symptoms following canal plugging. The transmastoid approach also reduces the risk associated with middle fossa surgery, and can be performed as an outpatient procedure.

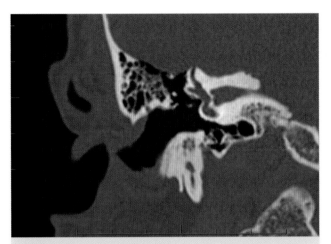

Fig. 28.11 Coronal CT scan demonstrates a right-sided superior semicircular canal dehiscence.

28.4.2 Labyrinthine Concussion and Temporal Bone Fractures

Following a head injury with a concussion, patients may experience position- and motion-induced vertigo and unsteadiness, in addition to high-frequency sensorineural hearing loss.[21] This can occur even in the absence of visible temporal bone fractures on CT scans. These patients have findings that are characterized as a labyrinthine concussion, and are thought to be due to damage to the membranous labyrinth through shearing forces.

A more severe head injury may result in a temporal bone fracture, which may produce both immediate and delayed vestibular symptomatology. The two types of temporal bone fractures encountered are capsular and extracapsular.

Capsular fractures run transverse across the petrous ridge, and are most often due to a severe blow to the occiput. A Battle sign often accompanies this type of fracture, and this sign is indicative of the severity of the injury. Total loss of hearing and the abrupt onset of severe vertigo accompany this type of fracture, which disrupts the cochlea or the semicircular canals. Because these patients are often comatose for several weeks following their injury, the vestibular system may be partly compensated when the problem is first discovered on regaining consciousness. Most of these patients experience unsteadiness and disequilibrium for up to 6 months, as the membranous labyrinth becomes fixated by labyrinthitis ossificans and as vestibular compensation occurs. The hearing loss is permanent.

Extracapsular fractures of the temporal bone usually run longitudinal or vertical to the petrous ridge. These fractures are more common, and occur in association with a blow to the temporoparietal region of the skull. The vestibular complaints and findings with this fracture are much less severe than those found with capsular fractures. If severe vertigo occurs, a PLF due to ossicular disruption should be suspected. The hearing loss associated with this fracture is usually conductive in nature, although high-frequency sensorineural loss can occasionally be seen. The usual vestibular complaints with this type of fracture are positional vertigo, motion-induced vertigo, and disequilibrium. Most of these symptoms resolve spontaneously, although vestibular rehabilitation and particle repositioning maneuvers may be indicated in some cases. A more complete discussion of temporal bone trauma can be found in Chapter 22.

28.4.3 Syphilitic Labyrinthitis

The incidence of syphilitic labyrinthitis has diminished considerably with improved treatments for human immunodeficiency virus as well as other sexually transmitted diseases. A recent Medline search found no new articles concerning the disease since 1997. However, it is imperative to consider syphilis as the possible etiology of any rapidly progressive hearing loss, with or without vertigo. In the early stages of syphilitic labyrinthitis, vestibular symptoms are uncommon and these cases may be characterized by progressive sensorineural hearing loss only. Steckelberg and McDonald[82] found in 38 cases of syphilitic labyrinthitis that the hearing loss was bilateral in 82% of cases and unilateral in 18%. Episodic vertigo was present in 42% of these cases.

As the patient ages into the 40s and 50s, syphilitic labyrinthitis is characterized not only by progressive hearing loss but also by episodic disequilibrium and vertigo. Wilson and Zoller[83] found that 80% of these patients had vestibular disturbances. Many of these patients have symptoms indistinguishable from Ménière syndrome.

The pathophysiology in these cases is related to the progression of vasculitis and obliterative endarteritis of the otic capsule.[84] If the bone overlying the semicircular canal is necrosed and sequestered, the patient develops signs indicative of a fistula of the lateral canal. These symptoms include a positive Hennebert sign as well as a positive Tullio sign. If the endarteritis involves the endolymphatic duct, a gumma or reactive fibrosis can block the duct with resultant symptoms of ELH.

The diagnosis of syphilitic labyrinthitis should be considered in any case of episodic vertigo with progressive hearing loss. Either the fluorescent treponemal antibody absorption test (FTA-Abs) or the rapid plasma reagin (RPR) test should be obtained during the initial evaluation. If either of these tests is positive, the patient should be treated for syphilis. The treatment in syphilitic labyrinthitis includes a combination of intramuscular (IM) and oral penicillin and corticosteroids. Because the spirochete replicates very slowly, prolonged therapy is necessary. Initially benzathine penicillin 2.4 million units IM is given weekly for 3 weeks.[16] This dose is then followed with oral Pen VK 500 mg q.i.d. for 3 months. Alternatively, intravenous penicillin G in high doses can be used in place of the benzathine penicillin. To this antibiotic regimen is added prednisone 40 to 60 mg per day. Surprising recovery of hearing can accompany this treatment. After 3 months, the prednisone can be tapered, depending on the stability of the hearing threshold. Vestibular symptoms are also improved in the vast majority of these patients.

28.4.4 Vascular Occlusion of the Labyrinthine/Cerebellar Artery

Occlusion of the labyrinthine artery leads to sudden profound loss of both cochlear and vestibular function. Although this condition tends to occur in older patients, it can also be seen in younger individuals with atherosclerotic vascular disease or with hypercoagulation disorder. Prior to the occlusion, patients often complain of episodic vertigo, which can herald the onset of transient ischemic attacks (TIAs). Baloh[85] reported that 62% of TIA patients experience episodic vertigo, and for 18% an isolated episode of vertigo was the initial symptom. TIAs are manifested by a variety of neurologic findings, including visual difficulties or amaurosis fugax, syncope, ataxia, extremity weakness, slurred speech or aphasia, and confusion. Early recognition of this possibility may allow preventive measures to prevent a stroke.

Lee[86] has further defined the various cerebellar stroke syndromes, including superior cerebellar, and inferior cerebellar. Inferior cerebellar strokes are due to occlusions of the posterior inferior cerebellar artery (PICA) or to occlusion of the anterior inferior cerebellar artery (AICA). Although cerebellar strokes are usually associated with other neurologic sequelae, some strokes can mimic acute peripheral vestibulopathy, or as Lee has termed it "pseudo-acute peripheral vestibulopathy." This can present with only peripheral vestibular findings and is most often due to occlusion of the medial branch of the PICA. Similarly, occlusion of the AICA can cause mild hearing loss and acute vertigo.

Once labyrinthine artery is occluded, the hearing loss is usually total and permanent. The acute vertigo episode subsides, leaving the patient with residual unsteadiness and disequilibrium. Over 4 to 6 months, the patient typically improves as the vestibular system undergoes compensation. Pathological studies of these cases reveal widespread necrosis of the membranous structures as well as labyrinthitis ossificans.[85] As the inner ear ossifies, the membranous structures become fixated, further aiding the compensation of these cases. If the labyrinthine artery occlusion is suspected, these patients should be referred for consultation with their internist, as this condition might represent a sentinel event in the development of atherosclerotic vascular disease.

Occlusion of the anterior vestibular artery also causes hearing loss and vertigo. Occlusion of the anterior vestibular artery usually results in the loss of hearing in the higher frequencies. Because the posterior vestibular circulation remains intact, these patients can experience benign paroxysmal positional vertigo (BPPV). After these patients are started on a management plan for their vestibular complaints, they should also be referred for evaluation and further therapy to their internist.

Medical management of suspected TIAs and stroke should include timely evaluation and initiation of therapy, ideally in less than 1 hour. Initial treatments before thrombolytic therapy, may include treatment of hypoglycemia or hyperglycemia, treatment of blood pressure abnormalities, cardiac monitoring, administration of fluids, and oxygen or respiratory assistance if indicated. Thrombolytic therapy usually includes intravenous or endovascular administration of tissue-type plasminogen activator (t-PA), depending on CT angiography findings. Further evaluation of possible cardiac arrhythmias should be considered in acute stroke patients, as embolic disease is often the etiology.

Once the patient is stabilized and thrombolytic therapy begun, the clinician should focus on controlling risk factors. Most patients who have had occlusions of the various cerebellar or labyrinthine arteries are treated with antiplatelet therapy such as aspirin, clopidogrel bisulfate, or, in some cases, warfarin.

Cholesterol lowering agents such as simvastatin or atorvastatin calcium as well as appropriate antihypertensive agents may also be indicated. Vestibular suppressants, antiemetics, and vestibular rehabilitation are also prescribed to further enhance recovery.

28.5 Labyrinthine Fistulas and Labyrinthitis

Erosion of the bony labyrinth by a cholesteatoma leads to the development of a labyrinthine fistula. Fistulas can develop over the lateral, superior, or posterior semicircular canal, as well as over the stapes footplate and cochlea. The symptoms that occur depend on the location and rate of growth of the fistula. If the fistula develops over the stapes footplate or the cochlea, the patient usually experiences mild unsteadiness or vertigo with a sensorineural hearing loss. If the fistula develops over a semicircular canal, vertigo and a positive fistula test are the predominant symptoms, although a mild sensorineural loss is often found. Ear drainage, conductive hearing loss, inflammation, and pain are superimposed on both conditions in the majority of cases. Evaluation of these patients should include microscopic examination and cleaning of the ear to identify the pathology, audiometric examination, and CT scans of the temporal bones. Labyrinthine fistula is a strong indication for surgery in these cases.

Labyrinthitis can develop if bacterial toxins, tissue fluids, or bacteria enter the labyrinthine fluid compartments. Labyrinthitis can be further subdivided into serous labyrinthitis and suppurative labyrinthitis.

Serous labyrinthitis occurs during the course of an episode of acute otitis media or mastoiditis. These patients present with vertigo of varying degrees as well as sensorineural hearing loss. Prompt treatment results in rapid recovery to normal status. In serous labyrinthitis, only bacterial toxins enter the fluid compartments, so that damage is usually not permanent, and therefore serous labyrinthitis is only diagnosed retrospectively, when there is recovery following treatment. Evaluation of serous and suppurative labyrinthitis is essentially the same as that described for labyrinthine fistula.

Suppurative labyrinthitis, on the other hand, presents with more severe vertigo and severe hearing loss in association with the acute otitis media. Suppurative labyrinthitis seems to occur in patients who have extremely intense pain and pressure in the ear. Following bacterial invasion of the inner ear, white blood cell invasion, fibrous exudate formation, membranous destruction, and labyrinthitis ossificans can occur in the inner ear. Bacterial invasion usually occurs through the round or oval window, and can follow surgical procedures such as stapedectomy. Unlike serous labyrinthitis, the hearing loss does not recover following suppurative labyrinthitis, although the vertigo improves with the development of labyrinthitis ossificans and with vestibular compensation. Treatment for both serous and suppurative labyrinthitis is aimed at drainage of the inflammatory focus, which might include myringotomy, mastoidectomy, or tympanomastoidectomy. Proper antibiotic coverage with corticosteroids is also indicated in these conditions.

28.6 Acoustic Tumors

Acoustic tumors most often present with unilateral progressive sensorineural hearing loss, tinnitus, and disequilibrium. Rarely these patients present with true episodic vertigo, which may be a reflection of either ELH or possibly a sudden change in the tumor size.

28.7 Episodic Vertigo Without Hearing Loss

The differential diagnosis of episodic vertigo without hearing loss includes vestibular neuritis, BPPV, vestibulotoxicity due to drugs, and migraine-associated vertigo (MAV). To rapidly differentiate these entities, vestibular neuritis present as sudden-onset acute vertigo without hearing loss, usually as a single episode; BPPV presents as multiple brief episodes of vertigo brought on by changing head positions; vestibulotoxicity is a chronic unsteadiness and ataxia that follows the intravenous administration of antibiotics; MAV presents with multiple episodes of vertigo without hearing change, and is often accompanied by chronic disequilibrium and positional vertigo. MAV usually has associated headaches.

28.7.1 Vestibular Neuritis

Vestibular neuritis presents as a sudden episode of vertigo without hearing loss in an otherwise healthy patient. It can occur in a single-attack form as well as multiple-attack form, and can affect one or both ears.

Clinical Presentation

Vestibular neuritis has been referred to as viral labyrinthitis, epidemic vertigo, neurolabyrinthitis epidemica, acute labyrinthitis, acute vestibular deficit syndrome, vestibular neuronitis, and Scarpa ganglionitis.[87] It occurs most often in the spring and early summer months. As a result, vestibular neuritis is often associated with upper respiratory infections, occurring 2 to 3 weeks afterward. Vestibular neuritis shows no specific sex predilection, but it is noted more often in patients in their 30 s and 40 s.

Three forms of vestibular neuritis can be differentiated: superior nerve, inferior nerve, and combined superior and inferior nerve. This differentiation is based on utilizing both ENG and VEMP data, because the ENG measures the integrity of the superior nerve and the VEMP measures the integrity of the inferior nerve.

Superior vestibular neuritis is characterized by the sudden onset of vertigo accompanied by nausea and vomiting. The vertigo can be prolonged, the severe episode lasting for several days and gradually improving over several weeks. The hearing is not usually affected by vestibular neuritis, but when it is, it is a high-frequency sensorineural loss that occurs. Vestibular neuritis is sometimes followed by positional vertigo and even BPPV. Recurrent irregular episodes of severe vertigo can also occur with this disorder, a circumstance that may be confused with vestibular Ménière disease, recurrent vestibulopathy, and vascular loop syndrome. The vertigo and disequilibrium gradually resolve over the first month or two after the initial episode.

Inferior vestibular neuritis is much more subtle in onset. Most patients complain of floating sensation, rocking motion, or a pulling sensation. BPPV from the posterior canal is very rare following inferior vestibular neuritis, as the reflex arc is disrupted. Movement triggered symptoms and visual sensitivity to movement are also frequent complaints. According to Murofushi et al,[88] inferior vestibular neuritis represents one third of all cases of vestibular neuritis. Because many patients do not seek treatment, the actual course of this illness is uncertain, but in most cases gradual improvement occurs with physical therapy and vestibular supplements.

Combined superior and inferior vestibular neuritis is characterized by severe, catastrophic vertigo ("vestibular crisis"). These patients are extremely ill with nausea, vomiting, and dehydration. Even after significant dosages of vestibular suppressives, these patients may be incapacitated by the acute vertigo. Gradually, over the next few months, they improve and are able to resume work, driving, and other activities. The management of these patients is similar to those undergoing a TML, including vestibular rehabilitation therapy and vestibular suppressives.

Histopathology and Pathophysiology

Histopathological studies have been performed on the temporal bones of patients with clinical histories consistent with vestibular neuritis. The vestibular nerves in these cases have axonal loss, endoneurial fibrosis, and atrophy.[87] These findings suggest that vestibular neuritis is due to a viral infection in the vestibular nerve, rather than to an inflammation of the labyrinth. The pathophysiology of this condition suggests that the acute vertigo accompanies the acute viral inflammation of the vestibular nerve, and may involve one or both ears, either simultaneously or sequentially. If only part of the vestibular nerve is fibrosed following an episode of vestibular neuritis, the remaining axons can be affected again and cause significant symptoms. On the other hand, if most of a vestibular nerve is fibrosed, only minimal symptoms would occur if the nerve were affected again. Several human viruses have been shown to affect the vestibular nerve and the membranous labyrinth, including rubeola, herpes simplex virus 1 (HSV1), reovirus, cytomegalovirus, and neurotropic strains of influenza and mumps virus.[89]

More recently, Roehm et al[90] have demonstrated experimentally that latent HSV1 can reactivate in vestibular ganglion cells, suggesting that HSV1 reactivation is indeed the etiologic mechanism in these cases.

Evaluation

The clinician is often asked to see a patient with vestibular neuritis in the emergency department. At that time, the history should focus on the presence or absence of hearing loss, tinnitus, ear fullness or pain, or ear drainage. Other neurologic symptoms should be sought also, including other cranial nerve deficits, weakness, visual deficits, and ataxia or lack of coordination, as well as a history of prior otologic surgery.

The ear, nose, and throat examination and the neurologic examinations are then performed. Usually with acute vestibular neuritis, spontaneous nystagmus away from the affected side can be seen without Frenzel glasses. The symptoms and nystagmus worsen with the affected ear in the down position. The seated Romberg test, also known as the Quix test, demonstrates a drift or rotation toward the affected side.

The evaluation of these patients includes audiogram, ENG, VEMP, and MRI scans. Audiograms are most often normal, although occasionally they do show a unilateral high-frequency sensorineural hearing loss. The patient in "vestibular crisis" will not tolerate caloric testing. The crisis must first be treated. ENG, if performed shortly after the onset of symptoms, will show spontaneous nystagmus and usually a caloric weakness. ENGs performed after the acute episode has subsided often show a unilateral or a bilateral decrease in caloric excitability, as well as a directional preponderance. The VEMP may show a decrease in amplitude. MRI scans with gadolinium contrast are usually unremarkable, although occasionally an acoustic tumor or a cerebellar infarction can present in an unusual fashion, and these will be detected.

Medical Treatment

Vestibular neuritis is treated initially with vestibular suppressives, such as diazepam 5 to 10 mg IV or p.o. To this regimen is added an antiemetic such as diphenhydramine 25 mg IM or ondansetron 4 to 8 mg IV every 6 to 8 hours until symptoms subside. A short course of steroid therapy is also begun in these patients, specifically using prednisone 60 mg per day for 7 to 10 days or using a methylprednisolone dose pack. Vestibular rehabilitation is also recommended for these cases.

Most cases of vestibular neuritis resolve over the next 2 to 4 weeks, though some may take up to 4 months for complete recovery. It is unclear whether steroid therapy influences the ultimate outcome in these cases.[91] Although the caloric responses in the involved ear do recover more rapidly with treatment, the ultimate symptomatic recovery does not appear to be changed by steroid therapy. This is due to either compensation or the fact that the vestibular nerve inflammation recovers over time without steroids. In addition, Strupp et al[92] have reported that antivirals, such as valacyclovir, have no effect on the recovery of function in vestibular neuritis.

28.8 Benign Paroxysmal Positional Vertigo

Benign paroxysmal positional vertigo is the most common cause of vertigo of peripheral origin, accounting for nearly 20% of all vestibular complaints.

28.8.1 Clinical Presentation

Patients with this condition typically complain of brief episodes of vertigo brought on by head positioning, especially on getting in and out of bed. The condition is usually worse in the mornings and evenings and it is also characterized by symptomatic and asymptomatic episodes. The average age of onset is 54 years, and the condition typically takes one of three forms: (1) the acute form, which typically resolves spontaneously over 3 months; (2) the intermittent form, which has active and inactive periods that may span several years; and (3) the chronic form, which has continuous symptoms over long durations.[93] In addition to the BPPV, many of

these patients also complain of prolonged unsteadiness and light-headedness.

The specific characteristics of BPPV are critical provocative positioning with the affected ear dependent, rotary nystagmus toward the dependent ear, a brief 1- to 5-second latency prior to onset, limited duration of 10 to 30 seconds, reversal on assuming an upright position, and fatigability of the response.[94] The presence of these findings essentially confirms the diagnosis.

28.8.2 Pathophysiology

Benign paroxysmal positional vertigo can be seen following head injury, vestibular neuritis, stapes surgery, or Ménière disease, and without any antecedent event. BPPV due to idiopathic causes appears to be the most common. The pathophysiology of BPPV is thought to be due to two proposed mechanisms.[94] The first, called canalolithiasis, proposes that the movement of endolymphatic densities or otoconia during positional testing subsequently causes displacement of the cupula of the posterior semicircular canal. The second, called cupulolithiasis, proposes that otoconia are bound into the cupula, the so-called cupulolithiasis, and with position testing the cupula is deflected. These mechanisms are based on temporal bone histopathology that reveals an agglomeration of basophilic material on the surface of the cupula in BPPV cases, as well as the response of patients to deafferentation of the posterior semicircular canal. Furthermore, Parnes and McClure[94] have noted free-floating particles on opening the posterior semicircular canal for an occlusion procedure.

28.8.3 Evaluation

The evaluation of patients with suspected BPPV includes a history and an ear, nose, and throat examination. The neurotologic examination should also be performed, including the Dix-Hallpike maneuver. An audiogram should be obtained to search for other disorders of the inner ear. In the early phase of BPPV, an ENG probably adds very little information. However, if symptoms persist, the ENG should be obtained to determine if a vestibular weakness exists and to document the presence of positional vertigo. Also, the VEMP can be used to document that the inferior vestibular nerve is indeed intact. If the VEMP is absent in the affected ear, the posterior canal is probably not the canal causing the symptoms. MRI scans should also be obtained if the condition persists after therapy or lasts longer than 2 to 3 months.

28.8.4 Management

Management of BPPV begins with a careful explanation to the patient of the nature of the illness. Not only does this alleviate anxiety, but also it provides background information to the patient prior to the inception of various treatments. Vestibular suppressives do not have a significant effect in this condition, although antiemetics can be useful. If the patient has significant symptom-free intervals, fatiguing exercises can be useful as initial therapy. These are performed by asking the patient to sit on the side of the bed and to quickly assume the position that will trigger the vertigo. This should be repeated until the response fatigues.

If the symptoms of BPPV have lasted more than 1 to 2 weeks, the patient should undergo the particle positioning maneuver.[95] In this maneuver, the patient is moved through a sequence of head positions that are thought to cause the movement of the free-floating particles from the posterior canal into the utricle. On completing the particle positioning maneuver, the patient is placed into a soft cervical collar and is advised to avoid bending or moving into a horizontal position for 48 hours. The maneuver is easy to perform, and resolves the BPPV in more than 90% of cases with one to two treatments.[95] A mastoid vibrator or oscillator can also be used in an effort to encourage the movement of the particles into the utricle.

Cases of horizontal canal BPPV have also been recognized. The main differentiating feature is that the provocative position triggers horizontal nystagmus toward the affected ear, as opposed to rotary nystagmus. These cases are treated by a "log rolling" maneuver, which is very similar to the particle positioning maneuver.

An alternative to the particle positioning maneuver is an exercise program that the patient performs, such as the Brandt-Daroff exercise. The objective of this exercise is the same, that is, to reposition the otoconia, and the results are by and large the same as for the office-based maneuvers.

If the symptoms of BPPV do not relent with particle positioning maneuvers over 1 year, posterior semicircular canal occlusion can be performed to stop the vertigo.[96] In this procedure, the posterior canal is identified through a transmastoid approach. The posterior canal is carefully opened (▶ Fig. 28.12), the perilymph wicked away, and the canal filled with bone *pâté* and a fascial plug. The procedure does seem to stop the vertigo of BPPV, although a sensorineural hearing loss can occur in 5% of cases. Because of the simplicity and effectiveness of the procedure as well as the low incidence of hearing loss, posterior canal occlusion is currently the surgical procedure of choice for BPPV. Parnes's group[81] has recently reported their large series of 65 cases with durable long-term results.

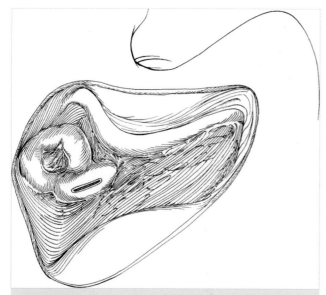

Fig. 28.12 Posterior canal occlusion, right ear, surgical position. Fenestra in the bony canal reveals the membranous duct.

28.9 Vestibulotoxicity

Patients who receive ototoxic drugs often suffer from debilitating illnesses that leave them bedridden for prolonged periods of time.[21] Vestibulotoxicity is usually not appreciated until the patient attempts to ambulate, and then notices a severe loss of balance. Vestibulotoxicity, or bilateral vestibular deficits, causes severe ataxia and oscillopsia and usually develops after a long course of intravenous aminoglycoside antibiotic therapy. However, vestibular ototoxicity can develop after a single dose of aminoglycoside antibiotic. In these cases, the diagnosis can be easily made by reviewing the medical record to determine if a potentially vestibulotoxic drug has been administered. If a bilateral vestibular deficit is suspected, it is necessary to obtain an audiogram and ENG with ice-water calorics. Rotary chair testing can confirm the bilateral vestibular weakness as well as evaluate the higher frequency range. Some regeneration of vestibular sensory neuroepithelia likely will occur, and that, coupled with vestibular rehabilitation, can improve the daily function of these patients.

28.10 Migraine-Associated Vertigo

Migraine-associated vertigo (MAV) is a syndrome characterized by episodic vertigo, positional vertigo, imbalance and unsteadiness, and motion intolerance.[97] It can be very difficult to differentiate MAV from recurrent vestibular neuritis, the main differentiating factor being a history of severe headache before or during the vertigo episode. MAV can occur during headache-free intervals, further confusing the issue.

Migraine is extremely common in the general population, with a 3:1 female predominance and affecting approximately 10% of the population. About one third of migraine sufferers have episodic vertigo.[98] Common migraine is characterized by a one-sided pulsating headache that severely limits daily activity. It usually occurs without premonition or aura and is often accompanied by nausea and vomiting as well as light and sound sensitivity. Classic migraine has an aura that may include ataxia, visual field cuts, difficulty speaking, as well as numbness or weakness of the extremities. These symptoms may be brief, and usually the headache, nausea, vomiting, and photophobia begin within a few minutes of onset. The exact cause of these symptoms is unclear at this time, but triggers include diet, stress, and anxiety.[99]

Several pathophysiological mechanisms for MAV have been proposed. One theory is that the vertigo represents an aura of the headache, due to a spreading wave of electrical depression over the cortex, perhaps as a result of decreased cerebral blood flow. Alternatively, it has been proposed that a neuropeptide is released from the cortex that circulates through the CSF to irritate the sensory epithelium of the vestibular system or the vestibular nuclei.[100] Another theory is that these neuropeptides cause vasospasm of the labyrinthine artery.

Migraine-associated vertigo patients typically present with a history of prolonged dizziness that may have been present for several months. There may be worsening by visual motion or head movement, and typically car sickness is described also. True vertigo occurs in two thirds of these patients, lasting for 2 to 24 hours in most cases. In fact, prolonged vertigo lasting over 24 hours is usually MAV, rather than other vestibular disorders. Hearing loss is uncommon in MAV.

The physical examination in these patients is usually unremarkable except for the presence of a rotary nystagmus, much like benign positional vertigo.

There are no specific diagnostic tests that clearly define MAV. Audiograms are usually normal, although a unilateral sensorineural loss would likely point to a different diagnosis. MRI scans are obtained to rule out internal auditory canal pathology, and do occasionally demonstrate white matter disease consistent with migraine. Normal findings on ENG, or hyperactive caloric tests, both suggest MAV, as opposed to recurrent vestibular neuritis. Rarely, a caloric weakness can be found in MAV patients, making the ENG less specific. VEMPs and ECochG are usually normal in MAV patients. After reviewing these studies, some clinicians then attempt to further clarify MAV into definite or probable MAV. Eggers et al[101] have clearly demonstrated that probable MAV is not a coherent diagnostic entity, so that this differentiation now seems artificial.

Migraine-associated vertigo patients usually respond to the same treatments that common and classic migraine patients respond to. The first level of treatment is to initiate a migraine-type diet avoiding smoked meats, cheeses, and other products thought to be triggers. A low dose of vestibular suppressant such as meclizine 25 mg b.i.d. or diazepam 2 mg t.i.d. may be helpful in these patients. A course of vestibular therapy is also helpful in MAV patients.

The second level of therapy by most otolaryngologists is to start prophylactic medications including nortriptyline, 10 mg at night, or a calcium channel blocker such as verapamil, 40 mg daily, up to three times daily. Most otolaryngologists refer MAV patients not responding to first- and second-level therapy to a neurologist. Other therapies that neurologists typically prescribe and monitor include topomirate, endomethacin, as well as a variety of triptan drugs to abort acute migraine episodes.

The otolaryngologist has a continuing role, however. Specifically, the clinician should monitor the MAV patient's status and response to vestibular therapy and vestibular suppression.

References

[1] Committee on Hearing and Equilibrium. Committee on Hearing and Equilibrium guidelines for the diagnosis and evaluation of therapy in Meniere's disease. Otolaryngol Head Neck Surg 1995; 113: 181–185

[2] Friberg U, Rask-Andersen H, Bagger-Sjöbäck D. Human endolymphatic duct. An ultrastructural study. Arch Otolaryngol 1984; 110: 421–428

[3] Peng L, Xiang-li Z, Yongqi L, Ge-hau Z, Xue-kun H. Clinical analysis of benign paroxysmal positional vertigo secondary to Meniere's disease. Scientific Research and Essays. 2010; 5: 3672–3675

[4] Rassekh CH, Harker LA. The prevalence of migraine in Ménière's disease. Laryngoscope 1992; 102: 135–138

[5] Parker W. Ménière's disease. Etiologic considerations. Arch Otolaryngol Head Neck Surg 1995; 121: 377–382

[6] Paparella MM, Mancini F. Vestibular Meniere's disease. Otolaryngol Head Neck Surg 1985; 93: 148–151

[7] Schuknecht HF, Suzuka Y, Zimmermann C. Delayed endolymphatic hydrops and its relationship to Meniére's disease. Ann Otol Rhinol Laryngol 1990; 99: 843–853

[8] Wladislavosky-Waserman P, Facer GW, Mokri B, Kurland LT. Meniere's disease: a 30-year epidemiologic and clinical study in Rochester, MN, 1951–1980. Laryngoscope 1984; 94: 1098–1102

[9] Futaki T, Semba T, Kudo Y. Treatment of hydropic patients by immunoglobulin with methyl B12. Am J Otol 1988; 9: 131–135

[10] Derebery MJ, Rao VS, Siglock TJ, Linthicum FH, Nelson RA. Ménière's disease: an immune complex-mediated illness? Laryngoscope 1991; 101: 225–229

[11] Morrison AW, Mowbray JF, Williamson R, Sheeka S, Sodha N, Koskinen N. On genetic and environmental factors in Ménière's disease. Am J Otol 1994; 15: 35–39

[12] Ylikoski J. Delayed endolymphatic hydrops syndrome after heavy exposure to impulse noise. Am J Otol 1988; 9: 282–285

[13] Derebery MJ, Valenzuela S. Ménière's syndrome and allergy. Otolaryngol Clin North Am 1992; 25: 213–224

[14] Hallpike CS, Cairns H. Observations on the pathology of Meniere's syndrome. J Laryngol Otol 1938; 53: 625–631

[15] Yamakawa K. Ueber die pathologische Veraenderung bei einem Meniere Krnaken. J Otolaryngol Soc Jpn. 1938; 44: 2310–2312

[16] Schuknecht HF. Pathology of the Ear, 2nd ed. Philadelphia: Lea & Febiger, 1993:449–529

[17] Shimizu S, Cureoglu S, Yoda S, Suzuki M, Paparella MM. Blockage of longitudinal flow in Meniere's disease: A human temporal bone study. Acta Otolaryngol 2011; 131: 263–268

[18] Altmann F, Kornfeld M. Histological studies of Ménière's disease. Ann Otol Rhinol Laryngol 1965; 74: 915–943

[19] Ichimiya I, Adams JC, Kimura RS. Changes in immunostaining of cochleas with experimentally induced endolymphatic hydrops. Ann Otol Rhinol Laryngol 1994; 103: 457–468

[20] Masutani H, Takahashi H, Sando I. Stria vascularis in Ménière's disease: a quantitative histopathological study. Auris Nasus Larynx 1992; 19: 145–152

[21] Borjab DI, Bhansali SA, Battista RA. Peripheral vestibular disorders. In: Jackler RK, Brackmann DE, eds. Neurotology. St. Louis: Mosby, 1994:629–650

[22] Rauch SD, Merchant SM, Thedinger BA. Meniere's syndrome and endolymphatic hydrops double-blind temporal bone study. Ann Otol Rhinol Laryngol 1989; 98: 973–883

[23] Swart JG, Schuknecht HF. Long-term effects of destruction of the endolymphatic sac in a primate species. Laryngoscope 1988; 98: 1183–1189

[24] Arenberg IK, Marovitz WF, Shambaugh GE, Jr. The role of the endolymphatic sac in the pathogenesis of endolymphatic hydrops in man. Acta Otolaryngol Suppl 1970; 275: 1–49

[25] Arenberg IK, Norback DH, Shambaugh GE, Jr. Distribution and density of subepithelial collagen in the endolymphatic sac in patients with Meniere's disease. Am J Otol 1985; 6: 449–454

[26] Gussen R. Meniere syndrome. Compensatory collateral venous drainage with endolymphatic sac fibrosis. Arch Otolaryngol 1974; 99: 414–418

[27] Bagger-Sjöbäck D, Friberg U, Rask-Anderson H. The human endolymphatic sac. An ultrastructural study. Arch Otolaryngol Head Neck Surg 1986; 112: 398–409

[28] Paparella MM. Pathogenesis of Meniere's disease and Meniere's syndrome. Acta Otolaryngol Suppl 1984; 406: 10–25

[29] Ikeda M, Sando I. Endolymphatic duct and sac in patients with Meniere's disease. A temporal bone histopathological study. Ann Otol Rhinol Laryngol 1984; 93: 540–546

[30] Erwall C, Friberg U, Bagger-Sjöbäck D, Rask-Andersen H. Degradation of the homogeneous substance in the endolymphatic sac. Acta Otolaryngol 1988; 105: 209–217

[31] Wackym PA. Histopathologic findings in Ménière's disease. Otolaryngol Head Neck Surg 1995; 112: 90–100

[32] Welling DB, Daniels RL, Brainard J, Western LM, Prior TW. Detection of viral DNA in endolymphatic sac tissue from Ménière's disease patients. Am J Otol 1994; 15: 639–643

[33] Dornhoffer JL, Waner M, Arenberg IK, Montague D. Immunoperoxidase study of the endolymphatic sac in Ménière's disease. Laryngoscope 1993; 103: 1027–1034

[34] Lee FP, Ho TL, Huang TS. Endolymphatic hydrops in animal experiments. A confirmation of mechanical and immunological methods of inducement. Acta Otolaryngol Suppl 1991; 485: 18–25

[35] Masutani H, Takahashi H, Sando I, Sato H. Vestibular aqueduct in Ménière's disease and non-Ménière's disease with endolymphatic hydrops: a computer aided volumetric study. Auris Nasus Larynx 1991; 18: 351–357

[36] Gartner M, Bossart W, Linder T. Herpes virus and Ménière's disease. ORL J Otorhinolaryngol Relat Spec 2008; 70: 28–31, discussion 31

[37] Andrews JC, Strelioff D. Modulation of inner ear pressure in experimental endolymphatic hydrops. Otolaryngol Head Neck Surg 1995; 112: 78–83

[38] Horner KC. Auditory and vestibular function in experimental hydrops. Otolaryngol Head Neck Surg 1995; 112: 84–89

[39] Zenner HP, Reuter G, Zimmermann U, Gitter AH, Fermin C, LePage EL. Transitory endolymph leakage induced hearing loss and tinnitus: depolarization, biphasic shortening and loss of electromotility of outer hair cells. Eur Arch Otorhinolaryngol 1994; 251: 143–153

[40] Gibson WP. Hypothetical mechanism for vertigo in Meniere's disease. Otolaryngol Clin North Am 2010; 43: 1019–1027

[41] Long CH, III, Morizono T. Hydrostatic pressure measurements of endolymph and perilymph in a guinea pig model of endolymphatic hydrops. Otolaryngol Head Neck Surg 1987; 96: 83–95

[42] Kitahara M, Takeda T, Yazawa Y, Matsubara H, Kitano H. Pathophysiology of Meniere's disease and its subvarieties. Acta Otolaryngol Suppl 1984; 406: 52–55

[43] Juhn SK, Ikeda K, Morizono T, Murphy M. Pathophysiology of inner ear fluid imbalance. Acta Otolaryngol Suppl 1991; 485: 9–14

[44] Cohen J, Morizono T. Changes in EP and inner ear ionic concentrations in experimental endolymphatic hydrops. Acta Otolaryngol 1984; 98: 398–402

[45] Salt AN, DeMott JE. Endolymph Calcium increases with time in hydropic guinea pigs. In: Abstracts of the Fifteenth Midwinter Meeting. St. Petersburg Beach, FL: Association for Research in Otolaryngology, 1992:128

[46] Ikeda K, Morizono T. Ionic activities of the inner ear fluid and ionic permeabilities of the cochlear duct in endolymphatic hydrops of the guinea pig. Hear Res 1991; 51: 185–192

[47] Morgenstern C, Mori N, Amano H. Pathogenesis of experimental endolymphatic hydrops. Acta Otolaryngol Suppl 1984; 406: 56–58

[48] Van de Water SM, Arenberg IK, Balkany TJ. Auditory dehydration testing: glycerol versus urea. Am J Otol 1986; 7: 200–203

[49] Schwaber MK, Hall JW, Zealear DL. Intraoperative monitoring of the facial and cochleovestibular nerves in otologic surgery: part II. Insights Otolaryngol. 1991; 6: 108

[50] Margolis RH, Rieks D, Fournier EM, Levine SE. Tympanic electrocochleography for diagnosis of Ménière's disease. Arch Otolaryngol Head Neck Surg 1995; 121: 44–55

[51] Moffat DA, Baguley DM, Harries MLL, Atlas M, Lynch CA. Bilateral electrocochleographic findings in unilateral Ménière's disease. Otolaryngol Head Neck Surg 1992; 107: 370–373

[52] Keim RJ. Clinical comparisons of posturography and electronystagmography. Laryngoscope 1993; 103: 713–716

[53] O'Leary DP, Davis LL. Vestibular autorotation testing of Menière's disease. Otolaryngol Head Neck Surg 1990; 103: 66–71

[54] de Waele C, Huy PT, Diard JP, Freyss G, Vidal PP. Saccular dysfunction in Menière's disease. Am J Otol 1999; 20: 223–232

[55] Seo T, Yoshida K, Shibano A, Sakagami M. A possible case of saccular endolymphatic hydrops. ORL J Otorhinolaryngol Relat Spec 1999; 61: 215–218

[56] Lin MY, Timmer FCA, Oriel BS et al. Vestibular evoked myogenic potentials (VEMP) can detect asymptomatic saccular hydrops. Laryngoscope 2006; 116: 987–992

[57] Nakashima T, Naganawa S, Sugiura M et al. Visualization of endolymphatic hydrops in patients with Meniere's disease. Laryngoscope 2007; 117: 415–420

[58] Gürkov R, Flatz W, Louza J, Strupp M, Ertl-Wagner B, Krause E. In vivo visualized endolymphatic hydrops and inner ear functions in patients with electrocochleographically confirmed Ménière's disease. Otol Neurotol 2012; 33: 1040–1045

[59] Ruckenstein MJ, Rutka JA, Hawke M. The treatment of Menière's disease: Torok revisited. Laryngoscope 1991; 101: 211–218

[60] Barrs DM, Keyser JS, Stallworth C, McElveen JT, Jr. Intratympanic steroid injections for intractable Ménière's disease. Laryngoscope 2001; 111: 2100–2104

[61] Doyle KJ, Bauch C, Battista R et al. Intratympanic steroid treatment: a review. Otol Neurotol 2004; 25: 1034–1039

[62] Piu F, Wang X, Fernandez R et al. OTO-104: a sustained-release dexamethasone hydrogel for the treatment of otic disorders. Otol Neurotol 2011; 32: 171–179

[63] Gates GA, Green JD, Jr, Tucci DL, Telian SA. The effects of transtympanic micropressure treatment in people with unilateral Meniere's disease. Arch Otolaryngol Head Neck Surg 2004; 130: 718–725

[64] Nedzelski JM, Schessel DA, Bryce GE, Pfleiderer AG. Chemical labyrinthectomy: local application of gentamicin for the treatment of unilateral Ménière's disease. Am J Otol 1992; 13: 18–22

[65] Pyykkö I, Ishizaki H, Kaasinen S, Aalto H. Intratympanic gentamicin in bilateral Ménière's disease. Otolaryngol Head Neck Surg 1994; 110: 162–167

[66] Telischi FF, Luxford WM. Long-term efficacy of endolymphatic sac surgery for vertigo in Ménière's disease. Otolaryngol Head Neck Surg 1993; 109: 83–87

[67] Goldenberg RA, Justus MA. Endolymphatic mastoid shunt for Ménière's disease: do results change over time? Laryngoscope 1990; 100: 141–145

[68] Bretlau P, Thomsen J, Tos M, Johnsen NJ. Placebo effect in surgery for Ménière's disease: nine-year follow-up. Am J Otol 1989; 10: 259–261

[69] Silverstein H, Norrell H. Retrolabyrinthine vestibular neurectomy. Otolaryngol Head Neck Surg 1982; 90: 778–782

[70] Plontke SK. Evaluation of the round window niche before local drug delivery to the inner ear using a new mini-otoscope. Otol Neurotol 2011; 32: 183–185

[71] Crane BT, Minor LB, Della Santina CC, Carey JP. Middle ear exploration in patients with Ménière's disease who have failed outpatient intratympanic gentamicin therapy. Otol Neurotol 2009; 30: 619–624

[72] Fiorino F, Pizzini FB, Barbieri F, Beltramello A. Magnetic resonance imaging fails to show evidence of reduced endolymphatic hydrops in gentamicin treatment of Ménière's disease. Otol Neurotol 2012; 33: 629–633

[73] Fiorino F, Pizzini FB, Barbieri F, Beltramello A. Variability in the perilymphatic diffusion of gadolinium does not predict the outcome of intratympanic gentamicin in patients with Ménière's disease. Laryngoscope 2012; 122: 907–911

[74] Kemink JL, Telian SA, el-Kashlan H, Langman AW. Retrolabyrinthine vestibular nerve section: efficacy in disorders other than Ménière's disease. Laryngoscope 1991; 101: 523–528

[75] Giddings NA, Shelton C, O'Leary MJ, Brackmann DE. Cochleosacculotomy revisited. Long-term results poorer than expected. Arch Otolaryngol Head Neck Surg 1991; 117: 1150–1152

[76] Schwaber MK, Whetsell WO. Cochleovestibular nerve compression syndrome. II. Vestibular nerve histopathology and theory of pathophysiology. Laryngoscope 1992; 102: 1030–1036

[77] Schwaber MK, Hall JW. Cochleovestibular nerve compression syndrome. I. Clinical features and audiovestibular findings. Laryngoscope 1992; 102: 1020–1029

[78] Weider DJ. Treatment and management of perilymphatic fistula: a New Hampshire experience. Am J Otol 1992; 13: 158–166

[79] Ikezono T, Shindo S, S , e , kine K et al. Cochlin-tomoprotein (CTP) detection test identifies tramatic perilymphatic fistula due to penetration middle ear injury. Acta Otolaryngol 2011; 131: 937–944

[80] Minor LB. Clinical manifestations of superior semicircular canal dehiscence. Laryngoscope 2005; 115: 1717–1727

[81] Beyea JA, Agrawal SK, Parnes LS. Transmastoid semicircular canal occlusion: a safe and highly effective treatment for benign paroxysmal positional vertigo and superior canal dehiscence. Laryngoscope 2012; 122: 1862–1866

[82] Steckelberg JM, McDonald TJ. Otologic involvement in late syphilis. Laryngoscope 1984; 94: 753–757

[83] Wilson WR, Zoller M. Electronystagmography in congenital and acquired syphilitic otitis. Ann Otol Rhinol Laryngol 1981; 90: 21–24

[84] Shih L, McElveen JT, Jr, Linthicum FH, Jr. Management of vertigo in patients with syphilis: is endolymphatic shunt surgery appropriate? Otolaryngol Head Neck Surg 1988; 99: 574–577

[85] Baloh RW. Vertebrobasilar insufficiency and stroke. Otolaryngol Head Neck Surg 1995; 112: 114–117

[86] Lee H. Neuro-otological aspects of cerebellar stroke syndrome. J Clin Neurol 2009; 5: 65–73

[87] Schuknecht HF, Kitamura K. Vestibular neuritis. Ann Otol Rhinol Laryngol Suppl 1981; 90: 1–19

[88] Murofushi T, Halmagyi GM, Yavor RA, Colebatch JG. Absent vestibular evoked myogenic potentials in vestibular neurolabyrinthitis. An indicator of inferior vestibular nerve involvement? Arch Otolaryngol Head Neck Surg 1996; 122: 845–848

[89] Gacek RR. Further observations on posterior ampullary nerve transection for positional vertigo. Ann Otol Rhinol Laryngol 1978; 87: 300–305

[90] Roehm PC, Camarena V, Nayak S et al. Cultured vestibular ganglion neurons demonstrate latent HSV1 reactivation. Laryngoscope 2011; 121: 2268–2275

[91] Fishman JM. Corticosteroids effective in idiopathic facial nerve palsy (Bell's palsy) but not necessarily in idiopathic acute vestibular dysfunction (vestibular neuritis). Laryngoscope 2011; 121: 2494–2495

[92] Strupp M, Zingler VC, Arbusow V et al. Methylprednisolone, valacyclovir, or the combination for vestibular neuritis. N Engl J Med 2004; 351: 354–361

[93] Parnes LS, Price-Jones RG. Particle repositioning maneuver for benign paroxysmal positional vertigo. Ann Otol Rhinol Laryngol 1993; 102: 325–331

[94] Parnes LS, McClure JA. Posterior semicircular canal occlusion in the normal hearing ear. Otolaryngol Head Neck Surg 1991; 104: 52–57

[95] Schwaber MK, Hall JW. Cochleovestibular nerve compression syndrome. I. Clinical features and audiovestibular findings. Laryngoscope 1992; 102: 1020–1029

[96] Epley JM. The canalith repositioning procedure: for treatment of benign paroxysmal positional vertigo. Otolaryngol Head Neck Surg 1992; 107: 399–404

[97] Brantberg K, Trees N, Baloh RW. Migraine-associated vertigo. Acta Otolaryngol 2005; 125: 276–279

[98] Stewart WF, Shechter A, Rasmussen BK. Migraine prevalence. A review of population-based studies. Neurology 1994; 44 Suppl 4: S17–S23

[99] Headache Classification Committee of the International Headache Society. Classification and diagnostic criteria for headache disorders, cranial neuralgias and facial pain. Cephalagia. 1988; 8 Suppl 7: 1–96

[100] Viirre ES, Baloh RW. Migraine as a cause of sudden hearing loss. Headache 1996; 36: 24–28

[101] Eggers SDZ, Staab JP, Neff BA, Goulson AM, Carlson ML, Shepard NT. Investigation of the coherence of definite and probable vestibular migraine as distinct clinical entities. Otol Neurotol 2011; 32: 1144–1151

29 Facial Nerve Disorders

Bruce J. Gantz and Pamela C. Roehm

29.1 Introduction

Proper management of facial nerve disorders requires an appreciation for the wealth of knowledge about this cranial nerve and for the gaps in our understanding of its pathophysiology. Many facial nerve disorders are extremely rare and their natural history is poorly documented. Other disorders, such as Bell palsy, are common and the natural history well known. Unfortunately, this knowledge does little to decrease the controversy regarding appropriate management of the disorder. It is unlikely that there will be a consensus regarding management of all the diseases and disorders described in this chapter. However, when a patient presents with a disorder of the facial nerve, the clinician must advise and provide management, or refer to those with the appropriate expertise. In many cases it is appropriate to offer more than one treatment plan and allow the patient to choose, based on the known risks and benefits of that plan. In these situations the patient must be aware of the unknowns inherent in any approach.

29.2 Anatomy of the Facial Nerve

The facial nerve has a complex three-dimensional course from its motor nucleus in the anterior pons to its insertion into the muscles of facial expression. After exiting posteriorly from the motor nucleus, fibers of the facial nerve turn abruptly around the abducens nucleus and exit from the brainstem at the ponto-medullary junction. At its exit from the brainstem, the facial nerve lies 1.5 mm anterior to cranial nerve VIII. The nervus intermedius, which is composed of parasympathetic fibers that become the greater superficial petrosal and chorda tympani nerves, exits the brainstem between cranial nerves VII and VIII. The facial nerve is about 1.8 mm in diameter at its root entry zone. After leaving the brainstem, it has a 15- to 17-mm course through the cerebellopontine angle (CPA) prior to entering the porus of the internal auditory canal (IAC). Within the CPA the facial nerve is in close proximity to the anterior inferior cerebellar artery (AICA), which provides the vascular supply to this segment of the nerve. The AICA may lie anterior to or between cranial nerves VII and VIII. Occasionally, a loop of AICA may course laterally to the fundus of the IAC.

After entering the IAC, the facial nerve travels 8 to 10 mm prior to entering the meatal foramen (▶ Fig. 29.1). In the IAC it occupies the anterosuperior quadrant, and at the fundus it is separated from the superior vestibular nerve by the vertical crest (Bill's bar) and from the cochlear nerve by the transverse crest. On entering the meatal foramen, the facial nerve narrows to its smallest diameter, 0.61 to 0.68 mm. The ratio of the fallopian canal diameter to the facial nerve diameter is at its lowest as well. Adour[1] has questioned the concept of meatal entrapment as a mechanism for facial nerve injury, but there are now substantial data demonstrating that entrapment at the meatal foramen and labyrinthine segment plays a role in the pathogenesis of at least some facial nerve disorders as detailed below.[2-13]

The labyrinthine segment is 4 mm in length between the meatal foramen and the geniculate ganglion. It is located immediately posterior and slightly superior to the basal turn of the cochlea. The labyrinthine segment is just anterior to the ampulla of the superior semicircular canal and courses superiorly as it

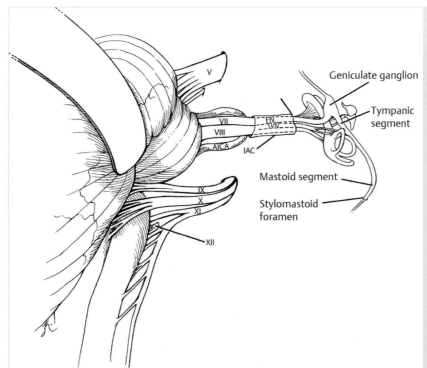

Fig. 29.1 Course and relationships of the left facial nerve from the pontomedullary junction to the stylomastoid foramen. AICA, anterior inferior cerebellar artery; FN, facial nerve; IAC, internal auditory canal; SVN, superior vestibular nerve.

Geniculate ganglion

Tympanic segment

Mastoid segment

Stylomastoid foramen

travels laterally, a position of importance for middle fossa surgery. At the geniculate ganglion, the nerve takes a 75-degree turn posteriorly into the tympanic segment. The greater superficial petrosal nerve (GSPN) exits the fallopian canal via the facial hiatus with the superficial petrosal artery (a branch of the middle meningeal artery), which is the vascular supply to this region of the nerve.

The tympanic segment is about 11 mm long and lies between the takeoff of the GSPN and the second genu. It forms the superior aspect of the oval window niche and is readily injured by pathological processes and unwary middle ear surgeons, due to its frequently occurring dehiscences.[14,15]

After passing between the stapes and the lateral semicircular canal, the nerve turns inferiorly into the mastoid segment. This measures 13 mm in length down to the stylomastoid foramen.

The stylomastoid artery, a branch of the postauricular artery, supplies this portion of the nerve. Dense connective tissue envelops the nerve as it exits the stylomastoid foramen. During procedures that require mobilization of this portion of the facial nerve, nerve injury can be avoided by including a margin of the connective tissue with the nerve during mobilization.[16]

29.3 Grading of Facial Weakness

Assessment of treatment efficacy requires a consistent system for grading facial weakness. The House-Brackmann scale[17] was originally developed for assessment of outcome in Bell palsy but has proven useful in management of all acute facial nerve disorders except when grading outcomes following grafting of the nerve (▶ Table 29.1).

Table 29.1 The House-Brackmann Scale

Grade	Description	Characteristics
I	Normal	Normal facial function in all areas
II	Mild dysfunction	Gross: slight weakness noticeable on close inspection; may have very slight synkinesis
		At rest: normal symmetry and tone
		Motion
		Forehead: moderate to good
		Eye: complete closure with minimum effort
		Mouth: slight asymmetry
III	Moderate dysfunction	Gross: obvious but not disfiguring difference between two sides; noticeable but not severe synkinesis, contracture, or hemifacial spasm
		At rest: normal symmetry and tone
		Motion
		Forehead: slight to moderate movement
		Eye: complete closure with effort
		Mouth: slightly weak with maximum effort
IV	Moderately severe dysfunction	Gross: obvious weakness or disfiguring asymmetry
		At rest: normal symmetry and tone
		Motion
		Forehead: none
		Eye: incomplete closure
		Mouth: asymmetric with maximum effort
V	Severe dysfunction	Gross: only barely perceptible motion
		At rest: asymmetry
		Motion
		Forehead: none
		Eye: incomplete closure
		Mouth: slight movement
VI	Total paralysis	No movement

Adapted with permission from House JW, Brackmann DE. Facial nerve grading system. Otolaryngol Head Neck Surg 1985;93:146–147.

29.4 Facial Nerve Disorders in Adults

29.4.1 Bell Palsy

One should expect that any fairly common disorder with a well-described natural history, multiple placebo-controlled treatment trials, a wealth of intraoperative observation, and morphological, histopathological, electrophysiological, and molecular data would be treatable with a minimum of controversy. This is far from true in the case of the acute facial paralysis first described by Sir Charles Bell. The debate over the efficacy of any medical or surgical therapy has changed its focus over time, but the fundamental disagreements have not changed in 30 years. Nevertheless, much is known about the natural history, possible etiologies, pathogenesis, and clinical evaluation of the patient with Bell palsy, so that a treatment algorithm may be formed and allows for unknown and debatable issues. An excellent review of these issues is available.[18]

Diagnosis

Although Bell palsy may not be idiopathic,[1] it remains a diagnosis of exclusion. The clinician must exclude all identifiable causes of facial paralysis that may be determined by history, physical examination, or radiological study. It is not uncommon for CPA tumors, skull base neoplasms, otitis media, or parotid lesions to be misdiagnosed as Bell palsy. These errors should be rare, as history and physical examination point to the correct diagnosis the vast majority of the time. A partial or total unilateral facial paralysis with onset over a 48-hour period without hearing loss, vertigo, or other cranial neuropathy and with a normal head and neck examination is likely to be Bell palsy. Other than audiometric evaluation, it does not require further diagnostic workup except for HIV testing or Lyme titers in appropriate circumstances. Some recovery should be noted within 3 to 6 months in all patients. If the patient presents with a typical acute-onset facial paralysis consistent with Bell palsy, magnetic resonance imaging (MRI) or computed tomography (CT) imaging is not necessary unless there is no return of function by 6 months postparalysis.

Occasionally, a sudden total facial paralysis occurs that does not resolve in 6 months. This situation requires thorough imaging and possibly surgical exploration prior to any attempt at reanimation. Parotid malignancy has been reported as long as 10 years after acute facial palsy.[19] A case of fluctuating facial paralysis has been seen in our institution in association with negative enhanced MRI and high-resolution temporal bone CT. An occult parotid malignancy was diagnosed 6 months later. Another case of acute facial paralysis 6 months after excision of a squamous cell carcinoma of the cheek skin proved to be metastatic carcinoma despite multiple negative imaging studies. These cases are unusual but point to the necessity of aggressive evaluation of all progressive facial pareses, segmental pareses, pareses associated with facial twitching prior to onset, pareses associated with other cranial neuropathies, and those acute palsies that do not show some recovery within 6 months.

Pathogenesis

May[20] suggested that Bell palsy begins with involvement of the sensory fibers of the facial nerve and subsequently involves the motor fibers. This process is consistent with the notion that the disease begins as a viral ganglionitis of the geniculate ganglion.[21] Nasopharyngeal cultures,[22] circulating antibodies,[23] biopsy,[24] polymerase chain reaction (PCR) of the geniculate ganglion from archived temporal bone,[25] and PCR of intraoperative washings of the facial nerve[26] from patients with Bell palsy all point to herpes simplex virus as the main etiologic agent. Ischemic and autoimmune injury have been proposed as the subsequent means of nerve degeneration, but it is now clear that entrapment at the meatal foramen and labyrinthine segment is critical in this process as originally described by Fisch and Esslen.[27] The evidence for this includes the following:

1. Temporal bone histopathological demonstration of a sharp demarcation between a normal nerve in the IAC and a severely degenerated nerve beyond the meatal foramen in a case of herpes zoster oticus[6]
2. Clear and convincing electrophysiological evidence[3,5] of conduction block at the meatal foramen and labyrinthine segment
3. Dramatic improvement in conduction across the labyrinthine segment after decompression[3]
4. Intraoperative observation at this institution and others[10] of an edematous-appearing nerve in the IAC and a cadaveric-appearing nerve distally
5. Return of some facial movement in a small number of patients immediately after middle cranial fossa (MCF) decompression[2]
6. Clinical series demonstrating the efficacy of MCF decompression in cases of recurrent facial paralysis[4,12]
7. Gadolinium enhancement of the labyrinthine segment in Bell palsy and herpes zoster oticus (HZO)[7–9,11,13]

None of these data imply that MCF decompression is indicated for Bell palsy, but it has convincingly implicated the meatal foramen and labyrinthine segment in the pathological process. Temporal bone morphometric evidence that the facial nerve is not as tightly constrained at the meatal foramen in young children may account for the lower incidence and better prognosis in this population.[28]

Prognosis

Several large studies have outlined the natural history of Bell palsy.[29,30] Generally, patients older than age 65 at onset of idiopathic facial paralysis have a worse recovery of facial function than younger patients.[29–31] Likewise, patients with diabetes not only have an increased incidence of Bell palsy but also have a poorer prognosis.[30,31]

The majority of patients have good recovery of facial function within 3 to 6 months without medical or surgical intervention (except, of course, eye care as needed). Identification of those patients who will not recover grade I or II function, therefore, should be the next goal after a diagnosis is made. Several important prognostic factors have been noted. Patients who never progress to complete paralysis and those with signs of recovery within the first 2 months have an excellent prognosis, with almost all returning to normal function. Electromyographic (EMG) evidence of voluntary activity[32,33] or an intact stapedial reflex[34] also portends an excellent prognosis. Finally, electroneurography (ENoG) findings of less than 90% degeneration of the electrically evoked compound muscle action potential during the first 2 weeks after onset of paralysis indicate almost certain near-normal or normal recovery. Patients with greater than 90% degeneration in the first 2 weeks have less than a 50% chance of good recovery.[32,33,35] These patients should be the focus of aggressive treatment efforts.

Unfortunately, there is no electrophysiological test that discriminates between nerve fibers that have undergone axonotmesis,[36,37] which should recover fully, and those that have more severe injury.[21] Further complicating this issue is intraoperative evidence of nerve fibers that are not stimulable distal to a pathological process, but that become stimulable shortly after removal of the pathology. This represents injury more severe than neurapraxia, but clearly is not axonotmesis because the recovery is too fast to allow time for regeneration. This phenomenon may explain the rapid recovery reported after some MCF decompressions[2] in which response to electrical stimulation was absent preoperatively. It is hoped that laboratory study of this process will improve clinical prognostication.

Eye Care

Eye care is the single most important treatment for any patient with grade II or worse facial function. Drying of the eye secondary to decreased eye closure and lacrimation rapidly leads to exposure keratopathy with breakdown of the cornea.[38,39] To prevent this complication, artificial tears are applied at least every 2 hours during the day. At bedtime, ophthalmic ointment is applied and a moisture chamber of plastic wrap is used to cover the eye. Use of a temporary tarsorrhaphy, gold weight, or other oculoplastic techniques provides better eye protection when either facial nerve function is not expected to return or when exposure keratopathy cannot be prevented by medical treatment alone.[38,39] Gold weights have almost entirely replaced tarsorrhaphies.

Medical Treatment

Multiple placebo-controlled trials of glucocorticoid therapy for Bell palsy have demonstrated mixed results, with some studies demonstrating benefit and others showing none. For summaries of these studies with conflicting conclusions see Limb and Niparko,[18] Selesnick and Patwardhan,[40] and Salinas et al.[41] The combination of prednisone and the antiviral acyclovir is also controversial. Adour et al[42] claimed a statistically significant benefit for the addition of acyclovir in combination with prednisone. However, a systematic review of this study and two other randomized controlled trials revealed a lack of consistent evidence for improved recovery from Bell palsy in patients treated with antivirals.[43] Acyclovir has low toxicity and, as noted above, there are good theoretical reasons for its use. Recently, there have been several new randomized trials directed at managing Bell palsy. Sullivan et al[44] performed a double-blind, placebo-controlled, randomized, factorial trial involving 496 patients with Bell palsy who were recruited within 72 hours after the onset of symptoms. Patients were randomly assigned to receive 10 days of treatment with either prednisolone or acyclovir, or with both agents, or with a placebo. The primary outcome was recovery of facial function, as rated on the House–Brackmann scale. The authors concluded that early treatment with prednisolone significantly improves the chances of complete recovery at 3 and 9 months. There is no evidence of a benefit of acyclovir given alone or an additional benefit of acyclovir in combination with prednisolone. Following this publication in the *New England Journal of Medicine*, an editorial in the same journal appeared by Gilden and Tyler[45] titles, "Bell's Palsy—Is Glucocorticoid Treatment Enough?" The authors state that lack of benefit from antiviral therapy by Sullivan et al conflicts with the results of a study by Hato et al[46] that compared a combination of valacyclovir (at a dose of 500 mg twice daily for 5 days) and prednisolone with placebo and prednisolone. A complete recovery was seen in 96.5% of 114 patients who received valacyclovir and prednisolone, as compared with 89.7% of 107 patients who received placebo and prednisolone (an absolute risk reduction of 6.8%). The authors state,

More striking was the report of the full recovery of 90.1% of patients with complete facial palsy who were treated with valacyclovir and prednisolone, as compared with 75.0% of those treated with placebo and prednisolone. The study by Sullivan et al clearly indicates that the addition of acyclovir provides no additional benefit to treatment with glucocorticoids alone. Both Hato et al and Sullivan et al show no benefit of antiviral therapy in patients with moderate palsy (paresis) and thus provide no rationale for treating these patients with valacyclovir. Although the study by Hato et al was methodologically flawed, the use of valacyclovir in combination with glucocorticoids could still be considered in patients with severe or complete facial palsy.

This is an important concept that most evidence-based studies have not recognized.

Finally, an editorial in *Lancet Neurology* in 2009 also raises the issue that those with complete paralysis might benefit from antiviral therapy.[47] De Ru et al[47] address the conclusions of another randomized clinical trial by Engström and colleagues,[48] who concluded that early treatment with prednisolone alone shortened the time to facial recovery and that valacyclovir did not affect recovery:

The investigators tried to include large numbers of patients in these drug trials, but in doing so they might have lost sight of the clinically important question of whether recovery rate can be improved in patients who are less likely to recover spontaneously— those with House-Brackmann scores of V or VI—who should be the target group. The answer to the question of whether each patient who presents with Bell's palsy should be given antiviral medication is not necessarily the same as the answer to the question of whether patients with a serious paralysis would benefit from antiviral medication. We are concerned that the report by Engström and colleagues will lead to unjustifiably inadequate treatment for patients with severe paralysis, and we are of the opinion that the pendulum still remains in a position that favors combination therapy for patients with Bell's palsy.

It was the opinion of de Ru et al that the use of antivirals should still be considered in patients with a severe or complete palsy, particularly those who have a high risk of herpes zoster infection even if they do not have the typical zoster rash.

For the reasons stated above, for patients presenting within 3 weeks of onset of complete paralysis, the authors currently recommend the use of a combination of prednisone 1 mg/kg/day for 10 to 14 days and acyclovir 1,000 mg t.i.d. The study by Murakami et al[26] strongly supports the addition of antiviral treatments.

Surgical Treatment

Surgical management of Bell palsy has evolved along with our understanding of the pathophysiology of the disease. May et al[49] clearly demonstrated the futility of transmastoid decompression. Only MCF decompression of the meatal foramen, labyrinthine segment, and geniculate ganglion can be expected to offer any benefit. Although we perform the MCF approach frequently for acoustic neuroma and vestibular nerve section with minimal morbidity, it is technically challenging even for experienced temporal bone surgeons and has significant potential for complications. Thus, even with proof of the efficacy of decompression, we would only advocate its performance in centers experienced with the MCF approach.

Fisch's[50] landmark study of MCF decompression demonstrated statistically significant improvements in outcome with surgery, but it is difficult to assess the degree of improvement in this study. Use of the House-Brackmann scale in subsequent reports makes this much easier. All patients had > 90% degeneration on ENoG within 14 days of onset of total paralysis and no voluntary EMG potentials. Fisch's[32] prognostic studies show at best a 50% rate of spontaneous "satisfactory" recovery when degeneration exceeds 90%. Sillman and coworkers[33] studied ENoG prognostication using the House-Brackmann scale and verified Fisch's result, demonstrating less than 50% recovery to grade I or II function when ENoG degeneration exceeded 90%. Thus the patients who would be expected to spontaneously return to grade I or II less than 50% of the time were treated with MCF decompression.

A multicenter prospective clinical trial of patients with Bell palsy showed that patients who did not reach 90% degeneration on ENoG within 14 days of paralysis ($n = 54$) all had return of function to House-Brackmann grade I or II (► Table 29.2). Patients with ≥ 90% degeneration on ENoG and no EMG motor unit potentials were offered surgical decompression of the facial nerve through an MCF approach. Thirty-four elected to have the decompression, whereas 36 were managed with steroids only. The results of the comparison were statistically significant in favor of decompression ($p < 0.0002$ stratified exact permutation test). The surgical decompression group exhibited House-Brackmann grade I or II results in 91% of those undergoing MCF decompression within 14 days of onset of acute paralysis. Of the 36 patients who chose not to undergo surgical decompression and were treated solely with steroids, 58% had a poor outcome at 7 months follow-up (House-Brackmann grade III or IV). Only 9% of the patients who did have MCF facial nerve compression had a poor outcome (► Table 29.2).[51]

Facial nerve decompression for Bell palsy is rarely necessary, as severe degeneration is uncommon. However, when severe degeneration does occur within 14 days of the onset of acute

Table 29.2 Bell Palsy Management[a]

House-Brackmann Grade	MCF Decompression (n)	Steroids Only (n)
I	14	5
II	17	10
III	2	19
IV	1	2
I/II	31 (91%)[b]	15 (42%)
III/IV	3 (9%)	21 (58%)

[a]ENoG: ≥ 90% degeneration by 14 days; EMG: no voluntary motor unit potentials.
[b]$p < 0.0002$ stratified exact permutation test MCF, middle cranial fossa.

paralysis, and there are no voluntary EMG motor units active, MCF surgical decompression is worthwhile.

Facial nerve decompression for the management of severe Bell palsy has also been controversial. A recent editorial in *Otology and Neurology* helps to clarify this approach; de Ru and colleagues[52] stated:

If we dive into the literature of the past 10 years, we only come across 1 study that attempts to appropriately assess the basic question, namely, the study by Gantz et al[51] in 1999. This study shows that when patients were given the option to either have surgery or not, the difference between the 2 groups turned out to be very significant: poor to average recovery in 58% of the nonsurgical group compared with 9% in the surgical group.

For many practitioners of evidence-based medicine, it is easy to devalue a decompression study, not double-blind randomized, long inclusion period, varying groups, etc. However, what kind of a study does one actually expect with regard to such a rare topic? Rare, because the group with such a severe degree of nerve failure rendering decompression an option is very small indeed.

If we try to not send the entire study to the bottom but instead try to extract the good stuff, then it turns out to be a fairly good study after all. You could not actually hope for more. We think we lack the necessary expertise in this area to perform the surgery; however, we do want to be able to refer our patients. Would we have this surgery performed if we were the patient? Yes! When considering the usefulness of evidence, the quality of the medical content and clinical relevance are at least of equal importance to the quality of the methodology. When confronted with rare cases, one should not jump to generalized conclusions.

The above leads to the conclusions that (1) although all evidence is equal, some evidence is more equal than other, and (2) a decompression can in certain cases, when performed by a skilled surgeon, lead to a better outcome then the conservative attitude. More research in carefully selected centers is necessary to establish further conclusive evidence.

Management Algorithm

Our approach to management of Bell palsy is displayed in ► Fig. 29.2. We perform an ENoG when the patient has a total paralysis and is seen within the first 14 days. If the patient has

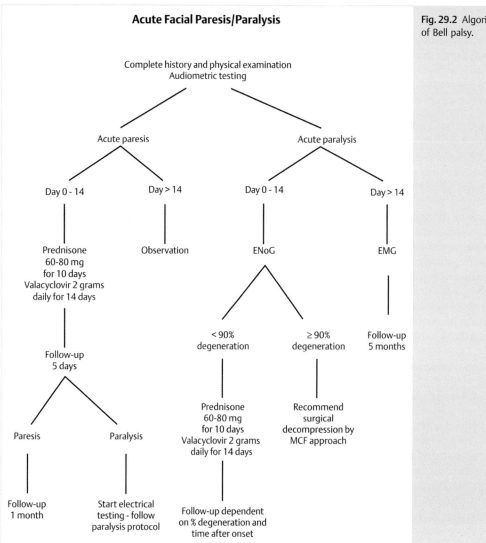

Acute Facial Paresis/Paralysis

Complete history and physical examination
Audiometric testing

Acute paresis

Acute paralysis

Day 0 - 14

Day > 14

Day 0 - 14

Day > 14

Prednisone
60-80 mg
for 10 days
Valacyclovir 2 grams
daily for 14 days

Observation

ENoG

EMG

Follow-up
5 days

< 90%
degeneration

≥ 90%
degeneration

Follow-up
5 months

Paresis

Paralysis

Prednisone
60-80 mg
for 10 days
Valacyclovir 2 grams
daily for 14 days

Recommend
surgical
decompression by
MCF approach

Follow-up
1 month

Start electrical
testing - follow
paralysis protocol

Follow-up dependent
on % degeneration and
time after onset

Fig. 29.2 Algorithm for evaluation and treatment of Bell palsy.

nearly 90% degeneration or is degenerating quickly, frequent follow-up ENoGs are performed.[32] If the 90% threshold is reached within 14 days and no voluntary EMG activity is seen, MCF decompression of the labyrinthine segment and geniculate ganglion is advised. Contraindications to MCF decompression would include general medical contraindications to surgery and age greater than 65. Beyond this age, the middle fossa dura is thinner and more tightly adherent to the tegmen, making elevation of the temporal lobe substantially more difficult. Some groups use the MCF approach for patients over this age limit for attempted hearing preservation in acoustic neuroma surgery. One group has reported a trend toward lower hearing preservation and increased cerebrospinal fluid (CSF) leak rates in patients over the age of 60 with the MCF approach.[53]

Surgical Technique

Facial nerve monitoring is performed routinely, as the facial nerve may be electrically stimulable with direct contact even when percutaneous stimulation suggests total absence of electrical response. EMG and visual monitoring of facial function require that the anesthesia team avoid the use of paralytic agents. A Foley catheter is inserted. Mannitol is given and hyperventilation is performed to reduce intracranial pressure. The hair is shaved above the ear and a posteriorly based 6 × 6 cm skin flap is elevated as shown in ▶ Fig. 29.3. An anteriorly based temporalis flap is raised after harvesting a large piece of temporalis fascia for use in closing. A 4 × 5 cm bone flap centered over the zygomatic root is drilled. Carefully raising the bone flap prevents dural tears, which must be closed to prevent CSF leaks. Bleeding from branches of the middle meningeal artery is controlled with bone wax and bipolar cautery. The vertical cuts must be parallel to facilitate subsequent placement of the middle fossa retractor. The bone flap is wrapped in moist gauze, and the skin and muscle flaps are retracted with care to avoid injury to the frontal branch of the extratemporal facial nerve.

The middle fossa dura is elevated off the tegmen using a combination of blunt and sharp dissection, and bipolar cautery. Elevation proceeds from posterior to anterior to avoid injuring an exposed GSPN or geniculate ganglion. The scrub technician watches for facial movement while working near the facial hiatus. The petrous ridge is identified posteriorly and the GSPN anteriorly. Elevation of the dura superiorly, posteriorly, and anteriorly from the surrounding cranium more evenly distributes pressure from the retractor and makes retractor placement significantly easier. The House-Urban retractor is placed with its tip at the petrous ridge medial to the arcuate eminence once sufficient exposure has been gained. Identification of the arcuate eminence can be one of the most difficult aspects of the procedure. Preoperative Stenver's views can be helpful, but

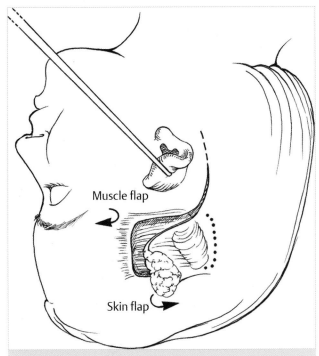

Fig. 29.3 Surgical position illustrating the skin incision (*solid line*) for the MCF approach. *Dashed line:* mastoid extension if transmastoid exposure is planned. *Dotted line:* temporalis muscle, fascia, and periosteal flap.

experience is the ultimate guide to the location of the superior semicircular canal. Until this critical landmark has been precisely located, slow bone removal broadly over the arcuate eminence and tegmen mastoideum is performed until the yellow-ivory bone of the otic capsule is uncovered. The superior canal is always perpendicular to the petrous ridge. The superior canal is blue-lined, and the IAC is then easily found at a 60-degree angle from the superior canal (▶ Fig. 29.4).

The GSPN will also be at a 60-degree angle from the IAC, but frequently it is covered with bone, limiting its usefulness as a landmark. Unlike MCF surgery for acoustic neuromas, the medial aspect of the IAC should not be widely opened, as this unnecessarily increases the risk of CSF leak. Approximately 120 degrees of the lateral IAC is blue-lined with diamond burs and the facial nerve is identified anterior to the vertical crest. It is then traced laterally to the geniculate ganglion and the tympanic segment. The fallopian canal is thinned with diamond burs and copious irrigation. The final layer of bone is removed with blunt elevators or picks. On exposing the middle ear, care must be taken to avoid injury to the ossicles.

The final step of the procedure is neurolysis with a 59–10 Beaver disposable microscalpel. Possible surgical findings include a nerve that is so edematous proximal to the meatal foramen that it obscures the superior vestibular nerve. Sometimes fibers "billow" out after the epineurium is split.[10] In cases where intraoperative electrical responses can be obtained, it is not unusual to see substantial decreases in threshold to electrical stimulation in the IAC after bony decompression, with further decreases after neurolysis.

Closure is accomplished by placing a free muscle graft in the IAC and repairing the tegmen tympani with a small bone graft harvested from the bone flap (▶ Fig. 29.5). This must be placed to prevent herniation of the temporal lobe into the middle ear and must be positioned to avoid interference with ossicular motion. The temporalis fascia graft is placed under the bone to seal the IAC defect. All exposed air cells are plugged with bone wax. Hyperventilation is stopped, and the temporal lobe is

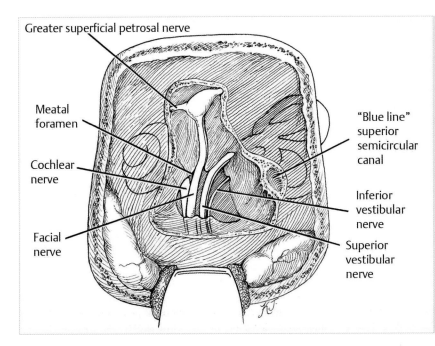

Fig. 29.4 Surgical view of the left middle cranial fossa exposure after craniotomy, temporal lobe retraction, and bony exposure are complete.

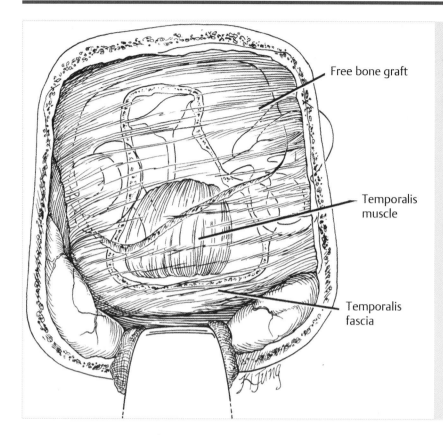

Free bone graft

Temporalis muscle

Temporalis fascia

Fig. 29.5 Temporalis muscle is placed within the IAC defect at the conclusion of decompression. A free bone graft is placed perpendicular to the axis of the IAC to prevent herniation of the temporal lobe into the middle ear or IAC. Temporalis fascia is then used to seal the temporal lobe dura and IAC.

allowed to settle into anatomic position. Two 4–0 Neuralon sutures are used to tack the dura to the pericranium inferiorly to prevent epidural hematoma. The bone flap is replaced and a watertight closure of the temporalis, galea, and skin is performed. A mastoid dressing is applied and the patient is observed in surgical intensive care overnight. At least 48 hours of perioperative steroids, antibiotics, and fluid restriction are routine. If there are no complications, the patient may be discharged as early as postoperative day 3. Potential complications include all of those associated with middle fossa surgery.

The most important management guidelines for "idiopathic" acute facial (Bell) paralysis are as follows: (1) Administer eye care to all patients. (2) Prescribe high-dose oral glucocorticoids (prednisone) to all patients unless there is a contraindication. (3) Prescribe valacyclovir, at least 1 g orally t.i.d. The duration and benefit of this treatment regimen depends on when the patient is first seen, with day 1 defined as the first day of observed weakness. Obviously, the sooner treatment is begun, the more likely it is to help. This latter point is especially true for antiviral medication, which works best when started within the first 3 days and somewhat also if started in the first 7 days. After 7 days, prednisone still might be helpful, but antivirals might or might not be helpful. (4) When the patient develops total facial paralysis, electrophysiological testing with ENoG should be initiated on day 3 or 4 following the onset of total paralysis. The electrophysiological testing should guide further surgical intervention. The criteria that appears to be the most appropriate are greater than 90% degeneration on ENoG before 15 days of total paralysis and there are no voluntary motor unit potentials on EMG. If surgical intervention is required, the approach should be through the middle fossa for decompression of the tympanic, geniculate ganglion, and meatal foramen portions of the facial nerve.

Assume a patient with "idiopathic" acute facial palsy (not Ramsay Hunt) presents on day 2. The landmark study of natural history by Peitersen[29] proved that eye care alone achieved 71% grade I results and a total of 84% grade I or II results. A grade II result is very acceptable. If a patient is treated promptly and aggressively with prednisone-valacyclovir, the grade I or II outcome rises even higher. Obviously, specialty clinics with qualified neuro-otologists see these "worst-case scenario" patients in whom surgery can be very appropriate. However, when emergency physicians, family doctors, internists, and neurologists learn that the standard of initial care is eye care, prednisone, and valacyclovir, the need for surgical intervention will be significantly reduced.[29,54]

29.4.2 Herpes Zoster Oticus

Herpes zoster oticus (HZO), or Ramsay Hunt syndrome, is characterized by severe pain, vesicles in the conchal bowl and sensory distribution of the facial nerve, and facial paralysis that tends to be more severe than that found in Bell palsy (▶ Fig. 29.6; ▶ Fig. 29.7). It is caused by the varicella zoster virus and not infrequently involves the vestibular and cochlear nerves causing hearing loss and vertigo. Involvement of cranial nerves V, IX, X, XI, and XII can also occur, prompting the alternative name "herpes zoster cephalicus."[55] The frequency of complete electrical degeneration of the facial nerve is much higher than with Bell palsy, and the prognosis for spontaneous, complete recovery is much lower (22 to 31%).[29,56,57] Even with the administration of steroids, facial nerve recovery rates are low.[57,58]

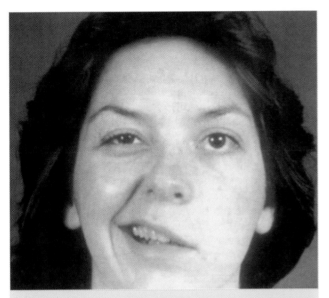

Fig. 29.6 Grade IV left facial paralysis from herpes zoster oticus.

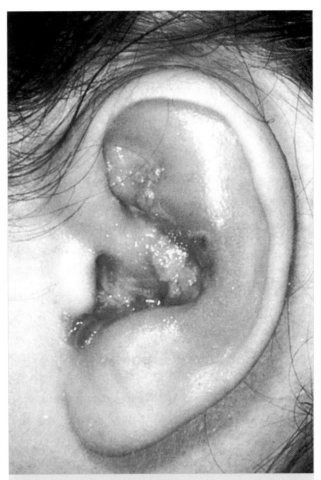

Fig. 29.7 Appearance of the left ear in the same patient as in ▶ Fig. 29.6. Note the vesicles characteristic of herpes zoster oticus.

Two uncontrolled studies of intravenous acyclovir therapy involving a total of 12 patients have demonstrated dramatic improvement of facial function as compared with historical controls.[59,60] Nine of 12 had grade I or II recoveries. Of the three who had grade III recoveries, one had only 1-month follow-up, one was elderly and missed multiple doses, and one began treatment 5 days following onset of paralysis. Other uncontrolled studies have looked at either intravenous or oral acyclovir therapy combined with steroids.[61-64] In the third study, of 91 patients who were treated within 7 days of onset of paralysis, 93% recovered to a grade I or II. In this study, a group of patients treated with steroids alone due to late onset of vesicles showed 68% recovered to a grade I or II.[61] Recovery to grade I or II in the remaining three studies was 36%, 74%, and 82.6%.[61,62,64] These differences appear to reflect both variation in treatment protocols and duration of symptoms prior to presentation.

Although there are good theoretical reasons to perform MCF decompression for this disease, the outcome appears to be so improved by medical therapy alone that this does not appear to be justified. Other studies have shown that HZO is characterized by multiple "skip" lesions throughout the course of the nerve, and so MCF decompression would be inadequate to address all areas of facial nerve compression.[65-70] Finally, ENoG prognostication appears unreliable in HZO. We have had a patient with grade VI facial movement and no response on ENoG recover function after 7 days of IV acyclovir. Again, this may occur because the nerve is more diffusely affected in HZO than in Bell palsy. A couple of studies still advocate surgical decompression, whether through the mastoid alone[65] or through a combined mastoid-MCF approach.[71]

For patients presenting within 3 weeks of onset of paralysis, we treat with a 2-week course of valacyclovir at zoster dosages of 1.5 g twice daily and 1 mg/kg/day prednisone for 14 days. Patients who have a medical contraindication to oral steroids are treated with weekly transtympanic injections of Solu-Medrol 0.3 to 0.4 cc of 40 mg/cc solution (Pfizer Inc.).

29.4.3 Facial Neuroma

Typically a schwannoma of the facial nerve, facial neuroma is a rare problem. Treatment decisions are hampered by an incomplete understanding of the disease's natural history. In their review, Lipkin and coworkers[72] identified 248 cases in the world literature and discussed seven cases managed at Baylor University over a 20-year period. In a survey of 1,400 temporal bones at the University of Minnesota, metastatic and contiguous malignant tumor involvement of the facial nerve was 16 times more common than primary neurogenic tumors, of which there was only one case.[73]

In the Baylor review,[72] facial weakness was a presenting symptom in about two thirds of cases. Approximately one in seven of them experienced sudden facial paresis, with the remainder having a gradual or unspecified onset. Hearing loss was present in half of patients at presentation, with tinnitus, ear canal mass, pain, vestibular symptoms, and otorrhea each occurring in 10 to 15% of cases. Tumor location was also variable, with 19% in the CPA, 30% in the IAC, 42% in the labyrinthine segment and geniculate, 58% in the tympanic segment, 48% in the vertical segment, and 14% peripheral to the stylomastoid foramen. Many tumors involved multiple segments of the nerve. Some cases of tympanic segment neuroma may reflect a reparative response to chronic inflammation.[74]

When the facial neuroma is confined to the IAC or CPA and no facial nerve symptoms are present, misdiagnosis as acoustic neuroma is not uncommon. Fagan et al[75] reported that an MRI showing the bulk of the tumor mass projecting posteriorly into the CPA, rather than concentric within the IAC, is highly suggestive of a facial neuroma. Unfortunately, this relationship is not present in all cases of facial neuroma, especially when the tumors are small.[76,77] Brackmann and colleagues[77,78] suggest using a combination of ENoG and auditory brainstem response (ABR) to help determine whether a tumor is an acoustic neuroma or a facial neuroma. However, tumors located primarily within the CPA may not affect facial function or ENoG even if quite large.[79]

Management options for facial neuromas include observation, microsurgery, and radiotherapy. Observation is recommended by many authors while the patient continues to have good facial nerve function (grade I or II) due to the risk of definitive treatment to nerve function and the certainty that a graft will yield a grade III or worse outcome.[76,80,81] Others recommend decompression without resection to allow the facial neuroma "room to grow" without compression of the nerve or its blood supply.[77] This technique was used in four patients with intraoperatively discovered facial schwannomas; three patients retained their preoperative facial nerve function and one showed improved function from grade V to grade II.[77] Pulec[82] first showed that some tumors can be dissected off facial nerve fascicles with preservation of facial nerve function at levels better than those expected after facial nerve grafting, and these findings have been confirmed by others.[79,83,84] Unfortunately, there is no current preoperative method to determine which facial neuromas would be amenable to fascicle preservation. Some authors have recommended resection soon after diagnosis, regardless of facial nerve function, because they feel that continued compression of the nerve by the tumor will cause damage to the uninvolved ends of the nerve, yielding poorer results during nerve grafting.[85] Radiotherapy has also been used in the primary treatment of these rare tumors in at least two cases.[86] One patient had a decrease in her tumor size following radiotherapy but no improvement in her facial function, and the second showed improvement in facial function without a decrease in tumor size.[86]

Until there is some means to predict which tumors will grow quickly and which can be treated without increased facial nerve dysfunction, the controversy regarding treatment of small facial schwannomas is unlikely to be resolved. Brainstem compression from a large CPA mass would mandate immediate resection, but within the temporal bone a facial neuroma could become quite sizable without threatening life. Decisions must be made based on the patient's age, degree of facial function, tumor locations, hearing status, and his or her own desires. ▶ Fig. 29.8 shows normal facial function of a 48-year-old man who had a tympanic facial neuroma diagnosed at exploratory tympanotomy 18 years earlier. ▶ Fig. 29.9 shows an enhanced MRI demonstrating no growth of the tumor. Cases such as this make it difficult to recommend surgery for a nonthreatening facial neuroma until at least grade III weakness is present.

The MRI scans in ▶ Fig. 29.10 and ▶ Fig. 29.11 demonstrate a contrasting case of a large facial neuroma of the descending segment in a 50-year-old woman with a 6-month history of slowly progressive facial weakness. She had grade III weakness and was not willing to undergo resection and grafting. It is often unwise to biopsy facial neuromas as noted by O'Donoghue et al,[85] but it would have been imprudent to leave a mass of this

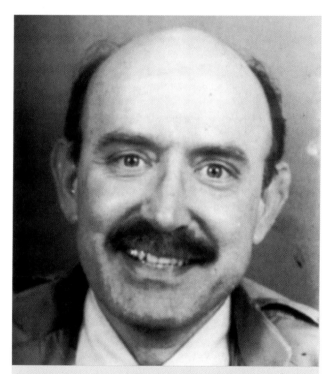

Fig. 29.8 Normal facial function in a patient known to have a neuroma of the right tympanic segment for 18 years. This was identified on exploratory tympanotomy for conductive hearing loss.

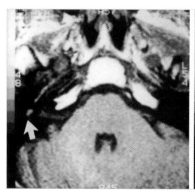
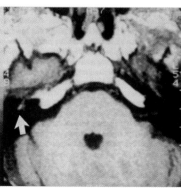

Fig. 29.9 Axial MRI with gadolinium on the same patient as in ▶ Fig. 29.8. The *white arrows* point to the facial neuroma on the right side.

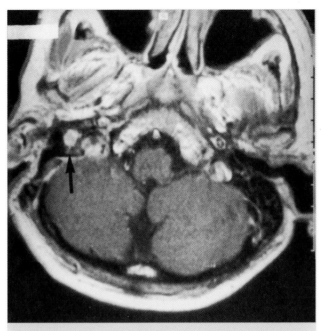

Fig. 29.10 Axial MRI with gadolinium. The *black arrow* points to a large facial neuroma of the descending segment of the right facial nerve.

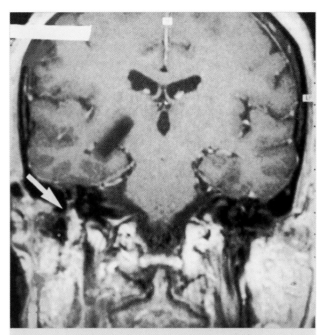

Fig. 29.11 Coronal MRI with gadolinium (same case as in ▶ Fig. 29.11). The *white arrow* points to a massively enlarged right facial nerve.

size in the patient without biopsy. She underwent a transmastoid decompression and biopsy of this mass, which proved to be a facial schwannoma from the second genu through the stylomastoid foramen. She awoke with grade IV facial function, and after 6 months was back to her preoperative grade III function. She was subsequently followed with serial MRI scans.

We have seen five cases of facial neuromas coexisting with vestibular schwannomas in patients with neurofibromatosis type II. In three patients, MCF excision of the acoustic neuroma was planned and the facial neuroma was identified intraoperatively. In the other two patients, who had no residual hearing and larger tumors compressing the brainstem, translabyrinthine excision was performed. The vestibular schwannoma was excised in all cases and the facial neuromas were left in place. In the patients receiving MCF excisions, facial nerve function was preserved in all three. Hearing was initially preserved in two of these patients. In one of the two, hearing was noted to be lost at 6 months, and the facial neuroma had enlarged on follow-up MRI. In the patients who had translabyrinthine excisions of their tumors, facial nerve function was lost postoperatively despite preservation of the facial neuroma. Obviously, decision making in such cases remains a complex problem.

29.5 Facial Nerve Disorders in Children

Orobello[87] has divided pediatric facial nerve disorders into three categories: congenital paralysis, prenatal acquired paralysis, and postnatal acquired paralysis. Congenital facial paralysis consists of developmental errors occurring during embryogenesis. Prenatal acquired paralysis is due to factors extrinsic to the fetus such as intrauterine trauma and maternal exposure to teratogens. Postnatal acquired paralysis includes many of the same diseases that affect adults as well as congenital disorders that manifest later in life. The incidence of newborn facial paralysis is 0.2% of all live births.[88]

29.5.1 Congenital Disorders

Möbius Syndrome

This rare syndrome (▶ Fig. 29.12) is characterized by congenital facial diplegia in association with unilateral or bilateral sixth nerve paralysis. Multiple modes of inheritance have been proposed, and there are three known loci for the syndrome.[89] Exposure of the fetus in utero to cocaine,[90] ergotamine,[91] or misoprostol (a synthetic analogue of prostaglandin E_1)[90] has been associated with the development of Möbius syndrome as well. There may be associated deformities of the extremities, other cranial nerve deficits, musculoskeletal deficiencies, and mental retardation.[89] The exact site of the lesion is disputed; see Orobello[87] or Gantz and Wackym[92] for summaries. Some studies have noted nuclear abnormalities of cranial nerve VI and VII; others have noted normal facial nuclei and failure of muscle development. One temporal bone study of an affected patient demonstrated normal facial nerve anatomy to the tympanic segment, where the nerve terminated in a manner consistent with an intrauterine "necrotic lesion" of the temporal bone.[93]

Treatment of these patients mandates ophthalmologic consultation. If motor end plates are absent, then XII to VII hypoglossal-to-facial nerve anastomosis or cross-facial reinnervation procedures would not be expected to be of benefit. If motor end plates are present, then the above-mentioned temporal bone findings would suggest exploration to identify the termination of the horizontal segment and subsequent grafting. Temporalis transposition may be helpful regardless of muscle status, as it implants a new neuromuscular system. Other studies have shown that bilateral gracilis free muscle transfers with

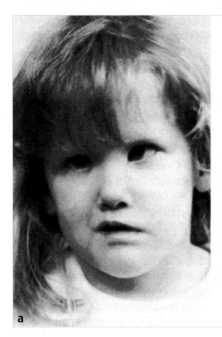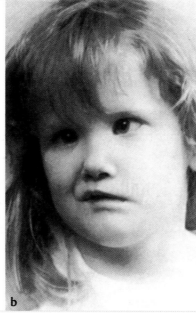

Fig. 29.12 Möbius syndrome. (a) Left facial paralysis and right facial paresis photographed at rest. (b) With smiling and rightward gaze, the right facial paresis and sixth nerve paralysis are apparent.

innervation from a branch of the trigeminal can restore smiling[94,95] and improve speech intelligibility,[96] even in the absence of biting in some patients.[97]

Hemifacial Microsomia

Hemifacial microsomia entails unilateral hypoplasia of the first and second branchial arches with resultant microtia, microstomia, and hypoplasia of the mandible. Neurogenic facial paresis is not uncommonly associated with this disorder, and has been reported in 22% of these patients.[98,99] Other congenital syndromes, particularly those with first and second arch abnormalities, may be associated with facial paresis or paralysis.

Congenital Unilateral Lower Lip Palsy

This disorder is characterized by autosomal dominant inheritance of congenital hypoplasia of the depressor anguli oris muscle and is manifested by asymmetric crying facies and asymmetry with smiling. Other congenital otologic and cardiovascular anomalies may be associated with this syndrome.[100] Facial symmetry and function almost always recover spontaneously.

29.5.2 Prenatal Acquired Paralysis

This category includes intrauterine trauma typically associated with difficult delivery. Cephalopelvic disproportion and high-forceps delivery are typically the cause when the site of lesion is in the extratemporal facial nerve, unless temporal bone fracture or intracranial injury has occurred. The trauma may be caused by forceps, but also can occur without forceps presumably from pressure from the maternal sacrum.[101] ENoG within the first 3 days of life should show no degeneration, with the subsequent degree of degeneration depending on the degree of injury. The absence of an evoked response within the first 3 days suggests either a congenital abnormality or earlier intrauterine trauma. EMG can help distinguish the latter two possibilities with the absence of fibrillations or of an evoked response suggesting congenital absence of the nerve-muscle unit. These are important distinctions because facial paralysis associated with delivery has an excellent prognosis, with 90% incidence of spontaneous recovery.[101] Teratogenic causes of facial paralysis include maternal thalidomide exposure and maternal rubella.

29.5.3 Postnatal Acquired Paralysis

This category includes all facial nerve disorders found in adults, but specific mention is made of two disorders that typically manifest in childhood, one hereditary and the other idiopathic.

Osteopetrosis

This disorder, also known as Albers-Schönberg disease, has dominant and recessive forms of varying severity. It is a bony dysplasia that can cause multiple cranial neuropathies secondary to entrapment at neural foramina. Progressive or fluctuating involvement of cranial nerves II, V, VII, and VIII is common. Complete intratemporal facial nerve decompression should be considered if there is radiological evidence of facial nerve entrapment by osteopetrosis associated with facial dysfunction (see also Chapter 23).

Melkersson-Rosenthal Syndrome

This is a triad consisting of recurrent facial or labial edema, fissured tongue (lingua plicata), and recurrent facial paralysis.[102] One or two components of the triad may be present without complete manifestation of the disease. The disease is inherited as an autosomal dominant trait with variable penetrance. The pathophysiology is unknown. Pathologically the disease is characterized by noncaseating granulomas.[103] Clinically, facial paralysis is seen in less than 40% of patients with the disorder. Typically episodes of paralysis become more severe and frequent over time, leading to synkinesis and incomplete recovery.[103] Graham and Kartush[4] reported MCF decompression of six patients for frequently recurring facial paralysis. None had recurrent attacks, including the one patient with Melkersson-Rosenthal syndrome who continued to have attacks of facial edema without weakness. In a second report, a patient had recurrent episodic facial paralysis following a transmastoid decompression. Following MCF decompression, this patient continued to have episodic transient paresis associated with facial edema on the operated side. However, these episodes lasted less than 24 hours, compared with preoperative episodes of facial paresis that would last 6 months at each occurrence.[12]

29.6 Facial Paralysis Secondary to Inflammatory Middle Ear Disease

29.6.1 Chronic Otitis Media

The management of facial paralysis secondary to chronic otitis media is perhaps the only topic of this chapter that does not evoke controversy.[104] Facial paralysis or paresis can be a complication of chronic ear disease with or without cholesteatoma. It presents an urgent indication for surgical intervention. In Takahashi and coworkers'[105] series of 1,600 patients with facial paralysis, only 50 were secondary to inflammatory middle ear disease. A mastoidectomy appropriate for the type of chronic ear disease present, followed by decompression of the involved portion of the facial nerve, must be performed promptly. Cholesteatoma adherent to the nerve is preferably removed, but it can be exteriorized if this cannot be done safely. Few would argue against a canal-wall-down technique in the setting of cholesteatomatous involvement of the facial nerve.

29.6.2 Acute Otitis Media

Facial paresis secondary to acute otitis media is not uncommon, although its exact incidence is uncertain. Standard treatment consists of myringotomy, intravenous antibiotics, and a high-resolution temporal bone CT to rule out coalescent mastoiditis. If there is no coalescence or other indications for mastoidectomy, the role of surgery for the facial paralysis is poorly defined. Limb and Niparko[18] advocate mastoidectomy without nerve decompression if facial function does not return in 1 week. Hughes and Pensak[106] advocate mastoidectomy and decompression from the cochleariform process to the stylomastoid foramen "if nerve dysfunction persists or progresses." Glasscock et al[107] suggest simple mastoidectomy if facial paralysis lasts 2 weeks. Harris[108] advocates mastoidectomy and nerve decompression if significant degeneration is apparent on ENoG.[108] Selesnick and Patwardhan[40] argue against surgical intervention at all. None of these sources relies on any case series because myringotomy and medical therapy are usually effective. In these cases we perform an ENoG if total paralysis is present for 3 days and perform mastoidectomy and nerve decompression from the cochleariform process to the stylomastoid foramen if degeneration exceeds 90%. If degeneration does not reach 90% and no other surgical indication is present, intravenous antibiotics and steroids are continued.

▶ Fig. 29.13 demonstrates the CT scan of a 40-year-old woman who presented with acute otitis media and facial paralysis. Myringotomy and intravenous antibiotics were begun, but an

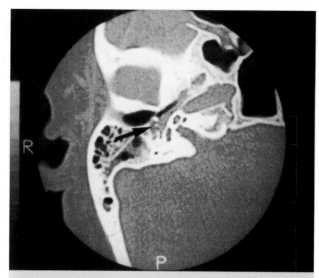

Fig. 29.13 Acute otitis media and facial paralysis with complete degeneration on ENoG. Note absence of coalescence. *Arrow* points to soft tissue mass enveloping stapes. At surgery this was found to be a granuloma compressing the dehiscent tympanic segment. Intraoperative electrophysiological findings are described in the text.

ENoG at 72 hours following paralysis showed no response. Canal-wall-up mastoidectomy demonstrated a granuloma compressed between the stapes and a widely dehiscent tympanic segment. Intraoperative electrical stimulation at 1 V prior to removing the granuloma demonstrated no response from the tympanic segment proximal to the granuloma and small EMG potentials without observable facial movement from the distal mastoid segment.

After removing the granuloma and decompressing vertical and tympanic segments, EMG potentials and facial motion were obtained with proximal stimulation at 0.25 V. A neurolysis was not performed. The patient was continued on intravenous antibiotics and discharged on postoperative day 4 with some detectable movement of the midface. Follow-up at 10 days showed grade IV movement; 1-month follow-up revealed a grade II result. Although we cannot be certain that she would not have had this same result without decompression, the pressure of the granuloma on the dehiscent nerve was sufficient to indent it halfway into the fallopian canal. The intraoperative electrophysiological changes after decompression were impressive. This case demonstrates that there is clearly a degree of facial nerve injury between neurapraxia and axonotmesis where a focal pathological process causes a rapidly reversible interference with distal conduction. For more discussion of facial nerve pathology from inflammatory middle ear disease, see Chapter 18.

29.6.3 Hemifacial Spasm and Essential Blepharospasm

Hemifacial spasm (HFS) is unilateral involuntary contraction of the facial musculature,[109] most commonly associated with a vessel contacting the root exit zone of the facial nerve.[110,111] Many studies suggest that HFS results not only from compression of root exit zone by the nerve but also from increased excitability of the facial nucleus.[112] HFS has also been found in several families, and so may be inherited with low penetrance.[113] Patients presenting with HFS rarely (< 1%) have a variety of other compressive lesions, including CPA lipomas,[114,115] meningiomas,[116] epidermoids,[117] arachnoid cysts,[118] and aneurysms.[119] Infrequently, these mass lesions may be located on the contralateral side.[120] Thus, the use of MRI to detect potential mass lesions is necessary in the evaluation of HFS.

Treatment options for HFS include serial Botox injections to affected musculature and microvascular decompression. Elston[121] first used Botox injections for treatment of this disorder and reported relief of involuntary eye contractions in six patients for 15 weeks. In a prospective randomized crossover controlled study of 11 patients with HFS, Yoshimura et al[122] found objective improvement following 84% of injections with Botox, and no objective improvement in patients who received placebo injections. The main complication was facial weakness, although bruising, diplopia, and ptosis were also reported. Over time, decreased responsiveness to Botox can develop. In a series of 45 patients treated for a mean of 15.8 years with serial Botox A injections, 49% eventually showed a decreased response.[123] The majority of these patients responded to dose adjustment; however, 27% did not respond to increased dosage and 18% had blocking antibodies to Botox A. These patients were treated successfully with Botox B.[123] Microvascular decompression (MVD), typically via suboccipital approach, is also effective in the treatment of HFS, with long-term cure rates in several large studies ranging from 80 to 90.5%.[124–128] Complications of MVD include CSF leak, hearing loss, cerebellar injury, and, rarely, brainstem infarct and death.[124,129]

Although not a disorder of the peripheral facial nerve, essential blepharospasm (EB) may be seen in patients referred for facial nerve disorders and should be distinguished from HFS. EB is a focal dystonia characterized by involuntary bilateral orbicularis oculi closure that can be severe enough to interfere with vision. EB may present along with other focal dystonias or as a component of Meige syndrome (EB plus dystonia of the lower face and jaw). Although the cause of EB is unknown, this condition is sometimes associated with traumatic injury in the area of the eye. The cornerstone of treatment is serial Botox injections[130] with oculoplastic procedures reserved for patients whose EB is resistant to this therapy.[131]

29.7 Nerve Repair

Nerve grafting is frequently required when facial neuromas are excised. It is commonly necessary in cases of facial paralysis following penetrating trauma to the facial nerve as well, and is less commonly needed in acoustic neuroma surgery. When a tension-free end-to-end anastomosis can be performed, this is the preferred technique. Most cases require an interposition graft. Either the greater auricular nerve or the sural nerve may be used for this purpose. Whenever there is a proximal and distal facial nerve stump, grafting is much preferred over any other reanimation technique. This is as true in the CPA as it is in the parotid. Suture anastomosis in the CPA is technically challenging, but yields gratifying results with excellent facial tone and good oral sphincter function returning after 6 to 8 months, albeit with significant synkinesis. If no proximal stump is

Table 29.3 The Repaired Facial Nerve Recovery Scale (RFNRS)

Grade	Description
A	Normal function
B	Independent motion of the eye and mouth, strong eye closure and mouth sphincter, mass motion, and possible slight forehead movement
C	Strong closure of eye and mouth with mass motion and no forehead movement
D	Incomplete eye closure and mouth movement, mass movement, and good tone
E	Minimal movement of any branch and poor tone
F	No movement

Data from Gidley PW, Gantz BJ, Rubinstein JT. Facial nerve grafts: from cerebellopontine angle and beyond. Am J Otol 1999;20:781–788.

available, a split XII–to–VII anastomosis is our preferred approach. Three 10–0 nylon epineural sutures are placed at anastomoses in the CPA and four are used in the temporal bone or parotid (see Chapter 21). Alternatively, collagen splints can be used to establish the anastomosis in the CPA,[132,133] and tissue glue can be used to anastomose the nerve more distally within the temporal bone or in the periphery.[134]

Grading the function of a facial nerve graft is difficult to fit into the House/Brackmann facial nerve grading scale. With a graft there is always mass motion and it is very rare to have any forehead movement, but there is usually very strong eye closure and smile. It is unfair to characterize this function of no forehead movement and strong eye closure as a III/VI result, but it is also unfair to claim it is IV/VI! For this reason a separate classification for facial nerve grafts was devised.[135] The Repaired Facial Nerve Recovery Scale (RFNRS) (► Table 29.3) employs a six-point scale similar to the House/Brackmann grading scale, but uses letters to differentiate it from the House/Brackmann scale. Class A is normal function and Class F is no movement. Class B is rare and indicates independent movement of the eye and mouth, strong eye closure and mouth sphincter, mass motion, and possible slight forehead movement. Class C is most common, strong closure of eye and mouth with mass motion and no forehead movement. Class D indicates incomplete eye closure and mouth movement, mass movement, and good tone. Class E is minimal movement of any branch and poor tone. This grading scale clarifies movement following grafting of the facial nerve. There is usually better function with a graft compared to a substitution procedure such as a VII–XII. There is also more spontaneity with a graft.

References

[1] Adour KK. Medical management of idiopathic (Bell's) palsy. Otolaryngol Clin North Am 1991; 24: 663–673

[2] McCabe BF. Some evidence for the efficacy of decompression for Bell's palsy: immediate motion postoperatively. Laryngoscope 1977; 87: 246–249

[3] Gantz BJ, Gmür A, Fisch U. Intraoperative evoked electromyography in Bell's palsy. Am J Otolaryngol 1982; 3: 273–278

[4] Graham MD, Kartush JM. Total facial nerve decompression for recurrent facial paralysis: an update. Otolaryngol Head Neck Surg 1989; 101: 442–444

[5] Niparko JK, Kileny PR, Kemink JL, Lee HM, Graham MD. Neurophysiologic intraoperative monitoring: II. Facial nerve function. Am J Otol 1989; 10: 55–61

[6] Jackson CG, Johnson GD, Hyams VJ, Poe DS. Pathologic findings in the labyrinthine segment of the facial nerve in a case of facial paralysis. Ann Otol Rhinol Laryngol 1990; 99: 327–329

[7] Tien R, Dillon WP, Jackler RK. Contrast-enhanced MR imaging of the facial nerve in 11 patients with Bell's palsy. AJNR Am J Neuroradiol 1990; 11: 735–741

[8] Schwaber MK, Larson TC, III, Zealear DL, Creasy J. Gadolinium-enhanced magnetic resonance imaging in Bell's palsy. Laryngoscope 1990; 100: 1264–1269

[9] Korzec K, Sobol SM, Kubal W, Mester SJ, Winzelberg G, May M. Gadolinium-enhanced magnetic resonance imaging of the facial nerve in herpes zoster oticus and Bell's palsy: clinical implications. Am J Otol 1991; 12: 163–168

[10] Marsh MA, Coker NJ. Surgical decompression of idiopathic facial palsy. Otolaryngol Clin North Am 1991; 24: 675–689

[11] Girard N, Poncet M, Chays A et al. MRI exploration of the intrapetrous facial nerve. J Neuroradiol 1993; 20: 226–238

[12] Dutt SN, Mirza S, Irving RM, Donaldson I. Total decompression of facial nerve for Melkersson-Rosenthal syndrome. J Laryngol Otol 2000; 114: 870–873

[13] Kinoshita T, Ishii K, Okitsu T, Okudera T, Ogawa T. Facial nerve palsy: evaluation by contrast-enhanced MR imaging. Clin Radiol 2001; 56: 926–932

[14] Schuknecht HF, Gulya AJ. Anatomy of the Temporal Bone with Surgical Implications. Philadelphia: Lea & Febiger, 1986

[15] Takahashi H, Sando I. Facial canal dehiscence: histologic study and computer reconstruction. Ann Otol Rhinol Laryngol 1992; 101: 925–930

[16] Brackmann DE, Arriaga MA. Surgery for glomus and jugular foramen tumors. In: Brackmann DE, ed. Otologic Surgery, 2nd ed. Philadelphia: WB Saunders, 2001

[17] House JW, Brackmann DE. Facial nerve grading system. Otolaryngol Head Neck Surg 1985; 93: 146–147

[18] Limb CJ, Niparko JK. The acute facial palsies. In: Jackler RK, Brackmann DE, eds. Neurotology, 2nd ed. Philadelphia: Elsevier Mosby, 2005

[19] Sclafani AP, Conley JJ. Occult parotid malignancy discovered 10 years after acute onset of complete facial paralysis. Otolaryngol Head Neck Surg 1994; 110: 235–238

[20] May M. Facial nerve disorders. Update 1982. Am J Otol 1982; 4: 77–88

[21] May M, Schaitkin BM. The Facial Nerve, 2nd ed. New York: Thieme, 2000

[22] Djupesland G, Berdal P, Johannessen TA, Degré M, Stien R, Skrede S. Viral infection as a cause of acute peripheral facial palsy. Arch Otolaryngol 1976; 102: 403–406

[23] Vahlne A, Edström S, Arstila P et al. Bell's palsy and herpes simplex virus. Arch Otolaryngol 1981; 107: 79–81

[24] Mulkens PS, Bleeker JD, Schröder FP. Acute facial paralysis: a virological study. Clin Otolaryngol Allied Sci 1980; 5: 303–310

[25] Burgess RC, Michaels L, Bale JF, Jr, Smith RJ. Polymerase chain reaction amplification of herpes simplex viral DNA from the geniculate ganglion of a patient with Bell's palsy. Ann Otol Rhinol Laryngol 1994; 103: 775–779

[26] Murakami S, Mizobuchi M, Nakashiro Y, Doi T, Hato N, Yanagihara N. Bell palsy and herpes simplex virus: identification of viral DNA in endoneurial fluid and muscle. Ann Intern Med 1996; 124: 27–30

[27] Fisch U, Esslen E. Total intratemporal exposure of the facial nerve. Pathologic findings in Bell's palsy. Arch Otolaryngol 1972; 95: 335–341

[28] Eicher SA, Coker NJ, Alford BR, Igarashi M, Smith RJ. A comparative study of the fallopian canal at the meatal foramen and labyrinthine segment in young children and adults. Arch Otolaryngol Head Neck Surg 1990; 116: 1030–1035

[29] Peitersen E. The natural history of Bell's palsy. Am J Otol 1982; 4: 107–111

[30] Adour KK, Byl FM, Hilsinger RL, Jr, Kahn ZM, Sheldon MI. The true nature of Bell's palsy: analysis of 1,000 consecutive patients. Laryngoscope 1978; 88: 787–801

[31] Devriese PP, Schumacher T, Scheide A, de Jongh RH, Houtkooper JM. Incidence, prognosis and recovery of Bell's palsy. A survey of about 1000 patients (1974–1983). Clin Otolaryngol Allied Sci 1990; 15: 15–27

[32] Fisch U. Prognostic value of electrical tests in acute facial paralysis. Am J Otol 1984; 5: 494–498

[33] Sillman JS, Niparko JK, Lee SS, Kileny PR. Prognostic value of evoked and standard electromyography in acute facial paralysis. Otolaryngol Head Neck Surg 1992; 107: 377–381

[34] Citron D, III, Adour KK. Acoustic reflex and loudness discomfort in acute facial paralysis. Arch Otolaryngol 1978; 104: 303–306

[35] May M, Blumenthal F, Klein SR. Acute Bell's palsy: prognostic value of evoked electromyography, maximal stimulation, and other electrical tests. Am J Otol 1983; 5: 1–7

[36] Seddon H. Three types of nerve injury. Brain 1943; 66: 237

[37] Sunderland S. Nerves and Nerve Injuries. Edinburgh: E & S Livingstone, 1968

[38] Seiff SR, Chang J. Management of ophthalmic complications of facial nerve palsy. Otolaryngol Clin North Am 1992; 25: 669–690

[39] Kinney SE, Seeley BM, Seeley MZ, Foster JA. Oculoplastic surgical techniques for protection of the eye in facial nerve paralysis. Am J Otol 2000; 21: 275–283

[40] Selesnick SH, Patwardhan A. Acute facial paralysis: evaluation and early management. Am J Otolaryngol 1994; 15: 387–408

[41] Salinas RA, Alvarez G, Ferreira J. Corticosteroids for Bell's palsy (idiopathic facial paralysis). Cochrane Database Syst Rev 2004; 4: CD001942

[42] Adour KK, Ruboyianes JM, Von Doersten PG et al. Bell's palsy treatment with acyclovir and prednisone compared with prednisone alone: a double-blind, randomized, controlled trial. Ann Otol Rhinol Laryngol 1996; 105: 371–378

[43] Allen D, Dunn L. Aciclovir or valaciclovir for Bell's palsy (idiopathic facial paralysis). Cochrane Database Syst Rev 2004; 3: CD001869

[44] Sullivan S, Donnan M. Smith, McKinstry, Davenport, Vale, Clarkson, Hammersley, Hayavi, McAteer, Stewart, Daly. N Engl J Med 2007; 357: 1598–1607

[45] Gilden DH, Tyler KL. Bell's palsy—is glucocorticoid treatment enough? N Engl J Med 2007; 357: 1653–1655

[46] Hato N, Yamada H, Kohno H et al. Valacyclovir and prednisolone treatment for Bell's palsy: a multicenter, randomized, placebo-controlled study. Otol Neurotol 2007; 28: 408–413

[47] de Ru JA, van Benthem PP, Janssen LM. Is antiviral medication for severe Bell's palsy still useful? Lancet Neurol 2009; 8: 509–, author reply 509–510

[48] Engström M, Berg T, Stjernquist-Desatnik A et al. Prednisolone and valaciclovir in Bell's palsy: a randomised, double-blind, placebo-controlled, multicentre trial. Lancet Neurol 2008; 7: 993–1000

[49] May M, Klein SR, Taylor FH. Idiopathic (Bell's) facial palsy: natural history defies steroid or surgical treatment. Laryngoscope 1985; 95: 406–409

[50] Fisch U. Surgery for Bell's palsy. Arch Otolaryngol 1981; 107: 1–11

[51] Gantz BJ, Rubinstein JT, Gidley P, Woodworth GG. Surgical management of Bell's palsy. Laryngoscope 1999; 109: 1177–1188

[52] de Ru JA, van Benthem PPG, Janssen LM. All evidence is equal, but some is more equal than others. Otol Neurotol 2010; 31: 551–553

[53] Oghalai JS, Buxbaum JL, Pitts LH, Jackler RK. The effect of age on acoustic neuroma surgery outcomes. Otol Neurotol 2003; 24: 473–477

[54] Murakami S. Yamano K. Hamajima Y. Evidence-based practical treatments for Bell's palsy. Presented at the annual meeting of the Academy of American Otolaryngology—Head and Neck Surgery, Toronto, Canada, September 19, 2006

[55] Adour KK. Otological complications of herpes zoster. Ann Neurol 1994; 35 Suppl: S62–S64

[56] Devriese P. Herpes zoster causing facial paralysis. In: Fisch U, ed. Facial Nerve Surgery. Amstelveen, Netherlands: Kugler, 1976

[57] Robillard RB, Hilsinger RL, Jr, Adour KK. Ramsay Hunt facial paralysis: clinical analyses of 185 patients. Otolaryngol Head Neck Surg 1986; 95: 292–297

[58] Kinishi M, Hosomi H, Amatsu M, Tani M, Koike K. [Conservative treatment of Hunt syndrome] Nippon Jibiinkoka Gakkai Kaiho 1992; 95: 65–70

[59] Dickins JR, Smith JT, Graham SS. Herpes zoster oticus: treatment with intravenous acyclovir. Laryngoscope 1988; 98: 776–779

[60] Uri N, Greenberg E, Meyer W, Kitzes-Cohen R. Herpes zoster oticus: treatment with acyclovir. Ann Otol Rhinol Laryngol 1992; 101: 161–162

[61] Murakami S, Hato N, Horiuchi J, Honda N, Gyo K, Yanagihara N. Treatment of Ramsay Hunt syndrome with acyclovir-prednisone: significance of early diagnosis and treatment. Ann Neurol 1997; 41: 353–357

[62] Ko JY, Sheen TS, Hsu MM. Herpes zoster oticus treated with acyclovir and prednisolone: clinical manifestations and analysis of prognostic factors. Clin Otolaryngol Allied Sci 2000; 25: 139–142

[63] Kinishi M, Amatsu M, Mohri M, Saito M, Hasegawa T, Hasegawa S. Acyclovir improves recovery rate of facial nerve palsy in Ramsay Hunt syndrome. Auris Nasus Larynx 2001; 28: 223–226

[64] Uri N, Greenberg E, Kitzes-Cohen R, Doweck I. Acyclovir in the treatment of Ramsay Hunt syndrome. Otolaryngol Head Neck Surg 2003; 129: 379–381

[65] Honda N, Yanagihara N, Hato N, Kisak H, Murakami S, Gyo K. Swelling of the intratemporal facial nerve in Ramsay Hunt syndrome. Acta Otolaryngol 2002; 122: 348–352

[66] Maybaum JL, Druss JG. Geniculate ganglionitis (Hunt's syndome). Clinical features and histopathology. Arch Otolaryngol 1934; 19: 574–581

[67] Aleksic SN, Budzilovich GN, Lieberman AN. Herpes zoster oticus and facial paralysis (Ramsay Hunt syndrome). Clinico-pathologic study and review of literature. J Neurol Sci 1973; 20: 149–159

[68] Guldberg-Moller J, Olsen S, Kettel K. Histopathology of the facial nerve in herpes zoster oticus. AMA Arch Otolaryngol 1959; 69: 266–275

[69] Blackley B, Friedmann I, Wright I. Herpes zoster auris associated with facial nerve palsy and auditory nerve symptoms: a case report with histopathological findings. Acta Otolaryngol 1967; 63: 533–550

[70] Etholm B, Schuknecht HF. Pathological findings and surgical implications in herpes zoster oticus. Adv Otorhinolaryngol 1983; 31: 184–190

[71] Pulec JL. Total facial nerve decompression: technique to avoid complications. Ear Nose Throat J 1996; 75: 410–415

[72] Lipkin AF, Coker NJ, Jenkins HA, Alford BR. Intracranial and intratemporal facial neuroma. Otolaryngol Head Neck Surg 1987; 96: 71–79

[73] Jung TT, Jun BH, Shea D, Paparella MM. Primary and secondary tumors of the facial nerve. A temporal bone study. Arch Otolaryngol Head Neck Surg 1986; 112: 1269–1273

[74] Babin RW, Harker LA, Kavanaugh KT. Traumatic intratympanic facial neuroma. A clinical report. Am J Otol 1984; 5: 365–367

[75] Fagan PA, Misra SN, Doust B. Facial neuroma of the cerebellopontine angle and the internal auditory canal. Laryngoscope 1993; 103: 442–446

[76] Kania RE, Herman P, Tran Ba Huy P. Vestibular-like facial nerve schwannoma. Auris Nasus Larynx 2004; 31: 212–219

[77] Angeli SI, Brackmann DE. Is surgical excision of facial nerve schwannomas always indicated? Otolaryngol Head Neck Surg 1997; 117: S144–S147

[78] Brackmann DE, House JW, Selters W. Auditory brainstem responses in facial nerve neurinoma diagnosis. In: Graham MD, House WF, eds. Disorders of the Facial Nerve: Anatomy, Diagnosis, and Management. New York: Raven Press, 1982

[79] Nadeau DP, Sataloff RT. Fascicle preservation surgery for facial nerve neuromas involving the posterior cranial fossa. Otol Neurotol 2003; 24: 317–325

[80] Liu R, Fagan P. Facial nerve schwannoma: surgical excision versus conservative management. Ann Otol Rhinol Laryngol 2001; 110: 1025–1029

[81] Kim CS, Chang SO, Oh SH, Ahn SH, Hwang CH, Lee HJ. Management of intratemporal facial nerve schwannoma. Otol Neurotol 2003; 24: 312–316

[82] Pulec JL. Facial nerve neuroma. Laryngoscope 1972; 82: 1160–1176

[83] Perez R, Chen JM, Nedzelski JM. Intratemporal facial nerve schwannoma: a management dilemma. Otol Neurotol 2005; 26: 121–126

[84] Sherman JD, Dagnew E, Pensak ML, van Loveren HR, Tew JM, Jr. Facial nerve neuromas: report of 10 cases and review of the literature. Neurosurgery 2002; 50: 450–456

[85] O'Donoghue GM, Brackmann DE, House JW, Jackler RK. Neuromas of the facial nerve. Am J Otol 1989; 10: 49–54

[86] Hasegawa T, Kobayashi T, Kida Y, Tanaka T, Yoshida K, Osuka K. [Two cases of facial neurinoma successfully treated with gamma knife radiosurgery] No Shinkei Geka 1999; 27: 171–175

[87] Orobello P. Congenital and acquired facial nerve paralysis in children. Otolaryngol Clin North Am 1991; 24: 647–652

[88] Falco NA, Eriksson E. Facial nerve palsy in the newborn: incidence and outcome. Plast Reconstr Surg 1990; 85: 1–4

[89] Kniffen CL, McCusick VA. Moebius syndrome 1. In: McCusick V, ed. Online Mendelian Inheritance in Man. Baltimore: Johns Hopkins University, 2005:157900

[90] Kankirawatana P, Tennison MB, D'Cruz O, Greenwood RS. Möbius syndrome in infant exposed to cocaine in utero. Pediatr Neurol 1993; 9: 71–72

[91] Graf WD, Shepard TH. Uterine contraction in the development of Möbius syndrome. J Child Neurol 1997; 12: 225–227

[92] Gantz BJ, Wackym PA. Facial nerve abnormalities. In: Smith JD, Bumsted RM, eds. Pediatric Facial Plastic and Reconstructive Surgery. New York: Raven Press, 1993

[93] Gonzalez CH, Vargas FR, Perez AB et al. Limb deficiency with or without Möbius sequence in seven Brazilian children associated with misoprostol use in the first trimester of pregnancy. Am J Med Genet 1993; 47: 59–64

[94] Saito H, Takeda T, Kishimoto S. Neonatal facial nerve defect. Acta Otolaryngol Suppl 1994; 510: 77–81

[95] Terzis JK, Noah EM. Dynamic restoration in Möbius and Möbius-like patients. Plast Reconstr Surg 2003; 111: 40–55

[96] Goldberg C, DeLorie R, Zuker RM, Manktelow RT. The effects of gracilis muscle transplantation on speech in children with Moebius syndrome. J Craniofac Surg 2003; 14: 687–690

[97] Lifchez SD, Matloub HS, Gosain AK. Cortical adaptation to restoration of smiling after free muscle transfer innervated by the nerve to the masseter. Plast Reconstr Surg 2005; 115: 1472–1479, discussion 1480–1482

[98] Carvalho GJ, Song CS, Vargervik K, Lalwani AK. Auditory and facial nerve dysfunction in patients with hemifacial microsomia. Arch Otolaryngol Head Neck Surg 1999; 125: 209–212

[99] Bassila MK, Goldberg R. The association of facial palsy and/or sensorineural hearing loss in patients with hemifacial microsomia. Cleft Palate J 1989; 26: 287–291

[100] McCusick VA. Depressor anguli oris muscle, hypoplasia of. In: McCusick VA, ed. Online Mendelian Inheritance in Man. Baltimore: Johns Hopkins University, 2005:125520

[101] Smith JD, Crumley RL, Harker LA. Facial paralysis in the newborn. Otolaryngol Head Neck Surg 1981; 89: 1021–1024

[102] Kelley J, McCusick VA. Melkersson-Rosenthal syndrome. In: McCusick VA, ed. Online Mendelian Inheritance in Man. Baltimore: Johns Hopkins University, 2005:155900

[103] Hornstein OP. Melkersson-Rosenthal syndrome. A neuro-muco-cutaneous disease of complex origin. Curr Probl Dermatol 1973; 5: 117–156

[104] Greene RM, Rogers RS, III. Melkersson-Rosenthal syndrome: a review of 36 patients. J Am Acad Dermatol 1989; 21: 1263–1270

[105] Takahashi H, Nakamura H, Yui M, Mori H. Analysis of fifty cases of facial palsy due to otitis media. Arch Otorhinolaryngol 1985; 241: 163–168

[106] Hughes GB, Pensak ML, eds. Clinical Otology, 2nd ed. New York: Thieme, 1997

[107] Glasscock ME, Shambaugh GE Jr, Johnson GD, eds. Surgery of the Ear. Philadelphia: WB Saunders, 1990

[108] Harris JP, Kim DP, Darrow DH. Complications of chronic otitis media. In: Nadol JB Jr, McKenna MJ, eds. Surgery of the Ear and Temporal Bone, 2nd ed. Philadelphia: Lippincott Williams & Wilkins, 2004

[109] Costa J, Espírito-Santo C, Borges A et al. Botulinum toxin type A therapy for hemifacial spasm. Cochrane Database Syst Rev 2005; 1: CD004899

[110] Bernardi B, Zimmerman RA, Savino PJ, Adler C. Magnetic resonance tomographic angiography in the investigation of hemifacial spasm. Neuroradiology 1993; 35: 606–611

[111] Hosoya T, Watanabe N, Yamaguchi K, Saito S, Nakai O. Three-dimensional-MRI of neurovascular compression in patients with hemifacial spasm. Neuroradiology 1995; 37: 350–352

[112] Møller AR. Vascular compression of cranial nerves: II: pathophysiology. Neurol Res 1999; 21: 439–443

[113] Miwa H, Mizuno Y, Kondo T. Familial hemifacial spasm: report of cases and review of literature. J Neurol Sci 2002; 193: 97–102

[114] Sade B, Mohr G, Dufour JJ. Cerebellopontine angle lipoma presenting with hemifacial spasm: case report and review of the literature. J Otolaryngol 2005; 34: 270–273

[115] Sprik C, Wirtschafter JD. Hemifacial spasm due to intracranial tumor. An international survey of botulinum toxin investigators. Ophthalmology 1988; 95: 1042–1045

[116] Gómez-Perals LF, Ortega-Martínez M, Fernández-Portales I, Cabezudo-Artero JM. [Hemifacial spasm as clinical presentation of intracranial meningiomas. Report of three cases and review of the literature] Neurocirugia (Astur) 2005; 16: 21–25, discussion 26

[117] Kobata H, Kondo A, Iwasaki K. Cerebellopontine angle epidermoids presenting with cranial nerve hyperactive dysfunction: pathogenesis and long-term surgical results in 30 patients. Neurosurgery 2002; 50: 276–285, discussion 285–286

[118] Takano S, Maruno T, Shirai S, Nose T. Facial spasm and paroxysmal tinnitus associated with an arachnoid cyst of the cerebellopontine angle—case report. Neurol Med Chir (Tokyo) 1998; 38: 100–103

[119] Nagata S, Matsushima T, Fujii K, Fukui M, Kuromatsu C. Hemifacial spasm due to tumor, aneurysm, or arteriovenous malformation. Surg Neurol 1992; 38: 204–209

[120] Matsuura N, Kondo A. Trigeminal neuralgia and hemifacial spasm as false localizing signs in patients with a contralateral mass of the posterior cranial fossa. Report of three cases. J Neurosurg 1996; 84: 1067–1071

[121] Elston JS. Botulinum toxin treatment of hemifacial spasm. J Neurol Neurosurg Psychiatry 1986; 49: 827–829

[122] Yoshimura DM, Aminoff MJ, Tami TA, Scott AB. Treatment of hemifacial spasm with botulinum toxin. Muscle Nerve 1992; 15: 1045–1049

[123] Mejia NI, Vuong KD, Jankovic J. Long-term botulinum toxin efficacy, safety, and immunogenicity. Mov Disord 2005; 20: 592–597

[124] Barker FG, II, Jannetta PJ, Bissonette DJ, Shields PT, Larkins MV, Jho HD. Microvascular decompression for hemifacial spasm. J Neurosurg 1995; 82: 201–210

[125] Illingworth RD, Porter DG, Jakubowski J. Hemifacial spasm: a prospective long-term follow up of 83 cases treated by microvascular decompression at two neurosurgical centres in the United Kingdom. J Neurol Neurosurg Psychiatry 1996; 60: 72–77

[126] Chung SS, Chang JH, Choi JY, Chang JW, Park YG. Microvascular decompression for hemifacial spasm: a long-term follow-up of 1,169 consecutive cases. Stereotact Funct Neurosurg 2001; 77: 190–193

[127] Yuan Y, Wang Y, Zhang SX, Zhang L, Li R, Guo J. Microvascular decompression in patients with hemifacial spasm: report of 1200 cases. Chin Med J (Engl) 2005; 118: 833–836

[128] Moffat DA, Durvasula VS, Stevens King A, De R, Hardy DG. Outcome following retrosigmoid microvascular decompression of the facial nerve for hemifacial spasm. J Laryngol Otol 2005; 119: 779–783

[129] McLaughlin MR, Jannetta PJ, Clyde BL, Subach BR, Comey CH, Resnick DK. Microvascular decompression of cranial nerves: lessons learned after 4400 operations. J Neurosurg 1999; 90: 1–8

[130] Hallett M. Blepharospasm: recent advances. Neurology 2002; 59: 1306–1312

[131] Patel BC. Surgical management of essential blepharospasm. Otolaryngol Clin North Am 2005; 38: 1075–1098

[132] Fisch U, Dobie RA, Gmür A, Felix H. Intracranial facial nerve anastomosis. Am J Otol 1987; 8: 23–29

[133] Arriaga MA, Brackmann DE. Facial nerve repair techniques in cerebellopontine angle tumor surgery. Am J Otol 1992; 13: 356–359

[134] Murray JA, Willins M, Mountain RE. A comparison of glue and a tube as an anastomotic agent to repair the divided buccal branch of the rat facial nerve. Clin Otolaryngol Allied Sci 1994; 19: 190–192

[135] Gidley PW, Gantz BJ, Rubinstein JT. Facial nerve grafts: from cerebellopontine angle and beyond. Am J Otol 1999; 20: 781–788

30 Immunologic Disorders of the Inner Ear

Jason A. Brant and Michael J. Ruckenstein

30.1 Introduction

In 1979, McCabe[1] described a group of patients who demonstrated bilateral sensorineural hearing loss (SNHL) that progressed over a period of weeks to months and who responded to immunosuppressive agents. He proposed that these patients suffered from an autoimmune mechanism for their hearing loss. Although the precise underlying pathophysiology for these patients remains unknown, and is likely varied, there is a large body of evidence supporting the immune hypothesis. Elucidating the underlying immune mechanism is important because immune-mediated hearing loss is one of the few causes of SNHL that is reversible.

Autoimmune inner ear disease (AIED) can be broken down into primary and secondary types. Primary AIED entails pathology restricted to the ear, whereas secondary AIED entails multisystemic autoimmune diseases that also involve the ear, such as Cogan syndrome, Wegener granulomatosis, systemic lupus erythematosus (SLE), and systemic vasculidities.

30.2 Epidemiology

Autoimmune inner ear disease is a rare disorder in both its primary and secondary forms. The precise incidence is difficult to determine given the lack of a standard diagnostic test; however, it has been estimated to account for less than 1% of hearing impairment or dizziness.[2] There appears to be a female preponderance, and symptoms often occur between the ages of 20 and 50.[2] With a few exceptions, inner ear involvement in systemic autoimmune disorders is also rare. Cogan syndrome, described below, represents the archetypal autoimmune inner ear disease and universally includes SNHL.

An entity of sympathetic autoimmune hearing loss has also been proposed. Damage to the structures of one ear is thought to expose antigens that can elicit an immune response directed against the contralateral ear.[3–5]

30.3 Pathology and Pathogenesis

A significant amount of research has helped to elucidate the immune status of the inner ear, and abnormalities that may contribute to immune-mediated inner ear disease. No model, however, has been created that is definitively analogous to human pathology.

For many years the inner ear was felt to be an immune-privileged site; however, research performed during the 1980s and 1990s showed that the inner ear was capable of mounting a locally mediated immune response.[6–9] The endolymphatic sac appears to be critical to the formation of this immune response as elimination of the sac blunts the reaction.[10–15] Cells mediating this response appear to gain access to the perilymphatic space (scala tympani) via the spiral modiolar vein.[16] The inflammatory cascade that results can cause decreased function secondary to loss of sensory cells, fibrosis, and eventually osteoneogenesis within the cochlea.[16,17]

Although a classic, cell-mediated immune response is certainly one mechanism of pathogenesis of AIED, other potential mechanisms are also relevant. Vasculitis within the labyrinthine vasculature, including the stria vascularis, is a likely mechanism of pathogenesis, particularly in cases of systemic vasculitides.[18] A cochlear neuritis theoretically could result in pathology that responds to immunosuppressive treatment. There is also evidence that antibodies can mediate a noninflammatory pathology, resulting in inner ear dysfunction.[19–21]

These various models have more than just a theoretical importance. The clinical entity known as AIED likely represents a group of disorders with heterogeneous mechanisms of pathogenesis. This has immense clinical significance for developing accurate diagnostic tests and effective treatment regimens for AIED. Thus, it is likely that a single test will never be developed that is highly accurate in diagnosing inner ear disorders that respond to immunosuppressive treatment. Furthermore, treatment strategies will likely have variable efficacy depending on the site of lesion and the underlying mechanism of pathogenesis. For example, intrascalar inflammation might be expected to respond to intratympanic therapy that is absorbed through the round window. Conversely, a vasculitis or neuritis would be unlikely to respond to this form of treatment.

30.4 Diagnosis

30.4.1 Clinical Presentation

The clinical hallmark of AIED is bilateral SNHL progressing over weeks to months.[1] This description is complicated by the fact that patients may present with unilateral hearing loss, and their course may fluctuate.[22] Vestibular symptoms can be present in up to 79% of patients.[22,23] These may include ataxia, imbalance, positional or episodic vertigo, and motion intolerance. Aural fullness and tinnitus may also be present.[2] There may be systemic manifestations of autoimmune disease apparent on examination of the middle and external ear such as effusion (Wegener), skin lesions, chondritis, chronic sinusitis or cough (Wegener), and visual loss (Cogan or Susac syndrome); however, most patients have normal physical examinations.

30.4.2 Differential Diagnosis

A broad differential must be maintained in a patient suspected of having AIED, which can be confused with sudden sensorineural hearing loss (SSNHL); however, they represent two distinct clinical entities. The hearing loss in AIED progresses over weeks to months, whereas SSNHL develops suddenly and is not progressive. Additionally, SSNHL is almost uniformly unilateral, whereas AIED initially may present with unilateral loss but eventually both ears are involved.

Ménière disease may also mimic AIED, and many patients eventually diagnosed with AIED were originally thought to have Ménière disease.[24] Similarly, many patients thought to initially have AIED actually have Ménière disease. The fluctuating course of the hearing in patients with Ménière disease may add to this confusion, as patients may appear to improve after steroid treatment. In these patients with recurrent unilateral hearing loss that appears to have responded to steroid treatment, the senior author has found it worthwhile to withhold steroid treatment for up to 2 weeks, to see if the hearing loss resolves spontaneously. Ultimately, the progressive course of AIED becomes apparent, facilitating clear differentiation of these diseases.

Otosyphilis can closely mimic AIED and must be ruled out.[25] Additionally, retrocochlear pathology, including acoustic neuroma, may present with similar symptoms. More rarely, meningitis, multiple sclerosis, and malignancy involving the dura may manifest as hearing loss similar to AIED.[24,26,27]

Given the broad differential for hearing loss, and the prevalence of systemic autoimmune diseases associated with AIED, a complete review of systems including questions directed at ocular disease, neurologic dysfunction, nephritis, arthritis, pneumonitis, sinusitis, and inflammatory bowel disease is necessary.

30.4.3 Laboratory Testing

Unfortunately, despite much study, a laboratory test that confirms the diagnosis of AIED has yet to be elucidated. The lymphocyte migration inhibition test (MIT)[1] and the lymphocyte transformation test (LTT)[28] are of historical interest, but neither was validated and thus neither is in clinical use. In 1990, Harris and Sharp[29] used Western blot analysis of serum from patients with steroid-responsive SNHL and from guinea pigs immunized with bovine cochlear extract, and found that both patients and animals demonstrated an antibody that bound to a 68-kd bovine inner ear antigen. Two later studies offered encouraging data indicating that detection of this antibody might offer an accurate way of confirming the diagnosis of AIED.[23,30] Identification of the precise idiotype of the antibody proved difficult. It clearly bound to heat shock protein 70 (HSP70), and this has served as the basis for the commercially available human test.[31] Others have proposed that it may be directed against a membrane transport molecule.[32] Regardless of the actual idiotype of the antibody, the weight of the current evidence indicates that the anti–68-kd anticochlear antibody (anti-HSP70) lacks the diagnostic accuracy (mean sensitivity = 0.48; mean sensitivity = 0.57) to rule in or rule out the diagnosis of AIED.[33]

Because AIED may be a harbinger of multisystemic autoimmune disease, laboratory testing to help in detecting such autoimmune disorders should be obtained and include a complete blood count (CBC) with differential, erythrocyte sedimentation rate, C-reactive protein, rheumatoid factor, antinuclear antibodies, antineutrophil cytoplasmic antibodies, anti–double-stranded DNA antibodies, anti–Sjögren syndrome (SS) A/B antibodies, antiphospholipid antibodies, complement levels, thyroid-stimulating hormone (TSH), and free thyroxine (T_4) levels. Otosyphilis must be ruled out with a test for tertiary syphilis [fluorescent treponemal antibody absorption (FTA-Abs) or microhemagglutination–*Treponema pallidum* (MHA-TP)]. In North America, Lyme disease does not seem to result in inner ear pathology, but in Europe, Lyme testing should be done.[25] HIV testing can be obtained in selected cases. Imaging should include a magnetic resonance imaging (MRI) scan with enhancement of the temporal bones to search for retrocochlear lesions.

It must be emphasized that the diagnosis of AIED remains a clinical one. The diagnosis of primary AIED can only be made in the presence of a clinical scenario of rapidly progressive SNHL that definitely responds to the administration of corticosteroids. We have no valid serologic/immunologic tests to diagnose primary AIED. Tests for multisystemic autoimmune or infectious diseases that can secondarily affect the inner ear are necessary.

30.5 Treatment of Primary AIED

Corticosteroids (prednisone or dexamethasone) remain the standard of care for patients with primary AIED, and a prospective, randomized clinical trial validated their use as empirical treatment.[34] Initial therapy for adults consists of a therapeutic trial of prednisone 1 mg/kg/day for 4 weeks and must be started as soon as possible, as irreversible damage can occur within 3 months of onset. Therapeutic response may occur at any time during this period. Patients who do not respond are tapered rapidly over a week to 10 days. Patients who do respond are tapered slowly over 4 weeks to a maintenance dose of 10 to 20 mg/day. Steroid treatment may have to be continued for extended periods of time, and repeated cycles might be necessary for relapses. A long-term follow-up of patients receiving steroid treatment showed an average of 9 years of treatment for those who were eventually able to be weaned.[35] If a patient has a relapse of symptoms, the regimen should be restarted with high-dose steroids for 4 weeks.

Diabetes mellitus, peptic ulcer disease, glaucoma, and hypertension represent common medical conditions that must be monitored closely in patients undergoing treatment with corticosteroids. Patients with uncontrollable diabetes or hypertension, or patients with a history of aseptic necrosis of the femoral head, severe osteoporosis, or psychosis should not be placed on corticosteroid therapy. Patients with a history of glaucoma should have a consultation with an ophthalmologist before starting high-dose corticosteroids. Additional common side effects include insomnia, gastritis, changes in mood, and changes in appearance.

30.5.1 Cyclophosphamide

In 1989 McCabe[36] urged that cyclophosphamide, not prednisone, should be the cornerstone of treatment for AIED. He described his treatment of using low-dose cyclophosphamide with low-dose prednisolone as a test treatment for AIED for 3 weeks, followed by 3 months of treatment for responders. Cyclophosphamide was discontinued first, and then the steroids tapered as long as hearing was maintained. The full treatment cycle was repeated as necessary for relapses. Currently, cyclophosphamide remains a therapeutic alternative for patients whose disease becomes refractory to prednisone or who cannot wean from steroids. It carries a high risk of side effects including infection, myelosuppression, hemorrhagic cystitis, infertility, and malignancy. Blood counts should be monitored at regular intervals. Because of these side effects, some patients may elect to allow the disease to take its natural course and then undergo cochlear implantation, rather than sustain the risks associated with chronic immunosuppression.

30.5.2 Methotrexate

Given the morbidity of cyclophosphamide and sustained high-dose corticosteroids, methotrexate was proposed as an alternative for maintenance following initial steroid treatment. It has been used in the management of other autoimmune diseases with favorable toxicity profiles,[37] and initially showed promising results.[38,39] A large, prospective, randomized controlled trial designed to look at maintenance of hearing following stabilization with steroids did not support the use of methotrexate.[34] Nonetheless, because patients with AIED may manifest different mechanisms of pathogenesis (see above), and because the response to immunosuppressives can be somewhat idiosyncratic, many clinicians still use methotrexate as a first-line prednisone-sparing treatment.

30.5.3 Etanercept

Etanercept is a genetically engineered antibody to tumor necrosis factor (TNF). An important inflammatory mediator throughout the body, TNF is found at high levels in the spiral ligament fibrocytes when they are stimulated by inflammatory cytokines.[40] It has proven to be both safe and relatively effective for patients with rheumatoid arthritis, and several small uncontrolled studies have demonstrated return of hearing and a positive safety profile in AIED patients. Animal studies have supported its use with reduced cochlear inflammation and improved hearing as well.[41–44] Two later trials confirmed its safety, but did not show etanercept to be efficacious for preserving or restoring hearing.[45,46] Other biological agents have also been evaluated, but remain experimental.[47]

Other treatments have been tried with variable efficacy, but have not become the standard of care, including intratympanic steroids and azathioprine.[48,49] Mycophenolate mofetil (CellCept, Roche, San Francisco, CA) inhibits both T- and B-cell synthesis, is well tolerated, and has favorable toxicity profile. Its use in AIED warrants further study.[50]

Plasmapheresis has also been shown to improve hearing in some patients with AIED. In two small uncontrolled studies, 50% and 75% of patients were able to wean from immunosuppresion.[51,52] This method remains experimental and carries high costs in both time and money. Its use as an adjunct for patients not responding to, or intolerant of, immunosuppression has been proposed.

Eventually, for patients who have failed medical management, or cannot tolerate medical treatment due to comorbidities or side effects, cochlear implantation becomes an option. As noted earlier, fibrosis and osteoneogenesis may be present in patients with autoimmune diseases, and preoperative evaluation should be undertaken with care.

30.6 Systemic Autoimmune Diseases Associated with Hearing Loss

30.6.1 Cogan Syndrome

Cogan syndrome is an autoimmune disease characterized by nonsyphilitic ocular keratitis and vestibuloauditory dysfunction. It often presents in the fourth decade of life with sudden hearing loss as the presenting symptom in 50% of patients.[53,54] Ocular and vestibulocochlear symptoms may present concomitantly or separately. Both will generally present within several months, and 85% of patients showed signs of both within 2 years.[53–55] The cochleovestibular symptoms include hearing loss, vertigo, and tinnitus in most patients, ataxia in about half, and oscillopsia in 25%. Hearing loss is sudden, bilateral, fluctuating, and progressive, and is most often downsloping. Vestibular symptoms are generally sudden onset and last for days.[53,54]

Ocular symptoms result from interstitial keratitis, are often bilateral, and include pain, scleral redness, and photophobia. Visual acuity is decreased secondary to corneal clouding. Generalized symptoms consistent with a systemic inflammatory state are common.[55]

Diagnosis is based on clinical examination and exclusion of other autoimmune diseases. Ocular manifestations are treated with topical steroids. Half of patients progress to bilateral class D hearing, with an additional 20% showing unilateral class D hearing. A small number of patients showed hearing improvement with systemic steroids; however, there are no controlled trials of steroids in this population.[54]

Vogt-Koyanagi-Harada syndrome is similar to Cogan syndrome in presentation, but also includes alopecia, vitiligo, and meningeal findings. It is thought to be secondary to sensitization to melanocytic antigens.[56]

30.6.2 Wegener Granulomatosis

Wegener granulomatosis (WG) is a systemic immune disorder characterized by necrotizing granulomas of the upper and lower respiratory tracts, and glomerulonephritis. Although most commonly involving the paranasal sinuses, WG can have otologic manifestations, which can comprise the patient's primary presenting complaints.[57,58] Diagnostic criteria were established in 1990, and subsequently cytoplasmic-staining antineutrophil cytoplasmic antibody (c-ANCA) in peripheral blood was found to have high sensitivity and specificity.[59] Ear involvement in WG is occurs in 20 to 60% of cases, and is unique among the autoimmune diseases, in that both the middle and inner ears may be involved.[60] The middle ear can be either involved directly, with inflammation of the middle ear space or mastoid, or indirectly, through inflammation of the eustachian tube or nasopharynx.[57] Hearing loss in WG is most commonly conductive and secondary to effusion of the middle ear. SNHL presents in up to one third of patients with hearing loss, is progressive over days to weeks, and can be present in up to 10% of all WG patients.[60] The underlying etiology is unknown, but several mechanisms have been proposed: inflammatory toxins entering through the round window, direct granulomatous involvement of the inner ear, or vasculitis of the vessels of the cochlear nerve or of the cochlea itself. Patients rarely report vestibular symptoms.[58,61] Improvement of the hearing loss with systemic treatment of the disease is variable.[57,62,63] A high index of suspicion must be maintained, as WG can be fatal in patients who are left untreated.

30.6.3 Systemic Vasculitides/Connective Tissue Disorders

Systemic lupus erythematous (SLE) is a common autoimmune disease characterized by excessive production of antinuclear antibodies that can form immune complexes in the blood. SNHL has been reported in 15 to 66% of patients with SLE and is often asymptomatic. The hearing loss is most commonly bilateral, symmetric, high frequency, and is not necessarily related to the severity of underlying disease or treatment.[64-67] Reports of vestibular symptoms are variable, ranging from 5 to 70%.[64,66,67]

Hearing loss has also been reported in ankylosing spondylitis, systemic sclerosis, rheumatoid arthritis, polyarteritis nodosa, and Sjögren syndrome.[68-72]

30.6.4 Susac Syndrome

Although the underlying pathophysiology is not entirely known, Susac syndrome, or retinocochleocerebral vasculopathy, is thought to be an autoimmune vasculopathy.[73-75] It is also known as RED-M syndrome for its clinical manifestations of retinopathy, encephalopathy, and deafness associated with microangiopathy. Progression of symptoms can last from weeks to years, and neuropsychological symptoms often dominate the clinical picture. The inner ear pathology results from cochlear end-arteriole occlusion. Hearing loss generally fluctuates and is asymmetric. It is worse in the low to middle frequencies, reflecting the predominance of arteriopathy at the cochlear apex. Vestibular symptoms may also be present, indicating involvement of the labyrinth. Women are disproportionately affected, presenting most commonly between 20 and 40 years of age. Neurologic symptoms are self-limiting with resolution over 2 to 4 years; however, some patients follow a polycyclic course with multiple remissions. Vestibular symptoms often resolve, but most patients show residual hearing loss. Immunosuppressive treatment regimens form the foundation of treatment, with antiplatelet agents serving as adjuvants.[74,75]

30.7 Conclusion

Although much effort has been exerted in the search for underlying mechanisms of autoimmune inner ear disease, no clear cause has been elucidated. Complicating the picture is the lack of strict diagnostic tests that can define a clear population of patients with the disease. There are likely multiple causes of this disease, and individuals may exhibit a wide range of clinical signs and symptoms. Clearly there remains significant work to be done.

References

[1] McCabe BF. Autoimmune sensorineural hearing loss. Ann Otol Rhinol Laryngol 1979; 88: 585–589
[2] Bovo R, Aimoni C, Martini A. Immune-mediated inner ear disease. Acta Otolaryngol 2006; 126: 1012–1021
[3] ten Cate WJ, Bachor E. Autoimmune-mediated sympathetic hearing loss: a case report. Otol Neurotol 2005; 26: 161–165
[4] Harris JP, Low NC, House WF. Contralateral hearing loss following inner ear injury: sympathetic cochleolabyrinthitis? Am J Otol 1985; 6: 371–377
[5] Richards ML, Moorhead JE, Antonelli PJ. Sympathetic cochleolabyrinthitis in revision stapedectomy surgery. Otolaryngol Head Neck Surg 2002; 126: 273–280
[6] Harris JP, Ryan AF. Immunobiology of the inner ear. Am J Otolaryngol 1984; 5: 418–425
[7] Harris JP, Ryan AF. Fundamental immune mechanisms of the brain and inner ear. Otolaryngol Head Neck Surg 1995; 112: 639–653
[8] Mogi G, Lim DJ, Watanabe N. Immunologic study on the inner ear. Immunoglobulins in perilymph. Arch Otolaryngol 1982; 108: 270–275
[9] Harris JP. Immunology of the inner ear: evidence of local antibody production. Ann Otol Rhinol Laryngol 1984; 93: 157–162
[10] Rask-Andersen H, Stahle J. Immunodefence of the inner ear? Lymphocyte-macrophage interaction in the endolymphatic sac. Acta Otolaryngol 1980; 89: 283–294
[11] Tomiyama S, Harris JP. The endolymphatic sac: its importance in inner ear immune responses. Laryngoscope 1986; 96: 685–691
[12] Rask-Andersen H, Danckwardt-Lillieström N, Friberg U, House W. Lymphocyte-macrophage activity in the human endolymphatic sac. Acta Otolaryngol Suppl 1991; 485: 15–17
[13] Yeo SW, Gottschlich S, Harris JP, Keithley EM. Antigen diffusion from the perilymphatic space of the cochlea. Laryngoscope 1995; 105: 623–628
[14] Rask-Andersen H, Stahle J. Immunodefence of the inner ear? Lymphocyte-macrophage interaction in the endolymphatic sac. Acta Otolaryngol 1980; 89: 283–294
[15] Altermatt HJ, Gebbers JO, Müller C, Arnold W, Laissue JA. Human endolymphatic sac: evidence for a role in inner ear immune defence. ORL J Otorhinolaryngol Relat Spec 1990; 52: 143–148
[16] Harris JP, Fukuda S, Keithley EM. Spiral modiolar vein: its importance in inner ear inflammation. Acta Otolaryngol 1990; 110: 357–365
[17] Ma C, Billings P, Harris JP, Keithley EM. Characterization of an experimentally induced inner ear immune response. Laryngoscope 2000; 110: 451–456
[18] Yoon TH, Paparella MM, Schachern PA. Systemic vasculitis: a temporal bone histopathologic study. Laryngoscope 1989; 99: 600–609
[19] Ruckenstein MJ, Hu L. Antibody deposition in the stria vascularis of the MRL-Fas(lpr) mouse. Hear Res 1999; 127: 137–142
[20] Nair TS, Prieskorn DM, Miller JM, Dolan DF, Raphael Y, Carey TE. KHRI-3 monoclonal antibody-induced damage to the inner ear: antibody staining of nascent scars. Hear Res 1999; 129: 50–60
[21] Calzada AP, Balaker AE, Ishiyama G, Lopez IA, Ishiyama A. Temporal bone histopathology and immunoglobulin deposition in Sjogren's syndrome. Otol Neurotol 2012; 33: 258–266
[22] Broughton SS, Meyerhoff WE, Cohen SB. Immune-mediated inner ear disease: 10-year experience. Semin Arthritis Rheum 2004; 34: 544–548
[23] Moscicki RA, San Martin JE, Quintero CH, Rauch SD, Nadol JB, Jr, Bloch KJ. Serum antibody to inner ear proteins in patients with progressive hearing loss. Correlation with disease activity and response to corticosteroid treatment. JAMA 1994; 272: 611–616
[24] Ruckenstein MJ. Autoimmune inner ear disease. Curr Opin Otolaryngol Head Neck Surg 2004; 12: 426–430
[25] Abuzeid WM, Ruckenstein MJ. Spirochetes in otology: are we testing for the right pathogens? Otolaryngol Head Neck Surg 2008; 138: 107–109
[26] Cox E, Kleiman M, Gelfand I. Acute deafness as the presenting symptom of bacterial meningitis. Pediatr Infect Dis J 2009; 28: 342–343
[27] Oh Y-M, Oh D-H, Jeong S-H, Koo J-W, Kim JS. Sequential bilateral hearing loss in multiple sclerosis. Ann Otol Rhinol Laryngol 2008; 117: 186–191
[28] Hughes GB, Kinney SE, Barna BP, Calabrese LH. Practical versus theoretical management of autoimmune inner ear disease. Laryngoscope 1984; 94: 758–767
[29] Harris JP, Sharp PA. Inner ear autoantibodies in patients with rapidly progressive sensorineural hearing loss. Laryngoscope 1990; 100: 516–524
[30] Gottschlich S, Billings PB, Keithley EM, Weisman MH, Harris JP. Assessment of serum antibodies in patients with rapidly progressive sensorineural hearing loss and Ménière's disease. Laryngoscope 1995; 105: 1347–1352
[31] Billings PB, Keithley EM, Harris JP. Evidence linking the 68 kilodalton antigen identified in progressive sensorineural hearing loss patient sera with heat shock protein 70. Ann Otol Rhinol Laryngol 1995; 104: 181–188
[32] Nair TS, Kozma KE, Hoefling NL et al. Identification and characterization of choline transporter-like protein 2, an inner ear glycoprotein of 68 and 72 kDa that is the target of antibody-induced hearing loss. J Neurosci 2004; 24: 1772–1779
[33] Lobo D, López FG, García-Berrocal JR, Ramírez-Camacho R. Diagnostic tests for immunomediated hearing loss: a systematic review. J Laryngol Otol 2008; 122: 564–573

[34] Harris JP, Weisman MH, Derebery JM et al. Treatment of corticosteroid-responsive autoimmune inner ear disease with methotrexate: a randomized controlled trial. JAMA 2003; 290: 1875–1883

[35] Kanzaki J, Kanzaki S, Ogawa K. Long-term prognosis of steroid-dependent sensorineural hearing loss. Audiol Neurootol 2009; 14: 26–34

[36] McCabe BF. Autoimmune inner ear disease: therapy. Am J Otol 1989; 10: 196–197

[37] Matteson EL, Fabry DA, Facer GW et al. Open trial of methotrexate as treatment for autoimmune hearing loss. Arthritis Rheum 2001; 45: 146–150

[38] Sismanis A, Thompson T, Willis HE. Methotrexate therapy for autoimmune hearing loss: a preliminary report. Laryngoscope 1994; 104: 932–934

[39] Sismanis A, Wise CM, Johnson GD. Methotrexate management of immune-mediated cochleovestibular disorders. Otolaryngol Head Neck Surg 1997; 116: 146–152

[40] Yoshida K, Ichimiya I, Suzuki M, Mogi G. Effect of proinflammatory cytokines on cultured spiral ligament fibrocytes. Hear Res 1999; 137: 155–159

[41] Rahman MU, Poe DS, Choi HK. Etanercept therapy for immune-mediated cochleovestibular disorders: preliminary results in a pilot study. Otol Neurotol 2001; 22: 619–624

[42] Wang X, Truong T, Billings PB, Harris JP, Keithley EM. Blockage of immune-mediated inner ear damage by etanercept. Otol Neurotol 2003; 24: 52–57

[43] Rahman MU, Poe DS, Choi HK. Autoimmune vestibulo-cochlear disorders. Curr Opin Rheumatol 2001; 13: 184–189

[44] Satoh H, Firestein GS, Billings PB, Harris JP, Keithley EM. Tumor necrosis factor-alpha, an initiator, and etanercept, an inhibitor of cochlear inflammation. Laryngoscope 2002; 112: 1627–1634

[45] Cohen S, Shoup A, Weisman MH, Harris J. Etanercept treatment for autoimmune inner ear disease: results of a pilot placebo-controlled study. Otol Neurotol 2005; 26: 903–907

[46] Matteson EL, Choi HK, Poe DS et al. Etanercept therapy for immune-mediated cochleovestibular disorders: a multi-center, open-label, pilot study. Arthritis Rheum 2005; 53: 337–342

[47] Cohen S, Roland P, Shoup A et al. A pilot study of rituximab in immune-mediated inner ear disease. Audiol Neurootol 2011; 16: 214–221

[48] Pyykkö I, Ishizaki H, Peltomaa M. Azathioprine with cortisone in treatment of hearing loss in only hearing ear. Acta Otolaryngol Suppl 1997; 529: 83–85

[49] Saraçaydin A, Katircioglu S, Katircioglu S, Karatay MC. Azathioprine in combination with steroids in the treatment of autoimmune inner-ear disease. J Int Med Res 1993; 21: 192–196

[50] Hautefort C, Loundon N, Montchilova M, Marlin S, Garabedian EN, Ulinski T. Mycophenolate mofetil as a treatment of steroid dependent Cogan's syndrome in childhood. Int J Pediatr Otorhinolaryngol 2009; 73: 1477–1479

[51] Luetje CM. Theoretical and practical implications for plasmapheresis in autoimmune inner ear disease. Laryngoscope 1989; 99: 1137–1146

[52] Luetje CM, Berliner KI. Plasmapheresis in autoimmune inner ear disease: long-term follow-up. Am J Otol 1997; 18: 572–576

[53] Gluth MB, Baratz KH, Matteson EL, Driscoll CLW. Cogan syndrome: a retrospective review of 60 patients throughout a half century. Mayo Clin Proc 2006; 81: 483–488

[54] Grasland A, Pouchot J, Hachulla E, Blétry O, Papo T, Vinceneux P Study Group for Cogan's Syndrome. Typical and atypical Cogan's syndrome: 32 cases and review of the literature. Rheumatology (Oxford) 2004; 43: 1007–1015

[55] Antonios N, Silliman S. Cogan syndrome: an analysis of reported neurological manifestations. Neurologist 2012; 18: 55–63

[56] Read RW, Holland GN, Rao NA et al. Revised diagnostic criteria for Vogt-Koyanagi-Harada disease: report of an international committee on nomenclature. Am J Ophthalmol 2001; 131: 647–652

[57] Wierzbicka M, Szyfter W, Puszczewicz M, Borucki L, Bartochowska A. Otologic symptoms as initial manifestation of wegener granulomatosis: diagnostic dilemma. Otol Neurotol 2011; 32: 996–1000

[58] Rasmussen N. Management of the ear, nose, and throat manifestations of Wegener granulomatosis: an otorhinolaryngologist's perspective. Curr Opin Rheumatol 2001; 13: 3–11

[59] Leavitt RY, Fauci AS, Bloch DA et al. The American College of Rheumatology 1990 criteria for the classification of Wegener's granulomatosis. Arthritis Rheum 1990; 33: 1101–1107

[60] McDonald TJ, DeRemee RA. Wegener's granulomatosis. Laryngoscope 1983; 93: 220–231

[61] Stone JH, Francis HW. Immune-mediated inner ear disease. Curr Opin Rheumatol 2000; 12: 32–40

[62] Illum P, Thorling K. Otological manifestations of Wegener's granulomatosis. Laryngoscope 1982; 92: 801–804

[63] Bradley PJ. Wegener's Granulomatosis of the ear. J Laryngol Otol 1983; 97: 623–626

[64] Maciaszczyk K, Durko T, Waszczykowska E, Erkiert-Polguj A, Pajor A. Auditory function in patients with systemic lupus erythematosus. Auris Nasus Larynx 2011; 38: 26–32

[65] Roverano S, Cassano G, Paira S et al. Asymptomatic sensorineural hearing loss in patients with systemic lupus erythematosus. J Clin Rheumatol 2006; 12: 217–220

[66] Karatas E, Onat AM, Durucu C et al. Audiovestibular disturbance in patients with systemic lupus erythematosus. Otolaryngol Head Neck Surg 2007; 136: 82–86

[67] Sperling NM, Tehrani K, Liebling A, Ginzler E. Aural symptoms and hearing loss in patients with lupus. Otolaryngol Head Neck Surg 1998; 118: 762–765

[68] Eryilmaz A, Dagli M, Karabulut H, Sivas Acar F, Erkol Inal E, Gocer C. Evaluation of hearing loss in patients with ankylosing spondylitis. J Laryngol Otol 2007; 121: 845–849

[69] Amor-Dorado JC, Arias-Nuñez MC, Miranda-Filloy JA, Gonzalez-Juanatey C, Llorca J, Gonzalez-Gay MA. Audiovestibular manifestations in patients with limited systemic sclerosis and centromere protein-B (CENP-B) antibodies. Medicine (Baltimore) 2008; 87: 131–141

[70] Kastanioudakis I, Skevas A, Danielidis V, Tsiakou E, Drosos AA, Moustopoulos MH. Inner ear involvement in rheumatoid arthritis: a prospective clinical study. J Laryngol Otol 1995; 109: 713–718

[71] Alatas N, Yazgan P, Oztürk A, San I, Iynen I. Audiological findings in patients with ankylosing spondylitis. J Laryngol Otol 2005; 119: 534–539

[72] Joglekar S, Deroee AF, Morita N, Cureoglu S, Schachern PA, Paparella M. Polyarteritis nodosa: a human temporal bone study. Am J Otolaryngol 2010; 31: 221–225

[73] Susac JO, Hardman JM, Selhorst JB. Microangiopathy of the brain and retina. Neurology 1979; 29: 313–316

[74] García-Carrasco M, Jiménez-Hernández C, Jiménez-Hernández M et al. Susac's syndrome: an update. Autoimmun Rev 2011; 10: 548–552

[75] Bitra RK, Eggenberger E. Review of Susac syndrome. Curr Opin Ophthalmol 2011; 22: 472–476

Part 4

Rehabilitation

31 Adult Audiological Rehabilitation

Stephanie Lockhart and John Greer Clark

"... and I have heard there is in Spain an instrument in use to be set to the ear that helpeth the thick of hearing."
—Sir Francis Bacon (1561–1626)

31.1 Introduction

The concept and practice of hearing loss rehabilitation has a long history, predating audiology itself by hundreds of years. But the greatest success in this endeavor awaited the 20th century, when electroacoustic improvements placed hearing instrumentation at the forefront of the management of hearing loss that was not amenable to medical intervention. The current literature suggests that the past avenues of aural rehabilitation that encompassed speech reading instruction and auditory training have largely given way to communication strategies training, development of enhanced listening skills, better recognition of barriers to successful communication, and instruction toward an improved management of the communication setting.[1–3] It is unfortunate, however, that rehabilitative practices at the audiology profession's core are frequently abandoned in hearing care delivery, relying instead on the allure of a purely technological fix to diminished hearing.[4,5]

The American Speech-Language-Hearing Association describes audiological rehabilitation is an ecological, interactive process that facilitates one's ability to minimize or prevent the limitations and restrictions that auditory dysfunctions can impose on personal well-being and communication, including interpersonal, psychosocial, educational, and vocational functioning. Given this working definition, it is apparent that there is overlap between the role of the audiologist and the speech pathologist in working with a person to improve total communication.[5]

The skill sets and scopes of practice of audiologists and speech pathologists share all nontechnological aspects of aural rehabilitation. Interestingly, audiologists are recognized more for their diagnostic abilities than their rehabilitation abilities. In fact, Medicare and many third-party payers do not recognize or reimburse for the treatment efforts of audiologists. Unfortunately, lack of reimbursement often helps to determine what is or is not routinely practiced, the consequence of which is that many audiologists do not provide audiological rehabilitation as it is defined above. To address this dilemma and afford patients a more comprehensive rehabilitation package, there is a movement by professional organizations to recognize audiologists for their treatment efforts and not just for diagnostics.

This chapter uses the term *audiological rehabilitation* (as opposed to *aural rehabilitation*) because it centralizes the role of the audiologist in the rehabilitation process. Some audiologists do, and rightfully so, bill patients directly for audiological rehabilitation. The more common model is to bundle the costs of rehabilitation along with the purchase price of hearing instrumentation. It is important to bear in mind that the audiological evaluation is most often only the beginning of a hearing treatment journey that does not end following a surgical audio-prosthetic implant or the selection and fitting of hearing aids. Audiologists in all employment settings should be appropriately compensated for their efforts at rehabilitation, as it is the provision of these treatment services that leads to documented higher levels of success.

This chapter focuses on adult audiological rehabilitation. Tinnitus and auditory implants are discussed elsewhere (see Chapters 32, 33, 37, and 38) and thus are not discussed here. The audiological rehabilitation needs of children with hearing loss are very different from those of adults; therefore, pediatric audiological rehabilitation is not addressed here. The following topics relative to adult audiological rehabilitation are discussed: consequence and prevalence of hearing loss, hearing aid styles and features, other amplification devices, hearing aid consultation, communication partner involvement, fitting process and post-fitting verification, and assistive listening devices. We fully acknowledge that the greatest successes in audiological rehabilitation occur when technology and communication training are provided together.[6] However, this chapter only provides a nod toward this more global approach to hearing care. When reading this chapter, the reader should bear in mind that successful communication with hearing loss is enhanced when physicians advise their patients that hearing loss treatment is a process and that the hearing aid fitting is often only a single component of that process.

31.2 Prevalence and Consequences of Hearing Loss

Prevalence of Adult Hearing Loss and Hearing Aid Use in the United States[44]

- 17% of American adults (36 million) report some degree of hearing loss
- Men are more likely than women to experience hearing loss
- The prevalence of hearing loss increases with age: 18% of Americans age 45 to 64 years, 30% of age 65 to 74 years, and 47% of age 75 years and over have a hearing impairment
- An estimated 26 million American adults age 20–69 have a noise-induced high-frequency hearing loss
- Only one in four people who could benefit from hearing aids actually wear them

It has been estimated that the number of people over 65 years of age with hearing loss in the United States will reach nearly 13 million by the year 2015. The impact of untreated hearing loss is well documented. A frequently cited survey by the National Council on Aging found significant consequences of untreated hearing loss, including worry, anxiety, sadness, depression, paranoia, emotional turmoil, insecurity, a tendency to withdraw from social situations, and strained relationships with family members.[7] Recent research has indicated that hearing loss has a negative impact on earnings and unemployment rates. In fact, a large-scale survey reported that those who fail to treat their hearing loss are collectively losing at least $100 billion in annual income.[8] Hearing is an important part of communication in the workplace, and thus, for many jobs, lack of hearing becomes a safety issue. Working individuals with untreated hearing loss may suffer losses in compensation, make mistakes on the job, and experience higher rates of unemployment. Additionally, the previously mentioned psychosocial effects of hearing loss may negatively affect job performance.[9] Fortunately, these negative impacts can be mitigated in large degree by the use of amplification.[10,11] The National Council on Aging study reported that benefits of hearing loss treatment include better relationships with family members, improved self-concept, improved mental health, and greater independence and security.[7]

The fact that hearing aids can improve the quality of life may seem intuitive. Even so, the adoption rate for hearing aids has remained surprisingly low, with only about one in four adults with hearing loss currently using hearing aids.[12] There are many reasons cited for the nonuse of amplification, including previous negative experience with hearing aids, the "stigma" of hearing aids, lack of perceived need, "only" unilateral hearing loss, negative word of mouth, and cost. Some patients are under the impression that hearing aids will not help "nerve deafness," tinnitus, or high-frequency hearing loss.[13] Audiologists, physicians, and professional organizations need to work together to raise awareness about both the significant advances in hearing aid technology and the documented improvements to quality of life afforded by amplification.

31.3 Hearing Aids

On the simplest level, hearing aids are miniature public address systems with the same basic components including microphone, amplifier, speaker (receiver), and power source. Electronic hearing aids have been available for over 100 years. However, it was not until the development of the transistor that head-worn amplification in the form of the first behind-the-ear (BTE) hearing aids appeared on the market in the 1950s:

A Brief History of Hearing Aids: 1950 to the Present[45]

- 1950s: first behind-the-ear (BTE) hearing aids using transistors; first in-the-ear (ITE) hearing aids became available; eyeglass hearing aids were popular
- 1960s: integrated circuits; size reduction; directional microphones introduced
- 1970s: miniaturization of microphones and receivers; zinc air batteries invented; ITE devices smaller and more popular
- 1980s: first in-the-canal (ITC) hearing aids; digital hearing aids in experimental form; computer programmable analog hearing aids; improved circuits with low distortion at high input levels
- 1990s: wide dynamic range compression (WDRC); first completely-in-canal (CIC) hearing aid; first commercially available digital hearing aids
- 2000s: Advanced digital signal processing; continued miniaturization

---

A proliferation of hearing aid styles has become available through the intervening years (▶ Fig. 31.1) and it is style consideration and the available technologies within a given instrument that guide hearing aid selection today.

31.3.1 Hearing Aid Styles

Hearing aids are available today in a wide variety of styles and sizes with a common misconception among patients that the larger behind-the-ear devices are "old fashioned" and that smaller hearing aids house better and newer technology. Yet each hearing aid style has its position in the marketplace, with no single style best addressing the particular needs of a given patient.

Behind-the-Ear

With a traditional behind-the-ear device (▶ Fig. 31.1a), the hearing aid is worn behind, or perhaps more correctly worded, over the ear and is coupled via a tube to an earmold that fits within the ear concha bowl and ear canal. The most severe losses require power behind-the-ear hearing aids, but patients often choose this style for durability and even cosmetics as the earmold piece may be less conspicuous than an in-the-ear style hearing aid. In spite of their wide fitting range from mild to profound hearing losses, for many years only approximately 20% of dispensed hearing aids have been traditional BTE instruments.

Open Fits

Another form of BTE hearing aid is the "open fit" hearing aid (▶ Fig. 31.1b). An open fit may be accomplished using a slim tube to route sound from the hearing aid down into the ear canal or by placing the receiver (speaker) directly within the canal. Open fits are indicated for people with normal or near-normal low-frequency hearing. The patient generally does not wear a custom earmold, but rather a tip or dome with openings for natural sound to enter and escape the ear canal. Open fittings are good for high-frequency losses. Essentially no low-frequency amplification is achieved because any low-frequency amplification escapes back through the openings in the tip or dome. The benefit of this style is comfortable use without occlusion. These devices are also very cosmetically appealing as the hearing aids are usually quite small as is the slim tube or receiver wire. These instruments can be fit in a "closed" fashion with a small ("micro") mold allowing for the delivery of greater amplification to the ear and a wider hearing loss fitting range.

In-the-Ear

In-the-ear (ITE) hearing aids (▶ Fig. 31.1c) are also called full shell hearing aids and are the largest of the devices that fit within the ear. Thus, they have advantages such as room for a volume control or push button for the patient to adjust the sound; an increased fitting range; room for directional microphones; larger, longer-life batteries; and better ease of use for patients with visual or dexterity issues.

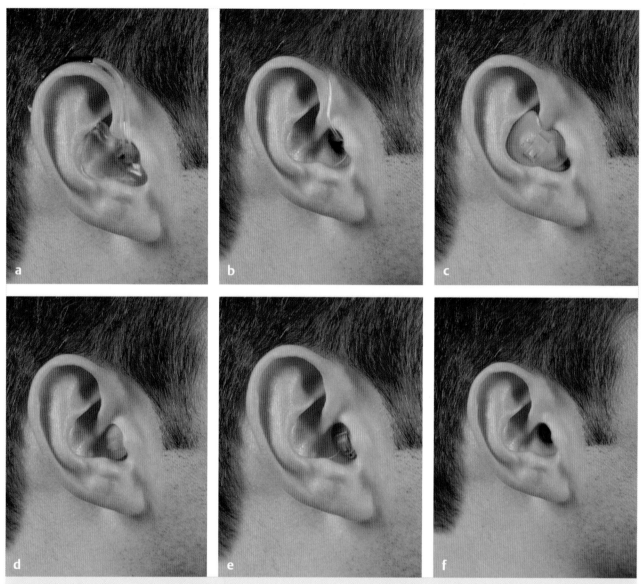

Fig. 31.1 Hearing aid styles. (a) BTE. (b) Open fit. (c) Full shell. (d) In the canal. (e) Completely in the canal. (f) Invisible in the canal. (Courtesy of Phonak, LLC.)

In–the-Canal

The in-the-canal (ITC) hearing aids (▶ Fig. 31.1d) are much smaller than ITE devices. They may have room for a push button or volume control, but usually not both. They may have room for directional microphones. ITCs are more cosmetically appealing than ITE devices, but ITC hearing aids do not, as a rule, have room for telephone circuitry (see Telecoils, below).

Completely–In-the-Canal

The completely-in the-canal (CIC) hearing aids (▶ Fig. 31.1e) were, until recently, the smallest in-the-ear aids available. They are seated completely in the ear canal with no part of the hearing aid extending into the concha bowl with removal made possible with an attached removal line. When audiometrically appropriate, the cosmetic appeal of these hearing aids makes them a popular choice, even with reduced battery life due to smaller size. CICs do not have room for directional microphones or telephone circuits. Although there is no room for user controls, a user may control hearing aid function if desired or needed through a remote control.

Invisible-In-Canal

The invisible-in-canal (IIC) hearing instrument (▶ Fig. 31.1f) is the smallest of the hearing aid styles, fitting past the second bend of the ear canal with the receiver just millimeters from the tympanic membrane. When properly fitted, these devices are virtually invisible. An extended wear version of the IIC hearing instrument is also available. IIC devices are suitable for mild to moderate hearing losses and the fitting is limited to ear canals with sufficient depth and width to accommodate the devices.

31.4 Hearing Aid Features

31.4.1 Telecoils

Telecoils are an important feature for many hearing aid users. In simplest terms, a telecoil is a metal coil within the hearing aid that picks up electromagnetic signal that emanates from a telephone's casing. When the telecoil is activated, the hearing aid will pick up the electromagnetic signal coming from the phone, allowing the user to hear the transmitted voice without acoustic feedback. The telecoil may be activated via a switch or button or may automatically turn on when the telephone is held close to the hearing aid. Telecoils are also used for hearing with an induction loop. An induction loop may be as small as one's own living room or as large as an auditorium. If the room is "looped," then users need only to activate their telecoil to hear the public address, television, etc. clearly without interference from background noise. Currently the American Academy of Audiology and the Hearing Loss Association of America (a hearing loss consumer advocacy organization) have an active initiative to "Loop America." Their efforts have led to a number of information kiosks at airports, bank teller windows, and shopping checkout aisles being wired for telecoil use, allowing patrons to hear without interfering background sounds. Telecoils do take up space within hearing aids and, therefore, are not available in the smaller hearing aid styles.

31.4.2 Directional Microphones

Directional microphones were used in hearing aids long before the advent of digital technology but they have become much more sophisticated. Directional microphones are used to create an area of focus for the listener. For example, at a busy restaurant, it is desirable to be able to focus on the person across from you and not pick up so much of the surrounding noise. The most basic directional microphones provide a fixed area of focus, directly in front of the wearer. More sophisticated systems will work in an adaptive manner to change the focus of the hearing aids, which is helpful in situations where there are multiple speakers. In very advanced systems, users may even manually select an area of focus that is directly to their right or left or even behind them. The use of directional microphones improves the signal-to-noise ratio for the hearing aid user, thus improving the ability to hear speech in noisy environments.

31.4.3 User Controls

Volume controls are available on most styles of hearing aid, either with a button or wheel on the device itself or via remote control. Volume controls in general allow patients to raise and lower the overall amplification level, although today's circuits allow for automatic volume adjustments so that many users choose instruments that do not have volume controls. Another type of user control is a multimemory control, which again may be an ear-level button or a remote control. A hearing aid with multiple memories allows the user to change to different "programs" for different listening situations much like progressive lenses allow for different prescriptions for different vision needs. For instance, there may be a setting for speech in noise, music, telephone, comfort in noise, and others. Some patients prefer "automatic" function and others prefer more control. Banerjee[14] studied the use of volume and multimemory controls and concluded that both may increase user satisfaction with hearing aids.

31.5 Digital Technology

The vast majority of hearing aids dispensed today are digital, as opposed to analog, devices. If a hearing aid is digital, it simply means that the incoming sound has passed through an analog-to-digital converter, which changes the sound from an acoustic signal to a digital signal. The frequency, intensity and temporal patterns of the signal are then analyzed and manipulated and changed back to an acoustic signal to be received by the ear. The most important part of the process is what happens in the analysis and manipulation of the sound. During the signal processing, various algorithms are applied to the sound in order to improve the listening experience for the user. The list of digital features is quite lengthy but generally includes noise reduction, feedback management, and wireless connectivity.

Most digital hearing aids employ some type of noise reduction. This may be approached in different ways, but in general the spectral and temporal aspects of incoming sound in individual frequency bands (analogous to the graphic equalizer on a home stereo) are analyzed by the hearing aid, and if the incoming signal is deemed likely to be noise, it is reduced. If the signal is deemed likely to be speech, it is left alone or even enhanced. It is important to note that a key word here is reduction and not elimination. It is easy to over-promise when it comes to discussing technology, and noise reduction is no exception.

Hearing professionals need to be careful not to give the impression that hearing aids will "cancel" all background noise. There is little argument that noise reduction improves listening comfort. Whether noise reduction actually improves speech understanding in noise is more questionable.[15] Although some research has shown a small degree of improvement in speech understanding with the use of noise reduction, this effect is minimal unless the noise reduction is combined with a directional microphone.[16,17]

Another key digital feature is feedback reduction. Acoustic feedback is a whistling sound that is created when amplified sound makes its way back out of the ear canal, reaches the hearing aid microphone, and is re-amplified. As the amount of gain in the hearing aid is increased, particularly in the higher frequencies, there is more risk of feedback. Also, the more open the fitting the more likely feedback is to occur. With older technology, one answer to feedback was to turn down high-frequency gain. This reduced feedback but also reduced audibility for critical high-frequency speech sounds. The other means to prevent unwanted feedback was to close any venting or "opening" that had originally been designed into the hearing aid to help reduce the echo perception of the user's own voice (occlusion effect) when low-frequency hearing sensitivity is near normal. Closing the venting helped reduce feedback but made the fit much more occluded.

The current anti-feedback algorithms utilize phase cancellation to reduce or eliminate feedback in most ears. The effectiveness of these systems varies among hearing aid manufacturers and even among individual patients using the same manufacturer due to physical differences in ear canals. However, current feedback reduction technology often can provide up to about 15 dB more stable gain without feedback.[18]

Current digital technology provides analysis of the user's acoustic environment. The hearing aid circuit can then adjust to accommodate different situations. For example, the hearing aid may switch to a directional mode if it determines that there is speech present in front of the listener and noise present behind. Or the hearing aid's digital circuit may determine that the only input is loud noise with no speech present, in which case the volume may be reduced automatically. The hearing aid may even change to a different program or memory to provide a different frequency response for music. Some patients prefer this level of automatic function, whereas others prefer traditional push button or volume controls, allowing an individual greater control over the hearing aid.

There are many other digital algorithms that function to improve comfort for reverberant environments, windy situations, and for environments containing impulse noise such as dishes clanging.

A rather recent addition to hearing aid technology is wireless capability. This allows for the hearing aid to receive a wireless signal that may be transmitted from a cell phone, television, computer, or any Bluetooth audio device. Remote controls are optional and allow the patient to control the hearing aid volume or change programs using a small hand-held device. These devices range from very simple to more complex. The list of available features is extensive, and thus it is incumbent on the audiologist to fully assess the patient's needs and lifestyle to determine the necessary level of technology.

31.6 Other Amplification

31.6.1 CROS/BiCROS

CROS is an acronym for contralateral routing of signals—a fitting paradigm that is appropriate for patients with one normal ear and one ear that cannot be aided. CROS hearing instruments consist of two parts: a transmitter worn on the unaidable ear that transmits sound to a receiver worn on the good ear. In the past, this transmission was accomplished via a cord worn across the back of the neck that physically connected the transmitter and receiver. Today's CROS systems are wireless and are available in both behind-the-ear and in-the-ear styles.

A BICROS hearing instrument is used for patients who have one unaidable ear and one impaired but aidable ear. BICROS differs from CROS in that the device on the better ear functions as a hearing aid as well as a receiver so that the device on the better ear not only receives a signal from the poorer ear but it also amplifies.

31.6.2 Bone Conduction Hearing Solutions

For patients with single-sided deafness (SSD), an alternative to the CROS is a bone conduction device. With CROS, the signal is transmitted wirelessly to the receiver on the good ear. With a bone conduction solution, the signal is transmitted through the skull from the poor side to the cochlea on the good ear. This may be accomplished surgically through implantable bone

conduction devices as discussed in Chapter 32. Bone conduction hearing aids may be indicated for patients with conductive hearing losses if it is not possible to wear a traditional hearing aid or for patients with SSD. The nonsurgical options for bone conduction also allow for sound transmission via bone conduction to stimulate the cochlea. One nonsurgical option is a traditional bone conduction hearing aid (▶ Fig. 31.2), which uses a bone oscillator attached to a headband which vibrates against the skull to stimulate the cochlea through the bone.

Another option for bone conduction transmission from a non-functioning ear to a normal ear is the transcranial CROS, in which a powerful hearing aid is fitted in the bony portion of the canal on the bad side and the sound is transmitted via bone conduction to the better cochlea. A more recently developed bone conduction hearing system consists of a small BTE device that wirelessly transmits to a second device worn in the mouth, affixed to the teeth. The in-the-mouth device delivers the sound that is conducted through the teeth to the bone and through the bone to the cochlea.

31.7 Hearing Aid Consultation

The advent of digital sound processing has greatly improved hearing loss management possibilities. Yet the importance of many of these technological advances available to audiologists often wanes in comparison to the importance of the effective delivery of patient services. The success of this delivery is based on a greater understanding of the patients being served and the most effective means to engage them in the rehabilitative process. Before the audiologist can proceed with the ordering of selected hearing aids and the subsequent fitting, patients must be psychologically prepared for a life change that they may be reluctant to undertake.

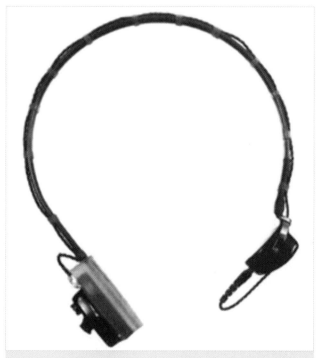

Fig. 31.2 A bone conduction aid with headband.

31.7.1 Patient Counseling Toward Improved Hearing Aid Acceptance

The patient's level of trust toward the health care professional is a precursor to the acceptance of hearing care recommendations and the establishment of the internal motivation to take action toward better hearing. Although not as strong as one or two generations ago, there remains an implicit trust between physicians and patients that fosters adherence to recommendations. Audiologists working within a physician's practice benefit from this implicit trust and often face less patient resistance to the acceptance of hearing aid recommendations than do audiologists in other settings. However, audiologists cannot fully guide and appropriately challenge those with hearing loss until they have a greater understanding of the impact of hearing loss on the individual.

Although 41.5% of surveyed practicing audiologists have stated that they believe they can predict treatment needs based on routine audiometrics,[19] there is far too much variability in human psychology and the hearing loss impact on different lifestyle demands to make this possible. The only means to truly understand the effect of hearing loss on patients is to encourage them to tell their "story."[2] A successful means to guide patients through this process is to make use of one of the many self-assessment tools available to audiologists. Unfortunately, these tools are used far too infrequently (▶ Table 31.1). Yet it is the sincere attempt to fully understand the patient's specific impact of hearing loss that bolsters requisite trust.

There is a long-observed social stigma to the use of hearing aids that was described by Blood et al[20] as the "hearing aid effect." These researchers found that subjects shown images of individuals wearing hearing aids rated the hearing aid user significantly lower in the areas of intelligence, achievement, personality, and appearance than they did images of individuals who were not wearing hearing aids. For many adult patients the acceptance of the need for hearing assistance can be closely tied to their own perception of body image and how this impacts their self-concept.[2] Wishing to maintain a positive self-concept is normal and generally healthy. It only becomes negative when it impedes progress toward a desired goal.

While coming to terms with a change in self-concept, many adults with acquired hearing loss must also confront the stress of living with a chronically challenging condition. For many, the hearing loss itself can be a major contributor to the level of experienced stress. Unless one has a hearing loss, it is difficult to appreciate fully the chronic stress experienced by those who do. Understanding this stress helps explain the levels of frustration, anger, and even despair expressed by many patients.

Demonstrating recognition of the impact of hearing loss on an individual's life in areas beyond the loss of effective commu-

nication can bolster trust. It can also position the hearing care provider to help the patient discover, when lacking, the internal motivation needed to be a successful user of hearing aids.

31.7.2 Building Motivation

As has long been recognized in health care, change does not occur without motivation. This has been found to be true in areas of medication adherence, substance abuse, eating disorders, dietary change, smoking cessation, exercise regimens, and any of a number of health-related issues.[21] Some adults with adventitious hearing loss arrive for a hearing evaluation without exercising the self-introspection required to appreciate fully the communication challenges presented by their hearing loss. Patients frequently operate on their own internal timetable and are only ready to proceed when they feel the necessity. The hearing care provider, like patients' family members, may be baffled that these patients fail to see the same communication frustrations so evident to others. Some patients with mild, or even moderate, hearing loss may not evidence significant hearing difficulties when in a consultation room with minimal auditory distractions and speaking one on one with a health care provider on a specific, prearranged topic. These individuals may be experiencing significant hearing difficulty in other situations, and it is important that unexpressed concerns about hearing not be overlooked. It becomes the audiologist's role to help patients recognize the negative impact of untreated hearing loss and to articulate their own reasons for change.

As is true for all, motivation that arises from within the patient is far more sustainable and leads to greater success than motivation that another may attempt to instill. Outward sources of motivation include descriptions of hearing loss findings that fail to speak directly to patients' perceived difficulties or their perceptions of the source of communication difficulties. Although test result discussions may be a sufficient springboard toward action for patients who arrive with sufficient motivation to accept recommendations, a better approach when motivation is lacking is often one that guides patients to reflect on the impact of hearing loss, helps patients to explore their willingness to make positive changes in their lives and to explore their perceived abilities to make these changes, and invites patients to look at the costs and benefits of action or inaction toward effective remediation. The use of simple tools for motivational engagement can often result in desired outcomes.[2,22,23]

31.7.3 Determining Needs

Although motivation may be a key to success, another important factor that can impact hearing aid success is the patient's speech understanding capability. If the word recognition score is very poor, the prognosis for success with hearing aids decreases greatly. Although poor speech recognition alone may not preclude success with hearing aids, it must be considered that patients with severe and profound hearing losses, along with very poor word recognition, may be candidates for cochlear implantation rather than traditional amplification. Additionally, any potential medical contraindications to the use of amplification must be evaluated by a physician (preferably an otolaryngologist) prior to proceeding with a hearing aid fitting.

Table 31.1 Audiologists' Use of Self-Assessment Measures[19]

	Au.D. Audiologists	Master's Audiologists
Never use	28%	33%
Use less than 25% of the time	31%	34%
Use more than 75% of the time	10%	7%

Once candidacy is determined, from an audiological as well as medical standpoint, the next step is to select the style and technology level of the hearing aids. The audiogram is one tool that helps guide the decision process. For example, a BTE hearing aid will likely be most appropriate for severe or profound losses. An open fitting is best suited for a high-frequency hearing loss with good hearing sensitivity in the lower frequency range.

With the features available today, the lifestyle of the patient has become a critical part of the decision process. As discussed earlier, hearing aids may employ noise reduction, directionality, multiple memories, wireless capability, and other features. However, not every patient needs every available feature. The audiologist must have a discussion with the patient that assesses the individual's situation and determines the needs of that particular patient. For example, patients who are frequently in challenging listening environments have very different needs than patients who spend most of the day watching television and who have a more limited social life. Someone with good dexterity may opt for a manual volume control, whereas someone with arthritis may prefer a device that adjusts automatically. Or a frequent cell phone user may want a Bluetooth interface for the hearing aids. The preferences of the patient also cannot be ignored. Given the choice, most patients would select a device that is cosmetically appealing, whereas for others this is not a concern.

The cost of a pair of hearing aids today ranges from approximately \$2,000 to \$6,000 depending on the level of technology. Given these figures, the patient's budgetary constraints must be taken into consideration in hearing aid selection. Wireless accessories (for remote control, and TV, telephone, or remote microphone connectivity) will further add to hearing aid cost by approximately \$150 to \$600 depending on the number and complexity of the accessories. In the United States, Medicare does not provide coverage for hearing aids, nor do most private insurance companies. For the majority of patients, hearing aids are an out-of-pocket expense; therefore, the budget of the patient needs to be part of the consultation.

The task of the audiologist is to consider the degree and configuration of the hearing loss as well as the lifestyle, style preference, and budget for the patient so that the patient and audiologist together can determine the best hearing management solution. If all patients stated that they wanted the best technology available regardless of style or cost, this task would be easy. But as is most often the case, the best recommendation for the hearing loss may not match the patient's style preference, or the recommended technology level may cost more than the patient's budget can accommodate.

31.8 Communication Partner Involvement

Involving the patient's primary communication partner in the rehabilitation process can aid in attempts to gain and sustain motivation. It is the fact that hearing loss creates difficulties not only for hearing others but also difficulties for others when they want to be heard that causes remediation of hearing loss to be an issue at all. The important others in the life of the person with hearing loss, by necessity, become significant partners in the rehabilitation process.

It is helpful when communication partners accompany patients to hearing aid consultations. When partners actively participate in early discussions of hearing difficulties, patients are more likely to report perceived benefit from amplification.[24]

Inclusion of a primary communication partner in the consultation and subsequent hearing loss treatment process is beneficial to both the communication partner and the patient. Both parties need to understand that hearing aids can typically restore only about one half of the degree of lost hearing, which results in a certain amount of residual deficit. They also need to appreciate the importance of speech recognition loss and that if only 80% of words are understood under ideal hearing evaluation conditions one cannot expect perfect speech understanding in the real world. Equally important is the patient's appreciation of the difficult communication task the communication partners have in delivering their message effectively to the patient with hearing loss. Finally, including a primary communication partner provides an opportunity for effective communication training for both parties.

31.9 Hearing Aid Fitting and Verification

Effective hearing aid fittings are inseparable from a verification of hearing aid performance. Once the hearing aids have been selected, programmed, and fitted on the patient, how do we know that the hearing aids are performing as they are supposed to perform? It would seem that a simple way to get this answer is to ask the patient, "How does it sound?" Although the perception of sound is important to acceptance of amplification, the patient's response to this direct question cannot be allowed to fully override the electroacoustic needs of the hearing loss. For instance, a new user may report that the hearing aid sounds too loud or tinny. Another user with an identical audiogram but with years of experience with hearing aids may report that the same hearing aid is too soft. If adjustments are made solely based on the patient's first reports, hearing aids may be modified to achieve comfort at the expense of audibility.

The use of objective measures as a tool to help determine the appropriateness of hearing aid settings is paramount. Probe microphone measures (also known as "real-ear measures") are considered by all major audiology associations to be the best practice for objectively measuring hearing aid performance. These measures are performed by placing a thin silicone tube attached to a microphone in the patient's ear, just past the speaker of the hearing aid. This allows measurement of the actual amount of amplified sound in the ear canal in response to an input signal allowing the audiologist, the patient, and the patient's primary communication partner to see just how much amplification is taking place. As these measures are frequency-specific, adjustments can be made to fine tune the hearing aids.

Other objective measures involve putting the patient in the sound booth and using recorded speech materials with and without the presence of background noise. Although this does not provide frequency-specific information, it does offer objective evidence as to the efficacy of the hearing aids for hearing in an environment that mimics the real world. Self-assessment tools were discussed earlier as being an important tool in hearing aid selection. They are equally useful to provide a "before and after" picture of hearing aid success or subjective ratings of hearing aid satisfaction.

A large-scale survey of hearing aid users attempted to determine the factors that contribute to success with hearing aids.[25] The survey included questions about whether certain procedures were completed as part of the hearing aid fitting and follow-up. The following measures were found to contribute positively to success with hearing aids: (1) objective measures, such as assessment of hearing speech in noise; (2) subjective measures of hearing aid benefit; (3) loudness discomfort measures, which determine the maximum comfortable loudness with the hearing aids in place; (4) probe microphone measures; and (5) patient satisfaction measures.

There is little argument that using verification tools is considered best practice. In particular, probe microphone measures have been called a "gold standard" when it comes to fitting, but fewer than half of audiologists use the technology.[26] Research has repeatedly documented the efficacy of this approach to documenting hearing aid performance in a time-efficient manner.[27,28] A recent checklist of recommended procedures given in a Consumer Reports buying guide for hearing aids included the use of real-ear testing to properly adjust hearing aids as well as other tests of speech understanding in quiet and noise.[29] Patients are now coming to appointments requesting these procedures. Third-party payers are also expecting objective documentation of received benefits from amplification. It is paramount that audiologists in all employment settings be prepared to provide proper services.

31.10 Hearing Aid Orientation

Once the hearing aids have been properly fitted and the performance has been verified, a full orientation of hearing aid use and care is necessary to ensure successful use of hearing instrumentation. Unfortunately, the amount of health-related information retained by adult patients is far less than health professionals may expect. Kessels[30] found that 40 to 80% of information provided by health care professionals is forgotten by the patient almost immediately, and nearly half of the information that is remembered is often remembered incorrectly. One can expect that as the amount of information presented increases, the ability to remember all pertinent details of that information will decrease.[31] Given the demographics of hearing aid fittings, these findings take on a greater impact, as Anderson et al[32] found information recall is even poorer for patients 70 years of age or older.

One must add to the potential for cognitive overload during the hearing aid orientation process the reported tendency that verbal instruction frequently overshoots patients' functional literacy levels.[33] Indeed, patient comprehension of supplemental printed material may also be compromised through a poor match of a patient's literacy levels and the reading level of the printed information.[34]

Given the documented deficiencies in the information transfer process within hearing aid orientations, Pichora-Fuller and Singh[35] suggest that current approaches to rehabilitative audiology need to be revamped. Reese and Hnath-Chisolm[36] found that several key factors may influence the retention of information, including the amount of information provided, the organization of the information, the use of written and visual information, and the delivery characteristics of the health care provider. Kessels[30] reports that only 14% of spoken health care information is typically remembered by patients, whereas over 80% may be remembered when a visual aid is used during discussions. In addition to using visual aids during the office appointment, a supplemental DVD viewed later at home has been shown to increase information retention.[37] These findings indicate that more than the spoken word alone should be used during the hearing aid orientation and indeed when conveying any health-related information to patients. To aid information retention, it becomes important for the hearing aid orientation process to incorporate different styles of learning that may include (1) auditory learning, (2) supplemental visual learning, (3) kinesthetic learning, and (4) off-site learning. As discussed by Clark and English,[2] the problem of poor information retention is frequently exacerbated by ineffective clinical communication practices of health practitioners themselves.

> **Health Care Provider Practices that Hinder Effective Patient Education[2]**
>
> - Use of professional jargon and words patients may not understand
> - Explanations with more detail than patients can remember
> - Providing information unrelated to patients' questions
> - Failure to ask if information is understood
> - Providing information without helping patients apply it to their lives

Frequently, health professionals operate under the assumption that all needed information should be provided at once. However, the vast amount of information that must be relayed to patients during the hearing aid orientation can be simply overwhelming. New hearing aid users are reportedly presented with 61 to 135 "information bits" during the hearing aid orientation, with sometimes as many as five information bits given in less than a minute.[38,39] To prevent cognitive overload, one might consider prioritizing information delivery, leaving some portions of the hearing aid orientation process to be given within a subsequent visit.

Hearing Aid Orientation Topics: To Aid Information Retention, Checked Items Can Be Considered for Presentation at a Subsequent Visit[2]

- Components of hearing aids
- Battery insertion and removal
  - ○ √ Battery life and battery toxicity
- Insertion and removal of hearing instruments
- Recommended wearing schedule and acclimatization
  - ○ √ Cleaning and moisture protection of hearing aids
- Overnight storage of hearing aids
  - ○ √ Basic troubleshooting
  - ○ √ Basic hearing aid maintenance
  - ○ √ Telephone and other device coupling
  - ○ √ Potential assistive listening device needs
  - ○ √ Hearing aid insurance, loss and damage policies, and loaner hearing aid programs
- Recommended follow-up and monitoring

31.11 Assistive Listening Devices

Properly selected and verified hearing instrumentation can markedly improve hearing and enhance one's life, employment status, and overall health status.[8,10,40–42] Yet, the physiological effects of a cochlear hearing loss limit the degree of sound amplification that can be delivered to the ear, with frequently no more than one half of the measured hearing loss being restored. This inherent limitation of hearing aids along with the degradation of received auditory signals due to the distance from the speaker, background noise, and room reverberation often necessitate the use of a variety of technologies to better receive desired signals.

Assistive listening devices (ALDs), also known as hearing assistance technologies (HATs), are designed to improve the reception of speech or to ensure that warning or alerting signals are received by those with hearing loss. Examples of these devices include FM or Bluetooth transmission of a talker's voice directly into one's hearing aids, captioned telephones, telephone ringer and doorbell alerts (through flashing lights or vibration), television sound transmission directly to hearing aids, closed captioning for TV and movies, headset sound reception at movies or live theater, and smoke alarm alerts. The Americans with Disabilities Act mandates that many public places, including hotel rooms, be equipped with these assistive devices. In spite of the long-time availability of these valuable assistive items, Stika et al[43] reported that fewer than 35% of audiologists informed their patients of assistance available through augmentative technologies. Clinical observations would suggest that this number has not improved greatly in the intervening years.

31.12 Conclusion

The goal of audiological rehabilitation is to help patients minimize the interpersonal, psychosocial, educational, and vocational limitations imposed by hearing loss. Hearing loss treatment is a journey, not an event. Technology is part of that journey, but equally important are communication training and counseling. It is important that audiologists are able to provide all aspects of audiological rehabilitation in order to maximize results for patients.

References

[1] Clark JG, English KE. Counseling in Audiologic Practice: Helping Patients and Their Families Adjust to Hearing Loss. Boston: Allyn & Bacon, 2004

[2] Clark JG, English KE. Counseling-Infused Audiologic Care. Boston: Pearson Education, 2014

[3] Montano JJ, Spitzer JB. Adult Audiologic Rehabilitation. San Diego: Plural Publishing Group, 2009

[4] Clark JG, Kricos P, Sweetow R. The circle of life: a possible rehabilitative journey leading to improved patient outcomes. Audiology Today 2010; 22: 36–39

[5] American Speech-Language-Hearing Association. Knowledge and skills required for the practice of audiologic/aural rehabilitation [knowledge and skills], 2001. www.asha.org/policy

[6] Sweetow RW. Instead of a hearing aid evaluation, let's assess functional communication ability. Hearing Journal 2007; 60: 26–31

[7] National Council on Aging. The Consequences of Untreated Hearing Loss in Older Persons. (Study conducted by the Senior Research Group, an alliance between the National Council on Aging and Market Strategies, Inc.) Washington, DC: National Council on the Aging, 1999

[8] National American Precis Syndicated. Money matters: hearing loss may mean income loss, 2007. www.napsnet.com/health/70980.html

[9] Kochkin S. Marke Trak VIII: patients report improved quality of life with hearing aid usage. Hearing Journal 2010; 64: 25–32

[10] Chisolm TH, Johnson CE, Danhauer JL et al. A systematic review of health-related quality of life and hearing aids: final report of the American Academy of Audiology Task Force On the Health-Related Quality of Life Benefits of Amplification in Adults. J Am Acad Audiol 2007; 18: 151–183

[11] Kochkin S. Marke Trak VIII: patients report improved quality of life with hearing aid usage. Hearing Journal 2011; 64: 25–32

[12] Kochkin S. Marke Trak VIII: 25 year trends in the hearing health market. Hearing Review 2009; 16: 12–31

[13] Kochkin S. Marke Trak VII: obstacles to adult non-user adoption of hearing aids. The Hearing Journal 2007; 60: 27–43

[14] Banerjee S. Hearing aids in the real world: use of multimemory and volume controls. J Am Acad Audiol 2011; 22: 359–374

[15] Yuen KC, Kam AC, Lau PS. Comparative performance of an adaptive directional microphone system and a multichannel noise reduction system. J Am Acad Audiol 2006; 17: 241–252

[16] Peeters H, Kuk F, Lau CC, Keenan D. Subjective and objective evaluation of noise management algorithms. J Am Acad Audiol 2009; 20: 89–98

[17] Nordrum S, Erler S, Garstecki D, Dhar S. Comparison of performance on the hearing in noise test using directional microphones and digital noise reduction algorithms. Am J Audiol 2006; 15: 81–91

[18] Ricketts T, Johnson E, Federman J. Individual differences within and across feedback suppression hearing aids. J Am Acad Audiol 2008; 19: 748–757

[19] Pietrzyk PD. Counseling Comfort Levels of Audiologists (AuD Capstone). Cincinnati, OH: University of Cincinnati, 2009

[20] Blood GW, Blood IM, Danhauer J. The hearing aid effect. Hearing Instruments 1977; 28: 12–16

[21] Tønnesen H. Engage in the Process of Change. Bispebjerg, Denmark: World Health Organization European Regional Office, 2012

[22] Clark JG. Sisyphus personified: audiology's attempts to rehabilitate adult hearing loss. The Hearing Journal 2010; 63: 26–28

[23] Clark JG, Maatman C, Gailey L. Moving patients forward: motivational engagement. Semin Hear 2012; 33: 35–45

[24] Hoover-Steinwart L, English K, Hanley JE. Study probes impact on hearing aid benefit of earlier involvement by significant other. Hearing Journal 2001; 54: 56–59

[25] Kochkin S, Beck DL, Christensen LA et al. Marke Trak VIII: The impact of the hearing healthcare professional on hearing aid user success. The Hearing Review 2010; 17: 12–34

[26] Dillon H. Audiologists Use of Real Ear Measurements, 2008. www.docstoc.com/docs/479565/Real-Ear-Measures

[27] American Academy of Audiology. Guidelines for the Audiologic Management of Adult Hearing Impairment, 2011. http://www.audiology.org/resources/documentlibrary/Documents/haguidelines

[28] Mueller HG, Hawkins DB, Northern JL. Probe Microphone Measurements: Hearing Aid Selection and Assessment. San Diego, CA: Singular Publishing, 1992

[29] Reports C. Hearing Well in a Noisy World: Hearing Aids, Hearing Protection, and More, 2009. http://www.consumerreports.org/cro/2012/12/hear-well-in-a-noisy-world/index.htm

[30] Kessels RPC. Patients' memory for medical information. J R Soc Med 2003; 96: 219–222

[31] McGuire LC. Remembering what the doctor said: organization and adults' memory for medical information. Exp Aging Res 1996; 22: 403–428

[32] Anderson JL, Dodman S, Kopelman M, Fleming A. Patient information recall in a rheumatology clinic. Rheumatol Rehabil 1979; 18: 18–22

[33] Nair EL, Cienkowski KM. The impact of health literacy on patient understanding of counseling and education materials. Int J Audiol 2010; 49: 71–75

[34] Shieh C, Hosei B. Printed health information materials: evaluation of readability and suitability. J Community Health Nurs 2008; 25: 73–90

[35] Pichora-Fuller MK, Singh G. Effects of age on auditory and cognitive processing: implications for hearing aid fitting and audiologic rehabilitation. Trends Amplif 2006; 10: 29–59

[36] Reese JL, Hnath-Chisolm T. Recognition of hearing aid orientation content by first-time users. Am J Audiol 2005; 14: 94–104

[37] Locaputo A, Clark JG. Increasing hearing aid orientation information retention through use of DVD instruction. The Hearing Journal 2011; 64: 44–50

[38] Tirone M, Stanford LS. Analysis of the hearing aid orientation process. Paper presented at the annual meeting of the American Speech-Language-Hearing Association, San Antonio, TX, 1992

[39] Lesner SA, Thomas-Frank S, Klinger MS. Assessment of the effectiveness of an adult audiologic rehabilitation program using a knowledge-based test and a measure of hearing aid satisfaction. J Acad Rehabilitative Audiol 2001; 34: 29–39

[40] Crandell CC. Hearing aids: Their effects on functional health status. The Hearing Journal 1998; 51: 22–30

[41] Kochkin S, Rogin CM. Quantifying the obvious: The impact of hearing instruments on quality of life. The Hearing Review 2000; 7: 2–34

[42] Larson VD, Williams DW, Henderson WG et al. NIDCD/VA Hearing Aid Clinical Trial Group. Efficacy of 3 commonly used hearing aid circuits: a crossover trial. JAMA 2000; 284: 1806–1813

[43] Stika CJ, Ross M, Cuevas C. Hearing Aid Services and Satisfaction: The Consumer Viewpoint. Hearing Loss 2002;25–31

[44] National Institute on Deafness and Other Communication Disorders. Quick Statistics, 2010. http://www.nidcd.nih.gov/health/statistics/pages/quick.aspx

[45] Deafness in Disguise. Timeline of Hearing Devices and Early Deaf Education. Washington University School of Medicine. Bernard Becker Medical Library, 2012. http://beckerexhibits.wustl.edu/did/timeline

32 Implantable Hearing Devices

Jeffery J. Kuhn and Angel J. Perez

32.1 Introduction

Recent advances in conventional hearing aid technology have resulted in improvements in functionality and cosmesis. The miniaturization of components, advances in digital signal processing, addition of directional microphones, and improvements in the ease of use (e.g., selective programming, automatic telecoil, Bluetooth capabilities, data logging, remote control) have led to greater acceptance of these devices by the hearing-impaired consumer. Despite these advances, only approximately 25% of individuals who would benefit from conventional amplification actually own hearing aids. Of hearing aid users, approximately 45% are either dissatisfied with or neutral about their experience, and about 12% have abandoned their aids to the dresser drawer.[1]

Historically, the various reasons for dissatisfaction or noncompliance include acoustic feedback, occlusion, adverse effects on the ear canal such as dermatitis and cerumen buildup, and inherent limitations of the device such as limited amplification above frequencies 4 to 6 kHz, sound distortion, and poor speech intelligibility in noisy environments. Although less problematic in the age of Bluetooth cell phone ear sets, some hearing aid candidates perceive a social stigma associated with hearing aid use. Other patients may have clinical conditions that make conventional aiding or surgical treatment difficult or impractical (e.g., chronic ear disease with persistent otorrhea; aural atresia; and single-sided deafness [SSD], defined as severe to profound sensorineural hearing loss [SNHL]).

Implantable hearing device manufacturers have made considerable strides in the past two decades in addressing the problems encountered by hearing aid users with the development of partially and fully implantable middle ear hearing devices. Conventional acoustic hearing aids function by receiving environmental sounds through a microphone and converting the vibratory information into an electrical signal that is processed, amplified, and delivered to the ear canal as acoustic energy. In contrast to conventional hearing aids, middle ear implantable hearing devices (MEIHDs) transmit acoustic energy directly to a mobile structure within the middle ear space (ossicle or round window membrane [RWM]) through the use of a vibrational transducer, thereby bypassing the external auditory canal. These devices are either partially or totally implantable.

The impetus for the development of MEIHDs has been centered primarily on the need to fulfill the amplification needs of patients with moderate to severe SNHL. This segment of the hearing-impaired population (approximately 7.3 million) have gain requirements in the mid- to high-frequency range that would increase the risks of acoustic feedback and sound distortion with the use of conventional hearing aids. Reducing feedback may necessitate a tighter fitting ear mold, which may lead to discomfort and a more pronounced occlusion effect. Although open fit/receiver-in-canal technology has virtually eliminated the problems of occlusion and feedback, this hearing aid design is best suited for individuals with mild to moderate hearing loss. The currently available implantable devices have the advantage of amplifying high frequencies without creating feedback, tend to improve sound fidelity by directly stimulating the ossicular chain, and eliminate discomfort and the occlusion effect by leaving the external auditory canal open.

Conceptually, MEIHDs are niche products that are meant to fill the hearing rehabilitation void between hearing aids and cochlear implants. Because the use of these devices involves surgical risks not associated with the fitting of traditional hearing aids, candidates for MEIHDs should be compelled to first try conventional hearing aids. Unlike with conventional hearing aids, MEIHDs can only be prescribed and placed by a physician. Patients should be free of infection and have a relatively normal middle ear anatomy in order to properly anchor the transducer. Hearing loss should be stable, and word recognition scores should meet the device manufacturer's candidacy criteria. Most importantly, the patient's expectations of benefit should be reasonable. MEIHDs are expensive and the cost is typically not covered by health insurance.

Technological advancements in implant design and processor capability, and the expansion of the marketplace to include a transcutaneous system, have made bone conduction implantable hearing devices (BCIHDs) an attractive alternative for patients with conductive or mixed hearing loss or SSD. Since the first application of an osseointegrated titanium implant in the temporal bone for the purpose of auditory rehabilitation,[2] the indications for use have evolved to include a wide variety of clinical situations. Patients with conductive or mixed SNHL who are not surgical candidates or are unable to tolerate a conventional hearing aid may benefit from the use of a BCIHD. This subset of patients includes those with a chronically draining ear due to chronic otitis media or otitis externa and those with a problematic chronically draining mastoid cavity. In addition, patients with otosclerosis, tympanosclerosis, or aural atresia who are poor candidates for, or have previously failed, surgical correction may benefit from the use of a BCIHD.

Patients who have had external auditory canal closure in conjunction with a skull base surgical procedure are suitable candidates based on any one of the three clinical indications: conductive hearing loss, mixed hearing loss, or SSD. The currently available implantable bone conduction systems have become an attractive alternative to the use of contralateral routing of signal (CROS) hearing aids and conventional bone conduction hearing aids. The use of traditional bone conduction hearing aids may lead to complaints of excessive pressure and pain, or headache, or may cause skin irritation due to the firm placement of the bone oscillator on the mastoid process. Furthermore, the attenuation of sound transfer due to intervening soft tissue and the variability in bone conductor placement may lead to inadequate gain. Current designs include the percutaneous implantable systems (Baha 3 System, Cochlear Bone Anchored Solutions, Gothenburg, Sweden; Ponto Bone Anchored Hearing System, Oticon Medical, Askim, Sweden), and a transcutaneous system (Alpha 1 System, Sophono, Inc., Boulder, CO).

32.2 Middle Ear Implantable Hearing Devices

32.2.1 Middle Ear Transducer Technology

The currently available MEIHDs in the United States and in Europe use one of two types of transducers: electromagnetic or piezoelectric. Electromagnetic devices function by transmitting an electrical current through an induction coil that is in proximity to a magnet. The magnetic field that is produced with this configuration causes the magnet to vibrate, resulting in movement of the ossicular chain. The induction coil may be located separate from the implanted magnet or integrated with the magnet in an assembly attached to the ossicular chain or in contact with the RWM (round window application approved for use in the European Union). The implant design that has the induction coil and magnet at a distance from one another requires considerable fitting accuracy, as the power delivered from the coil to the magnet decreases by as much as the cube of the distance between the two components.

Piezoelectric devices function by transmitting an electrical current through a piezoceramic crystal. The ceramic crystal consists of layers of lead, zirconium, and titanium oxide with the property of reversible electromechanical transduction: when a force is applied to the material, a voltage is generated; when a voltage is applied, motion is created. More specifically, by applying a sinusoidal input to a piezoelectric biomorph (two layers of lead-zirconate-titanate crystal on either side of a stiffening material, typically carbon fiber), the tip of the biomorph will oscillate according to the input frequency. Mechanical flexion of the biomorph, at a given rate, produces a characteristic electrical sinusoid. Conversely, by applying a direct current voltage to the biomorph ceramic crystal, one side of the crystal will expand while the other side contracts producing a bending motion. Therefore, attaching a probe or rod to one end of the crystal serves to either collect sound energy for the purpose of transmitting an electrical signal or to transmit vibrational energy as a result of an incoming electrical signal.

Electromagnetic and piezoelectric technologies have their advantages and disadvantages. Common to both designs, however, is the accuracy required for placement of the transducer. Although the implementation of an extra-coil electromagnetic system (induction coil and magnet separate from one another) is relatively simple from a surgical standpoint, the distance between the coil and magnet must adhere to strict guidelines to maintain optimal magnetic field strength. Attaching an electromagnetic transducer to the ossicular chain adds weight and, therefore, may attenuate vibration at high frequencies by a mass loading effect. If the transducer shifts or is placed at an angle relative to the coincident axis of stapes movement, sound energy transfer will be reduced and optimal performance is lost. Coupling the tip of an electromagnetic or piezoelectric transducer to the ossicular chain demands precision. Insufficient pressure at the point of contact with the ossicle will reduce acoustic energy transfer, whereas excessive tension may result in a conductive loss.[3] Electromagnetic transducers tend to have high power consumption and, therefore, require a rechargeable battery for the fully implantable device. Piezoelectric transducers consume less power and are highly sensitive, but generate limited voltage and displacement.[4] Whether electromagnetic or piezoelectric, both types of transducers should be able to generate forces corresponding to acoustic sound pressure levels (SPLs) of at least 110 to 120 dB SPL in order to provide adequate amplification to patients with hearing loss (HL) in the 50- to 90-dB HL range.[5]

32.2.2 Currently Available Middle Ear Implantable Hearing Devices

The middle ear implantable hearing device manufacturing community has evolved rapidly over the past 15 years as new technologies and designs have become available. Regardless of the specific marketing agenda of a given manufacturing firm, a common goal exists among the various research and development teams that have contributed to the advancement of these devices: amplify sound without sacrificing fidelity, and do it with a device that is biocompatible, invisible, and reliable. Although certain middle ear implantable devices are no longer available [partially implantable Rion Ehime (E)-type device; Totally Integrated Cochlear Amplifier (TICA), Implex American Hearing Systems, now owned by Cochlear Corp., Sydney, Australia; partially implantable Soundtec Direct System, formerly marketed by Soundtec, Inc., Oklahoma City, OK], their influence in the hearing rehabilitation marketplace has led to improvements in later designs. The following section reviews the semi- and fully implantable middle ear hearing devices that are currently available in the United States and Europe. Although each manufacturer has slightly different audiometric criteria for determining candidacy for their device, in general these devices have been designed for patients with moderate to severe SNHL with a minimum speech discrimination of 40 to 60%. Expanded criteria have been established in the European Union for the use of certain devices in patients with conductive and mixed hearing loss.

32.3 Electromagnetic Devices

32.3.1 Vibrant Soundbridge

The Vibrant Soundbridge (VSB), developed and formerly marketed by Symphonix Devices, Inc., San Jose, CA), was the first MEIHD to be approved by the Food and Drug Administration (FDA) (received in 2000) for use in patients with moderate to severe SNHL (▶ Fig. 32.1).

The device was acquired by Vibrant MED-EL (MED-EL Corp., Innsbruck, Austria) in 2003, and has since seen little change in the design of its implantable components. However, since commercial release of the device in the Europe in 1998, there have been several upgrades to the speech processor circuitry. Currently, an eight-channel digital processor (Vibrant Signia) is available and has been shown to significantly improve functional gain and speech intelligibility in noise as compared to the preimplant hearing aid condition that used the same eight-channel digital processor.

The VSB consists of an implanted component, the vibrating ossicular prosthesis (VORP) (▶ Fig. 32.2), which contains an internal coil and magnet and receiver module that is connected

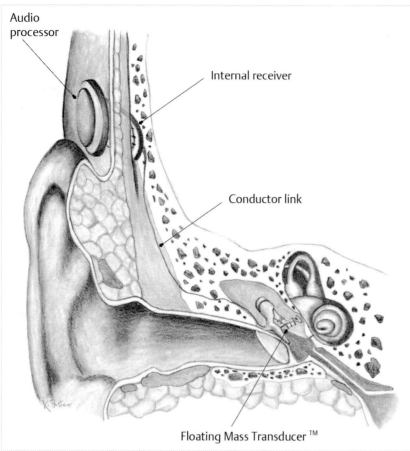

Fig. 32.1 The MED-EL Vibrant Soundbridge.

Audio processor

Internal receiver

Conductor link

Floating Mass Transducer ™

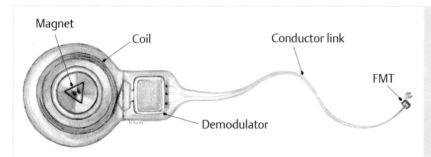

Fig. 32.2 Vibrating ossicular prosthesis (VORP).

Magnet

Coil

Conductor link

FMT

Demodulator

by a conductor link to the floating mass transducer (FMT) (▶ Fig. 32.3), and an externally worn audio processor. The VORP is implanted posterosuperior to the pinna on the temporal bone, similar to the technique used in cochlear implant surgery. The conductor link exits the VORP and traverses the mastoid cavity and the facial recess opening to the FMT that is attached to the long process of the incus with a titanium attachment clip (▶ Fig. 32.4).

The FMT is placed such that its orientation is coincident with the axis of stapes movement. The FMT is an electromagnetic transducer that consists of an electromagnetic coil that encases a small permanent magnet. The design of the FMT takes advantage of the natural vibratory motion of the ossicular chain and provides certain advantages as a "direct drive" system in terms of frequency response and fidelity.[6–9] The external audio processor contains the microphone, signal processor, transmitting coil, centering magnet, and battery. It is held in place by

transcutaneous magnetic attraction to the magnet in the implanted receiver coil. The auditory signal is collected by the microphone and transmitted via an amplitude-modulated carrier to the implanted internal receiver in the VORP. The signal is then demodulated and sent via the conductor link to the FMT.

Although the VSB has not been shown to be superior to conventional hearing aids in all studies that have assessed benefit in terms of audiometric criteria, many clinical studies have reported overall improved patient satisfaction. Subjective benefit as measured by validated questionnaires has shown reduced problems with feedback, occlusion effect, reverberation, and sound distortion, and at least equivalent amplification of sound as compared to traditional hearing aids.[10–13] In terms of functional gain and speech recognition in quiet and noise, several studies have demonstrated a significant benefit over conventional hearing aids.[10,11,14,15] This is especially notable given the technological advances in conventional hearing aid manufac-

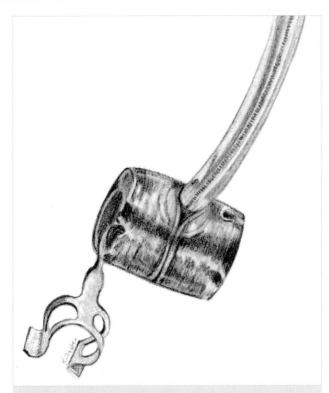

Fig. 32.3 Floating mass transducer (FMT).

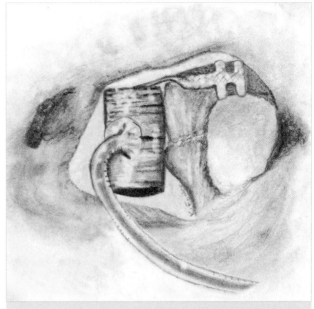

Fig. 32.4 The FMT attached to the incus.

turing in the last 10 years. Even in those studies that have shown no significant difference with regard to audiometric criteria and standardized or nonstandardized satisfaction surveys,[16,17] the VSB was declared a "good option" for patients with moderate to severe SNHL who could not tolerate a conventional aid and in those with chronic otitis externa. Long-term reliability of the VSB has been demonstrated in two recent studies that have shown stability of functional gain and speech recognition.[18,19] Both studies recognized few long-term problems, such as local skin irritation, and there were no internal devices failures in those patients implanted within the last 10 years. These studies help to confirm the long-term safety and efficacy of the VSB. The device has also been found to be a cost-effective solution for managing SNHL in patients with chronic external otitis media as determined by a quality-adjusted life-year outcome measure.[20]

Since 2008, the indications for the VSB have been expanded in Europe to include treatment of conductive and mixed hearing loss. As a result of considerable research efforts that have included a mathematical middle ear simulation model,[21] cadaveric temporal bone studies,[22–24] and clinical studies,[25–30] the placement of the FMT onto vibratory structures within the middle ear space other than the incus may be equally efficacious. Previous animal studies have demonstrated that the placement of a transducer against the RWM is capable of producing evoked responses equivalent to sound stimulation levels of 85 to 110 dB SPL across a broad frequency range. By modifying the FMT to fit into the round window niche, Colletti et al[25] were able to demonstrate favorable results in seven patients with severe mixed hearing loss. The wide interindividual difference in postoperative hearing results, however, suggested that there was migration of the FMT over time.

A more recent study reported favorable results with a similar wide variability in hearing benefit, suggesting either inadequate interface between the FMT and the RWM at the time of placement or eventual migration.[29] Cadaveric temporal bone studies using laser Doppler vibrometric measurements of stapes movement with the FMT subjected to various orientations and soft tissue cover conditions concluded that the best orientation of the FMT was perpendicular to the RWM and that a supporting soft tissue cover was important.[23,24] These studies disagreed, however, as to the benefit of soft tissue interposed between the FMT and RWM. The results in a recent clinical study demonstrated favorable coupling efficiency between the FMT and RWM, whether there was complete or partial contact as opposed to a reduced coupling efficiency and transfer of vibratory energy if coupling required the interposition of autologous tissue.[30] A round window (RW) coupler prosthesis (vibroplasty-RW coupler) has been developed by the manufacturer to facilitate placement of the FMT against the RWM (▶ Fig. 32.5).

Intraoperative electrocochleography has recently been shown to be a valuable tool for ensuring precise placement of the FMT in patients with moderate to severe conductive or mixed hearing loss.[31] Although some have found considerable variability in hearing outcomes in a limited number of patients using the RW vibroplasty technique,[32] others have demonstrated consistent efficacy with respect to postimplant aided thresholds, speech perception, and functional gain in both short- and long-term studies.[33–35] Although the round window insertion technique has been used primarily in patients with chronic otitis media and otosclerosis, favorable results have also been shown in patients with congenital aural atresia.[36–38] Other applications reported include the use of a titanium partial ossicular replacement prosthesis (PORP) or total ossicular replacement prosthesis (TORP) coupled to the FMT (vibroplasty PORP and TORP) for use in patients with moderate to severe mixed hearing loss.[26,39,40] The FMT has been coupled to different sites on the stapes and within the oval window niche including the

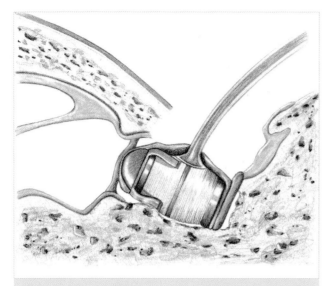

Fig. 32.5 FMT and vibroplasty–round window (RW) coupler in position against round window membrane.

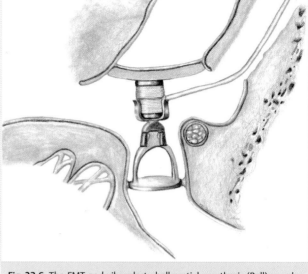

Fig. 32.6 The FMT and vibroplasty-bell partial prosthesis (Bell) coupler in position between the cartilage block and the stapes capitulum.

stapes head,[41,42] the footplate,[43] the oval window,[44] and in combination with a stapedotomy procedure.[45,46]

A vibroplasty-TORP assembly has also been placed through a stapedotomy opening in patients with moderate to severe mixed hearing loss.[47] The sound transfer efficiency of the vibroplasty-PORP and –TORP configurations as compared to the RW application has been studied in the temporal bone model.[48] Acoustic gain was found to be superior at all test frequencies, as measured by a third window laser Doppler vibrometry technique, for the FMT-PORP and -TORP assemblies as compared with RW placement. The manufacturer has since made available several titanium vibroplasty couplers, as a result of the work in Europe, including the vibroplasty–oval window (OW) coupler, vibroplasty-bell partial prosthesis (Bell) coupler (▶ Fig. 32.6), and vibroplasty-clip partial prosthesis (CliP) coupler. The VSB had received the Communauté Européene (CE) mark for conductive and mixed hearing loss in adults in 2008 and for the same indication in children in 2009. The device had also received the CE mark for moderate to severe SNHL in children in 2009. The phase II trial for mixed and conductive hearing loss indications is currently underway in the United States.

Magnetic resonance imaging (MRI) compatibility studies in the temporal bone model have demonstrated stability of the ossicular chain with an attached FMT both from a theoretic standpoint[49] and based on direct exposure to a 1.5-tesla (T) MRI scanner.[50,51] Although magnetization and functional integrity were maintained following 1.5-T exposures, positional changes of the FMT occurred in five of 18 temporal bone specimens when coupled to the incus. A recent retrospective review assessed subjective complaints and audiometric results in 12 VSB recipients who had previous inadvertent exposure to either a 1.0- or 1.5-T MRI scanner.[52] In nine of 12 patients with pre-MRI hearing tests available, there was no evidence of change in bone conduction thresholds following MRI exposure. However, two of the nine patients required repositioning of the FMT due to loss of transfer function and four of 12 patients described a change in the magnet strength of the sound processor, necessi-

tating an adjustment. There was no correlation between MRI scanner magnet strength (1.0 or 1.5 T) and reported symptoms during scanning (e.g., pain, noise) or during the refitting procedure.

32.3.2 Otologics Middle Ear Transducer Fully Implantable Hearing System (Carina)

The Otologics Fully Implantable Hearing System (Carina) (Otologics LLC, Boulder, CO) consists of four primary components: the implant, the programming system, the charger, and the remote control. The original implant design consists of the electronics capsule that contains the rechargeable battery, digital signal processor, microphone, and transmission coil, and is implanted entirely beneath the skin behind the auricle. The electronics capsule is connected to an electromagnetic transducer that is placed in contact with the incus (▶ Fig. 32.7).

The programming system consists of a NOAHlink programming interface that is worn around the neck. Using the OtoFit software, the NOAHlink interface receives signals from the computer through a wireless connection and sends the signals to the implant site through a radiofrequency coil that is held in place magnetically. Programming the implant is similar to the programming techniques used for conventional digital hearing aids. The programming system also provides the means for extensive testing and diagnostics of the middle ear transducer (MET) fully implantable ossicular stimulator. The charger system consists of a base station, charging coil, and charger body. The charging coil is placed over the implant site and held in place magnetically. Charging time is typically 1 hour if charging occurs on a daily basis. While charging the implant, the patient can conduct normal daily activities, adjust the volume, and turn the implant on and off. The remote control may be used to adjust the volume and turn the implant on and off by placing the remote against the skin over the implant site. The IS-1

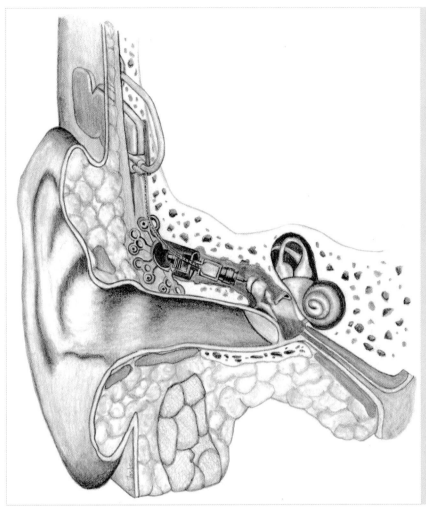

Fig. 32.7 Otologics MET Fully Implantable Hearing System (Carina).

connector between the electronics package (processor) and the MET stimulator allows for the implanted device to be exchanged with a minor surgical procedure. The processor must be exchanged when the rechargeable battery has reached its lifetime use, which is specified as 8 years with daily charging. The implantable microphone is permanently connected to the processor and must be exchanged with the processor.

A semi-implantable version of the device (MET), further developed by Otologics LLC from 1996 to 2000, received the CE mark in 2000 for moderate to severe SNHL in adults. FDA approval was not sought for the semi-implantable device in the United States in favor of developing and testing the fully implantable version. The semi-implantable device consists of an ear-level audio processor (button processor) that contains the microphone, signal processor, transmitting coil, and battery. The auditory signal is converted to an electrical signal that is transmitted transcutaneously to an internal coil and receiver stimulator. The receiver stimulator is connected to an electromagnetic transducer that is secured to the body of incus in a similar manner to that of the fully implantable device.

The fully implantable MET (marketed as the Carina) received the CE mark for moderate to severe SNHL in 2006 and for conductive and mixed hearing loss in 2007. Studies conducted in Europe have demonstrated benefit in small groups of patients with placement of the transducer against the RWM in those

with moderate to severe mixed hearing loss due to either sclerotic disease of the oval window niche or otosclerosis, and with placement of the transducer coupled to a partial titanium prosthesis on the stapes capitulum in patients with congenital aural atresia.[53–56] The device has also been implanted in conjunction with a stapedotomy procedure and following previous stapes surgery in patients with mixed hearing loss due to otosclerosis.[57] The phase I clinical trial in the United States, which included 20 patients with moderate to severe SNHL and speech recognition scores greater than 40%, demonstrated no significant benefit over the preoperative hearing aid condition as measured by monaural and binaural speech discrimination using consonant/nucleus/consonant (CNC) words and phonemes and hearing-in-noise testing (HINT). HINT scores improved substantially, however, after refitting at 12 months. The general perception of benefit as measured by subjective questionnaires showed that the implant performed at least as well as, if not significantly better than, the preimplant hearing aid condition in nearly every category.[58]

Of the various problems identified in the phase I trial, microphone position and migration were significant factors influencing hearing outcome and perceived benefit. Microphone migration contributed to feedback, limited functional gain, and deterioration of speech recognition and microphone position as the mastoid tip tended to accentuate anatomic noise (e.g.,

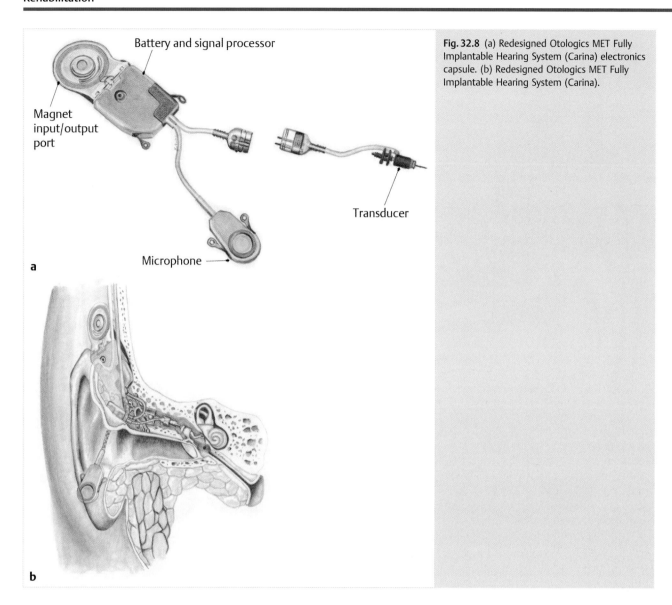

Battery and signal processor

Magnet
input/output
port

Transducer

Microphone

a

b

Fig. 32.8 (a) Redesigned Otologics MET Fully Implantable Hearing System (Carina) electronics capsule. (b) Redesigned Otologics MET Fully Implantable Hearing System (Carina).

skin movement, chewing, voicing). Phase II trials have been completed and the manufacturer has since revised the implant design to include a hermetically sealed titanium casing for the transducer, a smaller electronics capsule with modified connector, and new processor algorithms to eliminate feedback and reduce biological noise (▶ Fig. 32.8). Twenty additional patients will be implanted with the new device in order to meet FDA requirements. The redesigned device is currently available in Europe, Latin America, and Asia.

32.3.3 Ototronix MAXUM

The MAXUM system (Ototronix, LLC, Houston, TX) is a partially implantable device with a design based on Soundtec Direct System technology acquired by Ototronix in 2009 (▶ Fig. 32.9).

The MAXUM middle ear implant consists of a neodymium-iron-boron (NdFeB) magnet encased in a titanium housing, which is attached to the incudostapedial joint at the level of the neck of the stapes. The external processor is available in either a behind-the-ear (BTE) or in-the-canal integrated processor coil (IPC) configuration and consists of a digital sound processor

and electromagnetic coil. The sound processor receives the auditory signal, amplifies it, and transmits the electrical signal to the transceiver coil located near the tympanic membrane. The transceiver coil converts the electrical signal to electromagnetic energy that drives the middle ear implant, thereby causing the ossicles to vibrate. Although the transceiver coil is located in the external auditory canal, energy transfer occurs through electromagnetic induction and direct drive of the ossicular chain, therefore obviating the need for an acoustic seal and the generation of sound pressure energy in the canal. This design reduces the potential for occlusion, sound distortion, and feedback. The BTE configuration contains an electromagnetic coil embedded in an acrylic mold that is seated at an optimal distance of 2 mm from the tympanic membrane. The fully digital sound processor features directional microphones, noise cancellation capabilities, and a wide dynamic range of compression. The audio processor and implantable components were FDA approved in October 2009.

Ototronix has developed a new fitting protocol that provides a means for establishing accuracy and consistency in the fitting distance between the transceiver coil and the implanted

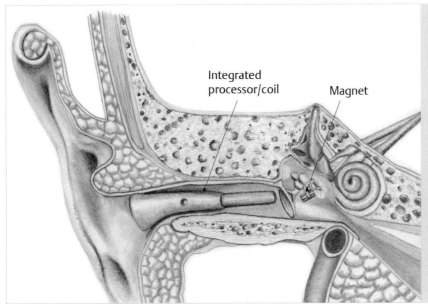

Fig. 32.9 The Ototronix MAXUM partially implantable device.

Integrated processor/coil

Magnet

magnet. The IPC component is manufactured with a malleable housing to allow re-fitting of the processor without the need for a new impression and subsequent remake of the IPC. The company has also redesigned the implantable magnet in order to allow placement without separating the incudostapedial joint and to secure the magnet with a glass-ionomer cement. Clinical studies conducted for the Soundtec Direct device demonstrated statistically significant improvement in various parameters measured including functional gain, speech discrimination in quiet, and perceived aided benefit (Abbreviated Profile of Hearing Aid Benefit or APHAB) compared to the best conventionally aided condition.[59,60]

Magnet instability and noise were frequent complaints of implanted subjects, although occlusion and feedback were greatly reduced or eliminated. The interposition of adipose tissue between the neck of the stapes and the collar of the magnet served to reduce the potential for magnet movement in subsequent patients. The MAXUM device has been redesigned to allow for placement of the magnet without separating the incudostapedial joint. Previous MRI compatibility studies conducted with the Soundtec device in cadaveric temporal bone specimens and in patients have demonstrated retained stability and integrity of the implant and the ossicular chain in a 0.3-T open MRI using a modified protocol.[61,62]

32.4 Piezoelectric Device

32.4.1 Envoy Esteem

The Esteem Totally Implantable Middle Ear Hearing System (Envoy Medical Corp., St Paul, MN) consists of three implantable components: the piezoelectric sensor and driver that are implanted in the middle ear, and the sound processor that is implanted on the temporal bone behind the auricle (▶ Fig. 32.10).

The piezoelectric sensor tip is attached to the incus using a bioactive glass-ionomer cement through a transmastoid atticotomy approach. The sensor "senses" vibrations from the tympanic membrane via its attachment to the incus and converts the mechanical vibrations into electrical signals that are transmitted to the sound processor. The sound processor amplifies and filters the signal and then sends it to the piezoelectric driver, which is coupled to the stapes capitulum using bone cement. The driver converts the modified electrical signal back to mechanical energy and vibrates the stapes. The incus and stapes are disarticulated and 1 to 2 mm of the distal aspect of the incus is resected to prevent feedback to the sensor. In short, the device uses the tympanic membrane as the microphone and amplifies acoustic energy delivered through the natural pathway of the external auditory canal.

The Esteem has three external instruments that are used for programming and testing the device after implantation. The esteem programmer is used by the audiologist to program the settings in the sound processor, and the personal programmer is used by the patient to adjust volume, select preset environmental modes, and turn the device on or off. The intraoperative system analyzer is used to perform diagnostics of system components intraoperatively and to verify proper performance of the implanted system postoperatively. The system contains a nonrechargeable lithium-iodide battery with an average useful life of 6 to 9 years. Battery replacement requires surgical replacement of the sound processor.

The phase I trial in the United States identified several problems with the original implant design (Envoy System, St. Croix Medical, Minneapolis, MN), including breaches in transducer hermaticity and limited functional gain in the high frequencies.[63] The manufacturer addressed these issues in the development of the second generation of the device (Esteem II) prior to phase II clinical trials. The phase II trial enrolled 57 adults with mild to severe SNHL and speech discrimination scores greater than 40%.[64] The postoperative audiometric results demonstrated significant improvements in mean speech reception threshold (SRT) and word recognition score (WRS), and the quality of life measures showed a statistically significant improvement in mean benefit with the implanted device over hearing aids on the APHAB assessment. There was no postoperative decline in bone thresholds as compared to the

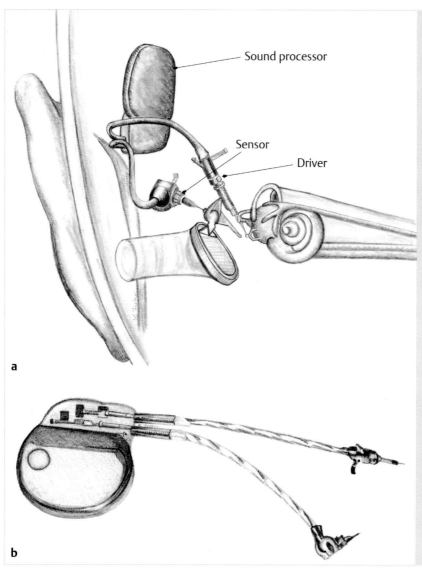

Sound processor

Sensor

Driver

a

b

Fig. 32.10 (a) Envoy Esteem Totally Implantable Middle Ear Hearing System. (b) Envoy Esteem sound processor and piezoelectric sensor and driver.

preimplant condition. The results of the phase II trial led to FDA approval of the device for moderate to severe SNHL in adults (age ≥ 18 years) in March 2010. The Envoy Esteem had previously received the CE mark for moderate to severe SNHL in 2006.

Notable postoperative adverse events during the phase II trial included taste disturbance (40%), tinnitus (14%), disequilibrium (19%), and transient facial paresis or paralysis (7%). Revision surgery was necessary in three patients due to fibrotic tissue interference at the transducer site. A 1-year follow-up study demonstrated sustained hearing outcomes and provided some insight as to the postoperative adverse events and the nuances with respect to device placement.[65] Hearing outcomes in a subset of patients (five of 57) in the phase II trial with profound high-frequency SNHL were reported in a separate study.[66] The WRS at 50 dB HL improved from a baseline unaided (10%) and aided (23%) average to 78% at 12 months postimplantation. All subjects had a statistically significant improvement in WRS.

The mean speech reception threshold improved from baseline unaided (65 dB) and aided (48 dB) conditions to 26 dB with the Esteem implant. Hearing in noise evaluation using the QuickSIN test was improved in four of five patients, but the

scores did not reach statistical significance. Envoy Medical plans to conduct a postapproval study that will include additional patients in order to address the postoperative adverse events in the phase II trial. The manufacturer has recently developed a smaller transducer size (25% reduction) that is currently under review by the FDA. There are currently no studies that address the MRI compatibility of the Envoy Esteem. The manufacturer warns against exposure of the device to an MRI scanner.

32.5 Investigational Devices

32.5.1 Direct Acoustical Cochlear Stimulation

The Direct Acoustical Cochlear Stimulation (DACS) system (Phonak Acoustic Implants SA, Sonova Holding AG, Lausanne, Switzerland) is based on the principle of a power-driven stapes prosthesis, and therefore it is intended for use in patients with severe mixed hearing loss due to advanced otosclerosis. It consists of an externally worn audio processor, an implanted electromagnetic transducer, a percutaneous plug and fixation system, and an "off-the-shelf" stapes prosthesis.[67] The external audio processor contains two microphones, a digital signal processing unit, and battery. The electrical output of the audio processor is delivered to the transducer via a percutaneous plug secured to the temporal bone. The vibrational energy is transferred to a coupling rod extending from the transducer onto which is placed a stapes wire-piston prosthesis. In order to allow for the natural transmission of sound energy when the device is turned off, a second stapes prosthesis is attached to the incus and placed into the stapedectomy opening.

The device was originally developed as a joint venture between Cochlear Ltd., Sydney, Australia, and Phonak AG, Stäfa, Switzerland. Clinical results in four patients at 2 years postimplantation demonstrated substantial improvements in sound field thresholds and speech intelligibility in quiet and noise (statistical analysis not conducted). Monosyllabic word recognition scores in quiet improved by 40 to 100% at 75 dB SPL. Postoperative unaided air conduction thresholds were improved by 14 to 28 dB pure-tone average (PTA) by virtue of the second stapes prosthesis. Subjective assessment by the APHAB in three patients at 12 months postimplantation showed significant improvements in three of four subscales in two patients and in all four in one patient.[5] Because of patient complaints regarding the percutaneous coupling of the external and internal device components, the manufacturer has replaced the percutaneous plug with a transcutaneous radiofrequency transmission component similar to that found in a cochlear implant. Despite further research and development efforts in Europe, the parent company, Sonova Holding AG, decided to close the manufacturing site in Switzerland in October 2011. Cochlear Ltd. plans to continue developing its version of the device.

32.5.2 Fully Implantable Hearing System

The Fully Implantable Hearing System (FIHS) (OtoKinetics, Salt Lake City, UT) is an investigational device that is being developed for use in individuals with conductive or mixed hearing loss or SNHL. The device consists of fully implanted microphone and sound processor that transmits the signal to a piezoelectric microtransducer implanted into the wall of the cochlea. Research and development of the microactuator and the implantable microphone has been completed, and an anatomic noise cancellation feature has been added. Safety studies, with respect to the cochleostomy in the lateral wall of the scala tympani and the histological response to the microactuator, have been completed in an animal model (George S. Lesinski, MD, personal communication). There are currently no clinical outcomes data available for this device.

32.6 Bone Conduction Implantable Hearing Devices

32.6.1 History

The concept of sound conduction through bone and body tissues had been described as early as the first century AD. Sound

transmission through the teeth was proposed as a potential tool for auditory diagnosis and treatment for deafness during the Renaissance period. During the early 20th century, the first dedicated bone oscillators were being designed in conjunction with the development of microphone and earphone technology. The early designs were worn secured to the mastoid bone with a headband, or alternatively, integrated into eyeglass frames. The inherent technological limitations of these early devices could not overcome the attenuation of sound transmission by scalp soft tissue, resulting in suboptimal high-frequency sound delivery. Other device-related problems included pressure and discomfort, low cosmetic appeal, and the stigma of wearing a bulky device. This eventually led to the overwhelming preference for air conduction devices.[68]

The concept of "bone-anchored" implants was first developed in Sweden in the 1960s when Dr. Per-Ingvar Branemark, an orthopedic surgeon, serendipitously discovered the biological fusion of metal to living bone while investigating bone marrow microcirculation through titanium optical chambers inserted in rabbit tibias. He described the process of osseointegration and found its application in the development of dental restorative implants.[69,70] Seeking to objectively evaluate osseointegration using acoustic parameters, he, along with Dr. Anders Tjellstrom and other otolaryngologists, designed a bone vibrator coupled to a maxillary dental implant. This assembly was then connected to an audiometer. Although the study yielded little information regarding osseointegration, the patient involved noticed very clear and loud sound transmission. This unexpected finding led to further interest in the development of bone-anchored hearing devices.[68] The first three patients were implanted in 1977, and results for the initial 13 recipients were published in 1981.[2] The average gain for early devices was 15 dB, patients were uniformly satisfied, and there were no instances of implant loss at 5 years postimplantation.

32.7 Concept of Osseointegration

Osseointegration is defined as a direct functional connection between living bone and a load-carrying implant without an intervening fibrous capsule and without relative movement.[71] Titanium has long been established as a transition metal uniquely suited for integration with living bone. Pure titanium forms a thin oxide layer when in contact with secreted cellular enzymes and superoxides, which in turn act as a matrix for the implant-to-tissue interaction. Other metals and alloys have failed to fully replicate this seemingly unique property.[72]

Load-bearing capacity is determined by the integrity of the connection between an implant and living bone and is a function of its primary stability and subsequent osseointegration. Primary stability refers to the baseline stability at implant placement, whereas osseointegration is the development of structural and functional contacts between bone and implant.[73] Primary stability is a function of the implant shape, diameter, and degree of insertion and thickness of the recipient bone bed.[74] Osseointegration is influenced by the biological quality of the bone,[75] and therefore factors such as patient age, osteoporosis, diabetes,[76] and prior radiation therapy[77] may have a detrimental effect on bone fixation. Peri-implant healing begins

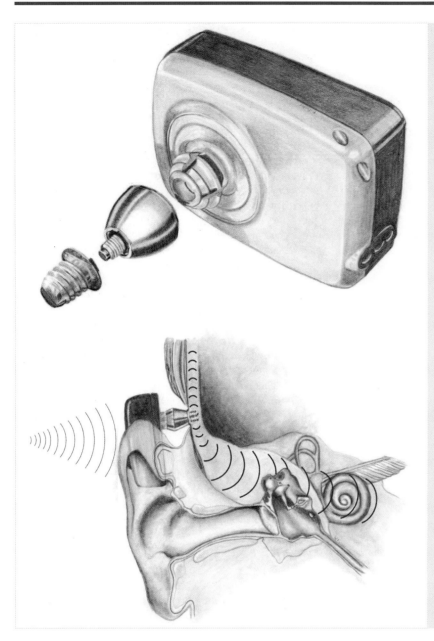

Fig. 32.11 (a) Baha 3 System: implant fixture, abutment, and sound processor. (b) Sound processor attached to implanted component.

with an early inflammatory response, followed by the formation of an afibrillar calcium layer.[78]

Within 24 hours following implantation, osteogenic cells make contact at the implant surface and begin producing fibrous osteoid, and then reparative woven bone. Osteogenesis proceeds from the host bone to the implant surface as well as from the implant surface to the host bone—a process termed "contact osteogenesis."[71] Trabecular bone is gradually substituted by mature lamellar bone during the final stage of osseointegration. Implant stability increases steeply during the first 2 weeks, and then tends to plateau and stabilize after the third week.[79] Although implant manufacturers continue to reinforce a long waiting period prior to loading the implant with the sound processor, it is not uncommon for adult patients to receive their sound processor at 4 to 6 weeks postimplantation.

32.8 Bone Conduction Implantable Hearing Devices

32.8.1 Percutaneous Implantable Systems

Baha 3 System

The Bone Anchored Hearing Aid (BAHA) system (Cochlear Bone Anchored Solutions, Gothenburg, Sweden) became commercially available in Europe in 1984[80] following the work of investigators in Sweden in the development of the implant and the technique for placement. The Baha System later received approval from the FDA in 1995 for conductive and mixed hearing losses. The device was approved for use in children 5 years of age and older in 1999, was then approved for bilateral fittings in 2001, and subsequently received approval for SSD in 2002. Since its inception, both the implant and audio processors have undergone several upgrades and changes.

The Baha system consists of a percutaneous, osseointegrated titanium implant and an abutment that couples to an externally worn sound processor (▶ Fig. 32.11). The most current generation of the implantable component, the Baha BI300, has a wider diameter (4.75 mm, versus 3.75 mm for the previous generation), a modified thread pattern, and a rough titanium oxide blasted (TiOblast) surface. This new design has been shown to provide improved stability over the prior design,[73,79,81] although advantages in the rate of osseointegration were not found. The redesigned, flask-shaped abutment (BA300) assumes a more narrow angle interface with the skin, therefore improving skin stability and reducing the incidence of skin reaction complications.[79] The Baha BI300 implantable fixture is available in 3- and 4-mm lengths and the BA300 abutment is available in 6- and 9-mm lengths. A hydroxyapatite coated abutment (Dermalock System) has recently been made available in 6, 8, 10, and 12 mm lengths.

There are three Baha 3 processors available that feature different power outputs and signal processing. Audiometric fitting is based primarily on bone conduction PTA in cases of mixed hearing loss, and this determines the processor selection for the system.

The BP100, which replaces its predecessor, the Baha Divino, is a digitally programmable sound processor that is worn behind the ear and provides adequate gain for patients with normal to mild loss on bone conduction threshold testing (less than 35 dB HL for the Divino and 45 dB HL for the BP100, respectively) in an ipsilateral ear with a conductive hearing loss. The BP100, released in 2009, features fully digital signal processing, automatic directional microphones, improved noise reduction capabilities, and a 12-channel analyzer.[82,83] For patients with bone conduction thresholds up to 55 dB HL, the Baha BP110 (which replaces the Baha Intenso) provides the most gain and highest output of the ear-worn sound processors.[84] The Baha Cordelle is a body-worn processor that is an appropriate choice for patients with bone conduction PTA thresholds up to 65 dB HL. When the mean bilateral bone conduction PTA threshold is higher than 65 dB HL, cochlear implant candidacy should be considered for hearing rehabilitation.[85] The SSD criteria include a profound SNHL in the implanted ear and air conduction (AC) PTA ≤ 20 dB HL (0.5, 1, 2, 3 kHz) in the contralateral ear.

Accessories available for the Baha System include a connector link for MP3 players and Bluetooth adapters, an FM receiver, and telecoil. The sound processor is manufactured with a Gore-Tex membrane cover over the microphone to reduce the potential for moisture penetration. The device is also available in a soft band version for children younger than 5 years of age. The company has recently released the Baha 4 Processor that will serve as an upgrade for the BP100 and Divino processors. The new processor accessories include wireless television streaming, built-in blue tooth capability, and a wireless remote microphone.

Although there is, typically, little concern for displacement of a titanium fixture when exposed to an MRI scanner, there is a 0.5% impurity of iron in the composition of the titanium metal.

An MRI compatibility study, using an earlier version of the BA-HA System fixture with attached abutment, showed no evidence of movement of the implant when placed flat onto its abutment top surface in a 9.4-T MRI scanner.[86] The degree of image distortion and artifact is typically minimal and limited to within 1 cm of the implant site with exposures to either a 1.5- or 3.0-T magnet.

Ponto Bone-Anchored Hearing System

The Ponto System (Oticon Medical, Askim, Sweden) was approved by the FDA in 2009 for conductive and mixed hearing loss, SSD, and bilateral fitting in patients 5 years of age and older. The Ponto and Ponto Pro sound processors are suitable for mixed losses with bone conduction PTA thresholds up to 40 dB HL. The new Ponto Pro Power sound processor (FDA approved in 2011) can provide benefit for patients with bone conduction (BC) PTA losses up to 50 dB HL. The implantable component consists of a 4.5-mm width, 3- or 4-mm length titanium fixture with an attached 6-mm abutment. Abutment lengths of 9 and 12 mm are also available. The company has recently introduced an angled (10-degree) abutment to accommodate situations where the sound processor may come in contact with an edge of the intact scalp.

The Ponto sound processors have a 10-channel frequency response shaping capability of 125 to 8,000 Hz and are digitally programmable. Additional features include an automatic adaptive directional microphone (Ponto Pro and Ponto Pro Power), noise management, wind noise reduction, and dynamic feedback cancellation. Data logging and a learning volume control are available on the Ponto Pro and Ponto Pro Power processors. The company has also recently introduced software to enable in-situ bone conduction audiometry for fitting and feedback management. The Ponto System accessories include an adapter for personal listening devices and FM receiver and telecoil adapters. The device is also available in a soft band version for infants and young children.

32.9 Transcutaneous Implantable System

32.9.1 Alpha 1 System

The Alpha 1 transcutaneous osseointegrated bone conduction hearing device (Sophono, Inc., Boulder, CO) received FDA approval in 2011 for conductive and mixed hearing losses and for SSD. The device had received the CE mark in Europe in 2010 and was acquired from Otomag GMbH (Rödinghausen, Germany) by Sophono, Inc. that same year. The age indications and the SSD criteria are the same as for the percutaneous systems. The current sound processor is suitable for mixed hearing loss with BC PTA thresholds up to 45 dB HL. The company plans to introduce a power option sound processor for BC PTA thresholds up to 55 dB HL and a body worn system for BC PTA thresholds up to 65 dB HL. The digitally programmable sound processor operates with 8 channels at 16 frequency bands with a range of 280 to 5,400 Hz. Maximum gain is 38 dB at 1,600 Hz with a peak output of 115 dB at 1,000 Hz. Processor features include customizable program switching, automatic noise reduction,

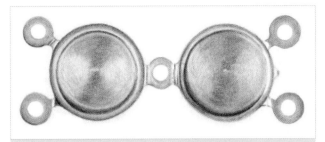

Fig. 32.12 Alpha 1 implantable component.

and feedback suppression. Accessories available include adapters for FM receiver, telecoil, and personal listening devices. The processor connects to a set of external magnets encased in an acrylic polymer. The processor and external magnet assembly is coupled magnetically to a set of magnets implanted beneath the scalp. The implantable component consists of two titanium encased magnets integrated into a single assembly (▶ Fig. 32.12). The device has recently received FDA approval for 1.5 and 3.0 Tesla MRI exposures.

32.10 Clinical Indications and Outcomes

32.10.1 Chronic Ear Disease

Patients with conductive or mixed hearing loss due to chronic ear disease who have otherwise failed, are poor candidates for, or are unwilling to undergo corrective procedures may be candidates for a BCIHD. Furthermore, patients who do not tolerate or receive inadequate benefit from conventional hearing amplification may also benefit from a bone conduction implantable device. The latter group includes patients with chronic otorrhea, keratosis obturans, and those who have undergone canal-wall-down procedures and have developed chronic otitis externa from a draining mastoid cavity. Patients with chronic ear disease composed the majority of subjects in a multicenter retrospective study that showed an average functional gain of 33 dB following implantation.[87] A direct audiometric comparison between conventional hearing aids and BCIHDs in patients with either chronic otorrhea or pain from ear mold occlusion demonstrated a significant signal-to-noise audiometric advantage after implantation in those with an air–bone gap of greater than 25 to 30 dB HL.[88] This may be explained by the need for increased power with conventional amplification at this level, which is inherently limited by feedback and saturation. Patients with lower conductive losses tended to benefit at least as well with conventional amplification as with a bone conduction hearing device. Nevertheless, the majority of patients reported a significant reduction in the number of episodes of otorrhea following implantation.

32.10.2 Congenital Aural Atresia

Options for hearing rehabilitation in patients with congenital aural atresia include surgical correction (atresiaplasty), use of a conventional bone conduction hearing aid, or placement of a BCIHD. Candidacy for atresiaplasty is traditionally determined using the Jahrsdoerfer computed tomography (CT) scoring guidelines. Scores less than 7 suggest a guarded optimism for success. This procedure is technically challenging, complications involving the neo-external auditory canal are relatively common, and long-term hearing benefits are inconsistent. Significant complications such as facial nerve injury and SNHL, however, are rare. Furthermore, the best hearing outcomes reported in terms of residual air–bone gap is between 25 and 35 dB HL in 60 to 75% of patients.[89,90] Current evidence supports a significant audiological advantage, shorter operative time, lower overall complication rate, and lower cost of BCIHDs over atresiaplasty surgery. Some consider it a superior option in patients with complete atresia or a Jahrsdoerfer score less than 5.[91,92] Despite the known binaural benefit of the head shadow effect when hearing in noise, studies have shown that sound localization skills in individuals with congenital conductive hearing loss do not improve consistently in those who have received a BCIHD as compared to patients with acquired unilateral conductive losses.[93,94]

Atresiaplasty continues to be an attractive option for patients with partial atresia and those with Jahrsdoerfer CT scores of at least 8. Experienced atresiaplasty surgeons may suggest that a superior cosmetic outcome is possible in optimal candidates when paired with microtia reconstruction and that further improvements in hearing are still possible with conventional amplification postoperatively.[95]

32.10.3 Bilateral Conductive Hearing Loss

Patients with bilateral conductive hearing loss, particularly those with complete canal atresia, may benefit from a single bone conduction implant, as transmitted sounds will reach both cochleas. However, studies have shown that interaural attenuation for bone-conducted sound is highly variable among individuals, potentially as high as 20 dB in the higher frequencies.[96,97] This finding, in addition to the potential benefit of having one functioning device in the case of a complication or malfunction in a contralateral device, supports the use of bilateral implantation. As compared with unilateral implantation, the use of bilateral implants has been shown to improve speech perception in quiet environments, sound localization, overall sound quality, and lifestyle subjective measures.[98] The advantage of the head shadow effect in binaural hearing may be less of a benefit in patients with bilateral bone conduction hearing devices because sound pressure energy will transmit, with little attenuation, to both cochleas from a single side. Therefore, some patients can experience difficulty hearing in noise and localizing sound in a complex listening environment.

Candidacy for bilateral implantation is determined by the audiometric criteria established by the individual manufacturer. For the Baha 3 System, the criteria include symmetric BC thresholds with less than 10 dB HL PTA difference across the frequency range of 0.5 to 3 kHz, or less than 15 dB HL difference at individual frequencies. The criteria established for the Ponto Bone Anchored Hearing System is the same except that BC PTA calculations are made using thresholds at 4 kHz versus 3 kHz.

32.10.4 Single-Sided Deafness

Single-sided deafness, which entails unilateral acquired sensorineural hearing loss, is associated with a number of clinicopathological conditions including vestibular schwannoma and other cerebellopontine angle tumors, idiopathic sudden SNHL, Ménière disease, and autoimmune inner ear disease. Surgical resection of temporal bone or lateral skull base lesions may result in ipsilateral profound deafness. The outcome of the specific disease process and the untoward effect of medical or surgical treatment can lead to a significant degree of hearing handicap. If contralateral hearing is intact, traditional rehabilitation efforts for these patients included contralateral routing of sound (CROS) amplification or the use of bilateral contralateral routing of sound (BiCROS). For BiCROS, the better ear receives amplified input from bilateral sources to compensate for an ipsilateral deficit. Although beneficial when sound is presented to the impaired site, CROS outcome studies uniformly report a relative hearing impairment on the better ear due to the occlusion effect of the ear mold and limited hearing in noise benefit.[99]

The benefit of a BCIHD over CROS amplification in SSD has been demonstrated in several studies in which speech perception in quiet and noise has been measured and subjective benefits ascertained.[100–102] As in patients with unilateral conductive losses, bone conduction implants do not appear to provide a significant benefit in terms of sound localization.[103] The audiometric criteria established for SSD is uniform among the three implant manufacturers and include profound SNHL (> 90 dB HL PTA) in the affected ear and normal hearing in the contralateral ear (< 20 dB HL AC PTA). Recent reports suggest that the audiometric criteria guiding the use of a bone conduction implantable device in SSD be expanded to include patients with contralateral mild to moderate SNHL and patients with less than profound loss, including those with moderate to profound losses who have not received benefit from conventional amplification.[101,102]

32.11 Surgical Procedure

The surgical technique for placement of the percutaneous BCIHD (e.g., Baha and Ponto Systems) was initially described in 1985 as a two-stage procedure in which the implant was secured to the temporal bone with overlying scalp tissue closure in the first stage.[8,1] A second-stage procedure was conducted 3 months later in which the abutment was placed and skin thinning took place. The rationale was to enhance osseointegration while minimizing the possibility of early accidental traumatic loss of the implant. Since then, several modifications to the procedure have resulted in a variety of options regarding skin flap design, staging of the procedure, and postoperative processor loading time. A comparison of single- versus two-stage implantation in adults found no statistically significant difference in the rate of implant failure or loss between the two techniques.[104] Single-stage implantation is currently recommended for most adults. In adults, the procedure can be safely performed under local anesthesia, depending on surgeon preference, patient characteristics, and surgical center factors.

The implant site is located behind the auricle, typically at a distance of 50 to 55 mm from the external auditory canal, and

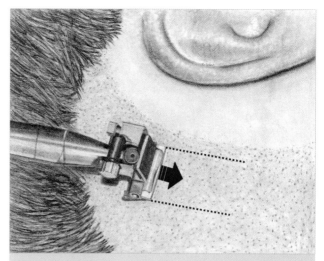

Fig. 32.13 Dermatome technique.

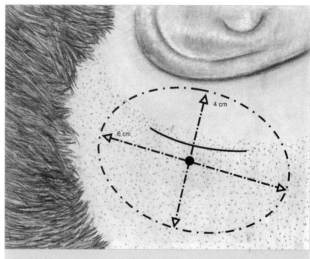

Fig. 32.14 Linear incision technique.

in a radius superior to the lateral sinus curve. The planned incision can be measured and marked after infiltration of local anesthetic and the hair removal in the immediate surrounding area. A dummy external processor aids with location and incision planning.

Various methods for managing the skin have been described for this procedure.[81,105–109] Until recently, the most popular method for managing the skin initially was to raise a rectangular, inferiorly or anteriorly based flap with a dermatome (▶ Fig. 32.13).

The subcutaneous tissue is then removed and the surrounding intact skin is undermined at a distance of 2 cm from the rectangular defect. Alternatively, a vertical linear or curvilinear incision (4 to 5 cm in length) just behind the postauricular hairline can be performed over the planned implant site with subsequent undermining and thinning of the surrounding skin (▶ Fig. 32.14).[110]

A shorter 1.5-cm horizontal incision technique has also been described.[111] The linear incision technique appears to be associated with fewer major skin and implant complications compared to the free graft and pedicled skin techniques.[112] Regardless of which incision type is used, the overlying objective in soft tissue preparation is to prevent overgrowth of hair and skin during wound healing and beyond. An area of subcutaneous tissue of at least 25 mm should be undermined and resected, taking care to eliminate all hair follicles from the underside of the skin.[106]

Following soft tissue preparation, the periosteum is incised and bluntly elevated. Drilling of the bone is performed perpendicular to the bone surface and to an initial depth of 3 mm. Copious irrigation is used to prevent overheating, as excessive heat and trauma is known to induce osteocyte death, which may potentially compromise osseointegration.[113] If the underlying bone is of adequate thickness after the initial depth, the well may be deepened to 4 mm. The bony well is then widened to 4.5 mm using a countersink drill bit to the appropriate depth (3 or 4 mm). The implant fixture is then carefully drilled at low speeds (15 rpm) and torque (10 to 50 N-cm). The torque settings are governed primarily by whether the procedure is performed in a child or an adult (higher torque settings of 45 to 50 N-cm in an adult). In the single-stage technique in which a skin flap has been developed, a skin punch is used to create a hole in the flap through which the abutment is exteriorized. If a linear incision technique is used, the implant is exteriorized either through the incision itself or through a separate opening in the intact scalp. The skin edges of the thinned, undermined area are approximated and secured directly to the underlying periosteum. A healing cap is placed on top of the abutment and a pressure dressing with antibiotic gauze provides light compression to prevent hematoma formation. A mastoid type dressing is then placed for 24 hours.

The surgical procedure for placing the transcutaneous BCIHD (i.e., Alpha 1) starts with a curvilinear incision approximately 7 cm posterosuperior to the external auditory canal meatus at an angle of 45 degrees in the sagittal plane. The position of the implant will be located 6 cm from the meatus. After elevation of an anteriorly based subperiosteal flap, a template is used to mark the proposed location of the twin magnets. Two recess wells are drilled to a depth of 2.6 mm using standard cutting and coarse diamond drill bits, and the magnets are seated. Shallow 0.5-mm wells are created to accommodate the anchoring brackets flush to the bone, and the implant is secured to the skull with low-profile 4-mm titanium screws. Preferably, the skin thickness overlying the magnet should be 4 to 5 mm to allow for optimal magnetic coupling and transmission of sound. Thicker flaps may be thinned as necessary.[114] The skin is then closed in layers. Most patients can be successfully fitted with the processor 3 to 4 weeks postimplantation.

32.11.1 Surgical Considerations for Pediatric Patients

The fact that bone composition in children is relatively softer (lower mineral-to-water ratio) and thinner than in adults, recommendations for the use of a BCIHD is restricted to children of at least 5 years of age. In general, a minimum thickness of 2.5 mm is recommended for implantation of a 3-mm-long fixture.[115] Stimulation of bony tissue expansion under a semipermeable membrane at the implant site has been described

for patients lacking adequate temporal bone thickness.[116] Implantation has been successfully accomplished in children as young as 3 years of age.[73,117] A European consensus statement on the use of these devices recommends that the procedure be performed in two stages in children, followed by processor loading 3 to 6 months after implantation.[118] Failure of implant osseointegration in children has been reported to be as high as 15% in a large retrospective series.[119] A two-stage procedure would protect the implant from accidental trauma during the critical period of osseointegration and reduces the potential for wound complications and lengthy aftercare. Placement of an ipsilateral "sleeper" fixture during the original procedure has been advocated for children under 10 years of age in order to account for the potential failure of the primary fixture.[120]

Single-stage implantation has been successfully attempted in selected pediatric patients,[121] and the viability of processor loading as early as 3 weeks has also been supported by studies involving pediatric patients with the redesigned Baha implant (BI300). Implant stability has been shown to increase steeply over the first 2 weeks postoperatively in both children and adults and then to plateau over a period of up to 6 months.[73,79] Further clinical studies are needed to support these findings. Manufacturer recommendations continue to support implant loading at 3 months for adults and at least 4 months for children, despite what may occur in clinical practice.

32.11.2 Complications

Complications arising from the implantation of a BCIHD are primarily related to the inherent foreign body inflammatory reaction involving the immediate adjacent skin.[122] These reactions can be further classified as local inflammation, infection, or skin and soft tissue overgrowth. Overall skin reaction rates have been reported between 7.5 and 30%,[87,123–125] although improvements in surgical technique and equipment over the past three decades may have lowered this rate 7.5 to 10%.[125] A classification system, devised by Holgers et al[123] and later modified by Wazen et al,[125] grades soft tissue reactions in an attempt to standardize reporting. Soft tissue reactions resulting in skin overgrowth of the abutment (i.e., grade 3 or above) are infrequent and have been reported to occur in 2% or less of all postoperative skin complications.[112,123] Skin reactions can be addressed with local wound care, typically in the form of topical antibiotic ointments, steroid containing creams, and frequent gentle cleansing around the abutment. Granulation tissue may be cauterized with silver nitrate. More severe reactions may necessitate systemic antibiotics and debridement of devitalized tissues.

Growth of skin over the abutment tends to be a late complication, occurring, on average, 12 months postimplantation, although it has been noted to occur as early as 3 months.[126] Chronic local inflammation and partial skin flap loss appear to precede this phenomenon. Prevention of skin overgrowth requires a meticulous surgical technique that includes removal of all subcutaneous tissues at the implant site immediately above the periosteum. Excessive skin flap mobility over remnant soft tissues may contribute to chronic inflammation. Patients should also be encouraged to wear the processor as often as possible and may wear an abutment cap when the processor is removed.

Once local inflammation occurs, prompt and aggressive treatment is recommended to prevent further sequelae. Clobetasol gel has been shown to effectively treat mild cases of skin overgrowth.[127] In-office excision of excess skin and placement of a longer 9-mm abutment should also be considered. Patients who do not respond to conservative measures should undergo operative skin flap revision. Revision surgery for skin overgrowth includes complete circumferential removal of skin and soft tissue in the immediate area of the abutment, application of a steroid cream, and placement of a Xeroform petrolatum gauze dressing and healing cap. For extensive skin regrowth and associated areas of necrosis, a wider radius of skin resection is recommended followed by replacement with a split-thickness skin graft.[128]

Failure of osseointegration with eventual loss of the implant is a rare but troublesome complication. Reports of implant failure rates range from 1 to 5%.[125,126,129,130] Children tend to have a higher rate of failure, ranging from 10 to 26%, with rates as high as 40% having been reported in children younger than 5 years of age.[119,120,131–133] Higher failure rates in children may be attributed to the thinner, softer composition of bone and limitations on the length of fixture that can be placed. This may predispose to incomplete insertion and potential instability. Bone thickness and implant length are key factors that determine an implant's primary stability.[73] Additionally, the increased propensity for accidental trauma in this population may contribute to the higher rate of failure.[120] Patients with medical conditions that may influence wound healing such as chronic local infection, poorly controlled diabetics, and chronic steroid use, and those who have previously received radiation therapy to the area, are also at a relatively increased risk for implant failure.[91,126,130] The cause of failure should be addressed and the underlying predisposing condition(s) (e.g., infection) should be treated prior to revision surgery. Intuitively, failures due to trauma and improper insertion appear more amenable to revision than those due to infection or poor wound healing.[128]

The potential for intracranial complications is quite low but must be included during the preoperative discussion with the patient. The risk of injury to the dura or sigmoid sinus may be greater in cases where the available temporal bone is thinner. In a series of adult patients, 8.5% of fixtures were noted to be in contact with dura during placement.[134] In a separate review of pediatric patients, 21% of fixtures were placed against exposed dura.[135] Bleeding from a dural sinus can be controlled with bone wax or plugging with muscle or fascia, and then an adjacent site is located for insertion of the implant.[131] Other intracranial complications reported as single-case reviews include the delayed development of an intracerebral abscess following an unsuccessful abutment change,[136] and the formation of an epidural hematoma at the implant site.[137]

32.12 Alternative Bone Conduction Hearing System

32.12.1 SoundBite System

The SoundBite Hearing System (Sonitus Medical, San Mateo, CA) is a bone conduction hearing device that utilizes direct bone conduction from the teeth to the cranium. This device does not require a surgical procedure for placement. It consists of an external microphone located in the ear canal that is connected to a BTE digital signal processor. This component transmits a wireless signal to a piezoelectric actuator embedded in a removable oral appliance seated against the distal maxillary dentition on the side of the poorer hearing ear. Dental evaluation of oral health, X-rays, and a dental impression are completed prior to fashioning a custom-fit oral appliance. The manufacturer guidelines stipulate that at least two contiguous maxillary molar or premolar teeth be present and that there is no evidence of dental decay or alveolar bone loss $\geq 35\%$. A preliminary study in a small group of patients with SSD showed significant improvements in speech intelligibility, and although two of five subjects complained of uncomfortable vibrotactile sensation on the teeth for frequencies up to 500 Hz, none of the subjects experienced this sensation for frequencies from 2,000 to 12,000 Hz.[138] The results of hearing in noise testing (HINT) in a short-term follow-up study in 28 patients showed a statistically significant improvement in average HINT advantage scores.[139]

A long-term follow-up study in 22 patients with SSD demonstrated statistically significant improvements in subjective hearing benefit as measured by APHAB and found no significant dental side effects, even in patients with complex dental restorations.[140] Eight of 22 patients (36%), however, were dissatisfied with their ability to eat while wearing the appliance. The device received FDA approval for SSD in January 2011 and for CHL in September 2011 for patients 18 years of age and older. The fitting criteria established for this device includes a BC PTA ≤ 25 dB HL for both CHL and SSD indications. The sound processor has a wide frequency bandwidth of response from 250 to 12,000 Hz with a maximum gain of 40 dB at 1,600 Hz and a peak output of 90 dB SPL. Output may be limited to 85 dB SPL for frequencies of 250 to 500 Hz due to the potential for vibrotactile sensation. Battery life is limited to 4 to 6 hours for the oral appliance and 12 to 16 hours for the BTE processor. Therefore, the cost of the device is influenced by the need for two in-the-mouth transducers due to the short battery life.

32.13 Future Directions

Efforts to further improve the technology of implantable bone conduction devices and circumvent the need for a percutaneous post are proceeding. A new device currently being developed, the bone conduction implant (BCI), consists of an electromagnetic transducer that is attached to the mastoid process and connected to an implanted receiver coil that receives the converted auditory signal transcutaneously from an external sound processor.[141] A preliminary study in cadaveric whole-head specimens demonstrated higher power outputs measured at the ipsilateral promontory, but lower transcranial contralateral outputs than a traditional percutaneous bone conduction implant. Another device, currently in the investigational stage of development, uses a subcutaneously implanted piezoelectric transducer to collect signals from an external sound processor. High-efficiency transmission to the cochlea has been demonstrated in embalmed cadaver heads.[142] The Med-El Corporation is currently developing its version of a semi-implantable bone conduction device that consists of an implantable component that uses an electromagnetic transducer similar in design to that of the FMT in the Vibrant Soundbridge. It is reasonable to assume that clinical studies will determine the efficacy and marketability of these newer devices.

32.14 Disclaimer

The authors are employees of the United States Government. This work was prepared as part of our official duties. Title 17 U.S.C. 105 provides that "copyright protection under this title is not available for any work of the United States Government." Title 17 U.S.C. 101 defines United States Government work as work prepared by a military service member or employee of the United States Government as part of that person's official duties. The views expressed in this chapter are those of the authors and do not necessarily reflect the official policy or position of the Department of the Navy, Department of Defense, or the United States Government.

References

[1] Kochkin S. MarkeTrak VIII: consumer satisfaction with hearing aids is slowly increasing. Hear J. 2010; 63: 19–32

[2] Tjellström A, Lindström J, Hallén O, Albrektsson T, Brånemark PI. Osseointegrated titanium implants in the temporal bone. A clinical study on bone-anchored hearing aids. Am J Otol 1981; 2: 304–310

[3] Jenkins HA, Pergola N, Kasic J. Intraoperative ossicular loading with the Otologics fully implantable hearing device. Acta Otolaryngol 2007; 127: 360–364

[4] Javel E, Grant IL, Kroll K. In vivo characterization of piezoelectric transducers for implantable hearing AIDS. Otol Neurotol 2003; 24: 784–795

[5] Backous DD, Duke W. Implantable middle ear hearing devices: current state of technology and market challenges. In: Donald PJ, Gluckman JL, Pensak ML, Doyle KJ, eds. Curr Opin Otolaryngol-Head Neck Surg. Philadelphia: Lippincott Williams & Wilkins, 14:314–318

[6] Dietz T, Ball G, Katz B. Partially implantable vibrating ossicular prosthesis. In: Transducers '97: 1997 International Conference on Solid-State Sensors and Actuators, Chicago, pp. 433–436

[7] Fredrickson JM, Coticchia JM, Khosla S. Ongoing investigations into an implantable electromagnetic hearing aid for moderate to severe sensorineural hearing loss. Otolaryngol Clin North Am 1995; 28: 107–120

[8] Hough J, Vernon J, Himelick T, Meikel M, Richard G, Dormer K. A middle ear implantable hearing device for controlled amplification of sound in the human: a preliminary report. Laryngoscope 1987; 97: 141–151

[9] Kartush JM, Tos M. Electromagnetic ossicular augmentation device. Otolaryngol Clin North Am 1995; 28: 155–172

[10] Todt I, Seidl RO, Gross M, Ernst A. Comparison of different vibrant soundbridge audioprocessors with conventional hearing AIDS. Otol Neurotol 2002; 23: 669–673

[11] Uziel A, Mondain M, Hagen P, Dejean F, Doucet G. Rehabilitation for high-frequency sensorineural hearing impairment in adults with the Symphonix Vibrant Soundbridge: a comparative study. Otol Neurotol 2003; 24: 775–783

[12] Sterkers O, Boucarra D, Labassi S et al. A middle ear implant, the Symphonix Vibrant Soundbridge: retrospective study of the first 125 patients implanted in France. Otol Neurotol 2003; 24: 427–436

[13] Fraysse B, Lavieille JP, Schmerber S et al. A multicenter study of the Vibrant Soundbridge middle ear implant: early clinical results and experience. Otol Neurotol 2001; 22: 952–961

[14] Truy E, Philibert B, Vesson JF, Labassi S, Collet L. Vibrant soundbridge versus conventional hearing aid in sensorineural high-frequency hearing loss: a prospective study. Otol Neurotol 2008; 29: 684–687

[15] Boeheim K, Pok SM, Schloegel M, Filzmoser P. Active middle ear implant compared with open-fit hearing aid in sloping high-frequency sensorineural hearing loss. Otol Neurotol 2010; 31: 424–429

[16] Schmuziger N, Schimmann F, à Wengen D, Patscheke J, Probst R. Long-term assessment after implantation of the Vibrant Soundbridge device. Otol Neurotol 2006; 27: 183–188

[17] Verhaegen VJO, Mylanus EAM, Cremers CWRJ, Snik AFM. Audiological application criteria for implantable hearing aid devices: a clinical experience at the Nijmegen ORL clinic. Laryngoscope 2008; 118: 1645–1649

[18] Mosnier I, Sterkers O, Bouccara D et al. Benefit of the Vibrant Soundbridge device in patients implanted for 5 to 8 years. Ear Hear 2008; 29: 281–284

[19] Rameh C, Meller R, Lavieille JP, Deveze A, Magnan J. Long-term patient satisfaction with different middle ear hearing implants in sensorineural hearing loss. Otol Neurotol 2010; 31: 883–892

[20] Snik AFM, van Duijnhoven NTL, Mylanus EAM, Cremers CWRJ. Estimated cost-effectiveness of active middle-ear implantation in hearing-impaired patients with severe external otitis. Arch Otolaryngol Head Neck Surg 2006; 132: 1210–1215

[21] Bornitz M, Hardtke HJ, Zahnert T. Evaluation of implantable actuators by means of a middle ear simulation model. Hear Res 2010; 263: 145–151

[22] Huber AM, Ball GR, Veraguth D, Dillier N, Bodmer D, Sequeira D. A new implantable middle ear hearing device for mixed hearing loss: a feasibility study in human temporal bones. Otol Neurotol 2006; 27: 1104–1109

[23] Arnold A, Stieger C, Candreia C, Pfiffner F, Kompis M. Factors improving the vibration transfer of the floating mass transducer at the round window. Otol Neurotol 2010; 31: 122–128

[24] Pennings RJE, Ho A, Brown J, van Wijhe RG, Bance M. Analysis of Vibrant Soundbridge placement against the round window membrane in a human cadaveric temporal bone model. Otol Neurotol 2010; 31: 998–1003

[25] Colletti V, Soli SD, Carner M, Colletti L. Treatment of mixed hearing losses via implantation of a vibratory transducer on the round window. Int J Audiol 2006; 45: 600–608

[26] Hüttenbrink KB, Zahnert T, Bornitz M, Beutner D. TORP-vibroplasty: a new alternative for the chronically disabled middle ear. Otol Neurotol 2008; 29: 965–971

[27] Linder T, Schlegel C, DeMin N, van der Westhuizen S. Active middle ear implants in patients undergoing subtotal petrosectomy: new application for the Vibrant Soundbridge device and its implication for lateral cranium base surgery. Otol Neurotol 2009; 30: 41–47

[28] Dumon T, Gratacap B, Firmin F et al. Vibrant Soundbridge middle ear implant in mixed hearing loss. Indications, techniques, results. Rev Laryngol Otol Rhinol (Bord) 2009; 130: 75–81

[29] Beltrame AM, Martini A, Prosser S, Giarbini N, Streitberger C. Coupling the Vibrant Soundbridge to cochlea round window: auditory results in patients with mixed hearing loss. Otol Neurotol 2009; 30: 194–201

[30] Rajan GP, Lampacher P, Ambett R et al. Impact of floating mass transducer coupling and positioning in round window vibroplasty. Otol Neurotol 2011; 32: 271–277

[31] Colletti V, Mandalà M, Colletti L. Electrocochleography in round window Vibrant Soundbridge implantation. Otolaryngol Head Neck Surg 2012; 146: 633–640

[32] Verhaegen VJO, Mulder JJS, Cremers CWRJ, Snik AFM. Application of active middle ear implants in patients with severe mixed hearing loss. Otol Neurotol 2012; 33: 297–301

[33] Yu JKY, Tsang WSS, Wong TKC, Tong MCF. Outcome of vibrant soundbridge middle ear implant in cantonese-speaking mixed hearing loss adults. Clin Exp Otorhinolaryngol 2012; 5 Suppl 1: S82–S88

[34] Baumgartner WD, Böheim K, Hagen R et al. The vibrant soundbridge for conductive and mixed hearing losses: European multicenter study results. Adv Otorhinolaryngol 2010; 69: 38–50

[35] Böheim K, Mlynski R, Lenarz T, Schlögel M, Hagen R. Round window vibroplasty: long-term results. Acta Otolaryngol 2012; 132: 1042–1048[Epub ahead of print]

[36] Frenzel H, Hanke F, Beltrame M, Steffen A, Schönweiler R, Wollenberg B. Application of the Vibrant Soundbridge to unilateral osseous atresia cases. Laryngoscope 2009; 119: 67–74

[37] Colletti L, Carner M, Mandalà M, Veronese S, Colletti V. The floating mass transducer for external auditory canal and middle ear malformations. Otol Neurotol 2011; 32: 108–115

[38] Mandalà M, Colletti L, Colletti V. Treatment of the atretic ear with round window Vibrant Soundbridge implantation in infants and children: electrocochleography and audiologic outcomes. Otol Neurotol 2011; 32: 1250–1255

[39] Colletti V, Carner M, Colletti L. TORP vs round window implant for hearing restoration of patients with extensive ossicular chain defect. Acta Otolaryngol 2009; 129: 449–452

[40] Huber AM, Mlynski R, Müller J et al. A new vibroplasty coupling technique as a treatment for conductive and mixed hearing losses: a report of 4 cases. Otol Neurotol 2012; 33: 613–617

[41] Beleites T, Neudert M, Beutner D, Hüttenbrink KB, Zahnert T. Experience with vibroplasty couplers at the stapes head and footplate. Otol Neurotol 2011; 32: 1468–1472

[42] Hüttenbrink KB, Beutner D, Bornitz M, Luers JC, Zahnert T. Clip vibroplasty: experimental evaluation and first clinical results. Otol Neurotol 2011; 32: 650–653

[43] Hüttenbrink KB, Beutner D, Zahnert T. Clinical results with an active middle ear implant in the oval window. Adv Otorhinolaryngol 2010; 69: 27–31

[44] Zehlicke T, Dahl R, Just T, Pau HW. Vibroplasty involving direct coupling of the floating mass transducer to the oval window niche. J Laryngol Otol 2010; 124: 716–719

[45] Kontorinis G, Lenarz T, Mojallal H, Hinze AL, Schwab B. Power stapes: an alternative method for treating hearing loss in osteogenesis imperfecta? Otol Neurotol 2011; 32: 589–595

[46] Dumon T. Vibrant soundbridge middle ear implant in otosclerosis: technique –indication. Adv Otorhinolaryngol 2007; 65: 320–322

[47] Schwab B, Salcher RB, Maier H, Kontorinis G. Oval window membrane vibroplasty for direct acoustic cochlear stimulation: treating severe mixed hearing loss in challenging middle ears. Otol Neurotol 2012; 33: 804–809

[48] Shimizu Y, Puria S, Goode RL. The floating mass transducer on the round window versus attachment to an ossicular replacement prosthesis. Otol Neurotol 2011; 32: 98–103

[49] Jesacher MO, Kiefer J, Zierhofer C, Fauser C. Torque measurements of the ossicular chain: implication on the MRI safety of the hearing implant Vibrant Soundbridge. Otol Neurotol 2010; 31: 676–680

[50] Todt I, Rademacher G, Wagner F et al. Magnetic resonance imaging safety of the floating mass transducer. Otol Neurotol 2010; 31: 1435–1440

[51] Todt I, Seidl RO, Mutze S, Ernst A. MRI scanning and incus fixation in vibrant soundbridge implantation. Otol Neurotol 2004; 25: 969–972

[52] Todt I, Wagner J, Goetze R, Scholz S, Seidl R, Ernst A. MRI scanning in patients implanted with a Vibrant Soundbridge. Laryngoscope 2011; 121: 1532–1535

[53] Martin C, Deveze A, Richard C et al. European results with totally implantable carina placed on the round window: 2-year follow-up. Otol Neurotol 2009; 30: 1196–1203

[54] Siegert R, Mattheis S, Kasic J. Fully implantable hearing aids in patients with congenital auricular atresia. Laryngoscope 2007; 117: 336–340

[55] Tringali S, Pergola N, Berger P, Dubreuil C. Fully implantable hearing device with transducer on the round window as a treatment of mixed hearing loss. Auris Nasus Larynx 2009; 36: 353–358

[56] Lefebvre PP, Martin C, Dubreuil C et al. A pilot study of the safety and performance of the Otologics fully implantable hearing device: transducing sounds via the round window membrane to the inner ear. Audiol Neurootol 2009; 14: 172–180

[57] Venail F, Lavieille JP, Meller R, Deveze A, Tardivet L, Magnan J. New perspectives for middle ear implants: first results in otosclerosis with mixed hearing loss. Laryngoscope 2007; 117: 552–555

[58] Jenkins HA, Atkins JS, Horlbeck D et al. Otologics fully implantable hearing system: phase I trial 1-year results. Otol Neurotol 2008; 29: 534–541

[59] Hough JVD, Matthews P, Wood MW, Dyer RK, Jr. Middle ear electromagnetic semi-implantable hearing device: results of the phase II SOUNDTEC direct system clinical trial. Otol Neurotol 2002; 23: 895–903

[60] Silverstein H, Atkins J, Thompson JH, Jr, Gilman N. Experience with the SOUNDTEC implantable hearing aid. Otol Neurotol 2005; 26: 211–217

[61] Dyer RK, Jr, Nakmali D, Dormer KJ. Magnetic resonance imaging compatibility and safety of the SOUNDTEC Direct System. Laryngoscope 2006; 116: 1321–1333

[62] Dyer RK, Jr, Dormer KJ, Hough JVD, Nakmali U, Wickersham R. Biomechanical influences of magnetic resonance imaging on the SOUNDTEC Direct System implant. Otolaryngol Head Neck Surg 2002; 127: 520–530

[63] Chen DA, Backous DD, Arriaga MA et al. Phase 1 clinical trial results of the Envoy System: a totally implantable middle ear device for sensorineural hearing loss. Otolaryngol Head Neck Surg 2004; 131: 904–916

[64] Envoy Medical Corp 2009

[65] Kraus EM, Shohet JA, Catalano PJ. Envoy Esteem Totally Implantable Hearing System: phase 2 trial, 1-year hearing results. Otolaryngol Head Neck Surg 2011; 145: 100–109

[66] Shohet JA, Kraus EM, Catalano PJ. Profound high-frequency sensorineural hearing loss treatment with a totally implantable hearing system. Otol Neurotol 2011; 32: 1428–1431

[67] Häusler R, Stieger C, Bernhard H, Kompis M. A novel implantable hearing system with direct acoustic cochlear stimulation. Audiol Neurootol 2008; 13: 247–256

[68] Mudry A, Tjellström A. Historical background of bone conduction hearing devices and bone conduction hearing aids. Adv Otorhinolaryngol 2011; 71: 1–9

[69] Brånemark PI, Adell R, Breine U, Hansson BO, Lindström J, Ohlsson A. Intra-osseous anchorage of dental prostheses. I. Experimental studies. Scand J Plast Reconstr Surg 1969; 3: 81–100

[70] Brånemark PI, Hansson BO, Adell R et al. Osseointegrated implants in the treatment of the edentulous jaw. Experience from a 10-year period. Scand J Plast Reconstr Surg Suppl 1977; 16: 1–132

[71] Brånemark PI. Osseointegration and its experimental background. J Prosthet Dent 1983; 50: 399–410

[72] Bjursten LM, Emanuelsson L, Ericson LE et al. Method for ultrastructural studies of the intact tissue-metal interface. Biomaterials 1990; 11: 596–601

[73] Marsella P, Scorpecci A, D'Eredità R, Della Volpe A, Malerba P. Stability of osseointegrated bone conduction systems in children: a pilot study. Otol Neurotol 2012; 33: 797–803

[74] Ivanoff CJ, Gröndahl K, Sennerby L, Bergström C, Lekholm U. Influence of variations in implant diameters: a 3- to 5-year retrospective clinical report. Int J Oral Maxillofac Implants 1999; 14: 173–180

[75] Aparicio C, Lang NP, Rangert B. Validity and clinical significance of biomechanical testing of implant/bone interface. Clin Oral Implants Res 2006; 17 Suppl 2: 2–7

[76] Drinias V, Granström G, Tjellström A. High age at the time of implant installation is correlated with increased loss of osseointegrated implants in the temporal bone. Clin Implant Dent Relat Res 2007; 9: 94–99

[77] Granström G, Tjellström A, Brånemark PI, Fornander J. Bone-anchored reconstruction of the irradiated head and neck cancer patient. Otolaryngol Head Neck Surg 1993; 108: 334–343

[78] Marco F, Milena F, Gianluca G, Vittoria O. Peri-implant osteogenesis in health and osteoporosis. Micron 2005; 36: 630–644

[79] D'Eredità R, Caroncini M, Saetti R. The new Baha implant: a prospective osseointegration study. Otolaryngol Head Neck Surg 2012; 146: 979–983

[80] Håkansson B, Tjellström A, Rosenhall U, Carlsson P. The bone-anchored hearing aid. Principal design and a psychoacoustical evaluation. Acta Otolaryngol 1985; 100: 229–239

[81] Dun CA, de Wolf MJ, Hol MK et al. Stability, survival, and tolerability of a novel baha implant system: six-month data from a multicenter clinical investigation. Otol Neurotol 2011; 32: 1001–1007

[82] Dun CA, Faber HT, de Wolf MJ, Cremers CW, Hol MK. An overview of different systems: the bone-anchored hearing aid. Adv Otorhinolaryngol 2011; 71: 22–31

[83] Flynn MC. Challenges and recent developments in sound processing for Baha®. Adv Otorhinolaryngol 2011; 71: 112–123

[84] Bosman AJ, Snik FM, Mylanus EA, Cremers WR. Fitting range of the BAHA Intenso. Int J Audiol 2009; 48: 346–352

[85] Verhaegen VJ, Mulder JJ, Mylanus EA, Cremers CW, Snik AF. Profound mixed hearing loss: bone-anchored hearing aid system or cochlear implant? Ann Otol Rhinol Laryngol 2009; 118: 693–697

[86] Fritsch MH, Naumann IC, Mosier KM. BAHA devices and magnetic resonance imaging scanners. Otol Neurotol 2008; 29: 1095–1099

[87] Lustig LR, Arts HA, Brackmann DE et al. Hearing rehabilitation using the BAHA bone-anchored hearing aid: results in 40 patients. Otol Neurotol 2001; 22: 328–334

[88] Mylanus EA, van der Pouw KC, Snik AF, Cremers CW. Intraindividual comparison of the bone-anchored hearing aid and air-conduction hearing aids. Arch Otolaryngol Head Neck Surg 1998; 124: 271–276

[89] Yeakley JW, Jahrsdoerfer RA. CT evaluation of congenital aural atresia: what the radiologist and surgeon need to know. J Comput Assist Tomogr 1996; 20: 724–731

[90] Teufert KB, De la Cruz A. Advances in congenital aural atresia surgery: effects on outcome. Otolaryngol Head Neck Surg 2004; 131: 263–270

[91] Granström G, Tjellström A. The bone-anchored hearing aid (BAHA) in children with auricular malformations. Ear Nose Throat J 1997; 76: 238–240, 242, 244–247

[92] Bouhabel S, Arcand P, Saliba I. Congenital aural atresia: bone-anchored hearing aid vs. external auditory canal reconstruction. Int J Pediatr Otorhinolaryngol 2012; 76: 272–277

[93] Hol MK, Bosman AJ, Snik AF, Mylanus EA, Cremers CW. Bone-anchored hearing aids in unilateral inner ear deafness: an evaluation of audiometric and patient outcome measurements. Otol Neurotol 2005; 26: 999–1006

[94] Kunst SJ, Leijendeckers JM, Mylanus EA, Hol MK, Snik AF, Cremers CW. Bone-anchored hearing aid system application for unilateral congenital conductive hearing impairment: audiometric results. Otol Neurotol 2008; 29: 2–7

[95] Yellon RF. Atresiaplasty versus BAHA for congenital aural atresia. Laryngoscope 2011; 121: 2–3

[96] Kaga K, Setou M, Nakamura M. Bone-conducted sound lateralization of interaural time difference and interaural intensity difference in children and a young adult with bilateral microtia and atresia of the ears. Acta Otolaryngol 2001; 121: 274–277

[97] Setou M, Kurauchi T, Tsuzuku T, Kaga K. Binaural interaction of bone-conducted auditory brainstem responses. Acta Otolaryngol 2001; 121: 486–489

[98] Janssen RM, Hong P, Chadha NK. Bilateral bone-anchored hearing aids for bilateral permanent conductive hearing loss: a systematic review. Otolaryngol Head Neck Surg 2012; 147: 412–422

[99] Kenworthy OT, Klee T, Tharpe AM. Speech recognition ability of children with unilateral sensorineural hearing loss as a function of amplification, speech stimuli and listening condition. Ear Hear 1990; 11: 264–270

[100] Baguley DM, Bird J, Humphriss RL, Prevost AT. The evidence base for the application of contralateral bone anchored hearing aids in acquired unilateral sensorineural hearing loss in adults. Clin Otolaryngol 2006; 31: 6–14

[101] Zeitler DM, Snapp HA, Telischi FF, Angeli SI. Bone-anchored implantation for single-sided deafness in patients with less than profound hearing loss. Otolaryngol Head Neck Surg 2012; 147: 105–111

[102] Wazen JJ, Van Ess MJ, Alameda J, Ortega C, Modisett M, Pinsky K. The Baha system in patients with single-sided deafness and contralateral hearing loss. Otolaryngol Head Neck Surg 2010; 142: 554–559

[103] Lin LM, Bowditch S, Anderson MJ, May B, Cox KM, Niparko JK. Amplification in the rehabilitation of unilateral deafness: speech in noise and directional hearing effects with bone-anchored hearing and contralateral routing of signal amplification. Otol Neurotol 2006; 27: 172–182

[104] Tjellström A, Håkansson B. The bone-anchored hearing aid. Design principles, indications, and long-term clinical results. Otolaryngol Clin North Am 1995; 28: 53–72

[105] de Wolf MJ, Hol MK, Huygen PL, Mylanus EA, Cremers CW. Clinical outcome of the simplified surgical technique for BAHA implantation. Otol Neurotol 2008; 29: 1100–1108

[106] Mudry A. Bone-anchored hearing aids (BAHA): skin healing process for skin flap technique versus linear incision technique in the first three months after the implantation. Rev Laryngol Otol Rhinol (Bord) 2009; 130: 281–284

[107] Wilkinson EP, Luxford WM, Slattery WH, III, De la Cruz A, House JW, Fayad JN. Single vertical incision for Baha implant surgery: preliminary results. Otolaryngol Head Neck Surg 2009; 140: 573–578

[108] Van Rompaey V, Claes G, Verstraeten N et al. Skin reactions following BAHA surgery using the skin flap dermatome technique. Eur Arch Otorhinolaryngol 2011; 268: 373–376

[109] Mylanus EA, Cremers CW. A one-stage surgical procedure for placement of percutaneous implants for the bone-anchored hearing aid. J Laryngol Otol 1994; 108: 1031–1035

[110] Bovo R. Simplified technique without skin flap for the bone-anchored hearing aid (BAHA) implant. Acta Otorhinolaryngol Ital 2008; 28: 252–255

[111] Gudis DA, Ruckenstein MJ. Baha surgery: evolution, techniques, and complications. In: Ruckenstein MJ, ed. Cochlear Implants and Other Implantable Hearing Devices. San Diego: Plural Publishing, 2012:375–387

[112] van de Berg R, Stokroos RJ, Hof JR, Chenault MN. Bone-anchored hearing aid: a comparison of surgical techniques. Otol Neurotol 2010; 31: 129–135

[113] Arnold A, Caversaccio MD, Mudry A. Surgery for the bone-anchored hearing aid. Adv Otorhinolaryngol 2011; 71: 47–55

[114] Siegert R. Partially implantable bone conduction hearing aids without a percutaneous abutment (Otomag): technique and preliminary clinical results. Adv Otorhinolaryngol 2011; 71: 41–46

[115] Tjellström A, Håkansson B, Granström G. Bone-anchored hearing aids: current status in adults and children. Otolaryngol Clin North Am 2001; 34: 337–364

[116] Granström G, Tjellström A. Guided tissue generation in the temporal bone. Ann Otol Rhinol Laryngol 1999; 108: 349–354

[117] Kohan D, Morris LG, Romo T, III. Single-stage BAHA implantation in adults and children: is it safe? Otolaryngol Head Neck Surg 2008; 138: 662–666

[118] Snik AF, Mylanus EA, Proops DW et al. Consensus statements on the BAHA system: where do we stand at present? Ann Otol Rhinol Laryngol Suppl 2005; 195: 2–12

[119] McDermott AL, Williams J, Kuo M, Reid A, Proops D. Quality of life in children fitted with a bone-anchored hearing aid. Otol Neurotol 2009; 30: 344–349

[120] McDermott AL, Sheehan P. Bone anchored hearing aids in children. Curr Opin Otolaryngol Head Neck Surg 2009; 17: 488–493

[121] Roman S, Nicollas R, Triglia JM. Practice guidelines for bone-anchored hearing aids in children. Eur Ann Otorhinolaryngol Head Neck Dis 2011; 128: 253–258

[122] Holgers KM, Thomsen P, Tjellström A, Bjursten LM. Immunohistochemical study of the soft tissue around long-term skin-penetrating titanium implants. Biomaterials 1995; 16: 611–616

[123] Holgers KM, Tjellström A, Bjursten LM, Erlandsson BE. Soft tissue reactions around percutaneous implants: a clinical study of soft tissue conditions around skin-penetrating titanium implants for bone-anchored hearing aids. Am J Otol 1988; 9: 56–59

[124] Håkansson B, Lidén G, Tjellström A et al. Ten years of experience with the Swedish bone-anchored hearing system. Ann Otol Rhinol Laryngol Suppl 1990; 151: 1–16

[125] Wazen JJ, Young DL, Farrugia MC et al. Successes and complications of the Baha system. Otol Neurotol 2008; 29: 1115–1119

[126] House JW, Kutz JW, Jr. Bone-anchored hearing aids: incidence and management of postoperative complications. Otol Neurotol 2007; 28: 213–217

[127] Falcone MT, Kaylie DM, Labadie RF, Haynes DS. Bone-anchored hearing aid abutment skin overgrowth reduction with clobetasol. Otolaryngol Head Neck Surg 2008; 139: 829–832

[128] Battista RA, Littlefield PD. Revision BAHA surgery. Otolaryngol Clin North Am 2006; 39: 801–813, viii

[129] Reyes RA, Tjellström A, Granström G. Evaluation of implant losses and skin reactions around extraoral bone-anchored implants: a 0- to 8-year follow-up. Otolaryngol Head Neck Surg 2000; 122: 272–276

[130] Shirazi MA, Marzo SJ, Leonetti JP. Perioperative complications with the bone-anchored hearing aid. Otolaryngol Head Neck Surg 2006; 134: 236–239

[131] Proops DW. The Birmingham bone anchored hearing aid programme: surgical methods and complications. J Laryngol Otol Suppl 1996; 21: 7–12

[132] Papsin BC, Sirimanna TK, Albert DM, Bailey CM. Surgical experience with bone-anchored hearing aids in children. Laryngoscope 1997; 107: 801–806

[133] Lloyd S, Almeyda J, Sirimanna KS, Albert DM, Bailey CM. Updated surgical experience with bone-anchored hearing aids in children. J Laryngol Otol 2007; 121: 826–831

[134] Tjellström A, Granström G. One-stage procedure to establish osseointegration: a zero to five years follow-up report. J Laryngol Otol 1995; 109: 593–598

[135] Granström G, Bergström K, Odersjö M, Tjellström A. Osseointegrated implants in children: experience from our first 100 patients. Otolaryngol Head Neck Surg 2001; 125: 85–92

[136] Scholz M, Eufinger H, Anders A et al. Intracerebral abscess after abutment change of a bone anchored hearing aid (BAHA). Otol Neurotol 2003; 24: 896–899

[137] German M, Fine E, Djalilian HR. Traumatic impact to bone-anchored hearing aid resulting in epidural hematoma. Arch Otolaryngol Head Neck Surg 2010; 136: 1136–1138

[138] Popelka GR, Derebery J, Blevins NH et al. Preliminary evaluation of a novel bone-conduction device for single-sided deafness. Otol Neurotol 2010; 31: 492–497

[139] Murray M, Popelka GR, Miller R. Efficacy and safety of an in-the-mouth bone conduction device for single-sided deafness. Otol Neurotol 2011; 32: 437–443

[140] Murray M, Miller R, Hujoel P, Popelka GR. Long-term safety and benefit of a new intraoral device for single-sided deafness. Otol Neurotol 2011; 32: 1262–1269

[141] Håkansson B, Reinfeldt S, Eeg-Olofsson M et al. A novel bone conduction implant (BCI): engineering aspects and pre-clinical studies. Int J Audiol 2010; 49: 203–215

[142] Adamson RB, Bance M, Brown JA. A piezoelectric bone-conduction bending hearing actuator. J Acoust Soc Am 2010; 128: 2003–2008

33 Cochlear Implants and Auditory Brainstem Implants

Ravi N. Samy

33.1 Introduction

The noted Helen Keller wrote, "Character cannot be developed in ease and quiet: only through experience of trial and suffering can the soul be strengthened, ambition inspired, and success achieved." This quotation typifies the challenges for patients who suffer severe to profound hearing loss. Cochlear implant (CI) and auditory brainstem implant (ABI) researchers have, for decades, worked to lessen such suffering. More than 200,000 patients worldwide have utilized CI and ABI since the 1970s. However, only relatively recently has their use dramatically increased in both adults and children who are hard of hearing or deaf. The increased use, particularly of CIs, is due in no small part to a combination of increased public awareness, coverage of costs of the device and surgical implantation (particularly in Asia), the option for bilateral devices, implantation with a significant amount of residual hearing, and improved performance and outcomes. These implants provide an effective form of rehabilitation, representing one end of a spectrum of options that typically begin with standard air-conduction hearing aids. Although the opposition of the deaf culture to CI placement has lessened, otologists should still be aware of the skepticism and bioethical debates present in the deaf community that can affect the community at large; thus, CIs are not appropriate for all potential recipients.[1]

This chapter reviews the currently available CIs and ABIs. A current PubMed search on cochlear and auditory brain implantation finds more than 7,000 published articles since the original 1957 study by Djourno and Eyries[2] describing electric current to stimulate the cochlear nerve. With rapid, continuing technological advancements in the field of cochlear and auditory brainstem implantation, readers can stay abreast of this large and expanding field by following the literature and presentations at clinical and research meetings.

33.2 Design Features of Cochlear and Auditory Brainstem Implants

Although CIs and ABIs vary in device size, function, and placement, their basic components are similar regardless of the manufacturer. With ongoing modifications and improvement related to all the device components (including software), three CI manufacturers approved by the United States Food and Drug Administration (FDA) are the Cochlear Corporation (Sydney, Australia), Advanced Bionics Corporation (Sylmar, California), and Med-El (Vienna, Austria). There are no clear-cut differences in implant performance among these three companies.[3]

The earliest generation of CIs consisted of a relatively simple electrode that was placed in the scala tympani to electrically stimulate the spiral ganglion cells and auditory nerve in patients with cochlear hair cell loss or dysfunction. After the initial CI studies were performed in the 1960s, the first portable implant system was placed in adults in 1972.[4,5] The FDA approved CIs in 1984 for adults with postlingual deafness;[5] following additional research and success, implantation was then approved for children in 1989. Compared with hearing aids in this patient population, these early devices provided some semblance of sound awareness and improvement in lip-reading skills, even in those with complete and profound deafness.

Since that time, hardware and software (i.e., sound processing strategies) have improved, delivering greater performance and the ability for recipients, both adults and children, to develop open-set word understanding.[6] The newest implants have pushed the envelope of hearing preservation, primarily in the low frequencies, allowing improved hearing in noise and music appreciation.[7] In addition, CIs have performed so well that bilateral implantation is increasing in both adults and children.

Cochlear implants function differently from the natural hearing mechanisms or hearing aids (whether air conduction, bone conduction, or implantable). (Hearing aids and implantable hearing aids are discussed in the other chapters in this section of the book.) A CI uses a microphone located in the sound processor, which is usually worn on the auricle; this external portion of the system resembles a behind-the-ear hearing aid. Sound processors can also be clipped to clothing or worn on the body (▶ Fig. 33.1; ▶ Fig. 33.2.[6]

The microphone receives analog acoustic energy, and converts it into electrical impulses that bypass the external auditory canal, tympanic membrane, ossicular chain, and cochlear hair cells; the impulses finally stimulate the cochlear portion of cranial nerve VIII. The CI processes and analyzes the electrical signal. Band-pass filters create separate and discrete frequency bands to provide for the narrow dynamic range of electric stimulation, which is much narrower than the dynamic range of the human ear (in ideal conditions, the ear functions from 20 to 20,000 Hz).[5] The electric signal is then sent via a radiofrequency

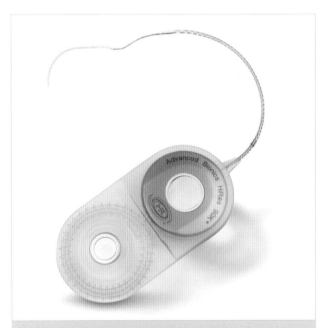

Fig. 33.1 Advanced Bionics Hi-Res 90K cochlear implant (internal receiver-stimulator). (Courtesy of Advanced Bionics LLC, Valencia, CA.)

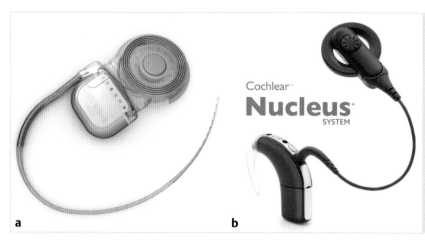

Fig. 33.2 (a) The Med-El Concert CI. (b) Cochlear Corp. Cochlea Nucleus CI24RE implant (Freedom) and external sound processor. (Courtesy of Med-El Corporation, Durham, NC, and Cochlear Ltd., Australia.)

signal from the transmitter coil of the external sound processor, which is attached to the internal implanted receiver stimulator via a magnet (i.e., transcutaneous connection).[5,6] In some devices, the magnet can be removed so that a magnetic resonance imaging (MRI) scan may be performed after implantation; however, some countries allow MRI scanning with the magnet in place. The electric signal is sent to the electrode array within the scala tympani of the cochlea, which then transmits current through the habenula perforata of the modiolus to the cochlear nerve.[6] At least two electrodes are needed to complete an electronic circuit (active and ground electrodes) in either a monopolar or bipolar fashion. Although scala vestibuli insertion can also be performed, this location does not function as effectively and can cause poorer postoperative results and outcomes.[5]

Each company's electrode array differs in design. Electrodes vary in length, in the number of electrode contacts, and in their spacing, flexibility, and stiffness. For example, some electrodes are designed to be placed perimodiolar to reduce power consumption and lengthen battery life. In addition, their performance may improve because of their proximity to the spiral ganglion cells, thus allowing lower psychophysical threshold and comfort levels.[8] As hearing preservation increases in importance, newer electrodes are smaller and softer, and can preserve hearing and be minimally traumatic.[9]

33.3 Audiological Evaluation

With improvements in CI performance, the criteria for their implantation have been relaxed. However, proper patient selection remains important to ensure good postoperative performance and device use, and the patient's expectations should be realistic. Typical candidates have bilateral moderate to severe/profound sensorineural hearing loss (SNHL) that does not benefit from hearing aids. Patients and their families must be motivated; patients must use the device as often as possible and be willing to undergo an auditory rehabilitation process that can take months to years.[6]

Successful cochlear implantation depends on a multidisciplinary team approach consisting of a dedicated CI audiologist who collaborates with an otologist who is well versed in the nuances of cochlear implantation, thus increasing the chances of surgical and audiological success. For children, additional personnel involved in evaluation of potential CI recipients include developmental pediatricians, psychologists, and speech-language

pathologists. The audiologist typically elicits a detailed case history that includes the duration of hearing loss, previous use of hearing aids, family history of hearing loss, etiology of hearing loss, phone use, interest in uni- or bilateral implantation, patient education about the CI, patient and family motivation, and social support systems.

Objective testing includes unaided ear-specific audiological testing—specifically, air conduction, bone conduction, and tympanometry. Ear-specific–aided warble-tone detection with hearing aids is also performed. A real-ear measure is done to verify if the hearing aid settings are appropriate. Further CI-evaluation–specific testing includes an aided (ear-specific) consonant-nucleus-consonant (CNC) word-recognition score (WRS) at 60 dBA (adjusted) and hearing-in-noise testing (HINT) in noise and quiet. A recent addition to the CI testing protocol is the AzBio sentence test, which measures speech recognition by using 10-talker babble to assess speech comprehension in noise; this can be used for audiological evaluation before and after implantation and is sometimes preferred because of the ceiling effects with HINT testing.[10] If a patient scores 50% or better in quiet with the AzBio, the AzBio test in noise is then used.

Next, the Bamford-Kowal-Bench speech-in-noise (BKB SIN) test can determine the signal-to-noise ratio in which a patient with a CI can understand sentences; this is measured pre- and postoperatively. If a patient complains of dizziness, a vestibular workup can be performed and may consist of videonystagmography (VNG), rotary chair testing, platform posturography, and vestibular-evoked myogenic potential (VEMP) evaluation. Potential adult CI recipients have a pure-tone average of > 50 dB, a WRS of < 50 to 60%, HINT in quiet < 60%, and CNC < 30%. Postlingual children may also undergo the above-mentioned tests; however, prelingual children often undergo age and developmental appropriate testing that includes an early speech perception (ESP) test, the Craig Lip Inventory, the Meaningful Auditory Integration Scale (MAIS), and the infant-toddler MAIS.[3]

33.4 Medical Evaluation

As the audiologist assesses whether the audiological criteria are met for implantation, the surgeon takes a history and performs a physical examination of the patient to identify any possible interference to the success of surgery or CI use. The information that the surgeon provides the patient supplements the information provided by the patient's consultation with the audiologist, by further detailing the surgical steps of CI placement. Additional patient education materials (i.e., written and video) are provided to the patient and family to improve comprehension and patient compliance, thereby reducing the risk of nonuse, which has been reported as high as 11%.[11] Patients must be able to tolerate a surgical procedure that lasts about 2 hours. Consultation should be sought with an anesthesiologist, who will assist when implantations are performed in patients with other comorbidities, particularly in the geriatric populations. Tobacco smokers are advised to stop smoking preoperatively to reduce the risk of wound complications, including wound infection or wound breakdown.[10] In addition, preoperative *Streptococcus pneumoniae* vaccination status is obtained and Prevnar and/or Pneumovax is given to reduce the risk of CI-related meningitis.[1,2]

Preoperative imaging is used to identify anatomic abnormalities. Historically, computed tomography (CT) scans were performed to evaluate temporal bone anatomy and certain cochleovestibular abnormalities (e.g., enlarged vestibular aqueduct and facial nerve course) before implantation. More recently, MRI with and without gadolinium has supplanted CT in the practice of most otologists who perform CI. The MRI provides a better evaluation of the cochlear nerve for assessment of aplasia (which precludes CI placement), detects retrocochlear lesions and brainstem/intracranial anatomy, and is more sensitive in detecting early labyrinthitis ossificans. Sometimes both scans are complementary, with CT scans superior for delineating bone and MRI scans superior for soft tissue evaluation.[1,3]

33.5 Surgical Procedure

After preoperative medical, radiological, and audiological clearance, the patient is ready for surgery. A thorough preoperative consent obtained from the patient or family reduces the likelihood of misunderstanding and adverse medicolegal consequences; risks, complications, hazards, and alternatives are discussed and documented. Treatments vary among surgeons for each patient, adult or pediatric. For example, a mastoidectomy with facial recess approach is typically performed in the United States, whereas transcanal, endaural/suprameatal, and even middle fossa approaches have been used in other parts of the world.[14-16] The procedure is performed in an outpatient setting or with 24-hour observation.

Preoperatively, the operative ear is marked. The surgeon should ensure the availability of a backup device in case of device failure or damage to the receiver stimulator package or electrodes during placement. In the operating room, the patient is given prophylactic antibiotics and intravenous steroids (dexamethasone 8 mg); steroids can reduce postoperative emesis and potentially aid in residual hearing preservation. Sequential compression devices reduce the risk of deep vein thrombosis (DVT). After intubation, rotation of the bed 180 degrees allows the surgeon to sit unimpeded at the head of the bed. Hair shaving is minimal. The incision site is marked and infiltrated with local anesthetic. Facial-nerve–monitoring needle electrodes are applied and tested for proper function using a tap test. To aid in the preservation of residual hearing, transtympanic steroid perfusion is also used as either dexamethasone or Solu-Medrol (Pfizer Inc.).[17] The patient is then prepped with Betadine and

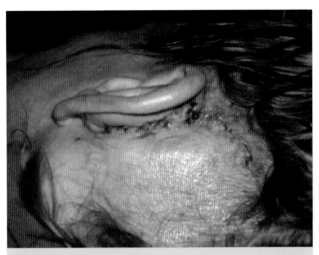

Fig. 33.3 Commonly used hockey-stick incision for cochlear implantation.

draped with a clear drape covering half the face to enable the surgeon to monitor facial movement.

A hockey-stick incision is commonly used; it begins a few millimeters behind the postauricular sulcus and extends varying lengths across the scalp (▶ Fig. 33.3).

The surgeon should avoid crossing the incision over the implanted, internal receiver stimulator. The Palva flap is designed and staggered from the skin incision; thus, in cases of flap necrosis, another layer of soft tissue protection is available for the implanted components. A complete mastoidectomy is performed. Some surgeons prefer to minimize saucerization and allow bony overhangs that reduce the chance of electrode migration. A well for the receiver-stimulator with suture tie-down holes is placed on a flat portion of the skull to minimize rocking of the receiver-stimulator; this is designed for each device type with templates specified by the manufacturer.[3] The well, drilled a couple of finger-breadths behind the postauricular sulcus, allows enough distance for the ear-level sound processor to be placed. In children, surgeons more often forgo a well in favor of subperiosteal pockets that hold the implant in position.[18] After the well is drilled, a trough created between the well and the mastoid permits the electrode(s) to pass unimpeded. This trough is smooth and without any sharp edges that could pierce the Silastic covering of the fragile, active electrode.

Next, a posterior tympanotomy/facial recess approach to the cochlea is most often used. It is imperative to avoid any damage to the ossicular chain, particularly in hearing preservation cases. The facial recess is broad enough to allow visualization of the incudostapedial joint, round window, and hypotympanic air cells. Ideally, the chorda tympani nerve is preserved to prevent postoperative dysgeusia but may be taken if needed. The round window overhang is then taken down, and the pseudomembrane is removed until the actual window/membrane is noted. Its proper identification reduces the risk of electrode placement into a hypotympanic air cell.

Once the implant package is opened, monopolar cautery should be taken off the field. If the patient has a pacemaker or contralateral implant, only bipolar cautery should be used from the start of the procedure. The receiver stimulator is then placed into the cochlear well with suture tie-down holes; the ground electrode is situated before the active electrode. Placing the active electrode last into the cochleostomy will minimize any intracochlear whiplash effect that could damage cochlear structures and also shortens the duration of perilymph leakage.

The electrode can be placed through the round window or a cochleostomy inferior to the round window, as long as the opening is large enough to pass the active electrode, which typically ranges from 0.8 to 1.2 mm.[3] Minimal suctioning of the perilymph is recommended when the scala tympani is opened. The skills to perform a proper and minimally traumatic cochleostomy/round window approach incorporate techniques learned during stapes surgery. Although both round window and cochleostomy approaches can be performed to place and insert the electrode array, the choice often depends on the surgeon's preference and electrode type (e.g., a contour array is meant to be placed via a cochleostomy). However, histological data increasingly show that the round window approach is less traumatic. In examining 12 temporal bones implanted from 1977 to 1997 via three different surgical approaches (cochleostomy, round window enlargement, standard round window), Richard et al[19] noted hydrops in five of 12 specimens that had a cochleostomy or enlargement approach; four of the five had blockage of the duct because of new tissue formation. Thus, the authors felt that implantation through the round window created the least amount of intracochlear trauma and tissue formation.

Before performing a cochleostomy, care is taken to stop any blood from accumulating around the cochlea by using Gelfoam and thrombin. The middle ear is irrigated and cleared of microscopic bony fragments. Avoiding either blood or bony fragments from entering the scala tympani can reduce the risk of labyrinthitis as well as intracochlear fibrosis and osteoneogenesis. Slowly inserting the electrode can minimize the trauma of insertion (e.g., basilar membrane penetration, damage to the osseous spiral lamina or spiral ligament). Excessive force should never be used. Temporal fascia harvested at the beginning of the procedure is used to seal the round window/cochleostomy. The wound is closed in layers with nonabsorbable monofilament sutures in the skin and absorbable sutures in the Palva flap and subcutaneous tissue. Intraoperative device testing involves impedance checks and telemetry. Telemetry, which can be used by all three systems, is known as neural-response telemetry (NRT) for Cochlear Corp. devices, auditory nerve response telemetry (ART) for Med-El devices, and neural response imaging (NRI) for Advanced Bionics devices.

Some surgeons advocate intraoperative radiological imaging (e.g., plain films or fluoroscopy), particularly in challenging cases, revision cases, or cases with anomalies of the cochlea.[20] After testing the device, a mastoid pressure dressing is applied. In the postoperative area, tuning-fork testing is performed to assess any residual hearing, if the recipient was a candidate for a hearing preservation approach. Facial nerve function is also assessed. The patient is then either discharged home when meeting postanesthesia care unit (PACU) criteria or admitted for overnight observation. Postoperatively, the patient is given oral antibiotics for 1 week to cover skin flora. Pain is usually mild and can be relieved by nonsteroidal antiinflammatory drugs and limited use of narcotics. Oral steroids can also be given to preserve residual hearing in select patients.

33.6 Complications

Today, complications are few, particularly when cochlear implantation is performed by an experienced surgeon. Depending on the patient's preoperative health status, potential systemic complications include pneumonia, DVT, stroke, and cardiopulmonary problems. The most common complications are minor and include temporary pain, dizziness, tinnitus, and taste changes. Wound infection, hematoma formation, wound dehiscence, and flap necrosis occur in fewer than 5% of patients and are preventable by attention to detail and meticulous skin closure; if these complications occur, they are usually treated conservatively.[22] Unfortunately, both the receiver-stimulator portion of the CI and the electrode arrays may be exposed after placement. The exposed electrode arrays can be managed conservatively with observation alone, whereas an exposed receiver-stimulator may require flap coverage and possible explantation (▶ Fig. 33.4).[22,23]

More serious complications of CI placement occur in < 1% of patients and include facial nerve paralysis, cerebrospinal fluid (CSF) leak, and meningitis. CSF leaks can occur during the cochleostomy, the mastoidectomy, or during creation of the well for the receiver-stimulator. Leaks are more often closed with soft tissue placement and rarely require the use of a postoperative lumbar drain or closure of the eustachian tube orifice, filling of the cavity with fat, and blind-sac external auditory canal closure. Prevnar (Pfizer Inc.) and/or Pneumovax (Merck & Co., Whitehouse Station, NJ) given preoperatively reduces the risk of meningitis from *S. pneumoniae;* however, meningitis can develop because of skin flora contamination (e.g., from *Staphylococcus aureus*). (See the U.S. Centers for Disease Control and Prevention website for up-to-date information on proper vaccination.) Both CSF leaks and meningitis are more common in patients with congenital ear malformations (e.g., common cavity deformity) and in those with earlier cochlear implants whose designs included a Silastic positioner placed after the active electrode was placed.[24] For any prolonged minor or major complications after implantation, CT scans can be obtained to determine if the device and electrode were properly placed.

Like all devices implanted in the human body, CIs have the potential for failure. Risks most often occur in younger children, particularly now that children as young as 4 to 6 months of age are receiving implants in countries outside the U.S. Overall, the cumulative survival rates for cochlear implants continue to improve.[25] However, there is still the risk of failure because of impact or trauma (common in the pediatric population), electronic dysfunction (impacting both the software and electronic circuitry), or leakage due to breaks in the hermetic seal. Fortunately, the cause of the failure can be identified in most patients who can then undergo explantation and reimplantation with the same or newer device, allowing success with continued use.[22,25]

33.7 Programming Strategies

The goals for programming include providing audibility for speech sounds, comfort with all sounds (music, environmental, speech), and a means for speech perception, language acquisition, and expression. The three FDA-approved manufacturers

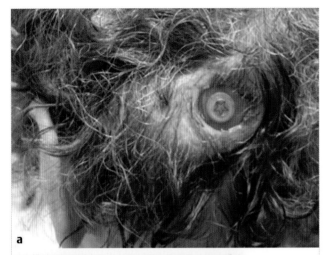

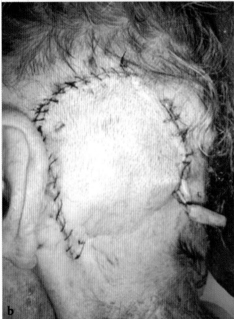

Fig. 33.4 A patient with an implant that has migrated. Explantation and flap rotation was performed to close the defect. (a) Preoperative. (b) Postoperative.

higher speeds to stimulate the electrodes and a limited number of electrodes instead of roving. Ongoing stimulation of these same electrodes one after another provide detail on the timing of speech. (3) Advanced Combined Encoder (ACE) combines the best features for optimal pitch and timing information, and provides roving capabilities like SPeak and high speed like CIS.[3,26]

Programming strategies vary for each user, and no single fitting-coding strategy (or map) is applicable for all.[27] Because recipients can have difficulty in noisy environments or face everyday listening challenges using telephones, additional technologies can improve performance, such as FM (frequency modulation) systems, telecoils, or induction loop systems.[28] Cochlear implants provide limited spectral and temporal information and have limited dynamic range, particularly with music. Efforts to model our complex acoustic environments into software algorithms are challenging.[29]

33.8 Postoperative Performance in Adults and Children

Numerous factors impact postoperative cochlear implant performance in adults and children. Although most individuals do well with the implant and develop open-set speech recognition, performance is difficult to predict for each patient.[3] Numerous prognostic factors have been evaluated to help the patient and family form realistic expectations. These include the cause of deafness (e.g., meningitis vs. aminoglycoside-induced deafness), the age of onset of deafness, the duration of hearing loss, the use of hearing aids, preoperative audiometric testing (e.g., HINT testing), family/social support, socioeconomic status, education level, and IQ.[30] In adults, self-motivation, positive attitudes, and even male sex have been associated with a greater self-satisfaction/subjective performance improvement with the CI.[31]

The ideal adult candidate has acquired postlingual SNHL. Postlingually deafened adults represent the majority of patients undergoing implantation. A period of auditory exposure, with the development of central nervous system (CNS) auditory pathways and associated normal speech production, speech perception, and expressive language, portends a good prognosis. However, in patients who have prolonged auditory deprivation, whether prelingual or postlingual, CI placement may allow sound awareness but not good sound recognition because of the degradation or underdevelopment of the central auditory pathways. Thus, the ability of the central nervous system to respond and adapt (i.e., neuroplasticity) to the implant signal is ultimately the determinant for solid performance.

Most CI recipients will improve their ability to hear, though some take longer to achieve satisfactory performance during a period of acclimatization after the initial activation. Clearly, pre-implant counseling by both the CI audiologist and CI surgeon is paramount. Adjustment of stimulation levels and other programming parameters improve performance and assist with trouble-shooting any patient complaints.[28] Postoperative auditory performance can also be improved with rehabilitation under the guidance of speech-language pathologists.[28]

Patients who have significant comorbidities, particularly conditions that affect the CNS, tend to have poorer results with CIs. In a report of 88 children who received CIs, Birman et al[32] noted that one third had additional disabilities, including but

have developed sound coding strategies; some are proprietary and used only in a particular implant (see more definitive audiological texts for a further discussion of such strategies). Coding strategies are software programs stored within the sound processor that convert the pitch, loudness, and timing of the analog acoustic signal into electrical impulses. Both simultaneous (activation of more than one electrode at a time) and nonsimultaneous stimulation strategies are available.[3]

Rates of stimulation also vary among implants, and no coding strategy is inherently superior to another in improving outcomes. Some of the available coding strategies are the following: (1) SPeak (spectral peak) is a roving strategy whose incoming signal roves across the 20 channels, stimulating up to 10 channels to best represent the incoming signal, which provides a rich detailed representation of sound yet minimizes the effects of noise. (2) CIS (continuous interleaved sampling) uses not limited to developmental delay, autism spectrum disorder, attention deficit disorder, cerebral palsy, and visual impairment. The main conditions associated with these disabilities included cochleovestibular dysplasia, cytomegalovirus, syndromal/chromosomal abnormalities, prematurity, and jaundice, and resulted in poorer implant performance.

For CIs in children, the FDA requires a minimum age of 1 year (unless the patient is at risk of developing labyrinthitis ossificans after an episode of meningitis), have profound SNHL, demonstrate a lack of benefit from hearing aids, and have no medical conditions that would contraindicate implantation. Family support and postoperative education, speech-language enrichment, and rehabilitation can lower nonuse rates and maximize speech reception and production. Cochlear implants have been shown to improve not only hearing but also speech production and quality of vocal function. Among pediatric implant recipients, normal or near-normal speech and language milestones show significant variability in outcomes. Such variations are possibly due to underlying neurocognitive/neuroplasticity issues, which could benefit from targeted interventions to improve outcomes.[33]

Although CI studies often focus on children and young or middle-aged adults, the elderly can also gain significant improvements in quality of life. In discussing issues of neuroplasticity and cognitive, social, and physical functioning, Lin et al[34] speculated that 150,000 elderly Americans may be candidates for CI, with numbers increasing with the aging of the population. In their center's 12-year experience with patients over the age of 60 years, Lin et al noted a 60% mean improvement in HINT-Q (hearing-in-noise testing in quiet); they realized that such gains decreased with increasing age and that higher preoperative HINT scores were associated with better postoperative performance. In a comparison of 28 patients 79 years of age or older and those 20 to 60 years of age, Lundin et al[35] reported no peri- or postoperative complications in the elderly group and a statistically significant improvement in performance after surgery ($p < 0.001$). However, the authors noted that rates of nonuse were higher in patients with postoperative dizziness, tinnitus, and limited social support.[35]

In a series of more than 1,000 patients, Lenarz et al[36] divided their patients into four age groups, with the oldest group 70 years of age and older. Based on speech and sentence tests in quiet and noise, they noted that learning curves and performance were comparable for geriatric patients and younger patients with cochlear implants, but that performance suffered in noise for geriatric patients, possibly owing to central auditory processing abnormalities associated with age. The authors questioned whether additional rehabilitation or cognitive training could be developed to improve performance in noisy settings for this population.

33.9 Electroacoustic Stimulation/ Hybrid Condition

Although the majority of adults and children eventually achieve open-set speech recognition with cochlear implants in quiet, device performance in noisy environments or with music is lacking.[37,38] Strategies such as multiple microphones in the sound processor or bilateral placement can improve sound localization and noise reduction strategies. Novel methods are needed to improve performance with music. In a review of music perception with standard CIs, McDermott[39] described numerous problems and noted that implant users (1) perceive rhythm as well as normal hearing listeners; (2) have poor melody recognition; (3) have unsatisfactory timbre perception; (4) rate musical sound quality as being less pleasant than normal-hearing listeners; (5) may improve subjective appreciation for music with auditory music training; and (6) could improve pitch perception by sound processors that incorporate temporal and spatial patterns of electrical stimulation. Finally, preservation of low-frequency residual hearing, particularly when amplified, can improve performance benefits for recipients, especially in noise.[39–41]

The hybrid or electroacoustic stimulation (EAS) type of CI facilitates the preservation of low-frequency hearing (250–1,000 Hz) when amplified with an air-conduction hearing aid and combined with electrical stimulation in middle to high frequencies (▶ Fig. 33.5). Using either standard length or short array electrodes, researchers have discovered that the human auditory system can integrate both low-frequency acoustic signals and high-frequency electrical stimulation.[38] This combined approach increases the potential population for CI placement. In short-term findings, these patients performed better in noisy situations and could appreciate music. Although EAS/hybrid

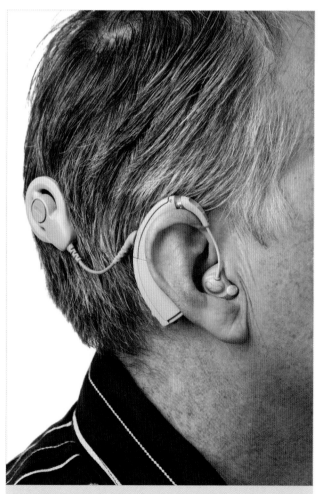

Fig. 33.5 A combined in-the-ear hearing aid and sound processor implanted in a patient implanted with a hybrid CI.

implants are approved for use in some parts of the world, the FDA continues to evaluate data in the United States.

Considerations of hearing preservation for the EAS/hybrid encompasses not only the surgical details but the individual's cochlear anatomy relative to electrode design (i.e., size, stiffness/flexibility); the goal is to minimize insertion trauma, which can cause a loss of spiral ganglion cells through fibrosis and osteoneogenesis, thus degrading CI performance.[42] The surgeon should avoid injury to the basilar membrane, osseous spiral lamina, spiral ligament, and the Reissner membrane. In a computational model, Kha and Chen[43] used the finite element method to design electrodes with better stiffness properties, specifically to reduce this significant factor as a cause of injury during insertion.

33.10 Costs

It has been demonstrated that CIs are cost-effective to the society in general, especially when used in children. With implantation, children can be mainstreamed in school and progress socioeconomically after high school, and adults can be gainfully employed. However, a CI is expensive technology (typically costing $25,000 for the device alone or nearly $50,000 per implantation when including surgery, anesthesia, and hospital costs). Therefore, it is financially prudent to avoid a high nonuse rate by predicting ahead of time which patients will benefit from implantation. Eppsteiner et al[44] suggested that 7% of patients with severe-to-profound hearing loss would not benefit from CI and estimated that the lifetime cost of the surgical and clinical management of a CI in such a patient at $1 million.

In a systematic review of articles addressing the economics of CI, Turchetti et al[47] showed that unilateral implantation was cost-effective in prelingually deafened children but with caveats in postlingually deafened adults. That is, unilateral CIs were less cost-effective in those with > 40 years of hearing impairment and those > 70 years in age; bilateral CIs were also less cost-effective. In the United Kingdom, only about 10,000 people have CIs, mostly unilateral CIs in adults. In a systematic review of bilateral CI placement, Crathorne et al[45] demonstrated clinical effectiveness but not cost-effectiveness within their health care system. In the United States, CI programs have been closed or limit the number of surgeries performed because of the financial losses incurred with implantation, particularly among Medicaid patients. Therefore, surgeons should understand supply-chain-and-revenue management principles to achieve financial sustainability and prevent patients from losing access to CI.[46]

One potential cost reduction is the development of a low-cost CI destined for India and other developing countries. The Defence Research and Development Organisation of India is planning clinical trials at five centers in India; the implant is projected to cost approximately one tenth that of what is currently available. This cost reduction could increase CI usage worldwide, even among indigent populations in the U.S.[48]

33.11 Auditory Brainstem Implantation

As ABI undergoes a renaissance in use, more than 1,000 patients have been implanted worldwide since 1979 when House

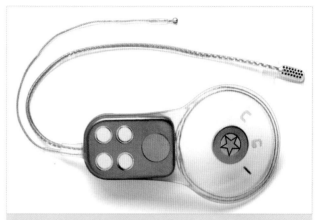

Fig. 33.6 Auditory brainstem implant. (Courtesy of Cochlear Ltd., Australia.)

and Hitselberger implanted the first patient with what was initially called a cochlear nucleus implant.[50] The patient wore it daily for more than 20 years with no long-term adverse sequelae.[51] The original FDA indication for ABI placement specified adults who had neurofibromatosis-2 (NF2). Similar in design to a CI, the ABI that is FDA approved and manufactured by Cochlear Corp. includes a 3- × 8-mm Silastic paddle and 21 platinum electrodes placed in the lateral recess of the fourth ventricle to stimulate the dorsal cochlear nucleus (▶ Fig. 33.6).

The device is intended to improve lip-reading skills and sound awareness in patients who had no other option and were not candidates for CI. Recently, ABIs have been used internationally in pediatric patients who would not benefit from cochlear implantation, such as those with bilateral cochlear nerve aplasia, complete labyrinthitis ossificans precluding CI placement, or bilateral cochlear nerve avulsion (e.g., temporal bone fractures).[49,52] Surprisingly, some children with ABIs developed open-set speech recognition rivaling that of CI recipients. The NF2 recipients have also demonstrated excellent performance, including speaking on the telephone. Many now believe that ABI outcomes differ based on patient pathology, surgical technique, coding strategy, and implant device.[52] As understanding of ABIs and the central auditory pathways improve, recipients should continue to have improved performance. In the U.S., the House Research Institute and the Children's Hospital of Los Angeles have partnered with the University of Verona to submit an FDA application allowing ABI placement in children.[53]

33.12 Future Considerations

Cochlear implants and ABIs continue to advance in hardware technology, software algorithms, and sound processor design. For example, Advance Bionics offers a waterproof external sound processor called Neptune. As animal and clinical studies evolve, some advances are ready for immediate adoption whereas others will take years to come to fruition in patient care.

Because steroids have been shown to improve the success rate of hearing preservation approaches, future electrode arrays may be coated with steroids or other materials (e.g., neurotrophic growth factors, stem cells, mannitol) to preserve or recover

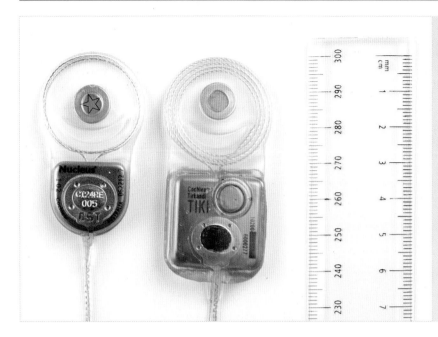

Fig. 33.7 Totally implantable cochlear implant (TIKI) implant to the right of the Cochlear Nucleus Freedom CI. (Courtesy of Cochlear Ltd., Australia.)

hearing,[54,55] or possibly reduce postoperative vestibular disorders. In a randomized clinical trial involving 43 adults, Enticott et al[56] noted that dizziness decreased in those who had topical methylprednisolone applied to the round window during CI placement versus controls (5% vs. 29%, respectively). However, safety must first be proven in animal models because of the concern about the immunosuppressive effects of steroids and the possible increased risks of wound and CI infection, even meningitis. Comparing two groups of guinea pigs (15 per group) with non-eluting or steroid-eluting electrode arrays, Niedermeier et al[57] exposed the animals to a virulent strain of *S. pneumoniae* and observed them for 5 days.[57] After clinical evaluation, CSF examination, culture, and histological examination of the brains and cochleas, the authors noted that meningitis developed in three of 15 animals with the non-eluting implants and four animals with dexamethasone-eluting arrays (the difference was not statistically significant).

Cochlear implants may be effective for the treatment of single-sided deafness.[58] The implant appears to improve sound localization and speech perception (especially in noisy environments) over the unaided condition, bone conduction hearing systems (including Baha, Oticon Ponto, Sophono, or Soundbite), or contralateral routing of signal (CROS) hearing aids.[59] Two independent acoustic systems are needed for interaural latency difference, time difference, and phase differences. Thus, for single-sided deafness, a CI can only help recover the unused auditory pathway, which assists with sound localization and uses squelch and summation to assist in speech perception in noisy environments. A CI can also reduce tinnitus in a patient with single-sided deafness.[58] Further studies are needed for widespread adoption in these patients, and hurdles of coverage by third-party payers and government agencies must be overcome.

Robotic and image-guided technology may also prove useful to reduce intracochlear damage and further provide more minimally invasive techniques. Using an automated image-guided microstereotactic frame for percutaneous cochlear implantation by a bone-attached parallel robotic system, Kratchman et al[60] achieved 0.38-mm accuracy at the cochlea in a cadaveric specimen. Meanwhile, Zhang et al[61] utilized scala tympani models to demonstrate that robot-assisted steerable electrode arrays could reduce intracochlear insertion forces; the authors plan to develop a second-generation robotic system that incorporates force-sensing capability with haptic/tactile feedback.

One of the most exciting developments in cochlear implantation is the concept of a totally implantable cochlear implant, such as the device used by Briggs et al[62] in three adults (▶ Fig. 33.7). The device, termed TIKI, has a lithium-ion rechargeable battery and an internal microphone. Its sound-processing strategies allow the TIKI to use either the internal microphone or an external sound processor.

After TIKI placement, no patient suffered any surgical or postoperative complications, and all performed better in speech-perception outcomes than before the operation; specifically, patients performed better in the external sound processor condition than with the internal microphone alone. However, patients complained of body noise interference (e.g., scalp moving over the microphone with head movements). When compared with the current semi-implantable devices, totally implantable devices have numerous benefits that could potentially increase the numbers of patients using implants, especially those who now opt out of a current-generation CI for various reasons. Totally implantable devices are more cosmetic, allow the auditory system to function 24 hours daily like the natural system, and can be used during bathing and swimming.[63]

33.13 Conclusion

Cochlear implants and ABIs are modern technological marvels that improve quality of life for severely to profoundly deaf individuals; their impact should not be underestimated. Although postoperative auditory performance varies for each recipient, CI and ABI are established and accepted rehabilitation options for select patients.[6] As the devices improve and our understanding about the auditory system increases (especially related to the neuroplasticity of the CNS), more patients will gain access to these remarkable technologies. Enthusiasm for the widespread use of CI and ABI are tempered by the underlying financial impediments that exist in the U.S. and worldwide. This chapter concludes with another Helen Keller quotation that exemplifies what many countless audiologists, surgeons, speech-language pathologists, researchers, and others have done to reduce the suffering and disability of deafness:

Although the world is full of suffering, it is full also of the overcoming of it.

References

[1] Kermit P. Enhancement technology and outcomes: what professionals and researchers can learn from those skeptical about cochlear implants. Health Care Anal 2012; 20: 367–384[Epub ahead of print]

[2] Djourno A, Eyries C. [Auditory prosthesis by means of a distant electrical stimulation of the sensory nerve with the use of an indwelt coiling] Presse Med 1957; 65: 1417

[3] Roland PS. Cochlear implants in adults and children. In: Gulya AJ, Minor LB, Poe DS, eds. Glasscock-Shambaugh Surgery of the Ear, 6th ed. Shelton, CT; PMPH, 2010:583–615

[4] Simmons FB. Cochlear implants. Arch Otolaryngol 1969; 89: 61–69

[5] Gantz BJ, Perry BP, Rubinstein JT. Cochlear Implants. In: Canalis RF, Lambert PR, eds. The Ear: Comprehensive Otology. Philadelphia: Lippincott Williams & Wilkins, 2000:633–646

[6] Toh EH, Luxford WM. Cochlear and brainstem implantation. Otolaryngol Clin North Am 2002; 35: 325–342

[7] Woodson EA, Reiss LA, Turner CW, Gfeller K, Gantz BJ. The Hybrid cochlear implant: a review. Adv Otorhinolaryngol 2010; 67: 125–134

[8] Runge-Samuelson C, Firszt JB, Gaggl W, Wackym PA. Electrically evoked auditory brainstem responses in adults and children: effects of lateral to medial placement of the nucleus 24 contour electrode array. Otol Neurotol 2009; 30: 464–470

[9] Mowry SE, Woodson E, Gantz BJ. New frontiers in cochlear implantation: acoustic plus electric hearing, hearing preservation, and more. Otolaryngol Clin North Am 2012; 45: 187–203

[10] Sørensen LT. Wound healing and infection in surgery. The clinical impact of smoking and smoking cessation: a systematic review and meta-analysis. Arch Surg 2012; 147: 373–383

[11] Schafer EC, Pogue J, Milrany T. List equivalency of the AzBio sentence test in noise for listeners with normal-hearing sensitivity or cochlear implants. J Am Acad Audiol 2012; 23: 501–509

[12] Parry DA, Booth T, Roland PS. Advantages of magnetic resonance imaging over computed tomography in preoperative evaluation of pediatric cochlear implant candidates. Otol Neurotol 2005; 26: 976–982

[13] http://www.cdc.gov/vaccines/vpd-vac/mening/cochlear/dis-cochlear-gen.htm

[14] Migirov L, Dagan E, Kronenberg J. Suprameatal approach for cochlear implantation in children: our experience with 320 cases. Cochlear Implants Int 2010; 11 Suppl 1: 195–198

[15] Jang JH, Song JJ, Yoo JC, Lee JH, Oh SH, Chang SO. An alternative procedure for cochlear implantation: transcanal approach. Acta Otolaryngol 2012; 132: 845–849

[16] Colletti V, Fiorino FG. New window for cochlear implant insertion. Acta Otolaryngol 1999; 119: 214–218

[17] Rajan GP, Kuthubutheen J, Hedne N, Krishnaswamy J. The role of preoperative, intratympanic glucocorticoids for hearing preservation in cochlear implantation: a prospective clinical study. Laryngoscope 2012; 122: 190–195

[18] Prager JD, Neidich MJ, Perkins JN, Meinzen-Derr J, Greinwald JH, Jr. Minimal access and standard cochlear implantation: a comparative study. Int J Pediatr Otorhinolaryngol 2012; 76: 1102–1106

[19] Richard C, Fayad JN, Doherty J, Linthicum FH, Jr. Round window versus cochleostomy technique in cochlear implantation: histologic findings. Otol Neurotol 2012; 33: 1181–1187

[20] Coelho DH, Waltzman SB, Roland JT, Jr. Implanting common cavity malformations using intraoperative fluoroscopy. Otol Neurotol 2008; 29: 914–919

[21] Spencer LJ, Gantz BJ, Knutson JF. Outcomes and achievement of students who grew up with access to cochlear implants. Laryngoscope 2004; 114: 1576–1581

[22] Samy RN, Rubinstein JT. Revision cochlear implant surgery. In: Edelstein DR, ed. Revision Surgery in Otolaryngology. New York: Thieme, 2009;125–132

[23] Walgama ES, Isaacson B, Kutz JW, Jr, Roland PS. Management of electrode exposure after cochlear implantation. Otol Neurotol 2012; 33: 1197–1200

[24] Lalwani AK, Cohen NL. Longitudinal risk of meningitis after cochlear implantation associated with the use of the positioner. Otol Neurotol 2011; 32: 1082–1085

[25] Battmer RD, Linz B, Lenarz T. A review of device failure in more than 23 years of clinical experience of a cochlear implant program with more than 3,400 implantees. Otol Neurotol 2009; 30: 455–463

[26] Agrawal D, Timm L, Viola FC et al. ERP evidence for the recognition of emotional prosody through simulated cochlear implant strategies. BMC Neurosci 2012; 13: 113[Epub ahead of print]

[27] Holmes AE, Shrivastav R, Krause L, Siburt HW, Schwartz E. Speech based optimization of cochlear implants. Int J Audiol 2012; 51: 806–816[Epub ahead of print]

[28] Wolfe J, Schafer EC. Programming Cochlear Implants. San Diego: Plural Publishing, 2010

[29] Desmond JM, Throckmorton CS, Collins LM. Using channel-specific models to detect and remove reverberation in cochlear implants. J Acoust Soc Am 2012; 132: 2050

[30] Roditi RE, Poissant SF, Bero EM, Lee DJ. A predictive model of cochlear implant performance in postlingually deafened adults. Otol Neurotol 2009; 30: 449–454

[31] Rekkedal AM. Assistive hearing technologies among students with hearing impairment: factors that promote satisfaction. J Deaf Stud Deaf Educ 2012; 17: 499–517[Epub ahead of print]

[32] Birman CS, Elliott EJ, Gibson WP. Pediatric cochlear implants: additional disabilities prevalence, risk factors, and effect on language outcomes. Otol Neurotol 2012; 33: 1347–1352

[33] Harris MS, Kronenberger WG, Gao S et al. Verbal short-term memory development and spoken language outcomes in deaf children with cochlear implants. Ear Hear 201 3; 34: 179–192

[34] Lin FR, Chien WW, Li L, Clarrett DM, Niparko JK, Francis HW. Cochlear implantation in older adults. Medicine (Baltimore) 2012; 91: 229–241

[35] Lundin K, Näsvall A, Köbler S, Linde G, Rask-Andersen H. Cochlear implantation in the elderly. Cochlear Implants Int 201 3; 14: 92–97

[36] Lenarz M, Sönmez H, Joseph G, Büchner A, Lenarz T. Cochlear implant performance in geriatric patients. Laryngoscope 2012; 122: 1361–1365

[37] Kokkinakis K, Azimi B, Hu Y, Friedland DR. Single and multiple microphone noise reduction strategies in cochlear implants. Trends Amplif 2012; 16: 102–116[Epub ahead of print]

[38] Gantz BJ, Turner C. Combining acoustic and electrical speech processing: Iowa/Nucleus hybrid implant. Acta Otolaryngol 2004; 124: 344–347

[39] McDermott HJ. Music perception with cochlear implants: a review. Trends Amplif 2004; 8: 49–82

[40] Tahmina Q, Bhandary M, Azimi B et al. The effect of visual information on speech perception in noise by electroacoustic hearing. J Acoust Soc Am 2012; 132: 2050

[41] Wang S, Liu B, Dong R et al. Music and lexical tone perception in Chinese adult cochlear implant users. Laryngoscope 2012; 122: 1353–1360

[42] Verbist BM, Ferrarini L, Briaire JJ et al. Anatomic considerations of cochlear morphology and its implications for insertion trauma in cochlear implant surgery. Otol Neurotol 2009; 30: 471–477

[43] Kha H, Chen B. Finite element analysis of damage by cochlear implant electrode array's proximal section to the basilar membrane. Otol Neurotol 2012; 33: 1176–1180

[44] Eppsteiner RW, Shearer AE, Hildebrand MS et al. Prediction of cochlear implant performance by genetic mutation: the spiral ganglion hypothesis. Hear Res 2012; 292: 51–58

[45] Crathorne L, Bond M, Cooper C et al. A systematic review of the effectiveness and cost-effectiveness of bilateral multichannel cochlear implants in adults with severe-to-profound hearing loss. Clin Otolaryngol 2012; 37: 342–354

[46] McKinnon BJ. Cochlear implant programs: balancing clinical and financial sustainability. Laryngoscope 201 3; 123: 233–238

[47] Turchetti G, Bellelli S, Palla I, Berrettini S. Systematic review of the scientific literature on the economic evaluation of cochlear implants in adult patients. Acta Otorhinolaryngol Ital 2011; 31: 319–327

[48] http://articles.timesofindia.indiatimes.com/2012-05-20/bangalore/31788114_1_cochlear-implant-drdo

[49] Colletti V, Carner M, Miorelli V, Guida M, Colletti L, Fiorino F. Auditory brainstem implant (ABI): new frontiers in adults and children. Otolaryngol Head Neck Surg 2005; 133: 126–138

[50] Hitselberger WE, House WF, Edgerton BJ, Whitaker S. Cochlear nucleus implants. Otolaryngol Head Neck Surg 1984; 92: 52–54

[51] House WF, Hitselberger WE. Twenty-year report of the first auditory brain stem nucleus implant. Ann Otol Rhinol Laryngol 2001; 110: 103–104

[52] Colletti L, Shannon R, Colletti V. Auditory brainstem implants for neurofibromatosis type 2. Curr Opin Otolaryngol Head Neck Surg 2012; 20: 353–357

[53] http://www.marketwatch.com/story/house-research-institute-and-childrens-hospital-los-angeles-partner-with-university-of-verona-hospital-to-bring-auditory-brainstem-implants-to-us-children-2012-09-07

[54] Infante EB, Channer GA, Telischi FF et al. Mannitol protects hair cells against tumor necrosis factor α-induced loss. Otol Neurotol 2012; 33: 1656–1663

[55] Hu Z, Ulfendahl M, Prieskorn DM, Olivius P, Miller JM. Functional evaluation of a cell replacement therapy in the inner ear. Otol Neurotol 2009; 30: 551–558

[56] Enticott JC, Eastwood HT, Briggs RJ, Dowell RC, O'Leary SJ. Methylprednisolone applied directly to the round window reduces dizziness after cochlear implantation: a randomized clinical trial. Audiol Neurootol 2011; 16: 289–303

[57] Niedermeier K, Braun S, Fauser C, Kiefer J, Straubinger RK, Stark T. A safety evaluation of dexamethasone-releasing cochlear implants: comparative study on the risk of otogenic meningitis after implantation. Acta Otolaryngol 2012; 132: 1252–1260[Epub ahead of print]

[58] Arts RA, George EL, Stokroos RJ, Vermeire K. Review: cochlear implants as a treatment of tinnitus in single-sided deafness. Curr Opin Otolaryngol Head Neck Surg 2012; 20: 398–403

[59] Kamal SM, Robinson AD, Diaz RC. Cochlear implantation in single-sided deafness for enhancement of sound localization and speech perception. Curr Opin Otolaryngol Head Neck Surg 2012; 20: 393–397

[60] Kratchman LB, Blachon GS, Withrow TJ, Balachandran R, Labadie RF, Webster RJ, III. Design of a bone-attached parallel robot for percutaneous cochlear implantation. IEEE Trans Biomed Eng 2011; 58: 2904–2910

[61] Zhang J, Wei W, Ding J, Roland JT, Jr, Manolidis S, Simaan N. Inroads toward robot-assisted cochlear implant surgery using steerable electrode arrays. Otol Neurotol 2010; 31: 1199–1206

[62] Briggs RJ, Eder HC, Seligman PM et al. Initial clinical experience with a totally implantable cochlear implant research device. Otol Neurotol 2008; 29: 114–119

[63] Cohen N. The totally implantable cochlear implant. Ear Hear 2007; 28 Suppl: 100S–101S

34 Rehabilitation of Peripheral Vestibular Disorders

Kelly S. Beaudoin, Kathleen D. Coale, and Judith A. White

34.1 Impairments Resulting from Peripheral Vestibular Disorders

Common impairments accompanying vestibular dysfunction include decreased gaze stability secondary to abnormal vestibulo-ocular reflex; abnormal motion perception caused by mismatch of sensory inputs affecting sensory integration necessary for balance; abnormal postural control (distorted labyrinthine and otolithic inputs cause impaired equilibrium and body alignment); decreased static and dynamic balance/gait secondary to vestibulospinal outputs responding incorrectly to mismatched sensory inputs; decreased sensory integration for balance (the balance system requires robust inputs from visual, vestibular, and sensory systems to make proper balance reactions); and anxiety. Movement increases instability in a vestibulopathic patient and yet is the absolute requirement for recovery. Physical deconditioning may develop when patients become fearful of movement and severely limit all mobility.

Patients with peripheral vestibular dysfunction present to rehabilitation with the following problems[1]: decreased vestibulo-ocular reflex (VOR) gain,[2] abnormal sensory integration for balance,[3] abnormal vestibulospinal reflex (VSR)/balance/gait,[4] vertigo provoked by position change,[5] limited community mobility,[6] and lack of knowledge regarding their diagnosis and prognosis.

Diagnoses seen by vestibular therapists commonly include both unilateral and bilateral disorders such as labyrinthitis/neuronitis, temporal bone fracture with concussion or benign paroxysmal positional vertigo (BPPV), Ménière syndrome (acute and chronic), acoustic neuroma (both resected and unresected), herpes zoster oticus/Ramsay Hunt syndrome, labyrinthine infarct, anteroinferior or posteroinferior cerebellar stroke, cervicogenic vertigo, BPPV by itself, phobic postural vertigo, aminoglygoside ototoxicity, and hereditary insidious vestibular loss. Central vestibular disorders are not addressed in this chapter.

34.2 Evaluation of Peripheral Vestibular Disorders

Clinical evaluation performed by the vestibular therapist consists of tests of gaze stability, static balance/sensory integration for balance, gait, postural control, and positional and positioning testing.

Oculomotor Exam

Room light:
- VOR to slow head movement
- Head impulse test
- Dynamic (with 2 Hz head movement) versus static visual acuity
- Pursuit eye movements
- VOR cancellation

Infrared goggles:
- Gaze holding: horizontal and vertical
- Head-shaking–induced nystagmus horizontal and vertical
- Tragal pressure induced nystagmus

Positional testing

Static Balance Exam

Modified clinical test of sensory integration and balance:
1. Eyes open on firm surface, feet together, timed trial of 30 seconds
2. Eyes closed on firm surface, feet together, timed trial of 30 seconds
3. Eyes open on foam surface, feet together, timed trial of 30 seconds
4. Eyes closed on foam surface, feet together, timed trial of 30 seconds
5. Eyes open on firm surface, feet in tandem stance, timed trial of 30 seconds
6. Eyes closed on firm surface, feet in tandem stance, timed trial of 30 seconds

Other static tests of balance:
1. Single limb stance, firm surface, eyes open
2. Single limb stance, firm surface, eyes closed
3. Eyes open, firm surface, head pitched up or down 45 degrees
4. Eyes closed firm surface, head pitched up or down 45 degrees

Findings from the initial vestibular assessment, along with vestibular laboratory testing results when available, assist the therapist with determining if the deficit is central or peripheral, unilateral or bilateral, or acute or chronic. Once impairments are identified, treatment planning and outcome prediction begins.

The static and dynamic balance tests are intertwined with the sensory integration examination, and information is gleaned about strategies used (ankle, hip, stepping) as well as ability to regain the center of mass over the base of support.[1] Determining which strategies the patient has available for balance recovery aids the therapist in treatment planning to facilitate safe community mobility and prevent falls. Computerized dynamic platform posturography (CDPP) is used in tertiary care centers to evaluate sensory integration for balance, center of mass, and sway information. These machines can also measure motor latencies for translational platform movements. Clinical gait examinations commonly employ the Dynamic Gait Index,[2] the Berg Balance Scale,[3] the Timed Up and Go test,[4] and more recently the Functional Gait Assessment.[5] Many of these tests have been shown to be specific for predicting fall risk and assessing outcomes in this patient population.[6–8]

Positional and positioning testing is performed using infrared video-oculography or Frenzel goggles to eliminate visual fixation and allow the examiner to directly visualize nystagmus patterns. The examiner must be knowledgeable in recognizing which nystagmus patterns indicate BPPV (▶ Table 34.1) and which patterns indicate other pathophysiology within or outside the peripheral vestibular system.

Other components of the clinical examination include strength, flexibility, and sensory testing of the lower extremities and careful consideration of cervical contributions. Manual segmental testing of the cervical spine can provide insight into the patient's problem when peripheral vestibular testing is nonlocalizing.[9] Careful attention must be paid to the patient's comorbidities for both treatment planning and outcome prediction. Knowledge of normal age-related changes in visual, sensory, and vestibular function should be employed when treating this population.

Self-perception of dizziness and resultant handicap is commonly measured with the Dizziness Handicap Inventory,[10] the Activities Specific Balance Control Questionnaire,[11] or the Vestibular Activities of Daily Living scale.[12] These questionnaires can be used before, during, and after treatment to evaluate results of rehabilitation intervention.

34.3 Treatment of Peripheral Vestibular Disorders

Once impairments and functional limitations are identified, research indicates treatment should begin promptly for optimal outcomes.[13] Recovery of function after vestibular loss involves three different mechanisms: (1) spontaneous recovery, (2) vestibular adaptation/plasticity, and (3) substitution of other strategies.[14]

Much of the static imbalance of vestibular dysfunction resolves spontaneously prior to the initiation of vestibular therapy. Vestibular rehabilitation usually takes place in the subacute stage and utilizes both adaptation and substitution to regain gaze and gait stability as well as community mobility recovery. An error signal is needed to stimulate compensation.[13] Therapists strive to elicit the error signal while treating patients by utilizing active head motion to present the brain with a reduced gain situation, causing retinal slip of the foveal visual image. Developing strategies for varied environments found in the community adds context specificity and improves outcome.[13]

Utilizing a variety of inputs—visual, vestibular, and somatosensory—enables the patient to develop new strategies for balance control and gaze stability in varying environments. Unilateral vestibular deficits recover gaze and gait stability quite well. Bilateral vestibular loss patients do not return to premorbid activity levels. Bilateral vestibular loss requires more substitution strategies, such as preprogrammed saccades, to facilitate gaze stability while the patient is in motion. Assistive devices, such as canes and walkers, are not often required long term for the unilateral peripheral vestibular patients. Bilateral vestibular patients have greater loss of vestibular input for balance, and therefore commonly require an assistive device for safe mobility. Recent research in the area of virtual reality is promising to promote treatment in multimodal sensory situations to facilitate better sensory integration for balance.[15]

Based on identified impairments and goals, treatments are provided one or two times per week for 4 to 6 weeks as outlined in ▶ Table 34.2, ▶ Table 34.3, ▶ Table 34.4, ▶ Table 34.5, and ▶ Table 34.6.

34.4 Gaze Stabilization Exercises

Given that the stimulus for vestibular adaptation is a retinal slip during head movement, exercises to correct the retinal slip and thereby allow the image to remain clear on the retina while the head is in motion have been described by Herdman and

Table 34.1 Extraocular Muscles and Nystagmus Direction in BPPV Affecting Various Canals

Canal	Ipsilateral Extraocular Muscle	Contralateral Extraocular Muscle	Direction of Nystagmus
Posterior canal	Superior oblique (depression, in-torsion)	Inferior rectus (depression, out-torsion)	Upbeat torsional
Anterior canal	Superior rectus (elevation, in-torsion)	Inferior oblique (elevation, out-torsion)	Downbeat torsional
Horizontal canal	Medial rectus (adduction)	Lateral rectus (abduction)	Geotropic = toward ground Ageotropic = away from ground

Table 34.2 Vestibular Rehabilitation Plan for Vestibulo-ocular Gain Deficit

Impairment	Goal	Treatment Options
Decreased gaze stability, decreased gain of VOR, greater than two-line drop from static visual acuity to dynamic visual acuity on Snellen chart	Allow clear vision when head is in motion	Treatment options: × 1, × 2 viewing exercises, full field × 1, × exercises, preprogrammed saccades, begin with static positions on level progressing to unstable surfaces

Table 34.3 Vestibular Rehabilitation Plan for Static Postural Control Deficits

Impairment	Goal	Treatment Options
Decreased static balance/decreased sensory integration for balance, < 30-second timed trials on Clinical Test and Sensory Intergration and Balance (CTSIB), 5–6 pattern on CDP	Redistribute weighting of preferred balance strategy to use remaining vestibular function, ability to use ankle/hip/stepping strategy as necessary to regain balance without a fall, static balance performance to match age-related norms	Vary surface: firm, foam, uneven, inside, outside; vary lighting/visual inputs, busy environments; vary base of support; vary head position

Table 34.4 Vestibular Rehabilitation Plan for Decreased Dynamic Balance

Impairment	Goal	Treatment Options
Decreased dynamic balance/gait	Safe community ambulation with least restrictive device	Initiate gait without assistive device where safe as early as possible
<45/56 on Berg Balance Scale, < 19 on Dynamic Gait Index (DGI)	Fall risk reduction/prevention	Vary surface: firm, foam, uneven, inside, outside, incline, decline
		Incorporate horizontal and vertical head turns
		Incorporate turns, pivots, circles
		Incorporate eyes opened/closed/dim lighting
		Increase visual flow/complexity: walk in closed mall, open mall, sidewalk with and against traffic
		Incorporate Tai Chi exercise[16,17]

Table 34.5 Vestibular Rehabilitation Plan for General Deconditioning

Impairment	Goal	Treatment Options
General deconditioning	Normalize community mobility, increase aerobic capacity	Initiate aerobic exercise: walking, stationary bike as early as possible
Decreased strength		Progressive strengthening exercises
Decreased cardiovascular conditioning		

Table 34.6 Vestibular Rehabilitation Plan for Decreased Cervical Mobility

Impairment	Goal	Treatment Options
Decreased cervical mobility	Normalize cervical segmental mobility to enhance proprioceptive input from the cervical receptors	Soft tissue massage, cervical manual therapy (joint mobilizations/neuromuscular reeducation), postural reeducation, proprioceptive retraining exercises

Whitney.[66] These exercises are designed to improve the gain, or ratio of eye to head motion, of the vestibular system. In × 1 viewing exercises, a target is held at arm's length from the individual's eyes and in plane with the eyes. The subject focuses the eyes on the target, such as an "X" on the card, and moves the head side to side approximately 45 degrees in each direction. The exercise is also completed in a vertical or up-and-down motion. Varied speeds of head movement are employed to correlate with the various speeds of head movements incurred over the day.[67] Exercises are performed in the home and at work to replicate daily environments a subject may encounter.

In × 2 viewing exercises, the head and card are moved in opposite directions so that the card is held at arm's length and as the card moves to the right the subject's head moves to the left, all the while maintaining the focus of the eyes on the card. Again, the head movement is approximately 45 degrees to either side, and the speed and environment are varied to achieve the best outcomes in daily environments. It is important to induce oscillopsia, or the retinal slip, to provide the error signal to the brain to facilitate an improvement in gaze stability. Both × 1 and × 2 viewing exercises should be performed with a near, or arm's-length, target, and a far, or 8 to 10 feet, target. Exercises are progressed from sitting to standing, to standing with a narrowed base of support, to standing on foam or unstable surfaces, to walking.[6,8] Full field viewing is described as performing the × 1 or × exercises with a visually "busy" background such as placing the "X" on a checkerboard for a near target, or in front of a patterned curtain for a far target.

34.5 Benign Paroxysmal Positional Vertigo

34.5.1 Etiology and Presentation

Benign paroxysmal positional vertigo is the most common peripheral vestibular disorder, resulting in complaints of vertigo.[22–24] A study in which patients were considered to have BPPV only if they presented with nystagmus during a Dix-Hallpike test established an incidence of 10.7 per 100,000 population per year.[22] A study performed by Oghalai et al[25] found that 9% of community-dwelling elderly randomly tested were found to have undiagnosed BPPV, suggesting that BPPV may be more common than estimated. In approximately one third of individuals BPPV does not spontaneously resolve. Many individuals may experience chronic or recurrent BPPV lasting for weeks and sometimes years. New research developments, as well as an increased understanding of vestibular physiology and the pathophysiology of BPPV, has directed new treatment protocols and maneuvers for the specific semicircular canals involved.

Benign paroxysmal positional vertigo is usually idiopathic and occurs spontaneously; however, it may occur following head trauma or in conjunction with vestibular neuritis or labyrinthitis.[26–28] BPPV is characterized by a brief episode of vertigo associated with a change in position of the head relative to gravity. Common changes in head position that may provoke BPPV include rolling over in bed, sitting up, lying down, looking up, and bending over. Functional activities that may provoke vertigo include going to the dentist or the hair salon, gardening, and bending forward. Subjective complaints associated with BPPV include nausea, light-headedness, and disequilibrium. BPPV is often associated with decreased balance and postural control.[29–31] Individuals may experience decreased balance lasting for hours to days following an episode of BPPV. In a study performed by Ruckenstein,[32] residual symptoms of light-headedness or imbalance were found to persist 2 weeks after resolution of vertigo in 47% of cases.

34.5.2 General Treatment Considerations

Intervention is directed at restoring the normal mechanisms of the inner ear and resolving symptoms associated with BPPV. It is also important to regard the complications related to single or recurrent episodes of BPPV. BPPV may be benign; however, the secondary comorbidities may be devastating to an individual. Decreased understanding of the cause of an individual's symptoms often results in anxiety and depression. Anxiety and depression may result in social isolation, which further leads to generalized weakness and deconditioning. Generalized weakness and deconditioning contributes to faulty gait mechanics, decreased balance strategies, and fear of falling, increasing an individual's overall risk for falls. Indirectly, BPPV may result in a greater occurrence of falls than reported.

Consideration should be given to patient safety education, static and dynamic balance assessment, and fall prevention. Proper education may significantly reduce patients' level of anxiety as well as increase their safety. Understanding the mechanism of BPPV will also enable patients to better self-manage their condition. Falls are one of the leading causes of injury and morbidity in individuals over age 65. Proper balance assessment assists in identifying factors contributing to an individual's risk for falls, which will aid in fall prevention.

Decreased postural stability has been documented in BPPV with the use of CDP.[29–31] Posterior canal BPPV (PC-BPPV) results in an impairment of the vestibular system to maintain postural control and balance.[31] Modification of the posterior canal dynamics, secondary to free-floating otoconia, may affect proper excitation of vestibular afferents, resulting in abnormal vestibulospinal output.[33] Horizontal canal BPPV (HC-BPPV) has not been found to make significant deficits in postural control compared with that of PC-BPPV.[34,35] However, a study performed by White et al[35] showed postural abnormalities in 80% of patients with apogeotropic HC-BPPV.

Postural instability in the elderly may result in falls, especially when combined with secondary comorbidities such as neuropathy, visual impairments, and generalized weakness. Treatment of BPPV using the canalith repositioning maneuver and liberatory maneuver results in improved postural stability in patients with posterior canal BPPV.[29,30] Not all patients immediately revert to normal postural stability after resolving BPPV. Younger individuals are more likely to present with increased stability immediately posttreatment.[30] Assessment and treatment of balance deficits may be necessary to restore balance in the elderly population, as underlying comorbidities may complicate recovery.

34.5.3 Posterior Canal BPPV

Posterior canal BPPV is the most common variant; it is estimated that 94% of BPPV cases involve the posterior canal.[36] An episode of PC-BPPV is precipitated by a change in head position relative to gravity such as lying down, looking up, and bending forward. Nystagmus can be evoked by performing the Dix-Hallpike positional maneuver. Identifying the mechanism (cupulolithiasis versus canalithiasis) as well as the involved canal is the first step in selecting the appropriate treatment maneuver.

Schuknecht[37] was the first to suggest that deposits adhering to the cupula of the posterior canal caused the canal to become sensitive to gravity, resulting in BPPV (cupulolithiasis). Changes in head position result in deflection of the cupula and stimulation of the receptors. Cupulolithiasis is characterized by a sensation of vertigo accompanied by upbeat ipsi-directional (toward the downward ear) torsional nystagmus in the Dix-Hallpike test position. The characteristic nystagmus has a short latency with prolonged duration (>60 seconds) and should diminish somewhat with repeated testing. The prolonged duration of positional nystagmus suggests cupulolithiasis as the mechanism. However, we now know that cupulolithiasis is the less frequent type of BPPV encountered.

Further research suggested that otoconia detach from the utricle and fall into the posterior canal where they are free-floating in the endolymph.[38,39] Changes in head position result in movement of the otoconia through the canal, consequentially exciting the receptors and causing the canal to become gravity sensitive (canalithiasis). Canalithiasis is characterized by a brief sensation of vertigo accompanied by upbeat ipsi-directional (toward the downward ear) torsional nystagmus in the Dix-Hallpike test position. The characteristic nystagmus may occur after a latency of several seconds, which then fatigues rapidly after 10 to 45 seconds. The paroxysmal, short duration of nystagmus suggests canalithiasis as the pathological mechanism. Typically, reversal of nystagmus is seen when the patient returns to the sitting position. Nystagmus should diminish markedly with repeated testing.

If the nystagmus does not fatigue with repeated testing but remains constant in the affected position, or if the nystagmus and symptoms do not diminish with repeated testing, the patient should be tested for a central etiology.

34.5.4 Dix-Hallpike Test

The Dix-Hallpike maneuver is the standard test for diagnosis of BPPV.[40] If the Dix-Hallpike maneuver fails to reproduce vertigo and nystagmus, it should be repeated. Otoconial debris may collect in the lateral head-hanging position, resulting in a positive test on the second trial.[41] If there is no success at eliciting vertigo or nystagmus in the posterior semicircular canals, the horizontal semicircular canals should be tested. Lest positional testing fail to reveal nystagmus and associated symptoms at the time of examination, BPPV should not be ruled out, as it may have fatigued. The patient should be instructed on self-testing as well as home repositioning therapy.

To perform the Dix-Hallpike test, the patient is positioned sitting on the exam table. The head is rotated 45 degrees. The patient is rapidly brought straight back with the head extended approximately 20 degrees. Nystagmus is recorded as well as the patient's subjective complaints. The patient is then brought back into the sitting positioning with the head maintained at 45-degree rotation. Reversal of nystagmus is noted (▶ Fig. 34.1).[40]

34.6 Treatment

The canalith repositioning procedure (CRP) was initially described by Epley to treat BPPV. This procedure was designed to stimulate the migration of free-moving otoconia in the endolymph of the semicircular canal back into the utricle. This procedure is effective in the treatment of PC-BPPV, and was achieved by the use of timed head maneuvers as well as applied vibration.[39] This procedure has been modified to exclude routine vibration. Studies suggest that the modified canalith repositioning procedure is as effective in the treatment of PC-BPPV, and that vibration applied during the maneuver provides no additional benefit and does not affect outcomes.[42–44]

In CRP (▶ Fig. 34.2) the patient is moved rapidly into the Dix-Hallpike position toward the direction of the affected ear. The patient's head is then kept in extension and rotated in the opposite direction 45 degrees toward the unaffected ear. The patient is then rolled into a side-lying position with the head turned 45 degrees downward toward the floor. Keeping the head rotated toward the unaffected ear with the chin tucked in 20 degrees, the patient slowly returns to a seated position.

The Semont liberatory maneuver is also successful in the treatment of BPPV.[45] The patient is sitting and the head is turned 45 degrees toward the unaffected side. The patient is then moved rapidly into a side-lying position on the affected side. After 1 to 2 minutes the patient is rapidly moved to the opposite side, maintaining the head in 45 degrees of rotation. This position is maintained for 1 to 2 minutes. The patient is then slowly brought back to a sitting position.

The Brandt-Daroff exercise is aimed at habituation. The patient is sitting and the head is maintained in 45 degrees of rotation. The patient moves quickly into a side-lying position, face up, and holds it for 30 seconds. If vertigo is induced, the patient must wait until the vertigo subsides plus an additional 30 seconds. The patient then returns to a seated position for 30 seconds. The procedure is then repeated to the opposite side.[46]

A recent evidence-based review by White et al[47] reports that the treatment efficacy for a single canalith repositioning session for posterior semicircular canal BPPV is 78%. Treatment efficacy increases with repetition of the maneuver and reaches an average of 90%.

34.7 Lateral Semicircular Canal BPPV

Lateral semicircular canal BPPV (LSC-BPPV) is thought to be rarer than posterior canal involvement. It is estimated that 2 to 15% of BPPV cases involve the lateral canal.[46] An episode of LSC-BPPV is precipitated primarily by rolling over in bed, and can be evoked by right and left positional maneuvers performed by rolling the patient's head from side to side in the supine position. Performing supine positional testing, in adjunct to the standard Dix-Hallpike test, improves the sensitivity in the identification and diagnosis of HC-BPPV.[35] If the LSC is not tested, BPPV may not be diagnosed and appropriately treated.

Geotropic LSC-BPPV was documented by McClure[48] in 1985. In geotropic LSC-BPPV, ampullopetal flow is stimulated, resulting in nystagmus beating toward the undermost ear when the head is turned from supine to a lateral position (▶ Fig. 34.3). Nystagmus is induced by otoconial debris from the utricular macula moving through the LSC, exciting the receptors. It is characterized by a brief sensation of vertigo with short latency and prolonged duration, accompanied by purely horizontal nystagmus. Reversal of nystagmus is seen when the patient is turned to the opposite side and typically does not diminish with repeated testing. Nystagmus and associated symptoms are typically worse when the head is turned toward the affected ear.

Apogeotropic LSC-BPPV was later documented by Baloh et al[49] in 1995. In apogeotropic nystagmus, ampullofugal flow is stimulated, resulting in nystagmus beating away from the

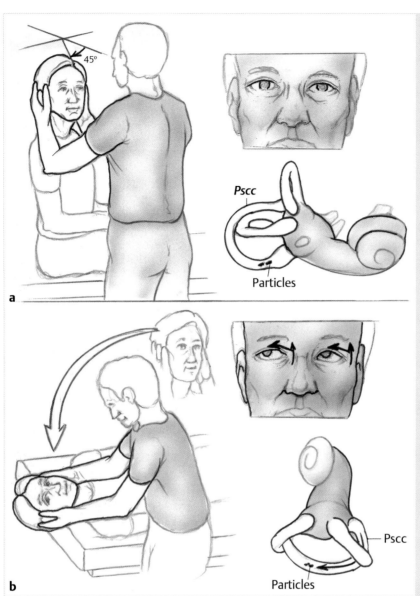

Fig. 34.1 (a,b) Dix-Hallpike positioning. PSCC, posterior semicircular canal.

undermost ear when the head is turned from a supine to a lateral position. Nystagmus is induced by otoconial debris adhering to the cupula, resulting in the cupula becoming gravity sensitive (► Fig. 34.4). Apogeotropic nystagmus may also be induced by the otoconial debris being trapped near the cupula, or proximal segment of the horizontal canal. Characteristics for apogeotropic LSC-BPPV are similar to geotropic LSC-BPPV; however, nystagmus is long lasting and beats away from the undermost ear. Nystagmus and associated symptoms are typically worse when the head is turned away from the affected ear. The apogeotropic variant is also more resistant to repositioning maneuvers. A study performed by White et al[47] utilized a combination of techniques for the treatment of apogeotropic LSC-BPPV with only a 50% success rate.

Identifying the involved ear is the first step in choosing the appropriate treatment for LSC-BPPV. The patient is lying supine with the head placed in approximately 20 degrees of flexion. The head is then turned to a lateral position. The direction and

degree of nystagmus is noted. The patient's head is then turned to the opposite side and reversal of nystagmus is noted. If the patient lacks appropriate cervical mobility, the patient should be rolled into a side-lying position to increase sensitivity of the test.

34.8 Treatment

34.8.1 Baloh-Lempert 360-Degree Roll

The treatment of choice for geotropic LSC-BPPV is the 360-degree barbeque roll maneuver. The maneuver starts with the patient in the supine position with the head flexed 0 to 30 degrees and consists of three 90-degree head rotations toward the unaffected ear. Each position is held for 30 to 60 seconds. The procedure may be repeated several times to promote the migration of free-moving otoconia in the endolymph of the horizontal canal back into the utricle. This procedure is effective in the

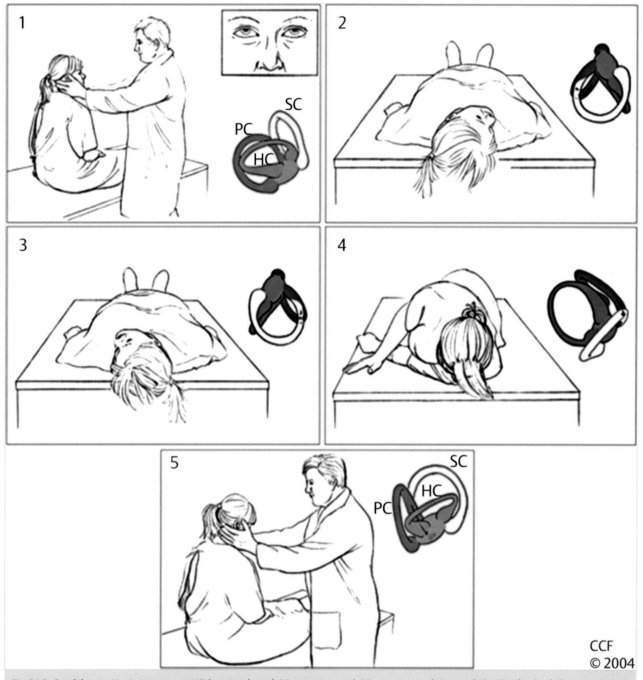

Fig. 34.2 Canalith repositioning maneuver. HC, horizontal canal; PC, posterior canal; SC, superior canal. (Copyright by The Cleveland Clinic Foundation. All rights reserved.)

treatment of LSC-BPPV and often results in the rapid cessation of positional vertigo and nystagmus.[35,50–52]

34.8.2 Vannucci-Asprella Maneuver

The patient begins in the sitting position on the exam table and is quickly moved into the supine position. Then the patient's head is quickly rotated toward the unaffected side. Maintaining cervical rotation, the patient is returned to the sitting position and the head is returned to midline. This is rapidly repeated five to eight times.[32] This procedure has been reported to be effective in relieving symptoms in 75 to 90% of patients with geotropic LSC-BPPV.[51,53–55]

The Vannucci-Asprella maneuver is also used in converting apogeotropic to geotropic LSC-BPPV. The procedure is used to attempt to detach or mobilize the otoconia from near the cupula in the posterior portion of the lateral canal.[54,55] Quick head thrusts away from affected ear may also mobilize the otoconia to the posterior portion of the canal.

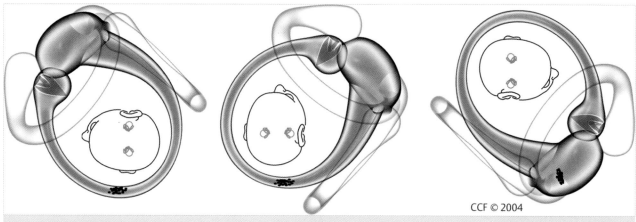

Fig. 34.3 Geotropic lateral canal BPPV. (Copyright by The Cleveland Clinic Foundation. All rights reserved.)

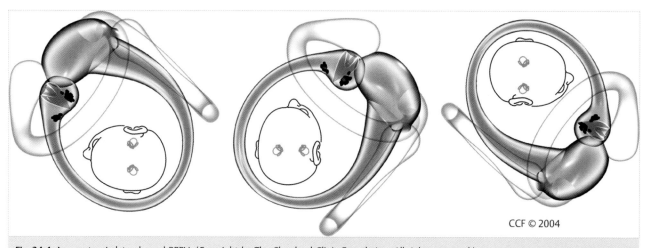

Fig. 34.4 Apogeotropic lateral canal BPPV. (Copyright by The Cleveland Clinic Foundation. All rights reserved.)

34.8.3 Gufoni Maneuver

The patient begins in the sitting position and is rapidly brought into the side-lying position toward the affected side in apogeotropic LSC-BPPV or toward the unaffected side in geotropic LSC-BPPV. The patient's head is then rotated 45 degrees downward for the treatment of geotropic LSC-BPPV or 45 degrees upward for the treatment of apogeotropic LSC-BPPV. This position is maintained for 2 to 3 minutes. Appiani et al[56] reported a success rate of 78% on the first trial and 100% with a repeated maneuver in patients with geotropic LSC-BPPV. This maneuver has also been found to be effective in the conversion of apogeotropic LSC-BPPV to geotropic.[54,57]

34.8.4 Modified Brandt Daroff Exercises

Habituation exercise is utilized if there is failure to resolve LSC-BPPV with canalith repositioning maneuver. The patient begins in the sitting position, keeping the head straight throughout the procedure, and rapidly lies down toward the affected ear. The patient remains in this position for 30 seconds after the vertigo stops and then repeats this procedure toward the opposite ear.[46]

34.8.5 Forced Prolonged Positioning

The patient is placed in the side-lying position on the unaffected side. This position is maintained for 12 hours to rid the horizontal semicircular canal of otoconial debris. A study performed by Vannucchi et al[58] found this to be effective in 90% of the patients.

34.9 Anterior Semicircular Canal BPPV

Anterior canal BPPV is a rare, little-known entity. There may be strong paroxysmal downbeat nystagmus in head-hanging positioning.[59,60] However, 75% of patients with this finding have explanatory central pathology, so this remains a diagnosis of exclusion. Paroxysmal downbeat nystagmus with a torsional component toward the affected side has been described in both contralateral[36] and ipsilateral[61,62] Dix-Hallpike positioning. This is explained by the gravitational movement of canaliths away from the ampulla during positioning that stimulates paroxysmal torsional downbeat nystagmus toward the affected ear. However, fluid dynamics may be complicated by the shared

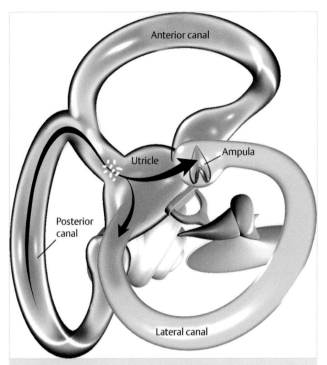

Fig. 34.5 Conversion of posterior to lateral canal BPPV. (Copyright by The Cleveland Clinic Foundation. All rights reserved.)

common crus, and some authors suggest considering the vertical canals (anterior and posterior) as a conjoint entity.

Numerous therapeutic maneuvers have been described for anterior canal BPPV, including a deep Dix-Hallpike to the ipsilateral or contralateral side with return to the sitting position,[63, 64] the modified Semont maneuver beginning with the nose down on the affected side,[62] and the Epley maneuver performed on the contralateral side.[36,41] Because the left anterior and right posterior semicircular canals are coplanar (and similarly the right anterior and left posterior), Dix Hallpike and canalith repositioning maneuvers are performed on the right side for left anterior canal involvement, and vice versa.

34.10 Complications and Recurrence

Complications associated with treatment of BPPV include the conversion of otoconial debris from one canal to another (▶ Fig. 34.5), combined posterior and horizontal canal BPPV, as well as recurrence of BPPV.[61,65]

34.11 Conclusion

The evidence basis of vestibular assessment and outcomes of vestibular rehabilitation is rapidly expanding.[5–8,18] Recent publications substantiate a decreased fall risk and improved dynamic visual acuity after vestibular rehabilitation.[7,19–21] Newer treatment approaches are attempting to enhance dynamic balance strategies in lifelike situations.[15] Although research in the area of dynamic balance recovery after vestibular insult is ongoing, challenges remain due to the complex multisystem contributions to balance.[16,22]

References

[1] Shumway-Cook A, Horak FB. Assessing the influence of sensory interaction on balance: Suggestion from the field. Phys Ther 1986; 66: 1548–-1550

[2] Shumway-Cook A, Woollacot M. Motor Control Theory and Practical Applications. Baltimore: Williams & Wilkins, 1995

[3] Berg KO, Wood-Dauphinee SL, Williams JI, Gayton DB. Measuring balance in the elderly. Physiotherapy Canada. 1989; 41: 304–311

[4] Podsiadlo D, Richardson S. The timed "up & go": a test of basic functional mobility for frail elderly persons. J Am Geriatr Soc 1991; 39: 142–148

[5] Wrisley D, Marchetti G, Kuharsky D, Whitney S. Reliability, internal consistency, and Validity of data obtained with the functional gait assessment. Phys Ther 2004; 84: 906–918

[6] Hall CD, Schubert MC, Herdman SJ. Prediction of fall risk reduction as measured by dynamic gait index in individuals with unilateral vestibular hypofunction. Otol Neurotol 2004; 25: 746–751

[7] Macias JD, Masingale S, Gerkin RD. Efficacy of vestibular rehabilitation therapy in reducing falls Otolaryngol Head Neck Surg 2005; 133: 323–325

[8] Whitney SL, Marchetti GF, Schade A, Wrisley DM. The sensitivity and specificity of the timed "up and go" and the dynamic gait index for self-reported falls in persons with vestibular disorders. J Vestib Res 2004; 14: 397–409

[9] Fitz-Ritson D. Assessment of cervicogenic vertigo. J Manipulative Physiol Ther 1991; 14: 193–198

[10] Jacobson GP, Newman CW. The development of the Dizziness Handicap Inventory. Arch Otolaryngol Head Neck Surg 1990; 116: 424–427

[11] Powell LE, Meyers AM. The Activities-specific Balance Confidence (ABC) Scale. J Gerontol A Bil Sci Med Sci 1995;50:M28–M34

[12] Cohen HS, Kimball KT, Adams AS. Application of the vestibular disorders activities of daily living scale. Laryngoscope 2000; 110: 1204–1209

[13] Zee DS. Adaptation to vestibular disturbances: some clinical implications. Acta Neurol Belg 1991; 91: 97–104

[14] Herdman SJ. Vestibular Rehabilitation. Philadelphia: F.A. Davis, 1994

[15] Sparto PJ, Whitney SL, Hodges LF, Furman JM, Redfern MS. Simulator sickness when performing gaze shifts within a wide field of view optic flow environment: preliminary evidence for using virtual reality in vestibular rehabilitation. J Neuroengineering Rehabil 2004; 1: 14

[16] McGibbon CA, Krebs , DE , Wolf , SL . et al Tai Chi and vestibular rehabilitation improve vestibulopathic gait via different neuromuscular mechanisms. Preliminary Report. BMC Neurol 2005; 5: 3

[17] McGibbon CA, Krebs DE, Wolf SL, Wayne PM, Scarborough DM, Parker SW. Tai Chi and vestibular rehabilitation effects on gaze and whole body stability J Vestib Res 2004; 14: 467–478

[18] Herdman SJ, Schubert MC, Tusa RJ. Strategies for balance rehabilitation: fall risk and treatment. Ann N Y Acad Sci 2001; 942: 394–412

[19] Badke MB, Shea TH, Miedaner JA, Grove CR. Outcomes after rehabilitation for adults with balance dysfunction. Arch Phys Med Rehabil 2004; 85: 227–233

[20] Herdman SJ, Schubert MC, Das VE, Tusa RJ. Recovery of dynamic visual acuity in unilateral vestibular hypofunction. Arch Otolaryngol Head Neck Surg 2003; 129: 819–824

[21] Cavanaugh JT, Goldvasser , D , McGibbon , CA , Krebs , DE . Comparison of head and body velocity trajectories during locomotion among healthy and vestibulopathic subjects . J Rehabil Res Dev 2005; 42: 191–198

[22] Mizukoshi K, Watanabe Y, Shojaku H et al. Epidemiological studies on benign paroxysmal positional vertigo in Japan. Acta Otolaryngol Suppl 1988; 447: 67–72

[23] Hotson JR, Baloh RW. Acute vestibular syndrome. N Engl J Med 1998; 339: 680–685

[24] Froehling DA, Silverstein MD, Mohr DN et al. BPPV: incidence and prognosis in a population based study in Olmsted County, Minnesota. Mayo Clin Proc 1991; 66: 596–601

[25] Oghalai JS, Manolidis S, Barth JL et al. Unrecognized benign paroxysmal positional vertigo in elderly patients. Otolaryngol Head Neck Surg 2000; 122: 630–634

[26] Bertholon P, Chelikh L, Timoshenko A et al. Combined horizontal and posterior canal benign paroxysmal positional vertigo in three patients with head trauma. Ann Otol Rhinol Laryngol 2005; 114: 105–110

[27] Baloh RW, Honrubia V, Jacobson K. Benign positional vertigo: clinical and oculographic features in 240 cases. Neurology 1987; 37: 371–378

[28] Pagnini P, Nuti D, Vannucchi P. Benign paroxysmal vertigo of the horizontal canal. ORL J Otorhinolaryngol Relat Spec 1989; 51: 161–170

[29] Di Girolamo S, Paludetti G, Briglia G et al. Postural control in benign paroxysmal positional vertigo before and after recovery. Acta Otolaryngol 1998; 118: 289–293

[30] Blatt PJ, Georgakakis GA, Herdman SJ et al. The effect of the canalith repositioning maneuver on resolving postural instability in patients with benign paroxysmal positional vertigo. Am J Otol 2000; 21: 356–363

[31] Black FO, Nashner LM. Postural disturbances in patients with benign paroxysmal positional nystagmus. Ann Otol Rhinol Laryngol 1984; 93: 595–599

[32] Ruckenstein MJ. Therapeutic efficacy of the epley canalith repositioning maneuver. Laryngoscope 2001; 111: 940–945

[33] Katsarkas A, Kearney R. Postural disturbances in paroxysmal positional vertigo. Am J Otol 1990; 11: 444–446

[34] Di Girolamo S, Ottaviani F, Scarano E et al. Postural control in horizontal benign paroxysmal positional vertigo. Eur Arch Otorhinolaryngol. 2000; 257: 372–375

[35] White J, Coale K, Catalano P et al. Diagnosis and management of lateral semicircular canal benign paroxysmal positional vertigo. Otolaryngol Head Neck Surg 2005; 133: 278–284

[36] Honrubia V, Baloh RW, Harris MR et al. Paroxysmal positional vertigo syndrome. Am J Otol 1999; 20: 465–470

[37] Schuknecht HF. Cupulolithiasis. Arch Otolaryngol 1969; 90: 765–778

[38] Hall SF, Ruby RR, McClure JA. The mechanism of benign paroxysmal vertigo. J Otolaryngol 1979; 8: 151–158

[39] Epley J. The canalith repositioning procedure: for treatment of benign paroxysmal positional vertigo. Otolaryngol Head Neck Surg 1992; 107: 399–404

[40] Dix MR, Hallpike CS. Pathology, symptoms and diagnosis of certain disorders of the vestibular system. Proc R Soc Med 1952; 45: 341–354

[41] Viirre E, Purcell I, Baloh RW. The Dix Hallpike test and the canalith repositioning manever. Laryngoscope 2005; 115: 184–187

[42] Hain TC, Helminski JO, Ries IL, Uddin MK. Vibration does not improve results of the canalith repositioning procedure. Arch Otolaryngol Head Neck Surg 2000; 126: 617–622

[43] Wolf JS. Boyey KP, Manokey BJ, Mattox DE. Success of the modified Epley maneuver in treating benign paroxysmal positional vertigo. Laryngoscope 1999; 109: 900–903

[44] Macias JD, Ellensohn A, Massingale S, Gerkin R. Vibration with the canalith repositioning maneuver: a prospective randomized study to determine efficacy. Laryngoscope 2004; 114: 1011–1014

[45] Semont A, Freyss G, Vitte E. Curing the BPPV with a liberatory maneuver. Adv Otorhinolaryngol 1988; 42: 290–293

[46] Herdman SJ, Tusa RJ. Assessment and treatment of patients with benign paroxysmal positional vertigo. In: Vestibular Rehabilitation. Philadelphia: FA Davis, 2000:451–475

[47] White J, Savvides P, Cherian N et al. Canalith repositioning for benign paroxysmal positional vertigo. Otol Neurotol 2005; 26: 704–710

[48] McClure JA. Horizontal canal BPV. J Otolaryngol 1985; 14: 30–35

[49] Baloh RW, Yue Q, Jacobson K et al. Persistent direction changing positional nystagmus. Neurology 1995; 45: 1297–1301

[50] Lempert T, Tiel-Wilck K. A positional maneuver for treatment of horizontal canal benign positional vertigo. Laryngoscope 1996; 106: 476–478

[51] Ciniglio Appiani G, Gagliardi M, Magliulo G. Physical treatment of horizontal canal benign positional vertigo. Eur Arch Otorhinolaryngol 1997; 254: 326–328

[52] Lempert T. Horizontal benign positional vertigo. Neurology 1994; 44: 2213–2214

[53] Asprella Libonati G, Gagliardi G, Cifarelli D, Larotonda G. Step by step treatment of lateral semicircular canal canolithiasis under videonystagmoscopic examination. Acta Otorhinolaryngol Ital 2003; 23: 10–15

[54] Casani AP, Vannucci G, Fattori B, Berrettini S. The treatment of horizontal canal positional vertigo: our experience in 66 cases. Laryngoscope 2002; 112: 172–178

[55] Vannucchi P, Asprella Libonati G, Gufoni M. Therapy of lateral semicircular canal canalithiasis. Audiological Med 2005; 3: 52–56

[56] Appiani GC, Catania G, Gargliardi M. A liberatory maneuver for the treatment of horizontal canal paroxysmal positional vertigo. Otol Neurotol 2001; 22: 66–69

[57] Appiani GC, Catania G, Gagliardi M et al. Repositioning maneuver for the treatment of the apogeotropic variant of horizontal canal benign paroxysmal positional vertigo. Otol Neurotol 2005; 26: 257–260

[58] Vannucchi P, Giannoni B, Pagnini P. Treatment of horizontal semicircular canal benign paroxysmal positional vertigo. J Vestib Res 1997; 7: 1–6

[59] Bertholon P, Bronstein AM, Davies RA, Rudge P, Thilo KV. Positional down beating nystagmus in 50 patients: cerebellar disorders and possible anterior semicircular canalithiasis. J Neurol Neurosurg Psychiatry 2002; 72: 366–372

[60] Crevits L. Treatment of anterior canal benign paroxysmal positional vertigo by a prolonged forced position procedure. J Neurol Neurosurg Psychiatry 2004; 75: 779–781

[61] Herdman SJ, Tusa RJ. Complications of the canalith repositioning procedure. Arch Otolaryngol Head Neck Surg 1996; 122: 281–286

[62] Brantberg K, Bergenius J. Treatment of anterior benign paroxysmal positional vertigo by canal plugging: a case report. Acta Otolaryngol 2002; 122: 28–30

[63] Semont A. BPPV, the liberatory maneuvers. In: Guidetti G, Pagnini P, eds. Labyrintholithiasis-related paroxysmal positional vertigo. Milan: Elsevier (Excerpta Medica), 2002

[64] Kim YK, Shin JE, Chung JW. The effect of canalith repositioning for anterior semicircular canal canalithiasis. ORL J Otorhinolaryngol Relat Spec 2005; 67: 56–60

[65] White JA, Oas JG. Diagnosis and management of lateral semicircular canal conversions during particle repositioning therapy. Laryngoscope 2005; 115: 1895–1897

[66] Herdman SJ, Whitney SL. Treatment of vestibular hypofunction. In: Herdman SJ, ed. Vestibular Rehabilitation (Contemporary Perspectives in Rehabilitation), 2nd ed. Philadelphia: F.A. Davis, 2000:387–423.

[67] Herdman, SJ. Role of vestibular adaptation in vestibular rehabilitation. Otolaryngol Head Neck Surg 1998:119:49–54.

[68] Tee LH, Chee NWC. Vestibular rehabilitation therapy for the dizzy patient. Ann Acad Med Singapore 2005;34(4):289–294.

35 Rehabilitation and Reanimation of the Paralyzed Face

David B. Hom

35.1 Introduction

Facial nerve paralysis is a significant functional and disfiguring deficit. It results from trauma, infection, tumor ablation, and Bell palsy. The facial nerve is one of the most commonly injured cranial nerves because of its long anatomic path from the brainstem to the facial musculature. The site of injury along the nerve's path determines the type of neurologic deficit seen clinically.

Facial paralysis impedes the normal facial functions for blinking, speaking, drinking, articulation, and nasal breathing (▶ Fig. 35.1).

In addition to giving voluntary facial movement, the facial nerve conveys facial expression. Specifically, emotions for fear, anger, happiness, and sadness are conveyed by facial expression from the facial nerve. This is important for communication and social interaction in humans.[1] Thus, facial paralysis also significantly compromises the ability to express oneself emotionally in society. Patients with facial paralysis frequently avoid appearing in family photos and avoid social functions, because they are embarrassed by their reduced nonverbal self-expression and worry that they will make others uncomfortable. These factors can lead to social isolation and hinder patients' interaction in society and the workplace. This chapter discusses the fundamentals of facial nerve injury and surgical methods to improve facial function of a paralyzed face.

35.2 Facial Nerve Anatomy

The facial nerve consists of sensory and motor nerve fibers. The facial nerve originates from the brainstem and takes a circuitous course through the temporal bone. It branches into the greater superficial petrosal nerve, giving taste to the upper palate, and tearing; the chorda tympani, giving taste to the tongue; and to the salivary submaxillary glands, with the main trunk exiting the stylomastoid foramen. The type of deficit seen depends on the area of the topographical nerve that is injured or transected (▶ Fig. 35.2).

As the facial nerve exits the stylomastoid foramen, most of the sensory nerve fibers have left the main trunk with the remaining fibers being motor. The cell body of each motor neuron originates at the brainstem, and this myelinated axon travels a circuitous course through the temporal bone. At the level of the stylomastoid foramen, the nerve has 6 to 10 fascicles with their topographical cross-sectional location debated.[2] The main branches of the facial nerve (temporal, zygomatic, buccal, mandibular, and cervical) can have various anatomic variations. ▶ Fig. 35.3 schematically shows these anatomic variations of the facial nerve branch patterns.[3]

Beyond the pes anserine, the multiple nerve branch interconnections between the divisions are most pronounced between the zygomatic and buccal branches. These nerve branch connections in this region help explain why midface muscle mobility remains when peripheral facial nerve injury occurs at this site and why aberrant nerve regeneration occurs more frequently during recovery (synkinesis) in this region. As the facial nerve branches travel more distally beyond a vertical axis line from the lateral canthus of the eye, many smaller nerve branches arborize. Thus, a laceration through the facial nerves medial to this vertical axis line at the lateral canthus usually does not require nerve repair.

In regard to the depth of the facial nerve, as it exits the stylomastoid foramen it remains underneath the superficial musculoaponeurotic system (SMAS). One of the most vulnerable areas

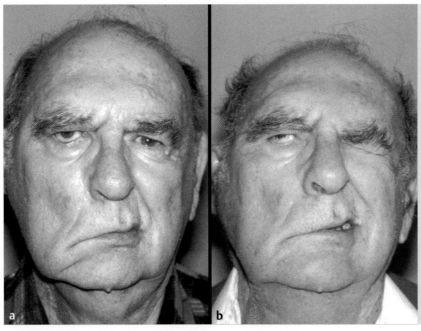

Fig. 35.1 A 65-year-old man with full facial paralysis in resting state (a) and attempting to close an eye with grimacing (b) following facial nerve sacrifice after tumor ablation.

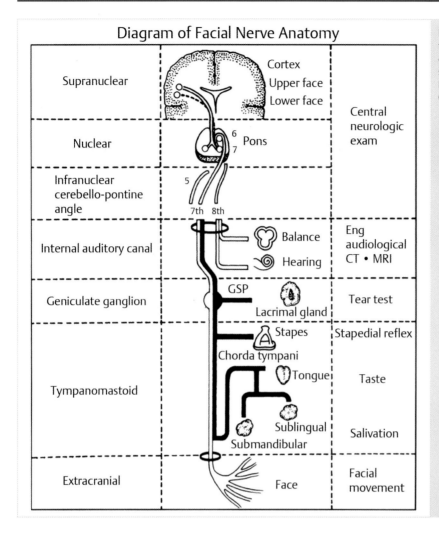

Diagram of Facial Nerve Anatomy

Fig. 35.2 Peripheral facial nerve path with its topographic distribution of functions. GSP, greater superficial petrosal. (Used with permission from May M, Fria TJ, Blumenthal F, et al. Facial paralysis in children: differential diagnosis. Otolaryngol Head Neck Surg 1981;89:841–848.)

of the facial nerve injury on the face is the frontal branch as it crosses over the middle third of the zygomatic arch. ▶ Fig. 35.4 shows anatomic locations of the facial nerve branches with respect to orientation and depth. The facial nerve innervates 23 paired muscles and one single muscle, the orbicularis oris (▶ Fig. 35.5).

35.3 Physiology of Facial Nerve Injury

When the facial nerve is injured, distinct histological and biochemical changes occur in the proximal nerve cell body, distal injured nerve, motor end plate, and muscle fibers. The degrees of these changes are secondary to the type of injury, patient age, nutritional status, soft tissue environment, and the distance the injury occurred from the injured cell body.[4]

During complete nerve transection, the neuron cell body undergoes marked metabolic changes in attempting to reestablish connections. Over a 3-week period, the cell body is converted into a regenerative state with increased protein and RNA synthesis. In the past, this has led to some clinicians advocating waiting 3 weeks before performing nerve repair or nerve grafting. However, now it is believed that the repair should be done as soon as possible. The proximal injured nerve stump begins to

sprout, growing peripherally at a rate of 1 to 3 mm per day. For example, nerve injury in the temporal bone will approximately require 140 days to travel 14 cm to the facial musculature.[5] In the distal nerve segment, wallerian degeneration occurs as the Schwann cells proliferate and transform into macrophages. These macrophages phagocytose the myelin and axon by-products. At the same time, the distal nerve and the motor endplates at the neuromuscular junction wait for the proximal nerve to grow into it.

During the nerve healing process, Schwann cells begin to proliferate, forming Bunger bands, which can be seen histologically waiting for the proximal nerve axon to grow into it for up to 2 years. ▶ Fig. 35.6 shows the degrees of nerve injury as classified by Sunderland. If no axons grow into the distal transected endoneural tubule after 2 years, the distal endoneural tubule disintegrates and scarring will occur at the neuromuscular junction. Thereafter, anastomosis of the peripheral nerve at this point would be futile.

It is important to note that a transected distal nerve can conduct nerve impulses up to 72 hours after injury; thus, it can be clinically electrically excitable up to this time period. For this reason, nerve repair of a transected nerve during this time interval is much easier to perform as the surgeon can more accurately identify the distal segment using the nerve stimulator. Even if nerve repair will have to be done at a later time, the

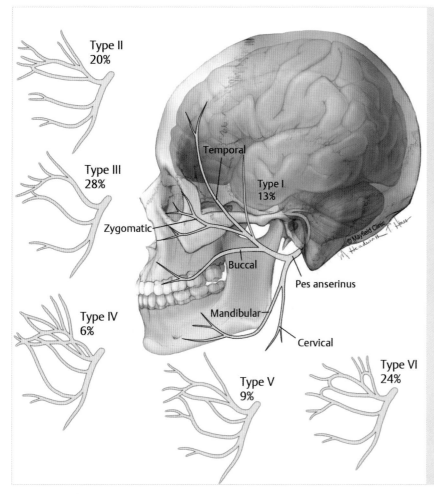

Fig. 35.3 In 90% of anatomic dissections, the facial nerve at the pes anserine divides into two major branches. In 6% of dissections, a pes trifurcation of nerve branches is present. (Adapted with permission from Davis RA, Budinger JM, Kurth LR. Surgical anatomy of the facial nerve and parotid gland based upon a study of 350 cervical facial halves. Surg Gynecol Obstet 1956;102:385–412.)

distal nerve can still be tagged with a colored nonabsorbable suture for later identification. For these reasons, early exploration within 3 days is recommended when acute nerve transection occurs.

35.4 Facial Muscle Degeneration

After denervation, the facial muscles follow a comparable physiological course to other muscles of the body. During the first month, the muscle fiber diameter progressive decreases to one half of the original diameter. A major question when performing a nerve graft or nerve transfer procedure is if the facial muscle is still capable of receiving reinnervation. If irreversible fibrosis at the motor endplate from muscle atrophy has occurred, then facial muscle reinnervation methods would be unsuccessful. A useful way to determine the status of the facial muscles is through electromyography.[6] If additional information is needed, a muscle biopsy can be performed to detect the presence of viable muscle.

35.5 Degrees of Facial Nerve Injury and Muscle Degeneration

Facial nerve paralysis can be classified by the degree of anatomic nerve disruption as described by Sunderland. With this classification, the different degrees of peripheral nerve injury correlate with the anatomic layers of the peripheral nerve that were injured.[7,8] This can be helpful to predict its prognostic recovery. When the facial nerve is paralyzed, the terms *neurapraxia, axonotmesis,* and *neurotmesis* are useful to describe its injured state. In each of these degrees of facial nerve injury, clinical facial paralysis is evident; however, depending on the degree of injury, the prognosis for recovery is different.

First-degree peripheral nerve injury (neurapraxia) is the least injured state of a paralyzed nerve. Neurapraxia is often described as "a bruised nerve." This state of nerve injury has an excellent prognosis, with recovery within a month. The nerve state displays a physiological nerve conduction blockade from myelin sheath injury. The nerve can still be electrically stimulated externally because the structural integrity of the nerve remains intact.

Axonotmesis is the next degree of peripheral nerve injury where disintegration of the axon has occurred with the endoneural tube remaining intact. Over time, as the proximal axon continues to elongate, it continues to grow into the distal endoneural tube.

Further degrees of nerve injury involve damage to the endoneural sheath and perineural sheath. It is important to note that once the endoneural tubule has been disrupted, the proximal nerve may sprout into other distal endoneural tubules, resulting in aberrant circuitry of the peripheral nerve, in turn resulting in synkinesis.

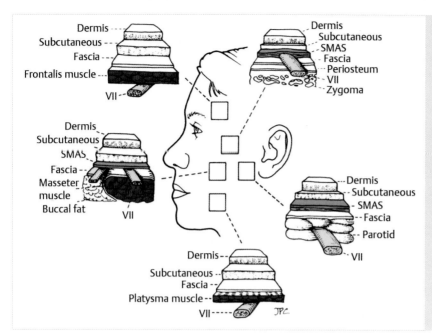

Fig. 35.4 Depth of main facial nerve branches with respect to the SMAS and facial muscles. (Used with permission from May M, Sobol S, Mester S. Managing segmental facial nerve injuries by surgical repair. Laryngoscope 1990;100:1062–1067.)

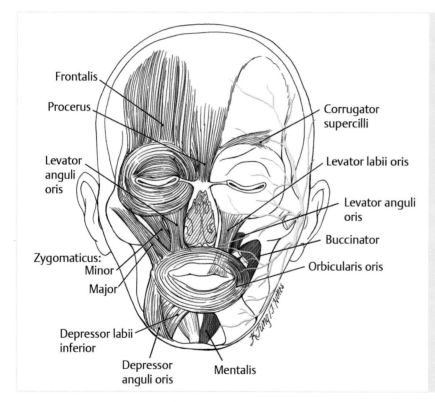

Fig. 35.5 Facial muscles with respect to the facial nerve. All but three muscles for facial expression lie superficial to branches of the facial nerve; the exceptions are the mentalis, buccinator, and levator anguli oris.

The highest degree of nerve injury is complete transection of the nerve, which is called neurotmesis. Because the epineurium (outer nerve sheath) is damaged, the regenerating proximal nerves sprout outside the nerve sheath, forming neuromas. A permanent neurologic deficit will result if it is not repaired or reinnervated. After many months, if a regenerating nerve reaches a different facial muscle motor endplate, abnormal innervations will result in uncoordinated facial movement (synkinesis). An example of this clinical state is when a patient attempts to close his eyes, his mouth also moves.

35.6 Diagnostic Tests to Determine Degree of Nerve Injury

When a patient presents with chronic facial nerve paralysis of unknown etiology, a computed axial tomography (CAT) scan of the temporal bone and parotid gland should be strongly considered. Another option in evaluating the parotid gland instead of a CAT scan is to perform a magnetic resonance imaging (MRI) scan of the parotid gland to search for lesions causing the facial paralysis.

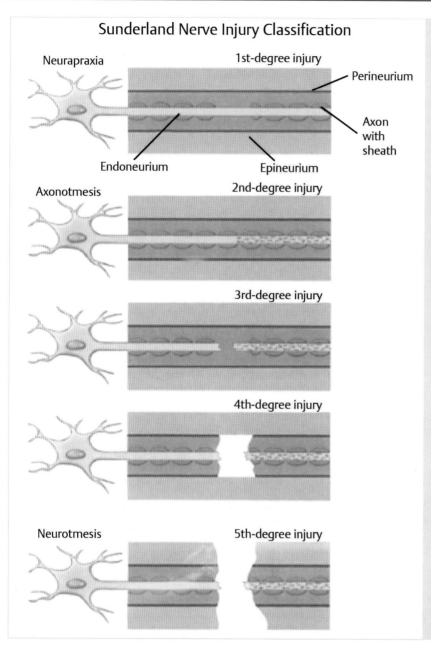

Sunderland Nerve Injury Classification

Neurapraxia — 1st-degree injury

Perineurium

Axon with sheath

Endoneurium — Epineurium

Axonotmesis — 2nd-degree injury

3rd-degree injury

4th-degree injury

Neurotmesis — 5th-degree injury

Fig. 35.6 Degrees of nerve injury are classified by Sunderland. (Used with permission from Campbell WW. Evaluation and management of peripheral nerve injury. Clin Neurophysiol 2008;119:1951–1965.)

Electrical diagnostic tests are helpful only if the nerve in question is in a complete paralysis state (no voluntary clinical movement). If the nerve shows any voluntary movement, electrical diagnostic tests are not useful. If the facial nerve paralysis has lasted over 1 year, electromyography (EMG) is very useful, as it can help determine what healing state the distal endoneural tubule of the facial nerve is in.[4] EMG findings of the injured facial nerve can show the following: normal action potentials, indicating that the nerve is intact; polyphasic action potentials, indicating that the nerve is attempting to recover; fibrillation potentials, indicating that the distal nerve is degenerating; and electrical silence, indicating that the distal nerve has degenerated or scarring has occurred at the motor endplate.

When a peripheral nerve shows fibrillation on EMG, disintegration of the muscle is occurring, with the distal endoneural tubule waiting for the proximal axon segment to grow into it. This nerve state is the best time to perform a nerve anastomosis procedure to try to restore the peripheral nerve. However, if the EMG shows electrical silence, either denervation muscular atrophy or endoneural tubule disintegration has occurred. If polyphasic action potentials are seen, reinnervation may be occurring and some facial movements may return over several months. Thus, with this finding, nerve reanimation procedures should be postponed. It should be emphasized that the single most useful prognostic indicator is voluntary facial movement on clinical exam. If voluntary movement persists or reappears within the first 3 weeks after nerve injury, the prognosis for a satisfactory recovery is good.

35.7 Anatomy and Function of Facial Muscles

35.7.1 Periorbital Region

The orbicularis oculi muscle is the key muscle for eyelid closure for corneal protection and blinking. The major movement during eyelid closure comes from the upper eyelid, with the lower eyelid moving slightly. The ability to close the eye rapidly and spontaneously is a major protective mechanism to protect the cornea and to spread the tears to maximize eye lubrication. The frontalis muscle is important in maintaining the eyebrow position and preventing ptosis of the brow, which can cause visual field impairment on superior gaze.

35.7.2 Perioral Region

The perioral muscles are important for maintaining upper and lower lip competence as a sphincteric action for mastication and speech. The facial expression of smiling is important in social interaction. The main muscle for controlling the oral sphincter is the orbicularis oris muscle. The major muscles affecting the corner of the mouth are the zygomaticus major and, to a lesser degree, the zygomaticus minor muscle (▶ Fig. 35.5).[9]

Smiles can be classified into three patterns: the "Mona Lisa" smile (in 67% of people), showing subtle elevation of the upper lip when the corners of the lip move laterally and superiorly; the "canine" smile (31%), showing a more superior elevation of the upper lip; and the "full denture" smile (2%), demonstrating more exposure of the upper teeth.

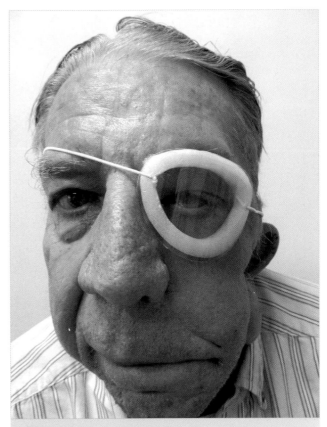

Fig. 35.7 Eye patch moisture chamber with an elastic strap to give comfort to the affected dry eye.

35.8 Medical Management of Facial Paralysis

Besides determining the etiology of the facial paralysis, maintaining protective eye care is crucial in patients with facial paralysis. If the cornea becomes scratched, it can lead to keratitis, ulceration, and later to blindness if not managed. Eye protective measures include an eye ointment at night and nonpreservative eyedrops every 2 to 3 hours during the day. Eye patch moisture chamber shields with an elastic strap add comfort to the affected dry eye and are very helpful to the patient (▶ Fig. 35.7). In addition, contact lenses, and Lacrisert (Merck & Co., Whitehouse Station, NJ) and hydroxypropyl cellulose ophthalmic insert may be beneficial in keeping the cornea moist. Sunglasses that curve around the temples or with side protector are also very helpful when it is windy outside.

35.8.1 Facial Reanimation and Timing of Surgical Treatment

The surgical goals for restoring facial function from facial paralysis are to achieve (1) facial symmetry at rest; (2) facial symmetry with voluntary motion; (3) separate and selective function of individual muscle groups; and (4) spontaneous facial motion during emotional expression.[4] Currently, no surgical procedure can achieve all of these goals. Also, no single surgical procedure is suitable for all patients. Thus, the surgical management of facial paralysis is tailored to the type of nerve injury and the goals of the patient.[10,11]

Surgical treatment strategies for facial nerve paralysis are based on the length of time of nerve paralysis and the site of injury. The timing for surgical repair of facial paralysis can be classified as immediate (0 to 3 weeks), delayed (> 3 weeks to 2 years), and late (> 2 years). Depending on these time periods, the optimal method to reanimate the facial paralysis can be determined. The importance of classifying such injuries is that procedures that involve nerve-to-nerve reattachment are usually most successful when performed within 2 years of injury, because after 2 years denervation muscular atrophy has likely occurred, preventing future reinnervations. In this circumstance, other surgical techniques such as muscular slings are required for facial movement.

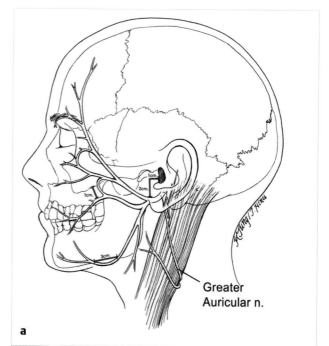

35.8.2 Immediate and Delayed Repair

The optimal method to repair a transected facial nerve is to directly connect its severed ends as soon as possible.[12] Once the nerve has been sutured together, the regenerating proximal nerve travels along its attached distal segment at 1 to 3 mm/day. Because the cell body of the facial nerve is located at the brainstem, the more proximal the facial nerve injury, the more time is needed for the regenerating nerve to reinnervate its facial musculature.

If there is a significant distance between severed nerve ends, resulting in nerve resection from tumor removal or trauma, this nerve gap is bridged with nerve grafts taken from the greater auricular nerve, sural nerve, medial antebrachial cutaneous nerve (anterior branch), or cervical plexus (▶ Fig. 35.8; ▶ Fig. 35.9; ▶ Fig. 35.10).[13]

In cases in which the nerve cannot be surgically reattached due to its location (i.e., facial nerve transection near the brainstem from an intracranial injury or tumor), other motor cranial nerves can be connected to the facial nerve distally. In this case, the hypoglossal nerve is commonly used to attach to the distal facial nerve. For facial movement, when such a patient wants to smile, he learns to push his tongue against his incisors. By connecting the hypoglossal nerve to the facial nerve, 90% of patients achieve good resting facial muscle tone, preventing a sagging face.

35.8.3 Late Repair

Two years after the onset of facial paralysis, denervation atrophy of the facial musculature has likely occurred.[12] To determine the condition of the distal facial nerve after 1 year, EMG is helpful in determining its physiological state. If the EMG shows electrical silence, the facial muscles have undergone denervation atrophy. Under these circumstances, nerve grafting or nerve reattachment using other cranial nerves will not be effective, but temporalis or masseter muscle slings can be rotated to give facial movement to the lower face. These dynamic muscle slings are innervated by the fifth cranial nerve. After this surgery, the patient is able to move his face by biting down.

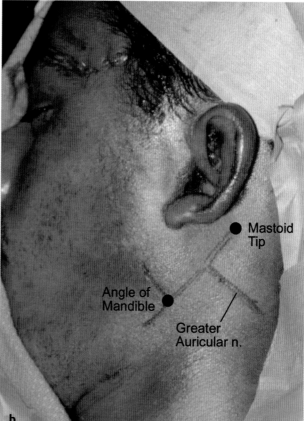

Fig. 35.8 Source of cable nerve grafts for facial interposition using the greater auricular nerve.

In cases where a patient requires facial support and cannot undergo a muscle sling procedure, static sling procedures are performed. Slings made from autogenous materials (fascia) and artificial materials (porous polytetrafluoroethylene [PTFE]) can be used to suspend sagging tissues of the lower eyelid, cheek, and lips.

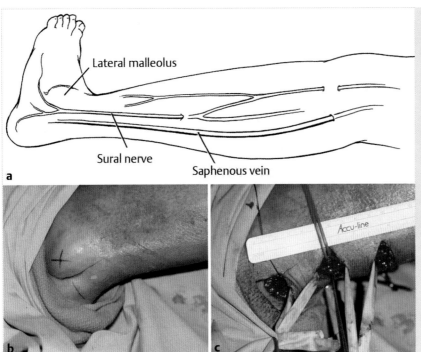

Fig. 35.9 Source of cable nerve grafts for facial interposition using the sural nerve.

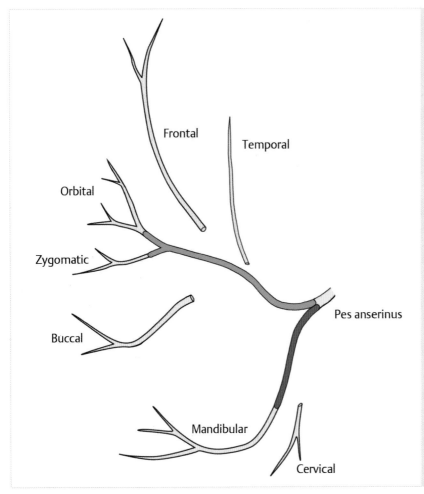

Fig. 35.10 Cable nerve grafts placed as interposition grafts.

35.9 Reinnervation Techniques

35.9.1 Primary Nerve Repair

The preferred method for nerve repair is tensionless nerve-to-nerve end-to-end anastomosis. Depending on the location on the nerve transection, the method of repair can vary. When the nerve at the brainstem has been transected, it is very difficult to perform an end-to-end repair due to the wound depth and decreased nerve mobility. Although a nerve repair is difficult at this site, surgeons feel it is worth attempting when a nerve transection is noted during a skull base procedure.[4]

Within the temporal bone portion of the nerve, the nerve cannot be mobilized until complete nerve decompression is performed. An option for repair at this site is to utilize various conduits to help guide the regenerating nerves from the proximal to distal nerve ends. Conduit materials include vein grafts, silicone grafting, and polyglycolic acid tubes. The conduit tubes have not been reported to give consistently better results than epineural repair and interpositional nerve grafting.[14] In addition, sutureless approximation of the nerve endings using fibrin glue, cyano-butyl-acrylate, nerve tubules, and laser neurorrhaphy has been proposed.[4] These techniques would be most beneficial in performing nerve anastomosis within the temporal bone when suture repair is difficult.

When a primary nerve anastomosis is currently performed, a meticulous epineural repair is done with three to seven sutures of 9–0 monofilament. There were earlier reports of attempting to reestablish fascicular repair to lessen synkinesis; however, it is difficult to determine the distinct topographical distribution of the nerves in each fascicle.[2]

35.9.2 Interposition Grafting

When a significant gap between the ends of a transected facial nerve is present, primary anastomosis is not possible. Interposition nerve grafting allows for the regenerating nerves from the proximal nerve to grow into the distal nerve stump by the graft's axons (▶ Fig. 35.8; ▶ Fig. 35.9; ▶ Fig. 35.10). During a radical parotidectomy, it is recommended that an attempt be made to reestablish continuity of the nerve with a nerve graft. In addition to using autogenous nerve grafts (greater nerve graft, sural nerve, median antebrachial nerve, cervical plexus), a variety of other materials for nerve conduits have been used (gold foil, collagen tubes, freeze thawed muscle). Currently, replacement of a segment of a missing facial nerve is most effective using autogenous interpositional nerve grafts.

The most commonly used donor nerve graft is the greater auricular nerve due to its proximity and diameter. The distal nerve branches of the greater auricular nerve graft may be helpful in anastomosing the individual branches of the facial nerve rather than trying to split the donor nerve. If a length greater than 10 cm is required, the sural nerve can be obtained. One must be careful in using the sural nerve in patients with diabetes or peripheral vascular disease due to their propensity for decreased sensitivity of their feet from trauma. It must be recognized that nerve grafts still result in synkinesis but they provide some degree of voluntary motion and natural resting tone. It has also been proposed that if no distal nerve is available to anastomose, one can consider directly implanting the proximal nerve into the viable target muscle (muscular neurotization).[15]

If the proximal nerve is transected close to the stylomastoid foramen, a mastoidectomy may be required to attain more access to the proximal nerve. It should be noted that within 1 cm above and below the stylomastoid foramen, the facial nerve trunk is closely adherent to the periosteum.

Another option using interpositional nerve grafting is cross–facial nerve grafting. A jump graft is connected to the contralateral functional facial nerve (usually buccal branch) and tunneled across the face to the paralyzed distal facial nerve. This option is based on the principle that the contralateral nerve pulses provide nerve input to the paralyzed facial nerve. Clinical trials using this cross–facial nerve method have been mixed, with some studies showing very weak movement. The results were improved when the cross–facial nerve was performed within 6 months of injury. Weakness of the donor facial nerve is minimized when very selective division of the redundant distal buccal zygomatic nerve branches is performed.[16] Currently, cross–facial nerve grafting is more often used to provide innervation for free muscle transfer.[17]

35.9.3 Hypoglossal to Facial Nerve Transposition

When the proximal nerve is not available, other cranial nerves can be used to serve as the neural input to the distal facial nerve as long as the distal nerve and muscles are intact. It is important to note that a functional deficit will result in sacrificing the donor cranial nerve.[18,19] Classically, the hypoglossal nerve is commonly used as the donor nerve input (▶ Fig. 35.11). However, if the patient has deficits in cranial nerves IX, X, or contralateral XII, it is not recommended to sacrifice the hypoglossal nerve because it will severely hinder the swallowing function. A hypoglossal facial nerve anastomosis is also contraindicated in patients with neurofibromatosis type 2 or developmental facial paralysis diseases, or in patients who lack sufficient extracranial facial nerve fibers and muscles.

In performing a hypoglossal to facial nerve transfer or nerve transposition procedure, the preferred preoperative EMG finding is fibrillation or denervation potentials of the target muscles showing that the distal nerve is degenerating but still intact. Other motor nerves have been proposed for innervating the distal facial nerve such as the masseter, phrenic, and spinal sensory nerves. However, the hypoglossal nerve has the advantage of maintaining good resting facial muscle tone. Mass movement of the face is present when the patient thrusts the tongue forward. However, selective movement of the different tissue regions cannot be performed. Improvement of resting facial tone begins at approximately 6 months after surgery, with voluntary motion starting several months later. Excellent results are seen in approximately 50% of cases, with setbacks being synkinesis, facial movement when eating and speaking, and facial tone hypertonicity leading to exaggerated voluntary movement.[19] Difficulty with eating and speaking with the classic hypoglossal facial nerve transfer may occur in up to 75% of patients.[20] It has been proposed that as strategic facial reanimation can be performed separating the upper and lower face, a hypoglossal facial nerve anastomosis can be performed just to the lower branches, with the upper face addressed separately (gold

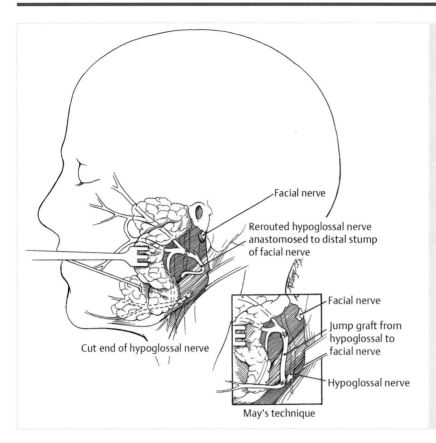

Fig. 35.11 Hypoglossal facial nerve crossover (classic technique) and hypoglossal facial nerve crossover jump graft (May's technique).

Facial nerve

Rerouted hypoglossal nerve anastomosed to distal stump of facial nerve

Cut end of hypoglossal nerve

Facial nerve

Jump graft from hypoglossal to facial nerve

Hypoglossal nerve

May's technique

weight, lower eyelid tightening, browlift) in order to minimize synkinesis and hypertonicity of the full face.

Being that the hypoglossal nerve crossover procedure can result in significant functional deficits in speech, mastication, and swelling, May et al[20] proposed the hypoglossal facial nerve jump graft to avoid tongue paralysis (▶ Fig. 35.11). By partially transecting the diameter of the hypoglossal nerve by one third, enough viable hypoglossal nerve is left intact to prevent tongue paralysis. The partially transected hypoglossal nerve is then anastomosed side-to-end to the proximal jump nerve graft, with the distal jump nerve graft sutured to the transected facial nerve. If the facial nerve transection has occurred proximal to the mastoid segment, the distal facial nerve can be mobilized from the mastoid to the partially transected hypoglossal nerve without a jump graft. The hypoglossal nerve crossover procedure can also be done in a staged fashion in patients who have bilateral facial paralysis.

Some proponents state that patients who underwent the hypoglossal facial nerve jump graft procedure compared to the classic 12–7 procedure had fewer problems with swallowing, mastication, and speech.[20] However, other surgeons who have performed this procedure report that the strength of the facial movement is weaker and requires a longer recovery period.[21]

35.10 Regional Muscle Transfer

35.10.1 Temporalis Muscle

When the facial nerve cannot be reanastomosed, the next option is to perform a regional muscle transfer to achieve facial movement. Major goals in improving facial function are to (1)

establish good resting tone to support of the face; (2) achieve eye protection with eyelid closure; and (3) elevate the corner of the mouth. When considering a temporalis muscle transposition, the trigeminal nerve must be intact for this procedure to be successful.[22] Determining whether it is intact is done by palpating the temporalis muscle while the patient bites down. Masseter muscle transposition has lost favor due to its nonoptimal vector pull, and thus we will describe just the temporalis muscle sling procedure.

The origin of the temporalis muscle attaches to the temporal crest of the temporal bone, with the muscle inserting on the mandibular coronoid process. In the classic approach, the temporalis muscle origin is transposed to the corner of the mouth by a lateral temporal incision approach. The preferred vector pull around the perioral region can be refined with extended fascial grafts (▶ Fig. 35.12).[23]

It should be emphasized that the pull using the temporalis sling in the conventional technique should be accentuated intraoperatively because stretching of the muscle and fascia occurs over time. The temporalis fossa donor defect can be filled with the remaining temporalis muscle or other implants. Over time, the patient learns that by biting on his posterior teeth, the motion is transmitted to the corner of the mouth. Another disadvantage of the conventional technique is that there is a lateral bulge of muscle over the zygomatic arch. If required, the muscle can be lengthened using temporalis fascia or a tensa fascia lata graft.

More recently, transposing the insertion site of the temporalis muscle attached to the coronoid process has been gaining popularity (orthodromic approach). With this technique, the temporalis muscle is approached through the melolabial crease

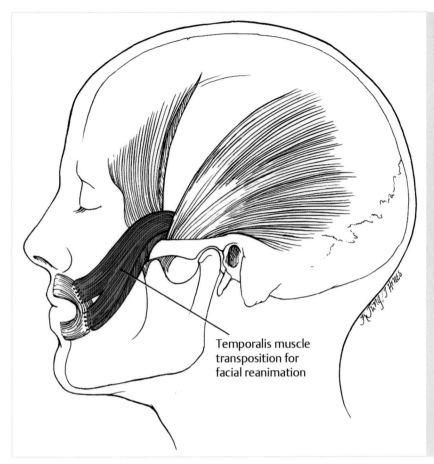

Fig. 35.12 A temporalis muscle sling created by transposing the origin site of the muscle on the temporal bone.

Temporalis muscle transposition for facial reanimation

or transoral approach to mobilize the temporalis muscle insertion site to the lateral corner of the mouth with or without tensor fascia lata grafts (▶ Fig. 35.13).[24,25]

Proponents of the orthodromic approach report that it is less invasive and requires less time to perform. In addition, there is no donor defect in the temporalis fossa and over the zygomatic arch. Further longitudinal studies will need to be performed to compare its results with those of the classic technique. With both techniques, functional temporalis muscle is required.

35.11 Static Suspension

35.11.1 Minimally Invasive Suspension Suture

If a patient is not a candidate for nerve repair, nerve transposition, or muscle transposition procedures due to the state of the facial nerve or the patient's medical condition, static suspension procedures are very beneficial. Establishing good resting support of the lower lip to improve lip competence is very important when eating or speaking; it also gives symmetry to the lower face at rest (▶ Fig. 35.14). In addition, static suspension procedures can be done in combination with the other procedures mentioned previously to give improved immediate lower facial support.

Traditionally, autogenous fascia lata strips have been used as the material of choice for suspension.[26] This straightforward technique can give significant improvement in supporting the

lower face and lateral commissure as an outpatient procedure under local anesthesia. A disadvantage is that fascia has a tendency to stretch over time, and thus the vector pulls needs to be overaccentuated at the time of surgery. To circumvent donor site morbidity, other materials can also be used for suspension such as PTFE (Gore-Tex) and cadaveric acellular human dermis (AlloDerm). These strips are placed in subcutaneous tunnels to the lateral commissure, melolabial crease lower lip, and nose, and anchored to the zygoma.[27] The implants can be placed through a preauricular, temporal, or melolabial approach. The disadvantage of using alloplast and allograft material is that later they can be rejected or cause a chronic inflammatory response, especially in a previously irradiated area.[28]

More recently, suspension sutures have also be used as a minimally invasive procedure to suspend the lateral commissure or external nasal valve to the zygoma as an outpatient procedure.[29,30] Suture suspension is a very useful procedure for a patient who is in poor medical condition or is not willing to undergo a more extensive procedure. The longevity of these sutures is yet to be determined (▶ Fig. 35.15).

35.11.2 Free Microvascular Muscle Transfer

In children, free gracilis microvascular muscle transfer is used for congenital facial paralysis. In acquired facial paralysis, this technique using gracilis, latissimus dorsi, and pectoralis minor muscles has also been reported. This technique is usually done

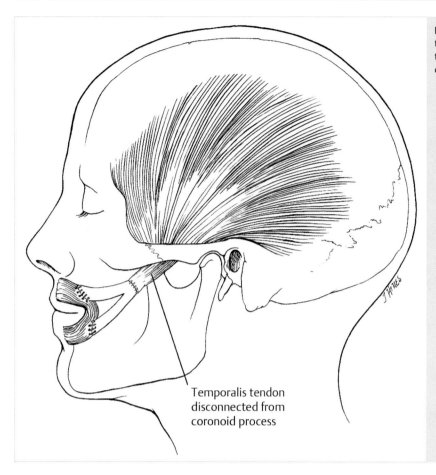

Temporalis tendon disconnected from coronoid process

Fig. 35.13 A temporalis muscle sling created by transposing the insertion site of the muscle from the coronoid process of the mandible (orthodromic approach).

in two stages in conjunction with a cross–facial nerve graft.[17,31] Overall, free microvascular muscle transfer with a cross–facial nerve graft has been reserved for younger patients who have no other alternative, because the success rate diminishes with advancing age.

35.12 Upper Face

35.12.1 Upper Eyelid Reanimation

Facial paralysis decreases the ability of the orbicularis oculi muscle to contract, decreasing the patient's ability to close the eye and blink. The blink reflex is essential in maintaining a healthy eye as it protects the eye from foreign bodies and facilitates the distribution of tears for lubrication. Without the blink response, eye dryness dramatically increases the risk of exposure keratitis, corneal abrasion, corneal ulcers, and possible blindness. This risk is further exacerbated if facial paralysis also leads to decreased tear production from injury to the greater superficial petrosal nerve.

The orbicularis oculi muscle acts as a sphincter to close the upper eyelid and to give tone to the lower eyelid. A tarsorrhaphy is the conventional procedure for corneal protection. What places the patient at extreme risk of having a corneal ulceration is when the BAD syndrome is present, in which the B stands for the lack of Bell's phenomena (when the eyes do not move superiorly on eyelid closure), the A stands for anesthesia of the cornea from fifth cranial nerve injury, and the D stands for dry eye. In most instances an ophthalmologist should be consulted

to monitor the status of the cornea and the globe. If there is a very high likelihood of corneal injury, a tarsorrhaphy may be indicated.

Aggressive eye care is required in keeping the eye moist at all times. We recommend ointment at night and eyedrops several times during the day. Depending on the patient's choice, the viscosity of the eyedrops can be adjusted during the day. Specifically, Lacri-Lube (Allergan) or HypoTears (Novartis) can be used at night and a less viscous ointment, such as methyl cellulose drops, 0.25 to 1%, during the day. By varying the concentration of the methylcellulose component in the eyedrops, one can adjust the viscosity of the eye solution. It also is recommended that nonpreservative eyedrops be used to reduce chronic irritation to the eye and sensitivity from the preservative. A transparent eye patch moisture chamber is also comforting to the patient (► Fig. 35.7).

In addition, when it is windy outdoors, the patient should wear sunglasses with lateral side protectors. One can also protect the eye by taping it in a downward lateral diagonal direction, making sure that the underside of the tape does not rub against the cornea. A temporary tarsorrhaphy using a 7-0 silk mattress suture could also be placed as a short-term means to protect the cornea.

The major goal in upper facial reanimation is to restore the ability to close the eye to protect the cornea. As long as cranial nerve III is intact, the patient still has the ability to open the eye. A variety of techniques has been used, with the mainstay of treatment over the years being a tarsorrhaphy (lid adhesion type); however, it has several shortcomings,

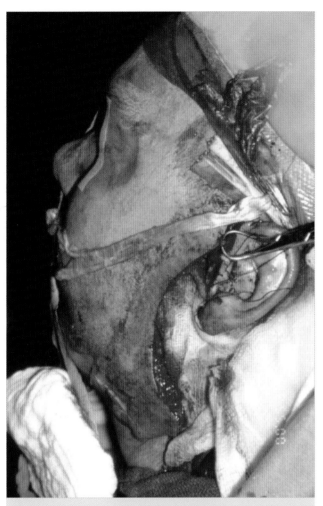

Fig. 35.14 Static facial sling using fascia lata for improving lower facial support.

including decreased lateral visual field, incomplete cornea coverage, no eyelid mobility during closure, and decreased cosmesis.

Over the last 20 years, the placement of gold weight implants in the upper eyelid has helped many patients improve functional eyelid closure. By having a tailored gold weight inserted within the upper eyelid, a patient is able to open and close his eyes spontaneously while being upright. These implants work by giving additional leverage to the upper eyelid, thus allowing the eyelid to spontaneously close by gravity (▶ Fig. 35.16). Eyelid opening is not impaired because cranial nerve III and the sympathetic nerves innervate eyelid levator function. In addition, procedures to tighten the lax lower eyelid can optimize functional eyelid closure and corneal protection.

Because gold weight implants are easily removed, their placement can be useful in patients who have an anticipated prolonged facial paralysis recovery (> 6 months).[32] If the patient is allergic to gold, then platinum weights can be used instead. Platinum weights have a lower profile, so some surgeons prefer a platinum weight to gold for better cosmesis. In addition, titanium chain link implants have been used in the upper eyelid as they conform to the shape of the eyelid.[33]

35.12.2 Rehabilitation of the Eye

The gold weight acts as leverage for the upper eyelid so that the patient is able to close the eye while sitting up at greater than a 45-degree angle. It does not work when the patient is lying supine. The muscles that allow the patient's eye to open are innervated by cranial nerve III (levator superioris, levator palpebrae superioris) and the sympathetic nervous system (Mueller's muscle).

Placement of weights in the upper eyelid is commonly performed. Optimally, the weight selected allows for eyelid closure that does not cause significant eyelid ptosis. This can be done preoperatively while the patient is sitting up, using double adhesive tape and various template sizes. Then the patient looks in a mirror and gives feedback on which weight looks best and which gives the greatest comfort.

A gold weight implant is performed in the following manner: an incision is made at the supratarsal crease and in a stair step through the orbicularis oculi muscle. A pocket is made in the pretarsal area, under the levator aponeurosis. Meticulous hemostasis must be achieved and the gold weight is secured. The inferior border of the weight should be approximately 3 mm superior to the lash line of the eyelid.

In fitting a patient with a gold weight template preoperatively, it should not impair the patient's visualize gaze when looking forward and should not cause a significant ptosis. It should give adequate closure while the patient is sitting up. Immediately after surgery in the operating room, one can test for adequate upper eyelid closure. If, at that time, additional weight is needed, the weight is removed, and a larger weight is placed in order to tailor the optimal weight for the patient. An upper eyelid weight, lower eyelid tightening procedure, and a direct brow can be performed concurrently in an outpatient setting under local anesthesia, with sedation to address the upper face in permanent facial paralysis.

Eyelid springs have also been used in the upper eyelid. Eyelid springs oppose the levator muscle to achieve eyelid closure; however, it can be difficult technically to maintain their proper positioning, and implant extrusion can result. This concept of eyelid springs was introduced approximately 30 years ago.[34] Orthodontic round wire (0.01-inch) is bent with needle-nosed pliers and placed in the upper eyelid. A Dacron patch is placed over one end to minimize extrusion.

The gold weight implant is made of 24-carat gold and is well tolerated by the tissues. The weights range from 0.6 to 2.8 g.

35.12.3 Approaching the Lower Eye

With facial paralysis, the orbicularis oculi muscle has less tonicity, resulting in a lax lower lid with sclera show and paralytic ectropion. If a patient has more than 6 mm of anterior traction from the lateral orbital rim to the lateral canthus, an increased lower eyelid laxity exists. This also holds true for the medial lid where the distance is greater than 5 mm from the inferior punctum to the sclera. For the mid-eyelid area, when the lower eyelid distance is greater than 12 mm from the sclera with the anterior traction test, a lax middle lower lid is evident. The most conservative way to tighten a lax lower lid is to make a small lateral lower eyelid incision, suspending the lower eyelid tarsal plate complex with a long-lasting 4–0 suture in the lateral orbital rim (tarsal tuck procedure). However, a longer lasting

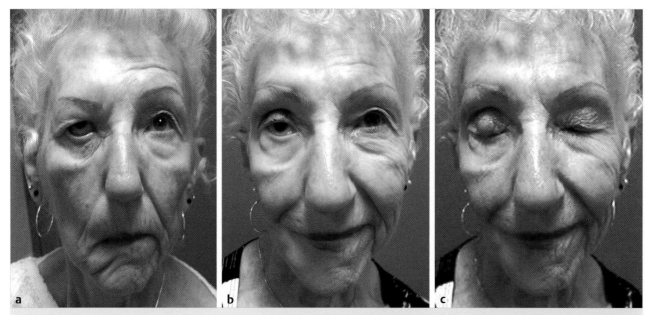

Fig. 35.15 Preoperative (a) and postoperative (b,c) photos of an 85-year-old woman with a permanent full facial nerve paralysis for 3 months following a radical parotidectomy for a cheek melanoma. She also had a history of pulmonary metastasis. Under local anesthesia with intravenous sedation as an outpatient, she underwent suture suspension of the oral commissure, gold weight implant, tarsal strip of the lower eyelid, and direct brow-lift procedure. The postoperative photos (b,c) were taken 12 months after surgery.

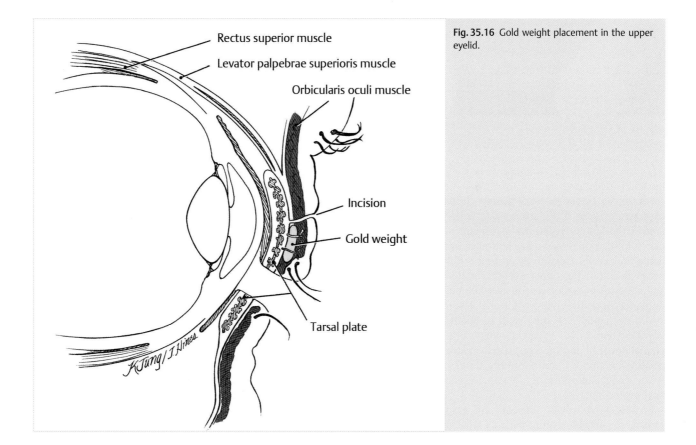

Rectus superior muscle

Levator palpebrae superioris muscle

Orbicularis oculi muscle

Incision

Gold weight

Tarsal plate

Fig. 35.16 Gold weight placement in the upper eyelid.

procedure is to shorten the eyelid by performing a wedge resection of all layers of the lower eyelid.

To address paralytic ectropion, a tarsal strip procedure is more commonly performed to achieve maximal lower eyelid suspension.[35] A lateral canthotomy is made followed by an inferior cantholysis, and the anterior lamella is separated from the posterior lamella. The conjunctiva is shaved on the inner aspect on the tarsal strip. The new lateral canthal tendon is created

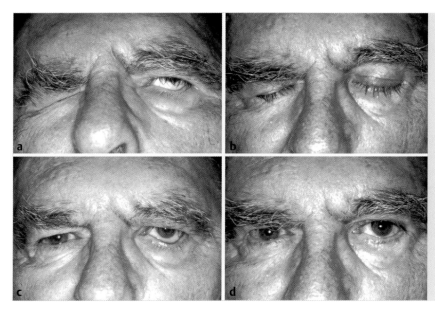

Fig. 35.17 Photos of a patient with facial paralysis before and after gold-weight implantation in the upper eyelid, lower eyelid tightening (tarsal strip), and a direct browlift: in the grimacing state (a) preoperatively and (b) postoperatively, and in the relaxed state (c) preoperatively and (d) postoperatively (12 months after surgery).

from the tarsal plate, making it 4 mm in width. The lateral tarsal complex is re-suspended laterally and superiorly. The excess amount of anterior lamella is excised, which includes the lashes, and it is re-suspended to the lateral orbital rim with 5-0 nylon suture.

The importance of lower eyelid positioning while tightening the suspension suture should be emphasized. The lower lash position should not cause an entropion or ectropion of the lashes, and the lower lid should slightly overlap the inferior limbus of the pupil. Placing 5-0 permanent sutures suspends the lower eyelid laterally and superiorly toward Whitnall's tubercle to give the maximal amount of lower eyelid support.

A medial canthoplasty can also be used to address medial lower eyelid laxity if needed. In order to diagnose a lax lower lid medially, the anterior traction test as described previously is most effective. A medial canthoplasty involves placing lacrimal probes through the superior and inferior canaliculi to preserve their patency and structure during the procedure. The gray line junction between the skin and conjunctiva is incised with a No. 64 Beaver blade and the medial canthal tendon is identified. The medial canthal tendons of the upper and lower eyelids are then opposed using a horizontal mattress of 5-0 (polydioxanone) monofilament synthetic absorbable suture. The skin is then closed, giving further support to the lower lid. The surgeon should stay at least 2 to 3 mm medial to the punctum when suturing to avoid occluding the canalicular ducts. In order to reinforce the closure, small Silastic bolsters can be placed for 2 weeks, protecting the medial canthal repair.

35.12.4 Approaching the Brow

Brow ptosis from facial paralysis commonly causes superior visual field defects. In performing a direct brow lift, one must recognize the optimal brow position. Ideally, the highest portion of the brow should be between the lateral limbus and the lateral canthal area. The brow length should be lined up between the ala and the medial canthus medially with the lateral limit being a line drawn from the nasal alar to the lateral canthus. In females, there should be more of a brow accentuation laterally. In males, the brow emphasis should be medially. The level of the brow should be at the supraorbital rims in males and above the supraorbital rims in females. A permanent suture (4-0 clear monofilament) is used to anchor the brow superiorly to the periosteum. Various approaches are used to lift the ptotic brow (direct, midforehead, pretrichial, coronal, and endoscopic). More commonly, the direct browlift is done because it is the most straightforward and gives the best long-term accurate positioning of the brow. A disadvantage is that a scar is present at the superior brow. Endoscopic browlift has been proposed; however, accurate brow positioning and the longevity of the procedure are more variable (▶ Fig. 35.17).

35.12.5 Combined Procedures for the Upper and Lower Face

In a patient with total facial paralysis, combined procedures addressing both the upper and lower face can be performed in the same surgery session.[36] However, if the patient has persistent upper facial swelling from an oncological resection, the lower face can be addressed first, and a week later the upper face can be addressed under intravenous sedation as an outpatient procedure (browlift, gold weight implant, lower eyelid tightening).

35.13 Ancillary Procedures

35.13.1 Botulinum Toxin and Selective Myectomy for Synkineses

To reduce synkinesis and hyperkinesis, botulinum toxin can be injected into targeted muscles to decrease their activity and thus reduce their aberrant movement on the paretic side.[37] Botulinum toxin induces paralysis by blocking acetylcholine release from the presynaptic terminal at the neuromuscular junction. The dosage is tailored to the targeted muscle, which lasts approximately 3 to 6 months. One report also described the beneficial facial results of injecting nonaffected facial muscles to reduce the antagonist muscle vector pull and improve facial symmetry.[38] After recurrent botulinum toxin injections and if a patient still desires permanent specific muscle paralysis, selective myectomy of the targeted muscle is an option.[39]

35.13.2 Physical Therapy Rehabilitation and Revision Surgery

Rehabilitation with facial exercises is beneficial in strengthening and retraining the facial muscles. Rehabilitation can be managed by a physical therapist, a speech pathologist, or an occupational therapist. The therapist should have expertise in treating facial paralysis patients. Patients are taught over time to train both agonistic and antagonistic muscle to coordinate preferred coordinated facial movement to diminish synkinesis. Thus, facial nerve rehabilitation and botulinum injection can be helpful in minimizing unwanted synkinesis movement.

In many cases, future surgical revisions after facial reanimation procedures are required to optimize results due to patient aging and tissue changes.[40] Thus, the comprehensive treatment of a patient with facial paralysis involves a long-term commitment to follow-up to maximize facial function and appearance.

35.14 Conclusion

In treating a patient with facial paralysis, a comprehensive and tailored approach is optimal to address the patient's functional, cosmetic, and psychological needs. In addition to facial reanimation procedures, facial paralysis rehabilitation is very helpful to maximize physical and mental recovery. Functional goals are to maximize eye protection, oral competency, facial movement, and facial symmetry. Due to dynamic facial aging changes, long-term follow-up is preferred because procedural adjustments following facial reanimation procedures may be required to maximize facial function and appearance.[15]

References

[1] Ishii L, Godoy A, Encarnacion CO, Byrne PJ, Boahene KD, Ishii M. Not just another face in the crowd: society's perceptions of facial paralysis. Laryngoscope 2012; 122: 533–538

[2] May M. Anatomy of the facial nerve (spatial orientation of fibers in the temporal bone). Laryngoscope 1973; 83: 1311–1329

[3] Davis RAAB, Anson BJ, Budinger JM, Kurth LR. Surgical anatomy of the facial nerve and parotid gland based upon a study of 350 cervicofacial halves. Surg Gynecol Obstet 1956; 102: 385–412

[4] Ridgway J, Crumley R, Kim J. Rehabilitation of facial paralysis. In: Flint PW, Haughey BH, Lund VJ, et al, eds. Otolaryngology–Head and Neck Surgery. Philadelphia: Mosby Elsevier, 2010:2416–2433

[5] May M. Microanatomy and Pathophysiology of the Facial Nerve. New York: Thieme, 1986:63–74

[6] May M, Schaitkin B. The Facial Nerve. New York: 2000

[7] Sunderland S. Nerve and Nerve Injuries. London: Churchill-Livingstone, 1978

[8] Sunderland S, Cossar DF. The structure of the facial nerve. Anat Rec 1953; 116: 147–165

[9] Kalliainen L. Salient healing features of muscles of the face and neck. In: Hom D, Hebda P, Gosain A, Friedman C, eds. Essential Tissue Healing of the Face and Neck. Shelton, CT: BC Decker and People's Medical Publishing House, 2009:66–82

[10] Barabás J, Klenk G, Szabó G et al. Modified procedure for secondary facial rehabilitation following total bilateral irreversible peripheral facial palsy. J Craniofac Surg 2007; 18: 169–176

[11] Tate JR, Tollefson TT. Advances in facial reanimation. Curr Opin Otolaryngol Head Neck Surg 2006; 14: 242–248

[12] Bascom DA, Schaitkin BM, May M, Klein S. Facial nerve repair: a retrospective review. Facial Plast Surg 2000; 16: 309–313

[13] Haller JR, Shelton C. Medial antebrachial cutaneous nerve: a new donor graft for repair of facial nerve defects at the skull base. Laryngoscope 1997; 107: 1048–1052

[14] Shumrick K. Rehabilitation and Reanimation of the Paralyzed Face. New York: Thieme, 2007:453–466

[15] Aitken JT. Growth of nerve implants in voluntary muscle. J Anat 1950; 84: 38–49

[16] Cooper TM, McMahon B, Lex C, Lenert JJ, Johnson PC. Cross-facial nerve grafting for facial reanimation: effect on normal hemiface motion. J Reconstr Microsurg 1996; 12: 99–103

[17] Shindo M. Facial reanimation with microneurovascular free flaps. Facial Plast Surg 2000; 16: 357–359

[18] Conley J, Baker DC. Hypoglossal-facial nerve anastomosis for reinnervation of the paralyzed face. Plast Reconstr Surg 1979; 63: 63–72

[19] Pensak ML, Jackson CG, Glasscock ME, III, Gulya AJ. Facial reanimation with the VII-XII anastomosis: analysis of the functional and psychologic results. Otolaryngol Head Neck Surg 1986; 94: 305–310

[20] May M, Sobol SM, Mester SJ. Hypoglossal-facial nerve interpositional-jump graft for facial reanimation without tongue atrophy. Otolaryngol Head Neck Surg 1991; 104: 818–825

[21] Atlas MD, Lowinger DS. A new technique for hypoglossal-facial nerve repair. Laryngoscope 1997; 107: 984–991

[22] May M, Drucker C. Temporalis muscle for facial reanimation. A 13-year experience with 224 procedures. Arch Otolaryngol Head Neck Surg 1993; 119: 378–382, discussion 383–384

[23] Sherris DA. Refinement in reanimation of the lower face. Arch Facial Plast Surg 2004; 6: 49–53

[24] Boahene KD, Farrag TY, Ishii L, Byrne PJ. Minimally invasive temporalis tendon transposition. Arch Facial Plast Surg 2011; 13: 8–13

[25] Sidle DM, Fishman AJ. Modification of the orthodromic temporalis tendon transfer technique for reanimation of the paralyzed face. Otolaryngol Head Neck Surg 2011; 145: 18–23

[26] Rose EH. Autogenous fascia lata grafts: clinical applications in reanimation of the totally or partially paralyzed face. Plast Reconstr Surg 2005; 116: 20–32, discussion 33–35

[27] Liu YM, Sherris DA. Static procedures for the management of the midface and lower face. Facial Plast Surg 2008; 24: 211–215

[28] Constantinides M, Galli SK, Miller PJ. Complications of static facial suspensions with expanded polytetrafluoroethylene (ePTFE). Laryngoscope 2001; 111: 2114–2121

[29] Alex JC, Nguyen DB. Multivectored suture suspension: a minimally invasive technique for reanimation of the paralyzed face. Arch Facial Plast Surg 2004; 6: 197–201

[30] Alam D. Rehabilitation of long-standing facial nerve paralysis with percutaneous suture-based slings. Arch Facial Plast Surg 2007; 9: 205–209

[31] Chuang DC. Free tissue transfer for the treatment of facial paralysis. Facial Plast Surg 2008; 24: 194–203

[32] Kartush JM, Linstrom CJ, McCann PM, Graham MD. Early gold weight eyelid implantation for facial paralysis. Otolaryngol Head Neck Surg 1990; 103: 1016–1023

[33] Mavrikakis I, Beckingsale P, Lee E, Riaz Y, Brittain P. Changes in corneal topography with upper eyelid gold weight implants. Ophthal Plast Reconstr Surg 2006; 22: 331–334

[34] Levine RE, Shapiro JP. Reanimation of the paralyzed eyelid with the enhanced palpebral spring or the gold weight: modern replacements for tarsorrhaphy. Facial Plast Surg 2000; 16: 325–336

[35] Anderson RL, Gordy DD. The tarsal strip procedure. Arch Ophthalmol 1979; 97: 2192–2196

[36] Hadlock TA, Greenfield LJ, Wernick-Robinson M, Cheney ML. Multimodality approach to management of the paralyzed face. Laryngoscope 2006; 116: 1385–1389

[37] Borodic GE, Pearce LB, Cheney M et al. Botulinum A toxin for treatment of aberrant facial nerve regeneration. Plast Reconstr Surg 1993; 91: 1042–1045

[38] Salles AG, Toledo PN, Ferreira MC. Botulinum toxin injection in long-standing facial paralysis patients: improvement of facial symmetry observed up to 6 months. Aesthetic Plast Surg 2009; 33: 582–590

[39] Patel B, Anderson R, May M. Selective myectomy. In: May M, ed. The Facial Nerve. New York: Thieme, 2001:467

[40] Terzis JK, Olivares FS. Secondary surgery in adult facial paralysis reanimation. Plast Reconstr Surg 2009; 124: 1916–1931

36 Otalgia

John S. McDonald

36.1 Introduction

Otalgia may be primary, with the source being the ear or temporal bone, or it may be secondary, referred to the ear with or without signs or symptoms of the primary source of the pain. In 50% or more of patients who complain of otalgia, the pain emanates from a source other than the ear.[1] Otalgia may be described as aching, boring, sharp, throbbing, burning, itching, or pressure-like, with a sensation of fullness. Concomitant complaints of vertigo, tinnitus, and even the subjective sense of hearing degradation may be part of the clinical spectrum of either primary or referred otalgia and cannot be used as differentiating factors.

36.2 Nociception and Pain

Bonica[3] defined pain as an unpleasant sensory and emotional experience associated with actual or potential tissue damage or described in terms of such damage. Tissue injury, whether caused by trauma or disease, constitutes a noxious stimulus that will activate nociceptors (receptors preferentially sensitive to a noxious stimulus or to a stimulus that would become noxious if prolonged).[2] The noxious stimulus or tissue damage activates nociceptors at the termination of thinly myelinated Aδ (group III) and unmyelinated C (group IV) afferent nerve fibers in the skin, muscles, joints, fascia, and other deep somatic structures.[3,4] Cutaneous nociceptors may be activated by mechanical, thermal, chemical, or other algesic stimuli, and nociceptors in the deep somatic structures may be activated by disease, inflammatory processes, contraction, ischemia, rapid distention, or other visceral stimuli.

Central to the theme of understanding the mechanism by which pain may be referred to the ear is the concept of central convergence. Sessle et al[5,6] have shown extensive convergence of cutaneous, tooth pulp, visceral, neck, and muscle afferents onto nociceptive and nonnociceptive neurons in the trigeminal subnucleus caudalis or medullary dorsal horn (MDH), so named because of its many similarities to the spinal dorsal horn, and suggested a role for these neurons in mediating pain, its spread, and referral.

Sensory innervation to the ear and periaural region is derived from cranial nerves V, VII, IX and X as well as cervical nerves 2 and 3. Primary nociceptive afferent fibers from CNs V, VII, IX and X as well as C2, C3 and C4 have all been shown to converge centrally and synapse with second order neurons in the trigeminal oral subnucleus caudalis or medullary dorsal horn (MDH).[4,7,8] There is a high degree of nociceptive convergence of the upper cervical nerves and the trigeminal system, providing overlap of peripheral C2, C3, and C4 nociceptive fibers, as well as C5, C6, and C7 nociceptive neurons in trigeminal spinal nuclei and paratrigeminal nuclei with those from cephalic nociceptive nerves V, VII, IX, and X.[8]

There are three types of neurons in the MDH: low-threshold mechanoreceptors (LTMs), which respond to nonnoxious stimuli; wide dynamic range (WDR) neurons, which respond to both noxious and nonnoxious stimuli; and high-threshold nociceptive-specific (NS) neurons, which respond exclusively to noxious stimuli. A substantial number of the WDR and NS neurons show extensive convergence and can be excited by peripheral afferents from skin, mucosa, viscera (i.e., laryngeal), temporomandibular joint (TMJ), jaw and tongue muscle, tooth pulp, and neck, provoking the spread and referral of pain.[10] Convergence of nociceptive fibers from C2 through C7 with WDR and NS neurons in the MDH may explain referral of pain from noxious stimuli from these nociceptive fibers not only to the ear but to the preauricular region and other areas of the face.

36.3 Anatomy

The auriculotemporal branch of the mandibular or third division of the fifth cranial nerve (CN V$_3$) provides sensory innervations for the tragus, anterior and superior aspects of the auricle, and external auditory canal, as well as the anterosuperior portion of the lateral external canal wall and tympanic membrane. The tensor tympani muscle, derived from the mandibular or first branchial arch, is innervated by a small nerve derived from the medial pterygoid branch of CN V$_3$. Although primarily motor in function, skeletal muscles receive sensory innervations from thinly myelinated Aδ (group III) and unmyelinated C (group IV) afferent nociceptive nerve endings in muscle fascia, in tight spatial connection to muscle arterioles and capillaries, and in tendons, acting as muscle nociceptors.[3,10,11]

Electromyographic studies of the tensor tympani and stapedius muscles have demonstrated contraction of both muscles concomitantly with several complex facial movements including tight closure of the eyes, opening and closing of the jaws, speaking, and swallowing.[12] It has been pointed out that tonic contraction of the tensor tympani muscle may be accompanied by otalgia, a sense of pressure and fullness in the ear(s), and tinnitus, or other transient acoustic sensations.[12] Mechanical injury to muscle, which may be derived from repetitive situations such as overcontraction or overstretching muscle, may produce pain. Chronic contraction of the masticatory muscles in cases of temporomandibular dysfunction (TMD), worsened by bruxism, may result in tensor tympani–mediated otalgia.

The facial nerve (CN VII) supplies sensory innervations to a portion of the posterior and posterosuperior auricle and to adjacent portions of the external auditory canal and lateral aspect of the tympanic membrane, as well as to a small area of skin in the postauricular area.[1] CN VII also supplies innervations to the stapedius muscle in the middle ear.

The glossopharyngeal nerve (CN IX) provides sensory innervations to the part of the posterior portion of the external auditory canal and meatus as well as an adjacent portion of the lateral surface of the tympanic membrane, the majority of the mastoid air cells, and the eustachian tube.[1] The tympanic plexus, which is composed of the tympanic branch of the glossopharyngeal nerve (Jacobson nerve) and the superior and inferior caroticotympanic branches of the sympathetic plexus surrounding the carotid artery, provides sensory innervations to the middle ear, including the medial aspect of the tympanic membrane.[1] The auricular branch (Arnold nerve) of the vagus nerve (CN X) innervates a portion of the posterior wall and the floor of the external canal and the corresponding external surface of the tympanic membrane.[1] The upper cervical nerves (C2, C3) also supply sensory innervations to the ear or periauricular structures. The posterior branch of the greater auricular nerve supplies sensory innervations to the majority of the posterior portion of the auricle as well as a portion of the skin over the mastoid region, which also receives some overlapping communication with the lesser occipital nerve (C2) in the mastoid region.

Although pain may be referred to the ear by way of any of the cranial or cervical nerves just mentioned, the most common source of referred pain to the ear is through the trigeminal nerve, the longest cranial nerve with the most extensive distribution in the head and neck region.[13,14]

36.4 Mechanism of Referred Pain

The mechanism by which pain may be referred to the ear from distant anatomic sites can be found in the concept of central convergence, wherein nociceptive neurons in lower centers such as the MDH receive convergent inputs from various tissues, with the result that higher centers within the brain cannot identify the actual input source.[5,15] These convergent inputs may also be involved in so-called central sensitization or neuroplasticity of nociceptive neurons, a process thought to contribute (along with peripheral sensitization) to hyperalgesia.[16] It is thought that as a result of this nociceptive input, some of the afferent inputs to the nociceptive neurons may be "unmasked" and become more effective in exciting these second-order neurons, with the result that pain is perceived as coming from the tissue that the afferents supply.[17] For example, pain may be experienced in the external ear including part of the external auditory canal and the tympanic membrane by convergence of primary Aδ or C afferent nociceptive fibers from the auriculotemporal branch of CN V$_3$ with other primary Aδ or C nociceptive afferent nerve fibers (most commonly other branches of CN V), at WDR or NS neurons in the MDH. Also, under the influence of nociceptive input from muscle, many cells acquire new receptive fields in deep tissues away from the site of stimulation, with the result that following muscle injury the neurons can be stimulated from body regions somatotypically appropriate for that neuron.[18] Thus, it is also possible that pain may be referred to the middle ear or eustachian tube by convergence of primary afferent nociceptors from the tensor tympani and tensor palati muscles with other primary nociceptive afferents at WDR or NS neurons in the MDH.

It is likely, then, as illustrated in the preceding example of pain sensed in the ear through the auriculotemporal branch of CN V$_3$, that convergence of primary nociceptive afferent fibers from CNs V, VII, IX, and X with WDR and NS neurons in the MDH (trigeminal subnucleus caudalis) may be the means by which pain may be referred to the ear.[9] It is also thought that pain referred to the preauricular region from C3 may be facilitated through overlap of at least C2, C3, and C4 nociceptive fibers with primary afferent nociceptive fibers from cranial nerve CN V$_3$.[9,50]

36.5 Primary Otalgia

Pain in the ear or earache may be either primary or referred (secondary) otalgia. When the source of the pain and the site to which it is localized (i.e., the ear) are the same, then the patient is said to have primary otalgia. When the source of the pain is separate from the site in which it is perceived (e.g., the ear), then the pain is said to be referred. The differential diagnosis of pathological causes is enumerated in the list below:

Primary Otalgia

- Otitis externa (bacterial or fungal)
- Myringitis
- Cerumen impaction
- Foreign body in the ear canal
- Perichondritis or chondritis of the auricle
- Relapsing polychondritis
- Carbuncle or furuncle
- Frostbite or burn of pinna
- Trauma to the external canal
- Traumatic perforation of the tympanic membrane
- Hemotympanum
- Herpes simplex virus infection
- Herpes zoster oticus
- Eustachian tube dysfunction
- Eustachian tube obstruction
- Otitis media and mastoiditis, which may be complicated by:
  - Petrositis
  - Subperiosteal abscess
  - Extradural/subdural abscess
  - Venous sinus thrombosis
  - Brain abscess
- External canal, middle ear, or skull base neoplasms including metastatic disease

Although in most cases the cause of primary otalgia is readily obvious, potentially the most ominous disorder, primary malignancy of the external canal, may not be at all obvious in its early stage and may be overlooked. Conversely it is most important to keep in mind that mild erythema of the tympanic membrane or erythema or mild swelling in the external auditory canal should not preclude a thorough head and neck examination to rule out other diseases/disorders that may refer to the ear and be the true cause of the patient's symptoms. A classic example is the patient with TMD or a TMJ with referred otalgia who may rub the external ear canal with a finger or foreign object in attempts to alleviate the pain, resulting in the appearance of bacterial or fungal otitis externa.

36.6 Referred Otalgia

The underlying cause of pain referred to the ear may be either acute or chronic in nature. For the purposes of this chapter, acute causes of referred otalgia are conditions that may be readily diagnosed with well-defined treatment parameters. The majority of these cases will be inflammatory or traumatic in their origin. Below is a list of the most frequently encountered acute disorders that may produce the feeling of pain in the ear.

Orofacial region:
- Exposed tooth root surfaces
- Pulpitis or pulpal necrosis
- Periapical infection
- Periodontal infection (superficial or deep)
- Unerupted or impacted teeth
- Traumatic occlusion
- Ill-fitting dental appliance
- Recent adjustment of arch wires (orthodontic therapy)
- Primary or recurrent herpes simplex virus infection
- Acute herpes zoster
- Recurrent aphthous stomatitis
- Mucocutaneous disorders (i.e., lichen planus)
- Geographic tongue
- Burning mouth or burning tongue
- Maxillary sinusitis
- Nasal infections
- Parotitis

Pharynx:
- Inflammatory disorder involving the hypo-oro-nasopharynx
- Tonsillitis and peritonsillar abscess
- Posttonsillectomy pain
- Eagle syndrome

Larynx and esophagus:
- Laryngitis
- Perichondritis or chondritis
- Arthritis of cricoarytenoid joint
- Hiatal hernia
- Gastroesophageal reflux
- Infection or foreign body in esophagus

Other sources:
- Traction or inflammation involving cerebrovascular blood supply (carotidynia)
- Thyroiditis
- Angina
- Aneurysm of great vessels

- Orofacial pain (chronic)
  - Temporomandibular disorders (TMD, TMJ); includes myofascial pain dysfunction (MPD) and intraarticular TMJ/TMD pain
- Neurologic disorders
  - Continuous neuropathic pain
    - Atypical or idiopathic facial pain, atypical or idiopathic odontalgia)
    - Postherpetic neuralgia
  - Episodic neuropathic (neuralgic) pain
    - Trigeminal neuralgia
    - Glossopharyngeal neuralgia
    - Nervus intermedius (geniculate) neuralgia
    - Occipital neuralgia
    - Vagal and superior laryngeal neuralgia
- Headaches (International Classification of Headache Disorders, 2nd edition [ICHD-2])
  - Primary headache disorders
    - Tension-type headache now including cervical myalgia
    - Chronic paroxysmal hemicranias
    - Giant cell arteritis (Temporal arteritis)
  - Secondary headache disorders
    - Headache or facial pain attributed to disorders of cranium, neck, eyes, ears, nose, sinuses, teeth, mouth, or other facial or cranial structures
- Neoplastic disease
  - Carcinoma, sarcomas (including Hodgkin's and non-Hodgkin's lymphomas), and metastatic disease

36.6.1 Acute Referred Otalgia

Painful disorders arising in the orofacial region, innervated by the second and third divisions of CN V, are the most common cause of referred pain to the ear.[13,19] Common causes of dental pain in this region include inflammation and pulpal necrosis with or without periapical pathosis and inflammation or infection of the supporting periodontal structures (e.g., the periodontal ligament) including superficial or deep periodontal infections or periodontal abscess. Other dental factors such as unerupted or impacted teeth, traumatic occlusion, ill-fitting dental appliances, or recently adjusted archwires in patients undergoing orthodontic therapy may also be causative factors. Referred pain to the ear may also arise from a variety of nondental, painful, oral inflammatory disorders including primary or recurrent herpetic gingivostomatitis, acute herpes zoster infection, recurrent aphthous stomatitis (primarily the major scarring form), mucocutaneous disorders such as erosive lichen

Those disorders that more frequently present as chronic ongoing pain complaints are listed in the box below. The listed disorders will typically have continued to persist beyond the usual expected time for an injury to heal, or are associated with some chronic disorder causing continuous pain or recurrence of pain at intervals over months or years.[2]

planus, inflammatory lesions of the tongue such as geographic tongue, and burning tongue or burning mouth syndrome.

Other painful disorders of the orofacial region that may be the cause of referred pain to the ear include maxillary sinusitis, nasal infections, and parotitis caused by infection or obstruction of the Stensen duct by a stone. Although CN V_1 provides the majority of the sensory trigeminal vascular innervations, some of the dural blood vessels are innervated by fibers from CN V_3. As pain is the only sensation that may be evoked by inflammatory or traction stimuli to the cerebrovascular blood supply, then disease in this area will nonselectively present as pain. Also, although TMD has an acute phase, it is most notable for its chronic nature, and hence it is included in this chapter in the differential diagnosis of chronic referred otalgia.

A variety of benign (although not necessarily at all inconsequential) as well as malignant conditions may present with unilateral neck pain. One disorder, benign carotidynia (idiopathic carotiditis), so named because of its relatively benign clinical course, is mentioned here, as on palpation it is known to radiate to the ipsilateral ear.[51] From a vascular standpoint to make this diagnosis, two major entities must be ruled out: carotid dissection and giant call arteritis. Even though the pathogenesis of carotidynia remains clear, the disorder may represent a variant of inflammatory/traction stimuli. Although the pathogenesis remains unclear, it has been proposed that patient reassurance, stress management, and the use of nonsteroidal antiinflammatory drugs (NSAIDs) and low-dose benzodiazepines be employed.[51]

Disorders of the pharynx may also present with referred pain to the ear, with inflammatory disorders of the oro-, naso-, or hypopharynx, tonsillitis, peritonsillar abscesses, and posttonsillectomy pain being common causes of referred otalgia. Eagle's syndrome, caused by an elongated styloid process, may present as referred pain to the ear and also may be confused with, or mimic, glossopharyngeal neuralgia.

Inflammatory disorders of the larynx and esophagus may be referred to the ear through the vagus nerve. Laryngeal causes of referred otalgia include laryngitis, perichondritis, chondritis, and arthritis of the cricoarytenoid joint. Esophageal disorders that may refer to the ear include gastroesophageal reflux, hiatal hernia and inflammation, infection, or foreign body in the esophagus.[20,21] Inflammatory processes arising from visceral sources such as the thyroid gland may be a source of referred pain to the ear as may disorders such as angina and aneurysms of the great vessels.

36.6.2 Chronic Referred Otalgia

When considering the expansive range of innervations of the ear and periaural structures through cranial nerves V, VII, IX, and X in light of the differential diagnosis of chronic pain conditions in the head and neck, then it becomes immediately obvious that the majority of them have at least the potential to refer pain to the ear. Also, taking into consideration the fact that the primary complaint of pain may be in the ear, regardless of the source of the pain, and the fact that chronic pain conditions are frequently of mixed fiber origin, then the potential immensity of the diagnostic challenge becomes evident.

The differential diagnosis of conditions that may produce chronic pain in the head and neck is a broad one and includes orofacial pain, neurologic disorders, primary and secondary headache disorders, and pain due to cancer.

36.6.3 Orofacial Pain

Not very arguably the most common chronic orofacial pain conditions that may result in referred pain to the ear are the temporomandibular disorders (TMD, TMJ pain).

Temporomandibular Disorders

Temporomandibular disorders (TMDs) along with such conditions as fibromyalgia, irritable bowel syndrome, chronic headaches, interstitial cystitis, chronic pelvic pain, chronic tinnitus, whiplash associated disorders, and vulvar vestibulitis, are classed as idiopathic pain disorders.[52] They often come together as a group of comorbid conditions characterized by a complaint of pain as a complex of other abnormalities in motor function, autonomic balance, neuroendocrine function, and sleep disorders. Most importantly, they have been associated with a state of pain amplification and psychological distress.

Temporomandibular disorders as a group are often enigmatic from the standpoint of both diagnosis and management. In the differential diagnosis of TMD are nonarticular conditions mimicking this disorder; extraarticular causes of limitation of jaw movement; articular derangement of the TMJ, where the disorder in question begins primarily in the joint and remains limited to it; and myofascial pain dysfunction (MPD) with or without intraarticular dysfunction.

Myofascial pain is the most common cause of TMD pain and hence one of the most common causes of referred pain from the orofacial region to the ear. It has been estimated, for example, that approximately 40% of patients with referred otalgia have hyperactivity of the muscles of mastication.[13] In 1952, Travell and Rinzler[22] used the term *myofascial* to refer to pain in a muscle or muscles. Myofascial pain is defined as pain or autonomic phenomena referred from active myofascial trigger points with associated dysfunction.[23] Myofascial pain is the most frequently encountered type of chronic facial, head, and neck pain, and the most controversial. According to Laskin,[24] MPD accounts for as many as 90% of cases of TMD. Although regarded by many as a specific disease entity, others term it a wastebasket diagnosis for soft tissue complaints, and still others simply deny its existence.[25] MPD has been characterized as a regional pain syndrome, often with sudden onset and with trigger points causing locally referred pain.[26] It has been defined as pain, tenderness, or other referred phenomena, with the dysfunction attributed to myofascial trigger points.[23] The sine qua non of MPD is a tender muscle trigger point. Trigger points may be latent or active. Active trigger points produce a pain complaint or other abnormal sensory symptoms. Palpation of an active trigger point may produce or reproduce the complaint of pain or dysfunction. Latent trigger points present with tenderness on palpation but to a lesser extent and without referral of pain.[27,28] Both active and passive trigger points can cause significant motor dysfunction.[28]

Trigger points have been noted to occur primarily in the deep midportion of the muscle and are best located by examining a muscle or muscle group while it is relaxed and being passively stretched by the examiner.[26] To identify a tender muscle trigger point, the examiner must first establish the sensation of finger pressure as a point of reference by palpating a nonpainful area and instructing the patient to respond when pain or tenderness other than the pressure from finger palpation is noted. When a tender muscle trigger point is present, there is usually a nodule or taut band to be felt.[28] Identification of the trigger point is then best done by rolling the nodule or taut band transversely under the fingers. Frequently, a verbal response from the patient is unnecessary as the patient will exhibit an involuntary "jump sign" when a tender muscle trigger point is located.

Myofascial pain appears to occur most commonly in the third, fourth, and fifth decades of life, with women being affected more frequently than men. This is true for patients with TMD whose pain is of myofascial origin as well as for patients with tension type headache produced by active tender muscle trigger points. TMD patients with pain of myofascial origin may present with muscle tenderness, popping, or clicking in one or both TMJs, limitation or deflection of jaw movement, and otologic manifestations. They may have jaw pain; frontal, frontotemporal, or occipital headache pain; toothache; sinus pain; earache; pre- or postauricular pain; sore throat; dysphagia; a sense of an object in the throat; or periorbital pain.

Referred or secondary otalgia is a frequent consequence of both acute and chronic orofacial pain conditions, with approximately 45% of patients with such pain having diseases of the teeth, periodontium, or suffering from TMD.[19] Pharmacotherapy is usually initiated early to palliate some of the patients' symptoms but should not be the primary treatment in most cases. The NSAIDs are most frequently used, and there is seldom if ever an indication for the use of narcotic analgesics. Muscle relaxants such as chlorzoxazone, methocarbamol, metaxalone, baclofen, and tizanidine can be used on a relatively long-term basis. Additionally, tricyclic antidepressants are frequently effective analgesic agents in chronic facial pain as they are in tension-type headache. Physical therapy is usually employed and may be accompanied with myoneural block therapy on an adjunctive basis. Frequently, splint therapy using flat plane passive appliances is employed, although this is not indicated in every case. In many cases of severe chronic facial pain, as in other forms of chronic head and neck pain, behavioral medicine evaluation and therapy is indicated and is often as essential as pharmacotherapy and physical therapy in managing the patient's pain.

Neurologic Disorders

Neuropathic pain is defined as pain arising as a direct consequence of a lesion or disease affecting the somatosensory system either at the peripheral or central level.[53] This is as opposed to somatic pain, which occurs in response to noxious stimulation of normal neural receptors. Neuropathic pain may be episodic or continuous in nature and may be mediated either peripherally or centrally. Both central and peripheral sensitization may play a sustaining role in perpetuating this disorder.

36.6.4 Continuous Neuropathic Facial Pain

Atypical or Idiopathic Facial Pain, and Atypical or Idiopathic Odontalgia

Neuropathic pain arising in the face is often an idiopathic condition, which has also been termed atypical facial pain (AFP), and is characterized as a continuous, or nearly continuous, unilateral, poorly defined, diffuse, aching, boring or burning pain not limited to the distribution of the fifth or ninth cranial nerves. It may overlay the distribution of the cervical nerves. The term *atypical odontalgia* (AO), which again is idiopathic, applies when the pain is said to emanate from a tooth or from several teeth. Patients with AFP or AO may experience referred otalgia, or its diffuse nature may approximate the ear in the preauricular facial region. Although trigger zones are absent, physical examination may reveal hyperalgesia, allodynia, and sympathetic hyperfunction. Attacks of AFP may be set off by mechanical stimulation including percussion or chewing.

Atypical facial pain is one of several neuropathic orofacial pain states. In addition to mechanisms associated specifically with nerve injury, factors such as peripheral sensitization of nociceptors or central sensitization, which can occur after sufficient nociceptive input, can lead to neuropathic pain.[29,30] Potential etiologic factors include trauma (such as chronic irritation or inflammatory stimuli, endodontic, surgical, or other traumatic events), hormonal factors, psychological factors, and local irritation.[30,31] Loss of segmental inhibition from deafferentation following nerve injury or impairment or loss of inhibitory interneurons may also be possible pathogenetic factors in AFP.

A neuropsychiatric assessment of patients with AFP or AO should be pursued, as a number of patients with this disorder may be found to have a specific psychiatric diagnosis as classified by the *Diagnostic and Statistical Manual of Mental Disorders* (DSM-IV) criteria. In a study of 68 patients with AFP, 46 (68%) were found to have a specific diagnosis by DSM-IV criteria, covering a wide variety of disorders, predominantly somatoform, affective, adjustment, or personality disorders.[31]

Although AFP (including AO) is often refractory to both medical and dental therapies, including analgesic therapy, some patients may respond to antidepressants, anticonvulsants, or both in combination.

Postherpetic Neuralgia

Despite its name, the term *postherpetic neuralgia* is a misnomer, as it does not fit the definition of neuralgic pain. Although it may have an intermittent nature, most patients describe a constant deep, aching, or burning pain in addition to any paroxysmal or lancinating qualities with the majority of patients reporting mechanical allodynia.[54]

As is well known, acute herpes zoster (shingles) results from reactivation of dormant varicella zoster virus (VZV) that can remain latent in the dorsal root or cranial nerve ganglion for many years following the original infection. The Norwegians gave herpes zoster a most accurately descriptive name "a belt of roses from Hell," describing the despair to which it may drive the affected patient.[55] Although an apt term, it is a particularly accurate moniker for postherpetic neuralgia (PHN), which may occur as a sequelae of this disorder.

The orofacial region is a relatively common site of involvement for herpes zoster infections and hence PHN. Although the pain and vesicular eruption from a VZV infection usually resolve within 2 to 3 weeks, pain in the form of PHN, which is far and away the most portentous complication of shingles, may persist beyond resolution of these initial symptoms. Pain may be referred to the ear from involvement of both the cranial and cervical nerves by VZV and PHN through pathways previously described in this chapter and may mimic geniculate or nervus intermedius neuralgia. Although the primary goal in the treatment of acute herpes zoster is to palliate the patient's pain and to effect early resolution of the acute stage of the disease, it is believed that in patients 50 years or age or older, treatment for the prevention of PHN is essential because of its frequency of occurrence in this age group and its potentially debilitating nature.[41]

Most patients with PHN give a complaint of a constant deep aching or burning pain, a paroxysmal lancinating pain, and allodynia, although many complain of itching that may be more agonizing to the patient than the pain itself.[54][56] These are thought to be mediated by nonnociceptive Aβ fibers and small myelinated Aδ fibers and unmyelinated C-fiber activation.[54] It is essential that when the symptoms of postherpetic neuralgia are first noted, a regimen of early aggressive intervention be initiated in an attempt to prevent these neurophysiological changes from taking place.

Although there is no universally accepted treatment regimen to provide prophylaxis against or effect resolution of early cases of postherpetic neuralgia, a variety of treatment approaches have been pursued, and antiviral medications may prove helpful if given early in high dose.[40] In addition to pharmacotherapy, these treatments may include invasive procedures such as the use of sympathetic nerve blocks (in the case of VZV involving a branch of the trigeminal nerve, a cervicothoracic block at C6, i.e., stellate ganglion block), somatic nerve blocks, and subcutaneous infiltration of local anesthetic and steroid beneath the areas of acute vesicular eruption. Sympathetic nerve block therapy often may be useful in the early phases of postherpetic neuralgia to relieve pain and halt its progression.[40] Pharmacotherapeutic approaches in treating acute VZV may include the use of antiviral medication, corticosteroids, analgesics, antidepressants, or topical therapy. NSAIDs may be used for controlling mild pain in acute herpes zoster, with opioid therapy being reserved for severe pain exacerbations. Mixed mu-opioid agonists and norepinephrine reuptake inhibitors such at tramadol may be good substitutes for opioids and should likely be tried first. Tricyclic antidepressant medications such as amitriptyline, nortriptyline, or desipramine may be used for both their potential pain-relieving and sedative properties. Anxiolytic agents such as lorazepam, alprazolam, or diazepam may also be used on a short-term basis.[40]

There is no single therapy that has been shown to reliably treat PHN pain, with the use of multiple pharmacotherapeutic approaches generally being necessary. A variety of topical agents, such as capsaicin, and local anesthetic agents, such as the lidocaine skin patch, may be useful adjuncts to other therapies in some patients.[42][57] Several classes of medication may be used in treating the pain of PHN. These include antidepressants such as amitriptyline or nortriptyline, anticonvulsants such as gabapentin and pregabalin (although the use of other anticonvulsants such as carbamazepine, phenytoin, clonazepam, and valproic acid may be considered and employed), and opioids (long-acting oral forms of oxycodone, morphine, and the fentanyl skin patch may be of help)[41] or mu-opioid agonists and norepinephrine reuptake inhibitors such as tramadol.[42][57] A trial-and-error approach using anticonvulsants such as carbamazepine, phenytoin, clonazepam, and valproic acid may be used. Transcutaneous electrical nerve stimulation (TENS) may also be a useful adjunct.

It should be emphasized that time is of the absolute essence, and sympathetic blockage in the form of a series of stellate ganglion blocks should be performed at the first sign of PHN involving a branch of CN V, which should be treated within 6 months of onset, as the likelihood of achieving satisfactory pain relief after this time is considerably diminished.[40]

36.6.5 Episodic Neuropathic (Neuralgic) Facial Pain

The classification of neuralgias of the face, head, and neck is confounding to many practitioners. Neuralgic pain is characterized by paroxysmal painful attacks of sharp, stabbing, electric shock–like, or burning pain. It may occur spontaneously or be evoked by innocuous stimulus such as light touch to a trigger zone. Examples of cranial nerve neuralgias include trigeminal neuralgia, glossopharyngeal neuralgia, nervus intermedius, and vagal and superior laryngeal neuralgia. Other painful disorders in the head and neck that carry the moniker *neuralgia* include occipital neuralgia and postherpetic neuralgia.

Trigeminal Neuralgia

Trigeminal neuralgia (TN), or tic douloureux, is characterized by episodic attacks of agonizingly intense sharp, stabbing, burning, or electric shock–like pain in the trigeminal distribution. Although not encountered as commonly as TMD, TN is the most frequently occurring neuralgic condition in the head and neck. Attacks of pain frequently occur in close proximity to the ear and are not uncommonly the cause of referred pain to the ear. Because of the relative frequency of occurrence, the etiology, pathogenesis, and management of trigeminal neuralgia have been studied extensively. Painful episodes may last from a few seconds to a few minutes and are triggered by light touch to a trigger zone on the face or intraorally, including such light stimulus as a breeze or vibration. Trigger zones are particularly common around the mouth and nose, with pain often being exacerbated by such simple acts as washing the face, applying makeup, brushing the teeth, and eating or drinking. Paradoxically, pinching or pressing the trigger area is unlikely to provide an attack of pain.[32]

The ICHD-2 recognizes two distinctive forms of trigeminal neuralgia, classic trigeminal neuralgia (CTN) and symptomatic trigeminal neuralgia (STN).[33] Cases in which no etiology can be established (e.g., idiopathic trigeminal neuralgia) and cases with potential vascular compression of CN V are included under the term *classic trigeminal neuralgia*. This diagnosis requires that no neurologic deficit be present. When a demonstrable structural lesion other than vascular compression is demonstrated, the diagnosis of STN is made. These abnormalities may include multiple sclerosis plaques or the presence of mass lesions or disorders of the posterior fossa. Unlike CTN, STN does not demonstrate a refractory period after a painful attack, and there may be sensory impairment in that trigeminal division.

As stated above, in the absence of other concomitant disease, physical examination is unremarkable in CTN, with the absence of any detectable neurologic deficit within the distribution of the involved branch of the trigeminal nerve. Although in the majority of TN cases no identifying etiology may be evident at the time of examination, in as many as 15% of patients there may be an underlying cause such as a benign or malignant neoplasm in the posterior fossa or multiple sclerosis that will make its presence known at a later point in time.[34] Thus it is recommended that when the diagnosis of TN is considered, a magnetic resonance imaging (MRI) study with and without contrast be performed, paying particular attention to the posterior cranial fossa.

Diagnostically, TN is most commonly confused with TMD of myofascial origin. The chief differentiating factor here is that the primary pain in TN will be limited to a single branch of CN V, whereas pain of myofascial origin is typically diffuse. Other disorders that must be considered when making the diagnosis of TN include dental causes such as pulpal pathology, dental infection or cracked teeth, periodontal pathology, pain from pressure of a denture on the mental nerve, AFP including AO, glossopharyngeal neuralgia, postherpetic neuralgia, cluster headache, paroxysmal hemicrania, and temporal arteritis.

It is thought that 80 to 90% of cases of TN may arise from specific abnormalities of trigeminal afferent neurons in the trigeminal root or ganglion, resulting in hyperexcitable afferents that give rise to paroxysmal episodes of pain as a result of synchronized afterdischarge activity.[25,30]

Both medical and surgical modalities of therapy have been used to treat trigeminal neuralgia. Although trigeminal neuralgia may be an excruciatingly painful disorder, in the absence of a neoplasm as its primary cause it is a nonfatal one, and therefore the primary approach to treatment should be medical intervention with surgery being reserved for patients who become refractory to or are unable to tolerate available medications. Various medications that demonstrate nerve membrane stabilizing qualities are available for use singly or in combination and include baclofen, carbamazepine, gabapentin, lamotrigine, sodium valproate, clonazepam, and phenytoin. In view of its greater safety, it has been recommended that baclofen should be the initial drug of choice for treating glossopharyngeal or trigeminal neuralgia.[35,37] In those cases where baclofen is ineffective or not tolerated, carbamazepine, oxcarbazepine, or gabapentin is the next drug of choice. For patients who do not respond to therapy with a single medication, the combination of two or more of them may be needed and titrated on an individual basis as tolerated and needed to manage the symptoms.

Examples include the use of baclofen and gabapentin, and baclofen with carbamazepine.[58]

Tricyclic antidepressants such as amitriptyline, nortriptyline and desipramine, trazodone (an antidepressant/antineuralgic drug not related to tricyclic, tetracyclic, or other known antidepressants), clonazepam (a benzodiazepine), and NSAIDs are frequently helpful when used in combination with antineuralgic drugs. The clinician may find that, in the end, the combination of medications becomes very individualized for the individual patient, balancing the right "cocktail" of medications without producing intolerable side effects from any one of them. In my experience, neural blockade with local anesthetic may also be effective in breaking the cycle of pain when used in combination with antineuralgic medications. In those cases where medications are no longer effective, surgical intervention may then be indicated. Although invasive neurosurgical procedures may provide pain relief, they carry significant risks, potentially permanent sequelae, the potential for failure, and the recurrence of pain. Gamma knife radiosurgery is a potential option with low morbidity compared with other interventions and a good to excellent outcome reported in 77% or more of patients.[38] It should be stressed here that not all patients with trigeminal neuralgia will respond to medical intervention, just as not all patients will respond to surgical treatment, and, unfortunately, some patients may not respond well to either modality of treatment.

Glossopharyngeal Neuralgia

Glossopharyngeal neuralgia is a relatively uncommon disorder characterized by unilateral paroxysmal attacks of sharp, stabbing, burning, or electric shock-like pain that may be felt in the ear, base of the tongue, tonsil, lateral pharyngeal wall, nasopharynx, and beneath the angle of the jaw. As with trigeminal neuralgia, a trigger zone is present, usually located in the lateral pharyngeal wall, tonsillar fossa area, or in the area of the external ear posterior to the ramus of the mandible with pain referring outward from the trigger point. Painful episodes may be provoked by stimulation of the trigger zone during swallowing, yawning, or coughing, with some patients experiencing bradycardia, syncope, and seizure during an attack of pain.[39] Other than the presence of a trigger zone, physical examination is essentially unremarkable in the classical form with the absence of any detectable neurologic deficits. Before making the diagnosis of glossopharyngeal neuralgia, care should be taken to rule out the presence of neoplasm or other cause in the oro-, hypo-, or nasopharynx or at the cerebellopontine angle. When found, this is termed *symptomatic glossopharyngeal neuralgia,* and, when present, aching pain may persist between paroxysms and sensory impairment may be noted.[33] A technique useful in making the diagnosis of classical glossopharyngeal neuralgia is to perform a local anesthetic block of the trigger point. Medical intervention for the treatment of glossopharyngeal is the same as for trigeminal neuralgia.

Nervus Intermedius (Geniculate) Neuralgia

Nervus intermedius (geniculate) neuralgia is a rare potentially debilitating disorder characterized by paroxysmal attacks of pain deep in the depth of the ear not attributed to another disorder.[33] The posterior wall of the auditory canal may be a trigger zone.[33,59] Potential therapies have included therapeutic approaches such as medical management as in more common cranial neuralgias, and surgical approaches including microvascular decompression and nerve sectioning.[59]

Vagal and Superior Laryngeal Neuralgia

Vagal and superior laryngeal neuralgia is an uncommon disorder characterized by sudden severe episodic attacks of brief lancinating electric shock-like pain involving the thyroid cartilage, pyriform sinus, and angle of the mandible, but rarely involving the ear. Attacks of pain may be precipitated by swallowing, yawning, or coughing, and usually occur in combination with glossopharyngeal neuralgia.[42,43] As with the other neuralgias, physical examination is essentially unremarkable with no neurologic deficit being noted within the distribution of the vagus nerve. The diagnosis is established by clinical history and by identifying a trigger zone. Laryngeal topical anesthesia or blockade of the superior laryngeal nerve is said to alleviate the pain and is a useful diagnostic and prognostic procedure.[33,44]

Pharmacological therapy as described for trigeminal neuralgia is indicated for the management of this disorder, with surgical management being reserved for those cases in which pharmacotherapy has been unsuccessful.

36.6.6 Headaches

The classification of headache is complex and often controversial. In 1988 the International Headache Society (HIS) published the first-ever classification of headache establishing uniform terminology and consistent operational diagnostic criteria covering the entire range of headache disorders.[45] In 2004, ICHD-2 was published, providing a foundation for clinical practice and research.[46] The reader is referred to the new ICHD-2 classification for an in-depth look at the current classification of headaches, as only those headache disorders commonly known to present with referred pain to the ear are discussed here.

Tension-Type Headache

Tension-type headache (TTH) is the most common type of primary headache, with 80% of all patients who seek medical care for their headaches falling into this category.[33] Although tenderness of the pericranial muscles is an extremely common finding, some patients do not demonstrate this feature and hence TTH is subclassified as with or without pericranial tenderness. As currently classified, TTH is broken down primarily into infrequent episodic TTH, frequent episodic TTH, and chronic TTH. All three forms are further subclassified as being associated with pericranial tenderness or not. Episodic TTH usually responds to over-the-counter analegsics.[49] For the TTH to be classified as chronic, it must have been present for at least 15 days a month on average for more than 3 months (180 days per year or more), lasting hours or occurring continuously, and having two of the following characteristics: bilateral location, pressing/tightening nonpulsatile quality, mild or moderate intensity, and not aggravated by routine physical activity such as walking or climbing stairs.[47]

Tension-type headache is usually described as a steady nonpulsatile aching pain that may be unilateral but is most commonly bilateral, and it may be localized to a single region in the head or it may be generalized. Pain may be felt in the frontotemporal region including the face, occipital region, parietal region, or any combination of these sites, with patients often describing a feeling of tightness, a drawing sensation, or band-like pressure. The pain from TTH, especially headache involving the frontotemporal region, may refer to the ear, presenting as otalgia. As in TMD, the resulting ear pain may cause of the patient to seek medical attention. The severity of the headache pain may vary from soreness to gnawing, or a dull ache to a sharp episodic or continuous stabbing pain. The patient frequently complains of a feeling of tightness or cramping in the neck or shoulder regions (cervical myalgia) but may also be felt in the masseter muscles. TTH may be accompanied by symptoms such as photophobia or phonophobia (but not both), periorbital pain, lacrimation, tinnitus, vertigo, and referred otalgia.

Although the relationship between peripheral and central mechanisms is believed to be the basis for initiation of TTHs, the means by which this happens is uncertain, although the same causative factors are considered in TTH and masticatory muscle pain.[60] It is suggested that the mechanisms behind TTH relate to persistent nociceptive input, leading to central sensitization that is adversely affected by impaired central modulation. Hence, it may be difficult to differentiate TTH that includes occipital, parietal, or frontotemporal pain from TMD pain of myofascial origin. All of them may present as frontotemporal, temporal, or occipital pain, often with neck or shoulder tightness, and all may be a source of referred pain to the ear or periaural region.

It is also important to understand that patients with myofascial facial pain may relate a history of TTHs, just as patients with TTHs frequently mention a previous or concomitant history of facial pain. Another confounding issue is the frequent bias and lack of global perspective on the part of the clinician. Some physicians fail to examine the orofacial structures and musculature, and overdiagnose TTH, and some dentists do not examine beyond the orofacial region and overdiagnose TMD. Musculoskeletal examination of a patient with TTH or TMD of myofascial origin (i.e., muscle tenderness producing pain) will demonstrate nodular or band-like tender muscle trigger points as previously described, which reproduce or exacerbate the patient's pain complaint. The appropriate diagnosis should be made based on the region from which the primary pain or dysfunction emanates.

Cluster Headache and Other Trigeminal Autonomic Cephalalgias

As a group, the autonomic cephalalgias share the clinical features of headache and prominent cranial parasympathetic autonomic features. Although cluster headache is not known to present with secondary otalgia as one of its features, chronic paroxysmal hemicranias, one of the other trigeminal autonomic cephalalgias listed in the ICHD-2, has been reported to present with otalgia with the sensation of external acoustic meatus obstruction.[48]

Giant Cell Arteritis (Temporal Arteritis)

Giant cell arteritis (GCA) is a form of primary headache known for its variable clinical features. Common complaints include headache, hyperalgesia of the scalp, polymyalgia rheumatica, and jaw claudication.[33] Hence, patients with this disorder may experience pain on mastication and referred pain to the teeth, ear, jaw, zygoma, and nuchal and occipital regions. The major risk of GCA is blindness from anterior ischemic optic neuropathy, which can be prevented by immediate steroid therapy.[33] Diagnosis may be made by palpation of a swollen tender scalp artery and elevated erythrocyte sedimentation rate and/or C-reactive protein. Temporal biopsy will reveal the presence of giant cell arteritis in some but not all cases. Treatment consists of corticosteroids that should result in rapid significant to complete resolution of symptoms.

Secondary Headaches

Secondary headaches include headache or facial pain attributed to disorders of cranium, neck, eyes, ears, nose, sinuses, teeth, mouth, or other facial or cranial structures. The common denominator in headache from this diverse spectrum of disorders is stretching, compression, or inflammation of pain-sensitive structures in the skull, including the brain, meninges, arteries, veins, eyes, ears, teeth, nose, and paranasal sinuses. The underlying cause may be a mass lesion, hemorrhage, or inflammatory disease. For example, as the cerebrovascular innervation (which is selectively nociceptive specific) is supplied by cranial nerve V_1 and some V_3 fibers, pain may be referred to the ear by any event that produces traction or inflammation in structures innervated by these nerves.

Cervicogenic pain as originally described was a headache form deriving its origin from one of several structures in the neck or back of the head (including nerves, ganglia, nerve roots, uncovertebral joints, intervertebral joints, disks, bone, periosteum, muscle, and ligaments).[49] Headache associated with myofascial tenderness in the cervical musculature is now coded as infrequent episodic TTH, frequent episodic TTH, or chronic TTH, all associated with pericranial tenderness and is no longer included as a form of cervicogenic pain.[33] As its name implies, cervicogenic headache originates in the neck with a referral pattern to the head, frequently the ophthalmic division of the trigeminal nerve, presenting as retro-orbital and frontotemporal headache pain or preauricular pain. This pain referral pattern is explained by close proximity of the cervical spinal and medullary dorsal horn with apparent convergence of some cervical nociceptive afferent fibers in the MDH.[41] Through this pattern of convergence, pain may also be referred to the vertex along the midline, periaural region(s), pinna of the ear(s), and jaw(s), including occasionally the teeth.[9]

36.7 Discussion

When the otologic examination is normal but the patient complains of ear pain, the general otolaryngologic examination should be extended to include additional areas. If not already obtained, careful mirror or fiberoptic examinations of the nasopharynx and laryngopharynx should be performed. The TMJ, temporal arteries, tonsillar fossae, base of tongue, carotid artery, and neck muscles should be carefully palpated. The teeth and cervical spine can be percussed. Imaging studies of the skull, sinuses, teeth, TMJs, and cervical spine can be obtained in selected patients.

Two diseases cited in this chapter that require prompt diagnosis and management are temporal arteritis and head and neck malignancy. Although temporal arteritis is uncommon, recognition is vital to initiate corticosteroid treatment and prevent blindness. Classically the artery pulse may be absent and the erythrocyte sedimentation rate (ERS) elevated, but on occasion the pulse may be normal, tenderness to palpation minimal, and laboratory test normal. The physician should maintain a high index of suspicion and initiate corticosteroid therapy promptly.

Recognition of head and neck malignancy is not as urgent as temporal arteritis, but some of these masses can easily be missed, with disastrous results. Particularly, neoplasms in the nasopharynx, sinus, tonsil, base of tongue, and hypopharynx can spread dramatically and quickly if not treated promptly. Ear pain can be the only manifestation of these malignancies. Suspicious soft tissue lesions should be biopsied.

Many different causes of referred otalgia were reviewed in this chapter, and the clinician should be familiar with all of them. For practical purposes, however, the most common causes are TMD (most commonly myofascial-pain dysfunction), cervical myalgia, and dental disease. TMD usually refers pain to the preauricular area over the joint and also to the angle of the jaw just behind and deep to the ramus of the mandible. There may be a history of clenching the teeth, bruxism, and prolonged dental work. The TMJ(s) may be tender to palpation and the examiner may feel popping, clicking, or crepitus on wide opening. Cervical myalgia usually refers pain to the postauricular area where the muscles attach to the mastoid tip, although it may commonly refer to the temporal or preauricular regions and ear. The sternocleidomastoid or trapezius muscles may be tender to palpation or may be in spasm on the involved side. Dental abscess may present with tenderness to percussion of the affected tooth. A dentist can best manage TMD and dental disease, and a physical therapist can help manage orofacial and cervical myalgia.

When a patient with persistent ear pain has no identifiable primary or secondary source of pain, an MRI of the head (brain) with and without contrast should be obtained with special attention to the base of skull on the involved side, including coronal views of the infratemporal fossa. Although MRI results usually are normal, the patient and physician are reassured that there is no serious intracranial disease. Following an extensive evaluation, if no etiology is found for the otalgia and if there is no response to empiric trials of therapy, the patient should be referred to a pain management clinic, which offers medical therapy as well as behavioral medicine evaluation and counseling.

References

[1] Paparella MM, Jung TTK, Gluckman JC, Meyerhoff WL, eds. Otolaryngology, vol 2, 3rd ed. Philadelphia: WB Saunders, 1991:1237–1242

[2] Bonica JJ. Definitions and taxonomy of pain. In: Bonica JJ, ed. The Management of Pain, vol 1, 2nd ed. Philadelphia: Lea & Febiger, 1990:18–27

[3] Bonica JJ. Anatomic and physiologic basis of nociception and pain. In: Bonica JJ, ed. The Management of Pain, vol 1, 2nd ed. Philadelphia: Lea & Febiger, 1990:28–94

[4] Cross SA. Pathophysiology of pain. Mayo Clin Proc 1994; 69: 375–383

[5] Sessle BJ. Hu JW, Amano N, Zhon G. Convergence of cutaneous, tooth pulp, visceral, neck and muscle afferent onto nociceptive and non-nociceptive neurons in trigeminal sub-nucleus caudalis medullary dorsal horn (MDH) and its implications for referred pain. Pain 1986; 27: 219–235

[6] Sessle BJ. The neurobiology of facial and dental pain: present knowledge, future directions. J Dent Res 1987; 66: 962–981

[7] Poletti CE. C-2 and C-3 radiculopathies: anatomy, patterns of cephalic pain and pathology. APS 1992; 1: 272–275

[8] de Leeuw R. and Klasser G.D. Orofacial Pain: guidelines for assessment, diagnosis, and management, 5th ed. The American Academy of Orofacial Pain, Hanover Park II; Quintessence Books, 2013

[9] Fromm GH, Sessle BJ. Trigeminal Neuralgia: Current Concepts Regarding pathogenesis and Treatment. Boston: Butterworth-Heinemann, 1991:71–104

[10] Stacey MJ. Free nerve endings in skeletal muscle of the cat. J Anat 1969; 105: 231–254

[11] Gerwin RD. Neurobiology of the myofascial trigger point. Baillieres Clin Rheumatol 1994; 8: 747–762

[12] Jerger J. Handbook of Clinical Impedance Audiometry. Dobbs Ferry, NY: American Electromedics, 1975:85–126

[13] Bernstein JM. Otalgia: its not always what it seems to be. J Respir Dis 1987; 8: 71–82

[14] Thaller SR, De Silva A. Otalgia with a normal ear. Am Fam Physician 1987; 36: 129–136

[15] Mense S. Nociception from skeletal muscle in relation to clinical muscle pain. Pain 1993; 54: 241–289

[16] Sessle BJ. Masticatory muscle disorders: basic science perspectives. In: Sessle BJ, Bryant PS, Dionne RA, eds. Temporomandibular Disorders and Related Pain Conditions: Progress in Pain Research and Management, vol 4. Seattle: IASP Press, 1995:47–61

[17] Sessle BJ. Recent insights into brainstem mechanisms underlying craniofacial pain. J Dent Educ 2002; 66: 108–112

[18] Mense S. Mechanisms of pain in hind limb muscles: experimental findings and open questions. In: Sessle BJ, Bryant PS, Dionne RA, eds. Temporomandibular Disorders and Related Pain Conditions: Progress and Pain Research and Management, vol 4. Seattle: IASP Press, 1995:63–69

[19] Bernstein JM, Mohl ND, Spiller H. Temporomandibular joint dysfunction masquerading as disease of ear, nose, and throat. Trans Am Acad Ophthalmol Otolaryngol 1969; 73: 1208–1217

[20] Gaynor EB. Otolaryngologic manifestations of gastroesophageal reflux. Am J Gastroenterol 1991; 86: 801–808

[21] Gibson WS, Jr, Cochran W. Otalgia in infants and children—a manifestation of gastroesophageal reflux. Int J Pediatr Otorhinolaryngol 1994; 28: 213–218

[22] Travell J, Rinzler SH. The myofascial genesis of pain. Postgrad Med 1952; 11: 425–434

[23] Travell JG, Simons DG. Myofascial Pain and Dysfunction: The Trigger Point Manual. Baltimore: Williams & Wilkins, 1983

[24] Laskin DM. Current concepts in the management of temporomandibular joint disorders. Continuing education course presented at annual meeting of the American Academy of Oral Pathology, 1982

[25] Fricton JR, Kroening R, Haley D, Siegert R. Myofascial pain syndrome of the head and neck: a review of clinical characteristics of 164 patients. Oral Surg Oral Med Oral Pathol 1985; 60: 615–623

[26] Campbell SM. Regional myofascial pain syndromes. Rheum Dis Clin North Am 1989; 15: 31–44

[27] Fricton JR. Myofascial pain syndrome. Neurol Clin 1989; 7: 413–427

[28] Menses, Simons DG. Myofascial pain caused by trigger points. In: Muscle Pain: Understanding Its Nature, Diagnosis, and Treatment. Philadelphia: Lippincott Williams & Wilkins, 2001:205–288

[29] Woda A. Mechanisms of neuropathic pain. In: Lund JP, Lavigne GH, Dubner R, Sessle BJ, eds. Orofacial Pain: From Basic Science to Clinical Management. Chicago: Quintessence, 2001:67–78

[30] Lavigne G, Woda A, Truelove E, Ship JA, Dao T, Goulet JP. Mechanisms associated with unusual orofacial pain. J Orofac Pain 2005; 19: 9–21

[31] Remick RA, Blasberg B, Campos PE, Miles JE. Psychiatric disorders associated with atypical facial pain. Can J Psychiatry 1983; 28: 178–181

[32] Fromm GH. Trigeminal neuralgia and related disorders. Neurol Clin 1989; 7: 305–319

[33] Headache Classification Committee of the International Headache Society. The International Classification of Headache Disorders. Cephalalgia 2004; 24: 175–182

[34] Devor M, Amir R, Rappaport ZH. Pathophysiology of trigeminal neuralgia: the ignition hypothesis. Clin J Pain 2002; 18: 4–13

[35] Bullitt E, Tew JM, Boyd J. Intracranial tumors in patients with facial pain. J Neurosurg 1986; 64: 865–871

[36] Fromm GH, Terrence CF, Maroon JC. Trigeminal neuralgia. Current concepts regarding etiology and pathogenesis. Arch Neurol 1984; 41: 1204–1207

[37] Fromm GH, Terrence CF, Chattha AS. Baclofen in the treatment of trigeminal neuralgia: double-blind study and long-term follow-up. Ann Neurol 1984; 15: 240–244

[38] Petit JH, Herman JM, Nagda S, DiBiase SJ, Chin LS. Radiosurgical treatment of trigeminal neuralgia: evaluating quality of life and treatment outcomes. Int J Radiat Oncol Biol Phys 2003; 56: 1147–1153

[39] Chalmers AC, Olson JL. Glossopharyngeal neuralgia with syncope and cervical mass. Otolaryngol Head Neck Surg 1989; 100: 252–255

[40] Katz JA, Phero JC, McDonald JS, Green DB. Herpes zoster management. Anesth Prog 1989; 36: 35–40

[41] Watson CPN. Management issues of neuropathic trigeminal pain from a medical perspective. J Orofac Pain 2004; 18: 366–373

[42] Loeser JD. Cranial neuralgias. In: Bonica JJ, ed. The Management of Pain, vol 1, 2nd ed. Philadelphia: Lea & Febiger, 1990:676–686

[43] Chawla JC, Falconer MA. Glossopharyngeal and vagal neuralgia. BMJ 1967; 3: 529–531

[44] Bonica JJ, ed. The Management of Pain, vol 1. Philadelphia: Lea & Febiger, 1953:790–797

[45] Headache Classification Committee of the International Headache Society. Classification and diagnostic criteria for headache disorders, cranial neuralgias and facial pain. Cephalalgia 1988; 8 Suppl 7: 1–96

[46] Dalessio DJ. Wolff's Headache and Other Head Pain, 5th ed. New York: Oxford University Press, 1987

[47] Lipton RB, Bigal ME, Steiner TJ, Silberstein SD, Olesen J. Classification of primary headaches. Neurology 2004; 63: 427–435

[48] Boes CJ, Swanson JW, Dodick DW. Chronic paroxysmal hemicrania presenting as otalgia with a sensation of external acoustic meatus obstruction: two cases and a pathophysiologic hypothesis. Headache 1998; 38: 787–791

[49] Sjaastad O, Fredriksen TA, Pfaffenrath V. Cervicogenic headache: diagnostic criteria. Headache 1990; 30: 725–726

[50] De Leeuw R. Orofacial Pain Guidelines for Assessment, Diagnosis, and Management, 4th ed. Hanover Park, IL: American Academy of Orofacial Pain, Quintessence Books, 2008

[51] Stanbro M, Gray BH, Kellicut DC. Carotidynia: revisiting an unfamiliar entity. Ann Vasc Surg 2011;25:1144–1153

[52] Diatchenko L, Nackley AG, Slade G, Fillingim RB, Maixner W. Idiopathic pain disorders—pathways of vulnerability. Pain 2006;123:226–230

[53] Haanpaa M, Attal N, Backonja M, et al. NeuPSIG guidelines on neuropathic pain assessment. Pain 2011;152:14–27

[54] Truini A, Galeotti F, Haanpa M, et al. Pathophysiology of pain in postherpetic neuralgia: a clinical and neurophysiological study. Pain 2008;140:405–410

[55] BMJ 1979;1:5

[56] Oaklander AL, Cohen SP, Raju Shubha VY. Intractable postherpetic itch and cutaneous deafferentation after facial shingles. Pain 2002;96:9–12

[57] Sampathkumar P, Drage LA, Martin DP. Herpes zoster (shingles) and post herpetic neuralgia. Mayo Clin Proc 2009;84:274–280

[58] Fromm GH, Terrence CF, Chatthaas AS. Baclofen in the treatment of trigeminal neuralgia: double-blind study and long term follow-up. Ann Neurol 1984;15:240–244

[59] Tubbs RS, Steck DT, Mortazavi MM, Cohen-Gadol AA. The nervus intermedius: a review of its anatomy, function, pathology and role in neurosurgery. World Neurosurg 2013;79:763–767

[60] Benoliel R, Sharav Y. Masticatory myofascial pain, tension-type and chronic daily headache. In: Sharav Y, Benoliel R, eds. Orofacial Pain and Headache. Philadelphia: Mosby Elsevier, 2008:132–133

37 Evaluation and Management of Pulsatile Tinnitus

Aristides Sismanis

37.1 Introduction

Pulsatile tinnitus (PT) is an uncommon otologic symptom that often presents a diagnostic and management dilemma for the otolaryngologist–head and neck surgeon. This chapter discusses the recent advances in the evaluation and management of PT.

37.2 Pathophysiology and Classification

Pulsating tinnitus originates from vascular structures within the cranial cavity, head and neck region, and thoracic cavity. Eddies and associated bruits produced by increased blood flow through vessels or stenosis of vascular lumina are responsible for this symptom. Depending on the vessel of origin, PT can be classified as arterial or venous. Pulsatile tinnitus can be further classified as objective or subjective based on whether it is audible to both patient and examiner or to the patient only.

Rarely pulsating noises, but not true PT, originate from other structures that are classified as nonvascular. High-pitched tinnitus with a pulsatile component, often bilateral and associated with high-frequency sensorineural hearing loss (SNHL), should not be confused with arterial PT. This type of tinnitus is subjective and is considered to be related to the SNHL.

The following section describes the most common etiologies of PT.

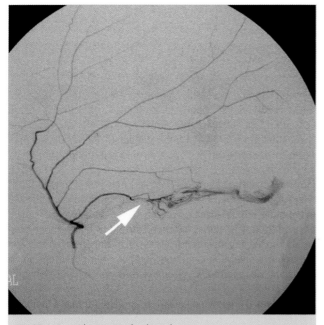

Fig. 37.1 Carotid angiography, lateral projection. An arteriovenous fistula (AVF) is shown (*arrow*) between a posterior meningeal branch of the middle meningeal artery and the transverse sinus.

37.3 Arterial Etiologies

37.3.1 Atherosclerotic Carotid Artery Disease

In patients older than 50 years of age, atherosclerotic carotid artery disease (ACAD) is a common cause of PT, and it is often associated with at least one of the following risk factors: hypertension, angina, hyperlipidemia, diabetes mellitus, and smoking. Pulsatile tinnitus may be the first manifestation of ACAD, and therefore the otolaryngologist may be the first to be consulted for this symptom.[1,2] Bruit(s) produced by turbulent blood flow at stenotic segments of the carotid system are responsible for the PT. In a series of 12 patients with PT secondary to ACAD, ipsilateral carotid bruit was present in all of them. Diagnosis can be confirmed in most patients by duplex ultrasound studies.[1] In patients with ACAD at the skull base or the cavernous sinus, duplex ultrasound studies might not be revealing, and magnetic resonance imaging (MRI) should be considered. Recently MRI has been shown to accurately identify carotid plaque features, including intraplaque hemorrhage, neovasculature, and vascular wall inflammation.[3]

37.3.2 Intracranial Vascular Abnormalities

Intracranial vascular abnormalities are uncommon etiologies of PT; however, a high index of suspicion and proper evaluation is required to avoid misdiagnosis and potential catastrophic consequences. The majority of these lesions are dural arteriovenous fistulas (AVFs) and malformations (AVMs), and PT is the most common manifestation. The transverse and sigmoid dural sinuses are the most commonly involved, followed by the cavernous sinus.[4,5] Dural AVFs make up approximately 15% of intracranial AVMs, which usually become symptomatic during the fifth or sixth decades of life.[6,7] In contrast to AVMs, AVFs are usually acquired and thought to result from dural sinuses, spontaneous or traumatic thrombosis, obstructing neoplasms, surgery, or infection. As the thrombosed segments recanalize, ingrowths of dural arteries occur and arterial to sinus anastomoses are formed.[6] PT in such patients is of the arterial type, and is always associated with a loud skull bruit over the involved area. ▶ Fig. 37.1 depicts a carotid angiogram of a patient with an AVF between a posterior meningeal branch of the middle meningeal artery and the transverse sinus.

According to a recent report, the most critical anatomic feature is the presence of cortical venous drainage, as this finding identifies lesions at high risk for future hemorrhage or ischemic neurologic injury.[8] It has been reported that patients presenting with PT have a less aggressive clinical course, with an estimated annual rate of intracerebral hemorrhage of 1.4 to 1.5%.[8] The mortality rate of a ruptured dural AVF has been reported between 10 and 20%.[6]

Aneurysms of the anterior inferior cerebellar artery, and dissecting aneurysms of the internal carotid and vertebral arteries,

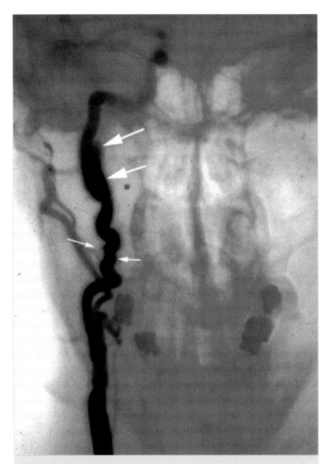

Fig. 37.2 Carotid angiography, anteroposterior view, of a 36-year-old woman with fibromuscular dysplasia. The "string of beads" is a pathognomonic finding (*arrows*).

although uncommon, can be associated with PT.[9,10] Other manifestations of dissecting aneurysms include pain, transient ischemic attacks, cranial neuropathies, Horner syndrome, and subarachnoid hemorrhage.[6,11–13] Sudden head rotation, especially when accompanied by extension (e.g., the ace serve in tennis), can be a precipitating event. Fibromuscular dysplasia (FMD), various arteriopathies such as Marfan syndrome, and osteogenesis imperfecta are predisposing factors.[14]

37.3.3 Glomus Tumors of the Jugular Foramen and Middle Ear

Subjective PT and conductive hearing loss are the most common manifestations of glomus jugulare and tympanicum tumors.[15] Diagnosis is based on otoscopic findings, and imaging studies of the temporal bone and skull base.

37.3.4 Fibromuscular Dysplasia

Fibromuscular dysplasia is a nonatherosclerotic, noninflammatory stenosing vascular disease that primarily affects women of ages 20 to 60 years. It most commonly involves the renal and internal carotid arteries, and hypertension, headache, and PT are the most common presenting symptoms.[16] Because of the PT, the otolaryngologist might be the first clinician to be

consulted. Cases with carotid or vertebral arteries involvement may develop dissection and/or aneurysms, and present with symptoms of transient ischemic attacks or stroke.[17,18] the typical angiographic finding is that of a "string of beads."[18] ▶ Fig. 37.2 is a carotid angiogram of a 36-year-old woman with FMD.

37.3.5 Tortuous Internal Carotid Artery

Pulsatile tinnitus secondary to a tortuous internal carotid artery is more common in older individuals and is often accompanied by an audible bruit over the involved vessel. Rarely, this entity may present as an abnormal sensation in the throat associated with a pulsating pharyngeal or cervical mass.[19,20] It is likely that aging carotid vessels become tortuous, resulting in turbulent blood flow and PT. Atherosclerosis and FMD have been reported in association with tortuous internal carotid arteries.[21]

In my experience this is a benign condition, and PT usually subsides spontaneously with time. Symptoms of cerebral ischemia warrant consultation with a vascular surgeon. Diagnosis is made with computed tomography angiography (CTA) or magnetic resonance angiography (MRA).[22] The box below summarizes the arterial etiologies.

Arterial Etiologies of Pulsatile Tinnitus

1. Dural, skull base, and cervical region AVMs/AVFs[5,85,128–132]
2. Atherosclerotic carotid and subclavian artery disease[1,2,107,133–136]
3. Glomus tumors of jugular foramen and middle ear[137,138]
4. Tortuous internal carotid artery[22]
5. Dehiscense superior semicircular canal[139]
6. Fibromuscular dysplasia of the carotid artery[16–18,140–143]
7. Increased cardiac output (anemia, thrombocythemia, thyrotoxicosis, pregnancy)[144,145]
8. Aneurysms of the anterior inferior cerebellar artery[9]
9. Extracranial carotid artery dissection[11–13,82,146]
10. Intrapetrous carotid artery dissection and aneurysm[83,147,148]
11. Brachiocephalic artery stenosis[149]
12. External carotid artery stenosis[150]
13. Vascular anomalies of the middle ear[116,151–156]
14. Aberrant artery in the stria vascularis[157]
15. Vascular compression of the eighth nerve[158–160]
16. Increased cardiac output (anemia, thrombocythemia, thyrotoxicosis, pregnancy)[144,145]
17. Aortic murmurs[161]
18. Paget disease[162–164]
19. Otosclerosis[48]
20. Hypertension or antihypertensive agents[48]

37.4 Venous Etiologies

37.4.1 Idiopathic Intracranial Hypertension Syndrome (Pseudotumor Cerebri)

In my experience, idiopathic intracranial hypertension (IIH) syndrome or pseudotumor cerebri is one of the most common etiologies of venous PT, which may be the first or only manifestation of this syndrome.[23,24] Other associated otologic symptoms may include hearing loss, dizziness, and aural fullness.[25] Due to the otologic presentations of this syndrome, the otolaryngologist might be the first clinician to be consulted.

This syndrome affects obese women of childbearing age in more than 90% of cases, and is characterized by increased intracranial pressure (ICP) without focal signs of neurologic dysfunction except for occasional fifth, sixth, and seventh cranial nerve palsies.[26-29] Rarely this syndrome may affect males and normal-weight individuals of any age.[30-32] Other common presenting symptoms include posture-dependent headaches, and visual changes (blurred vision, transient visual obscurations, retrobulbar pain, diplopia) due to papilledema, prompting patients to seek evaluation by a neurologist or an ophthalmologist.[33] Although papilledema is common in these patients, its absence does not exclude this entity.[34-36] Optical coherence tomography (OCT) has recently been reported to differentiate papilledema secondary to increased ICP from optic disk swelling secondary to optic neuropathy.[33,37] Diagnosis is established by lumbar puncture and documentation of elevated cerebrospinal fluid (CSF) pressure (greater than 200 mm H_2O) with normal CSF constituents.[38] In most patients, IIH syndrome has a benign and self-limiting course, but in up to 25% of patients chronicity has been reported.[26]

Despite a large number of hypotheses and publications over the past decade, the exact etiology of this syndrome remains unknown. Obesity and associated hormone secreting adipose tissue, vitamin A metabolism, and cerebral venous abnormalities are possible factors in the pathophysiology of this entity.[39,40] It has been reported that increased ICP in obese patients is secondary to associated elevated intraabdominal, pleural, cardiac filling, and cerebral venous pressures.[41-43] This pathophysiological mechanism has been further supported by an animal study demonstrating increased ICP upon acute elevation of intraabdominal pressure.[44] Increased cerebral blood flow secondary to cerebrovascular resistance changes and CSF hypersecretion induced by elevated estrogen levels, which are produced in excess by fat tissue in obese patients, have been reported as pathophysiological mechanisms as well.[45]

Pulsatile tinnitus in IIH syndrome is believed to result from the systolic pulsations of the CSF, which originate mainly from the arteries of the circle of Willis. These pulsations, which are increased in magnitude in the presence of intracranial hypertension, are transmitted to the exposed medial aspects of the dural venous sinuses (transverse and sigmoid), compressing their walls synchronously with the arterial pulsations.[24,46] The ensuing periodic narrowing of the dural venous sinuses lumen converts the laminar blood flow to turbulent and results in production of bruits, which are perceived by the patient as PT.[24] The low-frequency SNHL, present in many of these patients, is believed to result from the masking effect of the PT. This becomes evident by the fact that light digital compression applied over the ipsilateral internal jugular vein (IJV) abolishes the PT with immediate improvement or normalization of hearing.[24] Stretching or compression of the cochlear nerve and brainstem, caused by the increased ICP, may also play a role in the hearing loss and dizziness. This is supported by the presence of an abnormal auditory brainstem response (ABR) in one third of these patients.[47]

Magnetic resonance imaging and magnetic resonance venography (MRV) are necessary to rule out intracranial neoplastic lesions and dural sinus abnormalities.[37] Although MRI is normal in most patients, an empty sella, small ventricles, and flattening of the posterior aspect of the globe are suggestive of this entity.[48-50] Anatomic obstruction of the transverse venous sinuses has been reported in IIH syndrome. In a recent report, bilateral stenosis of the transverse sinuses with volume changes of the entire dural sinus system and associated cranial venous outflow obstruction was identified in 15 out of 17 (88%) of IIH syndrome patients and none in the control group of seven patients.[51] In another study, MRV identified bilateral dural venous sinus stenosis in 27 of 29 patients with IIH syndrome and only in four of the 59 controls. It was not clear whether stenosis was a cause or effect of the intracranial hypertension and this has been reported by others.[52,53] Direct retrograde cerebral venography with manometry has been recommended in order to establish diagnosis and treatment with stents.[54-57]

37.4.2 Sigmoid Sinus Dehiscence and Diverticula

Recently sigmoid sinus dehiscences and diverticula (SSDD) have been implicated as common etiologies of venous PT.[100-103] These abnormalities occur almost exclusevely in middle-aged females, and more often involve the right transverse-sigmoid sinus junction region. Many of these patients are obese and may have an audible mastoid bruit.[100-103] Although only in one study few patients had or were suspicious for IIH syndrome, a systematic evaluation for this syndrome had not been performed.[103] Since these cohorts of patients with SSDD strongly resemble that of patients with IIH syndrome, it is possible that increased intracranial pressure could have been an associated and perhaps a predisposing condition. Therefore it is imperative to properly investigate for IIH syndrome in high risk patients (obese, young or middle aged, females) presenting with venous PT and SSDD.

The role of intracranial hypertension in the pathogenesis of SSDD must be determined in future studies. Specifically the effect of chronic elevation of CSF pressure on the bony covering of the sigmoid sinus and potential formation of dehiscenses needs to be investigated. The author has seen several cases presenting with spontaneous CSF otorrhea or rhinorrhea due to skull base bony defects and associated IIH syndrome. In one case in particular, CSF rhinorrhea stopped spontaneously following bariatric surgery with weight reduction and normalization of CSF pressure.[104] As it has been previously mentioned in this chapter, elevated intra-abdominal and intrathoracic pressures are present in obese individuals and result in increased pressure of the venous intracranial structures.[84] The latter potentially may play a role in the formation of sigmoid sinus and jugular bulb diverticula.

37.4.3 Jugular Bulb Abnormalities

High-placed and dehiscent jugular bulbs are the most common reported jugular bulb abnormalities.[58-64] A bluish and inferiorly based retrotympanic lesion is the typical otoscopic finding.

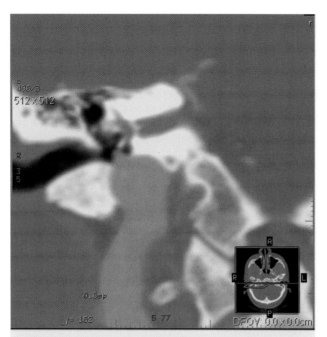

Fig. 37.3 Coronal computed tomography angiogram, venous phase, shows an enlarged dehiscent jugular bulb with an associated diverticulum.

▶ Fig. 37.3 shows a CTA scan of a patient with an enlarged dehiscent jugular bulb and an associated diverticulum.

37.4.4 Idiopathic or Essential Pulsatile Tinnitus

Idiopathic or essential PT and venous hum are terms used interchangeably in the literature to describe patients with PT of unclear etiology.[65,66] Diagnosis of this condition should be made only after appropriate evaluation and elimination of other disorders. Because the majority of studies on idiopathic PT were reported prior to the introduction of modern imaging techniques and the overall better understanding of the various etiologies of PT, it is possible that some of these patients may have had undiagnosed IIH syndrome or other pathologies such as AVFs, AVMs, and dural sinuses abnormalities. The box below summarizes the PT venous etiologies.

Venous Etiologies of Pulsatile Tinnitus

1. Idiopathic intracranial hypertension[24,165]
2. Jugular bulb abnormalities: high location, dehiscense, diverticula[105–110]
3. Transverse-sigmoid sinus stenosis and aneurysms[119,166–168]
4. Abnormal condylar and mastoid emissary veins[169,170]
5. Increased intracranial pressure associated with Arnold-Chiari syndrome or stenosis of the sylvian aqueduct[87]
6. Idiopathic or essential tinnitus[65,66,85,126]

37.5 Nonvascular Etiologies

37.5.1 Palatal, Stapedial, and Tensor Tympani Muscle Myoclonus

Most of the studies reported in the literature regarding palatal and middle ear muscles myoclonus are case reports or small case series, and therefore there is no evidence of a conclusive diagnostic test.[67,68] Myoclonic contractions of the tensor veli palatini, stapedial, levator veli palatini, salpingopharyngeus, and superior constrictor muscles can result in objective pulsating sounds.[69] These contractions are not synchronus with the arterial pulsations; rates can range between 10 and 240 pulses per minute, and occasionally can be confused with the arterial pulse. Most commonly, this type of tinnitus is described as being of clicking or buzzing quality, but this varies widely between patients.[70–72]

This disorder is often seen in young patients, usually within the first three decades of life, although it may be present in older individuals as well.[73–76] Involvement of the olivary tracts, posterior longitudinal bundle, dentate nucleus, and reticular formation has been identified in some of these cases. Associated neurologic disorders such as brainstem infarctions, multiple sclerosis, trauma, and syphilis have been reported as well.[65,77]

A tympanometric cogwheel or saw-toothed pattern has been reported for both stapedial and tensor tympani muscles, making it an unreliable diagnostic test for differenting the two entities.[76,78–81] Although visible tympanic movement on microscopy has been reported in association with tensor tympani myoclonus,[79] a definitive diagnosis can only be made by tympanotomy and direct visualization.[67]

37.6 Evaluation

The history, otoscopic examination, and auscultation are of utmost important in evaluating PT patients. In older patients with a previous history of cerebrovascular accident, transient ischemic attacks, hyperlipidemia, hypertension, diabetes mellitus, or smoking, a diagnosis of ACAD should be considered.[1] In obese females with associated hearing loss, headaches, aural fullness, dizziness, and visual disturbances, clinicians should suspect the IIH syndrome.[24,25] The body habitus of a morbidly obese patient with IIH syndrome is depicted in ▶ Fig. 37.4. Sudden onset of PT in association with cervical or facial pain, headache, and symptoms of cerebral ischemia is compatible with extracranial or intrapetrous carotid artery dissection.[82–84]

Otoscopy is essential for detection of a retrotympanic pathology such as high or exposed jugular bulb, aberrant carotid artery, glomus tumor, or Schwartze sign. Rhythmic movements of the tympanic membrane, soft palate, or pharynx can be present in patients with myoclonus of the tensor tympani, levator veli palatini, salpingopharyngeus, and superior constrictor muscles. Wide opening of the oral cavity during examination may eliminate the soft palate myoclonic contractions.[85] Transnasal fiberoptic inspection of the soft palate and pharynx may be more revealing in these patients.

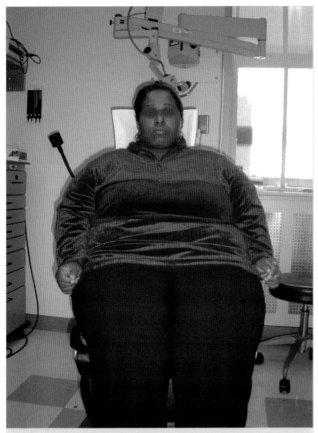

Fig. 37.4 Patient with idiopathic intracranial hypertension (IIH) syndrome.

Auscultation of the ear canal, periauricular region, orbits, cervical region, and chest is the most important aspect of the examination. This should be preferably performed with a modified electronic stethoscope in an audio booth.[86] ► Fig. 37.5 shows an electronic stethoscope.

Should objective PT be detected, its rate should be compared to the patient's pulse rate and the effect of light digital pressure over the ipsilateral IJV should be checked. PT of venous origin, such as the one present in patients with IIH syndrome, decreases or completely subsides with this maneuver.[24,25] In patients with arterial PT this maneuver is ineffective. The effect of head rotation on tinnitus intensity should also be checked. Venous PT decreases or completely subsides with head rotation toward the ipsilateral side, probably due to compression of the IJV between the contracting sternocleidomastoid muscle and the transverse process of the atlas.[25] A complete neurologic examination should be included in the examination.

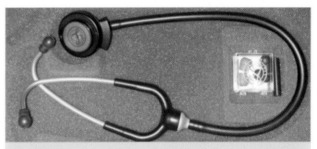

Fig. 37.5 Electronic stethoscope (Littmann, model 2000, 3 M, St. Paul, MN).

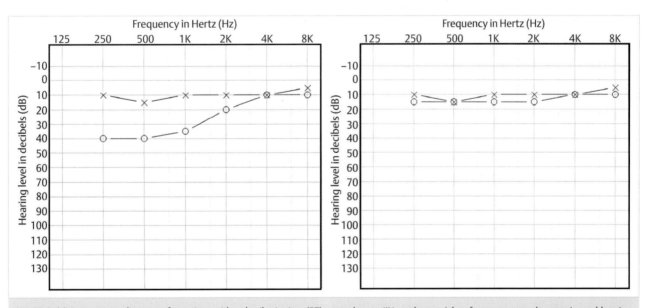

Fig. 37.6 (a) Pure-tone audiogram of a patient with pulsatile tinnitus (PT) secondary to IIH syndrome. A low-frequency pseudosensorineural hearing loss is present. (b) Repeated audiogram while the masking effect of the PT has been eliminated by digital pressure over the ipsilateral jugular vein reveals normalization of hearing.

37.6.1 Audiological and Electrophysiological Testing

Pure tone (air and bone conduction) and speech audiometry should be performed in all patients. When hearing loss of 20 dB or more is detected in the low frequencies, a repeat audiogram should be obtained while the patient is applying light digital pressure over the ipsilateral IJV. This maneuver typically results in improvement or normalization of pure tones in patients with venous PT, such as in IIH syndrome, due to elimination of the masking effect of tinnitus.[24] Discrimination is typically excellent in these patients. ► Fig. 37.6 depicts characteristic audiograms of a patient with IIH syndrome.

Impedance audiometry may be useful in patients suspected of tensor tympani myoclonus. Auditory evoked responses (such as ABRs) may be considered in selected cases only. Abnormalities of ABR, consisting mainly of prolonged interpeak latencies, have been detected in one third of patients with IIH syndrome, which may normalize following successful management.[47] Electronystagmography may be considered in patients with associated dizziness.[24]

37.6.2 Metabolic Workup

Metabolic workup is rarely revealing in these patients; however, complete blood count and thyroid function tests should be obtained in patients with increased cardiac output syndrome to exclude anemia and hyperthyroidism. Serum lipid profile and fasting blood sugar should be considered in patients in whom ACAD is suspected.

37.6.3 Ultrasound Studies

Duplex carotid ultrasound (including the subclavian arteries) and echocardiogram studies should be obtained in patients in whom ACAD is suspected and in valvular disease. These studies should be performed prior to any radiological evaluation because they may be the only tests required to establish diagnosis.[1]

37.6.4 Radiological Evaluation

The radiological evaluation is individualized based on the otoscopic findings and PT characterisitics (arterial/venous type).

Normal Otoscopy

- Patients with venous PT are scheduled for a CT of the temporal bones and brain MRI/MRV as initial imaging evaluation. Bony abnormalities of the jugular bulb/dural venous sinuses (Dehiscent sigmoid sinus/jugular bulb, diverticula sigmoid sinus/jugular bulb), and findings characteristic of IIH syndrome (empty sella, small ventricles, flattening of posterior aspect of globe) can be detected with these studies. ► Fig. 37.7 is an MRI of a IIH syndrome patient depicting an empty sella. Other rare congenital central nervous system abnormalities such as

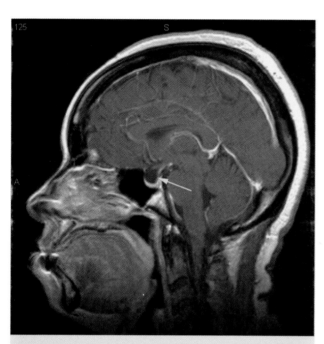

Fig. 37.7 Sagittal T1-weighted with gadolinium magnetic resonance imaging shows an empty sella (*arrow*).

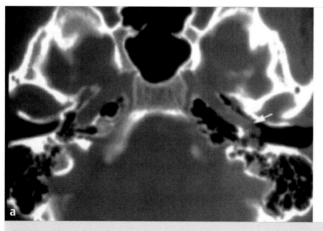
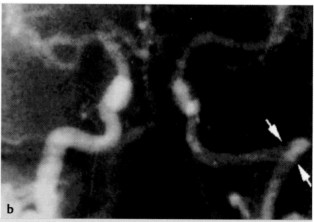

Fig. 37.8 (a) Axial CT of a patient with left middle ear aberrant internal carotid artery (*arrow*). (b) Same patient, anteroposterior skull view of an aortic arch injection, reveals the aberrant course of the left internal carotid (*arrows*) as compared with the normal right internal carotid artery.

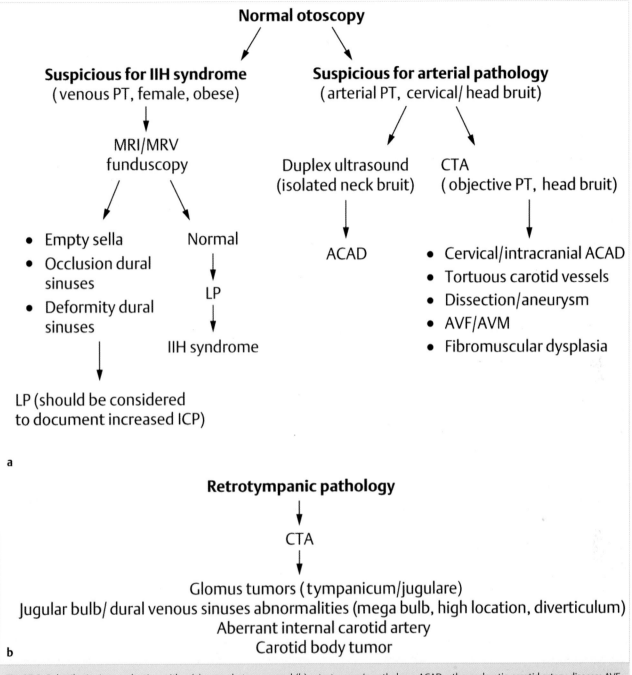

Fig. 37.9 Pulsatile tinnitus evaluation with a (a) normal otoscopy and (b) retrotympanic pathology. ACAD, atherosclerotic carotid artery disease; AVF, arteriovenous fistula; AVM, arteriovenous malformation; CT, computed tomography; CTA, computed tomography angiography; ICP, intracranial pressure; IIH, idiopathic intracranial hypertension; LP, lumbar puncture; MRA, magnetic resonance arteriography; MRI, magnetic resonance imaging; MRV, magnetic resonance venography; TB, temporal bone.

Chiari I malformation and stenosis of the sylvian aqueduct can be detected with brain MRI as well.[87]

• Patients with arterial PT are considered for a CTA as the initial evaluation. The literature as well as our experience with CTA suggest that this study is satisfactory in evaluating intracranial vascular lesions.[88–94] This is a fast imaging technique, and because the upper neck is included, cervical vascular pathol-ogy, such as a synchronous carotid body tumor, can be detected as well. Tortuous carotid vessels, AVF/AVMs, carotid artery dissections/aneurysms, cervical/intracranial ACAD, and FMD can be diagnosed with this study.[22]

• Patients with isolated cervical carotid bruits are considered for a carotid duplex ultrasound prior to a CTA. If ACAD is confirmed, no other imaging study is necessary.[95]

Abnormal Otoscopy/Retrotympanic Pathology

Patients with abnormal otoscopy/retrotympanic pathology should be considered for a CTA of the temporal bones and neck at the initial evaluation. For patients with glomus jugulare/tympanicum tumors, the presence of synchronous carotid body tumor(s) can easily be detected in the same study. Lesions of the temporal bones such as glomus tympanicum, ectopic carotid artery, and jugular bulb/dural venous sinuses abnormalities can easily be detected as well. ▶ Fig. 37.8a shows an axial CT of a patient with a left middle ear aberrant internal carotid artery, and ▶ Fig. 37.8b shows an angiogram of the same patient.

Carotid angiography is indicated only in cases in which there is strong suspicion of an AVF/AVM such as patients with loud retroauricular bruits, and for prospective surgical candidates in order to evaluate the collateral circulation of the brain (arterial and venous) in anticipation of possible vessel ligation or preoperative tumor embolization.[96] ▶ Fig. 37.9 depicts algorithms for evaluation of patients with PT.

37.7 Management

This section describes the management of the most common entities associated with PT. For obese patients with IIH syndrome, it is very important for them to comprehend the connection between their body weight and PT. Associated comorbidities such as hypertension, diabetes mellitus, gastroesophageal reflux, and obstructive sleep apnea are common in these patients, and appropriate referral to other specialists should be considered. Weight reduction is the most important aspect of management and will reduce or even eliminate PT in the majority of these patients.[28,97] Administration of acetazolamide (Diamox, Teva Pharmaceuticals USA, North Wales, PA) is thought to reduce CSF production and may be helpful in decreasing tinnitus intensity, although it rarely eliminates this symptom.[98] Lumbar-peritoneal shunt should be considered for patients with progressive deterioration of vision, persistent headaches, and disabling PT.[24,25,48,99] In morbidly obese patients, however, this procedure is often complicated by occlusion of the shunt secondary to increased intraabdominal pressure.[100] Weight reduction surgery in morbidly obese patients with PT is very effective in eliminating this symptom. Thirteen of 16 patients who underwent this procedure experienced complete resolution of their PT.[101] Evaluation and close follow-up by an ophthalmologist and neurologist are of outmost importance. Optic nerve sheath fenestration should be considered for patients with progressive visual loss.[102,103] Resolution of symptoms and papilledema has been reported following retrograde venography and stenting of the transverse sinus in IIH patients with associated stenosis/obstruction of this structure.[54,56,57,104] ▶ Fig. 37.10 is the venous phase of a CT angiogram of a female patient with IIH syndrome. A right hypoplastic transverse sinus and a stenotic left transverse sinus are present. This patient might be a candidate for sinus stenting.

Patients with ACAD and disturbing PT should be considered for surgical intervention.[105] Carotid endarterectomy (CEA) and carotid angioplasty with stenting (CAS) are the two procedures for treating ACAD. Randomized controlled trials comparing the efficacy of CEA to medical therapy have shown a clear benefit

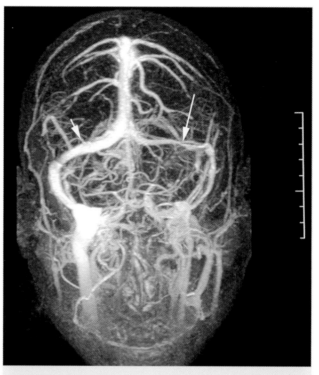

Fig. 37.10 The venous phase of a CT angiogram of a female patient with IIH syndrome. A right hypoplastic transverse sinus (*small arrow*) and a stenotic left transverse sinus (*large arrow*) are present.

for CEA in patients with symptomatic stenosis of greater than 70% and a lesser benefit in patients with 50% to 69% stenosis. More recent studies comparing CAS to CEA failed to reach conclusions regarding a clear neurologic outcome advantage of one method over the other.[106] Angioplasty has been reported to relieve PT secondary to atherosclerotic obstruction of the subclavian and intracranial carotid arteries.[107,108]

Glomus tympanicum tumors are amenable to surgical extirpation with excellent long-term results.[109,110] Treatment of glomus jugulare tumors should be individualized, and although the traditional management has been surgical removal, stereotactic radiosurgery has recently been demonstrated to be very effective with fewer complications.[111,112] In a recent meta-analysis study, tumor control was achieved in 97% of patients.[113] The study concluded that radiosurgery of glomus jugulare tumors should be considered as primary management.

Although there have been no prospective, randomized therapeutic trials for patients with carotid artery dissection, experience shows that anticoagulants such as heparin followed by coumadin are effective in preventing further artery-to-artery emboli.[82] In selected cases of carotid artery dissection with occlusion, stent-assisted angioplasty is effective.[114,115]

Surgical repair of symptomatic high/dehisced jugular bulbs and diverticula has been reported by using dust, perichondrium, tragal or conchal cartilage, and mastoid cortical bone.[51,107,168,169] Surgical repair of transverse and sigmoid sinus diverticula/dehiscences, and aneurysms is also effective in eliminating PT.[102,103,115,116,170] The majority of reports on medical therapy of myoclonus (benzodiazepine, orphenadrine citrate, carbamazepine, piracetam, and botulinum toxin) are case reports or studies with small number of cases and suggest a reduction in tinnitus; however, this improvement may have been caused by reporting bias.[67] Sectioning of the levator veli palatini muscle has been reported for cases with palatal myoclonus.[85] However, botulinum toxin injection seems to be a more appropriate treatment for this entity.[75,121,122] Tensor tympani and stapedial myoclonus may respond to sectioning of the respective muscles via tympanotomy.[81,123] My experience with three patients (four ears) has been very satisfactory with this technique.

Dural AVFs can be treated very effectively with combined transvenous coil occlusion of the venous sinus segment, and transarterial occlusion of supplying arteries.[124] Recently, an increasing number of reports support the use of stereotactic radiosurgery as the sole therapeutic modality or in combination with embolization and/or surgery.[125]

Finally, ligation of the IJV ipsilateral to the tinnitus has been recommended in the past for patients with idiopathic PT. The results of this procedure have been very inconsistent and poor overall. In a series of 13 patients with essential tinnitus, three underwent ligation of the ipsilateral IJV and only one benefited permanently. The other two patients experienced return of their PT within a few days.[126] This procedure should rarely if ever be performed for alleviating PT.[127]

References

[1] Sismanis A, Stamm MA, Sobel M. Objective tinnitus in patients with atherosclerotic carotid artery disease. Am J Otol 1994; 15: 404–407

[2] Daneshi A, Hadizadeh H, Mahmoudian S, Sahebjam S, Jalesi A. Pulsatile tinnitus and carotid artery atherosclerosis. Int Tinnitus J 2004; 10: 161–164

[3] Hatsukami TS, Yuan C. MRI in the early identification and classification of high-risk atherosclerotic carotid plaques. Imaging Med 2010; 2: 63–75

[4] Bink A, Berkefeld J, Kraus L, Senft C, Ziemann U. du Mesnil de RR. Long-term outcome in patients treated for benign dural arteriovenous fistulas of the posterior fossa. Neuroradiology 2010

[5] Bink A, Goller K, Lüchtenberg M et al. Long-term outcome after coil embolization of cavernous sinus arteriovenous fistulas. AJNR Am J Neuroradiol 2010; 31: 1216–1221

[6] Carmody RF. Vascular malformations. In: Zimmerman RA, Gibby WA, Carmody RF, eds. Neuroimaging Clinical and Physical Principles. New York: Springer-Verlag, 2000:833–862

[7] Hoang TA, Hasso AN. Intracranial vascular malformations. Neuroimaging Clin N Am 1994; 4: 823–847

[8] Zipfel GJ, Shah MN, Refai D, Dacey RG, Jr, Derdeyn CP. Cranial dural arteriovenous fistulas: modification of angiographic classification scales based on new natural history data. Neurosurg Focus 2009; 26: E14

[9] Zager EL, Shaver EG, Hurst RW, Flamm ES. Distal anterior inferior cerebellar artery aneurysms. Report of four cases. J Neurosurg 2002; 97: 692–696

[10] Vories A, Liening D. Spontaneous dissection of the internal carotid artery presenting with pulsatile tinnitus. Am J Otolaryngol 1998; 19: 213–215

[11] Depauw P, Defreyne L, Dewaele F, Caemaert J. Endovascular treatment of a giant petrous internal carotid artery aneurysm. Case report and review of the literature. Minim Invasive Neurosurg 2003; 46: 250–253

[12] Dehaene I, Meeus L. Vertebral artery dissection without ischemic events in the vertebro-basilar system. Acta Neurol Belg 1989; 89: 366–369

[13] Patel RR, Adam R, Maldjian C, Lincoln CM, Yuen A, Arneja A. Cervical carotid artery dissection: current review of diagnosis and treatment. Cardiol Rev 2012; 20: 145–152

[14] Medina DM, Carmody RF. Stroke. In: Zimmerman RA, Gibby WA, Carmody RF, eds. Neuroimaging Clinical and Physical Principles. New York: Springer-Verlag, 2000:833–863

[15] Fayad JN, Keles B, Brackmann DE. Jugular foramen tumors: clinical characteristics and treatment outcomes. Otol Neurotol 2010; 31: 299–305

[16] Olin JW, Sealove BA. Diagnosis, management, and future developments of fibromuscular dysplasia. J Vasc Surg 2011; 53: 826–836, e1

[17] Dufour JJ, Lavigne F, Plante R, Caouette H. Pulsatile tinnitus and fibromuscular dysplasia of the internal carotid. J Otolaryngol 1985; 14: 293–295

[18] Van Damme H, Sakalihasan N, Limet R. Fibromuscular dysplasia of the internal carotid artery. Personal experience with 13 cases and literature review. Acta Chir Belg 1999; 99: 163–168

[19] Hosokawa S, Mineta H. Tortuous internal carotid artery presenting as a pharyngeal mass. J Laryngol Otol 2010; 124: 1033–1036

[20] Beriat GK, Ezerarslan H, Kocatürk S, Mıhmanoğlu AF, Kuralay E. Pulsatile oropharyngeal and neck mass caused by bilateral tortuous internal carotid artery: a case report. Kulak Burun Bogaz Ihtis Derg 2010; 20: 260–263

[21] Aleksic M, Schütz G, Gerth S, Mulch J. Surgical approach to kinking and coiling of the internal carotid artery. J Cardiovasc Surg (Torino) 2004; 45: 43–48

[22] Sismanis A, Girevendoulis A. Pulsatile tinnitus associated with internal carotid artery morphologic abnormalities. Otol Neurotol 2008; 29: 1032–1036

[23] Sismanis A. Pulsatile tinnitus. A 15-year experience. Am J Otol 1998; 19: 472–477

[24] Sismanis A. Otologic manifestations of benign intracranial hypertension syndrome: diagnosis and management. Laryngoscope 1987; 97 Suppl 42: 1–17

[25] Sismanis A, Butts FM, Hughes GB. Objective tinnitus in benign intracranial hypertension: an update. Laryngoscope 1990; 100: 33–36

[26] Sørensen PS, Krogsaa B, Gjerris F. Clinical course and prognosis of pseudotumor cerebri. A prospective study of 24 patients. Acta Neurol Scand 1988; 77: 164–172

[27] Fishman RA. Benign intracranial hypertension. In: Cerebrospinal Fluid in Disease of the Nervous System. Philadelphia: WB Saunders, 1980:128–139

[28] Skau M, Sander B, Milea D, Jensen R. Disease activity in idiopathic intracranial hypertension: a 3-month follow-up study. J Neurol 2011; 258: 277–283

[29] Brackmann DE, Doherty JK. Facial palsy and fallopian canal expansion associated with idiopathic intracranial hypertension. Otol Neurotol 2007; 28: 715–718

[30] Bruce BB, Kedar S, Van Stavern GP et al. Idiopathic intracranial hypertension in men. Neurology 2009; 72: 304–309

[31] Bruce BB, Kedar S, Van Stavern GP, Corbett JJ, Newman NJ, Biousse V. Atypical idiopathic intracranial hypertension: normal BMI and older patients. Neurology 2010; 74: 1827–1832

[32] Dessardo NS, Dessardo S, Sasso A, Sarunić AV, Dezulović MS. Pediatric idiopathic intracranial hypertension: clinical and demographic features. Coll Antropol 2010; 34 Suppl 2: 217–221

[33] Heidary G, Rizzo JF, III. Use of optical coherence tomography to evaluate papilledema and pseudopapilledema. Semin Ophthalmol 2010; 25: 198–205

[34] Marcelis J, Silberstein SD. Idiopathic intracranial hypertension without papilledema. Arch Neurol 1991; 48: 392–399

[35] Digre KB, Nakamoto BK, Warner JE, Langeberg WJ, Baggaley SK, Katz BJ. A comparison of idiopathic intracranial hypertension with and without papilledema. Headache 2009; 49: 185–193

[36] Thurtell MJ, Newman NJ, Biousse V. Visual loss without papilledema in idiopathic intracranial hypertension. J Neuroophthalmol 2010; 30: 96–98

[37] Rougier MB. [Diagnosing bilateral papilledema] J Fr Ophtalmol 2010; 33: 424–429

[38] Wall M, George D. Idiopathic intracranial hypertension. A prospective study of 50 patients. Brain 1991; 114 Pt 1A: 155–180

[39] Biousse V, Bruce BB, Newman NJ. Update on the pathophysiology and management of idiopathic intracranial hypertension. J Neurol Neurosurg Psychiatry 2012; 83: 488–494

[40] Wall M. Idiopathic intracranial hypertension (pseudotumor cerebri). Curr Neurol Neurosci Rep 2008; 8: 87–93

[41] Sugerman HJ, DeMaria EJ, Felton WL, III, Nakatsuka M, Sismanis A. Increased intra-abdominal pressure and cardiac filling pressures in obesity-associated pseudotumor cerebri. Neurology 1997; 49: 507–511

[42] Johnston I, Paterson A. Benign intracranial hypertension. I. Diagnosis and prognosis. Brain 1974; 97: 289–300

[43] Felton WL, Marmarou A, Bandon K. Cerebrospinal fluid pressure dynamics in pseudotumor cerebri. Neurology 1991; 41: 348

[44] Josephs LG, Este-McDonald JR, Birkett DH, Hirsch EF. Diagnostic laparoscopy increases intracranial pressure. J Trauma 1994; 36: 815–818, discussion 818–819

[45] Gross CE, Tranmer BI, Adey G, Kohut J. Increased cerebral blood flow in idiopathic pseudotumour cerebri. Neurol Res 1990; 12: 226–230

[46] Langfitt TW. Clinical methods for monitoring intracranial pressure and measuring cerebral blood flow. Clin Neurosurg 1975; 22: 302–320

[47] Sismanis A, Callari RH, Slomka WS, Butts FM. Auditory-evoked responses in benign intracranial hypertension syndrome. Laryngoscope 1990; 100: 1152–1155

[48] Sismanis A, Smoker WR. Pulsatile tinnitus: recent advances in diagnosis. Laryngoscope 1994; 104: 681–688

[49] Agid R, Farb RI, Willinsky RA, Mikulis DJ, Tomlinson G. Idiopathic intracranial hypertension: the validity of cross-sectional neuroimaging signs. Neuroradiology 2006; 48: 521–527

[50] Passi N, Degnan AJ, Levy LM. MR Imaging of Papilledema and Visual Pathways: Effects of Increased Intracranial Pressure and Pathophysiologic Mechanisms. AJNR Am J Neuroradiol 2012

[51] Rohr A, Bindeballe J, Riedel C et al. The entire dural sinus tree is compressed in patients with idiopathic intracranial hypertension: a longitudinal, volumetric magnetic resonance imaging study. Neuroradiology 2012; 54: 25–33

[52] Farb RI, Vanek I, Scott JN et al. Idiopathic intracranial hypertension: the prevalence and morphology of sinovenous stenosis. Neurology 2003; 60: 1418–1424

[53] Lee SW, Gates P, Morris P, Whan A, Riddington L. Idiopathic intracranial hypertension; immediate resolution of venous sinus "obstruction" after reducing cerebrospinal fluid pressure to < 10 cmHO. J Clin Neurosci 2009; 16: 1690–1692

[54] Kumpe DA, Bennett JL, Seinfeld J, Pelak VS, Chawla A, Tierney M. Dural sinus stent placement for idiopathic intracranial hypertension. J Neurosurg 2012; 116: 538–548

[55] Donnet A, Metellus P, Levrier O et al. Endovascular treatment of idiopathic intracranial hypertension: clinical and radiologic outcome of 10 consecutive patients. Neurology 2008; 70: 641–647

[56] Higgins JN, Cousins C, Owler BK, Sarkies N, Pickard JD. Idiopathic intracranial hypertension: 12 cases treated by venous sinus stenting. J Neurol Neurosurg Psychiatry 2003; 74: 1662–1666

[57] Owler BK, Parker G, Halmagyi GM et al. Pseudotumor cerebri syndrome: venous sinus obstruction and its treatment with stent placement. J Neurosurg 2003; 98: 1045–1055

[58] Buckwalter JA, Sasaki CT, Virapongse C, Kier EL, Bauman N. Pulsatile tinnitus arising from jugular megabulb deformity: a treatment rationale. Laryngoscope 1983; 93: 1534–1539

[59] Bush ML, Jones RO, Given C. The value of CT venography in the diagnosis of jugular bulb diverticulum: a series of 3 cases. Ear Nose Throat J 2009; 88: E4–E7

[60] El-Begermy MA, Rabie AN. A novel surgical technique for management of tinnitus due to high dehiscent jugular bulb. Otolaryngol Head Neck Surg 2010; 142: 576–581

[61] Haupert MS, Madgy DN, Belenky WM, Becker JW. Unilateral conductive hearing loss secondary to a high jugular bulb in a pediatric patient. Ear Nose Throat J 1997; 76: 468–469

[62] Overton SB, Ritter FN. A high placed jugular bulb in the middle ear: a clinical and temporal bone study. Laryngoscope 1973; 83: 1986–1991

[63] Robin PE. A case of upwardly situated jugular bulb in left middle ear. J Laryngol Otol 1972; 86: 1241–1246

[64] Smythe GO. A case of protruding jugular bulb. Laryngoscope 1975: 669–672

[65] Chandler JR. Diagnosis and cure of venous hum tinnitus. Laryngoscope 1983; 93: 892–895

[66] Engstrom H, Graf W. On objective tinnitus and its recording. Acta Otolaryngol Suppl 1950; 95: 127–137

[67] Bhimrao SK, Masterson L, Baguley D. Systematic review of management strategies for middle ear myoclonus. Otolaryngol Head Neck Surg 2012; 146: 698–706

[68] Pulec JL, Hodell SF, Anthony PF. Tinnitus: diagnosis and treatment. Ann Otol Rhinol Laryngol 1978; 87: 821–833

[69] Costa de Araujo P, Savage J Costa de AP. Objective tinnitus from middle ear myoclonus. Arch Otolaryngol Head Neck Surg 2012; 138: 421

[70] Badia L, Parikh A, Brookes GB. Management of middle ear myoclonus. J Laryngol Otol 1994; 108: 380–382

[71] East CA, Hazell JW. The suppression of palatal (or intra-tympanic) myoclonus by tinnitus masking devices. A preliminary report. J Laryngol Otol 1987; 101: 1230–1234

[72] Zipfel TE, Kaza SR, Greene JS. Middle-ear myoclonus. J Laryngol Otol 2000; 114: 207–209

[73] Bjork H. Objective tinnitus due to clonus of the soft palate. Acta Otolaryngol Suppl 1954; 116: 39–45

[74] Crandall PH, Fang HC, Herrmann C, Jr. Palatal myoclonus; a new approach to the understanding of its production. Neurology 1957; 7: 37–51

[75] Daval M, Cohen M, Mari I, Ayache D. [Objective tinnitus and essential palatal tremor in children: report of a case] Rev Laryngol Otol Rhinol (Bord) 2009; 130: 117–119

[76] Oliveira CA, Negreiros Júnior J, Cavalcante IC, Bahmad F, Jr, Venosa AR. Palatal and middle-ear myoclonus: a cause for objective tinnitus. Int Tinnitus J 2003; 9: 37–41

[77] Heller MF. Vibratory tinnitus and palatal myoclonus. Acta Otolaryngol 1962; 55: 292–298

[78] Watanabe I, Kumagami H, Tsuda Y. Tinnitus due to abnormal contraction of stapedial muscle. An abnormal phenomenon in the course of facial nerve paralysis and its audiological significance. ORL J Otorhinolaryngol Relat Spec 1974; 36: 217–226

[79] Howsam GD, Sharma A, Lambden SP, Fitzgerald J, Prinsley PR. Bilateral objective tinnitus secondary to congenital middle-ear myoclonus. J Laryngol Otol 2005; 119: 489–491

[80] Golz A, Fradis M, Netzer A, Ridder GJ, Westerman ST, Joachims HZ. Bilateral tinnitus due to middle-ear myoclonus. Int Tinnitus J 2003; 9: 52–55

[81] Golz A, Fradis M, Martzu D, Netzer A, Joachims HZ. Stapedius muscle myoclonus. Ann Otol Rhinol Laryngol 2003; 112: 522–524

[82] Selim M, Caplan LR. Carotid Artery Dissection. Curr Treat Options Cardiovasc Med 2004; 6: 249–253

[83] Saeed SR, Hinton AE, Ramsden RT, Lye RH. Spontaneous dissection of the intrapetrous internal carotid artery. J Laryngol Otol 1990; 104: 491–493

[84] Sila CA, Furlan AJ, Little JR. Pulsatile tinnitus. Stroke 1987; 18: 252–256

[85] Ward PH, Babin R, Calcaterra TC, Konrad HR. Operative treatment of surgical lesions with objective tinnitus. Ann Otol Rhinol Laryngol 1975; 84: 473–482

[86] Sismanis A, Butts FM. A practical device for detection and recording of objective tinnitus. Otolaryngol Head Neck Surg 1994; 110: 459–462

[87] Wiggs WJ, Jr, Sismanis A, Laine FJ. Pulsatile tinnitus associated with congenital central nervous system malformations. Am J Otol 1996; 17: 241–244

[88] Giesel FL, Essig M, Zabel-Du-Bois A et al. High-contrast computed tomographic angiography better detects residual intracranial arteriovenous malformations in long-term follow-up after radiotherapy than 1.5-Tesla time-of-flight magnetic resonance angiography. Acta Radiol 2010; 51: 64–70

[89] Prestigiacomo CJ, Sabit A, He W, Jethwa P, Gandhi C, Russin J. Three dimensional CT angiography versus digital subtraction angiography in the detection of intracranial aneurysms in subarachnoid hemorrhage. J Neurointerv Surg 2010; 2: 385–389

[90] De Monti M, Ghilardi G, Caverni L et al. Multidetector helical angio CT oblique reconstructions orthogonal to internal carotid artery for preoperative evaluation of stenosis. A prospective study of comparison with color Doppler US, digital subtraction angiography and intraoperative data. Minerva Cardioangiol 2003; 51: 373–385

[91] Jayaraman MV, Mayo-Smith WW. Multi-detector CT angiography of the intra-cranial circulation: normal anatomy and pathology with angiographic correlation. Clin Radiol 2004; 59: 690–698

[92] Sanelli PC, Mifsud MJ, Stieg PE. Role of CT angiography in guiding management decisions of newly diagnosed and residual arteriovenous malformations. AJR Am J Roentgenol 2004; 183: 1123–1126

[93] Karamessini MT, Kagadis GC, Petsas T et al. CT angiography with three-dimensional techniques for the early diagnosis of intracranial aneurysms. Comparison with intra-arterial DSA and the surgical findings. Eur J Radiol 2004; 49: 212–223

[94] Perkins JA, Sidhu M, Manning SC, Ghioni V, Sze R. Three-dimensional CT angiography imaging of vascular tumors of the head and neck. Int J Pediatr Otorhinolaryngol 2005; 69: 319–325

[95] Buskens E, Nederkoorn PJ, Buijs-Van Der Woude T et al. Imaging of carotid arteries in symptomatic patients: cost-effectiveness of diagnostic strategies. Radiology 2004; 233: 101–112

[96] Remley KB, Coit WE, Harnsberger HR, Smoker WR, Jacobs JM, McIff EB. Pulsatile tinnitus and the vascular tympanic membrane: CT, MR, and angiographic findings. Radiology 1990; 174: 383–389

[97] Sinclair AJ, Burdon MA, Nightingale PG et al. Low energy diet and intracranial pressure in women with idiopathic intracranial hypertension: prospective cohort study. BMJ 2010; 341: c2701

[98] Ko MW. Idiopathic intracranial hypertension. Curr Treat Options Neurol 2011; 13: 101–108

[99] Abubaker K, Ali Z, Raza K, Bolger C, Rawluk D, O'Brien D. Idiopathic intracranial hypertension: lumboperitoneal shunts versus ventriculoperitoneal shunts—case series and literature review. Br J Neurosurg 2011; 25: 94–99

[100] Sugerman HJ, Felton WL, III, Salvant JB, Jr, Sismanis A, Kellum JM. Effects of surgically induced weight loss on idiopathic intracranial hypertension in morbid obesity. Neurology 1995; 45: 1655–1659

[101] Michaelides EM, Sismanis A, Sugerman HJ, Felton WL, III. Pulsatile tinnitus in patients with morbid obesity: the effectiveness of weight reduction surgery. Am J Otol 2000; 21: 682–685

[102] Corbett JJ, Nerad JA, Tse DT, Anderson RL. Results of optic nerve sheath fenestration for pseudotumor cerebri. The lateral orbitotomy approach. Arch Ophthalmol 1988; 106: 1391–1397

[103] Ko MW. Idiopathic intracranial hypertension. Curr Treat Options Neurol 2011; 13: 101–108

[104] Ogungbo B, Roy D, Gholkar A, Mendelow AD. Endovascular stenting of the transverse sinus in a patient presenting with benign intracranial hypertension. Br J Neurosurg 2003; 17: 565–568

[105] Singh DP, Forte AJ, Brewer MB, Nowygrod R. Bilateral carotid endarterectomy as treatment of vascular pulsatile tinnitus. J Vasc Surg 2009; 50: 183–185

[106] Perkins WJ, Lanzino G, Brott TG. Carotid stenting vs endarterectomy: new results in perspective. Mayo Clin Proc 2010; 85: 1101–1108

[107] Donald JJ, Raphael MJ. Pulsatile tinnitus relieved by angioplasty. Clin Radiol 1991; 43: 132–134

[108] Emery DJ, Ferguson RD, Williams JS. Pulsatile tinnitus cured by angioplasty and stenting of petrous carotid artery stenosis. Arch Otolaryngol Head Neck Surg 1998; 124: 460–461

[109] Forest JA, III, Jackson CG, McGrew BM. Long-term control of surgically treated glomus tympanicum tumors. Otol Neurotol 2001; 22: 232–236

[110] Rohit JY, Jain Y, Caruso A, Russo A, Sanna M. Glomus tympanicum tumour: an alternative surgical technique. J Laryngol Otol 2003; 117: 462–466

[111] Chen PG, Nguyen JH, Payne SC, Sheehan JP, Hashisaki GT. Treatment of glomus jugulare tumors with gamma knife radiosurgery. Laryngoscope 2010; 120: 1856–1862

[112] Navarro Martín A, Maitz A, Grills IS et al. Successful treatment of glomus jugulare tumours with gamma knife radiosurgery: clinical and physical aspects of management and review of the literature. Clin Transl Oncol 2010; 12: 55–62

[113] Guss ZD, Batra S, Limb CJ et al. Radiosurgery of glomus jugulare tumors: a meta-analysis. Int J Radiat Oncol Biol Phys 2011; 81: e497–e502

[114] Cohen JE, Gomori JM, Leker RR, Ben-Hur T, Grigoriadis S, Rajz G. Recanalization of symptomatic carotid artery dissections causing occlusion with multiple stents: the use of delayed double-contrast road map. Neurol Res 2010; 32: 293–296

[115] Donas KP, Mayer D, Guber I, Baumgartner R, Genoni M, Lachat M. Endovascular repair of extracranial carotid artery dissection: current status and level of evidence. J Vasc Interv Radiol 2008; 19: 1693–1698

[116] Glasscock ME, III, Dickins JR, Jackson CG, Wiet RJ. Vascular anomalies of the middle ear. Laryngoscope 1980; 90: 77–88

[117] Presutti L, Laudadio P. Jugular bulb diverticula. ORL J Otorhinolaryngol Relat Spec 1991; 53: 57–60

[118] Rouillard R, Leclerc J, Savary P. Pulsatile tinnitus: a dehiscent jugular vein. Laryngoscope 1985; 95: 188–189

[119] Gologorsky Y, Meyer SA, Post AF, Winn HR, Patel AB, Bederson JB. Novel surgical treatment of a transverse-sigmoid sinus aneurysm presenting as pulsatile tinnitus: technical case report. Neurosurgery 2009; 64: E393–E394, discussion E394

[120] Otto KJ, Hudgins PA, Abdelkafy W, Mattox DE. Sigmoid sinus diverticulum: a new surgical approach to the correction of pulsatile tinnitus. Otol Neurotol 2007; 28: 48–53

[121] Bryce GE, Morrison MD. Botulinum toxin treatment of essential palatal myoclonus tinnitus. J Otolaryngol 1998; 27: 213–216

[122] Penney SE, Bruce IA, Saeed SR. Botulinum toxin is effective and safe for palatal tremor: a report of five cases and a review of the literature. J Neurol 2006; 253: 857–860

[123] Golz A, Fradis M, Netzer A, Ridder GJ, Westerman ST, Joachims HZ. Bilateral tinnitus due to middle-ear myoclonus. Int Tinnitus J 2003; 9: 52–55

[124] Kirsch M, Liebig T, Kühne D, Henkes H. Endovascular management of dural arteriovenous fistulas of the transverse and sigmoid sinus in 150 patients. Neuroradiology 2009; 51: 477–483

[125] Loumiotis I, Lanzino G, Daniels D, Sheehan J, Link M. Radiosurgery for intracranial dural arteriovenous fistulas (DAVFs): a review. Neurosurg Rev 2011; 34: 305–315, discussion 315

[126] Hentzer E. Objective tinnitus of the vascular type. A follow-up study. Acta Otolaryngol 1968; 66: 273–281

[127] Jackler RK, Brackmann DE, Sismanis A. A warning on venous ligation for pulsatile tinnitus. Otol Neurotol 2001; 22: 427–428

[128] Woo HJ, Song SY, Kim YD, Bai CH. Arteriovenous malformation of the external ear: a case report. Auris Nasus Larynx 2008; 35: 556–558

[129] Mahmood A, Malik GM. Dural arteriovenous malformations of the skull base. Neurol Res 2003; 25: 860–864

[130] Bink A, Berkefeld J, Kraus L, Senft C, Ziemann U. du Mesnil de RR. Long-term outcome in patients treated for benign dural arteriovenous fistulas of the posterior fossa. Neuroradiology 2010

[131] Tylern RS, Babin RW. Tinnitus. In: Cummings CW, Frederickson JM, Harker LA, et al, eds. Head and Neck Surgery. St. Louis: CV Mosby, 1986:3201–3217

[132] Chen YJ, How CK, Chern CH. Cerebral dural arteriovenous fistulas presenting as pulsatile tinnitus. Intern Med J 2007; 37: 503

[133] Nishikawa M, Handa H, Hirai O et al. Intolerable pulse-synchronous tinnitus caused by occlusion of the contralateral common carotid artery. A successful treatment by aorto-carotid bypass surgery. Acta Neurochir (Wien) 1989; 101: 80–83

[134] Sonmez G, Basekim CC, Ozturk E, Gungor A, Kizilkaya E. Imaging of pulsatile tinnitus: a review of 74 patients. Clin Imaging 2007; 31: 102–108

[135] Daneshi A, Hadizadeh H, Mahmoudian S, Sahebjam S, Jalesi A. Pulsatile tinnitus and carotid artery atherosclerosis. Int Tinnitus J 2004; 10: 161–164

[136] Hatsukami TS, Yuan C. MRI in the early identification and classification of high-risk atherosclerotic carotid plaques. Imaging Med 2010; 2: 63–75

[137] Spector GJ, Ciralsky RH, Ogura JH. Glomus tumors in the head and neck: III. Analysis of clinical manifestations. Ann Otol Rhinol Laryngol 1975; 84: 73–79

[138] Pensak ML. Skull base surgery. In: Glasscock ME, Shambaugh GE, eds. Surgery of the Ear. Philadelphia: WB Saunders, 1990

[139] Hillman TA, Kertesz TR, Hadley K, Shelton C. Reversible peripheral vestibulopathy: the treatment of superior canal dehiscence. Otolaryngol Head Neck Surg 2006; 134: 431–436

[140] Gruber B, Hemmati M. Fibromuscular dysplasia of the vertebral artery: an unusual cause of pulsatile tinnitus. Otolaryngol Head Neck Surg 1991; 105: 113–114

[141] Wells RP, Smith RR. Fibromuscular dysplasia of the internal carotid artery: a long term follow-up. Neurosurgery 1982; 10: 39–43

[142] Foyt D, Carfrae MJ, Rapoport R. Fibromuscular dysplasia of the internal carotid artery causing pulsatile tinnitus. Otolaryngol Head Neck Surg 2006; 134: 701–702

[143] Olin JW, Froehlich J, Gu X et al. The United States Registry for Fibromuscular Dysplasia: results in the first 447 patients. Circulation 2012; 125: 3182–3190

[144] Cochran JH, Jr, Kosmicki PW. Tinnitus as a presenting symptom in pernicious anemia. Ann Otol Rhinol Laryngol 1979; 88: 297

[145] Cary FH. Symptomatic venous hum. Report of a case. N Engl J Med 1961; 264: 869–870

[146] Liess BD, Lollar KW, Christiansen SG, Vaslow D. Pulsatile tinnitus: a harbinger of a greater ill? Head Neck 2009; 31: 269–273

[147] Palacios E, Gómez J, Alvernia JE, Jacob C. Aneurysm of the petrous portion of the internal carotid artery at the foramen lacerum: anatomic, imaging, and otologic findings. Ear Nose Throat J 2010; 89: 303–305

[148] Le Reste PJ, Ferre JC, Gauvrit JY, Morandi X, Hamlat A. Spontaneous bilateral intrapetrous carotid dissection complicated by a ruptured dissecting aneurysm. J Neuroradiol 2011; 38: 193–195

[149] Campbell JB, Simons RM. Brachiocephalic artery stenosis presenting with objective tinnitus. J Laryngol Otol 1987; 101: 718–720

[150] Fernández AO. Objective tinnitus: a case report. Am J Otol 1983; 4: 312–314

[151] Bold EL, Wanamaker HH, Hughes GB et al. Magnetic resonance angiography of vascular anomalies of the middle ear. Laryngoscope 1994; 104: 1404–1411

[152] Steffen TN. Vascular anomalites of the middle ear. Laryngoscope 1968; 78: 171–197

[153] Soyka MB, Schuknecht B, Huber AM. [Aberrant internal carotid artery as a cause of pulsatile tinnitus: a difficult diagnosis in MRI?] HNO 2010; 58: 151–154

[154] Pirodda A, Sorrenti G, Marliani AF, Cappello I. Arterial anomalies of the middle ear associated with stapes ankylosis. J Laryngol Otol 1994; 108: 237–239

[155] Wang CH, Shi ZP, Liu DW, Wang HW, Huang BR, Chen HC. High computed tomographic correlations between carotid canal dehiscence and high jugular bulb in the middle ear. Audiol Neurootol 2011; 16: 106–112

[156] Abboud O, Saliba I. Middle ear carotid artery. Otolaryngol Head Neck Surg 2011; 144: 290–291

[157] Gulya AJ, Shuknecht HF. A large artery in the apical region of the cochlea of a man with pulsatile tinnitus. Am J Otol 1984; 5: 262

[158] Lesinski SG, Chambers AA, Komray R, Keiser M, Khodadad G. Why not the eighth nerve? Neurovascular compression—probable cause for pulsatile tinnitus. Otolaryngol Head Neck Surg 1979; 87: 89–94

[159] De Ridder D, De Ridder L, Nowé V, Thierens H, Van de Heyning P, Møller A. Pulsatile tinnitus and the intrameatal vascular loop: why do we not hear our carotids? Neurosurgery 2005; 57: 1213–1217, discussion 1213–1217

[160] Levine RA. Typewriter tinnitus: a carbamazepine-responsive syndrome related to auditory nerve vascular compression. ORL J Otorhinolaryngol Relat Spec 2006; 68: 43–46, discussion 46–47

[161] Remley KB, Harnsberger HR, Jacobs JM, Smoker WR. The radiologic evaluation of pulsatile tinnitus and the vascular tympanic membrane. Semin Ultrasound CT MR 1989; 10: 236–250

[162] Levine SB, Snow JB, Jr. Pulsatile tinnitus. Laryngoscope 1987; 97: 401–406

[163] Gibson R. Tinnitus in Paget's disease with external carotid ligation. J Laryngol Otol 1973; 87: 299–301

[164] Davies DG. Paget's disease of the temporal bone. A clinical and histopathological survey. Acta Otolaryngol 1968: 242: (Suppl):–3

[165] Sismanis A, Hughes GB, Abedi E, Williams GH, Isrow LA. Otologic symptoms and findings of the pseudotumor cerebri syndrome: a preliminary report. Otolaryngol Head Neck Surg 1985; 93: 398–402

[166] Zenteno M, Murillo-Bonilla L, Martínez S et al. Endovascular treatment of a transverse-sigmoid sinus aneurysm presenting as pulsatile tinnitus. Case report. J Neurosurg 2004; 100: 120–122

[167] Russell EJ, Wiet R, Meyer J, Meyer J, De Michaelis BJ. Objective pulse-synchronous "essential" tinnitus due to narrowing of the transverse dural venous sinus. Int Tinnitus J 1995; 1: 127–137

[168] Gard AP, Klopper HB, Thorell WE. Successful endovascular treatment of pulsatile tinnitus caused by a sigmoid sinus aneurysm. A case report and review of the literature. Interv Neuroradiol 2009; 15: 425–428

[169] Lambert PR, Cantrell RW. Objective tinnitus in association with an abnormal posterior condylar emissary vein. Am J Otol 1986; 7: 204–207

[170] Forte V, Turner A, Liu P. Objective tinnitus associated with abnormal mastoid emissary vein. J Otolaryngol 1989; 18: 232–235

38 Theory and Treatment of Tinnitus and Decreased Sound Tolerance

Marcia L. Dewey and David R. Friedland

38.1 Introduction

Tinnitus is the perception of sound in the absence of environmental stimuli. Subjective tinnitus is the most common form of tinnitus and is the result of sound generated within the auditory pathways and brain. Subjective tinnitus includes sounds often described as tones, ringing, buzzing, or crickets. It is almost always associated with sensorineural hearing loss and is present in approximately 10 to 15% of the general population with about 5% being severely disturbed by the percept. The prevalence is much higher in occupations involving noise exposure such as the military. The United States Department of Veterans Affairs annual report for fiscal year 2011 indicates tinnitus is the most prevalent service-connected disability, with 840,865 veterans receiving compensation.[1] In fiscal year 2006 the U.S. government spent $539 million in compensation for tinnitus alone and over $1 billion when including noise-induced hearing loss. The aging population is also leading to increases in the numbers of patients and costs associated with these disorders.

38.2 Neural Basis of Tinnitus

Tinnitus is postulated to represent a central nervous system pathology generated by activity within the primary auditory pathways or their associated connections. Failure to alleviate many cases of tinnitus after transection of the auditory nerve provides additional evidence that the percept is generated centrally.[2] Hyperactivity in the dorsal cochlear nucleus, inferior colliculus, and auditory cortex has been identified in humans with tinnitus and in animal models of tinnitus and hearing loss. The abnormal neural activity in the central auditory system is currently thought to be secondary to neural plastic mechanisms causing spontaneous activity along the auditory pathway. These changes may involve increases in spontaneous activity in excitatory neurons, alterations in activity in inhibitory neurons, or the formation of self-perpetuating feedback loops among several different cell classes or regions.[3–5]

Under normal circumstances, neural plasticity is the brain's ability to adapt to a changing environment by changing the weights of the connections between neurons or groups of neurons. However, these plastic changes can also result in dysfunction. This is postulated to be the case in peripheral hearing loss, with tinnitus being a secondary result of central compensation to deafferentation. Recent functional imaging evidence gives support for this model. Studies utilizing magnetoencephalography (MEG) have demonstrated a marked shift of the cortical representation of the tinnitus frequency into an area adjacent to the expected tonotopic location. In addition, a strong positive correlation was found between the subjective strength of the tinnitus and the amount of cortical reorganization, indicating that the amount of abnormal plasticity is directly related to tinnitus severity.[6]

Changes in expression of plasticity-related genes in the cochlear nucleus have been noted after deafferentation. Aminoglycoside-induced deafness results in the upregulation of specific α-amino-3-hydroxy-5-methyl-4-isoxazolepropionic acid (AMPA) and N-methyl-D-aspartate (NMDA) receptor subunits. Other investigators have observed regulatory changes in protein kinase C isoforms β1, δ, and γ. Glycine immunoreactivity and changes in potassium channel expression have been observed in the cochlear nucleus associated with specific neuronal classes after deafferentation. Higher auditory centers also show changes in protein expression after cochlea ablation or deafness including calbindin-D28k, GAP-43, and NMDAR1. Acoustic trauma has elicited changes in expression of the plasticity related genes *BDNF, c-Fos,* and *Arg3.1* in the auditory cortex. Some studies have reported genes that do not change expression but have alterations in their respective protein levels, thus indicating the presence of posttranscriptional modulation.

Llinás and colleagues[7] have proposed a model linking deafferentation with subsequent cortical plasticity in the generation of tinnitus. Under normal circumstances, thalamic cells fire in the beta and gamma frequency range in the awake state and in the theta band in the sleeping state. When thalamic auditory cells are deafferentated from loss of input due to peripheral damage to the auditory system, they begin to burst in the theta band much like they would in the sleeping state. This theta-band oscillation is in turn reflected at the cortical level via thalamocortical interactions. At the cortical level, plastic changes as a result of this now-dominant theta band oscillation result in the loss of lateral inhibition with a resultant halo of gamma-band activity, known as the edge effect. It is hypothesized that this spontaneous, and constant, gamma-band hyperactivity is inherent to the percept of tinnitus.

38.3 Decreased Sound Tolerance

Decreased sound tolerance is frequently observed with tinnitus patients in the presence of normal hearing as well as with hearing loss. There are several forms of sound intolerance all of which have both a physiological and psychological basis. There is some disagreement among professionals working with sound intolerance as to specific definitions. We prefer and utilize the following definitions, which have been previously described.[8]

Hyperacusis is sensitivity or intolerance to ordinary levels of sound associated with a component of distress. Everyday sounds that are tolerated by others will seem loud or not be tolerated by the hyperacusic patient. This is due to an abnormally strong reaction to sounds in the auditory system as well as the limbic system and autonomic nervous system. *Misophonia* is a dislike or even hatred of being exposed to certain sounds. This is also due to an abnormally strong reaction of the autonomic and limbic systems to the sounds, which are a result of the enhanced connections between these systems and the auditory system.[9,10] Misophonic patients report disliking a particular sound regardless of the loudness level. These sounds may be characterized as annoying and unpleasant and can trigger an intense reaction such that the patient will avoid the sound at great lengths. In these cases, the reaction to the sound may be labeled as *phonophobia.* These conditions should not be confused with *recruitment,* which is present in sensory hearing loss and is defined as an abnormal growth of loudness. More specifically, there is a rapid growth of perceived loudness in the frequency region where the hearing loss in present.[11]

Hyperacusis is the most common associated condition seen in tinnitus patients, in about 40%.[9,10] Hyperacusis is hypothesized to be a disruption in the central gain system.[12] There is an increase of neuronal activity within the subcortical areas of the brain and enhancement of sound by the central auditory pathways.[9] Often patients begin overuse of hearing protection, which only serves to increase the central gain and worsen the condition.[12] In cases of sound sensitivity, as with disturbing tinnitus, associated stimulation of the limbic and autonomic nervous systems creates a reflexive response.[9,10] The limbic system is designed to monitor the environment for potential threats. If a threat is detected, the autonomic nervous system is activated and a heightened state of arousal will result, leading to anxiety.

There are various conditions associated with hyperacusis/misophonia, but in the majority of cases etiology is unknown.[10] In some instances these conditions have been linked with trauma or diseases of the ear such as perilymph fistula, acoustic trauma, ototoxicity, and Bell palsy; diseases such as Lyme, Addison, and Tay-Sachs; syndromes such as Williams, Ramsay Hunt, and chronic fatigue; as well as psychiatric and neurologic injuries or disorders.[13]

Although it is not within the scope of this chapter to discuss the specifics of treatment for sound tolerance issues, similar management strategies outlined for tinnitus can be applied to hyperacusis/misophonia as well. Treatment of these sound tolerance issues involves the use of sound therapy in conjunction with counseling, similar to the approaches to tinnitus management that are discussed later. Misophonia and phonophobia are more difficult to treat, with some debate about the proper treatment protocol.

38.4 Evaluation of Tinnitus

38.4.1 Otologic Evaluation

Subjective tinnitus is largely associated with peripheral deafferentation. As such, physical examination and otologic assessment is critical to identifying temporal bone pathology that may cause hearing loss and the resultant tinnitus percept. Although this chapter focuses on the audiological evaluation of tinnitus, it is important that the clinician recognize and evaluate organic causes of hearing loss. In addition, this chapter does not discuss other forms of tinnitus such as pulsatile or myoclonic, but physical examination is critical to identifying causes of these associated conditions.

Otoscopy or microscopic otoscopy is essential in the tinnitus evaluation. Subjective tinnitus can consist of low-frequency noises, often described as a rumble, hum, or ocean sound. This is often indicative of low-frequency sensorineural loss (i.e., deafferentation in the low frequencies) such as seen in Ménière disease, but can also be seen in conductive losses.[14] This may be

seen in serous otitis media, tympanic membrane perforations, ossicular trauma, otosclerosis, otitis externa, or cerumen impaction. Resolution of these conditions can improve or eliminate the tinnitus percept.[15]

Most subjective tinnitus is secondary to sensorineural hearing loss. Although most cases are related to presbycusis or noise trauma, other causes of sensorineural hearing loss should be excluded. Asymmetric or unilateral tinnitus with associated asymmetric sensorineural hearing loss should be evaluated, as should most cases of unilateral hearing loss. A magnetic resonance imaging (MRI) scan may be considered to rule out retrocochlear pathology. Infectious etiologies such as chronic suppurative otitis media, labyrinthitis, or meningitis should be checked. Depending on the history and physical examination, further studies for syphilis or Lyme disease may be considered. Autoimmune conditions can be considered, especially if associated with problems in other systems, as in Cogan's syndrome.

Asymmetric hearing loss may also be secondary to vascular compromise, and the presence of bruits or other neurologic findings may prompt evaluation of the carotid and vertebral arteries. Neoplasms arising from, metastasizing to, or invading the temporal bone can involve the otic capsule and cause sensorineural hearing loss and subjective tinnitus. Trauma can also cause hearing loss and may involve transmission through the ossicular chain, leading to inner ear concussion or perilymph fistula (i.e., as in Q-tip trauma). Trauma to the petrous temporal bone has a high rate of sensorineural hearing loss.[16] Barotrauma can also lead to hearing loss and tinnitus.[17]

38.4.2 Audiological Evaluations

Audiometric Evaluation

The tinnitus evaluation includes several key factors but starts with a comprehensive audiometric assessment. Pure-tone air and bone conduction thresholds, speech audiometry, immittance measures, and loudness discomfort levels should be obtained. Extended high-frequency air conduction thresholds from 250 to 16,000 Hz should be measured to obtain a full assessment of the patient's auditory thresholds. The rationale for testing beyond the standard 8,000 Hz is twofold. First, there may be asymmetries exhibited in the ultrahigh frequencies that are not present at or below 8,000 Hz, suggesting additional pathology. Second, establishing ultrahigh frequency thresholds allows tinnitus pitch and loudness matching at ranges above the standard 8,000 Hz.[18,19] Immittance measurements allow for evaluation of middle ear status as well as the acoustic reflex pathway to assess seventh and eighth nerve function. Loudness discomfort levels assess the presence of hyperacusis or misophonia, and they can be reassessed at future appointments to identify improvement in tolerance levels following therapy.[18]

High-resolution distortion product otoacoustic emissions (DPOAEs) at 8 to 10 points/octave are performed to assess outer hair cell damage.[20] This provides an objective test of cochlear status as well as assessment of outer hair cell function. Because there is a strong correlation between cochlear function and tinnitus percept, measures of cochlear function with DPOAEs provide additional diagnostic information beyond standard thresholds measures.[20] In some cases damage to outer hair cells is observed in the presence of normal hearing on the standard audiogram.[21] In these cases, DPOAEs provide confirmation of cochlear damage, which can aid in counseling tinnitus patients as to the tinnitus trigger, especially in cases of normal hearing.[22]

Psychoacoustic Measures

A tinnitus evaluation is a recognized billable evaluation as of 2005, and audiologists are able to use Current Procedural Terminology (CPT) code 92625 titled "Assessment of Tinnitus." Three main components of the tinnitus evaluation must be completed to properly bill this code: pitch match, loudness match, and minimal masking level (MML).[23] Residual inhibition (RI) is a fourth component typically recognized as part of standard tinnitus evaluations. Psychoacoustic research in all four areas of tinnitus measurement present varying opinions on the proper methodology of assessment.[18,23,24] There is general consensus, however, that psychoacoustic measures do not correlate well with disturbance level, severity, or subjective loudness ratings of tinnitus. Despite this, measuring a patient's tinnitus is a useful clinical tool. It is often beneficial for patients to be able to quantify and objectify their tinnitus. This also provides a baseline measure, as pitch and loudness may alter during ongoing management.[25] Quantifying tinnitus is also critical when performing tinnitus research.

Tinnitus pitch measures can provide some diagnostic and counseling value. For example, Ménière disease typically presents with low-frequency roaring tinnitus rather than high-tone ringing. Similarly, in cases of sensorineural hearing loss the pitch match is often seen at the edge frequency of the audiogram, the frequency at which hearing loss worsens relatively abruptly.[26]

The minimal masking level (MML) is the minimal level at which a sound, typically broadband noise, just covers up or completely masks the patient's tinnitus so it is no longer detectible. The MML can be obtained using narrow-band noise or white noise. There has been some evidence to suggest that MMLs will be lower after management of tinnitus, and therefore may be valuable to measure before, during, and after treatment as a gauge of success.[27]

Residual inhibition (RI) testing is performed to assess any reduction in tinnitus following the cessation of a masker. Testing typically involves presentation of broadband noise for 1 minute at 10 dB above the MML. The phenomenon of residual inhibition has a high prevalence; in excess of 75% of patients exhibit some degree of RI.[24] The most effective masker has frequencies in the frequency region where hearing impairment is present.[28] These results are helpful in determining proper levels for sound therapy.

Questionnaires

Questionnaires are an important part of the tinnitus evaluation. They can be used to rate the severity of tinnitus disturbance, to assess the impact on quality of life, and to determine the efficacy of treatment with pre- and posttreatment administration. The Tinnitus Handicap Inventory (THI) is one of the most commonly used tinnitus questionnaires and has a corresponding severity rating.[29] This questionnaire is use to identify difficulties that a patient is experiencing because of the tinnitus.

Questionnaires such as the Tinnitus Function Index (TFI) look at a patient's report of distress in associated areas such as concentration, sleep, hearing, or socialization.[30]

The Tinnitus Reaction Questionnaire (TRQ) consists of 26 statements in four categories (general distress, interference, severity, and avoidance).[31] The patient rates each statement as occurring "not at all," "a little of the time," "some of the time," "a good deal of the time," and "almost all of the time." The TRQ is used to measure the psychological distress associated with tinnitus. A statement on suicide ideations is included in the TRQ. In our clinic all the audiologists specializing in tinnitus assessment and management have received training in appropriate questioning and counseling of patients expressing suicidal ideation. Such training is essential when working routinely with tinnitus patients. This training was provided by a staff psychologist with whom we routinely collaborate regarding tinnitus patients.

The Holmes-Rahe Stress Inventory is used to assess life events that contribute to a patient's stress levels. This inventory was developed after examining the medical records of over 5,000 medical patients with a positive correlation found between stressful life events and their illnesses.[32] Patients are asked to select from a list of 43 life events that have occurred within the past 12 months. Each life event is rated with a life change unit from 11 to 100, the more stressful the event the higher the rating. A total score is obtained by adding up the life change units for each event selected. A score of ≥ 300 means significant risk of illness, scores between 150 and 299 indicate moderate illness risk, and scores below 150 indicate slight risk of concomitant illness. This particular scale is used to help identify and counsel tinnitus patients on the correlation between tinnitus distress and life events that increase stress.

38.5 Treatment and Management

38.5.1 Somatic Conditions

Although tinnitus is a pathology of the auditory system, there is ample evidence to suggest significant interaction with the somatosensory system, which can modulate the tinnitus percept.[33–36] The most common somatic systems associated with tinnitus include trigeminal nerve disorders, temporomandibular joint (TMJ) disorders, and injuries of the upper cervical neck, head, or face.[37]

It is possible to have tinnitus in the presence of normal peripheral function in about 10% of cases.[37] This is typically associated with nonauditory factors, particularly somatic injuries or disorders. Trigeminal and other somatosensory inputs may influence neuronal activity in the cochlear nuclei of the brainstem. Anatomic evidence demonstrates connections between these regions such as the trigeminal nucleus and the ventral and dorsal cochlear nuclei.[38] This may explain tinnitus that is associated with facial problems (TMJ disorder, trigeminal nerve disorder, and dental pain) due to input from the trigeminal nerve to the dorsal cochlear nucleus. As a matter of fact, patients with TMJ disorder and tinnitus are more likely to have normal peripheral hearing.[39] Treatments shown to provide success with tinnitus include stretching, posture training, and auricular acupuncture.[40] Appropriate treatment for TMJ disorder and physical therapy for the neck and face often provide benefits for tinnitus sufferers.[37,39]

38.5.2 Audiometric and Psychoacoustic Intervention

The management of tinnitus includes two key components: sound therapy and counseling. Sound therapy provides stimulation to the brain, thereby reducing the overall strength of the tinnitus signal. Sound therapy alone, however, does not address the long-standing emotional issues seen with disturbing tinnitus. Counseling addresses the emotional aspect seen in disturbing tinnitus.[41] The key to success is to pair appropriate counseling techniques along with specific sound therapy.[42,43]

Sound Therapy

The first principle in tinnitus treatment is sound therapy, which is used to diminish the tinnitus perception. Sound therapy may offer some relief from tinnitus by increasing neural stimulation along the central auditory pathway and interacting with the tinnitus generator. Some theories of the efficacy of sound therapy suggest it may disrupt the synchronous neural firing in the central auditory pathway.[44,45] Sound stimulation of the auditory pathway may also stimulate and soothe the limbic system. In cases of hearing loss, sound therapy via amplification can compensate for hearing deficits.[46] Diminishing the tinnitus perception is achieved by providing contrast with background sound. By enhancing background sounds, the perceived strength of the tinnitus signal can effectively be decreased.

38.6 Tinnitus Retraining Therapy

The best known sound-based therapy is tinnitus retraining therapy (TRT) developed by Pawel Jastreboff. It is based on his neurophysiological model of tinnitus, which began with his work with Jonathan Hazell in the 1980s.[9,47] Over the years, Jastreboff has fine-tuned his approach to tinnitus management while maintaining the basic principles of TRT. The tenets of TRT include the concept of habituation along with counseling. Habituation is a decrease in response to a stimulus after repeated exposure. TRT incorporates acoustic stimulation, typically low-level broadband noise via ear level sound generators or hearing aid/sound generator combination devices, to disrupt the detection of tinnitus at subcortical levels.[48] The device(s) are worn daily when the tinnitus is bothersome, but at least for several hours, and treatment continues typically up to 9 months, longer in more severe cases. Treatment focuses on the behavioral retraining of the associations with the limbic and autonomic nervous systems and the tinnitus perception. Retraining affects both the subcortical and cortical centers involved in processing the tinnitus signal. Treatment reduces the strength of the connections involved in tinnitus, and thereby decreases the detectability of the tinnitus, leading to a reduced emotional response. The goal is to cause permanent change at the neuronal synapses involved in processing the tinnitus-related signal.[9]

38.7 Neuromonics Tinnitus Treatment

The Neuromonics tinnitus treatment (Neuromonics, Westminster, CO) is a management option that combines use of a proprietary sound-generating device with counseling. The device is similar to an MP3 player and delivers a neural stimulus embedded in music.[49] Patients are instructed to listen to the device 2 to 4 hours daily. The music consists of four 1-hour tracks; two are baroque (classical) and two are new age (spa music). The manufacturer uses the patient's audiogram and equalizes the sound to a patient's specific hearing levels. That is, it enhances frequency regions where the patient has hearing loss and reduces the sound level in frequency regions of better hearing. The music and stimulus are delivered via high-quality headphones such as the Bang & Olufsen A8. The neural stimulus is reported to "stimulate a wide range of auditory pathways as well as the limbic and autonomic nervous systems of the brain."[27] The recommended treatment length is 6 to 8 months, and after approximately 2 months the neural stimulus is removed. The embedded neural stimulus is a low-level broadband noise that is included to provide an increased sense of relief from the tinnitus. As with TRT, the concept is not to completely mask out the tinnitus at any point in the treatment, but rather to listen to the music at a low volume to promote long-term desensitization to the tinnitus disturbance. Several studies support and verify benefit with this treatment device.[49-54]

The Neuromonics tinnitus treatment uses basic principles of sound therapy and patients may find the music more acceptable than traditional sound therapy using white or pink noise ear-level sound generators.[27,49] Recent studies, however, have not shown significant differences between Neuromonics tinnitus treatment and ear-level sound generators.[53] The proprietary music with the embedded neural stimulus may not have any specific composition that provides any further benefit than white noise or possibly even soothing/pleasant music via an MP3 player. The main downside to the Neuromonics device is cost; it is sold only through practitioners for US$3,000 to $5,000. Further, it is not recommended for hearing loss greater than a pure-tone average (PTA) of 55 dB.

38.8 Generalized Sound Therapy

A wide range of sounds can be used to successfully manage tinnitus. These include fan noise, music, tabletop noise generators, white noise, and nature sounds. Such sound therapy involves using sounds, not based on the availability of various devices, but chosen specifically by patients based on their preferences. In our clinic we advise all patients with tinnitus to utilize "sound enrichment," which is a term coined by Jastreboff and Hazell.[48] This term, borrowed from TRT, describes the use of sound in the environment 24 hours a day, 7 days a week. The general rule is for patients with tinnitus to avoid silence. For most tinnitus patients tinnitus disturbance is greater in quiet; this is due to the contrast between the tinnitus and the background noise. We have had a great deal of success with patient-selected sounds. The best delivery method is an MP3 player, as it is ear level and presentation does not change as the patient moves to different environments. It is inexpensive and accessible to most patients. The sound selections can be customized for each person's preference, and, using audio editing software, other sounds may be embedded or the spectral characteristics may be altered. Further, residual inhibition can provide significant relief from tinnitus, and clinically we are able to investigate many different sounds to find what works best for each patient.

38.9 Sound Generators/Maskers

Sound generators or maskers are ear-level devices that emit a low-level, broadband "white" or "pink" noise. The difference between a sound generator and masker is only in the way the patient uses the device. In most management cases of tinnitus, sound therapy is not meant to be used to mask, or completely cover, the tinnitus. However, one approach of sound therapy is to entirely or partially mask the tinnitus. In some cases patients are able to use ear-level sound generators as maskers and successfully mask out the tinnitus completely.[55] Residual inhibition may also occur with such masking. The masker does not necessarily have to be located in the frequency region of the tinnitus pitch. Rather, the best masker quality may correspond to the frequency region of hearing loss.[28] However, in most cases tinnitus management involves habituating patients to their tinnitus perception, which requires patients to hear their tinnitus during the sound therapy. Therefore, partial masking rather than complete masking is usually preferable to allow habituation to the tinnitus percept, and thus the term *sound generator* is more appropriate.[48]

38.10 Amplification

38.10.1 Hearing Aids and Combination Devices

At least 70% of patients with tinnitus also have hearing loss.[56-58] As such, amplification is the preferred management in most cases, because this option addresses both the issue of hearing loss and tinnitus. There are four main benefits to amplification with tinnitus patients. First, amplification helps to relieve some of the frustration with hearing loss by improving communication ability and reducing fatigue and listening effort. Second, amplification of ambient background noise serves as a form of sound enrichment. Ambient noise can act as a partial masker of tinnitus. Third, the amplified signal helps to reduce the contrast between the tinnitus and silence, making the tinnitus easier to ignore. Fourth, amplification restores input to the auditory regions that are deprived by hearing loss. The input from hearing aids induces increased neural activity in the central auditory system.[45,59] This increased stimulation of the central auditory system can reduce the brain's "overcompensation" as a result of the lack of stimulation due to the hearing loss.[60-62]

The benefits of amplification with tinnitus are noted in 60 to 90% of patients.[60,63] It has been reported that hearing aids alone provide as much benefit as sound generators.[64] Patients fit with hearing aids combined with proper counseling had outcomes that were twice as successful as the benefit from counseling without amplification. Therefore, the best management strategy incorporates tinnitus-specific counseling with sound therapy.

Combination devices are hearing aids that incorporate a sound generator. The benefits of low-level noise with sound generators, the basis of TRT, has been well documented.[9,48] Combination devices have become increasingly popular in recent years, as several mainstream hearing aid manufacturers offer these options in a variety of hearing aid technologies. There is a popular trend among manufacturers to offer training and guidance to audiologists for fitting such devices. With digital technology the sound generators in these combination devices offer a variety of sounds such as white noise, pink noise, speech noise, fractal tones, and the ability to use low- and high-pass filters to adjust the frequency response of a broadband noise stimulus.[46,65] It is also possible to stream wirelessly to hearing aids and combination devices from MP3 players. With this technology the possibilities of sounds available are unlimited.

The main goal of employing these devices, whether hearing aids, sound generators, or combination devices, is to provide relief to the patient. The intention in adding the sound generator is to maintain a continuous background noise, whose purpose is to provide sound enrichment, reduce the perceived strength of the tinnitus signal, and increase the ambient noise that can act as a partial masker to the tinnitus. The principle is to make the tinnitus less noticeable acutely, and, over the long-term, enhance habituation to the perception of the tinnitus.[66]

38.10.2 Cochlear Implants

Recent studies have demonstrated most tinnitus patients will benefit from cochlear implantation, with up to 86% of patients showing significant reduction in their tinnitus percept after cochlear implantation.[67-69] The same principles that apply to amplification also apply to cochlear implantation: reduce the frustration of hearing loss, increase the ambient noise, reduce the contrast of tinnitus and silence, and restore auditory input to the central auditory pathway. Additionally, direct electrical stimulation of the auditory nerve may promote neural plastic changes in the central auditory system causing reduced representation of the tinnitus frequency.

38.10.3 Counseling

Counseling provides the patient with information about tinnitus and helps the patient to identify and address the maladaptive thoughts, beliefs, and behaviors that contribute to the negative reaction of the tinnitus. There are several counseling approaches that work well for tinnitus patients. They do not always need to be administered by professional counselors. Many tinnitus patients will benefit from appropriate counseling techniques provided by the clinician administering the sound therapy. That said, the clinician providing tinnitus management and sound therapy should be trained in such counseling techniques.

Counseling should include education on tinnitus, helping the patient recognize the involvement of the limbic and autonomic nervous systems in tinnitus disturbance. The use of standardized questionnaires to screen for depression and anxiety are helpful, as tinnitus distress is linked with emotional distress.[70]

Depression and anxiety are seen in 62% and 45%, respectively, of tinnitus patients.[71] Tinnitus patients also may exhibit somatoform disorders, obsessive compulsive disorder (OCD), post-traumatic stress disorder (PTSD), psychosis, or dementia.[70]

The Beck Depression Inventory or the Patient Health Questionnaire (PHQ) are easily administered screens for depression.[72,73] The Beck Anxiety Inventory or the Generalized Anxiety Disorder 7 (GAD) can be used to screen for anxiety disorder.[74,75] In case of suspicion of psychiatric disorder, further diagnostic evaluation by a specialist (e.g., psychiatrist, clinical psychologist) is warranted. For some patients it is more beneficial to have professional counseling using specific techniques. A collaborative approach between the clinician providing sound therapy and the professional counselor may be appropriate for patients with more severe disturbance or a history of depression/anxiety or other psychological issues.

38.10.4 Counseling in Tinnitus Retraining Therapy

Jastreboff's tinnitus retraining therapy recommends a direct counseling method.[48] The main approach to counseling is to demystify the tinnitus mechanisms. Retraining counseling involves educating the patients that the tinnitus is a normal compensatory mechanism. Counseling involves teaching sessions aimed at providing a new frame of reference by explaining potential mechanisms of tinnitus generation, detailed explanation of the neurophysiological model of tinnitus, as well as explanation of the activation of the limbic and autonomic nervous systems.

Cognitive Behavioral Therapy

There is close association between tinnitus disturbances and psychiatric disorders.[70,76,77] Cognitive behavioral therapy (CBT) has been shown to be helpful in treating tinnitus patients.[78] It is a form of psychotherapy based on the premise that emotions and behavioral disturbances are driven by the way we think about what we encounter in our life. Therapy includes both cognitive and behavioral components. Cognitive therapy seeks to identify and alter the negative thoughts and beliefs associated with emotional disturbance and destructive behavior. Behavioral techniques are used to reduce emotional distress and behavior patterns that are unproductive and counterproductive. CBT utilizes behavioral exercises, such as relaxation techniques or biofeedback, and cognitive restructuring, which involves challenging and remodeling negative thoughts to improve a patient's reactions.

Cognitive behavioral therapy was developed for use with depression and is frequently used for conditions such as anxiety, OCD, PTSD, and chronic pain. The strategies employed in CBT help people with life skills and coping skills, including patient education about the condition. Although many practitioners of CBT are not trained in treating tinnitus, benefits are still seen in patients with tinnitus, as the comorbid symptoms, such as depression, anxiety, and sleep problems, are often alleviated. Tinnitus disturbance is reduced when these related symptoms are treated successfully.[78–80]

Mindfulness-Based Stress Reduction

Mindfulness is a philosophy developed by a Vietnamese Buddhist monk, Thich Nhat Hanh, that addresses living in the present moment to attain enlightenment. John Kabat-Zinn began applying this and other Buddhist principles to a stress reduction program at the University of Massachusetts Medical School in 1979 to treat stress, anxiety, pain, and illness. The great success of his approach has gained acceptance in modern psychology and psychiatry as mindfulness based therapy, commonly called "mindfulness-based stress reduction" (MBSR).[81,82] The basis of mindfulness teaches the skill of dwelling fully in the present moment, being aware of what is going on within and around us. There are several tools to practice mindfulness, such as meditation, conscious breathing, mindful walking, and awareness of the present moment. Meditation is used to center the body and thoughts with posture and focused thinking on the breath. The practice of mindfulness is a goal for everyday existence, not only during times of meditation. Conscious breathing is an integral part of mindfulness therapy. Much like CBT, mindfulness suggests that patients recognize their feelings, thoughts, and ideas. However, the key to mindfulness is to acknowledge these thoughts without judgment, without allowing them to influence us in any way. There have been promising results with mindfulness-based therapy in the reduction in tinnitus disturbance. Mindfulness training may constitute a useful addition to educational counseling provided to tinnitus patients, with the goal of targeting the psychological consequences of tinnitus.[83,84]

Acceptance and Commitment Therapy

As the name suggests, acceptance and commitment therapy (ACT) involves accepting one's feelings and acting on them. Rather than fight the feeling attached to a behavior, the person observes and accepts the feelings, and changes the unwanted behavior. As with CBT, a change in attitude is needed to change a behavior. However, ACT focuses on changing behavior regardless of the emotion and accepting the emotion, without a focus on changing the emotion as with CBT. This approach encourages patients to engage in activities despite their negative feelings. For example, patients are encouraged to go to work despite their anxiety about their tinnitus, showing the patients that they can live with the anxiety and eliminate the control it has on their life. Patients are taught three main principles: to accept the effects of life's hardships, to choose directional values, and to take action. Some of these approaches are similar to mindfulness therapy, such as observing one's feelings and recognizing and accepting the feelings as natural responses to the circumstance. ACT is an empirically based psychological intervention.[85] As with CBT and mindfulness, these strategies have been shown to benefit the disturbance that tinnitus has on patients' lives.[86]

Our clinic offers an array of referral sources for our tinnitus patients, including counselors knowledgeable in CBT, ACT, and mindfulness training, as well as other stress-relieving approaches such as meditation, yoga, massage, and tai chi instruction. Stress is the most significant exacerbating factor for tinnitus, and when stress is contributing to the tinnitus disturbance it must be addressed.[87] We often provide patients with simple instructions on effective relaxation methods with handouts and audio tracks on progressive relaxation therapy, conscious and deep breathing exercises, imagery, and meditation.

38.10.5 Medications

As tinnitus is considered to involve a generator and/or perceiver in the peripheral or central auditory systems, recent research has focused on treatments acting on chemical transmission at the synaptic level, to alter activity in auditory pathway neurons. Various medications with specific effect on inhibitory or excitatory neurons have been trialed for tinnitus treatment.

GABAergic Medications

γ-Aminobutyric acid (GABA) is the chief inhibitory neurotransmitter in the central nervous system and is also expressed in the inner ear. GABA binds to specific transmembrane receptors in the plasma membrane of both pre- and postsynaptic neuronal processes. Therefore, GABA has been postulated to be a potential treatment for tinnitus by reducing the activity of spontaneously active auditory neurons. However, to date, there has been no supportive research for the successful use of GABA for tinnitus reduction.[88–92]

Acamprosate (Campral)

Acamprosate is a drug typically used to treat alcoholism. Alcoholism is postulated to disrupt the balance between excitation and inhibition in the brain. Similarly, tinnitus is hypothesized to be a result of neural plastic mechanisms along the auditory pathway that may involve alterations in excitatory and inhibitory neurons. Acamprosate regulates the effects of glutamate (excitatory) and GABA (inhibitory) neurotransmitter systems centrally. There is merit to the idea that this drug's dual mechanism may reestablish the balance between the excitatory and inhibitory neurons that cause tinnitus. There are a limited number of studies to date showing some success in tinnitus treatment. A double-blind study comparing 23 acamprosate recipients to 18 placebo controls showed a significant improvement in the subjective rating of tinnitus in the active drug group.[93] This study did not provide information on matching each group as to the duration and severity of their initial tinnitus. A recent double-blinded placebo-controlled crossover study also demonstrated a positive effect of acamprosate on tinnitus perception.[94] There was a reduction in tinnitus measures during the active drug period without a significant change in such measures during the placebo period, regardless of whether the subject experienced the active drug first or after the crossover. Further studies are needed to confirm these potential benefits seen with this drug treatment.

Antidepressants and Antianxiety Medications

As noted earlier, depression and anxiety are frequently found in tinnitus patients.[71] Treatment of the psychiatric condition can alleviate some of the issues that patients attribute to their tinnitus. These include insomnia and the inability to concentrate or even function in one's day-to-day routines, depending on the severity of the disorder. Some studies suggest there are benefits to tricyclic antidepressants and antianxiety medications for tinnitus patients without a diagnosis of major depressive disorder or anxiety disorder. However, long-term benefit (in excess of a placebo effect) has not been shown for any treatment. The most promising classes of drugs seem to be antidepressants and antianxiety agents (especially benzodiazepines). Unfortunately, benzodiazepines carry the risk of drug dependence and are not good choices for long-term relief. Psychotherapy represents a better option for long-term treatment of the comorbid psychiatric issues seen in tinnitus patients.

Sleeping Pills

Insomnia and fatigue are common in tinnitus patients. There is a strong correlation between tinnitus disturbance and insomnia.[95] Fatigue can exacerbate tinnitus and an increase in tinnitus will further disrupt sleep, causing a cycle of poor sleep and increased disturbance. For tinnitus patients with moderate or severe insomnia, it may be appropriate to prescribe "sleeping pills" temporarily until the tinnitus is better controlled so as not to disturb sleep. Sleep agents with antidepressive effects may be most beneficial.[96]

38.10.6 Other Treatments

The following subsections discuss various treatment/management options that are currently available but lack a scientific basis for their claims, or are just being developed and lack well-designed studies of clinical efficacy. Nevertheless, practitioners should know about them so that treatment decisions can be made with full knowledge of all available options.

Ti-Ex Tinnitus Therapy Device and the TinniTool Laser Therapy

The Ti-Ex tinnitus therapy device (Neuwirth, Spittal, Drau, Austria) reports stimulation of the inner ear and the auditory nerve using a weak electric current. The treatment is administered by the patient at home with a MP3 player like device and headphones worn for two 30-minutes sessions each day until improvement in tinnitus is seen. The claim is that the device "works from the understanding that the hair cells in the inner ear can regenerate."[97]

The TinniTool laser therapy device (DisMark Company, Maur, Switzerland) is also self-administered at home, 20 minutes daily for up to 10 weeks. The device utilizes low-level laser therapy (5-mW output and 650-nm wavelength) to reportedly relieve tinnitus. The claim is to reduce tinnitus by increasing blood flow in the inner ear by penetrating the subcutaneous layers, which allows the "regeneration of healthy inner ear cells."[98]

Both the Ti-Ex tinnitus therapy device and the TinniTool Laser therapy device report tinnitus benefits via regeneration of inner ear hair cells. It is difficult to accept these claims as adult human hair cells in the inner ear do not regenerate as they do in lower animals or in the perinatal period. Further, the claim that electrical or laser stimulation, administered externally, has direct effect on hair cells lacks support.

The Inhibitor

The Inhibitor (MEDMELtronics, Dallas, Texas, United States) is a handheld device that delivers an ultrasonic tone (reportedly 20 to 60 kHz) via bone conduction during a 1-minute application period. This device is developed and marketed by David Holmes, who provides his own unpublished data on presentations of various ultrasonic sounds with tinnitus patients. His data claims temporary inhibition of tinnitus occurs in 70 to 75% of patients treated, with the amount of relief time varying from a few minutes to up to 17 days. He hypothesizes the ultrahigh-frequency stimulation generates a harmonic that puts the frequency of the tinnitus 180 degrees out of phase. The Inhibitor is not meant to provide long-term reduction in tinnitus, and the amount of relief time varies. In our clinic we have found a similar 70–75% success rate, but reductions entail a minor change in tinnitus and for typically less than 5 minutes.

Tinnitus Phase-Out

The tinnitus phase-out treatment can be completed with a device or an application on a smartphone. This treatment reports benefit for predominantly tonal tinnitus on the basis of sound cancellation principles. Using proprietary software, tinnitus pitch and loudness matching are obtained and a "phase-shift audio technology is applied to create a program to significantly reduce or eliminate the perception of the tinnitus."[99]

The phase cancellation mechanism between two sounds out of phase by 180 degrees cannot be realized between an externally administered sound and an internally generated tinnitus percept. The concept in this device is that the cancellation will occur in the cortex, rather than peripherally, thus reducing the tinnitus percept. How such a device can determine the phase of a sound that cannot be heard outside the subject is not clear. It is possible that a tone-generating device could cause residual inhibition, due to disruption of the abnormal synchronous neural activity.[3] A follow-up study concluded that the tinnitus phase-out device did not lead to significant sound canceling of tinnitus.[100]

New Tinnitus "Apps" for Smartphones

There are many smartphone applications ("apps") that have a variety of options for tinnitus treatments. These may be as simple as various sounds that can be used as background noise or employed in generalized sound therapy. Others may include guided relaxation or hypnosis-type strategies that are beneficial in reducing the comorbid symptoms that often accompany tinnitus, thus providing some benefits. Others make additional claims, such as the tinnitus phase-out app that requires the input of a patient's tinnitus pitch match and that embeds or removes this frequency to aid in tinnitus relief or reduction. The information provided earlier in this chapter will allow the practitioner to make an informed decision about which of these apps may have merit in tinnitus management. As noted earlier, a good management approach always involves both sound therapy and counseling. In the hands of a knowledgeable practitioner, some of these programs may be part of a complete tinnitus management therapy plan.

Acupuncture

Acupuncture is not currently an accepted treatment for tinnitus. However, otoacoustic emissions in tinnitus patients following acupuncture showed a difference between the amplitude before and after acupuncture.[101] Another study showed improvement in subjective tinnitus, though no changes were seen in the audiogram.[102] These results may, in part, support the anecdotal reports of tinnitus improvement following acupuncture, but the effectiveness of acupuncture for tinnitus relief has not yet been established by rigorous randomized controlled trials.[103]

The National Institutes of Health (NIH) Consensus Panel concluded that there is evidence to recommend acupuncture for only two medical indications: dental pain and nausea. (The nausea can be postsurgical, chemotherapy induced, or related to pregnancy.) No other indications are included due to the lack of good-quality research on acupuncture outcomes, not secondary to studies showing lack of efficacy. Further trials in the effectiveness of acupuncture treatment on tinnitus are needed before it can be considered a reasonable treatment option.

Alternative Medications

Thus far there are no well-designed studies supporting the use of any specific medication, vitamin, or herbal supplement to cure tinnitus. As noted above, there are various medications that may be used to treat the comorbidities of tinnitus, such as depression, anxiety, and sleep disturbance. Tinnitus is a commonly reported side effect of many prescription and over-the-counter medications, and thus any medication or supplement may worsen symptoms. Obtaining a history that includes information about the onset of tinnitus and the intake of drugs is helpful in confirming or ruling out a possible drug side effect or interaction as the etiology of tinnitus.

Nutritional deficits as causes of tinnitus need further investigation.[104,105] However, there are several over-the-counter "medications" marketed for tinnitus such as Tinni-Fix, Total Tinnitus Solution, RingSTOP, Arches Tinnitus formula, and Quietus, to name a few. The ingredients include herbal extracts, amino acids, antioxidants, vitamins, and minerals. Some claim to boost the immune system and promote overall hearing function, but all claim to be able to reduce, relieve, or prevent tinnitus symptoms. There are also claims for ginkgo biloba, riboflavins, folic acid, zinc, magnesium, manganese, coenzyme 10, echinacea, and Vitamins B-3, B-6, B-12, and E. However, with all of them, no good randomized controlled studies have shown any significant improvement in tinnitus over placebo. Additionally, there can be side effects and prescription drug interactions when patients self-prescribe these over-the-counter supplements.

38.10.7 Surgery for Tinnitus

Vagal Nerve Stimulation

Vagal nerve stimulation appears to alter cortical activity and may reduce spontaneous activity through plastic reorganization. Vagal nerve stimulation has been studied for disorders of neural activity such as epilepsy and depression. Recent investigation demonstrated that rats with noise-induced tinnitus exposed to vagal nerve stimulation paired with tones showed an elimination of tinnitus behaviors and physiology.[106] These findings persisted weeks beyond treatment. Another animal study demonstrated acute effects on cortical excitability with vagal nerve stimulation.[107] The feasibility and safety of transcutaneous vagal stimulation are being explored.[108]

Eighth Nerve Rhizotomy

Prior to the understanding of central nervous system reorganization as a result of peripheral deafferentation, it was thought that tinnitus was generated peripherally. Various forms of rhizotomy and nerve sectioning of cranial nerve VIII have been employed to treat refractory tinnitus. There are only sporadic case reports of this technique in the literature, and it is often associated with vestibular schwannoma resections. Although successes are reported, there are also well-documented failures, including worsening of tinnitus symptoms, underscoring the primary role that deafferentation plays in the genesis of the tinnitus percept.[2] Cochlear nerve section is no longer a reasonable option for the treatment of tinnitus.

Microvascular Decompression for Tinnitus

One theory of tinnitus has been that the percept is generated by vascular compression of cranial nerve VIII, typically by the anterior inferior cerebellar artery (AICA). A few centers have studied microvascular decompression as a potential treatment for tinnitus.[109–111] Appropriate subjects appear to include those with narrow-band hearing loss that is presumably from focal compression of this tonotopy in the cochlear nerve. This audiometric finding is in contrast to most tinnitus patients who have a hearing loss across broader frequencies. Studies of this technique have demonstrated 33% of patients with significant improvement and 10% with worsening.[112] There remains controversy regarding the use of microvascular decompression for treating tinnitus and it is not widely employed.

Neuromodulation

The goal in tinnitus treatment is to reverse plastic changes in neural activity, reset baseline activity, or disrupt abnormal pathways. This has led to various techniques of neuromodulation to treat refractory tinnitus. For example, implantation of cochlear auditory prostheses has been demonstrated to significantly reduce tinnitus in patients. Studies have demonstrated that up to 86% of patients have a significant reduction in their tinnitus percept after cochlear implantation.[68,69] Limiting this approach is that many tinnitus sufferers have retained functional hearing in the affected ear, or have significant hearing in the opposite ear, and fall outside the criteria for candidacy for a cochlear implant. The recent attention paid to hearing preservation cochlear implantation may relax such criteria and allow for implantation for tinnitus.

Using a similar approach to the problem of peripheral deafferentation, a custom-designed ring electrode for chronic stimulation was placed on the cranial nerve VIII in six patients. Tinnitus symptoms improved in four of the patients, but the effect was not immediate, with clinically relevant changes seen after up to 6 months of chronic stimulation. This would suggest

central reorganization rather than acute interference with the tinnitus pathway. Interestingly, only two of the responders had a perceptible change in tinnitus loudness. Rather, all four responders described a change of their tinnitus percept into a less obtrusive, more pleasant sound, suggesting a stimulation-induced reorganization of the tonotopic or secondary auditory processing structures with downstream limbic influences.[113]

Although the source of the tinnitus percept has not been definitively localized, it is likely that the auditory cortex plays a major role in perception. As such, studies have examined the role of direct and indirect stimulation of the auditory cortex and associated brain regions for the suppression of tinnitus.[113–118] These include repetitive transcranial magnetic stimulation (rTMS) studies, which have shown the ability to suppress tinnitus perception acutely and to produce longer lasting effects after repetitive stimulation.[119–122]

Stimulation of cortical neurons can be accomplished transcranially by passing a large current through a coil, generating a brief magnetic field below the coil. The coil is held above the head and passes the brief magnetic pulse, unattenuated, into the cortex. A sufficient intensity will induce neural activity in the cortex. Low-frequency TMS (< 1 Hz) has been shown to result in decreased cortical excitability, whereas high-frequency TMS (5–20 Hz) results in an increase in excitability.[118] Repetitive application of TMS can alter neuronal activity within specific brain regions. Success has been seen using rTMS in various neurologic and psychiatric disorders associated with increased cortical activity.[123]

Because rTMS modulates cortical activity, this treatment may disrupt the tinnitus percept by interfering with cortical hyperexcitability associated with tinnitus. Various stimulation sites have been used including points along the auditory cortex and in brain areas responsible for attentional and emotional processing, such as the dorsolateral and ventrolateral prefrontal cortex, parietal area, and temporal cortex.[124–126] Some results suggest that greater tinnitus reduction is obtained with a combination of stimulation sites including both the auditory cortex and the prefrontal cortex.[117,127] These results support recent theories that suggest that tinnitus does not originate from one brain region, but rather involves several sites in the brain including both auditory and nonauditory areas.[128]

Brief periods of stimulation can block or inhibit brain function, in essence creating a virtual lesion. These stimulations have shown reduction in tinnitus during stimulation, and with repeated sessions long-term effects have been reported.[118,129] Improvement varies across studies, with some reporting positive effects that persist for up to 6 months after repeated treatments.[129] Short-term positive effects have been clearly demonstrated for tinnitus; however, long-term benefits are questionable. Greater benefit has been seen with tinnitus of shorter duration. Greater hearing loss has correlated with poorer outcomes with rTMS.[129]

Direct stimulation of target areas in the brain with implantable electric devices may also be a feasible approach to tinnitus management. For example, direct current stimulation along the superior temporal gyrus can acutely alter sound and tinnitus perception.[130] Further, stimulating electrodes at various locations along the auditory pathway from cochlear stimulation with cochlear implants, to brainstem implants, up to direct stimulation of the auditory cortex have all been shown to have some success in treating tinnitus.[116,131] Electrical stimulation of nonauditory areas of the brain has also shown promise in tinnitus treatment. Deep brain stimulation in the subthalamic or ventral intermediate nucleus, typically used for disease such as Parkinson's disease and essential tremor, have shown reduction or elimination of tinnitus in some patients.[132] The theory is that stimulation may be interrupting perceptual integration of phantom sensations generated in the central auditory system.

38.11 Conclusion

Tinnitus is a difficult clinical condition and each patient requires a tailored approach to management. The clinician can focus on a bottom-up approach and provide enriched auditory input with hearing aids, music generators, combination devices, or electrical implants. Alternatively, a top-down approach may be employed and includes pharmacological modifications of neural activity, behavioral interventions, or, in extreme cases, direct stimulation of cortical structures. In all cases, appropriate evaluation is essential to characterizing the quality of the tinnitus, the severity of the tinnitus percept, and the changes that occur with clinical intervention. Further, we cannot stress enough the importance and efficacy of educating and counseling patients regarding their condition and associated comorbidities.

References

[1] Veterans Benefits Administration Annual Benefits Report Fiscal Year 2011. Washington, DC: Department of Veterans Affairs. D.C., 2011:http://www.vba.va.gov/REPORTS/abr/2011_abr.pdf

[2] House JW, Brackmann DE. Tinnitus: surgical treatment. Ciba Found Symp 1981; 85: 204–216

[3] Bartels H, Staal MJ, Albers FW. Tinnitus and neural plasticity of the brain. Otol Neurotol 2007; 28: 178–184

[4] Kaltenbach JA, Zhang J. Intense sound-induced plasticity in the dorsal cochlear nucleus of rats: evidence for cholinergic receptor upregulation. Hear Res 2007; 226: 232–243

[5] Møller AR. Neural plasticity in tinnitus. Prog Brain Res 2006; 157: 365–372

[6] Mühlnickel W, Elbert T, Taub E, Flor H. Reorganization of auditory cortex in tinnitus. Proc Natl Acad Sci U S A 1998; 95: 10340–10343

[7] Llinás RR, Ribary U, Jeanmonod D, Kronberg E, Mitra PP. Thalamocortical dysrhythmia: a neurological and neuropsychiatric syndrome characterized by magnetoencephalography. Proc Natl Acad Sci U S A 1999; 96: 15222–15227

[8] Baguley D, Andersson G. Hyperacusis: Mechanisms, Diagnosis, and Therapies. San Diego: Plural Publishing, 2007

[9] Jastreboff PJ, Hazell JW. A neurophysiological approach to tinnitus: clinical implications. Br J Audiol 1993; 27: 7–17

[10] Jastreboff PJ, Jastreboff MM. Tinnitus retraining therapy for patients with tinnitus and decreased sound tolerance. Otolaryngol Clin North Am 2003; 36: 321–336

[11] Moore BC. Cochlear Hearing Loss, 1st ed. London: Whurr Publishers, 1998

[12] Formby C, Sherlock LP, Gold SL. Adaptive plasticity of loudness induced by chronic attenuation and enhancement of the acoustic background. J Acoust Soc Am 2003; 114: 55–58

[13] Jastreboff PJ, Jastreboff MM. Decreased sound tolerance and tinnitus retraining therapy (TRT). Aust N Z J Audiol 2002; 21: 74–81

[14] Crummer RW, Hassan GA. Diagnostic approach to tinnitus. Am Fam Physician 2004; 69: 120–126

[15] Oliveira CA. How does stapes surgery influence severe disabling tinnitus in otosclerosis patients? Adv Otorhinolaryngol 2007; 65: 343–347

[16] Ishman SL, Friedland DR. Temporal bone fractures: traditional classification and clinical relevance. Laryngoscope 2004; 114: 1734–1741

[17] Klingmann C, Praetorius M, Baumann I, Plinkert PK. Barotrauma and decompression illness of the inner ear: 46 cases during treatment and follow-up. Otol Neurotol 2007; 28: 447–454

[18] Henry JA, Meikle MB. Psychoacoustic measures of tinnitus. J Am Acad Audiol 2000; 11: 138–155

[19] Tinnitus Task Force 2001

[20] Zhou X, Henin S, Long GR, Parra LC. Impaired cochlear function correlates with the presence of tinnitus and its estimated spectral profile. Hear Res 2011; 277: 107–116

[21] Bartnik G, Hawley M, Rogowski M, Raj-Koziak D, Fabijanska A, Formby C. [Distortion product otoacoustic emission levels and input/output-growth functions in normal-hearing individuals with tinnitus and/or hyperacusis] Otolaryngol Pol 2009; 63: 171–181

[22] Bartnik G, Rogowski M, Fabijańska A, Raj-Koziak D, Borawska B. [Analysis of the distortion product otoacoustic emission (DPOAE) and input/output function (I/O) in tinnitus patient with normal hearing] Otolaryngol Pol 2004; 58: 1127–1132

[23] White S. Bottom line: tinnitus evaluation and intervention. The ASHA Leader 2009

[24] Vernon JA, Meikle MB. Tinnitus: clinical measurement. Otolaryngol Clin North Am 2003; 36: 293–305, vivi.

[25] Vernon JA, Meikle MB. Tinnitus masking. In: Tyler RS, ed. Tinnitus Handbook. Clifton Park, NJ: Delmar, 2000:313–356

[26] Moore BC, Vinay , Sandhya . The relationship between tinnitus pitch and the edge frequency of the audiogram in individuals with hearing impairment and tonal tinnitus. Hear Res 2010; 261: 51–56

[27] Davis PB, Paki B, Hanley PJ. Neuromonics tinnitus treatment: third clinical trial. Ear Hear 2007; 28: 242–259

[28] Roberts LE. Residual inhibition. Prog Brain Res 2007; 166: 487–495

[29] Newman CW, Jacobson GP, Spitzer JB. Development of the Tinnitus Handicap Inventory. Arch Otolaryngol Head Neck Surg 1996; 122: 143–148

[30] Meikle MB, Henry JA, Griest SE et al. The Tinnitus Functional Index: development of a new clinical measure for chronic, intrusive tinnitus. Ear Hear 2011; 12

[31] Wilson PH, Henry J, Bowen M, Haralambous G. Tinnitus reaction questionnaire: psychometric properties of a measure of distress associated with tinnitus. J Speech Hear Res 1991; 34: 197–201

[32] Holmes TH, Rahe RH. The Social Readjustment Rating Scale. J Psychosom Res 1967; 11: 213–218

[33] Shore SE. Plasticity of somatosensory inputs to the cochlear nucleus—implications for tinnitus. Hear Res 2011; 281: 38–46

[34] Lanting CP, de Kleine E, Eppinga RN, van Dijk P. Neural correlates of human somatosensory integration in tinnitus. Hear Res 2010; 267: 78–88

[35] Levine RA. Somatic (craniocervical) tinnitus and the dorsal cochlear nucleus hypothesis. Am J Otolaryngol 1999; 20: 351–362

[36] Pinchoff RJ, Burkard RF, Salvi RJ, Coad ML, Lockwood AH. Modulation of tinnitus by voluntary jaw movements. Am J Otol 1998; 19: 785–789

[37] Levine RA, Abel M, Cheng H. CNS somatosensory-auditory interactions elicit or modulate tinnitus. Exp Brain Res 2003; 153: 643–648

[38] Zhou J, Shore S. Projections from the trigeminal nuclear complex to the cochlear nuclei: a retrograde and anterograde tracing study in the guinea pig. J Neurosci Res 2004; 78: 901–907

[39] Levine RA, Nam EC, Oron Y, Melcher JR. Evidence for a tinnitus subgroup responsive to somatosensory based treatment modalities. Prog Brain Res 2007; 166: 195–207

[40] Latifpour DH, Grenner J, Sjödahl C. The effect of a new treatment based on somatosensory stimulation in a group of patients with somatically related tinnitus. Int Tinnitus J 2009; 15: 94–99

[41] Alpini D, Cesarani A, Hahn A. Tinnitus school: an educational approach to tinnitus management based on a stress-reaction tinnitus model. Int Tinnitus J 2007; 13: 63–68

[42] Cima RF, Maes IH, Joore MA et al. Specialised treatment based on cognitive behaviour therapy versus usual care for tinnitus: a randomised controlled trial. Lancet 2012; 379: 1951–1959

[43] Searchfield GD, Kaur M, Martin WH. Hearing aids as an adjunct to counseling: tinnitus patients who choose amplification do better than those that don't. Int J Audiol 2010; 49: 574–579

[44] Dominguez M, Becker S, Bruce I, Read H. A spiking neuron model of cortical correlates of sensorineural hearing loss: Spontaneous firing, synchrony, and tinnitus. Neural Comput 2006; 18: 2942–2958

[45] Kaltenbach JA, Zhang J, Finlayson P. Tinnitus as a plastic phenomenon and its possible neural underpinnings in the dorsal cochlear nucleus. Hear Res 2005; 206: 200–226

[46] Sweetow RW, Sabes JH. Effects of acoustical stimuli delivered through hearing aids on tinnitus. J Am Acad Audiol 2010; 21: 461–473

[47] Jastreboff PJ. Phantom auditory perception (tinnitus): mechanisms of generation and perception. Neurosci Res 1990; 8: 221–254

[48] Jastreboff PJ, Hazell JW. Tinnitus Retraining Therapy: Implementing the Neurophysiological Model. Cambridge, UK: Cambridge University Press, 2008

[49] Davis PB, Wilde RA, Steed LG, Hanley PJ. Treatment of tinnitus with a customized acoustic neural stimulus: a controlled clinical study. Ear Nose Throat J 2008; 87: 330–339

[50] Goddard JC, Berliner K, Luxford WM. Recent experience with the neuromonics tinnitus treatment. Int Tinnitus J 2009; 15: 168–173

[51] Hanley PJ, Davis PB. Treatment of tinnitus with a customized, dynamic acoustic neural stimulus: underlying principles and clinical efficacy. Trends Amplif 2008; 12: 210–222

[52] Hanley PJ, Davis PB, Paki B, Quinn SA, Bellekom SR. Treatment of tinnitus with a customized, dynamic acoustic neural stimulus: clinical outcomes in general private practice. Ann Otol Rhinol Laryngol 2008; 117: 791–799

[53] Newman CW, Sandridge SA. A comparison of benefit and economic value between two sound therapy tinnitus management options. J Am Acad Audiol 2012; 23: 126–138

[54] Vieira D, Eikelboom R, Ivey G, Miller S. A multi-centre study on the long-term benefits of tinnitus management using Neuromonics tinnitus treatment. Int Tinnitus J 2011; 16: 111–117

[55] Bentler RA, Tyler RS. Tinnitus management. ASHA 1987; 29: 27–32

[56] Nicolas-Puel C, Faulconbridge RL, Guitton M, Puel JL, Mondain M, Uziel A. Characteristics of tinnitus and etiology of associated hearing loss: a study of 123 patients. Int Tinnitus J 2002; 8: 37–44

[57] Ratnayake SA, Jayarajan V, Bartlett J. Could an underlying hearing loss be a significant factor in the handicap caused by tinnitus? Noise Health 2009; 11: 156–160

[58] Kuk FK, Peeters H. The hearing aid as a music synthesizer. Hearing Review 2008; 15: 28–38

[59] Eggermont JJ, Roberts LE. The neuroscience of tinnitus. Trends Neurosci 2004; 27: 676–682

[60] Beck DL. Hearing aid amplification and tinnitus: 2011 overview. The Hearing Journal 2011; 64: 12–14

[61] Schaette R, Kempter R. Development of tinnitus-related neuronal hyperactivity through homeostatic plasticity after hearing loss: a computational model. Eur J Neurosci 2006; 23: 3124–3138

[62] Willott JF. Physiological plasticity in the auditory system and its possible relevance to hearing aid use, deprivation effects, and acclimatization. Ear Hear 1996; 17 Suppl: 66S–77S

[63] Kochkin S, Tyler R. Tinnitus treatment and the effectiveness of hearing aids: hearing care professional perceptions. The Hearing Review 2008

[64] Parazzini M, Del Bo L, Jastreboff M, Tognola G, Ravazzani P. Open ear hearing aids in tinnitus therapy: an efficacy comparison with sound generators. Int J Audiol 2011; 50: 548–553

[65] Sweetow R, Mette Kragh Jeppesen A. A new integrated program for tinnitus patient managment: Widex Zen therapy. The Hearing Review 2012; 19: 20–26

[66] Henry JA, Zaugg TL, Schechter MA. Clinical guide for audiologic tinnitus management II: treatment. Am J Audiol 2005; 14: 49–70

[67] Pan T, Tyler RS, Ji H, Coelho C, Gehringer AK, Gogel SA. Changes in the tinnitus handicap questionnaire after cochlear implantation. Am J Audiol 2009; 18: 144–151

[68] Quaranta N, Fernandez-Vega S, D'elia C, Filipo R, Quaranta A. The effect of unilateral multichannel cochlear implant on bilaterally perceived tinnitus. Acta Otolaryngol 2008; 128: 159–163

[69] Quaranta N, Wagstaff S, Baguley DM. Tinnitus and cochlear implantation. Int J Audiol 2004; 43: 245–251

[70] Langguth B, Kleinjung T, Fischer B, Hajak G, Eichhammer P, Sand PG. Tinnitus severity, depression, and the big five personality traits. Prog Brain Res 2007; 166: 221–225

[71] Dobie RA. Depression and tinnitus. Otolaryngol Clin North Am 2003; 36: 383–388

[72] Beck AT, Steer RA, Garbin GM. Psychometric properties of the Beck Depression Inventory: twenty-five years of evaluation. Clin Psychol Rev 1988; 8: 77–100

[73] Kroenke K, Spitzer RL, Williams JB. The PHQ-9: validity of a brief depression severity measure. J Gen Intern Med 2001; 16: 606–613

[74] Beck AT, Steer RA. Beck Anxiety Inventory Manual. San Antonio, TX: Harcourt Brace & Company, 1993

[75] Spitzer RL, Kroenke K, Williams JB, Löwe B. A brief measure for assessing generalized anxiety disorder: the GAD-7. Arch Intern Med 2006; 166: 1092–1097

[76] Langguth B, Kleinjung T, Landgrebe M. Severe tinnitus and depressive symptoms: a complex interaction. Otolaryngol Head Neck Surg 2011; 145: 519–, author reply 520

[77] Zöger S, Svedlund J, Holgers KM. Relationship between tinnitus severity and psychiatric disorders. Psychosomatics 2006; 47: 282–288

[78] Martinez-Devesa P, Perera R, Theodoulou M, Waddell A. Cognitive behavioural therapy for tinnitus. Cochrane Database Syst Rev 2010: CD005233

[79] Martinez Devesa P, Waddell A, Perera R, Theodoulou M. Cognitive behavioural therapy for tinnitus. Cochrane Database Syst Rev 2007: CD005233

[80] Robinson SK, Viirre ES, Bailey KA et al. A randomized controlled trial of cognitive-behavior therapy for tinnitus. Int Tinnitus J 2008; 14: 119–126

[81] Baer RA, Carmody J, Hunsinger M. Weekly change in mindfulness and perceived stress in a mindfulness-based stress reduction program. J Clin Psychol 2012; 68: 755–765

[82] Zeidan F, Martucci KT, Kraft RA, Gordon NS, McHaffie JG, Coghill RC. Brain mechanisms supporting the modulation of pain by mindfulness meditation. J Neurosci 2011; 31: 5540–5548

[83] Philippot P, Nef F, Clauw L, Romree M, Segal Z. A randomized controlled trial of mindfulness-based cognitive therapy for treating tinnitus. Clin Psychol Psychother 2011: 12

[84] Gans JJ. Mindfulness-based tinnitus therapy is an approach with ancient roots. The Hearing Journal 2010; 63: 52–56

[85] Dewane C. The ABCs of ACT—acceptance and committment therapy. Social Work Today 2008; 8: 34

[86] Westin VZ, Schulin M, Hesser H et al. Acceptance and commitment therapy versus tinnitus retraining therapy in the treatment of tinnitus: a randomised controlled trial. Behav Res Ther 2011; 49: 737–747

[87] Folmer RL, Griest SE, Meikle MB, Martin WH. Tinnitus severity, loudness, and depression. Otolaryngol Head Neck Surg 1999; 121: 48–51

[88] Dehkordi MA, Abolbashari S, Taheri R, Einolghozati S. Efficacy of gabapentin on subjective idiopathic tinnitus: a randomized, double-blind, placebo-controlled trial. Ear Nose Throat J 2011; 90: 150–158

[89] Aazh H, El Refaie A, Humphriss R. Gabapentin for tinnitus: a systematic review. Am J Audiol 2011; 20: 151–158

[90] Bakhshaee M, Ghasemi M, Azarpazhooh M et al. Gabapentin effectiveness on the sensation of subjective idiopathic tinnitus: a pilot study. Eur Arch Otorhinolaryngol 2008; 265: 525–530

[91] Witsell DL, Hannley MT, Stinnet S, Tucci DL. Treatment of tinnitus with gabapentin: a pilot study. Otol Neurotol 2007; 28: 11–15

[92] Bauer CA, Brozoski TJ. Effect of gabapentin on the sensation and impact of tinnitus. Laryngoscope 2006; 116: 675–681

[93] Azevedo AA, Figueiredo RR. Tinnitus treatment with acamprosate: double-blind study. Braz J Otorhinolaryngol 2005; 71: 618–623

[94] Sharma DK, Kaur S, Singh J, Kaur I. Role of acamprosate in sensorineural tinnitus. Indian J Pharmacol 2012; 44: 93–96

[95] Alster J, Shemesh Z, Ornan M, Attias J. Sleep disturbance associated with chronic tinnitus. Biol Psychiatry 1993; 34: 84–90

[96] Belli H, Belli S, Oktay MF, Ural C. Psychopathological dimensions of tinnitus and psychopharmacologic approaches in its treatment. Gen Hosp Psychiatry 2012; 34: 282–289

[97] Bentsen P. Electrical suppression of tinnitus with the TI-EX. Norwegian Congress for Otolaryngology—Head and Neck Surgery. Frederikstad, Norway, 2001

[98] Cuda D, De Caria A. Effectiveness of combined counseling and low-level laser stimulation in the treatment of disturbing chronic tinnitus. Int Tinnitus J 2008; 14: 175–180

[99] Vermeire K, Heyndrickx K, De Ridder D, Van de Heyning P. Phase-shift tinnitus treatment: an open prospective clinical trial. B-ENT 2007; 3 Suppl 7: 65–69

[100] Meeus O, Heyndrickx K, Lambrechts P, De Ridder D, Van de Heyning P. Phase-shift treatment for tinnitus of cochlear origin. Eur Arch Otorhinolaryngol 2010; 267: 881–888

[101] de Azevedo RF, Chiari BM, Okada DM, Onishi ET. Impact of acupuncture on otoacoustic emissions in patients with tinnitus. Braz J Otorhinolaryngol 2007; 73: 599–607

[102] Wang K, Bugge J, Bugge S. A randomised, placebo-controlled trial of manual and electrical acupuncture for the treatment of tinnitus. Complement Ther Med 2010; 18: 249–255

[103] Park J, White AR, Ernst E. Efficacy of acupuncture as a treatment for tinnitus: a systematic review. Arch Otolaryngol Head Neck Surg 2000; 126: 489–492

[104] Cevette MJ, Barrs DM, Patel A et al. Phase 2 study examining magnesium-dependent tinnitus. Int Tinnitus J 2011; 16: 168–173

[105] Coelho CB, Tyler R, Hansen M. Zinc as a possible treatment for tinnitus. Prog Brain Res 2007; 166: 279–285

[106] Engineer ND, Riley JR, Seale JD et al. Reversing pathological neural activity using targeted plasticity. Nature 2011; 470: 101–104

[107] Nichols JA, Nichols AR, Smirnakis SM, Engineer ND, Kilgard MP, Atzori M. Vagus nerve stimulation modulates cortical synchrony and excitability through the activation of muscarinic receptors. Neuroscience 2011; 189: 207–214

[108] Kreuzer PM, Landgrebe M, Husser O et al. Transcutaneous vagus nerve stimulation: retrospective assessment of cardiac safety in a pilot study. Front Psychiatry 2012; 3: 70

[109] Brookes GB. Vascular-decompression surgery for severe tinnitus. Am J Otol 1996; 17: 569–576

[110] De Ridder D, Ryu H, Møller AR, Nowé V, Van de Heyning P, Verlooy J. Functional anatomy of the human cochlear nerve and its role in microvascular decompressions for tinnitus. Neurosurgery 2004; 54: 381–388, discussion 388–390

[111] Møller MB, Møller AR, Jannetta PJ, Jho HD. Vascular decompression surgery for severe tinnitus: selection criteria and results. Laryngoscope 1993; 103: 421–427

[112] Vasama JP, Moller MB, Moller AR. Microvascular decompression of the cochlear nerve in patients with severe tinnitus. Preoperative findings and operative outcome in 22 patients. Neurol Res 1998; 20: 242–248

[113] Bartels H, Staal MJ, Holm AF, Mooij JJ, Albers FW. Long-term evaluation of treatment of chronic, therapeutically refractory tinnitus by neurostimulation. Stereotact Funct Neurosurg 2007; 85: 150–157

[114] De Ridder D, De Mulder G, Verstraeten E et al. Primary and secondary auditory cortex stimulation for intractable tinnitus. ORL J Otorhinolaryngol Relat Spec 2006; 68: 48–54, discussion 54–55

[115] De Ridder D, De Mulder G, Walsh V, Muggleton N, Sunaert S, Møller A. Magnetic and electrical stimulation of the auditory cortex for intractable tinnitus. Case report. J Neurosurg 2004; 100: 560–564

[116] Friedland DR, Gaggl W, Runge-Samuelson C, Ulmer JL, Kopell BH. Feasibility of auditory cortical stimulation for the treatment of tinnitus. Otol Neurotol 2007; 28: 1005–1012

[117] Kleinjung T, Eichhammer P, Landgrebe M et al. Combined temporal and prefrontal transcranial magnetic stimulation for tinnitus treatment: a pilot study. Otolaryngol Head Neck Surg 2008; 138: 497–501

[118] Kleinjung T, Vielsmeier V, Landgrebe M, Hajak G, Langguth B. Transcranial magnetic stimulation: a new diagnostic and therapeutic tool for tinnitus patients. Int Tinnitus J 2008; 14: 112–118

[119] Folmer RL. Repetitive transcranial magnetic stimulation for tinnitus. Arch Otolaryngol Head Neck Surg 2011; 137: 730–, author reply 730–732

[120] Folmer RL, Carroll JR, Rahim A, Shi Y, Hal Martin W. Effects of repetitive transcranial magnetic stimulation (rTMS) on chronic tinnitus. Acta Otolaryngol Suppl 2006: 96–101

[121] Langguth B, Hajak G, Kleinjung T, Pridmore S, Sand P, Eichhammer P. Repetitive transcranial magnetic stimulation and chronic tinnitus. Acta Otolaryngol Suppl 2006: 102–105

[122] Langguth B, Kleinjung T, Marienhagen J et al. Transcranial magnetic stimulation for the treatment of tinnitus: effects on cortical excitability. BMC Neurosci 2007; 8: 45

[123] Walsh V, Rushworth M. A primer of magnetic stimulation as a tool for neuropsychology. Neuropsychologia 1999; 37: 125–135

[124] De Ridder D, Song JJ, Vanneste S. Frontal cortex TMS for tinnitus. Brain Stimul 2013; 6: 355–362

[125] Vanneste S, De Ridder D. The involvement of the left ventrolateral prefrontal cortex in tinnitus: a TMS study. Exp Brain Res 2012; 221: 345–350

[126] Vanneste S, van der Loo E, Plazier M, De Ridder D. Parietal double-cone coil stimulation in tinnitus. Exp Brain Res 2012; 221: 337–343

[127] Langguth B, Landgrebe M, Frank E et al. Efficacy of different protocols of transcranial magnetic stimulation for the treatment of tinnitus: pooled analysis of two randomized controlled studies. World J Biol Psychiatry 2012: 22

[128] Kreuzer PM, Landgrebe M, Schecklmann M et al. Can temporal repetitive transcranial magnetic stimulation be enhanced by targeting affective components of tinnitus with frontal rTMS? A randomized controlled pilot trial. Front Syst Neurosci 2011; 5: 88

[129] Peng Z, Chen XQ, Gong SS. Effectiveness of repetitive transcranial magnetic stimulation for chronic tinnitus: a systematic review. Otolaryngol Head Neck Surg 2012; 147: 817–825

[130] Fenoy AJ, Severson MA, Volkov IO, Brugge JF, Howard MA, III. Hearing suppression induced by electrical stimulation of human auditory cortex. Brain Res 2006; 1118: 75–83

[131] Soussi T, Otto SR. Effects of electrical brainstem stimulation on tinnitus. Acta Otolaryngol 1994; 114: 135–140

[132] Cheung SW, Larson PS. Tinnitus modulation by deep brain stimulation in locus of caudate neurons (area LC). Neuroscience 2010; 169: 1768–1778

39 Medical-Legal Aspects of Otology

Benjamin H. Pensak and Myles L. Pensak

39.1 Introduction

The medical-legal environment within which physicians practice today is vastly different from the world in which medicine was practiced a generation ago. The training of residents and fellows, the daily practice rules for documentation and execution, and the guidelines within which physicians practice now are defined by increasingly complex mandates, regulations, and guidelines, many of which enhance patient safety and practice efficiency. Unfortunately, many of these same rules and guidelines are, in practice and application, poorly articulated encumbrances that inhibit effective and efficient care of patients. Moreover, physicians, as the front line in patient contact, are responsible for complying with such rules and guidelines in the context of their most important charge: caring for the patient. Understanding the fundamentals of the legal framework within which a physician practices is important and necessary to practice contemporary medicine today. This chapter focuses on four specific medical-legal concepts: confidentiality, the Stark law, consent, and medical malpractice.

As a result of the introductory level at which the following concepts are presented, consult with local counsel if you have specific questions, if you are confronted with litigation regarding any of the matters discussed in this chapter, or if you desire additional information specifically addressing how the matters discussed herein affect your practice.

39.2 Confidentiality, Privacy Regulation, and Compliance

Confidentiality is the principle of medical ethics that states that the information a patient reveals to a physician is private and is limited in how and when it can be disclosed to a third party.[1] The physician's obligation to maintain confidentiality serves as a cornerstone of the physician–patient relationship, fostering an environment that encourages the free sharing of relevant information without fear that such information may become public knowledge. The importance of this concept is embodied in modern American jurisprudence by the general ability to prevent one's physician from testifying in court regarding the content of discussions related to health conditions and treatment.[2] In the technological world that we live in today, and with the ever-increasing number of individuals with potential access to confidential health information, the United States government has instituted certain rules and guidelines intended to protect confidential health information, primarily through the Health Insurance Portability and Accountability Act (HIPAA) of 1996 and the Health Information Technology for Economic and Clinical Health Act (HITECH), enacted as part of the American Recovery and Reinvestment Act (ARRA) of 2009. HITECH requires HIPAA-covered entities to report data breaches affecting 500 or more individuals to the Department of Health and Human Services (DHHS) and the media, in addition to notifying the affected individuals, and extends the requirements of HIPAA to business

associates (e.g., service providers supporting a clinical trial) of covered entities.[3]

The information covered by HIPAA is known as protected health information (PHI) and includes information created or received by a covered entity and related to a person's health or condition and the provision of health care or payment related to health care.[4] A further related term covering a subset of PHI is *individually identifiable health information* (IIHI), which is PHI that identifies the patient or could reasonably lead to the identification of the patient.[5] The rules and guidelines enacted under HIPAA are intended to ensure confidentiality, availability, and protection against threats and information disclosure. Although there is certain flexibility among the covered entities, and as between rural practitioners and complex quaternary health care systems, certain principles remain consistent. DHHS, the department responsible for drafting many of the rules and guidelines under HIPAA, has addressed both required standards and aspirational standards for implementation and maintenance of related regulations.

The HIPAA legislation comprises two parts. The first part addresses health insurance matters, which are not discussed here. The second part requires "covered entities" (i.e., health plans, health care clearinghouses, and health care providers), including physicians, to protect the privacy and ensure the security of patients' medical information. The obligations to protect privacy and ensure security are described in two rules promulgated by DHHS under HIPAA and are referred to respectively as the privacy rule and the security rule. Note that although the privacy aspects of HIPAA apply to all health care providers, the security rules impact only those health care providers who transmit PHI by electronic means.[6]

Failure to comply with HIPAA regulations may result in civil or criminal penalties as established by ARRA. Civil penalties typically accrue to negligent violations of HIPAA, whereas criminal penalties are applied to knowing violations of HIPAA. The American Medical Association (AMA) on its website, http:// www.ama-assn.org/ama/pub/physician-resources/solutions-managing-your-practice/coding-billing-insurance/hipaahealth-insurance-portability-accountability-act/hipaa-violations-enforcement.page, succinctly summarizes the minimum and maximum civil liabilities associated with HIPAA violations under current law (▶ Table 39.1).

The penalties are not applied to individuals who are found to be criminally liable for violating HIPAA or who did not know, or could not have known, of a HIPAA violation despite exercising reasonable diligence to ensure compliance.[7] In addition, such civil liability may be avoided if a person is found to be noncompliant through reasonable cause and corrects such deficiency within 30 days.[8]

Covered entities may also be subject to criminal penalties as defined by the law in the event that a covered entity knowingly obtains or discloses PHI in violation of HIPAA requirements. Criminal liability can result in a fine of not more than $50,000 and imprisonment of not more than 1 year, or both; if the underlying cause of action included false pretenses, then a fine

Table 39.1 Penalties for Violations of HIPAA

HIPAA Violation	Minimum Penalty	Maximum Penalty
Individual did not know (and by exercising reasonable diligence would not have known) that he/she violated HIPAA	$100 per violation, with an annual maximum of $25,000 for repeat violations (the maximum that can be imposed by state attorneys general regardless of the type of violation)	$50,000 per violation, with an annual maximum of $1.5 million
HIPAA violation due to reasonable cause and not due to willful neglect	$1,000 per violation, with an annual maximum of $100,000 for repeat violations	$50,000 per violation, with an annual maximum of $1.5 million
HIPAA violation due to willful neglect, but violation is corrected within the required time period	$10,000 per violation, with an annual maximum of $250,000 for repeat violations	$50,000 per violation, with an annual maximum of $1.5 million
HIPAA violation is due to willful neglect and is not corrected	$50,000 per violation, with an annual maximum of $1.5 million	$50,000 per violation, with an annual maximum of $1.5 million

of not more than $100,000 and imprisonment of not more than 5 years, or both; and finally, if the underlying act was committed with the intent to sell, transfer, or use PHI for commercial advantage, personal gain, or malicious harm, then a fine of not more than $250,000 and imprisonment of not more than 10 years, or both.[9]

Although HIPAA protects information, it does not create a private course of action (i.e., an individual whose PHI has been improperly disclosed or used may not sue based solely on the violation of HIPAA); however, the violation of HIPAA may be used as evidence to establish other tort claims related to a failure to comply with a standard of care.[10] However, once a penalty is applied as a result of a HIPAA violation, it will be publicly announced by DHHS, in such manner as the secretary of the DHHS deems appropriate, to the public and to certain identified organizations and agencies involved in licensure and overseeing the conduct of health care programs and medical practices.[11]

The HIPPA security information can be obtained in detail at www.hhs.gov/ocr/privacy/hipaa/understanding/, and a detailed understanding of HIPAA violations, rules, and enforcements can be found at www.hhs.gov/ocr/privacy/hipaa/adminstration/. Finally, a useful summary of the HIPAA privacy rules can be found at http://www.hhs.gov/ocr/privacy/hipaa/understanding/summary/privacysummary.pdf.

Although HIPAA establishes the baseline level for protection of PHI, in any given state the state law may preempt the federal HIPAA requirements if the state law is more stringent than HIPAA by way of providing "greater privacy protection for the individual who is the subject of the individually identifiable health information,"[12] so it is imperative that physicians familiarize themselves with state-specific rules that may preempt HIPAA. Note that HIPAA permits the patient to whom the PHI relates to access his or her own information and to determine to whom such information may be disclosed.[13]

39.3 HIPAA Security Principles

Risk assessment and management is the cornerstone for compliance and will reflect variability among covered entities depending on an organization's size, scope of practice, and other attributes. All covered entities are required to establish defined policies, supported by appropriate written documentation, that restrict access to and use of PHI, allow for evaluating breaches

and developing response tools, provide for security and a compliance function to monitor such access and use, address workforce training, and provide for emergency contingency plans.[14] In addition to the general requirements of HIPAA, because of the fluidity of electronic PHI, additional safeguards are required, including policies covering work stations, disposal procedures for hardware or outdated computers, limiting access to software, and control of programs containing or related to electronic PHI.[15] Each covered entity is obligated to provide a notice of its privacy practices to each patient, and a covered entity (including physicians) that has a direct treatment relationship with the patient must use good faith efforts to obtain the patient's acknowledgment that such privacy notice has been received, and if such acknowledgment cannot be obtained, the covered entity should document the reason for failing to obtain such acknowledgment.[16] Covered entities are obligated to reasonably mitigate the harmful effects caused by a breach of HIPAA or its own internal privacy policies.[17]

When a covered entity is permitted (by way of a written consent from the patient) or required (because of an overriding obligation) to disclose PHI, HIPAA requires that the covered entity disclose the minimum PHI necessary under the applicable circumstances. HIPAA permits disclosure of PHI: "1) To the Individual (unless required for access or accounting of disclosures); 2) [in connection with] Treatment, Payment, and Health Care Operations; 3) [in order to permit an] Opportunity to Agree or Object; 4) [in connection with] Incident to an otherwise permitted use and disclosure; 5) Public Interest and Benefit Activities; and 6) [in connection with a] Limited Data Set for the purposes of research, public health or health care operations."[18]

39.4 The Stark Law

The Stark law is complex, but the crux of its focus has been described as follows: "A physician is prohibited from referring a patient for any [designated health service] to an entity in which the physician (or an immediate family member) has a financial interest, unless an exception applies."[19] The "financial interests" specifically identified by the legislation are generally described as (1) "an ownership or investment interest in the entity [to which a referral is made]" or (2) "a compensation arrangement between the physician (or an immediate family member of such physician) and the entity [to which a referral is made]."[20] The ownership interest includes debt or equity (although this prohibition does not apply to publicly traded debt or equity in regulated companies with assets exceeding $75 million).[21] On the other hand, a compensation interest includes instances where anything of value is exchanged (e.g., cash, gift, or meal).[22]

The Stark law is really two distinct pieces of legislation: first, as the Ethics in Patient Referral Act of 1989, which was included in the Omnibus Budget Reconciliation Act (OBRA) of 1989 and is commonly referred to as Stark I, and second, as part of OBRA of 1993 and is commonly known as "Stark II" (with a third, three-piece set of rules and comments that were undertaken based on the second of the aforementioned pieces of legislation). The Stark law, as these distinct pieces of legislation are known, collectively prohibits physicians self-referring for Medicare and Medicaid patients. This ostensibly simple concept has proven more complicated than it might seem, because the Stark law is a strict liability law, meaning any violation is enforceable immediately, and because it is stated as a flat prohibition despite the myriad situations that can trigger its applications, the exceptions to the prohibition are quite extensive and complicated in their application.[23]

This law is named after the California congressmen, Pete Stark, who sponsored the initial bill; however, Congressman Stark, as recently as 2007, expressed regret regarding the complexity of the Stark law.[24] In addition to its complexity, opinion is divided regarding physician self-referral and whether implicit self-interest drives physicians to make patient-care decisions on the basis of the physician's financial interests.[25] Furthermore, the Stark law arguably impedes a physician's ability to respond to patient need, service, and convenience if the physician himself may be rendering services and, given the myriad forms in which medical services are delivered today, all the Stark law may be accomplishing in practice is to exempt physicians from the ownership ranks of medical facilities.[26]

The Stark law grew out of, and still has heavy overlap with, the Federal False Claims Act (FFCA), which prohibits fraudulent claims against the government. It is because of its relation to the FFCA that the Stark law is limited to self-referrals in the context of Medicare and Medicaid (i.e., programs pursuant to which the federal government is billed for medical services). Stark I barred self-referrals to clinical laboratories under Medicare rules. Stark II expanded restrictions to referrals of Medicaid patients and added several services, in addition to laboratory services, that would be subject to the prohibition against self-referral. The services subject to the Stark law are known as designated health services (DHS) and include clinical laboratory services; physical therapy services; occupational therapy services; radiology services, including magnetic resonance imaging, computed axial tomography scans, and ultrasound services; radiation therapy services and supplies; durable medical equipment and supplies; parenteral and enteral nutrients, equipment, and supplies; prosthetics, orthotics, and prosthetic devices and supplies; home health services; outpatient prescription drugs; and inpatient and outpatient hospital services.[27]

Interestingly, although the Stark law focuses on physicians, it is frequently hospitals that are the subject of Stark law violation claims. Penalties for violating the Stark law include denial of payment, refund of amounts collected in violation of the Stark law, and fines.[28] If the violation of the Stark law is intentional,

then fines can also be levied up to $15,000 per claim and up to $100,000 per general arrangement.[29] In addition, violations of the Stark law can lead to exclusion from federal programs (e.g., Medicare and Medicaid), which is effectively a death sentence for a health care provider. Finally, as noted above, the Stark law is closely related to the FFCA, and violations of the Stark law may also lead to liability under the FFCA (note, however, that compliance with the Stark law does not necessarily mean that an individual is in compliance with the FFCA).

The concept of "whistleblower" actions applies to Stark law violations. Whistleblower actions, known formally as *qui tam* actions, arise when a person with knowledge of a violation of law brings suit on behalf of the government.[30] Someone bringing a *qui tam* action can receive 15 to 20% of any recovery made by the government, and may well feel incentivized to do so if there is a dispute between the claimant and defendant.[31]

As noted above, multiple exceptions to the Stark law exist that need to be considered under applicable circumstances. Stark law guidelines can be found online at several sites, including the websites of the Office of the Inspector General (at http://oig.hhs.gov/compliance/physician-education/index.asp) and the Centers for Medicare and Medicaid (at http://www.cms.gov/Medicare/Fraud-and-Abuse/PhysicianSelfReferral/index.html).

39.5 Consent

Consent is a process whereby an *informed* patient or legal surrogate is expected and required to participate in the medical decision-making process. The concept of informed consent has its foundation in the ethical doctrine that human beings have the right to control decisions that affect them and, in particular in the medical context, the notion of autonomy and agency principles that underlie fiduciary law that patients, as principals, have the inherent right to direct activities that impact their body, on the basis of information and guidance provided by their physician, as agent.[32] These precepts were established in American jurisprudence in the seminal *Schloendorff* case in 1914, which described the relevant precept as follows: "Every human being of adult years and sound mind has a right to determine what shall be done with his own body; and a surgeon who performs an operation without his patient's consent commits an assault [*sic*] for which he is liable in damages."[33]

Schloendorff functioned to mark in the legal world a moment in the evolution of the physician–patient relationship. Historically, the relationship was perceived to be parental in nature, with the physician entrusted to make determinations regarding the proper course of care and the extent of information to be provided to patients regarding both their condition and the treatment path.[34] That relationship has evolved to the current state that is more closely rooted in the principal/agent construct, and the notion that patients should be making the ultimate decision regarding the course of their care, with the physician providing appropriate and necessary information for the patient to make a choice regarding such care.

Beyond the evolution of the concept of how the physician–patient relationship is supposed to work, from a legal perspective the necessity for informed consent derives from the law of battery, which protects individuals against unwanted touching.

Thus, if a doctor fails to obtain consent from a patient, the treatment or diagnosis, presumably requiring some level of physical interaction, would constitute an unwanted touching and hence commission of battery by the doctor. The consent of the patient therefore constitutes the granting of permission to be touched.[35] In order for the consent to be valid, and for precepts of the doctrine of informed consent to be satisfied, several elements must be addressed in obtaining informed consent.

Certain states require a written informed consent document, whereas others permit oral consent; however, for liability purposes, a written informed consent provides the physician clearer evidence that consent was obtained.[36] The elements of consent include a reasonable understanding of the nature of the treatment or procedure, including the probability of success, acceptable or reasonable alternatives to the proposed intervention, the consequences of forgoing the proposed treatment, and the risks, benefits, and recognized uncertainties of the aforementioned treatment and the alternatives thereto (because a patient cannot assess the risks and benefits of the proposed treatment without understanding the risks and benefits of the alternative treatment methods).[37] In addition to these commonly accepted and recognized disclosures relevant to obtaining informed consent, there are trends to expecting additional disclosures regarding the physician's success and experience with proposed treatment.[38]

We believe that even where not required by state law, it is advisable to obtain written consent. A useful reference for all of the matters we discuss in this chapter, as well as other legal questions you might have, is a series of books published by West Publishing in its Nutshell Series. Two of the books in that series are particularly relevant to the matters at hand: *Health Care Law and Ethics in a Nutshell* and *Medical Liability in a Nutshell*. The authors of the latter book propose 15 pieces of information that should be covered in all consent forms:

1. Patient's name
2. Date and time of consent
3. Patient's condition in layman's language to the extent feasible
4. Proposed procedure and details related thereto in layman's language to the extent feasible
5. Name of physician explaining procedure and obtaining consent
6. All material risks of the proposed treatment
7. Treatment alternatives, including no treatment
8. Prognosis and treatment alternative risks
9. Disclaimer regarding outcomes
10. Name of physician performing procedure
11. Consent of patient to treatment
12. Consent of patient to deviate from proposed procedure related to unforeseen circumstances, including any limitations
13. Acknowledgment that patient has asked questions and has received answers to them
14. Consent of patient regarding proposed handling of any removed organs or tissue
15. Signature of patient or legal guardian (if applicable) and a witness[39]

A written consent form cannot ensure that a patient will not subsequently claim that consent was not obtained, whether because of a failure to disclose all risks or any of a variety of other reasons; however, a clearly structured form, that is adapted for the specific patient and that contains descriptions that the patient can understand, decreases the likelihood that a patient could, or would, claim that consent was not obtained.[40]

The physician should undertake to ensure that the patient understands the contents of the consent and related matters (e. g., the patient's condition and comprehension of the proposed intervention) before consent may be accepted. Note that the elements of informed consent must be considered collectively as well as individually; thus, if a physician describes and obtains consent regarding one procedure, but then proceeds to perform another procedure, or even the described procedure but in a way far exceeding the manner described, then informed consent would not be considered to have been obtained. However, this does not mean that a physician needs to cover each and every piece of information relevant to treatment.[41]

In any event, the courts commonly accept that a physician should not be expected to disclose risks that are common knowledge or risks that the patient is already aware of. This is particularly relevant in the context of a physician who goes beyond the consent because of situations faced once in the course of performing the procedure, which could result in liability. A physician is typically justified in undertaking such expanded scope when the patient's life is in jeopardy or the patient faces serious harm if the scope is not expanded; however, if a reasonable physician should have foreseen the expansion as a reasonable possibility, then it should have been disclosed in obtaining the patient's initial consent.[42]

Each of the elements of informed consent can be complex and not clearly defined. A degree of reasonable latitude is extended such that it allows for the tailoring of individual circumstances and is further nuanced by the standard employed in a given state to determine the threshold for providing the information underlying the informed nature of the consent. Such threshold is typically based on either the reasonable physician or the reasonable patient standard. In other words, what information would a physician, or patient, as the case may be, reasonably believe the patient requires in order to make an informed decision? Both standards are based on the "reasonable" person, meaning that the assessment is with respect to an ideal "reasonable" patient, not the particular patient relevant to the procedure at hand (i.e., a physician will not fail in his disclosure obligations if a reasonable person would find the information provided adequate to make an informed decisions, even if a specific patient were to allege that he or she required additional information).

Presumed or implied consent occurs only in limited circumstances, such as when a patient is not capable of consenting (whether because of emergency, incompetence, or being an unemancipated minor) and no surrogate or guardian is available to provide consent, in which case consent will be "presumed" if the treatment is necessary to save a life or prevent serious harm or when a reasonable physician would conclude that the patient has in fact provided consent to the treatment based on the patient's voluntary actions and apparent knowledge of the circumstances (a classic example is the cruise ship passenger who receives an inoculation after waiting in a line with other passengers, and then alleges that he did not consent to the inoculation).[43] Here, the principle of beneficence may require a physician to act on the patient's behalf in a lifesaving measure.

In addition, in states that permit oral consent (i.e., a signed informed consent document is not required), silence may constitute consent if a reasonable person would be expected to verbally object to the proposed treatment if she did not consent to the proposal.[44]

It is worth noting that rarely are physicians subject to legal liability related purely to informed consent, or the lack thereof; rather, informed consent–related claims are coupled with claims related to negligence and medical malpractice.[45] However, in the unlikely event that the physician faces a suit related solely to the failure to obtain consent, a patient would have to prove (1) there was an attendant risk that was not disclosed; (2) the physician violated the applicable disclosure standard by not disclosing such risk; (3) the undisclosed risk arose; and (4) the failure to disclose such risk caused the patient's injury.[46]

39.6 Malpractice and Negligence

Medical malpractice claims are most commonly based on the legal concept of negligence.[47] The typical negligence claim is pursued through a tort action, which refers to when one person has caused a harm to another that justifies the harmed in recovering from the harmer, whereas malpractice specifically refers to a tort committed by a professional acting in his or her professional capacity.

Negligence is defined as "conduct which falls below the standard established by law for the protection of others against unreasonable risk or harm."[48] To meet the fundamental requirements of negligence, a case must prove (1) that the physician and patient established a formal relationship pursuant to which the physician owed the patient a duty of care; (2) that there was negligence by the physician; (3) the negligence resulted in a cause of injury or death; and (4) that damages result from such negligence. We expand briefly on each of the facets of a negligence claim below.

39.6.1 Formation of Physician/Patient Relationship

Regardless of the Hippocratic oath, physicians do not have an affirmative obligation to treat someone; rather, the physician–patient relationship is formed through the consent of both parties and constitutes an implied or express contract to provide and receive medical services.[49] Once that relationship is formed, the physician owes the patient a duty of care, but until formation of the relationship occurs the physician cannot be liable for an archetypal negligence claim because the plaintiff cannot establish the existence of the first element of such a claim.

The physician–patient relationship is established on "spell of illness" basis; thus, once the treatment has run its course, the relationship is deemed finished, until the next one is formed.[50] Typically, the relationship is formed as one might expect: consultation is scheduled, meeting occurs, and treatment is begun. At any or all of these steps the parties may expressly state the relationship exists or in the parties' conduct the relationship is implied. Based on the contractual nature of the relationship, including prior to entering a formal relationship, the physician–patient relationship can typically be terminated at any time by either party, subject to the physician remaining obligated to ensure that patient receives adequate care until the patient is transitioned to another, appropriate, physician; however, there are certain circumstances where courts have found that a physician did not have the right to terminate the relationship (e.g., the full treatment has not been performed), in which case the patient plaintiff may pursue a breach of contract claim or a claim of abandonment, and a physician is never permitted to terminate the physician–patient relationship on the basis of the patient's race, gender, national origin, or because of a particular indication.[51]

39.6.2 Negligence

In the medical malpractice context, negligence is established by reference to a standard based on the skill and care that a "reasonable practitioner" would exercise under like circumstances.[52] In other words, did the defendant physician exercise the skill and care that a "reasonable practitioner" would under similar circumstances? It is also worth bearing in mind that "reasonable" care will depend on the resources available, which historically have correlated with geography (inasmuch as a rural practitioner may not have access to the same technology as an urban practitioner), this concept is known as the "locality rule," although it has been given ever-decreasing weight.[53]

39.6.3 Causation

Causation is the perhaps self-evident concept that the physician's failure to exercise the appropriate level of care was the cause of the patient's injury, which must be established by a preponderance of the evidence and frequently requires expert testimony.[54] This evidentiary standard is lower than the more commonly referenced beyond a reasonable doubt standard, which applies in criminal cases, but in civil cases (which include all tort claims), only more than 50% of the evidence must support the position at hand. In addition, to carry a medical malpractice negligence claim, the plaintiff must demonstrate that the physician's actions were the "but for" cause of the injury. In other words, "but for" the physician's conduct, the patient would not have suffered the injury. A related concept that can underlie a physician's defense is that of superseding causes, which means that another intervening event actually resulted in the injury, a concept that the defendant would have to prove and that requires its own legal analysis.[55]

39.6.4 Damages

A medical malpractice claim finally also requires that the patient have suffered compensable harm. Such harm is typically remedied by two types of damages: compensatory and punitive. Compensatory damages are meant to compensate the patient for the harm suffered (including the costs of the failed treatment and additional treatment required by the underlying negligence), whereas punitive damages are meant to punish the defendant for his or her misconduct and typically are only awarded when the defendant acted willfully or recklessly.

Recognizing that a charge of negligence or malpractice can arise, there are several well-recognized measures that all physicians can take to reduce the likelihood of a lawsuit, especially in situations where there is poor outcome regarding the management of a patient. Active participation within your working institution (this can be a large medical center or ambulatory surgical center) in minimizing risk is vital. By enhancing outcomes and creating a culture of safety and accountability, the physician begins to work within an environment that is patient centered. This culture of safety will optimize the likelihood that will dramatically reduce errors resulting from wrong-sided surgery, medication errors, surgical positioning errors, errors of ignorance, errors of omission, and errors of commission.

In situations wherein an untoward outcome does occur, it has been clearly demonstrated that the most important act that a physician can take is to be forthright, compassionately understanding, and above all truthful with both the patient and the family. Spending time answering questions directly, and framing the patient's general health and welfare, will maximize the likelihood that there will not be an erosion of confidence by the patient or family member. Seeking appropriate legal counsel within both the physician's practice and work environment will ensure optimal outcome.

In considering liability directly related to patient treatment, we mention briefly that a physician who fails to obtain consent, or obtains inadequate consent in light of the treatment undertaken, can face civil and criminal charges for the common law tort, and current crime, of battery. Battery involves an unwanted touching, and given that most physician–patient interactions involve some physical contact, it is not necessary that implied consent, or overt consent, to such touching must be obtained to avoid liability associated with battery.

39.7 Conclusion

In a litigious society such as in the United States, knowledge of fundamental rules of engagement with patients, third-party insurers, institutions, organizations, and the general population is requisite. Much has been made of practicing defensive medicine, and clearly this has led to a marked increase in the overall cost of health care. Following the admonition of *primurn nonnocere*, above all do no harm, should remain a guidepost for physician practice. Upholding standards of empathy, compassion, integrity, preparedness, and discipline, as outlined well over a century ago by Osler, will most assuredly minimize issues related to violation of law by the practicing physician.

References

[1] Hall M, Ellman I, Orentlicher D. Health Care Law and Ethics In a Nutshell, 3rd ed. St. Paul, MN: West Publishing, 2011:111

[2] Ruebner R, Reis LA. Hippocrates to HIPAA: a foundation for a federal physician-patient privilege. Temple Law Rev 2004; 77: 505–575

[3] Dahm L.L. Carrots and sticks in the hitech act: should covered entities panic Health Law. 2009–2010; 22: 1–12

[4] Drumke MWA. HIPAA primer. HeinOnline The Brief 2008; 37: 34–43

[5] DeWitt RE, Harton AE, Hoffman WE, et al. Patient Information and Confidentiality. Treatise on Health Care Law. New York: Matthew Bender, Lexis Nexis Group, 2011:3–16: §16.01

[6] Scheutzow S. HIPAA. A primer. GPSolo 2004; 21: 39–42

[7] 42 U.S.C. Section 1320d-5

[8] 42 U.S.C. Section 1320d-5

[9] 42 U.S.C. Section 1320d-6

[10] Drumke MWA. HIPAA primer. HeinOnline The Brief 2008; 37: 34–43

[11] 45. C.F.R. Section 160.426

[12] 45 C.F.R. Section 160.202

[13] DeWitt RE, Harton AE, Hoffman WE, et al. Patient Information and Confidentiality. Treatise on Health Care Law. New York: Matthew Bender, Lexis Nexis Group, 2011:3–16: §16.01

[14] Medical Records Privacy Under HIPAA. Administrative Requirements and Compliance Dates. Treatise on Health Care Law. New York: Matthew Bender, Lexis Nexis Group, 2011: Chapter 13

[15] Buttell PC. The Privacy and Security of Health Information in the Electronic Environment Created by HIPAA. Kans J Law Public Policy 2000; 10: 399–410

[16] United States Department of Health and Human Services. OCR Privacy Breach: Summary of HIPAA Privacy Rul. http://www.hhs.gov/ocr/privacy/hipaa/understanding/summary/privacysummary.pdf

[17] Wachler AB, Fehn A, Pendleton A. Final HIPAA security rule allows greater flexibility. Health Lawyer 2003; 15: 1–13

[18] United States Department of Health & Human Services. OCR Privacy Breach: Summary of HIPAA Privacy Rul. http://www.hhs.gov/ocr/privacy/hipaa/understanding/summary/privacysummary.pdf

[19] Sutton PA. The Stark law in retrospect. Ann Health Law 2011; 20: 15–48, 8, 1

[20] 42 U.S.C. 1877(a)(2); 42 U.S.C. 1395(nn)(a)(2); 42 C.F.R. Section 411.354

[21] Wagner IH. The difficulty of doing business with Stark in an ever-changing and overly complex regulatory environment: after twenty years, where are we heading? Ann Health Law 2010; 19 1 Spec No: 241–247

[22] Wagner IH. The difficulty of doing business with Stark in an ever-changing and overly complex regulatory environment: after twenty years, where are we heading? Ann Health Law 2010; 19 1 Spec No: 241–247

[23] Sutton PA. The Stark law in retrospect. Ann Health Law 2011; 20: 15–48, 8, 1

[24] Sutton PA. The Stark law in retrospect. Ann Health Law 2011; 20: 15–48, 8, 1

[25] Wales SD. The Stark law: boon or boondoggle? An analysis of the prohibition on physician self-referrals. Law Psychol Rev 2003; 27: 1–28

[26] Wales SD. The Stark law: boon or boondoggle? An analysis of the prohibition on physician self-referrals. Law Psychol Rev 2003; 27: 1–28

[27] 42 U.S.C. 1395(nn)(h)(6)

[28] Veilleux JW. Catching flies with vinegar: a critique of the Centers for Medicare and Medicaid self-disclosure program. Health Matrix Clevel 2012; 22: 169–225

[29] Veilleux JW. Catching flies with vinegar: a critique of the Centers for Medicare and Medicaid self-disclosure program. Health Matrix Clevel 2012; 22: 169–225

[30] West RP. Being a Qui Tam whistleblower: it's not for everybody. Business Law Today 2008; 17: 31–37

[31] Hall M, Bobinski MA, Orentlicher D. Health Care Law and Ethics. New York: Aspen Publishing, 2007:1375

[32] Bartlett P. Doctors as fiduciaries: equitable regulation of the doctor-patient relationship. Med Law Rev 1997; 5: 193–224

[33] Schloendorff v. Society of New York Hospital. 105 N.E. 92 (NY 1914): 93

[34] King JS, Moulton BW. Rethinking informed consent: the case for shared medical decision-making. Am J Law Med 2006; 32: 429–501

[35] Grimm AD. Informed consent for all! No exceptions. N M Law Rev 2007; 37: 39–83

[36] Boumil MM, Hattis PA. Medical Liability in a Nutshell, 3rd ed. St. Paul, MN: West Publishing, 2011:112

[37] Ginsberg MD. Informed consent: no longer just what the doctor ordered? The "contributions" of medical associations and courts to a more patient friendly doctrine. Michigan State University Journal of Medicine and Law 2011; 15: 17–69

[38] Rado SGA. A patient's right to know: a case for mandating disclosure of physician success rate as an element of informed consent. Health Matrix Clevel 2008; 18: 501–530

[39] Boumil MM, Hattis PA. Medical Liability in a Nutshell, 3rd ed. St. Paul, MN: West Publishing, 2011:112–113

[40] Hall M, Bobinski MA, Orentlicher D. Health Care Law and Ethics. New York: Aspen Publishing, 2007:54–55

[41] Boumil MM, Hattis PA. Medical Liability in a Nutshell, 3rd ed. St. Paul, MN: West Publishing, 2011:117–119

[42] Boumil MM, Hattis PA. Medical Liability in a Nutshell, 3rd ed. St. Paul, MN: West Publishing, 2011: 117–119

[43] Grimm AD. Informed consent for all! No exceptions. N M Law Rev 2007; 37: 65–66

[44] Boumil MM, Hattis PA. Medical Liability in a Nutshell, 3rd ed. St. Paul, MN: West Publishing, 2011: 117–119

[45] Hall M, Bobinski MA, Orentlicher D. Health Care Law and Ethics. New York: Aspen Publishing, 2007:215

[46] Hall M, Bobinski MA, Orentlicher D. Health Care Law and Ethics. New York: Aspen Publishing, 2007:215

[47] Atwell BL. The modern age of informed consent. Univ Richmond Law Rev 2006; 40: 595

[48] Restatement (Second) of Torts. 1965. Section 282

[49] Hall M, Bobinski MA, Orentlicher D. Health Care Law and Ethics. New York: Aspen Publishing, 2007:113

[50] Hurley v. Eddingfield. 59 N.E. 1059 (Ind 1901)

[51] Boumil MM, Hattis PA. Medical Liability Medical Liability in a Nutshell, 3rd ed. St. Paul, MN: West Publishing, 2011:18–23

[52] Boumil MM, Hattis PA. Medical Liability in a Nutshell, 3rd ed. St. Paul, MN: West Publishing, 2011: 39–82

[53] Boumil MM, Hattis PA. Medical Liability in a Nutshell, 3rd ed. St. Paul, MN: West Publishing, 2011: 39–82

[54] Heydemann HW, Macdonald MG, Neely EJ. Medical Malpractice. Treatise on Health Care Law. New York: Matthew Bender, Lexis Nexis Group, 2011:3: Chapter 12

[55] Boumil MM, Hattis PA. Medical Liability in a Nutshell, 3rd ed. St. Paul, MN: West Publishing, 2011: 148–151

Index

Note: Page numbers set **bold** or *italic* indicate headings or figures, respectively.